Fetal and Neonatal Neurology
and Neurosurgery

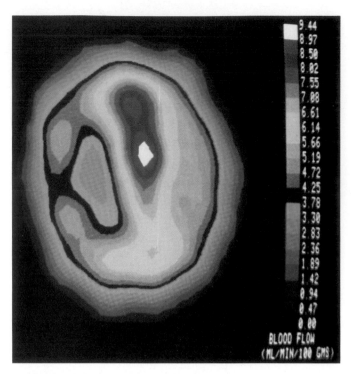

Frontispiece I *PET scan of a pre-term infant with a left-sided intracerebral haemorrhage. [^{15}O] water was used as an inert tracer for estimation of cerebral blood flow (CBF). The highest local CBF was 10 ml. 100 g^{-1}. min^{-1}. Most of the left hemisphere was perfused at less than half this rate. (Reproduced with permission from Volpe et al 1983.)*

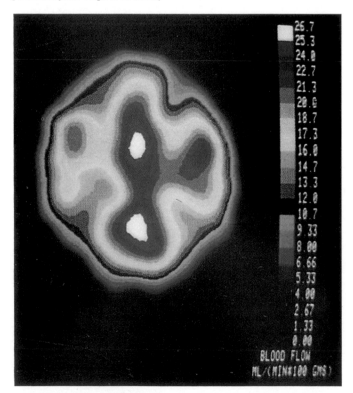

Frontispiece II *PET scan from an asphyxiated full-term infant showing reduction in blood flow to the watershed region between the middle and posterior cerebral artery distribution. (Reproduced with permission from Volpe 1987.)*

Fetal and Neonatal Neurology and Neurosurgery

EDITED BY

Malcolm I. Levene MD FRCP
Reader in Child Health and Honorary Consultant Paediatrician, Department of Child Health, Leicester University School of Medicine, UK

Michael J. Bennett MD FRCOG FRACOG
School of Obstetrics and Gynaecology, Royal Hospital for Women, University of New South Wales, Sydney, Australia

Jonathan Punt MB FRCS
Consultant Paediatric Neurosurgeon, University Hospital, Queen's Medical Centre, Nottingham, UK

CHURCHILL LIVINGSTONE
EDINBURGH LONDON MELBOURNE AND NEW YORK 1988

CHURCHILL LIVINGSTONE
Medical Division of Longman Group UK Limited

Distributed in the United States of America by
Churchill Livingstone Inc., 1560 Broadway, New York,
N.Y. 10036, and by associated companies, branches
and representatives throughout the world.

First published 1988

ISBN 0 443 03713 2

British Library Cataloguing in Publication Data
Fetal and neonatal neurology and neurosurgery
  1. Man. Foetuses and newborn babies.
  Nervous system. Diseases
  I. Levene, Malcolm I. (Malcolm Irvin)
  II. Bennett, M. J. (Michael Julian), *1942*–
  III. Punt, Jonathan
  618. 3'268

Library of Congress Cataloging in Publication Data
Fetal and neonatal neurology and neurosurgery.
  1. Brain—Diseases. 2. Fetus—Diseases. 3. Infants
(Newborn)—Diseases. 4. Central nervous system—
Diseases—Treatment. 5. Parental diagnosis. I. Levene,
Malcolm I. II. Bennett, M. J. (Michael Julian)
III. Punt, Jonathan. [DNLM: 1. Brain—embryology.
2. Brain Diseases—in infancy & childhood. 3. Fetal
Diseases—therapy. 4. Neurosurgery—in infancy &
childhood. 5. Prenatal Diagnosis—methods. 6. Ultra-
sonic Diagnosis—methods. WQ 211 F41916]
RG629.B73F46 1989   612'.64018   88–6145

Printed at The Bath Press, Avon

Foreword

Twenty-nine of the fifty-five contributors to this comprehensive and authoritative work are drawn from overseas; I hope that they, in particular, will be prepared to forgive a brief, but parochial and personal comment.

Specialisation within paediatrics in Britain only began after World War II. In those days it was possible to 'specialise' in more than one sub-division of paediatrics. The writer, as a Founder Member both of the Neonatal Society (1959) and of the British Paediatric Neurology Association (1975), could once claim, however mistakenly, expert knowledge of the newborn and of disorders of the nervous system in infants and children.

This book may serve as a monument to such pretensions! On April 18th, 1775 James Boswell quoted Johnson as saying "Knowledge is of two kinds. We know a subject ourselves, or we know where we can find information upon it." *Fetal and Neonatal Neurology and Neurosurgery* will become an invaluable work of reference for obstetricians, paediatricians and other specialists concerned with the care of newborn babies, including – dare one say it – for the three distinguished Editors themselves.

Emeritus Professor Sir Peter Tizard

Preface

Neurological disability is the most feared complication of pregnancy, labour and the early months of life. The earliest recognizable neural tissue develops approximately 18 days after fertilization and development of the central nervous system proceeds to maturity some 6 years later. The developing brain is an extremely vulnerable organ and is subject to a wide range of insults that may alter structure or function. Problems affecting the immature brain may come under the care of the obstetrician, neonatologist, general paediatrician or paediatric neurologist and neurosurgeon. Investigations may encompass a wide range of other specialists including radiologists, physicists, pharmacologists, microbiologists, physiologists, pathologists, biochemists and ophthalmologists. These major cross-specialty links make it difficult to consider the developing central nervous system (CNS) for what it is: a complex but continuous process rather than a series of loosely related parts.

The basic aim of this book is to consider the developmental neurology and pathology of the developing CNS from conception to the end of the first year of life. We have approached the subject as specialists representing obstetrics, paediatrics and neurosurgery but with a particular interest in the immature brain. We have attempted to break down the constraints of our respective specialty training to produce a book that crosses these divisions and brings together all the aspects of brain development and pathology during the critical stages of early development. We have been supported in this aim by our 55 contributors who represent a wide range of disciplines and the experience of 10 different countries within Europe, Australia and North America.

The book is presented in three parts: morphological development, methods of investigation and management. Part 1 is a comprehensive review of embryology and developmental anatomy of the CNS and provides the basic foundation necessary to understand much of the pathology that may occur. Part 2 incorporates methods of investigating the immature brain, both fetal and neonatal. The rapid advance in our understanding of cerebral pathology is directly related to the recent introduction of these methods. We have drawn upon the experience of those responsible for developing these techniques to discuss their role and limitations. Some of these methods are already used in routine clinical practice and others are state-of-the-art and unlikely to ever come into routine use but give important information on both structure and function. Part 3 involves the management of disorders of the developing brain and this is further subdivided into sections related to particular areas of clinical interest.

We hope that this book will provide all those involved in the management of the fetus and infant with the information necessary to understanding better the delicate mechanisms that exist within the central nervous system. Perhaps better understanding of these fragile tissues will, in the future, enable more effective treatment or prevention of neurological handicap.

Leicester, 1988   M.I.L., M.J.B., J.P.

Contributors

Dr L. N. J. Archer MA MRCP
Consultant Paediatric Cardiologist
John Radcliffe Hospital
Headington
Oxford
UK

Dr P. Barbor MB FRCP
Consultant Paediatrician
Queen's Medical Centre
Nottingham
UK

Dr A. Beaugerie MD
Department of Paediatric Neurology
Catholic University of Louvain
Brussels
Belgium

Professor M. J. Bennett MD FRCOG FRACOG
School of Obstetrics and Gynaecology
Royal Hospital for Women
University of New South Wales
Sydney
Australia

Professor J. C. Birnholz MD
Rush-Presbyterian-St Luke's Medical Center
Chicago, Illinois
U.S.A.

Dr G. K. Brown MB PhD
Senior Lecturer
Department of Paediatrics and Murdoch Institute
Royal Children's Hospital
Melbourne
Australia

Dr J. K. Brown MB FRCP
Consultant Paediatric Neurologist
Royal Hospital for Sick Children
Edinburgh
UK

Professor A. Calame MD
Division of Neonatal Medicine and Developmental Unit
Department of Paediatrics
CHUV
Lausanne
Switzerland

Dr J. Connell BM MRCP
Research Fellow
Department of Paediatrics and Neonatal Medicine
Royal Postgraduate Medical School
Hammersmith Hospital
London
UK

Professor D. M. Danks MD
Director
The Murdoch Institute for Research into Birth Defects
Royal Children's Hospital
Melbourne
Australia

Dr Pamela A. Davies MD FRCP
London
UK

Formerly: Reader in Paediatrics
Institute of Child Health
Guilford Street
London *and* Honorary Consultant Paediatrician
Hammersmith Hospital
London

Dr L. S. de Vries MD
Research Fellow
Department of Paediatrics & Neonatal Medicine
Royal Postgraduate Medical School
Hammersmith Hospital
London
UK

Dr L. M. S. Dubowitz MD
Lecturer
Department of Paediatrics & Neonatal Medicine
Royal Postgraduate Medical School
Hammersmith Hospital
London
UK

Professor V. Dubowitz MD PhD FRCP
Department of Paediatrics & Neonatal Medicine
& Jerry Lewis Muscle Research Centre
Royal Postgraduate Medical School
Hammersmith Hospital
London
UK

Dr M. S. B. Edwards MD
Director of Paediatric Neurosurgery
Associate Professor of Neurosurgery and Paediatrics
University of California
San Francisco
USA

Dr Marjorie A. England PhD
Senior Lecturer
Department of Anatomy
Leicester University School of Medicine
UK

Dr D. H. Evans PhD
Principal Physicist & Honorary Reader
Department of Medical Physics
Leicester Royal Infirmary
UK

Dr C-L. Fawer MD
Research Fellow
Division of Neonatal Medicine and Developmental Unit
Department of Paediatrics
CHUV
Lausanne
Switzerland

Professor A. R. Fielder MB FRCS
Professor
Department of Ophthalmology
Leicester University School of Medicine
UK

Professor O. Flodmark MD PhD
Professor
Department of Radiology
University of British Columbia
Vancouver
British Columbia
Canada

Dr W. J. Garrett
Director
Department for Medical Imaging
Royal Hospital for Women
Sydney
Australia

Dr N. Gibson MB MRCP
Research Fellow
Department of Child Health
Leicester University Medical School
UK

Dr R. W. Gill PhD
Head of Doppler Section
Ultrasonics Institute
Chatswood, Sydney
Australia

Dr M. S. Golbus MD
Obstetrics, Gynaecology and Reproductive Sciences
School of Medicine
University of California
San Francisco
USA

Dr S. H. Green MA MB FRCP
Senior Lecturer in Paediatrics and Child Health
Honorary Paediatric Neurologist
Institute of Child Health
University of Birmingham
Birmingham Children's Hospital
Birmingham
UK

Dr G. Greisen MD
Research Fellow
Department of Paediatrics
Rigshospitalet
Copenhagen
Denmark

Dr J. E. Haddow MD
Associate Medical Director
Foundation for Blood Research
Scarborough
Maine
USA

Dr S. Hall MSc MB MFCM
PHLS Communicable Surveillence Centre and
Paediatric Epidemiology Department
Institute of Child Health
London
UK

Dr P. A. Hamilton MB MRCP
Senior Lecturer and Consultant Paediatrician
St George's Hospital
Tooting
London
UK
Formerly: Lecturer
Department of Paediatrics
University College London

Dr J. Heckmatt MD MRCP
Lecturer
Department of Paediatrics and Neonatal Medicine and
Jerry Lewis Muscle Research Centre
Royal Postgraduate Medical School
Hammersmith Hospital
London
UK

Professor J. C. Hobbins MD
Department of Obstetrics and Gynaecology
Yale University School of Medicine
New Haven
USA

Dr P. Hope MB MRCP
Consultant Paediatrician
John Radcliffe Hospital
Oxford
UK
Formerly: Senior Lecturer
Department of Paediatrics
University College London
UK

Dr R. J. Hudgins MD
Assistant Professor of Neurological Surgery and Paediatrics
University of California
San Francisco
USA

Professor I. Kjellmer MD
Department of Paediatrics I
East Hospital
Gothenburg University
Sweden

Dr J-C. Larroche MD
Director of Research (CNRS)
Hôpital Port-Royal
Paris
France

Dr S. Lary PhD
Research Fellow
Department of Paediatrics and Neonatal Medicine
Royal Postgraduate Medical School
Hammersmith Hospital
London
UK

Dr L. R. Leader ChB FRACOG
Senior Lecturer
School of Obstetrics and Gynaecology
Royal Hospital for Women
Paddington
Sydney
Australia

Dr M. I. Levene MD FRCP
Reader in Child Health and Honorary Consultant
Paediatrician
Leicester University School of Medicine
UK

Professor G. Lyon MD
Department of Paediatric Neurology
Catholic University of Louvain
Brussels
Belgium

Dr R. A. Minns MB PhD
Department of Paediatric Neurology
Royal Hospital for Sick Children
Edinburgh
UK

Dr M. Mirmiran MD
Netherlands Institute for Brain Research
Amsterdam
Netherlands

Dr J. Mushin MB
Research Fellow
Department of Paediatrics & Neonatal Medicine
Royal Postgraduate Medical School
Hammersmith Hospital
London
UK

Mrs R. Oozeer
Department of Neurophysiology
Hammersmith Hospital
London
UK

Professor C. S. Peckham MD
Paediatric Epidemiology Department
Institute of Child Health
London
UK

Dr G. Pilu MD
Section of Prenatal Pathophysiology
2nd Department of Obstetrics and Gynecology
Bologna University School of Medicine
Italy

Professor H. F. R. Prechtl MD
Department of Developmental Neurology
University Hospital
Groningen
Netherlands

Mr J. Punt MB FRCS
Consultant Paediatric Neurosurgeon
University Hospital
Queen's Medical Centre
Nottingham
UK

Professor E. O. R. Reynolds MD FRCP
Professor of Neonatal Paediatrics
Department of Paediatrics
University College London
Rayne Institute
London
UK

Professor R. W. Smithells MD FRCP
Department of Paediatrics & Child Health
Clarendon Wing
Leeds General Infirmary
Leeds
UK

Professor D. F. Swaab MD PhD
Director
Netherlands Institute for Brain Research
Amsterdam
Netherlands

Dr K. Thiringer MD
Senior Lecturer in Paediatrics,
Consultant Neonatologist
University of Gothenburg
Department of Paediatrics I
Gothenburg
Sweden

Dr J. Q. Trounce MB MRCP
Research Fellow
Department of Child Health
Leicester University School of Medicine
UK

Dr D. I. Tudehope MB FRACP
Director of Neonatology and Reader in Child Health
Mater Misericordiae Mothers' Hospital
Brisbane
Australia

Dr A. Vacca MB FRACOG
Director of Obstetrics and Gynaecology
Mater Misericordiae Mothers' Hospital
Brisbane
Australia

Dr D. A. Viniker MD MRCOG
Department of Obstetrics and Gynaecology
Whipps Cross Hospital
London
UK

Dr P. S. Warren PhD
Senior Specialist
Department of Medical Imaging
Royal Hospital for Women
Sydney
Australia

Dr J. E. Wraith MB
Fellow in Medical Genetics
Murdoch Institute for Research into Birth Defects
Royal Children's Hospital
Melbourne
Australia

Dr I. D. Young MD MRCP
Senior Lecturer
Department of Child Health
Leicester University School of Medicine
UK

Contents

PART 1

Normal development of the central nervous system

1. Normal development of the central nervous system

Dr Marjorie A. England

At birth, the brain and spinal cord are already highly developed and exhibit considerable functional ability, although anatomical development continues for a further two years after birth (Dobbing & Sands 1973). This chapter describes the embryological and fetal development of the central nervous system indicating the age at which structures have been reported to develop. Unfortunately the ageing and subsequent staging of embryos and fetuses is a source of confusion amongst embryologists. The age of the developing child has been referred to in postconceptual and postmenstrual (gestational) weeks or lunar months. Crown–rump (CR) length is also commonly described. A more accurate method of assessing maturity is based on a series of developing external and internal features combined with CR measurements. Streeter (1942, 1948) presented a series of Horizons, 1–23, which described embryos until day 47 after fertilization. When true age is based on a fertilization date, full-term is at week 38 (266 completed days of gestation). Recently O'Rahilly (1973) has made

slight alterations to Streeter's Horizons. These comprise modifications between stages 14 to 23; they have been incorporated in the Carnegie Staging System and extend to 56 days. Tables 1.1 and 1.2 indicate the relationship between stages, crown–rump length and age of the embryo and fetus. Throughout this chapter, wherever possible, the postconceptual age of the embryo (up to 56 days) is given, and thereafter the postmenstrual (gestational) age. In some cases it is not possible to know from the authors' original descriptions whether they were referring to postconceptual or gestational age and some confusion between these two is inevitable.

The newborn brain weighs 300–400 g at full-term and lies in a head whose circumference averages 34 cm (males) (Willis & Grossman 1981). Male brains weigh slightly more than those of females but, in either case, brain constitutes 10% of the body weight at birth (Crelin 1973). This chapter describes in a very general manner, how the central nervous system, comprising the brain and spinal cord, is formed.

Table 1.1 Embryological development of the central nervous system: relationship between postconceptual age of the embryo and the Carnegie stage (the crown-rump (CR) length and somite stages are also included).

	Postconceptual age (days)	Carnegie stage	CR length (mm)	Somite stage
Neurulation	18–19	8	1.0–1.5	2.5
	20–21	9	1.5–3.0	1–3
	22–23	10	2.0–3.5*	4–12
	24–25	11	2.5–4.5*	13–20
	26–27	12	3–5	21–29
Secondary canalization	28–30	13	4–6	30–35
	31–32	14	5–7	
	33–36	15	7–9	
	37–40	16	8–11	
	41–43	17	11–14	
	44–46	18	13–17	
	47–48	19	16–18	
	49–51	20	18–22	
Retrogressive differentiation (to 80 days)	52–53	21	22–24	
	54–55	22	23–28	
	56	23	27–31	

*refers to greatest length rather than crown–rump length

Table 1.2 Fetal growth: the approximate crown–rump (CR) length to gestational (postmenstrual) age

Gestational age (weeks)	CR length (mm)
9	50
10	61
12	87
14	120
16	140
18	160
20	190
22	210
24	230
26	250
28	270
30	280
32	300
36	340
38	360

For further reading the excellent book by Lemire et al (1975) is recommended.

An understanding of the normal development allows one to appreciate the structure of the central nervous system and to analyse its defective development.

GENERAL DEVELOPMENT

EARLY DEVELOPMENT (NEURULATION)

This stage covers post conceptual age 18–27 days. The first indications of the human central nervous system appear in the late primitive streak stages approximately 18 days after fertilization (stage 8 (O'Rahilly & Muller 1987), 1.0–1.5 mm CR). An area of thickened embryonic neuro-ectoderm initially lying cranial to the primitive streak is called the neural plate. This region will give rise to the brain and spinal cord. Experimental studies on lower vertebrates have shown that the underlying notochord and pre-axial mesoderm have induced the overlying ectoderm to thicken and form neuro-ectoderm. During elongation of the notochord in subsequent stages, the neural plate broadens and eventually extends to the oropharyngeal membrane.

Late in stage 8 and in early stage 9 (20–21 days) the neural plate forms a midline groove flanked on either side by a parallel neural fold (Fig. 1.1) (Ranson & Clark 1959, O'Rahilly 1973, O'Rahilly & Gardner 1979). These neural folds are largely cerebral (Fig. 1.2) and the future forebrain, midbrain and hindbrain are identifiable (O'Rahilly & Muller 1981). Towards the end of the third week (day 22, stage 10, 4–12 somites) (Fig. 1.3) the neural folds move toward one another and fuse to form the neural tube. The middle of the tube is called the central or neural canal. As the upper margins of the neural folds fuse, a group of ectoderm cells on either side of the developing neural tube migrates inwards to form the neural crest.

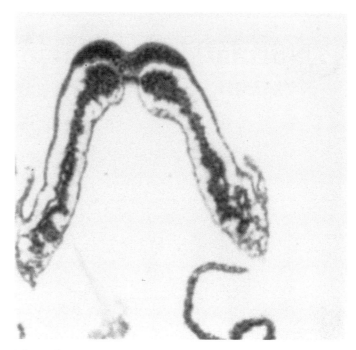

Fig. 1.1 Stage 9 (days 20–21): a transverse section of the neural folds and somites.

The neural folds initially fuse opposite somites 2–7 (O'Rahilly & Gardner 1977) in a 6–7 somite stage embryo. This is the future occipitocervical region (Muller & O'Rahilly 1985). The neural tube cephalic to the fourth pair of somites will form the brain and caudal to the fourth somites the spinal cord (Lemire et al 1975). Fusion proceeds both cephalically and caudally. Caudally, the neural tube is fused at the level of the most recently formed somite. By late stage 10 (22–23 days) the neural tube is fused the length of the embryo from the otic plate (region of the future ear) to the 12th somite. In stage 11 (24–25 days, 13–20 somites) fusion is present as far cranially as the level of the colliculi. Fusion continues both cephalically and caudally until only the ends of the tube remain open; the openings being the rostral (anterior) neuropore and the caudal (posterior) neuropore. This means that the central canal is in communication with the amniotic cavity and fluid. The closure of the rostral neuropore occurs on day 24 (stage 11) (O'Rahilly & Gardner 1979, O'Rahilly et al 1984) and this site corresponds to the lamina terminalis in older brains. In experimental animals, it has been shown that a temporary occlusion of the spinal central canal occurs before the caudal neuropore closing. This occlusion is concomitant with a rapid and substantial enlargement of the brain (Desmond & Schoenwolf 1986) and it is believed that these two events are linked, resulting in the brain ventricles being a sealed, closed-off system before caudal neuropore closure. The caudal neuropore closes about two days later than the rostral one (stage 12, 21–29 somites, 26 days) (O'Rahilly & Gardner 1979, O'Rahilly et al 1984) during the 24–25 somites stage. Closure is at the level of L1 to L2 (Ferner 1939).

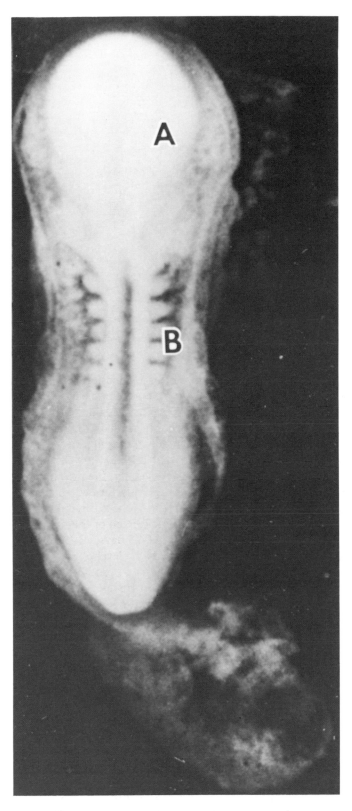

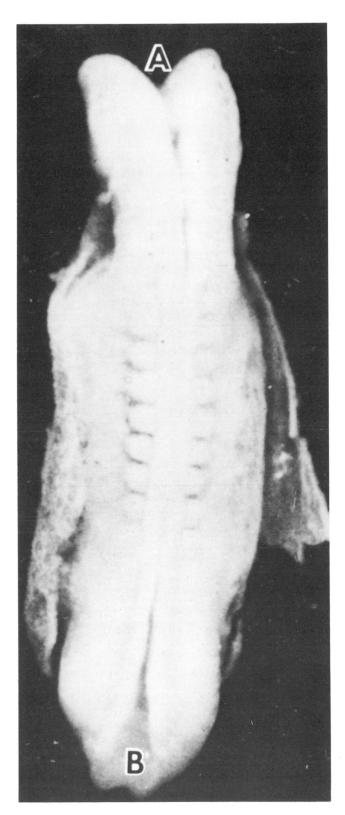

Fig. 1.2 Stage 10 (days 22–23): the cephalic end of the embryo can be clearly distinguished at this stage. Cephalic region (A), somites (B). (Reproduced with permission of Wolfe Medical Publications.)

Fig. 1.3 Stage 10 (days 22–23): the neural tube is fusing in the region of the somites. The cephalic (anterior) and caudal (posterior) neuropores are open at this stage. Cephalic neuropore (A), caudal neuropore (B). (Reproduced with permission of Wolfe Medical Publications.)

The formation of the remaining lower lumbar, sacral and coccygeal segments occurs during secondary caudal neural tube formation.

SECONDARY CAUDAL NEURAL TUBE FORMATION

Otherwise known as secondary canalization, this takes place during postconceptual days 30–50. At the caudal end of the neural tube (stage 12, 26–27 days, Muller & O'Rahilly 1985) there is a large aggregate of undifferentiated cells called the caudal cell mass. This mass is a blend of notochord and neural tube cells which extends into the end bud (Schoenwolf 1979, Muller & O'Rahilly 1985). In a short time, small vacuoles appear in the caudal cell mass in the vicinity of the neural tube. Cells lying adjacent to the vacuoles re-orient themselves around the perimeters of the vacuoles and assume the appearance of ependymal cells. As the vacuoles coalesce with one another, these cells take on the appearance of neural cells. Eventually the coalesced vacuoles connect with the central canal of the already-formed neural tube (stages 13 or 14, 28–32 days).

RETROGRESSIVE DIFFERENTIATION

Retrogressive differentiation occurs during postconceptual days 50–80. At about stage 16 (37–40 days) the tail and the structures within it begin to regress and ultimately the tail will disappear (Fallon & Simandl 1978, FitzGerald 1985). By stages 18–20 (44–51 days) the caudal-most part of the neural tube begins to regress and its central canal also begins to decrease in size. The central canal will remain as the ventriculus terminalis within the conus medullaris of the adult spinal cord. In some individuals it is found in the upper filum terminale. Its appearance has been described variously by Kunimoto (1918) in the 15.5 mm CR (stage 18, 44–46 days) embryo and by Kernohan (1925) in the stage 20 (49–51 days) embryo. There is a small dilation of the central canal at the level of the second coccygeal vertebra (the 32nd vertebra) which persists throughout life.

The filum terminale first appears at stage 23 (56 days) (Streeter 1919). As the caudal neural tube continues to atrophy, a small ependymal vestige is left which remains at the tip of the coccygeal segments, the coccygeal medullary vestige. Between this vestige and the ventriculus terminalis, the neural tube continues to atrophy. As it atrophies, a fibrous glial strand is formed called the filum terminale. Remains of ependyma may be found within the fetal filum terminale (Gamble 1967, 1969, 1971) and may persist postnatally. While the filum persists throughout life, the coccygeal medullary vestige disappears.

ASCENT OF THE SPINAL CORD

The spinal cord extends into the tail of the embryo until stages 18 to 20 (44–51 days) and the beginning of retrogressive differentiation. Once the filum terminale and conus medullaris have formed, the conus assumes a higher and higher position within the vertebral canal (Fig. 1.4). This phenomenon is believed to be due to the vertebrae growing more rapidly than the spinal cord. As a result, the spinal cord 'ascends' in the canal and may reach its adult level of L1–L2 as early as week 31. There is a great deal of variation, however, and more usually the L1–L2 level is reached within two weeks postnatally.

PRIMARY BRAIN VESICLES

The brain forms from the neural tube cranial to the fourth pair of somites.

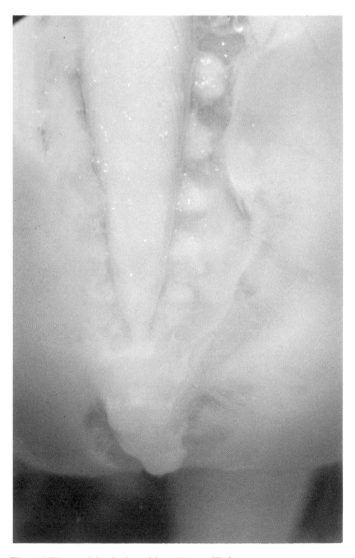

Fig. 1.4 The caudal spinal cord in a 60 mm CR fetus.

With the formation of the cranial neural tube and subsequent closure of the rostral neuropore, the three primary brain vesicles form in week 3 (stage 9, 20–21 days) (Muller & O'Rahilly 1983). From cranially–caudally the vesicles are the forebrain (prosencephalon), the midbrain (mesencephalon) and the hindbrain (rhombencephalon). These three areas can be identified, however, at the open neural groove stage two days before the neural tube forms (Muller & O'Rahilly 1983). The three primary vesicles are easily identifiable as the midbrain flexure occurs between the forebrain and midbrain regions (Bartelmez 1923), while the rhombencephalon dominates the brain (Muller & O'Rahilly 1983). The lumen of the rhombencephalon is the widest part of the neural tube by the end of stage 13 (28–30 days).

The hindbrain has four subdivisions or rhombomeres (Muller & O'Rahilly 1983). The first three rhombomeres (Bartelmez 1923) are related to the otic plates (future ear) while the fourth (Muller & O'Rahilly 1983) is opposite and slightly caudal to the somites. This fourth area represents the hypoglossal region. The floor of the hindbrain has six rhombic grooves related to the primordia of the 5th, 6th, 7th, 8th, 9th and 10th cranial nerves. The most rostral of the six rhombic grooves occurs at the level of the pontine flexure and is related to the trigeminal nerve. These grooves disappear by stage 15 (33–36 days).

Two constrictions appear in the brain. The first occurs at about stages 12–13 (26–30 days) immediately caudal to the midbrain and is termed the isthmus rhombencephali. A second isthmus appears at stages 22–23 (54–56 days) rostral to the midbrain, i.e. the isthmus prosencephali (Stroud 1900).

BRAIN FLEXURES

During week 3 (stage 9, 20–21 days) the brain grows more rapidly in the dorsal lamina than in the ventral lamina and as a result flexes ventrally. The first flexure, the cranial or mesencephalic flexure, is present at stage 9 (20–21 days) (O'Rahilly & Gardner 1977, Muller & O'Rahilly 1985) while the neural groove is still completely open. Ventrally this flexure marks the site of the future midbrain (Bartelmez & Evans 1926).

Ultimately, there are three flexures formed; the first, the cranial (midbrain, mesencephalic) flexure occurs between the midbrain and forebrain. Shortly, at stages 13 and 14 (28 to 32 days) the cervical flexure occurs between the hindbrain and spinal cord. This flexure is directed ventrally. The third flexure, the pontine flexure, arises from differential growth in the hindbrain (stages 13–16, 28–40 days) (Lemire et al 1975) and results in the hindbrain roof becoming very thin (see **Cerebellum** p. 18 and Figs. 1.5, 1.6). The cranial and cervical flexures occur due to orientation of the head, and ultimately the cervical flexure disappears.

The brain flexures also result in the white and grey matter greatly altering their positions at different levels in the brain. Originally the brain and spinal cord have a similar basic structure; but after the flexures develop the alar and basal plates (see p. 9 for definition) can only be distinguished in transverse sections of the midbrain and hindbrain (Lemire et al 1975). The sulcus limitans will extend as far as the junction of the forebrain and midbrain.

SECONDARY BRAIN VESICLES

During weeks 5–6 the forebrain subdivides to form two vesicles; the cranial telencephalon (endbrain) and

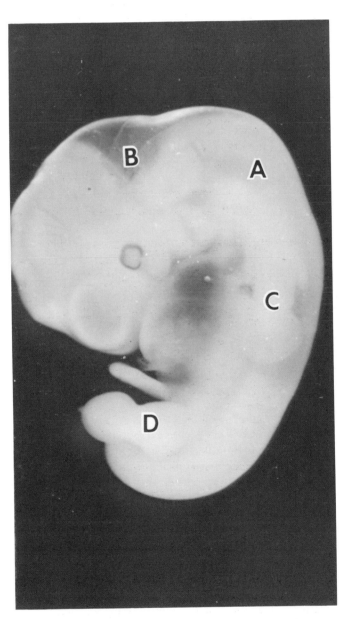

Fig. 1.5 Stage 15 (days 33–36): the cervical flexure (A) and pontine flexure (B), arm bud (C) and leg bud (D).

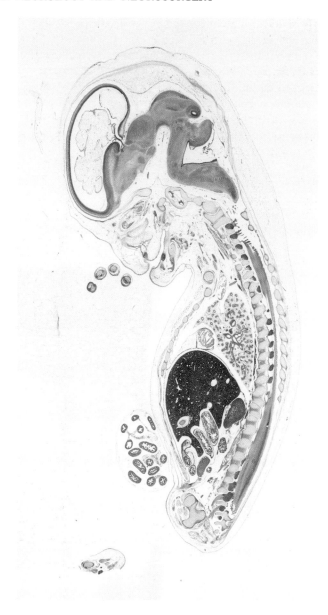

Fig. 1.6 Parasagittal section illustrating the brain flexures.

the diencephalon (between brain) (Gilbert 1935). The midbrain remains undivided. The hindbrain subdivides to form two areas; the cranial metencephalon (afterbrain) and the myelencephalon (marrow brain). There are now a total of five secondary brain vesicles.

Histology of the spinal cord

Early embryo

The development of the spinal cord has been studied extensively because it is the simplest model.

As the neural folds first fuse to form a tube, the walls are composed of a single layer of columnar epithelium.

These cells proliferate rapidly so that the neural tube walls soon become thickened and composed of a pseudostratified columnar epithelium. The central canal initially is relatively large but later, when the white and grey matter increase, it will become smaller. The epithelial layer is called the ventricular zone (germinal or ependymal layer or matrix) (Boulder Committee 1970). All of these cells synthesize DNA at this stage of development. At 17–21 days each cell is approximately wedge-shaped and attached at both ends to the outer and luminal surfaces of the neural tube (Sauer 1936, Sidman & Rakic 1973). During week 4, the cells successively retract to the luminal margin of the neural tube and divide. The daughter cell nuclei then migrate back into the layer and reconnect to the outer margin of the neural tube. The process is repeated so that these cells eventually give rise to all the neural and macroglial cells in the central nervous system.

Once the neural tube has closed, this ventricular layer will give rise to the immature neurones (neuroblasts or primitive neurones) (Fujita 1973). These cells, unlike the neuro-epithelial cells, are not connected to the luminal surface. While the neuro-epithelial cells are producing immature neurones, they are also producing glioblasts (spongioblasts or primitive neuroglia). As the earliest immature neurones migrate from the neuro-epithelial layer they are accompanied by glia. Radial glia are also present from the earliest stages and form the glia limitans. They may also guide neurones. During the early stages, neurone production predominates. Even when the neurones cease dividing, glia production continues throughout life (Sturrock 1982a). The most rapid increase in glial number occurs just before and during early myelination. This increase in glial cells is brought about by division of the glial cells already present in white matter (Sturrock 1982b). Finally, the neuro-epithelial cells produce ependymal cells. Ultimately, these cells will line the ventricular system of the brain, choroid plexuses and central canal of the spinal cord.

Soon (stages 15–17, 33–43 days) a second layer, the marginal zone (subpial or molecular layer), appears outside the ventricular zone. This relatively acellular layer is composed of the outer parts of the neuro-epithelial cells and will eventually form the white matter (Boulder Committee 1970). By 26–38 mm CR the marginal zone surrounds the entire cord (Lemire et al 1975).

As the neuro-epithelial cells proliferate, the lateral walls of the spinal cord thicken but the roof and floor plates remain thin. At stages 15–17 (33–43 days) a shallow groove (sulcus limitans) appears between the dorsal and ventral parts of the spinal cord. The dorsal part of the spinal cord becomes the alar plate (lamina) and the ventral part the basal plate (lamina). The alar and basal plates extend throughout the spinal cord as long columns (Fig. 1.7). The alar plates form the dorsal grey columns comprised of groups of afferent nuclei. The basal plates form the ventral and lateral grey columns. Axons from unipolar neurones in the spinal ganglia enter the spinal cord and form the dorsal roots of the spinal nerves whilst axons from ventral horn cells grow out of the spinal cord and form the ventral roots of the spinal cord. The relative thickness of the three layers of the spinal cord changes; by 38–55 mm CR the ependymal layer is thinner and by 55–75 mm CR the marginal zone is increasing in thickness at a greater rate than the mantle zone. The posterior median septum is now evident as a thin glial layer (Lemire et al 1975). By 75–105 mm CR there is a greater volume of white matter than grey matter and by 180–265 mm CR the thoracic cord is composed of over 60% white matter (Lemire et al 1975).

Beginning in week 12, ascending, descending and propriospinal fibres invade the marginal zone (FitzGerald 1985).

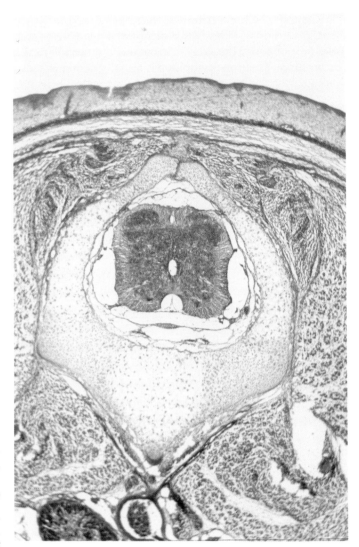

Fig. 1.7 The 120 mm CR lumbar spinal cord. The alar and basal plates are evident.

The third layer of the neural tube, the intermediate layer (middle or mantle layer), is present by 10 mm CR (38–40 days) and located between the ventricular and marginal zones. This layer forms from neuroblasts which have arisen in the ventricular zone and then move outwards. This thick cellular middle layer begins at stage 18 (44–46 days) and is destined to form the grey matter. The cells migrating to form this layer do not do so uniformly; there is a difference in pattern and intensity of migration from various parts of the neural tube (Kallen 1977). As a result, migration occurs in waves (Berquist & Kallen 1954). The ventral cells acquire their positions in the basal plate before the dorsal cells form the alar plates (His 1888, Kallen 1977). Initially the neuroblasts are apolar and lack processes. Later they develop processes at the opposite poles and are referred to as bipolar. Finally, the processes directed towards the lumen regress and the neuroblasts become unipolar. The remaining process becomes the axon and grows towards the periphery of the neural tube to contribute to the marginal layer. Subsequently, a group of outgrowths (primordial dendrites) form at the pole opposite the axon so becoming a multipolar cell. The multipolar neurone cytoplasm is initially homogeneous, although later large amounts of RNA and neurofibrils are present. The axon grows actively and either contacts other cells in the neural tube wall, usually via the marginal zone, or becomes motor by passing out of the neural tube to an effector organ. The dendrites become more complex by establishing contacts with adjacent nerve cells or their processes. Initially, the axons and dendrites arise independently but there is an interaction and correlation between dendritic tree formation and synaptic contacts. By stage 18 (44–46 days), the processes of the intermediate zone grow outwards into the narrow marginal zone.

Okado and Kojima in a recent study (1984) report that by 7 mm CR (32 days) the primary afferents, interneurones and motor neurones are identifiable, but not, as yet, connected. By 10–12 mm CR (38–42 days) the motor-cell columns in the cervical region are large and the first synapses are present in the motor nucleus between the motor neurone, dendrites and interneurones.

The first association neurones appear in the alar plate at 10 mm CR (Okado & Kojima 1984). By 22 mm CR (51–52 days) connections develop between sensory fibres and interneurones. When the fibrous components of the spinal reflex arc are complete at 22 mm CR, there is a rapid increase in the density of synapses in the motor nucleus at the level of the cervical spinal cord. Wozniak et al (1980) reported that synaptogenesis proceeds craniocaudally.

Late embryo and fetus

Okado & Kojima (1984) have identified three periods of synaptogenesis which coincide with descriptions of behavioural responses by other authors. These include spinal reflex activities at 8 weeks (Fitzgerald & Windle 1942), when the fibrous connections of the spinal reflex arc are complete; the onset of local activities (Humphrey 1964a & b) with a rapid increase in axodendritic synapses (9.5 weeks); and multiple responses at 13–15 weeks with a rapid increase in axosomatic synapses (Humphrey & Hooker 1959). Recent ultrasound studies (de Vries et al 1982) have shown that the first observable movements are at 7.5 weeks.

The spinal cord, like the brain, develops in identifiable spurts of growth and differentiation. Two periods have been identified in the first half of fetal development at 9.5–10.5 weeks and at 17.5–21 weeks (Okado & Yokota 1980).

Neuroglia

Macroglia

The supporting cells of the central nervous system form from the neuroepithelial cells of the ventricular zone. During the production of immature neurones, the supporting cells (glioblasts or spongioblasts) are also produced and migrate into the intermediate and marginal zones. Here they will differentiate to form astroblasts and then astrocytes (for review see Sturrock 1986); or oligodendroblasts and then oligodendrocytes. There is some controversy as to whether astrocytes and oligodendrocytes are two distinct cell types. In a recent paper, Choi et al (1983) proposed that oligodendrocytes in human fetal spinal cord form (with an intermediate astroglial form) from radial glial cells.

Microglia

There has been some controversy concerning the origins of the microglia. It was previously reported that they form from mesenchyme cells outside the central nervous system and then invade after the blood vessels form in the late fetal period (Barr 1979). However, microglia, which are small neuroglial cells, have been demonstrated in the human central nervous system from 5 to 8 weeks postconception by light microscopy (Kershman 1939), electron microscopy (Sturrock 1984) and by histochemical methods (Fujimoto & Mizoguti 1985). Blood vessels are present in the central nervous system from very early developmental stages. Embryonic human optic nerve has well-formed blood vessels, complete with tight junctions present at 8 weeks.

REGIONAL DEVELOPMENT

FOREBRAIN (TELENCEPHALON)

The telencephalon is composed of a median part and two lateral cerebral vesicles which, from the outset, grow more rapidly than the other areas of the brain (Desmond & O'Rahilly 1981).

Before rostral neuropore closure at stage 11 the optic diverticulae grow from the future diencephalon region of the forebrain (stage 10, 22 days), in front of which the future telencephalon can be identified (Muller & O'Rahilly 1985). In stage 14 (31–32 days) (O'Rahilly et al 1984), the telencephalon forms as two rostral, bilateral outpocketings, the cerebral vesicles, which are the future cerebral hemispheres. These vesicles, connected by a median region, appear in stage 14–15 (31–36 days) in the region of the foramen of Monro. The cerebellar plates and the commissural plates are present at stage 11 (24–25 days) (Gardner et al 1975, Muller & O'Rahilly 1984, 1985). As the cerebral hemispheres grow, they eventually cover the diencephalon, mesencephalon and hindbrain (Fig. 1.8).

The cavity of each hemisphere will form the lateral ventricles; and they are connected by the interventricular foramina (of Monro) to the lumen of the median region, the third ventricle (stage 16, 37–40 days).

The walls of the cerebral vesicles are composed of nervous tissue and ultimately form the cerebral hemispheres. As they

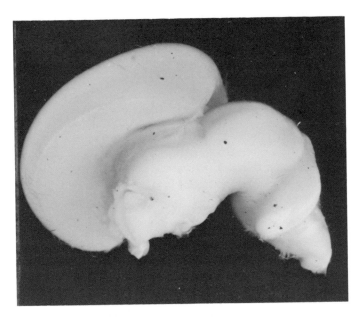

Fig. 1.8 The relationship of the cerebral hemispheres to the diencephalon and mesencephalon (one hemisphere has been dissected off).

expand forward, upwards and backwards their medial surfaces are separated by the longitudinal fissure. Eventually, however, the two hemispheres will meet in the midline, flattening against one another and trapping mesenchyme which forms the falx cerebri.

As the cerebral hemispheres grow, the rostral portion becomes the frontal pole. The posterior pole, which is growing caudo–ventrally forms the temporal pole. The new posterior part forms the occipital pole.

In the early stage 15 (33–36 days) the walls of the cerebral vesicles appear uniform, but rapidly begin to differentiate (stage 16, 37–40 days). The first area appears ventrally as two swellings in the floor of the lateral ventricle. These swellings form the corpus striatum in the inferior-lateral wall and will contribute to the formation of the amygdala (Humphrey 1968) (evident at stage 15, 33–36 days, O'Rahilly et al 1984), caudate nucleus, putamen (O'Rahilly & Gardner 1977) and with further development and migration to the pulvinar, nucleus lateralis posterior and possibly to other thalamic structures (Rakic & Sidman 1969, O'Rahilly & Gardner 1977).

The remaining cerebral vesicle in a suprastriatal position is referred to as the pallium and will form the cerebral cortex. Along its medial wall where the pallium is attached to the diencephalon, the wall of the pallium becomes very thin and projects into the lateral ventricle along a groove known as the choroidal fissure. This fissure extends from the level of the interventricular foramen posteriorly. Vascularization of the thin layer forms a tela choroidea and then the choroid plexus. The vascularization of cerebral cortex also starts at this embryonic age (Marin-Padilla in press a).

Immediately above the attachment of the choroid plexus there is a small thickening of the wall which bulges into the lateral ventricle. This area is the hippocampus and it appears as a longitudinal ridge in the ventricle and as a longitudinal groove, the hippocampal fissure on the medial surface of the hemisphere. The hippocampal fissure, therefore, runs parallel and above the choroidal fissure. The pallium above the hippocampal fissure and the dorsal and lateral walls are now referred to as the cortex of the neopallium. The neopallium adjacent to the corpus striatum forms the paleopallium (pyriform cortex) which is an olfactory cortex.

In stage 17 (41–43 days) the internal capsule is established (Marin-Padilla 1983), followed in stage 18 (44–46 days) by fibres from this area penetrating the superficial zones of the cerebral vesicle. As the fibres penetrate the superficial zones of the cerebral vesicles, they mark the establishment of an external white layer (a primordial plexiform lamina). By stage 20 (49–51 days) this lamina as well as the primitive corticipetal fibres extends through the entire surface of the cerebral cortex.

By stage 17 (41–43 days) the corpus striatum has thickened and fibres are running between it and the ventral thalamus. The floor of the cerebral hemisphere, including the corpus striatum, does not grow as rapidly as the remaining vesicle which expands and assumes a 'C' shape. The lateral ventricles within, also assume a 'C' shape to form the anterior and inferior horns. The 'C' shape is well-defined by 12 weeks but the posterior horn develops later. The final shape of the ventricles is assumed during months 5–6 of gestation. The hemisphere at the caudal end turns down and then forward to form the temporal lobe (Fig. 1.9). The inferior horn and the choroid

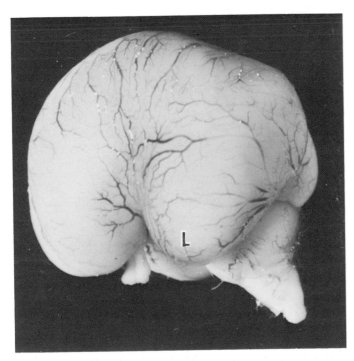

Fig. 1.9 The 18-week fetal brain; note the temporal lobe (L).

fissure are carried with the lobe. The choroid plexuses of the inferior horn will arise in the area of the choroid fissure. The surface of the hemisphere overlying the corpus striatum also grows slowly and is soon overtaken by the adjacent cortex growing more rapidly and is buried. This buried region is called the insula and is located deep in the lateral sulcus.

In stages 20–22 (49–55 days) descending internal capsule fibres passing between the diencephalon and telencephalon penetrate through the corpus striatum and divide it into two parts; medial and lateral areas (Fig. 1.10). The medial area appearing at 15–18 mm CR (Lemire et al 1975) is called the caudate nucleus and the lateral area the lentiform nucleus. This nucleus is subdivided into a lateral portion, the putamen, and a medial portion, the globus pallidus or pallidum, which is a derivative of the diencephalon. Not all the cortical fibres pass through the internal capsule, some pass lateral to the lentiform nucleus and form the external capsule. The internal capsule also becomes 'C'-shaped as the hemispheres expand. The caudate nucleus is influenced by this expansion and becomes elongated and horseshoe-shaped as it follows the outline of the lateral ventricle. The timing of the major events in human neocortical ontogenesis during the embryonic period is illustrated in Figure 1.11.

By the end of the embryonic period (stage 23, 8 weeks) the maximum brain diameter is 12–15 mm. The brainstem, however, is much better developed at this stage than the rest of the brain. During the fetal period, the weight of telencephalon doubles (expressed as a percentage of CNS weight); and by birth the cerebral vesicles weigh 305–345 g (Crelin 1973).

Histology of the cerebral cortex

The adult cerebral neocortex has six layers when examined histologically. They are numbered I–VI when looked at from superficial to deep. Traditionally these layers have been thought to arise from within and grow out towards the external surface. Three successive waves of cell migration were thought to form the neocortex, the earliest layers to form being layer V (ganglionic) and layer VI (multiform) in the first wave; followed by layer IIIa (pyramidal) and layer IV (inner granular) in the second wave; and layer I

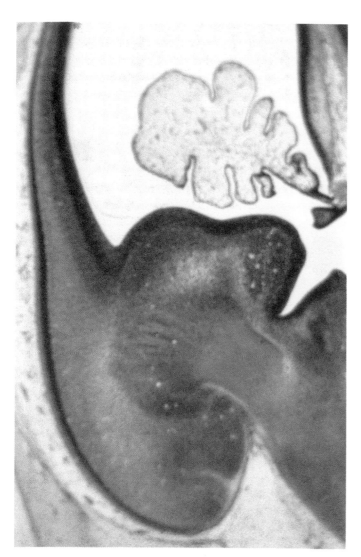

Fig. 1.10 The internal capsule dividing the corpus striatum into medial and lateral parts in a 27 mm CR embryo.

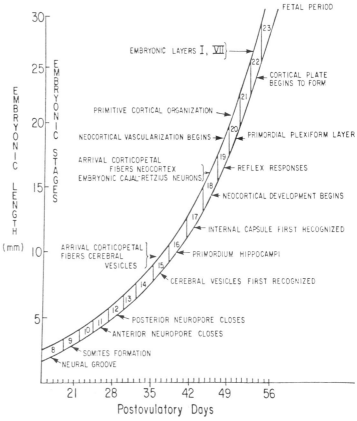

Fig. 1.11 Summary of the major events in human cortical ontogenesis. (Reproduced with permission of Dr Marin-Padilla.)

(plexiform) and layer II (outer granular) in the final wave (Warwick & Williams 1973).

Recently, however, Marin-Padilla in a series of studies has presented new and very convincing data which demonstrate that the reverse is true. By studying the formation of layer I, he established that it had a previously unrecognized importance in the overall organization of the cerebral cortex (Marin-Padilla 1984, in press b). He found that the undifferentiated telencephalic vesicle is first penetrated by primitive corticipetal fibres which extend throughout the layer. These fibres are believed to be monoaminergic and are possibly of mesencephalic origin. They course horizontally and establish a superficial or external white matter which is termed the marginal zone (Boulder Committee 1970) or primordial plexiform layer (Marin-Padilla 1978).

Larroche (1981) in a report on a 20 mm CR embryo observed that the cerebral hemisphere at this time is approximately 1 mm thick and is composed of two layers. The inner (ventricular) or matrix layer is a pseudostratified epithelium with numerous mitoses near the luminal (ependymal) surface. The outer, marginal or plexiform layer has an appreciable cell density whose nuclei are lighter than those of the matrix (ventricular zone). Neurones, stimulated by the presence of corticipetal fibres, appear and develop in this external white matter or marginal zone. Larroche (1981) describes them as large, well-differentiated neurones which she interpreted as Cajal–Retzius cells. This primitive layer is called the primordial plexiform layer (Marin-Padilla 1971, Larroche & Houcine 1982). It is well-established by stage 20 (50 days) (Marin-Padilla 1983) and is of short duration. O'Rahilly et al (1984) report this layer as early as stage 15 (33–36 days) near the corpus striatum. The primordial plexiform layer is functionally active, as shown by the fact that it is the first to contain synapses, so confirming its precocious development. At this stage the layer is 40 μm thick. The Cajal–Retzius cells form a special class whose maturation and development are in advance of the rest of the brain (Larroche 1981, Marin-Padilla & Marin-Padilla 1982). Duckett & Pearse (1968) reported that these cells are the first site of cholinesterase activity.

The cortical plate (pyramidal cell plate) is next to develop at stage 22 (25 mm CR, 54 days) as migrating neuroblasts guided by radial glial fibres (Rakic 1981) penetrate the primordial plexiform layer and accumulate within it (Marin-Padilla 1984, in press b). The cortical plate, which represents the mammalian neocortex, divides the primordial plexiform layer into a superficial layer I (external white matter) and a deep layer VII (layer VIb, subplate zone) of the future neocortex (Marin-Padilla 1978). This finding has been corroborated by Larroche et al (1981). The neurones remaining in layer I will form the embryonic, horizontally oriented Cajal–Retzius neurones. At this stage the neurones have a single, descending axonal process which becomes horizontal in the lower half of layer I as cortical development proceeds (Marin-Padilla &

Marin-Padilla 1982). As these processes become horizontal during the developmental expansion of the cortex, they lose their connection with layer VII.

Meanwhile, most neurones in layer VII become transformed into pyramidal-like and Martinotti neurones. The recurrent axonal collaterals of the first neurones and the ascending axons of the second establish connections with layer I. At this stage the pyramidal-like neurones represent the projection neurones and the Cajal–Retzius and Martinotti neurones the associative elements of this early cortical organization (Marin-Padilla 1971, 1984).

Just as the cortical plate divides the primordial plexiform layer into two layers, it also divides the primitive corticipetal fibres into two plexuses. One plexus is superficial to the cortical plate and the other lies below it. The first synapses which appear occur in relation to these two plexuses (Molliver et al 1973, Larroche 1981) and are believed to be functional at this stage.

As development proceeds the future pyramidal neurones of the cortical plate are attracted to layer I and make synaptic connections with it. As the neurones arrive at the superficial part of the cortical plate they contact layer I and grow apical dendritic bouquets which penetrate layer I and anchor themselves to it. At this stage the neurones are apparent as young pyramidal cells. Then, when new neuroblasts arrive to displace the young pyramidal cells these still retain their connection to layer I and this influences their subsequent growth (Marin-Padilla 1984, in press b). The apical dendrites of the pyramidal cells lengthen as the neuronal body becomes further removed from layer I. Synaptic contacts are established between the dendritic bouquets of all the pyramidal neurones and the horizontal axonal processes of the Cajal–Retzius neurones in layer I. The Cajal–Retzius neurones serve as a link between the primitive corticipetal fibres and young pyramidal neurones. This means that, regardless of their ultimate function, position, size, etc., all the cortical pyramidal neurones are receiving similar primitive information. In addition, as dual sets of pyramidal and Martinotti neurones are probably present at all levels of the cerebral cortex, the pyramidal cells may be inhibited by the axonal terminals of the Martinotti neurones at the level of their dendritic bouquets in layer I. Marin-Padilla (1984) suggests that the young neurones require this primitive information for their further growth and maturation. Ultimately, the specific functions of the young pyramidal cells are determined by the arrival of other afferent systems (thalamic fibres, both non-specific and specific fibres; callosal and cortico–cortical fibres). Regional differences in the architecture of the cerebral cortex are also related to the arrival of specific systems of afferent fibres.

The small neurones of layer I are recognized late in prenatal cortical formation. Their distribution is limited and their function may be local rather than generalized as that of the Cajal–Retzius neurones (Marin-Padilla 1984).

During development, layer I increases in thickness dramatically both vertically and horizontally; 25 to 250 μm between 11 weeks and birth, though the original plexiform arrangement is maintained (Marin-Padilla 1984). Marin-Padilla suggests that this dramatic increase in layer thickness is due to a progressive increase in the number of horizontal collateral branches of the Cajal–Retzius neurones and of the primitive corticipetal fibres. As the cortex develops, the horizontal axons of Cajal–Retzius neurones occupy the lower regions of layer I, while the corticipetal fibres and their collaterals occupy its upper region.

While layer I (primitive superficial plexiform) continues to play an important role in the organization of the adult cerebral cortex, layer VII (primitive deep plexiform or subplate zone) undergoes regressive changes and some of its neurones degenerate and eventually disappear (Marin-Padilla 1971, 1988b).

The remaining layers of the cerebral cortex evolve from the cortical plate and give rise to layers VI, V, IV, III and II. Together, they represent a recent mammalian innovation added to the more primitive (premammalian) cortical organization represented by layers I and VII (Fig. 1.12) (Marin-Padilla 1971, 1978, 1983, in press b). In the course of cortical ontogenesis, the differentiation and maturation of the neurones of the cortical plate, and hence of its various laminations, follow an ascending 'inside-out' progression. Neuronal differentiation (and maturation) starts at layer VI (Marin-Padilla 1970a, 1970b) and ascends progressively through layers V, IV, III and II. This ascending neuronal differentiation follows the sequential arrival of the various systems of corticipetal fibres. Corticipetal fibres (afferent) fibres arrive at the cortical plate sequentially and also follow an ascending progression. In general terms, non-specific thalamo–cortical fibres are first recognized at the level

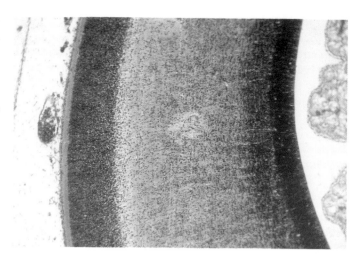

Fig. 1.12 The layers of the developing cerebral cortex of a 35 mm CR embryo; the choroid plexus appears at the right.

of layers VI–V, specific thalamo–cortical fibres at layers V–VI, callosal fibres at layer III and cortico–cortico fibres at layer II, respectively. The prenatal differentiation of each cortical layer is characterized by the maturation of its own pyramidal (projection) neurones which roughly represent 80% of its neuronal elements. On the other hand, the interneurones (short circuit, associative, Golgi type II neurones) of each lamina differentiate and become incorporated into the cortical organization much later in development. However, the origin, differentiation and functional incorporation of the various types of cortical interneurone have been insufficiently studied and remain poorly understood. The differentiation of the various cortical layers during the fetal period of human development are reproduced in Table 1.3.

Table 1.3 Development of the cerebral cortex during the fetal period; the thickness and differentiation of various laminations (layers I and VII as well as the cortical plate)

Age (wk)	Length (mm)	Layer I (μm)	Cortical plate (μm)	Development cortical plate	Layer VII (μm)
7	22 CR	PPL,30	No CP	—	PPL
11	40 CR	22–35	100–120	Undifferentiated CP	30–50
15–16	80–100 CH	50–60	300–500	Layers VI, V, undiff. CP	250–300
18–20	140–160 CH	90–100	700–800	Layers VI, V, IV, undiff. CP	Undetermined*
24–26	200–250 CH	125–135	900–1000	Layers VI, V, IV, IIIC, undiff. CP	Undetermined*
28–30	280–320 CH	150–170	1300–1500	Layers VI, V, IV, IIIC, IIIB, undiff. CP	Undetermined*
38–40	420–460 CH	250–300	1800–2100	Layers VI, V, IV, IIIC, IIIB, IIIA IIB, undiff. CP	Undetermined*

*As layer VII becomes progressively intermingled and incorporated into the expanding cortical white matter, its dimensions and limits are no longer recognizable.

wk, weeks of gestation; PPL, primordial plexiform layer; CP, cortical plate; CR, crown-rump; CH, crown-heel.

(Reproduced with permission from Marin-Padilla, in press b.)

Diencephalon

The posterior part of the forebrain is called the diencephalon. Its lumen is continuous with the lumen of the anterior part of the forebrain and together their lumena form the third ventricle.

Three swellings form on each side of the diencephalon; the future thalamus, epithalamus and the hypothalamus in the floor. Caudal to the thalamus, the lateral and medial geniculate bodies form. The epithalamus gives rise to the pineal body, the posterior commissure and the nucleus habenulae. The mammillary bodies, the tuber cinereum and part of the hypophysis (pituitary) arise in the hypothalamus.

The pineal body and subcommissural organ form at the junction of the diencephalon and mesencephalon.

The optic vesicles and second cranial nerve also form from the diencephalon.

Thalamus

The thalamus is located in the superior portion of the diencephalon. It contains the main afferent relay nuclei projecting onto the cerebral cortex. The auditory and visual pathways relay in the medial and lateral geniculate bodies respectively. The thalamic region can be identified as early as stage 10 (22–23 days) (Muller & O'Rahilly 1985).

The thalamus is further subdivided into a dorsal and a ventral part. The dorsal part forms the main portion of the thalamus. Although the epithalamus, ventral thalamus and hypothalamus differentiate first, and all four structures are present by stage 15 (33–36 days) (Lemire et al 1975), the growth of the dorsal thalamus overshadows that of the other three after stage 20 (49–51 days). The dorsal thalamus develops from two bulges, one on either side of the third ventricle, which grow rapidly (stages 20–21, 49–53 days). In approximately 80% of brains the two bulges fuse in the midline, forming a bridge of grey matter across the third ventricle called the massa intermedia. This is always present by 14–15 weeks gestation and almost fills the third ventricle (Lemire et al 1975). Although by 50–60 mm CR parts of the major subdivisions of the thalamus have appeared, the cephalic region of the dorsal thalamus remains undifferentiated (Lemire et al 1975).

The pulvinar appears at 70–90 mm CR and by 110–130 mm CR it overhangs the geniculate bodies.

As the dorsal thalamus grows caudally the geniculate bodies are carried caudally and ventrally and eventually by 250 mm CR (26 weeks gestational age) the lateral geniculate body has rotated into its final position. With further growth of the dorsal thalamus, the ventral thalamus is displaced laterally and away from the third ventricle (Kuhlenbeck 1948), which itself is reduced to a narrow canal (45–125 mm CR) and eventually a slit.

Also, as the thalamus grows the lateral part of its superior surface fuses with the thin wall of the cerebral vesicle overlying it. This part of the thalamus (diencephalon) is brought into close proximity to the corpus striatum (telencephalon) and eventually the two regions become continuous and provide a route for projection fibres to and from the cortex via the internal capsule.

The ventral thalamic nucleus gives rise to several nuclei. By mid-term the major nuclear subdivisions are identifiable (Lemire et al 1975).

The sulci separating the parts of the diencephalon appear in stage 18 (44–46 days), although two later fuse to form the hypothalamic sulcus of the adult brain (Lemire et al 1975).

The development of the thalamo–cortical connections has been described by Rakic (1981) as occurring in three phases. Initially, thalamic fibres grow into the intermediate zone of the cerebral wall and collect below the cortical plate. This is followed by the fibres entering the appropriate cortical region in a diffuse manner. In the final phase the fibres are distributed into specific terminal fields (Rakic 1981). For example, the somatic sensory pathways (touch, pain, temperature, conscious proprioception) relay in the ventral posterior nuclei of the thalamus and project to somatic sensory areas of the cortex, particularly the postcentral gyrus.

Epithalamus

The epithalamus forms in the caudal part of the roof and the dorsal lateral walls adjoining this region. Initially this swelling appears to be large, but with later development it becomes smaller in relative terms. Whilst the epithalamus can be identified early in development (stage 15, 33–36 days) it is shifted caudally by the tremendous growth of the dorsal thalamus.

Pineal gland (epiphysis cerebri)

The pineal gland develops from the midline in the caudal part of the roof of the diencephalon. High concentrations of serotonin and melatonin are present in this gland.

The pineal gland first becomes distinguishable at stage 14 (31–32 days) (O'Rahilly 1968, O'Rahilly et al 1982, O'Rahilly et al 1984) and appears at stage 15 (33–36 days) (Bartelmez & Dekaban 1962) as a thickening in the ependyma between the rostral habenular commissure and the caudal posterior commissure. This thickening in the ependyma is followed by the appearance of a slight recess. After approximately 10–15 weeks, the gland begins to increase in size (Dooling et al 1983a) and at the end of the first trimester consists of irregular tubules separated by loose mesenchymal cells (Dooling et al 1983a). By 16–23 weeks numerous large and small nests of epithelial cells are present and, at the end of the second trimester (24–27 weeks), there are numerous solid cords of cells. Melanin-pigment cells are present at this time particularly at the periphery, although they are also dispersed throughout the gland. At the beginning of the third trimester (28–31 weeks) the gland has an alveolar appearance but as the parenchymal cells enlarge the pigment cells are not as conspicuous (Dooling et al 1983a). From 32–39 weeks there is an increase in small hyperchromic cells. At term, the pineal contains large vesicular cells mixed with small hyperchromic cells (Dooling et al 1983a) but few pigment granules are present.

Posterior and habenular commissures

The posterior commissure is present at stage 15 (33–36 days) (O'Rahilly et al 1984) or stage 23, (56 days according to Dekaban 1954) and is formed when fibres invade the caudal part of the pineal recess from both sides (Warwick & Williams 1973).

The nucleus habenulae forms in the lateral wall of the diencephalon. Originally it lies close to the geniculate bodies but as the thalamus grows it becomes separated. The habenular commissure is present at stage 20, 49–51 days (O'Rahilly et al 1984) in the cranial pineal recess.

Hypothalamus

The hypothalamus is a suprasegmental area responsible for integrating autonomic and endocrine gland control. It lies in the inferior portion of the diencephalon ventral to the hypothalamic sulci, where it is formed by proliferating immature neurones of the intermediate layer. Later, nuclei concerned with homeostasis and endocrine functions develop and a pair of nuclei (mammillary bodies) develop on the ventral surface in stages 16–17 (37–43 days). The mammillary bodies originally arise as a single thickening which in the third month is divided by a furrow into two structures (Warwick & Williams 1973). The tuber cinereum develops anterior to the mammillary bodies.

Globus pallidus

The globus pallidus also forms from the diencephalon (Sidman & Rakic 1973, O'Rahilly & Gardner 1977) although others have thought that it is a derivative of the telencephalon. It arises as a longitudinally oriented bulge in the hypothalamus (Kuhlenbeck & Haymaker 1949). This region will give rise to the globus pallidus and subthalamic nucleus (Hewitt 1958, 1961). As the cerebral hemispheres enlarge, the globus pallidus shifts laterally (Sidman & Rakic 1973, O'Rahilly & Gardner 1977) and eventually it comes to lie medial to the putamen.

Pituitary gland (hypophysis cerebri)

The hypophysis is attached to the floor of the hypothalamus by the pituitary stalk. The pituitary gland has a dual origin; an anterior pituitary or glandular portion and a posterior pituitary or nervous portion. The anterior pituitary (also called the adenohypophysis) arises as a shallow diverticulum (Rathke's pouch) from the oral ectoderm and will contribute to the pars anterior (distalis), pars tuberalis and pars intermedia. The posterior pituitary (also called the neural lobe, pars neuralis or neurohypophysis) arises as an evagination (infundibulum) from the floor of the hypothalamus and is therefore a derivative of the neuro-ectoderm. This neural portion of the pituitary will form the pars nervosa, the infundibular stem and the median eminence.

The first indications of the adenohypophysis are evident at stage 10 (22–23 days) (Muller & O'Rahilly 1985), while Rathke's pouch appears during stage 12 (26–27 days) rostral to the notochord and during the next two stages (28–32 days) this pouch deepens and contacts the floor of the diencephalon (Lemire et al 1975). However, the first evagination of the diencephalic floor (the infundibulum), does not occur until stage 16 (37–40 days) and this region then assumes the appearance of a 'wrinkled sac' (Lemire et al 1975). By stage 21 (52–53 days) it is a deep sac whose lumen remains connected to the third ventricle. Tilney (1936), in a study of the hypophysis from the 11 mm CR embryo to the adult, presents a clear and comprehensive study of the development and appearance of this gland.

Recently O'Rahilly (1983) has claimed that instead of this interpretation, the hypophysis forms from a single locus.

Adenohypophysis (anterior pituitary) and the stalk of Rathke's pouch

At stage 17 (41–43 days) the stalk which connects Rathke's pouch with the stomodeal roof (primitive mouth cavity), begins to constrict in places so that the lumen is no longer continuous. Between stages 19–21 (47–53 days) the lumen of the stalk connecting Rathke's pouch with the foregut becomes largely obliterated. The stalk, which is initially thick and solid, becomes thinner and then thread-like. Finally, the centre portion of the stalk disappears leaving only a remnant at each end (Wislocki 1937) (stage 22, 54–55 days, O'Rahilly 1983). In the following stage the cranial portion disappears as the sphenoid cartilage appears but the caudal portion persists in the posterior nasopharynx as the pharyngeal hypophysis (Melchionna & Moore 1938, Boyd 1956, Lemire et al 1975).

The anterior pituitary is divided into three regions: pars tuberalis, pars intermedia and pars anterior (distalis).

The first indications of the pars tuberalis are seen late in stage 16 (37–40 days). Two lateral lobes (or tuberal processes) arise from Rathke's pouch near the mouth epithelium and in the following stage (17, 41–43 days) surround the infundibulum laterally. The bilateral lobes then begin to curve medially. By the end of stage 23 (56 days), the two pars tuberalis meet in the midline (behind the optic chiasma). They continue caudally to invest the median tuber cinereum by 45 mm CR (Lemire et al 1975), fuse with it at 55 mm CR, and completely invest the infundibulum between 120 and 170 mm CR.

By stage 18 (44–46 days) the second region, the pars intermedia, becomes identifiable as the anterior lobe cells adjacent to the infundibulum. In stage 19 (47–48 days) the pars intermedia grows laterally around the posterior lobe of the pituitary. The third region, the pars anterior enlarges dorsally in the midline, at the stage when the stalk of Rathke's pouch becomes threadlike (stage 21, 52–53 days). As a result the lumen of Rathke's pouch becomes smaller and is eventually reduced to a cleft (Rathke's cleft). This is not usually identifiable in the adult but cysts may form in its remnants.

At the same time (stages 19–21, 47–53 days), the floor of the third ventricle is becoming wider. By 55 mm CR, 'vascular grooves' in this region have formed blood vessels which have penetrated the pars distalis and pars tuberalis (Lemire et al 1975). All three regions of the adenohypophysis have now become glandular.

Neurohypophysis (posterior pituitary)

The neurohypophysis develops early functional activity, as evidenced by the detection of its hormones after 10 weeks (Dicker & Tyler 1953, Skowsky & Fisher 1973). Both the neurovascular contacts and the neurosecretory granules appear around 10 weeks. By 8.5 weeks (45 mm CR) the axon profiles contain accumulations of granular vesicles (Okado & Yokota 1980). Later in development these granular vesicles store hormones but it is not clear whether this is so at the earlier stages.

At 15.5–19 weeks there is a further increase in the number of vesicles. This is associated with an increase in the neurosecretory materials in the hypothalamic supra-optic and/or paraventricular nuclei which send axons into the neural lobe (Okado & Yokota 1980).

Between 170 and 200 mm CR the posterior pituitary differentiates further and the proximal cells resemble neuroglial cells while the distal cells are oval or fusiform. Nerve fibres from the hypothalamus grow into the pars nervosa.

Generally, the entire pituitary gland is well-formed by 110 days (Dicker & Tyler 1953).

Infundibular stem

During the fetal period (120 mm CR) the stem elongates and forms a backward angle of 20 degrees with the ventricular floor. By 170 mm CR the stalk assumes an angle of 45 degrees and by birth is nearly perpendicular (Lemire et al 1975).

Subcommissural organ

The subcommissural organ appears at the junction of the diencephalon and mesencephalon.

This organ was originally described by Dandy & Nichols (1910) as two bands of columnar epithelium united in the shape of a groove. Although this organ is present in the fetus (Wislocki & Roth 1958), it is vestigial at birth and disappears in the early adult (Rakic 1965). Dooling et al (1983a) describe the organ as a prominent secretory structure at 12–24 weeks, gradually becoming less distinct by 25–40 weeks. This change is brought about by atrophy and by the loss of specialized epithelial cells. However, it has been suggested that this rudiment is still an active cell population (Kelly 1982).

MIDBRAIN (MESENCEPHALON)

The midbrain originally has relatively thin walls and its lumen is a continuation of the third ventricle. As a result of the walls thickening, the lumen of the midbrain is eventually reduced to the narrow cerebral aqueduct (of Sylvius). This aqueduct connects the third and fourth ventricles. The dorsal midbrain roof (tectum) enlarges as two pairs of protuberances form, the rostral or superior colliculi and the inferior colliculi (Lund 1978). The superior colliculi are concerned with visual reflexes and the inferior colliculi with auditory transmission. Several nuclear groups also develop from the basal plates in the midbrain floor (tegmentum): the midbrain reticular formation, the red nucleus, the substantia nigra, and the oculomotor (III) and trochlear (IV) motor nuclei. The floor is additionally thickened by the base consisting of the cerebral peduncles — two large tracts conveying fibres from the cerebral cortex to subcortical areas.

In the early embryo (stage 10, 22–23 days) the rostral limit of the mesencephalon is a narrowing caudal to the optic primordium called the promesencephalic sulcus. The caudal limit is termed the isthmus rhombencephali (Warwick & Williams 1973). Later in development, the rostral limit is the mesmetencephalic sulcus (the future isthmus).

Neuromeres

As the rostral neuropore closes, two midbrain neuromeres appear in the midbrain floor — a large rostral one and a smaller caudal one. These landmarks are linked with the cephalic flexure which appears in this region (stage 12, 26–27 days) and caudal to the second neuromere is the mesmetencephalic sulcus.

Colliculi

The colliculi (tectum or corpora quadrigemina) form from

cells which migrate from the alar plates. The primordium of the colliculi is the collicular plate which appears at stage 11 (24–25 days). The two neuromeres described above have been equated with Streeter's pretectal and collicular areas (Bartelmez & Dekaban 1962). When the sulcus limitans appears (stages 13–14, 28–32 days) the corpora are separated from the tegmentum. Also during stage 14 (31–32 days) the isthmus grows rapidly. The tectum then thickens (7–9 mm CR) and the collicular plate is approximately equal in thickness throughout its area. In stage 16 (37–40 days) the borders of the colliculi are further established rostrally and caudally as the posterior commissure and the dorsal decussation of the trochlear nerve (IV) assume their positions in the midbrain. During stage 17 (41–43 days) the primordia of the paired bilateral superior colliculi and the paired bilateral inferior colliculi become visible as the collicular plate thickens. They become distinct by stage 18 (44–46 days).

Red nucleus

By stage 15 (33–36 days) the basal laminae are distinctly larger than the alar laminae of the same region. As the basal plate grows, the relative size of the midbrain lumen becomes smaller. At stage 16 (37–40 days) the two somatic efferent columns are present in the basal plate. The midventral region between the two columns contains collections of neuroblasts which will form the midventral proliferation. This structure is well-formed by stage 18 (44–46 days). By stage 20 (49–51 days) some of its lateral cells will separate and form the red nucleus together with cells from the lateral angle of the basal lamina. Fibres arrive from the cerebellum and contribute to the formation of the tegmentum. Fibres from the cerebellum running in the brachium conjunctivum (superior cerebellar peduncle) also arrive and invade the midventral proliferation. By the middle of week 9 (40 mm CR) they clearly demarcate the capsule of the red nucleus (Morrell 1985). The brachium conjunctivum is finely myelinated by 180 mm CR and by the eighth month it is heavily myelinated.

From stages 20–21 (49–53 days) up until stage 23 (56 days) several structures become evident in the red nucleus. By stages 20–21 the fasciculus retroflexus is seen passing through the medial aspect of the red nucleus, followed in stages 21–22 (52–55 days) by the appearance of the mamillotegmental tract. In stage 23, clusters of cells (pars magnocellularis) appear in the red nucleus at approximately the same time as the functionally linked dentate nucleus appears in the cerebellum.

By the end of the third month the red nucleus is clearly defined (Warwick & Williams 1973) and reaches its full size at 5 years of age.

Substantia nigra

The substantia nigra forms as cells from the ventrolateral aspect of the midventral proliferation spread and form a crescent-shaped mass (Cooper 1946, 1950, Lemire et al 1975) (stages 20–21, 49–53 days). This broad layer of grey matter is adjacent to the cerebral peduncle. The basis pontis also forms from the midventral proliferation and by stage 23 (56 days) its cells have established a continuity with the nigral cells. Later, at 60 mm CR, two zones are established in the substantia nigra; the corpus and the cauda. By 90 mm CR (12 weeks) the substantia nigra is pyramidal and by 190 mm CR (20 weeks) a third zone appears called the caput. It is possible to find some brown pigmentation at this stage, but it is not visible in gross specimens until 5 years of age. The 'adult' appearance is assumed at puberty (Lemire et al 1975).

By the eighth month (300 mm CR) myelinated fibres extend from the substantia nigra to the contralateral substantia nigra. They also extend to the subthalamic nucleus, into the medial lemniscus, descending corticospinal fibres and temporo-pontine pathway.

Cerebral peduncles

The cerebral peduncles develop as small thickenings from the ventral laminae. In the fourth month they increase rapidly in size and become more prominent as their fibre tracts appear in the marginal zone (Warwick & Williams 1973). These tracts are passing through the midbrain to the brain stem and spinal cord and they include the cortico–pontine, cortico–bulbar, and cortico–spinal tracts.

HINDBRAIN (METENCEPHALON)

The metencephalon is composed of a dorsal tissue mass, the cerebellum forming the roof, and a ventral tissue mass (the pons) forming the floor. The fourth ventricle lies between these two masses.

Cerebellum

The cerebellum (little brain) is an outgrowth of the hindbrain (metencephalon) and is located rostral to the developing trigeminal nerve (sensory). It appears at the same time as the pontine flexure. The flocculonodular lobes are the first to form and differentiate. They are also the first to have a mature cell population and to myelinate.

Initially the rhombencephalic region in the early embryo (stage 12, 26–27 days) has a very thin roof oriented longitudinally. With the appearance of the pontine flexure (stage 13–14, 28–32 days) the rhombencephalon is re-oriented from a longitudinal axis to a horizontal one. In this process, the very thin roof creases (plica chorioidea). Cranial to this landmark the cerebellum will develop, while the choroid plexus will form at its site.

The rhombencephalon is now diamond-shaped and at

its most lateral part (the alar plates) there is a burst of mitotic activity during the fourth week. This neuroblast activity causes the dorsal portion of the alar plates to enlarge and form the rhombic lips. The rhombic lips are a proliferative zone which contributes cells ventrally to the brainstem (pontine nuclei and inferior olive) and dorsally to the cerebellum. Initially the lips are small swellings which bulge into the fourth ventricle (40–90 mm CR) (Fig. 1.13). The cerebellum, which now has a large number of neuroblasts, bulges externally. This area continues to grow at the expense of the intraventricular portion. By stage 17 (41–43 days) the rhombic lips have differentiated rostrally from the level of the vestibular nuclei to the rostral end of the rhombic roof. Because the mitotic rate is high in the rhombic lips, and neuroblasts migrate into the lips, the pontine flexure continues to deepen. As a result, the rhombic lips fuse to the ventral portion of the alar plates. Initially these areas are parallel to the longitudinal axis of the neural tube. Then, as the pontine flexure forms, the rhombic lips come to run in an oblique line rostrally towards the midline. Eventually they fuse in the midline to form a dumb-bell shaped cerebellum. The lateral regions grow rapidly and form the lateral lobes.

The first fissure (posterolateral) appears early in the fourth month (50 mm CR), separating the nodule from the vermis, the floccules and the hemispheres. This fissure is separating the most primitive phylogenetic portion, the flocculonodular lobe (archicerebellum) from the remainder (trigeminal–spinal portion). The second fissure to appear is the primary fissure at 75 mm CR separating the culmen from the declive. Later, secondary fissures appear in the vermis and flocculonodular lobes which eventually extend into the hemispheres and give rise to the adult folia.

The dumb-bell shape of the cerebellum is acquired when the middle portions ultimately proliferate more than the rostral or caudal portions (Fig. 1.14). Then the hemispheres grow and almost obscure the vermis. The vermian lobules are present at 150 mm CR and their folia are beginning to form.

Finally, the cerebellum overgrows the fourth ventricle, the pons and the medulla. In the neonate, the cerebellum weighs 18–20 g and comprises 5–6% of the weight of the entire brain (Crelin 1973). Although by birth the cerebellum has the same shape as in the adult, cellular differentiation, migration and myelination continue.

Histology of the cerebellum

In the embryo, the cerebellar wall consists of three identifiable layers; the ventricular, intermediate and marginal zones. The first indications of the future cerebellar cortex are the development of Purkinje cells generated in the roof of the fourth ventricle (intermediate cells of the alar plates). These cells then migrate externally at 9–10 weeks, until they come to lie in the most superficial part of the marginal zone.

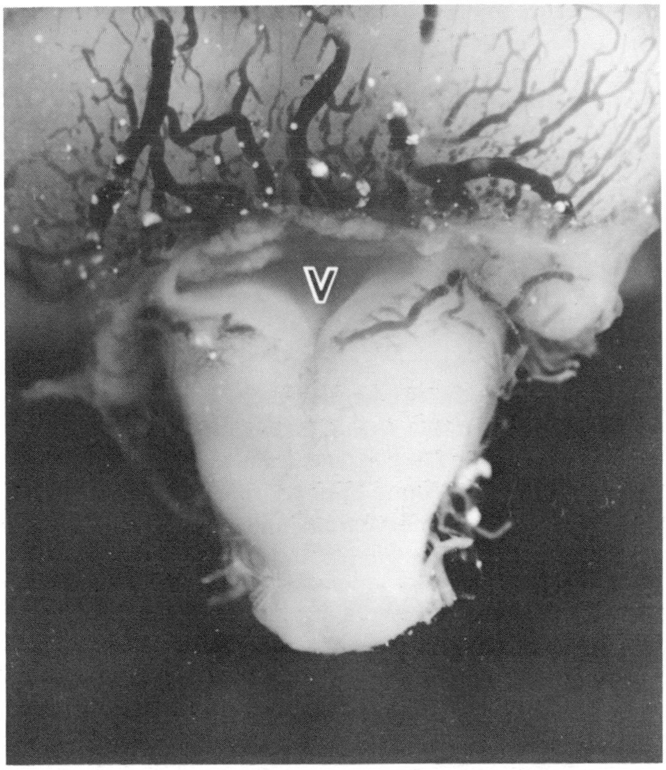

Fig. 1.13 The developing cerebellum. Fourth ventricle (v).

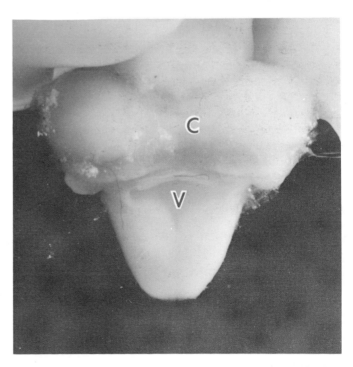

Fig. 1.14 The cerebellum of the week-15 fetus. Cerebellum (C), fourth ventricle (v).

At the same time, a subventricular zone forms (particularly prominent in the rhombic lip) and by 10–11 weeks granule cells derived from this layer migrate over the external surface of the cerebellum and form a transient layer, the external granular layer. Once the cells to which this layer gives rise are postmitotic, they migrate inward trailing a perpendicular axon and develop dendrites upon reaching their position below (internal to) the Purkinje cell layer. A transient layer, the lamina dissecans, separates the internal granular layer from the Purkinje cells. Ultimately this is filled by migrating granule cells and disappears (Rakic & Sidman 1970). At the same time as the postmitotic granule cells migrate inwards (16–25 weeks), the Purkinje cells enlarge and develop dendritic trees. Shortly following the appearance of the internal granular layer, basket cells also start to form.

The transient external granular layer normally regresses markedly between 2 and 4 months after birth (Friede 1973). It becomes progressively thinner as the number of cells in the layer decreases. By 18 months after birth the adult appearance is reached (Larroche 1966). Medulloblastoma, a brainstem tumour of childhood is thought to originate in malignant external granule cells (Kadin et al 1970).

Other intermediate-layer cells which did not migrate, give rise to the dentate and fastigial nuclei which are apparent at an early stage, as well as the globose and emboliform nuclei.

Pons

The pons forms from the basal lamina in the ventral metencephalon. Three groups of motor cell arise from the basal lamina. From medial to lateral these are: 1. somatic efferents giving rise to the nucleus of nerve VI; 2. the special visceral efferent (branchiomotor) nucleus of nerve VII (caudally), and 3. nerve V (cranially) and general visceral efferent (superior salivary nucleus) of nerve VII.

The nuclei pontis of the basilar part of the pons are formed by a contribution from the alar plate of the myelencephalon, as well as from cells of the metencephalon. Later, their axons grow transversely in the marginal zone to the cerebellum of the opposite side. These comprise the transverse fibres of the pons and the brachium pontis (middle cerebellar peduncle) (Hamilton & Mossman 1972).

HINDBRAIN (MYELENCEPHALON)

The myelencephalon forms the medulla (medulla oblongata) and is continuous cranially with the pons and caudally with the spinal cord. It is arbitrarily divided into two areas: the rostrally 'open' part of the medulla and the caudally 'closed' part continuous with the spinal cord (Moore 1982).

The 'open' part of the medulla is wide and flat due to the pontine flexure causing the walls to splay outwards. As a result, the roof is thinned and the medullary walls containing the alar plates flatten out and come to lie lateral to the basal plates. The cavity of the fourth ventricle is therefore diamond-shaped. As a result of the alar plates lying lateral to the basal plates, the motor nuclei which are derivatives of the basal plates form medially. The sensory nuclei from the alar plates generally form laterally. The motor nuclei form three columns, which are, from medial to lateral, the general somatic efferent, the special visceral (branchial) efferent and the general visceral efferent. The sensory nuclei form four columns, which are, from medial to lateral, the general visceral afferent, the special visceral afferent, the general somatic afferent and the special somatic afferent. The olivary nuclei form when some cells from the alar plates migrate ventrally.

The caudal 'closed' portion of the myelencephalon resembles the spinal cord structurally but unlike the spinal cord, islands of grey matter form in the marginal zone. These are principally the gracile nuclei located medially, and the cuneate nuclei located laterally. The pyramids containing the cortico–spinal fibres descending from the cerebral cortex are in the ventral area.

Association fibres, commissures and the pyramidal tract

Association fibres connect adjacent areas of the brain, while commissures connect equivalent areas on the opposite side of the brain. The pyramidal tract is the only tract to span the entire length of the central nervous system without synaptic relay.

Association fibres

The development and growth of the association fibres in the cerebral cortex is poorly understood.

Commissures

The forebrain roof is thickened by bundles of fibres crossing between the two hemispheres. The most important commissures cross the rostral end of the forebrain in the lamina terminalis. They extend from the roof plate of the diencephalon to the optic chiasma. Bartelmez & Dekaban (1962) divided the embryonic lamina terminalis (stage 22, 54–55 days) into four regions:

1. a ventral primordium for the optic chiasma (chiasmatic plate)
2. a short membranous portion dorsal to the chiasmatic plate which will become the adult lamina terminalis
3. a commissural plate for the anterior and hippocampal commissures and corpus callosum
4. a membrane to the velum transversum which is dorsal to the commissural plate.

The first commissures to form from the commissural plate are the anterior and hippocampal commissures (Rakic & Yakovlev 1968). The commissural plate enlarges caudally and axons from the cerebral cortex of each hemisphere begin to grow through the plate to form the commissures. The anterior commissure (week 10, 40 mm CR) has a large temporal component and connects the olfactory bulbs and areas related to it, while the hippocampal (or fornix) commissure (weeks 10–11, 45–55 mm CR) connects the hippocampal formations. These are phylogenetically older regions of the brain. After these commissures form, the corpus callosum begins to form and connects neocortical regions. Initially, the corpus callosum, the largest commissure to form from the commissural plate, lies in the lamina terminalis above the hippocampal commissure. As the cortex enlarges, more and more fibres are added and the corpus callosum gradually extends beyond the lamina terminalis and at birth extends over the diencephalic roof (pineal). As it spreads caudally it overrides the hippocampal commissure. The crossing over of the callosal fibres begins in the first trimester (50–60 mm CR, weeks 10–11), becomes distinct by 60–80 mm CR (weeks 12–13) and continues throughout most of the fetal period (Rakic & Yakovlev 1968, O'Rahilly & Gardner 1977).

While the cerebral commissures are forming, other commissures are also developing: the optic chiasma, the habenular (or superior) commissure and the posterior commissure (stage 15, 33–36 days) (O'Rahilly 1968, O'Rahilly et al 1984). The habenular commissure develops immediately rostral to the stalk of the pineal while the posterior develops behind the stalk at the junction of the di–mesencephalic boundary.

At 54 mm CR the anterior and posterior commissures and the corpus callosum are present.

As the corpus callosum connects the two hemispheres, the fornix is cut off from the rest of the hemisphere, as well as the tela choroidea, a horizontal sheet of pial mesenchyme adhering to a thin, ependyma-only area of the brain wall. This results in the choroid plexus of the lateral ventricle lying peripherally at the edge of the tela choroidea and the choroid plexus of the third ventricle lying on the ventral surface of the tela. The choroid plexus of the third ventricle lies in the roof of the third ventricle. The septum pellucidum may form from part of the medial hemispherical wall ventral to the corpus callosum.

Pyramidal tract

The pyramidal tract grows through an organized brainstem and spinal cord (Humphrey 1960). Pyramidal fibres have been identified in the cerebral peduncles at 32 mm CR and the pyramidal decussation is complete by 17 weeks (Humphrey 1960). Well-myelinated fibres are scattered above the pyramidal decussation by 23 weeks (220 mm CR) and some are also apparent below the decussation in the anterior and lateral cortico–spinal tracts. Well-differentiated glial cells are also identifiable among the tracts (Wozniak & O'Rahilly 1982). From 29 weeks on, an adult arrangement is apparent in the distal part of the tract. Yakovlev & Rakic (1966) have published a detailed account of the distribution and pattern of these fibres in the fetal and neonatal spinal cord. All of the tracts' fibres are myelinated by 18 months of life.

It should be remembered, however, that the presence of incoming fibres from the brainstem to the spinal cord does not necessarily indicate that they are functional (Okado & Kojima 1984).

Monoamine-synthesizing neurones

By the end of the embryonic period, the brainstem is more highly developed than more rostral structures (O'Rahilly & Gardner 1977). Monoamine-synthesizing neurones are present at this time in the brainstem and will have assumed a near-adult distribution in the spinal cord, cerebellum and forebrain by mid-term (Olson et al 1973). Generally, the cell bodies of noradrenaline-synthesizing neurones are located in the medulla oblongata (ventral and ventrolateral portions, dorsal and dorsomedial portions) and in the locus coeruleus and nucleus subcoeruleus. Dopamine neurones are present in the substantia nigra (pars compacta), in the tegmentum of the caudal mesencephalon and rostral pons and in the hypothalamus (arcuate nucleus).

Cell bodies of indoleamine-synthesizing neurones (5-hydroxytryptamine) are present cephalocaudally in the lateral reticular formation of the caudal portion of the mesencephalon, the rostral part of the pons and the raphe of the pons and medulla oblongata.

Cranial nerves

The 12 pairs of cranial nerves appear between weeks 5 and 6. O'Rahilly et al (1984) in an extensive study of 100 features of the brain and related structures report that the cranial nerves of the rhombencephalon, with one exception (abducent) develop more rapidly than those associated with the midbrain and forebrain.

They report that in stages 12 and 13 (26–30 days), the order of development of efferent, afferent, or both types of fibre is as follows: nerves XII, V, VII, VIII, IX/X and XI. Then the following nerves appear: during stage 13 (28–30 days), nerve III; stage 14 (31–32 days), nerve IV; and stage 15 (33–36 days), nerve VI. Late in stage 15, the first olfactory (nerve I) fibres develop and in stages 19–20 (47–51 days) the optic (nerve II) fibres are found.

Nuclei

The motor nuclei appear much earlier (stage 12, 26–27 days) than the sensory nuclei (stage 17, 41–43 days). This pattern of motor before sensory is true in the rhombencephalon, mesencephalon and diencephalon (O'Rahilly et al 1984).

A detailed analysis of the cranial nerves and nuclei is reported by O'Rahilly et al (1984) and is recommended for a more detailed account.

Sulci and gyri formation

Initially the cerebral hemispheres are smooth (Fig. 1.15), but as they grow, complex patterns of sulci and gyri develop. These patterns permit an increase in cerebral cortical volume without a concomitant increase in cranial volume. Hofman (1985) in a recent study of mammalian brains suggests that in addition to considerations of volume, there are also limitations on the degree of cortical folding based on the thickness of the cortex. By birth, the total surface area of cerebral cortex buried in the sulci and fissures is approximately twice that of the visible surface area of the cerebral cortex (Larroche 1966).

The sulci and fissures develop in a repeatable and recognizable pattern that can serve as an indicator of both developmental age and of normal development.

The fetal brain increases dramatically in weight at 24–25 weeks (Dooling et al 1983b) and many gyri become well-defined between 26 and 28 weeks. Fujimura & Seryu (1977), however, state that the brain growth (weight) is a smooth progression until week 33 in contrast to the findings of Dooling et al. Secondary and tertiary gyration occur late in gestation (weeks 40–44). The frontal and temporal areas become increasingly complex and a few weeks later similar changes occur in the orbital and occipital gyri.

The sulci begin to appear during month 4 with the lateral and central fissures among the earliest to form along

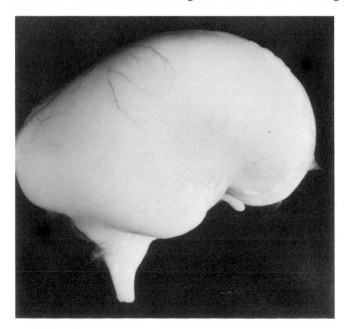

Fig. 1.15 External appearance of the cerebral hemispheres in a fetus at 130 mm CR length. Note the smooth cerebral surface.

with the pre- and postcentral sulci and the posterior portion of the superior temporal sulcus (Rorke & Riggs 1969).

The first primary fissure to appear is the longitudinal fissure at 8 weeks and this is very distinct by week 10. The transverse fissure and the hippocampal sulcus are evident at 9–10 weeks (Hines 1922, Humphrey 1967).

By week 14 the lateral sulcus (Sylvian fissure) appears as a shallow depression on the lateral surface of the hemispheres. This depression deepens as the surrounding frontal, parietal and temporal areas grow rapidly and by week 19 the tissue of the depression forms the insula (Fig. 1.16). There is also an associated thickening of the pia-arachnoid and an increasingly rich blood supply. As the insula remains exposed throughout most of gestation (Dooling et al 1983b) many other sulci and fissures are better indicators of gestational age.

The callosal sulcus appears around week 14 together with the corpus callosum. The olfactory sulcus appears as a shallow depression at week 16 and gradually becomes distinct at week 25. The parieto–occipital fissure appears at week 16. As it forms, a distinctive layer of cells appears in the molecular layer of the isocortex at the future site of the fissure. As the fissure develops, this layer of cells is carried down into the walls of the fissure and eventually disappears.

By week 16 the calcarine fissure is also present and appears on the right before the left. By week 27 this fissure indents the occipital horn of the lateral ventricle.

At 20 weeks the central sulcus (Rolandic sulcus) is a distinct groove and by 22–23 weeks a distinct sulcus. The right central sulcus appears before the left.

It is of interest that many areas appear on the right side of the brain before they appear on the left. Secondary gyri also appear earlier on the right side followed by those on the left side.

At birth the sulci and gyri are similar in arrangement to those of the adult. The central sulcus, however, is slightly more rostral and the lateral sulcus more oblique than in the adult (Fig. 1.17).

Choroid plexuses

Four choroid plexuses develop in the brain: one in the medial wall of each lateral ventricle, one in the roof of the third ventricle and one in the roof of the fourth ventricle (Streeter 1912, 1951). These plexuses secrete cerebrospinal fluid (CSF).

The choroid plexus of the fourth ventricle forms first at stage 18 (44–46 days). As the pontine flexure occurs, the thin rhombic roof of the fourth ventricle changes its greatest dimension from a longitudinal to a horizontal one. The transverse crease or plica choroidea which forms, is where the choroid plexus will develop in the roof of the fourth ventricle. Initially the choroid plexus has a horizontal orientation and this position ultimately corresponds to the location of the foramina of Luschka. The final position of

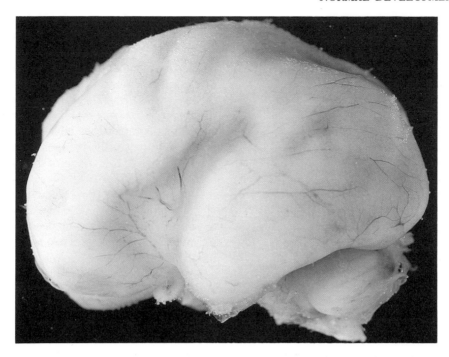

Fig. 1.16 The early insula. Note the central sulcus.

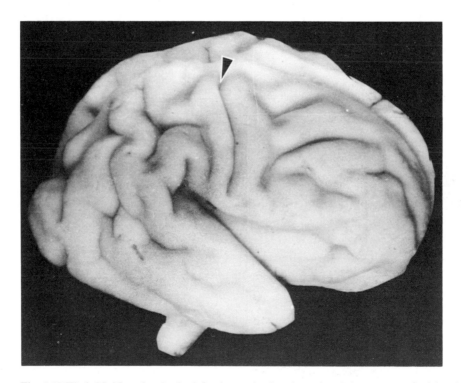

Fig. 1.17 Week 28. Note the clearly defined central sulcus (arrow) and the patterns of sulci and gyri. (Reproduced by permission of Wolfe Medical Publications.)

the choroid plexus is determined by the subsequent changes which occur in the rhombic roof (see **Cerebellum**). As the thin ependyma roof of the fourth ventricle loses its mitotic activity it forms a single epithelial layer. This layer has an external covering of very vascular pia mater which together with the epithelial layers is known as the tela choroidea. As the pia mater proliferates rapidly, the tela choroidea invaginates into the fourth ventricle (Brocklehurst 1969) to form the choroid plexus. In the 37 mm CR embryo the epithelium is columnar but by 59 mm CR it has become cuboidal (Hoyes & Barber 1976). The cellular elements of the choroid plexus become granulated and appear as a secretory epithelium. The histological structure of the fetal and adult choroid plexus is, therefore, different (Larroche 1966).

The first perforation to appear in the roof of the fourth ventricle is the midline foramen of Magendie. This foramen is the result of an active process of differentiation which occurs before the choroid plexus begins to function; perforation is not a result of the build-up of CSF pressure. Shortly after CSF appears outside the fourth ventricle, the thin arachnoid trabeculae differentiate. Laterally, two additional foramina (of Luschka) appear in the roof of the fourth ventricle, adjacent to cranial nerves VII and VIII. Although these foramina have been described as patent as early as 195 mm CR, week 21, their exact time of opening is not known. At birth, all three foramina are patent, although Alexander (1931) found that 20% of the population had no foramina of Luschka.

The choroid plexuses of the lateral ventricles form in a similar manner (stage 19, 47–48 days), whilst those of the third ventricle develop last (stage 21, 52–53 days) (Lemire et al 1975).

Myelination

The rate of myelination varies with the site and the fetal age. Some tracts myelinate early and rapidly, while others myelinate early and slowly. Those which function first tend to be myelinated first (Hamilton & Mossman 1972, Gilles et al 1983). Those with long phases of myelination are particularly at risk (Gilles et al 1983). In general, however, myelin accumulates slowly in the third trimester followed by a sudden, marked, increased deposition (Gilles et al 1983).

Myelin is formed in the CNS by oligodendrocytes. Immediately before the beginning of myelin deposition, there is a marked proliferation of oligodendrocytes and an increased vascularization of the area (Lemire et al 1975). Myelin is laid down first on the fibre close to the nerve cell body and then deposition proceeds along its axon (Keene & Hewer 1931, Gilles et al 1983). The oligodendrocyte wraps its lipoprotein plasma membranes repeatedly around the axon to produce the myelin sheath. An oligodendrocyte myelinates more than one axon (Bunge et al 1961). Generally, myelination proceeds in the direction of the major flow of information (Gilles et al 1983). The only major exception inside the central nervous system is the myelination of transpontine fibres and the middle cerebellar peduncle before the cortico–pontine fibres myelinate in the mesencephalic cerebral peduncle (Gilles et al 1983).

Spinal cord. As the cell tracts and columns differentiate their interrelationships are changing constantly. The formation of myelin in the spinal cord begins during the middle of the fetal period (11–14 weeks, 75–105 mm CR) (Hamilton & Mossman 1972) and continues until one year after birth. Myelination begins in the cervical cord and proceeds caudally. Okado & Kojima (1984) showed that myelination begins at 12 weeks but the growth patterns of the myelinated tracts and myelin deposition are labile and variable (Gilles et al 1983). Okado & Kojima's study (1984) also demonstrated that myelination and synaptogenesis occur simultaneously in some periods of development. Previously it had been thought that synaptogenesis preceded myelination (Bodian 1970).

Gilles et al (1983) reported that, with the exception of the cranial and spinal roots which were not examined, the earliest myelin in the CNS is deposited before week 20 in the rhombencephalic portion of the medial longitudinal fasciculus. They also observed that there are selected systems in the lower brainstem and rostral spinal cord which myelinate by mid-gestation and are heavily myelinated by birth. They include the fasciculus cuneatus, the caudal medial lemniscus, the trapezoid body and the lateral lemniscus, the inferior cerebellar peduncle and the spinal trigeminal tract.

Brain. Myelination reaches the cerebral hemispheres by birth and is completed 2–3 years after birth (Lemire et al 1975, Gilles et al 1983). The greatest quantity of myelin is deposited in the telencephalon during the third trimester and postnatally (Gilles et al 1983). The first to acquire myelin sheaths are neurones in the olfactory, optic and acoustic cortical areas and the motor cortex (pyramidal cells) (Crelin 1973). The last to be myelinated are the projection, commissural and association neurones of the cerebral hemispheres (Crelin 1973). The projection fibres begin myelination before the association fibres, whose myelination continues through adulthood.

Wozniak & O'Rahilly (1982) observed that myelination is in progress in the pyramidal tract at the level of the pyramidal decussation in a week 23 fetus (220 mm CR). Gilles et al (1983) reported that the optic tract is myelinated in week 29, the chiasma at 32 weeks, and the radiation in weeks 38–39. Myelination occurs in the posterior limb of the internal capsule at week 32, the corona radiata at week 34, the cingulum and the cerebral peduncle medial to the cortico–spinal tract at week 38 and the fornix at week 39. Later at week 46, the corpus callosum and anterior commissure become myelinated, with the mammilo–thalamic tract at either week 48 (Gilles et al 1983) or week 36 (according to Yakovlev & Lecours 1967).

The cranial nerves of the midbrain, pons and medulla begin myelination during the sixth month (Crelin 1973).

The cerebellar connections are myelinated and the afferent thalamic pathways are myelinated as far as the thalamus in the seventh month.

By 32 weeks of gestation (300 mm CR) myelinated fibres are found extending from the substantia nigra to the subthalamic nucleus, to the contralateral substantia nigra to the medial lemniscus, descending cerebro–spinal fibres and the temporo–pontine pathway (Lemire et al 1975).

However, it is clear when comparing the findings of different authors that there is a great deal of biological and methodological variation (Langworthy 1933, Larroche 1966, Yakovlev & Lecours 1967, Gilles et al 1983).

ACKNOWLEDGEMENTS

I am deeply grateful to Professor M. Marin-Padilla (Dartmouth College, USA), who generously read and commented upon this text. He also suggested the use of and contributed Figure 1.11 and Table 1.3. Dr A. R. Lieberman (University College London) also generously read and made extensive comments upon the chapter, Dr R. R. Sturrock and Dr I. H. M. Smart (University Dundee) and Dr J. Wakely (Leicester University) also very kindly read this chapter and made useful and constructive comments.

I would also like to express my gratitude to Dr G. Batcup (Leeds General Infirmary) to Dr E. C. Blenkinsopp (Watford General Hospital) and to Mr P. A. Runicles (The Middlesex Hospital Medical School) for allowing me to photograph materials.

Professor K. Carr (Department of Anatomy) generously allowed me to photograph Figure 1.7 from The Belfast Collection, the Queen's University of Belfast, Northern Ireland.

Dr K. Shiota (Department of Anatomy, Kyoto University) very kindly gave me permission to photograph Figure 1.1 from the Kyoto Embryology Collection, Japan. I am very grateful to Toa Medical Electronics Co., Ltd for their support.

The photographers whose assistance was invaluable are Mr K. Garfield, Central Photographic Unit and Mr G. L. C. McTurk both of Leicester University.

Figures 1.2 and 1.3 were originally produced by Professor H. Nishimura (Professor Emeritus of Anatomy, Kyoto University) and Figure 1.17 was photographed from the Royal Free Hospital School of Medicine, London.

REFERENCES

Alexander L 1931 Die Anatomie der Seitentaschen der vierten Hirnkammer. Zeitschrift fur die gesamte Anatomie 95: 531–707

Barr M L 1979 The human nervous system: an anatomic viewpoint. 3rd edn. Harper & Row, Hagerstown, Md.

Bartelmez G W 1923 The subdivisions of the neural folds in man. Journal of Comparative Neurology 35: 231–247

Bartelmez G W, Dekaban A S 1962 The early development of the human brain. Contributions to Embryology 37: 13–32

Bartelmez G A, Evans H M 1926 Development of the human embryo during the period of somite formation including embryos with 2 to 16 pairs of somites. Contributions to Embryology 17: 1–67

Berquist H, Kallen B 1954 Notes on the early histogenesis and morphogenesis of the central nervous system in vertebrates. Journal of Comparative Neurology 100: 627–660

Bodian D 1970 A model of synaptic and behavioural ontogeny. In: Schmitt F O (ed) The neurosciences second study program. Rockefeller University Press, New York. pp 129–140

Boulder Committee 1970 Embryonic vertebrate central nervous system: revised terminology. Anatomical Record 166: 257–262

Boyd J D 1956 Observations on the human pharyngeal hypophysis. Journal of Endocrinology 14: 66–77

Brocklehurst G 1969 The development of the human cerebrospinal fluid pathways with particular reference to the roof of the fourth ventricle. Journal of Anatomy 105: 467–475

Bunge M B, Bunge R P, Ris H 1961 Ultrastructural study of remyelination in an experimental lesion in adult cat spinal cord. Journal of Biophysical and Biochemical Cytology 10: 67–94

Choi B H, Kim R C, Lapham L W 1983 Do radial glia give rise to both astroglial and oligodendroglial cells? Developmental Brain Research 8: 119–130

Cooper E R A 1946 The development of the human red nucleus and corpus striatum. Brain 69: 34–44

Cooper E R A 1950 The development of the thalamus. Acta Anatomica 9: 201–226

Crelin E A 1973 Functional anatomy of the newborn. Yale University Press, London

Dandy A, Nichols G E 1910 On the occurrence of a mesocoelic recess in the human brain, and its relation to the sub-commissural organ of lower vertebrates; with special reference to the distribution of Reissner's fibre in the vertebrate series and its possible function. Proceedings of the Royal Society London 82: 515–529

Dekaban A 1954 Human thalamus: an anatomical, developmental, and pathological study. II. Development of the human thalamic nuclei. Journal of Comparative Neurology 100: 63–97

Desmond M E, O'Rahilly R 1981 The growth of the human brain during the embryonic period proper. I. Linear axes. Anatomy and Embryology 162: 137–151

Desmond M E, Schoenwolf G C 1986 Evaluation of the roles of intrinsic and extrinsic factors in occlusion of the spinal neurocoel during rapid brain enlargement in the chick embryo. Journal of Embryology and Experimental Morphology 97: 25–46

de Vries J I P, Visser G H A, Prechtl H F R 1982 The emergence of fetal behaviour. I. Qualitative aspects. Early Human Development 7: 301–322

Dicker S E, Tyler C 1953 Vasopressor and oxytocic activities of the pituitary glands of rats, guinea pigs and cats and of human foetuses. Journal of Physiology 121: 206–214

Dobbing J, Sands J 1973 The quantitative growth and development of the human brain. Archives of Disease in Childhood 48: 757–767

Dooling E C, Chi J G, Gilles F H 1983a Dorsal mesodiencephalic junction: pineal, subcommissural organ, and mesocoelic recess. In: Gilles F H, Leviton A, Dooling E C (eds) The developing human brain: growth and epidemiologic neuropathology. John Wright, London, pp 105–112

Dooling E C, Chi J G, Gilles F H 1983b Telencephalic development: changing gyral patterns. In: Gilles F H, Leviton A, Dooling E C (eds) The developing human brain: growth and epidemiologic neuropathology. John Wright, London, pp 94–104

Duckett S, Pearse A G E 1968 The cells of Cajal–Retzius in the developing human brain. Journal of Anatomy 102: 183–187

England 1983 A colour atlas of life before birth. Wolfe Medical Publications, London

Fallon J F, Simandl B K 1978 Evidence of a role for cell death in the disappearance of the embryonic human tail. American Journal of Anatomy 152: 111–129

Ferner H 1939 Zur Differenzierung der RumpfSchwanzknospe beim Menschen. Zeitschrift fur Mikroskopisch-Anatomische Forschung 45: 555–562

Fitzgerald J E, Windle W F 1942 Some observations on early human fetal movements. Journal of Comparative Neurology 76: 159–167

FitzGerald M J T 1985 Neuroanatomy: basic and applied. Bailliere Tindall, London

Friede R L 1973 Dating the development of human cerebellum. Acta Neuropathologica (Berlin) 23: 48–58

Fujimoto E, Mizoguti H 1985 The first appearance of microglia in human embryonic pallium. Proceedings of the XII International Anatomical Congress Abstract 218

Fujimura M, Seryu J I 1977 Velocity of head growth during the perinatal period. Archives of Diseases of Childhood 52: 105–112

Fujita S 1973 Genesis of glioblasts in the human spinal cord as revealed by Feulgen cytophotometry. Journal of Comparative Neurology 151: 25–34

Gamble H J 1967 Observations upon the human filum terminale. Journal of Anatomy 101: 631–632

Gamble H J 1969 Electron microscope observations on the human foetal and embryonic spinal cord. Journal of Anatomy 104: 435–453

Gamble H J 1971 Electron microscope observations upon the conus medullaris and filum terminale of human fetuses. Journal of Anatomy 110: 173–179

Gardner E, O'Rahilly R, Prolo D 1975 The Dandy–Walker and Arnold–Chiari malformations. Archives of Neurology (Chicago) 32: 393–407

Gilbert M S 1935 The early development of the human diencephalon. Journal of Comparative Neurology 62: 81–116

Gilles F H, Shankle W, Dooling E C 1983 Myelinated tracts: growth patterns. In: Gilles F H, Leviton A, Dooling E C (eds) The developing human brain: growth and epidemiologic neuropathology. John Wright, London, pp 117–183

Hamilton W, Mossman H W 1972 Hamilton, Boyd and Mossman's human embryology: prenatal development of form and function. 4th edn. Heffer, Cambridge

Hewitt W 1958 The development of the human caudate and amygdaloid nucleus. Journal of Anatomy 92: 377–382

Hewitt W 1961 The development of the human internal capsule and lentiform nucleus. Journal of Anatomy 95: 191–199

Hines M 1922 Studies in the growth and differentiation of the tel-encephalon in man: the fissura hippocampi. Journal of Neurology 34: 73–171

His W 1888 Zur Geschichte des Gehirns sowie der centralen und periferischen Nervenbahnen beim menschlichen Embryo. Abh. math.-phys. Kl. Kgl. Sachs. Ges. Wiss. 14: 339–392

Hofman M A 1985 Size and shape of the cerebral cortex in mammals. I. The cortical surface. Brain Behavioural Evolution 27: 28–40

Hoyes A D, Barber P 1976 Ultrastructure of the epithelium of the human fetal choroid plexus. Journal of Anatomy 122: 743

Humphrey T 1960 The development of the pyramidal tracts in human fetuses, correlated with cortical differentiation. In: Tower D B, Schade J P (eds) Structure and function of the cerebral cortex. Elsevier, Amsterdam, pp 93–103

Humphrey T 1964a Some correlations between the appearance of human fetal reflexes and the development of the nervous system. In: Purpura D P, Schade J P (eds) Growth and maturation of the brain. Elsevier, Amsterdam, pp 93–133

Humphrey T 1964b Some correlations between the appearance of human fetal reflexes and the development of the nervous system. Progress in Brain Research 4: 93–135

Humphrey T 1967 The development of the human hippocampal fissure. Journal of Anatomy (London) 101: 655–676

Humphrey T 1968 The development of the human amygdala during early embryonic life. Journal of Comparative Neurology 132: 135–166

Humphrey T, Hooker D 1959 Double simultaneous stimulation of human fetuses and the anatomical patterns underlying the reflexes elicited. Journal of Comparative Neurology 112: 75–102

Kadin M E, Rubinstein L J, Nelson J S 1970 Neonatal cerebellar medulloblastoma originating from the fetal external granular layer. Journal of Neuropathology and Experimental Neurology 29: 583–600

Kallen B 1977 Errors in the differentiation of the central nervous system. In: Vinken P J, Bruyn G W (eds) Handbook of clinical neurology, Vol 30. North Holland, New York, pp 41–83

Keene M F L, Hewer E E 1931 Some observations on myelination in the human central nervous system. Journal of Anatomy 66: 1–13

Kelly 1982 Circumventricular organs In: Haymaker, Adams (eds) Histology and histopathology of the nervous system, Vol II. Thomas, Springfield, Illinois, pp 1735–1800

Kernohan J W 1925 The ventricular terminalis; its growth and devel-opment. Journal of Comparative Neurology 38: 107–125

Kershman J 1939 Genesis of microglia in the human brain. Archives of Neurology and Psychiatry 41: 24–50

Kuhlenbeck H 1948 The derivatives of the thalamus ventralis in the human brain and their relation to the so-called subthalamus. Military Surgery 102: 433–447

Kuhlenbeck H, Haymaker W 1949 The derivatives of the hypothalamus in the human brain; their relation to the extrapyramidal and autonomic systems. Military Surgery 105: 26–52

Kunimoto K 1918 The development and reduction of the tail and of the caudal end of the spinal cord. Contributions to Embryology 8: 161–198

Langworthy O R 1933 Development of behavioural patterns and myelinations of the nervous system in the human fetus and infant. Contributions to Embryology 24: 1–57

Larroche J C 1966 Development of the nervous system in early life. II. The development of the central nervous system during intrauterine life. In: Falkner F (ed) Human development. Saunders, Philadelphia, pp 257–276

Larroche J C 1981 The marginal layer in the neocortex of a 7-week-old human embryo. Anatomy and Embryology 162: 301–312

Larroche J C, Houcine O 1982 Le neo-cortex chez l'embryon et le foetus humain: apport du microscope electronique et du Golgi. Reproduction, Nutrition, Developpement (Paris) 22: 163–176

Larroche J C, Privat A, Jardin L 1981 Some fine structures of the human fetal brain. In: Minkowsky A (ed) Sam Levine International Symposium, Paris. Karger, Basel, pp 350–358

Lemire R J, Loeser J D, Leich R W, Alvord E C 1975 Normal and abnormal development of the human nervous system. Harper & Row, London

Lund R D 1978 Development and plasticity of the brain: an introduction. Oxford University Press, New York

Marin-Padilla M 1970a Prenatal and early postnatal ontogenesis of the human motor cortex: a Golgi study. I. The sequential development of the cortical layers. Brain Research 23: 167–183

Marin-Padilla M 1970b Prenatal and early postnatal ontogenesis of the human motor cortex: a Golgi study. II. The basket-pyramidal system. Brain Research 23: 185–191

Marin-Padilla M 1971 Early prenatal ontogenesis of the cerebral cortex (neocortex) of the cat (Felis domestica): a Golgi study. I. The primordial neocortical organization Zeitschrift fur Anatomie und Entwicklungsgeschichte 134: 117–145

Marin-Padilla M 1978 Dual origin of the mammalian neocortex and evolution of the cortical plate. Anatomy and Embryology 152: 109–126

Marin-Padilla M 1983 Structural organization of the human cerebral cortex prior to the appearance of the cortical plate. Anatomy and Embryology 168: 21–40

Marin-Padilla M 1984 Neurons of layer I: a developmental analysis (ch 14). In: Peters A, Jones E G (eds) Cerebral cortex: cellular components of the cerebral cortex, Vol I. Plenum Press, London, pp 447–478

Marin-Padilla M 1984a Embryonic vascularization of the mammalian cerebral cortex. In: Jones E G, Peters A (eds) Cerebral cortex: cellular components of the cerebral cortex, Vol VII. Plenum Press, New York (in press)

Marin-Padilla M 1984b Early ontogenesis of the human cerebral cortex. In: Jones E G, Peters A (eds) Cerebral cortex: cellular components of the cerebral cortex, Vol VII. Plenum Press, New York (in press)

Marin-Padilla M, Marin-Padilla M T 1982 Origin, prenatal development and structural organization of layer I of the human cerebral (motor) cortex: a Golgi study. Anatomy and Embryology 164: 161–206

Melchionna R H, Moore R A 1938 The pharyngeal pituitary gland. American Journal of Pathology 14: 763–771

Molliver M E, Kostovic I, Van Der Loos H 1973 The development of synapses in cerebral cortex of the human fetus. Brain Research 50: 403–407

Moore K L 1982 The developing human clinically oriented embryology, 3rd end. Saunders, London

Morrell N W 1985 The development of the human midbrain tegmentum with particular reference to the red nucleus. Journal of Anatomy 140: 544

Muller F, O'Rahilly R 1983 The first appearance of the major divisions of the human brain at stage 9. Anatomy and Embryology 168: 419–432

Muller F, O'Rahilly R 1984 Cerebral dysraphia (future anencephaly) in a human twin embryo at stage 13. Teratology 30: 167–177

Muller F, O'Rahilly R 1985 The first appearance of the neural tube and optic primordium in the human embryo at stage 10. Anatomy and Embryology 172: 157–169

Okado N, Kojima T 1984 Ontogeny of the central nervous system: neurogenesis, fibre connection, synaptogenesis and myelination in the spinal cord in continuity of neural functions from prenatal to postnatal life. In: Prechtl H F R (ed) Clinics in developmental medicine No 94. Spastics International Medical/Blackwells, Oxford

Okado, N, Yokota N 1980 An electron microscopic study on the structural development of the neural lobe in the human fetus. American Journal of Anatomy 159: 261–273

Olson L, Boreus L O, Seiger A 1973 Histochemical demonstration and mapping of 5-hydroxytryptamine and catecholamine — containing neuron systems in the human brain. Zeitschrift fur Anatomie und Entwicklungsgeschichte 139: 259–282

O'Rahilly R 1968 The development of the epiphysis cerebri and the subcommissural complex in staged human embryos. Anatomical Record 160: 488–489

O'Rahilly R 1973 Developmental stages in human embryos including a survey of the Carnegie Collection. Embryos of the first three weeks (stages 1–9). Carnegie Institution of Washington, Washington, DC

O'Rahilly R 1983 The timing and sequence of events in the development of the human endocrine system during the embryonic period proper. Anatomy and Embryology 166: 439–451

O'Rahilly R, Gardner E 1977 The developmental anatomy of the human central nervous system. In: Vinken R J, Bruyn G W (eds) Handbook of clinical neurology: congenital malformations of the brain and skull Myrianthopoulos N C (ed) Amsterdam XXX, i, p 15–40

O'Rahilly R, Gardner E 1979 The initial development of the human brain. Acta Anatomica 104: 123–133

O'Rahilly R, Muller F 1981 The first appearance of the human nervous system at stage 8. Anatomy and Embryology 163: 1–13

O'Rahilly R, Muller F 1987 Developmental stages in human embryos. Carnegie Institution of Washington, no 637

O'Rahilly R, Muller F, Bossy J 1982 Atlas des stades du developpement du systeme nerveus chez l'embryon humain intact. Archives d'Anatomie, d'Histologie et d'Embryologie Normales et Experimentales 65: 57–76

O'Rahilly R, Muller F, Hutchins G M, Moore G W 1984 Computer ranking of the sequence of appearance of 100 features of the brain and related structures in staged human embryos during the first 5 weeks of development. American Journal of Anatomy 171: 243–257

Rakic P 1965 Mesocoelic recess in the human brain. Neurology (Minneapolis) 15: 708–715

Rakic P 1981 Developmental events leading to laminar and areal organization of the neocortex. In: Schmitt F O, Worden F G (eds) Organization of the cerebral cortex. MIT Press, London

Rakic P, Sidman R L 1969 Telencephalic origin of pulvinar neurons in the fetal human brain. Zeitschrift fur Anatomie und Entwicklungsgeschichte 129: 53–82

Rakic P, Sidman R L 1970 Histogenesis of cortical layers in human cerebellum, particularly the lamina dissecans. Journal of Comparative Neurology 139: 473–500

Rakic P, Yakovlev P I 1968 Development of the corpus callosum and cavum septi in man. Journal of Comparative Neurology 132: 45–72

Ranson S W, Clark S L 1959 The Anatomy of the nervous system its development and function. Saunders, London

Rorke L B, Riggs H E 1969 Myelination of the brain in the newborn. Lippincott, Philadelphia

Sauer F C 1936 The interkinetic migration of embryonic epithelial nuclei. Journal of Morphology 60: 1–11

Schoenwolf G C 1979 Histological and ultrastructural observations of tail bud formation in the chick embryo. Anatomical Record 193: 131–148

Sidman R L, Rakic P 1973 Neuronal migration with special reference to the developing human brain: a review. Brain Research 62: 1–35

Skowsky R, Fisher D A 1973 Immunoreactive arginine vasopressin (AVT) in the fetal pituitary of man and sheep. Clinical Research 21: 205

Streeter G L 1912 The development of the nervous system. In: Keibel F, Mall F P (eds) Manual of human embryology, Vol II. Lippincott, Philadelphia, pp 1–156

Streeter G L 1919 Factors involved in the formation of the filum terminale. American Journal of Anatomy 25: 1–11

Streeter G L 1942 Carnegie Institution of Washington Publications 30: 211–245

Streeter G L 1948 Carnegie Institution of Washington Publications 32: 133–203

Streeter G L 1951 Developmental horizons in human embryos, age groups XI–XXIII. Embryol. Reprint Vol II. Carnegie Institute of Washington, Washington DC. Contributions of Embryology 34: 165–196

Stroud B B 1900 If an 'isthmus rhombencephali' why not an 'isthmus prosencephali'? Proceedings of the American Association of Anatomists, pp 27–29

Sturrock R R 1982a Changes in cell number in the central canal ependyma and in the dorsal grey matter of the rabbit thoracic spinal cord during fetal development. Journal of Anatomy 135: 635–647

Sturrock R R 1982b Cell division in the normal central nervous system. Advances in Cellular Neurobiology, Vol 3. Academic Press, New York

Sturrock R R 1984 Microglia in the human embryonic optic nerve. Journal of Anatomy 139: 81–91

Sturrock R R 1986 Postnatal ontogenesis of astrocytes. Astrocytes, Vol 1. Academic Press

Tilney F 1936 The development and constituents of the human hypophysis. Bulletin of the Neurological Institute of New York 5: 387–436

Warwick R, Williams P L 1973 Gray's Anatomy, 35th edn. Churchill Livingstone, Edinburgh

Willis W D Jr, Grossman R G 1981 Medical neurobiology. 3rd edn. Mosby, London

Wislocki G B 1937 The meningeal relations of the hypophysis cerebri. II. An embryological study of the meninges and blood vessels of the human hypophysis. American Journal of Anatomy 61: 95–129

Wislocki G B, Roth W D 1958 Selective staining of the human subcommissural organ. Anatomical Record 130: 125–133

Wozniak W, O'Rahilly R 1982 An electron microscopic study of myelination of pyramidal fibres at the level of the pyramidal decussation in the human fetus. Journal fur Hirnforschung 23: 331–342

Wozniak W, O'Rahilly R, Olszewski B 1980 The fine structure of the spinal cord in human embryos and early fetuses. Journal fur Hirnforschung 21: 101–124

Yakovlev P I, Lecours A 1967 The myelogenetic cycles of regional maturation of the brain. In: Minkowski A (ed) Regional development of the brain in early life. Blackwells, Oxford, pp 3–70

Yakovlev P I, Rakic P 1966 Patterns of decussation of bulbar pyramids and distribution of pyramidal tracts on two sides of the spinal cord. Transactions of the American Neurological Association 91: 366–367

PART 2

Methods

Functional assessment

The assessment of neurological function is essential in following progress of the fetus, infant or growing child. Methods are based on clinical assessment and observation which in the newborn is considerably easier than in fetal life. Functional assessment of fetal behaviour (Ch. 2) is possible by a number of methods but direct observations by means of ultrasound gives information comparable to clinical assessment of the newborn infant. Methods of functional assessment must take account of the rapid development occurring in early life and it is necessary to develop standardized norms for the assessment of function at different stages of fetal and neonatal life. This section reviews the assessment of fetal and neonatal behaviour as well as the newborn neurological examination (Ch. 3). Less direct methods for studying aspects of fetal cerebral function are also considered including habituation (Ch. 4). Methods for the assessment of both normal and abnormal development in infants and children are essential for monitoring developmental or perinatal compromise likely to affect the maturing brain (Ch. 5). These methods provide the 'acid test' by which fetal and neonatal neurology can be measured and the effects of changes in management monitored.

2. Assessment of fetal neurological function and development

Prof H. F. R. Prechtl

HISTORICAL PERSPECTIVES

Throughout its history the study of fetal behaviour has been determined by two factors: 1. the development of new methods for detection, and 2. the current concepts of behaviour. The oldest method, reporting on fetal movements perceived by expectant mothers, was supplemented at the end of the last century by observations with the aid of the stethoscope. Preyer mentioned in his famous book *Die spezielle Physiologie des Embryo* (1885) that fetal movements could be heard at 12 to 16 weeks pregnancy. His approach was very much in the mould of nineteenth century natural history and in the tradition of close observations of embryos, such as those carried out and described by Carl Ernst von Baer in his book *Über die Entwicklungsgeschichte der Tiere-Beobachtung und Reflexion* (1828). Preyer's comparative approach led him to full acceptance of spontaneous motor activity in the human fetus, an idea which then got somewhat lost for nearly a century. A similar fate befell Ahlfeld's (1888) observation of fetal breathing movements which met fierce opposition despite his careful recordings (Ahlfeld 1905, Reifferscheidt 1911). At this time, however, the growing influence of the reflex arc resulted in little attention being paid to spontaneous activity, indeed this was often incorrectly interpreted and not recognized as having an endogenous origin. The influence is noted in the first systematic neurological studies of exteriorized fetuses by Minkowsky (1928), an adults' neurologist, and also in studies by the comparative anatomists Hooker and Humphrey (for comprehensive summary see Hooker 1952, Humphrey 1978) who devoted their life work to the study of neurological development of human fetuses. Much has been learned from their investigations of responses to stimulation by a hair aesthesiometer in fetuses who survived therapeutic abortions for a few minutes in an isotonic fluid bath at body temperature. Their findings have been described in detail and are widely quoted in the relevant literature. Until recently they were the only basis of knowledge of prenatal development of neural functions. However, when Hooker's motion-pictures of his experiments with fetuses are carefully compared with modern ultrasound recordings of the intact, unstimulated fetus, it becomes evident that the exteriorized fetuses were in a terminal condition and did not show the normal patterns. Moreover, it must not be forgotten that responses of the kind Hooker and Humphrey studied are artificial because in normal life the fetus is never exposed to such stimuli. One may conclude that these fetal reflex studies were dealing with latent capacities of the nervous system which never become overt under normal conditions and that these capacities were studied in anoxic and dying fetuses.

Renewed interest in fetal motility by American psychologists (for review see Carmichael 1970), occurred in the 1940s. Fetal movements were recorded with pneumatic tambours placed on the abdominal wall (Kellog 1941). Special interest was directed to the effects of maternal activities and position on the quantity of fetal activity (Richards et al 1938, Schmeidler 1941, Harris & Harris 1946). Most of these investigations were motivated by interest in the prenatal development of behaviour.

Considerable attention has been paid to maternal perception of fetal movements and Walters (1964) was able to study four types of movement, recorded weekly by 34 expectant mothers from 32 weeks until birth. Four types of movement were distinguished: 1. slow squirming, 2. quick kicks, 3. hiccups, and 4. wave-like ripples. Each of these movement types followed a different developmental course with respect to quantity and quality. Previously, Newbery (1941) had shown similar trends but also reported intra-individual stability of squirming movements and kicks during the last eight weeks of pregnancy. These investigations of fetal motility were followed by a host of obstetric studies with quite different aims. Mothers were asked to monitor daily, for 12 hours, all fetal movements they felt with the objective being an assessment of fetal well-being. Sadovsky & Yaffe (1973) developed such a method of a daily fetal movement record (DFMR) and have applied this in high-risk pregnancies as an alarm sign of fetal jeopardy. Fetal movements may stop 12 to 48 hours before fetal death.

What has euphemistically been called 'fetal well-being' actually means absence of an immediately life-threatening condition. The method is relatively simple and cheap, and the reliability of maternal perception is fairly good even though mothers consistently record less fetal movements than are recorded by more objective methods. When the maternal counts were checked by simultaneous recordings with electromagnetic coils (Sadovsky et al 1973), an overall agreement was obtained of 87% with range 64–100%. Later, these relationships were reported to be less favourable when ultrasound observations were employed (Gettinger et al 1978, Hertogs et al 1979, Sorokin et al 1981, Schmidt et al 1982). Despite the limited reliability of maternal perception of fetal activity, a drop below 10 movements per day may be treated as an alarm signal (Sadovsky et al 1974, Pearson & Weaver 1976, Sadovsky 1981, Liston et al 1982), but further investigations must precede any intervention.

A variety of recording methods of fetal movements has been employed in studies which focused on different aspects of fetal physiology. Strain gauges were used (Timor-Tritsch et al 1976) for the classification of fetal movements and for assessing activity cycles (Robertson et al 1982). For diagnostic purposes piezo-electric sensors were applied (Sadovsky et al 1977).

What all these methods have in common is their indirect way of assessing fetal activity. Even the subjective recordings by expectant mothers make use of only gross fetal movements. In a way these techniques are comparable to actograms of neonates which also record only gross motor effects and lack the necessary resolution to study detail. Mechanical or electrical methods and maternal perception are all restricted to the second half or to the last trimester of pregnancy.

The real advancement in studying the neurology of the fetus came from the introduction of modern linear array real-time ultrasound equipment. This methodological breakthrough now provides a tool to study fetal activity throughout pregnancy and the organization of behavioural states at the end of gestation, and helps to visualize motor responses to experimental stimuli. An approach within the conceptual context of developmental neurology is now available for detailed investigation of the prenatal development of neural functions. As this method is non-invasive and apparently safe (Stark et al 1984), studies of normal fetuses under natural conditions are possible and are an indispensable basis for diagnostic procedures of the abnormal and compromised fetus. Only if the normal patterns are sufficiently known can grave errors in interpreting and diagnosing abnormalities be avoided.

The era of ultrasound studies of fetal behaviour was opened by the pioneering work of Reinold in Vienna (Reinold 1971, 1976). Despite the limited quality of the early equipment, Reinold distinguished in the fetus of 8–16 weeks, strong and brisk movements involving the entire body and slow and sluggish movements confined to fetal parts. He also described episodes without spontaneous movements and possible displacement of the fetus by uter-

ine contractions or palpation. A very similar classification was made by Jouppila (1976): between 6 and 20 weeks he distinguished violent movements of the whole fetus from smaller movements of the limbs. In a more detailed study by van Dongen & Goudie (1980), four patterns were described but again they were global and did not specify distinct movement patterns. Similar classifications of movement patterns were put forward by Higginbottom et al (1976), Schillinger (1977), Shawker et al (1980) and Adamson et al (1980). There are two exceptions to this approach. The first was made by Birnholz et al (1978) who said that 'Fetal motion was categorized according to a scheme suggested by Hooker and Humphrey with particular attention to extension of the head or limbs relative to the trunk, rotation or dispacement of the torso, or individual phenomena related to specific limb, regional, or organ activity'. Their eight movement categories were rather difficult to relate to Hooker's work but it was the first attempt to classify observed fetal phenomena in the context of previous neurological investigations. The latter was even more so in the study of Ianniruberto & Tajani (1981) who state 'Our own systematic observations ... are mainly qualitative and based on the assumption that motoscopic examination of the fetus would allow specific investigation of neuromotor development; we were interested therefore mainly in pattern analysis'. This motoscopic method was described very briefly and was intended for neurological assessment of impaired older children. Ianniruberto & Tajani (1981) provided descriptions of movements they observed in fetuses of 6–28 weeks gestation but they were often too brief and interpretative and the authors did not specify what the fetus was actually doing (e.g. vermicular movements, creeping, climbing, hands exploring uterine wall, etc.). In addition to the normal fetus, these authors mention anecdotal observations of abnormal and compromised fetuses.

While early ultrasound observations of the fetus were carried out with the aim of providing an additional technique for the assessment of fetal well-being (a concept which was never defined and remains vague), the later studies had a more basic interest in neuromotor development, in providing a timetable of the developmental steps. In addition they hoped to recognize deviations in these motor patterns if, for example, the fetus became compromised, was malformed or had chromosomal defects. Recently a new approach to fetal studies emerged whereby the fetal neural functions were investigated in the context of developmental neurology. Fetal motor patterns were carefully compared (de Vries et al 1982, 1984, 1985) with the previously systematically studied pre-term (Prechtl et al 1979, Prechtl & Nolte 1984) and full-term infants (Prechtl 1974, 1977). It became appreciated that all the different kinds of fetal movement were practically identical to the motor patterns which can be seen in infants after birth, even though not all of them are present in the newborn but reappear some weeks after birth. On the other hand, the fetal repertoire is more limited as the newborn possesses motor patterns which are never observed in the fetus (see later). These observations provided strong evidence for a continuum of many neural functions from prenatal to postnatal life (Prechtl 1984). This also facilitates greatly the identification and categorization of fetal movements and their deviations from the norm. What is gained in the analysis and diagnostic procedure of neurological functions and dysfunctions of the fetus is consistency with the neonate, born either pre-term or at term. In the following text the description of fetal behaviour will be given within the context of developmental neurology.

FETAL BEHAVIOUR

Neurological assessment before birth

One of the fundamental aspects of developmental neurology is the notion of age-specific repertoires of neural functions. Throughout the development of an organism, neural functions appear to be adapted to the particular requirements of the environment to which the organism is exposed at particular stages (e.g. intra-uterine versus extra-uterine). Such ontogenetic adaptations (Oppenheim 1984) are brought about by developmental transformations which can be observed at particular ages. Although there exist, generally, wide variations between individuals, ontogenetic changes clearly follow a timetable. Emergence of new functions and regression of earlier functions are both essential developmental processes. As a consequence, the properties of the neural repertoire can differ so profoundly at different ages that they may be regarded as both qualitative and quantitative differences between these properties. Any technique of assessment of the neurological condition has therefore to start from an analysis of the age-specific repertoire of the developing nervous system (for details see Prechtl 1982). In this context, what is true for the infant and child is also valid for the fetus. Two aspects are candidates for fetal neurological assessment, as they are direct expressions of neurological integrity:

1. Distinct fetal motor patterns
   a. their temporal sequence of appearance
   b. the quality of the individual specific movement pattern
   c. the rate of their occurrence at various gestational ages
2. The emergence and organization of behavioural states.

Emergence of fetal motor patterns

The build-up of the fetal repertoire of distinct movement patterns follows closely a temporal sequence. The first movements appear at 7 weeks (gestational age) and consist of slow extension and flexion movements of the spine. From 8 weeks onwards slow general movements and jerky startles can be observed. Only a few days later, these generalized movements are followed by localized movements of an arm or leg. The localized movements may be either slow or fast. The previously held belief that the earliest fetal movements have a jerky character, followed later by slower movements, is incorrect. There is also no period of generalized amorphic movements which later 'individuate' (Coghill 1929, 1943) into specific localized movements. The short interval between the emergence of generalized movements (which continue nearly unchanged until after birth) and of isolated limb movements makes such a process most unlikely. From 10 to 12 weeks the repertoire expands rapidly and many new movement patterns appear (see Fig. 2.1). It should be stressed that all the fetal movements described up to now can also be seen postnatally. This greatly facilitates their categorization. In the following description of the different types of fetal movement (from Prechtl 1986) the same terminology is employed as has been used for the categorization of postnatal movement patterns.

Startles. Quick, generalized movements which always start in the limbs and often spread to trunk and neck. The duration of a startle is one second or less. Usually they occur singly but sometimes they may be repetitive. They can be superimposed incidentally on a general movement.

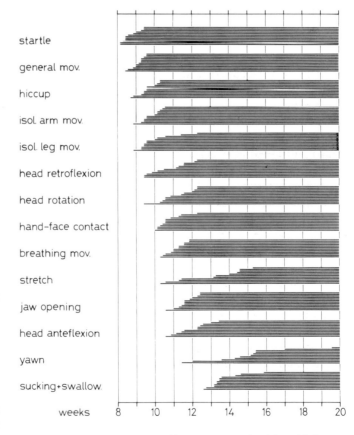

Fig. 2.1 Timetable of emergence of fetal movements in 12 low-risk fetuses. Data from longitudinal, weekly one-hour observations during first half of pregnancy. Ages in full weeks and days. Small scatter of onset age is seen in frequently occurring movements; wide scatter in movements with low incidence. (Modified from De Vries et al 1982.)

General movements. Gross movements which are slow and involve the whole body. They may last from a few seconds to a minute. What is particular about them is the indeterminate sequence of arm, leg, neck and trunk movements. They wax and wane in intensity, force and speed. Despite this variability, they must be considered as a distinct, easily recognized pattern.

Hiccup. A phasic contraction of the diaphragm, often repetitive at regular intervals. A bout may last up to several minutes. In contrast to the startle, this movement always starts in the trunk but may be followed by movement of the limbs.

Breathing movements. Fetal breathing movements are paradoxical. Every contraction of the diaphragm (which leads after birth to an inspiration) causes an inward movement of the thorax and a simultaneous movement of the abdomen outwards. The sequence of 'breaths' can be regular or irregular. No amniotic fluid enters the lungs during breathing movements. Isolated breaths may resemble a sigh.

Isolated arm or leg movements. An arm or a leg may be moved in isolation without other parts moving. The speed may vary and so may the amplitude of the movement.

Twitches. Quick extensions or flexions of a limb or the neck. They are never generalized and are not repetitive.

Cloni. Repetitive, tremulous movements of one or more limbs. Their rate is about 3 per second and there are rarely more than 3 or 4 at a time in normal fetuses.

Isolated hand movements. The fingers may flex or extend together repetitively or in isolation. Some hand postures may resemble hand gestures seen in later life and the hand may rotate outwards or inwards (supination or pronation).

Hand–face contact. The hand may accidentally touch the face either by an arm movement in the direction of the face or by a head movement in the direction of the hand. Hand–mouth contact occurs but it is often difficult to judge precisely where the hand makes contact.

Retroflexion of the head. Backward bending of the head may vary in speed from slow to jerky. The head may remain in a retroflexed position from one second to a minute, often accompanied by an over-extension of the spine.

Lateral rotation of the head. The head is rotated from the midline to a lateral position or vice versa. This movement occurs in isolation. The speed is usually slow; the amplitude may vary.

Rhythmical side-to-side movements of the head.
As in postnatal rooting, the regularity is not consistent. The movements are slow but always consist of a lift-off from the surface the fetus is resting on.

Opening of the mouth. Amplitude and speed may vary. Occurs in isolation. Sometimes tongue protrusion can be observed.

Yawn. A slow opening of the mouth followed by maintenance of the open position for several seconds ending with a quick closure.

Rhythmical mouthing. Small and rhythmical quiver of the jaws without opening of the mouth. Occurs in bursts of 5 to 10 movements which have a rate of about 4 or 5 per second.

Sucking. Bursts of rhythmical jaw movements with a rate of about one per second and of varying length. Sometimes they are followed by swallowing, indicating that the fetus is drinking amniotic fluid.

Stretch. This complex motor pattern consists of over-extension of the spine, retroflexion of the head, abduction, external rotation and elevation of the arms. The movement lasts several seconds and occurs singly.

Rotation of the fetus. The rotation may occur along the longitudinal axis or the transverse axis of the fetal body. These movements are always forceful. Alternating leg movements, when the feet are in contact with the uterine wall, may result in a somersault. Rotation around the sagittal axis is initiated by either a rotation of the head or of the hip.

Eye movements. Slow as well as rapid and repetitive (nystagmoid) eye movements can be distinguished. The displacement of the eye ball can be seen either as a flicker of the echo behind the orbit or as shifts in the position of the echos from the lenses. (See Chapter 6.)

The age-related sequence of the appearance of these movement patterns is dependent upon the structural maturation of the nervous system. Unfortunately, our knowledge of the structural development of the human fetal nervous system is lamentably limited when considering the emergence of most of the fetal movement patterns. An exception is the study of the ultrastructure of the cervical spinal cord by Okado & Kojima (1984). They demonstrate how minimal the requirement in synaptic density on the motor neurones is for providing the structural basis for the generation of the early movements. At the end of the first trimester a considerable increase in synapse formation is seen and this is associated with a considerable enrichment of the motor repertoire. Surprisingly, despite the relatively immature structure, the movements are fully co-ordinated and hardly change their form during further development of the structure.

The study of movements generated by anencephalic fetuses has added considerably to our understanding of the neural mechanisms underlying distinct motor patterns (Visser et al 1985a). The lack of normal patterns of movement in fetuses with major defects of the neural tube provides convincing evidence for the necessity of normally ordered neurones even if they are amazingly sparse and their connections limited in number. Results from electrical recordings of neural activity in tissue cultures corroborate these observations (Stafström et al 1980, Droge et al 1986). As soon as a minimal differentiation of connectivity is reached, organized activity in burst–pause patterns develops.

How much the timetable of the emergence of fetal movements depends on growth is illustrated by the delayed appearance of the motor patterns in fetuses of type I diabetic patients (Visser et al 1985). As fetal growth is retarded by about one week, the timetable of fetal movements is shifted for about the same time but the sequence remains the same as in normal fetuses.

Quality of individual specific movement

Not only have fetal movement patterns a distinct feature which makes them easily recognizable in the same fetus and also in different fetuses, the individual movement pattern of a general movement or startle or another type of movement has in addition to its form (co-ordination which makes the pattern recognizable) other characteristics which can be described. These aspects deal with more complex properties such as fluency and smoothness and also with variability in terms of changes in speed, amplitude, force and direction. This is especially important in the case of general movements. A general movement, lasting for example 25 seconds, will fluctuate in both waxing and waning during its course, which is most characteristic for the intact nervous system. There is a decay of this variability of fetal movements when the integrity of the nervous system is compromised. Such observations have been made in pre-term infants (Prechtl & Nolte 1984) and in full-term fetuses (Bekedam et al 1985). The best way to assess such changes is observation of these movements from replayed videotape recordings. The visual Gestalt-perception is a powerful instrument to detect such alterations in the complexity of movements. The interobserver agreement has been tested (Bekedam et al 1985) and found to be highly reliable. Although this method is still in its infancy, it is a most promising diagnostic tool in neurological assessment.

Rate of fetal movements and their developmental course

The quantitative aspects of fetal movements have received extensive attention (de Vries et al 1985). Not only do the various movement types differ in their incidence at a particular age of the fetus, they also show different trends during their developmental course. Even the features of the same type of movement show a wide scatter between individuals observed at a particular age. The intra-individual consistency from week to week turned out to be low in longitudinal studies, although the observation time was 60 minutes and thus relatively long (de Vries et al 1987). This all makes the quantitative assessment of fetal motility a poor diagnostic indicator of fetal neurological condition.

This conclusion is in agreement with previous findings in pre-term infants. In a longitudinal study, a carefully selected low-risk group, all of whom subsequently had normal development, was compared to a high-risk group, the majority of whom subsequently developed handicap.

There was no significant quantitative difference between the different movements (weekly 2-hour observations), with the exception of clonus (Prechtl & Nolte 1984).

Development and organization of behavioural states

The term behavioural states is used to describe temporary stable conditions of neural and autonomic functions, known as sleep and wakefulness. These states are characterized by distinct behaviour of certain variables acting in concert. Observation and recording of such variables which have been selected as criteria, provide a method for monitoring behavioural states over prolonged periods. Extensive studies of behavioural states have been carried out in newborn full-term and pre-term infants, based on recordings of eye movements, heart-rate pattern, breathing pattern, opening or closing of eyelids, motility and EEG-patterns. All these variables change their characteristics or parameters episodically (i.e. from present to absent, regular to irregular, high to low voltage, etc.). There are several classifications of behavioural states but the most widely used is that numbering from state 1 to 5, covering all sleep and awake states in the full-term newborn (see Table 2.1) and avoiding interpretative terminology (Prechtl 1974). This is discussed with reference to the newborn in Chapter 3.

States follow each other in a cyclical manner. Cycles of sleep states (stage 1 and 2) last about 50 minutes. In the healthy full-term newborn the co-ordination between the variables is such that transitions from one state to another do not last longer than 2 to 3 minutes (i.e. all variables have changed their parameters to those characteristic for the new state). It is this phenomenon of alignment between the variables at the transitions which develops at around 36 to 38 weeks gestational age. Before this age states are 'poorly organized' (Parmelee et al 1967) as the separate variables fluctuate more inconsistently than later. On the other hand, there are periods of congruency between state variables which fit the state definition but they do not start and end simultaneously. The possibility of coincidence of occurrence exists even if the separate

Table 2.1 Comparative behavioural states in newborn and fetus

Neonate	Eyes	Respiration	Movements
State 1	closed	regular	only startles
State 2	closed	irregular	episodic gross
State 3	open	regular	no
State 4	open	irregular	continual
State 5	open/closed	crying	continual

Fetus	Heart rate	Eye movements	Movements
State 1F	regular, low	no	only startles
State 2F	irregular	yes	episodic gross
State 3F	regular, high	yes	no
State 4F	irregular, high	yes	continual

variables oscillated completely independently from each other. Such an extreme condition does not usually appear to be the case since from about 30–32 weeks onwards a bias in the relationship between particular state variables may exist (see Prechtl et al 1979).

With regard to the ontogeny of behavioural states in the fetus, Nijhuis et al (1982) were able to show that fetuses of 36 and 38 weeks gestation had developed behavioural states which were fully comparable in their organization to those in full-term neonates. In this study the selection of the criteria of state had to be adapted to the particular situation in utero and differed in part from those employed in neonates. Three independent variables were chosen: 1. fetal heart-rate pattern (excluding accelerations during movements), 2. eye movements (present or absent) and, 3. gross body movements (present or absent). An important step was achieved by the differentiation between 'coincidence' and 'true behavioural state'. Coincidence was defined as any period in which the parameters of variables met the criteria of a particular state but without the simultaneity of changes during transitions from one state to another. With this distinction it became much easier to focus on the ontogenetic events in the emergence of true behavioural states. In this context there are two main questions: 1. What is the developmental course of the various types of coincidence?, 2. When do synchronized transitions occur and are there age differences between the different kinds of transition between certain states? The study by van Vliet et al (1985a) provides data from a group of fetuses of low-risk nulliparous women. There are certain minor differences from the previously studied multiparous group but the increase in the percentage of coincidences mimicking state 1 between 32 and 40 weeks was similar to that in the multiparous group. Surprisingly enough there was no prevalence in the synchronization of a certain type of transition before 36–38 weeks. The occurrence of well-aligned transitions is inconsistent within the same individual fetus and seemingly follows no particular rule. Future research will have to concentrate on these aspects rather than to argue about the existence of states before 36 weeks without convincing data. It is clear, however, that the choice of state variables is crucial. Single variables (e.g. fetal heart rate or eye movements) are insufficient to identify states and hence are misleading.

The developmental course of behavioural states can now be studied in the compromised fetus and compared to low-risk cases. van Vliet et al (1985b) have investigated the development of behavioural states of growth-retarded fetuses and found a delay in the onset of states in most of the cases. This was irrespective of the fact that the different kinds of coincidence were hardly altered in their occurrence. What was obviously different in these fetuses was the ability to synchronize their variables at the transitions. This finding emphasizes the importance of discriminating between coincidence and true behavioural state. The abnormalities in the development of behavioural states in growth-retarded fetuses would have been missed without their distinction.

CONCLUSION

For assessment of the fetal neurological condition, quantitative recordings of fetal motility are of limited value. Either subjective counting of movements felt by the expectant mother or instrumental recording through the abdominal wall are restricted to the second half of pregnancy. A rapid decline of fetal motility is an alarm sign of a life-threatening condition. Less dramatic conditions can be hardly detected. An analysis of motor patterns is also impossible.

Modern ultrasound equipment in combination with videotape recording provides a powerful tool to investigate fetal motor patterns and the emergence and organization of behavioural states. Both aspects are direct expressions of neural activity and are excellent candidates for the assessment of neurological dysfunctions of the fetal nervous system. As there exists a continuum of neural functions from prenatal to postnatal life, fetal movement patterns and behavioural states can be compared easily with those of the pre-term and full-term infant. In many respects such a comparison also holds true for the functional expressions of neural dysfunction.

REFERENCES

Adamson G D, Cousin A J, Gare D J 1980 Rhythmic fetal movements. American Journal of Obstetrics and Gynecology 136: 239–242

Ahlfeld F 1888 Über bisher noch nicht beschriebene intrauterine Bewegungen des Kindes. Verhandlungen der Deutschen Gesellschaft für Gynäkologie 2: 203–210

Ahlfeld F 1905 Die intrauterine Tätigkeit der Thorax- und Zwerchfellmuskulatur. Intrauterine Atmung. Monatschrift für Geburtshilfe und Gynäkologie 21: 143–163

Bekedam D J, Visser G H A, Vries J J de, Prechtl H F R 1985 Motor behaviour in the growth retarded fetus. Early Human Development 12: 155–166

Birnholz J C, Stephens J C, Faria M 1978 Fetal movement patterns: a possible means of defining neurological developmental milestones in utero. American Journal of Roentgenology 130: 537–540

Carmichael L 1970 The onset and early development of behavior. In: Mussen P H (ed) Manual of child psychology, Vol 1. Wiley, New York

Coghill G E 1929 Anatomy and the problem of behavior. Cambridge University Press, Cambridge, UK

Coghill G E 1943 Flexion spasms and mass reflexes in relation to the ontogenetic development of behavior. Journal of Comparative Neurology 76: 463–486

de Vries J I P, Visser G H A, Prechtl H F R 1982 The emergence of fetal behaviour. I. Qualitative aspects. Early Human Development 7: 301–322 de Vries J I P, Visser G H A, Prechtl H F R 1984 Fetal motility in the first half of pregnancy. In: Prechtl H F R (ed) Continuity of neural functions from prenatal to postnatal life. Clinics in Developmental Medicine, Vol 94. Blackwell, Oxford, pp 79–92

de Vries J I P, Visser G H A, Prechtl H F R 1985 The emergence of fetal behaviour. II. Quantitative aspects. Early Human Development 12: 99–120

Droge M H, Gross G W, Hightower M H, Czisny L E 1986 Multielectrode analysis of coordinated, multisite, rhythmic bursting in cultured CNS monolayer networks. Journal of Neuroscience 6: 1583–1592

Gettinger A, Roberts A B, Campbell S 1978 Comparison between subjective and ultrasound assessment of fetal movements. British Medical Journal 2: 88–90

Harris D B, Harris E S 1946 A study of fetal movements in relation to mother's activity. Human Biology 18: 221–237

Hertogs K, Roberts A B, Cooper D, Griffin D R, Campbell S 1979 Maternal perception of fetal motor activity. British Medical Journal 2: 1183–1185

Higginbottom J, Bagnall K M, Harris P F, Slater J H, Porter G A 1976 Ultrasound monitoring of fetal movements. Lancet 3: 719–721

Hooker D 1952 The Prenatal Origin of Behaviour. University of Kansas Press, Lawrence

Humphrey T 1978 Function of the nervous system during prenatal life. In: Stave U (ed) Perinatal physiology. Plenum, New York, pp 651–683

Ianniruberto A, Tajani E 1981 Ultrasonographic study of fetal movements. Seminars in Perinatology 5: 175–181

Jouppila P 1976 Fetal movements diagnosed by ultrasound in early pregnancy. Acta Obstetrica et Gynecologica Scandinavica 55: 131–135

Kellogg W N 1941 A method for recording the activity of the human fetus in utero with specimen results. Journal of Genetic Psychology 58: 307–326

Liston R M, Cohen A W, Mennuti M T, Gabbe S G 1982 Antepartum fetal evaluation by maternal perception of fetal movement. Obstetrics and Gynecology 60: 424–426

Milani-Comparetti A, Gidoni E A 1967 Pattern analysis of motor development and its disorders. Developmental Medicine and Child Neurology 9: 625–630

Minkowski M 1928 Neurobiologische Studien am menschlichen Foetus. Handbuch der Biologischen Arbeitsmethoden Abteilung V Teil 5B, pp 511–618

Newbery H 1941 Studies in fetal behavior. IV. The measurement of three types of fetal activity. Journal of Comparative Psychology 32: 521–530

Nijhuis J G, Prechtl H F R, Martin C B Jr, Bots R S G M 1982 Are there behavioural states in the human fetus? Early Human Development 6: 177–195

Okado N, Kojima T 1984 Ontogeny of the central nervous system: neurogenesis, fibre connection, synaptogenesis and myelination in the spinal cord. In: Prechtl H F R (ed) Continuity of neural functions from prenatal to postnatal life. Clinics in Developmental Medicine, Vol 94. Blackwell, Oxford, pp 79–92

Oppenheim R W 1984 Ontogenetic adaptations in neural development; towards a more 'ecological' developmental psychobiology. In: Prechtl H F R (ed) Continuity of neural functions from prenatal to postnatal life. Clinics in Developmental Medicine, Vol 94. Blackwell, Oxford, pp 16–30

Parmelee A H Jr, Wenner W H, Akiyama Y, Schultz M, Stern E 1967 Sleep states in premature infants. Developmental Medicine and Child Neurology 9: 70–77

Pearson J F, Weaver J B 1976 Fetal activity and fetal wellbeing: an evaluation. British Medical Journal 1: 1305–1307

Prechtl H F R 1974 The behavioural states of the newborn infant (a review). Brain Research 76: 1304–1311

Prechtl H F R 1977 The neurological examination of the full-term newborn infant, 2nd edn. Clinics in Developmental Medicine, Vol 63. Heinemann, London, p 65

Prechtl H F R 1982 Assessment methods for the newborn infant, a critical evaluation. In: Stratton P (ed) Psychobiology of the human newborn. Wiley, Chichester, pp 21–52

Prechtl H F R 1984 Continuity of neural functions from prenatal to postnatal life. Clinics in Developmental Medicine, Vol 94. Blackwell, Oxford, p 255

Prechtl H F R 1986 Prenatal motor development. In: Wade M A,

Whiting H T A (eds) Motor development in children: aspects of coordination and control. Nijhoff, Dordrecht, pp 53–64

Prechtl H F R, Fargel J W, Weinmann H M, Bakker H H 1979 Posture, motility and respiration in low-risk preterm infants. Developmental Medicine and Child Neurology 21: 3–27

Prechtl H F R, Nolte R 1984 Motor behaviour of preterm infants. In: Prechtl H F R (ed) Continuity of neural functions from prenatal to postnatal life. Clinics in Developmental Medicine, Vol 94. Blackwell, Oxford, pp 79–92

Preyer W 1885 Die spezielle Physiologie des Embryo. Grieben, Leipzig

Reifferscheid K 1911 Über intrauterine Atembewegungen des Foetus. Deutsche Medizinische Wochenschrift 37: 877–880

Reinold E 1971 Fetale Bewegungen in der Frühgravidität. Zeitschrift für Geburtshilfe und Gynäkologie 174: 220–225

Reinold E 1976 Ultrasonics in early pregnancy. Diagnostic scanning and fetal motor activity. Contributions to Gynaecology and Obstetrics, Vol 1. S. Karger, Basel, p 148

Richards T W, Newbery H, Fallgatter R 1938 Studies in fetal behavior. II. Activity of the human fetus in utero and its relation to other prenatal conditions, particularly the mother's basal metabolic rate. Child Development 9: 69–78

Robertson S S, Dierker L J, Sorokin Y, Rosen M G 1982 Human fetal movement: spontaneous oscillations near one cycle per minute. Science 218: 1327–1330

Sadovsky E 1981 Fetal movements and fetal health. Seminars in Perinatology 5: 131–143

Sadovsky E, Yaffe H 1973 Daily fetal movement recording and fetal prognosis. Obstetrics and Gynecology 41: 845–850

Sadovsky E, Polishuk W Z, Mahler Y, Malkin A 1973 Correlation between electromagnetic recording and maternal assessment of fetal movement. Lancet i: 1141–1143

Sadovsky E, Yaffe H, Polishuk W Z 1974 Fetal movement monitoring in normal and pathologic pregnancy. International Journal of Gynaecology and Obstetrics 12: 75–79

Sadovsky E, Polishuk W Z, Yaffe H, Adler D, Pachys F, Mahler Y 1977 Fetal movements recorder, use and indications. International Journal of Gynecology and Obstetrics 15: 20–24

Schillinger H 1977 Quantitative Untersuchungen zur embryonalen Motorik mit dem Ultraschall-time-motion-Verfahren. Archiv für Gynäkologie 222: 137–147

Schmeidler G R 1941 The relation of fetal activity to the activity of the mother. Child Development 12: 63–68

Schmidt W, Cseh I, Hara K, Neusinger J, Kubli F 1982 Die muetterliche Perzeption fetaler Bewegungen im letzten Schwangerschaftsdrittel. Geburtshilfe und Frauenheilkunde 242: 798–802

Shawker T H, Schuette W H, Whitehouse W, Rifka S M 1980 Early fetal movements: a real-time ultrasound study. Obstetrics and Gynecology 55: 194–198

Sorokin Y, Pillay S, Dierker L J, Hertz R H, Rosen M G 1981 A comparison between maternal, tocodynamometric and real time ultrasonographic assessments of fetal movement. American Journal of Obstetrics and Gynecology 140: 456–460

Stafström C E, Johnston D, Wehner J M, Sheppard J R 1980 Spontaneous neural activity in fetal brain reaggregate cultures. Neuroscience 5: 1681–1690

Stark C R, Orleans M, Haverkamp A D, Murphy J 1984 Short- and long-term risks after exposure to diagnostic ultrasound in utero. Obstetrics and Gynecology 63: 194–201

Timor-Tritsch I, Zador I, Hertz R H, Rosen M G 1976 Classification of human fetal movement. American Journal of Obstetrics and Gynecology 126: 70–77

van Dongen L G R, Goudie E G 1980 Fetal movement patterns in the first trimester of pregnancy. British Journal of Obstetrics and Gynaecology 87: 191–193

van Vliet M A T, Martin C B Jr, Nijhuis J G, Prechtl H F R 1985a Behavioural states in the fetuses of nulliparous women. Early Human Development 12: 121–136

van Vliet M A T, Martin C B Jr, Nijhuis J G, Prechtl H F R 1985b Behavioural states in growth retarded human fetuses. Early Human Development 12: 183–198

von Baer C E 1828 Über die Entwicklungsgeschichte der Thiere-Beobachtung und Reflexion. Teil I. Gebrüder Bornträger, Königsberg

Visser G H A, Bekedam D J, Mulder E J H, Ballegooie E van 1985b

Delayed emergence of fetal behaviour in type-1-diabetes women. Early Human Development 12: 167–172

Visser G H A, Laurini R N, Vries J I P de, Bekedam D J, Prechtl H F R 1985a Abnormal motor behaviour in anencephalic fetuses. Early Human Development 12: 173–182

Walters C E 1964 Reliability and comparison of four types of fetal activity and of total activity. Child Development 35: 1249–1256

3. Clinical assessment of the infant nervous system

Dr L. M. S. Dubowitz

Although the primary aim of modern intensive care has been to improve survival and reduce the incidence of neurodevelopmental handicap, until recently very few attempts were made to assess the neurological status of these infants in the neonatal unit. The reason for this apathy has partially been that in contrast to the examination in adults, abnormal neurological signs in the full-term and even more in the premature infant only rarely led to the localization of the lesion. The initial results correlating early neurological assessments with later outcome (Donovan et al 1962) have also been disappointing.

Early examinations of the newborn, as of older children, have followed the topography of the nervous system. The failure to diagnose by these conventional methods neurological lesions in the newborn infant provided an impetus to look for other methods of assessment. The aims of this chapter are:

1. To review some of the approaches to the neurological assessment of the newborn infant and the examinations which have been developed during the last few decades to achieve this.
2. To discuss a practical method for everyday assessment of pre-term and full-term infants in the neonatal nursery and follow-up clinics.
3. To delineate the clinical features of some of the most common problems in the neonatal nursery, such as asphyxia, infection, growth retardation, drug effects, and haemorrhagic and ischaemic brain lesions.

CURRENT APPROACHES TO THE EVALUATION OF THE NERVOUS SYSTEM

Peiper, in the first part of this century, developed a great interest in the behaviour of the newborn infant (Peiper 1928, 1963), particularly in neonatal reflexes. Some of these reflexes are similar to those observed in pathological states in adults or after experimental brain lesions in animals. From these observations the mistaken belief developed

that the young infant was similar to these experimental preparations. The young infant was also thought to lack the functional capacity of the cortex and the cerebellum. The newborn was considered to be a brainstem preparation and its neural function a bundle of reflexes. Peiper never developed a systematic examination for the newborn infant but he paved the way for André-Thomas.

André-Thomas also had a great interest in the development of the integrated reflexes. In addition he studied the development of various aspects of muscle tone (André-Thomas & de Ajuriaguerra 1949). He defined active tone, associated with voluntary or spontaneous movements of the infant; and passive tone associated with the capacity of the muscles to be lengthened when joints are moved passively. André-Thomas & Saint-Anne Dargassies (1952) developed a neurological examination based on these definitions (Saint-Anne Dargassies 1955, André-Thomas et al 1960). Saint-Anne Dargassies subsequently mapped these neurological features during the course of development in the premature infant by studying one infant born at 26 weeks gestation longitudinally and by studying infants born between 26 and 40 weeks gestation cross-sectionally (Saint-Anne Dargassies 1966). She noted that neurological maturity was primarily related to gestational age and not weight. She also showed that the trend in development of the infant born prematurely was similar outside and inside the uterus. She tried to define the various stages of muscle tone in terms of gestation, which made this examination rather subjective (Saint-Anne Dargassies 1977). Amiel-Tison further developed this method of assessment by making the descriptions more objective and quantitative (Amiel-Tison 1979, Amiel-Tison & Grenier 1980). Table 3.1 shows the items of this examination. Recently Amiel-Tison has also included assessment of vision and hearing (Amiel-Tison et al 1982).

In 1964 Prechtl saw a need for an examination which was not based primarily on the topography of the nervous system, as he felt that such an examination in the neurologically compromised newborn might not show any deviation at all or it might be impossible to interpret

Table 3.1 Items of French neurological examination

	Passive tone of limbs	Axial tone	Primary reflexes
Examination of the eyes	Lower limb	Spontaneous posture	Sucking
Hypertonic elevation of the eyelids	Heel to ear angle	Free space behind neck	Moro
Occular signs	Popliteal angle	Ventral flexion of the trunk	Palmar grasp
Pupils	Dorsiflexion angle of the foot	Dorsal extension of the trunk	Response to traction
Pupillary light reflex	Ankle clonus	Opisthotonos	Plantar grasp
Pursuit of light	Adductor angle	Response to repeated ventral	Automatic walking
	Symmetry of foot flapping	flexion of the head	Others
Acoustic blink reflex		Active contraction of neck flexors	
Alertness	Upper limb	Active contraction of neck extensors	
Crying	Full flexion at elbow	Straightening of trunk	
Jitteriness	Recoil of elbow		
Seizures	Scarf sign		
Motor activity	Symmetry of wrist flexion		
Facial palsy	Symmetry of hand flapping		
Limb palsy			

abnormal findings. He aimed to design an examination 'to obtain maximum amount of information about the complex neural functions in minimum time and with no risk to the patient' (Prechtl & Beintema 1964). In the second edition of his manual (Prechtl 1977) he outlined the sequence of decisions which were necessary to design such an examination (Fig. 3.1). He showed that it was not only necessary to standardize rigorously the method of eliciting the various responses but also the behavioural state for each component of the examination (Prechtl 1972). The basic examination can be divided into observed and elicited items. Whenever possible the responses are also described quantitatively or scored semi quantitatively (by + or −).

The examination is then summarized under the following headings: posture, motility, pathological movements, motor system (abnormal tonus), responses (intensity), threshold of responses, tendon reflexes, Moro response, state, cry, hemisyndrome, syndrome of abnormal reactivity. This examination takes about 30 minutes. Prechtl also devised a shorter examination suitable for screening (Prechtl 1977). It consists of a limited number of items thought to give the highest chance of differentiating between normal and suspect full-term infants. The items include the assessment of posture and motility in the supine position, resistance to passive movement, the traction test, sucking and the Moro response, and assessment of the position and movement of

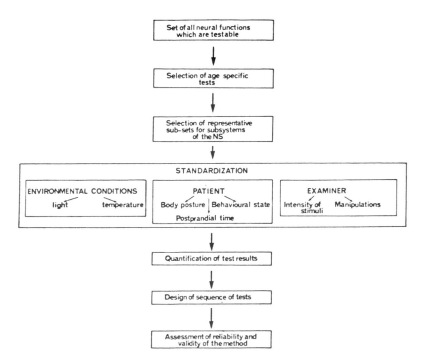

Fig. 3.1 Flow diagram indicating all decision steps for the design of the neurological examination. (Reproduced with permission from Prechtl 1977.)

the eyes. The screening examination was found to give many false positives compared with the full examination (Touwen et al 1977).

Prechtl's examination gives reliable information about the neurological status of full-term infants when the test is performed by experienced examiners. It can differentiate between central and peripheral involvement and allows description of system dysfunction. However, it presents various difficulties when ill infants in the neonatal unit are examined. The test is so designed that reliable information on the state of the nervous system can only be obtained if it is performed in full, under standard conditions. This might pose difficulties in ill infants. Considerable experience is required on the part of the examiner in grading the strengths of some of the responses. Examination items have been chosen to be most appropriate for full-term infants and are assumed to be equally suitable for premature infants reaching 40 weeks postmenstrual age. This hypothesis, however, has not been proven. There is evidence that not all aspects of neuronal maturation proceed in the same way inside and outside the uterus, thus infants reaching 40 weeks postmenstrual age might be different depending on their postnatal age and exposure to the extra-uterine environment (Howard et al 1976, Casaer et al 1982, Palmer et al 1982, Lacey et al 1985, Piper et al 1985). The importance of experience and environment in shaping neuronal development has often been stressed.

Parmelee & Michaelis (1971) tried to devise an examination based on the Prechtl approach. They gave more implicit instruction on grading the various responses and aimed at a total score. The main shortcoming of this approach has been that some of the responses in the abnormal infant tend to be weaker while others are exaggerated; thus many abnormal infants may come up with a normal total score. It is not surprising that the predictive power of this examination turned out to be poor.

The examinations reviewed so far have been aimed primarily at assessing neurological function and not interactive behaviour. For many years there has been a great interest in understanding the relative contribution of the infant to the nature–nurture equation. The first studies on interactive behaviour were in older infants but that such behaviour exists in the very young neonate was demonstrated by Graham as long ago as 1956 (Graham 1956, Graham et al 1956). In 1973 Brazelton introduced a more quantitative scheme based on 27 items of behaviour and 20 reflex items. In Brazelton's own words the scale was designed to score the babies' behavioural repertoire and use of states to manage his or her responsiveness. Such behaviour will to some extent depend on factors affecting the infant's neurological state, but not only on these. The examination has been frequently used as a neurological evaluation. However, it is not suitable for this purpose as it is a much more global and thus less-specific test to assess neurological integrity. In the early stages it was compared for its predictive value with

other neurological tests. While it gave better prediction for neurological outcome than neurological examinations which were not specifically geared to neonates, this was not the case when it was compared with examinations such as that of Prechtl (Leijon & Finnstrom 1982).

The examination was primarily designed as a research tool. It is most valuable when used repeatedly in the neonatal period. Under these circumstances the infant acts as its own control. This might then show the process of recovery following events which occurred in the perinatal period, such as growth retardation (Als et al 1976) and drug use. It may show differences in responses in relation to such diverse factors as noxious stimuli in the neonatal unit, attitudes of different care givers or ethnic influences (Brazelton et al 1977). By recording these changes in the neonatal period it is also possible to study the effect of these on later mother–infant interaction. The scope for it as a research tool is thus very wide. The present test, which is already fairly long, has been designed for full-term infants. The one which is developed presently for premature infants is even longer; thus to try to use these tests as a routine is impractical. In spite of this, the impact of the Brazelton test on the general approach and examination processes in the neonatal unit has been tremendous. It made clinicians aware of the interactive and emotional capabilities of very young infants. Many of the concepts have been incorporated not only in the evaluation of the neonates but also brought about change in the routine practices of neonatal intensive care units so that the development of the interactive processes of the newborn infant are least interfered with.

NEUROLOGICAL ASSESSMENT IN THE NURSERY

METHOD OF RECORDING

It is one of the paradoxes of neonatal care that infants whose neurological status we are most concerned about tend to be least evaluated. None of the above examinations are suitable for the assessment of ill infants on ventilators and all require considerable expertise, not only in interpretation but also in eliciting the responses and recording them.

The ideal neurological examination should be applicable soon after birth in order to try to document the effect of drugs, hypoxia, trauma and other environmental factors in the perinatal period and thereby identify and possibly prevent or reduce complications. It should be applicable to pre-term and full-term infants. The same examination should be suitable for sequential examination from birth at any gestation until 40 weeks postmenstrual age (Dubowitz & Dubowitz 1981). This should make possible:

1. documentation of the normal evolution of neurological behaviour in the pre-term infant after birth;

2. comparison of pre-term infants at various periods after birth with newborn infants of corresponding postmenstrual age;
3. detection of neurological signs and their subsequent evolution.

If the examinations can be carried out during the first week of life in premature infants one should be able to get information on infants in incubators and even on ventilators. A clinical assessment incorporating a good history, observation of abnormal external features, and an examination incorporating evaluation of the infant's state, tone and movement, primitive reflexes, sensory function (such as hearing and vision), as well as observations on how the infant responds to handling and stimulation can be obtained on most infants with minimum disturbance. Frequent evaluation will have to be performed by personnel without great expertise in neurological assessment, i.e. the resident staff. While they cannot be expected necessarily to interpret all the findings, if the instructions are explicit for both eliciting and recording signs then this is feasible even in most ill infants and good interobserver correlation can be achieved. In our experience, forms such as the one illustrated in Figure 3.2 can achieve this goal (Dubowitz & Dubowitz 1981). The speed of the examination will also be aided if the examiner only has to circle items or alter drawings.

The limitation is that the conditions under which the examination will be carried out will not be ideal and will not be absolutely standard. The factor which most influences not only neurological signs but also many vital functions is the infant's state (Prechtl 1977). To achieve comparable states infants should be examined about two-thirds between one feed and the next. If an infant is asleep it is useful to follow a sequence given in the proforma as items such as habituation will be performed while the infant is in the most suitable state for these. Often these stimuli, or turning the infant from a prone to supine position, will bring the infant to a higher state; thus tone, movement and primitive reflexes can be assessed. If one starts with a sleeping infant, it will usually be most alert after these items are elicited and will thus be in the most suitable state to examine eye movements and test vision and hearing. If the infant is fully awake at the beginning of the examination, it might be better to start with the last items first, as too much handling may upset the baby and it will be difficult to get it back to optimal state.

ASSESSMENT OF GESTATIONAL AGE

The importance of knowing the gestational age of the infant to be evaluated cannot be overstressed. First-ly, the findings for various aspects of the neurological examination will depend on the infant's maturity. Secondly, certain neurological findings are characteristic of small-for-gestational age infants born at full-term without necessarily being indicative of a neurological disturbance, while they would be indicative of this in an infant of appropriate weight (Dubowitz et al 1983). Third, the same insult will have a different impact on different parts of the nervous system and thus produce different clinical signs as a function of gestational age of the infant.

Actual gestational age can only be estimated from knowledge of the time of conception. In a woman with regular periods the time of ovulation and thus conception can be estimated with accuracy; unfortunately this is least likely in women who are at the greatest risk of perinatal insults, i.e. those with low social class status and premature birth. Thus, indirect measures have been used which depend on the fact that a number of factors in the fetus's growth development will be strongly but not solely dependent on gestational maturity. All these indirect estimates will also be dependent to variable degrees on the fetus's nutritional state, noxious influences and illness while the infant is still in the uterus and immediately after birth. (For example, anthropometric measures, such as head circumference, weight and length have been used but are imprecise when used at birth.) Fetal crown–rump measurement (Robinson & Fleming 1975) and estimation of the biparietal measurement (Campbell 1969) in early pregnancy are probably some of the most accurate guides for assessment of gestational age. However, after 16 weeks gestation they become increasingly inaccurate for this purpose.

Saint-Anne Dargassies showed over two decades ago that neurological maturation is dependent on gestational age and not on the size of the infant. Thus, a number of schemes estimating gestational age on the basis of neurological maturity evolved (Brett 1963, Koenigsberger 1966, Robinson 1966, Amiel-Tison 1968, Dubowitz et al 1970). The objection to this approach has been that the same criteria are used to assess maturity as are used to assess neurological abnormality.

The maturation of certain external characteristics (Mitchell & Farr 1965, Usher et al 1966) and hyaloid membrane in the eye (Hittner et al 1977) are also strongly related to gestational age. Various schemes use these to estimate gestational age. The argument in favour of this approach has been that these characteristics are not affected by neurological state. They are, however, affected by the nutritional state of the fetus (Mitchell & Farr 1965, Ounsted et al 1978), hormonal factors and some drugs. They also very rapidly change under certain manipulations of the extra-uterine environment, such as the use of radiant heaters. Some of the most favoured criteria, such as breast nodule, ear cartilage and nails, change only late in gestation. None of the criteria used, either neurological or external, have a very strong relation to gestational age; however, when a combination of them is employed a very high correlation can be shown (Dubowitz & Dubowitz 1977). This correlation is best if a combination of external characteristics and selected neurological criteria which are more dependent on maturity and not on normality is employed. As each criterion might be affected in one particular infant the error is least when a large number of criteria are summated. It also should be noted that in infants less than 29–30 weeks little change can be noted in either neurological or external characteristics with decreasing gestational age. The only suitable and reliable method for accurate estimation of gestational age in this population is the measurement of nerve conduction velocity (Dubowitz et al 1968, Schulte et al 1968, Moosa & Dubowitz 1971, Miller et al 1983). This is a relatively simple technique which can be taught to ancillary staff and will give the most reliable estimate of gestational age if performed within the first three weeks of life; after which it might be affected by such postnatal factors as low thyroid function (de Vries et al 1986).

INSPECTION

It is not in the scope of this chapter to describe all the possible markers for central nervous system abnormality which may be noted by inspection of an infant, as these are documented in great detail elsewhere. The examiner should always be on the look-out for dysmorphic features, abnormalities of the face and skull, as possible markers (Smith 1982).

NEUROLOGICAL EXAMINATION

Throughout the examination note should be taken of the infant's state; this is easily definable by observation as shown by concomitant EEG activity in infants above 36 weeks gestation, but is considerably less well differentiated in earlier gestation. In the older infant, the state of arousal will greatly modify the responses to any tests. Some of this dependence can also be demonstrated by the tone pattern, even in smaller infants. Prechtl suggests that all responses should be elicited in an optimal state only. We find this impractical in the intensive care nursery situation. Second best is to make a recording of the infant's state whenever a response is elicited, so that if sequential examinations are analysed this can be taken into account. We use Brazelton's grading of state as many small infants do appear to fit these better (Table 3.2). We start our examination by assessing the infant's responses and response decrement to light and auditory stimuli. This usually helps to arouse the infant. Neurologically intact infants show a response to these stimuli by 27–28 weeks gestation. Response decrement can also be noted in premature infants; however, whether this is due to fatigue or true habituation is difficult to establish. The most common cause for not being able to elicit a response is that the ambient noise or light in the nursery is too high. Irritable infants often show increasing response to repetitive stimuli.

Table 3.2 Comparison of grading of states by Prechtl and Brazelton

Prechtl and Beintema (1964)

State 1	Eyes closed, regular respiration, no movements
State 2	Eyes closed, irregular respiration, no gross movements
State 3	Eyes open, no gross movements
State 4	Eyes open, gross movements, no crying
State 5	Eyes open or closed, crying

Brazelton (1973)

State 1	Deep sleep with regular breathing, eyes closed, no spontaneous activity, no eye movements
State 2	Light sleep with eyes closed; rapid eye-movements, irregular respiration
State 3	Drowsy or semidozing; eyes open or closed, activity variable, movements usually smooth
State 4	Alert, with bright look; minimal motor activity
State 5	Eyes open, considerable motor activity
State 6	Crying

ASSESSMENT OF TONE AND POSTURE

Tone has been defined as the resistance of the muscle to stretch. It is one of the main determinants of resting posture and of the resistance one notices in the muscles when the position of any part of the body is changed. It can thus be best evaluated by observing resting posture and by assessing resistance of the limbs to passive movement or to changes in posture.

Posture

This should be observed with the infant's head in the midline and is best recorded with the aid of diagrams. With increasing maturity the infant passes from a predominantly extended posture to one with extension of the upper limbs but flexion in the lower limbs, to flexion in both upper and lower limbs and eventually to flexion and adduction in all four limbs. The gestational age range at which each phase occurs is fairly wide. These preference postures are often difficult to define at lower gestational ages (Prechtl et al 1979) when the infants tend to be active for long periods of time. They are, however, distinct and consistent enough to be easily recordable in a drowsy state. A distinct difference is also noted between the postures of full-term infants and premature infants reaching 40 weeks postmenstrual age (Fig. 3.3a,b). This difference is most noticeable in infants with the shortest gestation and in the ones who spend most of their time in the prone posture, suggesting an effect of the extra-uterine environment (Palmer et al 1982). Thus, a posture with strongly flexed arms is abnormal in a pre-term infant at 40 weeks postmenstrual age, with or without extended legs (Fig. 3.3c).

Tone

The assessment of tone by resistance to passive movement or to changes in posture can be very subjective and what

NAME	D.O.B./TIME	WEIGHT	E.D.D. L.N.M.P.	E.D.D. U/snd.	**STATES** 1. Deep sleep, no movement, regular breathing. 2. Light sleep, eyes shut, some movement. 3. Dozing, eyes opening and closing. 4. Awake, eyes open, minimal movement. 5. Wide awake, vigorous movement. 6. Crying.	STATE	COMMENT	ASYMMETRY
HOSP. NO.	DATE OF EXAM	HEIGHT						
RACE SEX	AGE	HEAD CIRC.	GESTATIONAL SCORE WEEKS ASSESSMENT					

HABITUATION (≤ state 3)

LIGHT Repetitive flashlight stimuli (10) with 5 sec. gap. Shutdown = 2 consecutive negative responses	No response	A. Blink response to first stimulus only. B. Tonic blink response. C. Variable response.	A. Shutdown of movement but blink persists 2-5 stimuli. B. Complete shutdown 2-5 stimuli.	A. Shutdown of movement but blink persists 6-10 stimuli. B. Complete shutdown 6-10 stimuli.	A. Equal response to 10 stimuli. B. Infant comes to fully alert state. C. Startles + major responses throughout.			
RATTLE Repetitive stimuli (10) with 5 sec. gap.	No response	A. Slight movement to first stimulus. B. Variable response.	Startle or movement 2-5 stimuli, then shutdown	Startle or movement 6-10 stimuli, then shutdown	A. B. Grading as above C.			

MOVEMENT & TONE — Undress infant

POSTURE (At rest — predominant) ✱			(hips abducted)	(hips adducted)	Abnormal postures: A. Opisthotonus. B. Unusual leg extension. C. Asymm. tonic neck reflex			
ARM RECOIL Infant supine. Take both hands, extend parallel to the body; hold approx. 2 secs. and release.	No flexion within 5 sec.	Partial flexion at elbow >100° within 4-5 sec.	Arms flex at elbow to <100° within 2-3 sec.	Sudden jerky flexion at elbow immediately after release to <60°	Difficult to extend; arm snaps back forcefully			
ARM TRACTION Infant supine; head midline; grasp wrist, slowly pull arm to vertical. Angle of arm scored and resistance noted at moment infant is initially lifted off and watched until shoulder off mattress. Do other arm.	Arm remains fully extended	Weak flexion maintained only momentarily	Arm flexed at elbow to 140° and maintained 5 sec.	Arm flexed at approx. 100° and maintained	Strong flexion of arm <100° and maintained			
LEG RECOIL First flex hips for 5 secs, then extend both legs of infant by traction on ankles; hold down on the bed for 2 secs. and release.	No flexion within 5 sec.	Incomplete flexion of hips within 5 sec.	Complete flexion within 5 sec.	Instantaneous complete flexion	Legs cannot be extended; snap back forcefully			
LEG TRACTION Infant supine. Grasp leg near ankle and slowly pull toward vertical until buttocks 1-2" off. Note resistance at knee and score angle. Do other leg.	No flexion	Partial flexion, rapidly lost	Knee flexion 140-160° and maintained	Knee flexion 100-140° and maintained	Strong resistance; flexion <100°			
POPLITEAL ANGLE Infant supine. Approximate knee and thigh to abdomen; extend leg by gentle pressure with index finger behind ankle.	180-160°	150-140°	130-120°	110-90°	<90°			
HEAD CONTROL (post. neck m.) Grasp infant by shoulders and raise to sitting position; allow head to fall forward; wait 30 sec.	No attempt to raise head	Unsuccessful attempt to raise head upright	Head raised smoothly to upright in 30 sec. but not maintained.	Head raised smoothly to upright in 30 sec. and maintained	Head cannot be flexed forward			
HEAD CONTROL (ant. neck m.) Allow head to fall backward as you hold shoulders; wait 30 secs.	Grading as above	Grading as above	Grading as above	Grading as above				
HEAD LAG Pull infant toward sitting posture by traction on both wrists. Also note arm flexion. ✱								
VENTRAL SUSPENSION Hold infant in ventral suspension; observe curvature of back, flexion of limbs and relation of head to trunk. ✱								
HEAD RAISING IN PRONE POSITION Infant in prone position with head in midline.	No response	Rolls head to one side	Weak effort to raise head and turns head to one side	Infant lifts head, nose and chin off	Strong prolonged head lifting			
ARM RELEASE IN PRONE POSITION Head in midline. Infant in prone position; arms extended alongside body with palms up.	No effort	Some effort and wriggling	Flexion effort but neither wrist brought to nipple level	One or both wrists brought at least to nipple level without excessive body movement	Strong body movement with both wrists brought to face, or 'press-ups'			
SPONTANEOUS BODY MOVEMENT during examination (supine). If no spont. movement try to induce by cutaneous stimulation.	None or minimal / Induced	A. Sluggish. B. Random, incoordinated. C. Mainly stretching.	Smooth movements alternating with random, stretching, athetoid or jerky	Smooth alternating movements of arms and legs with medium speed and intensity	Mainly: A. Jerky movement. B. Athetoid movement. C. Other abnormal movement.		1 2	
TREMORS Mark: Fast (>6/sec.) or Slow (<6/sec.)	No tremor	Tremors only in state 5-6	Tremors only in sleep or after Moro and startles	Some tremors in state 4	Tremulousness in all states			
STARTLES	No startles	Startles to sudden noise, Moro, bang on table only	Occasional spontaneous startle	2-5 spontaneous startles	6+ spontaneous startles			
ABNORMAL MOVEMENT OR POSTURE	No abnormal movement	A. Hands clenched but open intermittently. B. Hands do not open with Moro.	A. Some mouthing movement. B. Intermittent adducted thumb	A. Persistently adducted thumb. B. Hands clenched all the time.	A. Continuous mouthing movement. B. Abnormal toe posture. C. Abnormal finger posture. D. Convulsive movement.			

Fig. 3.2

REFLEXES

					STATE	COMMENT	ASYMMETRY

TENDON REFLEXES
Biceps jerk
Knee jerk
Ankle jerk

Absent		Present	Exaggerated	Clonus

PALMAR GRASP
Head in midline. Put index finger from ulnar side into hand and gently press palmar surface. Never touch dorsal side of hand.

Absent	Short, weak flexion	Medium strength and sustained flexion for several secs.	Strong flexion; contraction spreads to forearm	Very strong grasp. Infant easily lifts off couch
R L	R L	R L	R L	R L

PLANTAR GRASP
Press the thumb against the ball of the infants foot.

No response	Partial plantar flexion of toes.	Toes curl around examiners finger.		
R L	R L	R L		

ROOTING
Infant supine, head midline. Touch each corner of the mouth in turn (stroke laterally).

No response	A. Partial weak head turn but no mouth opening. B. Mouth opening, no head turn.	Mouth opening on stimulated side with partial head turning	Full head turning with or without mouth opening	Mouth opening with very jerky head turning

SUCKING
Infant supine; place index finger (pad towards palate) in infant's mouth; judge power of sucking movement after 5 sec.

No attempt	Weak sucking movement: A. Regular. B. Irregular.	Strong sucking movement, poor stripping: A. Regular. B. Irregular.	Strong regular sucking movement with continuing sequence of 5 movements. Good stripping.	Clenching but no regular sucking.

WALKING (state 4, 5)
Hold infant upright, feet touching bed, neck held straight with fingers.

Absent		Some effort but not continuous with both legs	At least 2 steps with both legs	A. Stork posture; no movement. B. Automatic walking.

PLACING
Lift infant in an upright position and allow dorsum of foot to touch protruding edge of a flat surface.

No response	Dorsiflexion of ankle only	Full placing response with flexion of hip and knee and placing sole of foot on surface.		
R L	R L	R L		

MORO
One hand supports infant's head in midline, the other the back. Raise infant to 45° and when infant is relaxed let his head fall through 10°. Note if jerky. Repeat 3 times.

No response, or opening of hands only	Full abduction at the shoulder and extension of the arm	Full abduction but only delayed or partial adduction	Partial abduction at shoulder and extension of arms followed by smooth adduction A. Abd>Add B. Abd=Add C. Abd<Add	A. No abduction or adduction; extension only. B. Marked adduction only.

STATE column for MORO: J / S

NEUROBEHAVIOURAL ITEMS

EYE APPEARANCES

Sunset sign Nerve palsy	Transient nystagmus. Strabismus. Some roving eye movement.	Does not open eyes	Normal conjugate eye movement	A. Persistent nystagmus. B. Frequent roving movement C. Frequent rapid blinks.

AUDITORY ORIENTATION (state 3, 4)
To rattle. (Note presence of startle.)

A. No reaction. B. Auditory startle but no true orientation.	Brightens and stills; may turn toward stimuli with eyes closed	Alerting and shifting of eyes; head may or may not turn to source	Alerting; prolonged head turns to stimulus; search with eyes	Turning and alerting to stimulus each time on both sides

ASYMMETRY column for AUDITORY ORIENTATION: S

VISUAL ORIENTATION (state 4)
To red woollen ball

Does not focus or follow stimulus	Stills; focuses on stimulus; may follow 30° jerkily; does not find stimulus again spontaneously	Follows 30-60° horizontally; may lose stimulus but finds it again. Brief vertical glance	Follows with eyes and head horizontally and to some extent vertically, with frowning	Sustained fixation; follows vertically, horizonally, and in circle

ALERTNESS/RESPONSIVENESS
Do not score appearance but responsiveness to visual stimulation.

Inattentive; rarely or never responds to direct stimulation	When alert, periods rather brief; rather variable response to orientation	When alert, alertness moderately sustained; may use stimulus to come to alert state	Sustained alertness; orientation frequent, reliable to visual stimuli.	Continuous alertness, which does not seem to tire, to visual stimuli.

DEFENSIVE REACTION
A cloth or hand is placed over the infant's face to partially occlude the nasal airway.

No response	A. General quietening. B. Non-specific activity with long latency.	Rooting; lateral neck turning; possibly neck stretching.	Swipes with arm	Swipes with arm with rather violent body movement

PEAK OF EXCITEMENT

Low level arousal to all stimuli; never > state 3	Infant reaches state 4-5 briefly but predominantly in lower states	Infant predominantly state 4 or 5; may reach state 6 after stimulation but returns spontaneously to lower state	Infant reaches state 6 but can be consoled relatively easily	A. Mainly state 6. Difficult to console, if at all. B. Mainly state 4-5 but if reaches state 6 cannot be consoled.

IRRITABILITY (states 3, 4, 5)
Aversive stimuli:
Uncover   Ventral susp.
Undress   Moro
Pull to sit   Walking reflex
Prone

No irritable crying to any of the stimuli	Cries to 1-2 stimuli	Cries to 3-4 stimuli	Cries to 5-6 stimuli	Cries to all stimuli

CONSOLABILITY (state 6)

Never above state 5 during examination, therefore not needed	Consoling not needed. Consoles spontaneously	Consoled by talking, hand on belly or wrapping up	Consoled by picking up and holding; may need finger in mouth	Not consolable

CRY

No cry at all	Only whimpering cry	Cries to stimuli but normal pitch	Lusty cry to offensive stimuli; normal pitch	High-pitched cry, often continuous

NOTES * If asymmetrical or atypical, draw in on nearest figure. Record any abnormal signs (e.g. facial palsy, contractures, etc.). Draw if possible.

CHECK LIST OF ABNORMAL SIGNS

Head and trunk control	Orientation & alertness
Limb tone	Irritability
Motility	Consolability
Reflexes	Deviant sign

Modified from *The Neurological Assessment of the Preterm and Full-term Newborn Infant*, by Lilly and Victor Dubowitz.
© 1981 Spastics International Medical Publications, 5A Netherhall Gardens, London NW3 5RN.

Record time after feed:

EXAMINER:

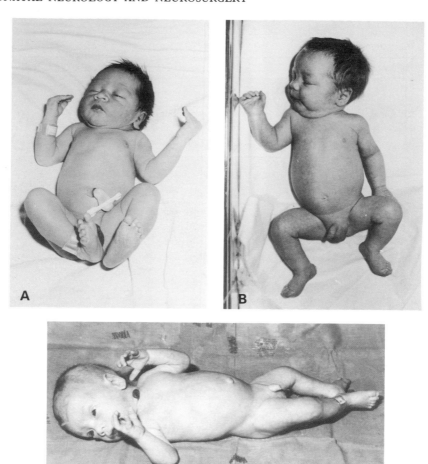

Fig. 3.3 Posture: (**a**) normal full-term infant, day 2; (**b**) normal pre-term infant born at 29 weeks gestation and examined at 40 weeks postmenstrual age (PMA); (**c**) abnormal pre-term infant born at 30 weeks gestation and examined at 40 weeks PMA. This infant later showed signs of cerebral diplegia. Note the reduced arm and leg flexion in the normal pre-term infant (**b**) examined at 40 weeks PMA compared with full-term infant (**a**). There is also strong arm flexion and extended legs in the infant which developed cerebral palsy.

is called strong or weak might vary considerably from one examiner to another. This becomes important if one wants to record changes in the same infant or compare lesser differences between different infants. Measuring the angle of resistance to passive movement in a similar way to that described by French workers or to traction will help to quantify some of these responses.

Limb tone

Before any assessment of this is made it is important to ascertain that there are no fixed contractures. Assessment of flexor tone in the upper and lower limbs can be made by testing the power of recoil of the limbs when they are rapidly extended and by measuring the angle at which resistance occurs when vertical traction is applied to the limbs (Fig. 3.4). Tone in the hamstring can be assessed by measurement of the popliteal angle. Additional information on limb tone will also be obtained by looking at the amount of flexion or

extension which might occur when an infant is put into ventral suspension or is pulled to sit. The traction response and recoil both increase with gestational age, reflecting the increase in flexor tone with increasing maturity; in normal premature infants, arm flexor tone is always less than that of the legs.

Trunk and neck tone

These are assessed by observing the infant in the supine posture and in ventral suspension by testing head control (Fig. 3.5). The tone of the anterior neck muscles is observed with the infant held by the shoulders in the sitting position and while the infant is pulled to sit. Tone in the posterior neck muscles is also observed in the sitting position and in ventral suspension. Flexor tone of the neck muscles can be demonstrated from about 28 weeks gestation onward but is not evident in the pull-to-sit manoeuvre until several weeks later. In normal infants, extensor tone in the neck muscles

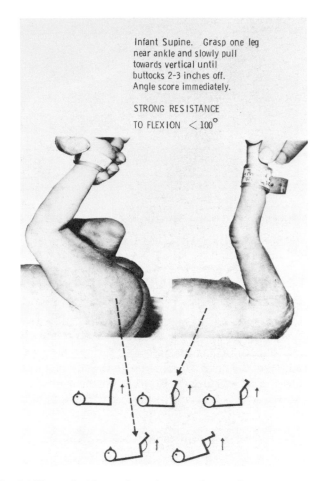

Infant Supine. Grasp one leg near ankle and slowly pull towards vertical until buttocks 2–3 inches off. Angle score immediately.

STRONG RESISTANCE TO FLEXION < 100°

Fig. 3.4 The method for scoring resistance to leg traction.

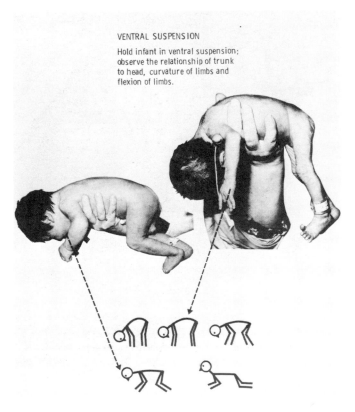

VENTRAL SUSPENSION

Hold infant in ventral suspension; observe the relationship of trunk to head, curvature of limbs and flexion of limbs.

Fig. 3.5 The method for scoring ventral suspension.

often cannot be demonstrated until full-term. Low-risk (but not high-risk) premature infants have better head control at 40 weeks postmenstrual age than newborn full-term infants (Palmer et al 1982). All premature infants also show more hip and knee extension at 40 weeks postmenstrual age (Fig. 3.6).

Generally increased or decreased tone can be a manifestation of a central nervous system (CNS) insult but the more common cause is systemic illness. In contrast, abnormal tone pattern is nearly always a sign of CNS insult. A disproportionally tight popliteal angle compared with the rest of the leg tone is frequently found in association with germinal matrix or intraventricular haemorrhages (Dubowitz et al 1981). A persistently asymmetrical popliteal angle from 40 weeks postmenstrual age onwards might be an early marker for hemiplegia (Fig. 3.7). Marked increase in arm flexor tone in association with increased leg extensor tone can be observed in normal crying infants. If noted in a quiet infant at any gestation it should raise the suspicion of CNS pathology. It is, however, non-specific and a sign of cerebral irritability. It is associated with a number of conditions, such as the onset of an intraventricular haemorrhage, hypoxic–

ischaemic encephalopathy, periventricular leukomalacia and progressive ventricular enlargement. Relative increase in the neck extensor muscles compared with the flexor ones is a similar abnormality first reported by Amiel-Tison et al (1977). This is often associated with hypoxic–ischaemic lesions, meningitis or increased intraventricular pressure. Again, it may be observed in the normal crying infant.

ABNORMAL FINGER AND TOE POSTURE

A number of characteristic abnormal finger and toe postures may be observed in newborn infants. Although the mechanisms underlying them are not clearly understood, they show such high correlations with abnormal neurological states that they may serve as useful markers (de Vries et al 1985).

Fisted hands, adducted thumbs

A tightly fisted hand with the thumb enclosed by the other fingers and which does not open spontaneously is one of the oldest signs noted in neurologically abnormal infants and has been considered a precursor of spasticity. While it should definitely be considered as a marker, as it occurs only rarely in an otherwise normal infant, its close association with spasticity is doubtful. Sequential

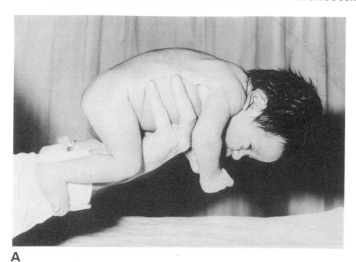
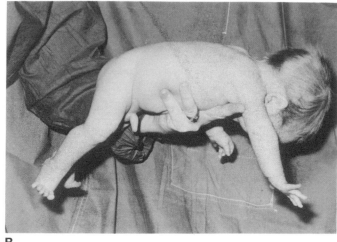

A   **B**

Fig. 3.6 Ventral suspension. (a) full-term infant examined on day 2; (b) normal pre-term infant born at 29 weeks of gestation and examined at 40 weeks postmenstrual age (PMA). Note that there is more extension of head, trunk, hip and knee in the prematurely born infant.

examinations have shown that this may be a transient sign in infants who later completely normalize. It also has not been observed in a number of infants examined regularly who later became quadriplegic. It is, however, one of the few signs which might help to localize a lesion. When present unilaterally, a lesion in the contralateral hemisphere can often be demonstrated on ultrasonography. In premature infants, tightly fisted hands are not seen but persistent strong thumb adduction, even without flexion of the other finger, has the same significance.

Flexed index finger

Isolated flexion of the index finger with the other fingers

extended may be seen in the crying full-term infant. However, persistence of this hand posture is rare. We observed this sign (Fig. 3.8) persistently in a quiet state in a number of premature infants around 40 weeks postmenstrual age. It showed frequent association with cystic leukomalacia.

Dorsiflexion of the big toe (spontaneous Babinski)

This again may occur transiently in the normal crying infant. When seen in a quiet baby in the supine position it is suggestive of an upper motor neurone lesion on the contralateral side (Fig. 3.9). It may be observed in all infants with large haemorrhages or infarcts on the opposite side to the lesion. We have observed this

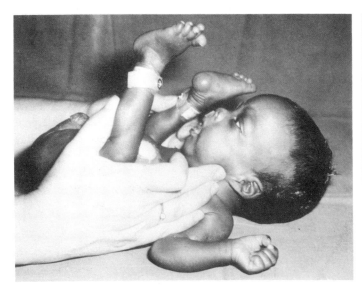
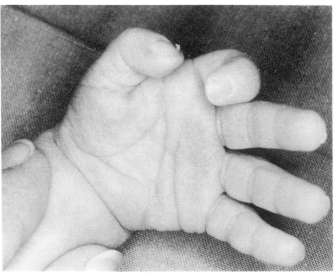

Fig. 3.7 Asymmetrical popliteal angle; This is often a marker for future hemiplegia.

Fig. 3.8 Abnormal finger posture; the flexed thumb and index finger are frequently seen in association with cystic leukomalacia.

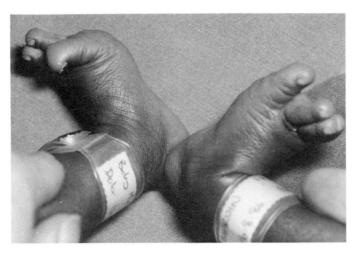

Fig. 3.9 Spontaneously up-going toe on the left; when asymmetrical, this is often an early neonatal sign on the affected side in infants who later show hemisyndrome or hemiplegia.

sign as early as 30 weeks postmenstrual age. It has also been noted by 40 weeks postmenstrual age in infants with extensive periventricular cystic leukomalacia, all of whom later developed cerebral palsy.

STRENGTH AND QUALITY OF MOVEMENT

Power

The power of the infant's movement as opposed to tone can be difficult to distinguish. The most useful way of differentiating the two is to observe the infant's capability of moving against gravity. While hypotonia without weakness may be seen in any ill infant, hypotonia in association with weakness is a sign of neurological dysfunction.

Movement

The quality, quantity and symmetry of spontaneous movements can easily be observed, even in the smallest and illest of infants. Both quality and quantity change with increasing age. The movement in the immature infant often consists of slow asymmetric twisting and stretching movements of the trunk and limb, often termed athetoid. This may be accompanied by rapid repetitive wide-amplitude movements of the limbs, resembling myoclonus. There is gradual change to smooth alternating movement of the arms with medium speed and intensity. The quantity of motor activity changes little from approximately 28 to 35 weeks but decreases rapidly thereafter. This maturational decline in motor activity is similar inside and outside the uterus.

Abnormal movements

The normal infant is characterized by its variable pattern of movement while stereotyped movements (repetitive suck-ing, chewing and bicycling) are associated with an abnormal neurological state. Abnormality of motor function may also be manifested by inappropriate quality and quantity of movement for the infant's maturity or by asymmetries.

Jitteriness, tremors and startles

High-frequency, low-amplitude tremors are normal in awake full-term infants during the first 2–3 days of life; they are, however, abnormal after this period, except when the infant is crying or is in REM sleep. Although they are seen relatively commonly in premature infants reaching 40 weeks postmenstrual age, they are often associated with other deviant clinical signs or abnormalities on ultrasound scans and should not be regarded as normal.

Startles are apparently spontaneous Moro reactions.

Jitteriness is a state with frequent startles and markedly tremulous limbs. In contrast to convulsions, these tremors are very stimulus-sensitive and can be inhibited by flexion of the limbs. Differentiation from convulsions, however, on clinical grounds can be difficult, as can be shown when simultaneous EEG recordings are available.

NEONATAL REFLEXES

A multitude of transitory 'reflexes' which are unique to the neonate have been described. In spite of the extensive literature on their description and development, little is known about the mechanism which produces them. Many are already present in early gestation and show a distinct developmental profile with increasing age of the infant. The reflexes which we found most useful were palmar and plantar grasp, the Moro reflex and placing reaction. Our original schemes also included the rooting reflex and automatic walking. The last two, however, have been of no value in the longitudinal assessment of premature infants. The orogastric tube interferes with the rooting reflex. The walking reflex cannot be elicited in infants who spend most of their time prone and thus have externally rotated hips and everted feet.

Palmar grasp

Stimulation of the palm of the hand produces weak flexion of the finger from 27 to 28 weeks postmenstrual age (PMA). With increasing maturity the contraction spreads to the arm until at 37–38 weeks PMA this is strong enough to allow the infant to be lifted off the cot.

Plantar grasp

This reflex, which produces curling of the toes over the examiner's finger when the ball of the foot is stimulated, is well developed even in infants of 26 weeks PMA and becomes only slightly stronger with increasing maturity.

Moro reflex

This response is most easily elicited by the sudden dropping of the baby's head in relation to its body. At 25–27 weeks PMA the only response to this manoeuvre is the opening of the hand. With increasing maturity, extension and abduction of the upper extremity can be noted, followed by some adduction at the shoulder from 33 to 34 weeks PMA. The adductive element gradually becomes stronger. In full-term infants at birth, abduction and adduction are equal, and in the weeks following the adductive element becomes weaker again. Neurologically optimal premature infants show much less adduction at 40 weeks PMA than full-term infants.

Placing reaction

When the dorsum of the foot is stroked with the edge of the table it provokes stepping-over-the-edge in the stimulated foot. An attempt at this can be seen from 34 weeks PMA onwards and matures to the full response in the next 2–4 weeks.

Abnormal responses

The neonatal reflexes tend to show certain common features in association with neurological insults. These can be considered together. Absent or high threshold responses will be found in apathetic non-alert infants. Newborns who are hyperexcitable due to biochemical or CNS disturbances will have low-threshold exaggerated response or inappropriately mature reactions for their postmenstrual age. Root, plexus and nerve injuries will always produce asymmetrical responses, while symmetrical responses will often be found in association with large asymmetrical cortical lesions. There are two notable exceptions: poor plantar (Fig. 3.10) and placing responses may be observed on the contralateral side of large parenchymal haemorrhages and infarction in the parietal areas. These may be the earliest and often only signs of a future hemiplegia, particularly in premature infants. The probable mechanism is reduced

afferent input to elicit the response. Reduced sensation on that side can often be demonstrated later in these infants, although it is difficult to elicit in the early neonatal period.

Sucking and feeding

Feeding requires the co-ordinated action of sucking, swallowing and breathing. Adequate co-ordination for this already exists at 28 weeks gestation. At this stage, however, sucking is not powerful enough nor is there sufficient synchrony with swallowing to allow adequate feeding. With increasing maturity sucking becomes more powerful and co-ordinated and by 32–34 weeks a normal infant is able to feed orally. With the development of sucking and swallowing there is also the development of a characteristic feeding posture. It has been shown that the maturation of oral feeding is more related to postnatal than postmenstrual age (Casaer et al 1982).

Abnormal sucking and swallowing

Isolated abnormalities of sucking and swallowing are often related to a non-neurological cause. Depression of the nervous system due to any cause may produce poor sucking and swallowing. However, contrary to general belief, severe neurological damage may co-exist with normal feeding behaviour, though apparently not with normal feeding posture. On the other hand, in an infant with a history of perinatal asphyxia severe sucking and swallowing difficulties out of proportion to the rest of the infant's neurological problems should raise the possibility of an underlying neuromuscular disorder.

OCULAR ABNORMALITIES
(See also Chapter 42).

Sunset sign has been associated with hydrocephalus in older infants. However, in the newborn period, particularly in premature infants, considerable ventricular dilatation might be present without any evidence of a sunset sign. Conversely, premature infants with a dolicocephalic head may show marked sunsetting without any evidence of ventricular dilatation.

Skew deviation of the eyes is usually associated with large haemorrhages or hypoxic encephalopathy (Volpe 1981).

Abnormal pupillary reactions. Although common in the presence of major insult, in contrast with adults, these have no localizing value.

Abnormal eye movements (nystagmus) may be seen in normal newborns but as a manifestation of neurological disease in this age group it is rare. The most common abnormalities are tonic deviation of the eye (usually a sign of convulsions) and roving eye movements which are frequent sequelae to intraventricular haemorrhage but have no clinical significance.

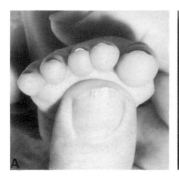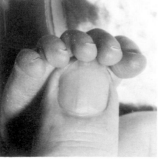

Fig. 3.10 Abnormal plantar grasp (a) in an infant with parenchymal extension in association with GMH–IVH. The leg movements were symmetrical. The normal response is shown in (b).

Visual orientation and alertness

This can and should be tested as part of the routine neurological assessment. A red woollen ball is an excellent stimulus which can be presented at a distance of 15–20 cm. Starting in the midline the ball is moved laterally in either direction, then vertically and finally in an arc. The infant's ability to focus and track this object is assessed (Dubowitz et al 1980).

From 29 to 30 weeks PMA infants are able to focus or track briefly horizontally (Fig. 3.11). With increasing maturity they can track the ball more smoothly and further. Later they will also be able to track it vertically and in an arc. These visual responses are delayed in many neurologically abnormal premature infants but more specifically in those with germinal matrix haemorrhage–intraventricular haemorrhage (GMH–IVH). The absence of visual tracking ability in a full-term infant by the end of the first week or in a preterm infant reaching 40 weeks PMA should be taken as an abnormal neurological sign indicating disturbance in alertness or in the visual pathway. Unfortunately, in contrast to previous claims (Miranda & Hack 1979), apparently good visual function cannot be regarded as proof of an intact visual pathway or as a marker of future neurological integrity (Fig. 3.12a,b). Infants with peripheral retinal lesions due to retrolental fibroplasia can track. However, these lesions might later involve more central parts of the retina and cause blindness. Also, infants with extensive subcortical cystic leukomalacia apparently involving the occipital cortex may also have excellent tracking abilities in the neonatal period which disappear around 48–58 weeks PMA, suggesting that early vision is not necessarily cortically mediated (Dubowitz et al 1986).

The newborn infant's visual function can be further evaluated clinically by testing pattern preference. (This is outside the scope of routine clinical examination and is fully discussed on p. 526.)

ALERTNESS

Alertness should not be based on the infant's appearance but on the ability to respond to stimulation. Staring eyes may, for instance, give the appearance of hyperalertness in moderately asphyxiated infants (Sarnat & Sarnat 1976) and in apnoeic infants treated with theophylline, although they may have poor responsiveness to stimuli.

HEARING

The assessment of hearing should be part of the routine neurological evaluation of the infant. It can easily be tested with a broad band (white noise) plastic telephone rattle of 60–80 dB similar to those supplied in a Denver kit. The rattle is used approximately 15–20 cm away from the ear. The presence or absence of the response can be tested while the infant is asleep, when it will usually respond either with a startle or just movement of the feet. Each ear can also be tested separately. The head is elevated about 20 degrees and is supported in the midline by the examiner's hand, leaving it free to rotate. The stimulus is presented on each side in turn with the hand and the rattle out of sight.

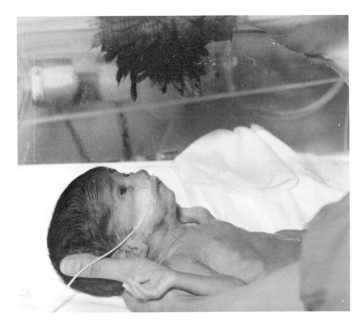

Fig. 3.11 Testing visual function inside the incubator; infant born at 29 weeks gestation and tested at 31 weeks postmenstrual age.

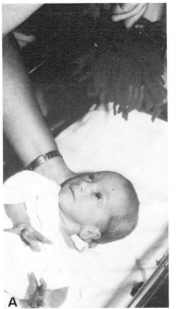
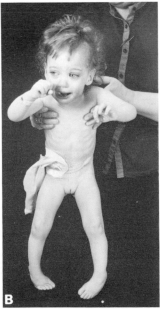

Fig. 3.12 Infant at full-term postmenstrual age showing good visual fixation and tracking (a); the same infant some months later (b) with no visual interest and apparently blind.

Infants in incubators and on ventilators can also be tested by this method.

The response can be persistently elicited in neurologically normal infants from 27 to 28 weeks PMA, it is reliable and correlates well with the presence of an Auditory Brainstem Response (ABR) at at least 80 dB. Asymmetrical responses with the rattle correspond to asymmetrical ABRs. A poor response, however, particularly in a noisy environment, should be treated with caution as 20–30% of infants with normal ABRs may have an absent response. A strong visual stimulus may inhibit the auditory response in a visually alert infant. Although a visual cue from the rattle could give an apparently positive response in a deaf infant, this is much more easily avoided in the neonate than in older infants where behavioural tests can be misleading unless performed under ideal conditions. In the newborn we found the rattle a reliable screening test when performed in the above manner (Fig. 3.13).

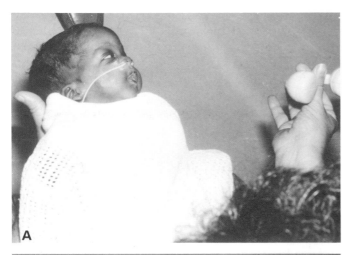

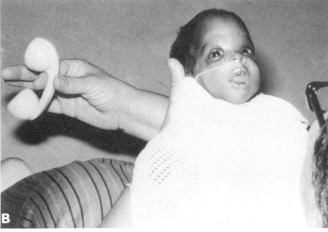

Fig. 3.13 Hearing response to rattle. The infant has a clear response (head and eye turning) to the left (**a**) but not to the right (**b**). ABR testing at this time showed normal response to 60 dB on the left but doubtful response to 60 dB on the right.

IRRITABILITY AND CONSOLABILITY

By recording the infant's peak of excitement and response to consoling during the examination its control of state can be assessed. When the infant's peak of excitement, irritability and consolability are considered together, one is able to get a clear impression of an infant who is unresponsive, apathetic and difficult to arouse or over-responsive, hyperirritable and possibly difficult to console.

NEUROLOGICAL PROFILES IN RELATION TO SPECIFIC INSULTS

In our experience, examinations performed in the above manner are repeatable and thus provide a means for recognition of the various abnormal neurological profiles related to specific insults. It has also been possible to map the developmental profile of the neurologically optimal infant and compare it with those who suffered neurological insults.

THE SMALL-FOR-GESTATIONAL AGE FULL-TERM INFANT

Small-for-gestational age (SGA) infants have often been described in the past as apathetic and hypotonic (Als et al 1976, Schulte et al 1971). These observations, however, have usually been made on infants born to pre-eclamptic mothers who received medication in late pregnancy and during delivery. When SGA infants who were the product of uncomplicated pregnancy and labour, and where the mother received no significant medication, were serially evaluated a different picture emerged (Dubowitz et al 1983). Soon after birth the infants were found to be hypertonic, hyperalert, had a low threshold for primitive reflexes and habituated poorly. Often the sucking response was tonic and the Moro response consisted of an extension reaction only. Many of the infants were also irritable but could be pacified easily. If their condition remained stable, this state persisted for about a week, after which they gradually normalized. If the infants were polycythaemic or hypoglycaemic or hypothermic the state of hypertonicity would suddenly disappear and would often be replaced by hypotonia. The jitteriness ceased and the infants often became less alert and even apathetic. The last picture was also seen soon after birth in SGA infants with perinatal asphyxia. At follow-up, infants who remained hypertonic were less likely to show abnormal signs during the first year of life than those who became hypotonic. It would thus appear that the hypertonic hyperexcitable state is optimal for the SGA infant and could indicate an adequate response to stress.

GERMINAL MATRIX HAEMORRHAGE–INTRAVENTRICULAR HAEMORRHAGE

Volpe (1978) recognized two characteristic syndromes in association with these lesions. 'Catastrophic deterioration' usually occurs in infants who do not survive the haemorrhage. The accompanying signs he described consisted of stupor → coma, apnoea, generalized tonic seizures, pupils fixed to light, flaccid quadriparesis. Volpe speculated that the syndrome reflects movement of blood through the ventricular system, sequentially affecting the diencephalon, midbrain, pons and medulla. With the advent of cranial ultrasonography it has been possible to try to find clinical correlates between the site, size and evolution of these haemorrhagic lesions. While these findings do accompany a number of the larger bleeds they can also be observed in the absence of any evidence of intraventricular bleeding.

The second clinical presentation Volpe described was the saltatory syndrome which consisted of alteration in level of consciousness, change in the quantity and quality of spontaneous movement and aberrations of eye position and movement. Deterioration and improvement continued over many hours.

By comparing ultrasound findings with repeated clinical evaluations we were able to identify haemorrhages clinically (Dubowitz et al 1981) which in the past have been considered silent (Papile et al 1978) and to map out three distinct clinical stages in infants with GMH–IVH (Dubowitz et al 1985). Preceding the haemorrhage or at the time of onset, hypertonicity (more marked in the arms), excessive motility with tremors and startles may be noted. Tendon reflexes are brisk, the Moro is abnormal. Visual and auditory orientations are absent. The infant is usually irritable. Stage 2 is seen with established haemorrhage. Tone and motility are decreased but the popliteal angle is relatively tighter. Tremors and startles are absent. There is generally poor reactivity. Visual orientation is absent. Stage 3 is the phase of recovery. Limb tone becomes normal first, including the popliteal angle. Motility improves next. First auditory then visual orientation recover. Head and trunk control are the last to normalize. During this phase roving eye movements are often noted. In infants who later show abnormal development a number of deviant signs may be noticeable at this stage. Interestingly the severity of the early clinical signs does not necessarily relate to the extent of the haemorrhagic lesion or to later outcome. There is, however, a correlation between the speed of recovery and the number of persistent deviant signs, as opposed to delayed maturation, during the phase of recovery (Dubowitz et al 1984). (See also Chapter 28.)

CYSTIC PERIVENTRICULAR LEUKOMALACIA

These lesions seem to follow either intra-uterine or extra-uterine ischaemic insults. If the insult occurred during fetal life the infant might show hardly any abnormal signs other than some degree of hypotonia and mild lethargy at birth. If the lesion is the result of a severe ischaemic insult during the neonatal period, the signs of that illness are likely to be the most prominent. The evolution of clinical signs associated with this pathological entity are initial hypotonia and some degree of lethargy; auditory and visual responses are age appropriate. The infants then improve and for a period they may appear normal. However, between 6 and 10 weeks after the insult a very characteristic clinical picture emerges. The infants gradually become more and more irritable but the cry is of normal pitch. Though they can be pacified with feeding very little else is of use. They exhibit markedly abnormal tone pattern with marked increase of flexor tone in the arms and extensor tone in the legs. Marked neck extensor hypertonia is usually present (Fig. 3.14). Movements may be normal or stereotyped. Tongue protrusion is often present giving the impression of hypothyroidism. Fisting and adducted thumbs are relatively rare at this stage but abnormal finger and toe postures are usually present bilaterally. The finger posture consists of flexion of the thumb and index finger with the other fingers extended. The big toe is spontaneously dorsiflexed. The placing reaction is poor. The Moro reaction is abnormal, consisting of forward extension only with hardly any abduction or adduction. Frequent tremors and startles may be noted. Visual and auditory functions are normal at this stage. There is no apparent difference in the neonatal period between

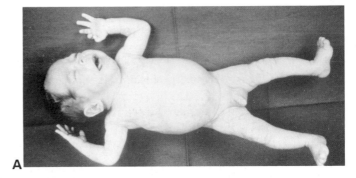

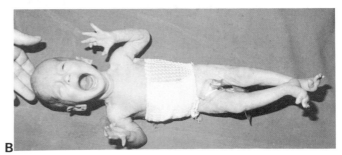

Fig. 3.14 Infants with leukomalacia at 42 weeks postmenstrual age. Note the extended neck, flexed arms, extended legs and abnormal finger posture in periventricular leukomalacia (**a**) and subcortical leukomalacia (**b**). Clinically the two conditions cannot be distinguished.

the infants with periventricular and subcortical lesions but the clinical picture is very different from the one seen in infants with large haemorrhage (Table 3.3). Later the infants with periventricular lesion develop signs of diplegia but maintain their vision. They become less irritable. The infants with subcortical lesion remain irritable; they frequently develop infantile spasms and become quadriplegic. In spite of their early good visual function they become cortically blind. The evolution of abnormal signs in these infants illustrates the importance of repeated evaluations. If these infants are only examined around the time of discharge from the unit (often around 36–38 weeks PMA) they would appear normal.

Table 3.3 Comparison of neurological patterns in intraventricular haemorrhage (IVH) and cystic leukomalacia (40 weeks postmenstrual age)

Neurological pattern	Large IVH	Cystic leukomalacia
Head/trunk tone	↓	normal or ↑
Neck ext > flexion	±	++
Limb tone abnormal	↓ or ↑	↑
Asymmetry	++	–
Fisting or abnormal toe/finger pattern	+	+++
Motility	variable	limited
Tremors and startles	+	+++
Moro abnormal	↓	↑
Irritability	+	+++

HYPOXIC–ISCHAEMIC ENCEPHALOPATHY IN FULL-TERM INFANTS

A number of distinct clinical stages can be recognized in infants who suffered anoxic fetal damage (Sarnat & Sarnat 1976, Dubowitz 1985). Table 3.4 shows the stages which might be observed in hypoxic–ischaemic encephalopathy. In the mildest form this consists of hyperalertness, a general increase in tone but in a normal distribution and general hyperexcitability. This stage lasts for less than 24 hours; the infants either recover or progress to the next stage.

Infants who exhibited abnormally good visual tracking responses did not tend to progress beyond the second stage. However, further progression was noted in infants who appeared hyperalert but were unable to track. The earlier stages might not be observed in all infants, as in some of them the insult occurs well before delivery and they might thus already have reached the unresponsive phase by the time they are delivered. Although none of the signs are specific for hypoxic–ischaemic encephalopathy their evolution and recovery are the best guides for prognosis in these infants.

In the hypoxic–ischaemic infant without any evidence of intracranial haemorrhage initially floppy unresponsiveness has a bad prognosis. However, the infant with a choroid plexus or subarachnoid haemorrhage, though often hypotonic and unresponsive for a prolonged period, has more potential for recovery. These clinical findings thus need to be considered in parallel with EEG and ultrasound findings. (See also Chapter 33.)

CONCLUSIONS

The value of the neonatal neurological examination compared with imaging has often been questioned in the past, both in relation to diagnosis and prognosis. Infants have often been said to be neurologically silent despite large intracranial lesions. We have been able to demonstrate that if age-appropriate techniques are used and the examinations are performed repeatedly, the impact of such lesions on the nervous system can be clearly demonstrated. In addition, one can also follow the process of recovery.

In contrast to older children, it is often not possible in the neonate to demonstrate any focal signs in relation to focal lesions. Imaging techniques are therefore more appropriate to diagnose the site of the lesion. However, the impact of a lesion will not only depend on the site and size but also on the biochemical and physiological changes which it produces. Apparently similar lesions

Table 3.4 Stages in hypoxic–ischaemic encephalopathy

Stage I	Stage II	Stage III	Stage IV
Poor habituation	Poor habituation	No habituation	Poor response to stimuli
Hypertonia (flexor)	Hypertonia (flexor)	Tone variable extended posture with flexed arms	Hypotonia ++
Neck extensor hypertonia ±	Neck extensor hypertonia	Neck extensor hypertonia	Hypotonia + intermittent "decerebrate" posture
Startles, tremors	Startles, tremors	Startles, tremors	No tremors or startles
±Irritable	Irritable but consolable	Irritable but not consolable	±Irritable when roused
–	±Adducted thumbs	Fisting, mouthing	Mouthing
±Abnormal Moro	±Abnormal Moro	Abnormal Moro (ext)	Moro absent
–	±Hyperalertness	Poor alertness	Stuporous
–	–	±Convulsions	–

on imaging may be associated with strikingly different neurological changes. Similarly, the outcome of an insult in the developing nervous system will also be dependent on the compensation and plasticity which the neonatal brain is capable of mounting. It is therefore not surprising that the best correlates with future outcome have been the speed of recovery and the persistence of abnormal signs, which can best be evaluated by repeated neurological assessments.

REFERENCES

Als H, Tronick F, Adamson L, Brazelton T B 1976 The behaviour of the full term but underweight newborn infant. Developmental Medicine and Child Neurology 18: 590–602

Amiel-Tison C 1968 Neurological evaluation of the maturity of newborn infants. Archives of Disease in Childhood 43: 89–93

Amiel-Tison C 1979 Birth injury as a cause of brain dysfunction in full term newborns. In: Korobkin R, Guilleminault C (eds) Advances in perinatal neurology. SP Medical and Scientific Books, pp 57–83

Amiel-Tison C, Grenier A 1980 Evaluation neurologique du nouveau-ne et du nourisson. Masson, Paris

Amiel-Tison C, Korobkin R, Esque-Vaucouloux M T 1977 Neck extensor hypertonia: a clinical sign of insult to the central nervous system of the newborn. Early Human Development 1: 181–190

Amiel-Tison C, Barrier G, Shnider S M, Levinson S C, Stefani S J 1982 A new neurologic and adaptive capacity scoring system for evaluating obstetric medications in full term newborn infants. Anesthesiology 56: 340–350

André-Thomas, de Ajuriaguerra J 1949 Etude semiologique du tonus musculaire. Editions Medicales Flammarion, Paris

André-Thomas, Saint-Anne Dargassies S 1952 Etudes neurologiques sur le nouveau-ne et la jeune nourisson. Masson, Paris

André-Thomas, Chesni Y, Saint-Anne Dargassies S 1960 The neurological examination of the infant. Little Club Clinics in Developmental Medicine, No 1. National Spastics Society, London

Brazelton T B 1973 Neonatal behavioural assessment scale. Clinics in Developmental Medicine, No 50. SIMP/Heinemann Medical, London

Brazelton T B, Tronick E, Lechting A, Lasky R E, Klein R E 1977 The behaviour of nutritionally deficient Guatemalan infants. Developmental Medicine and Child Neurology 19: 364–372

Brett E 1963 The estimation of foetal maturity by the neurological examination of the neonate. In: Dawkins M, MacGregor B (eds) Gestational age, size and maturity. Clinics in Developmental Medicine, No 19. SSMEIU/Heinemann, London, pp 105–114

Campbell S 1969 The prediction of fetal maturity by ultrasonic measurement of the biparietal diameter. Journal of Obstetrics and Gynaecology 76: 603–609

Casaer P, Daniels H, Devlieger H, de Cock P, Eggermont E 1982 Feeding behaviour in preterm neonates. Early Human Development 7: 331–346

de Vries L S, Dubowitz L M S, Dubowitz V et al 1985 Predictive value of cranial ultrasound in the newborn baby: a reappraisal. Lancet ii: 137–140

de Vries L S, Heckmatt J Z, Burrin J M, Dubowitz L M S, Dubowitz V 1986 Low serum thyroxine concentrations and neural maturation in preterm infants. Archives of Disease in Childhood 61: 862–866

Donovan D E, Coves P, Paine R S 1962 The prognostic implications of neurological abnormalities in the neonatal period. Neurology 12: 910–914

Dubowitz L M S 1985 Neurological assessment of the full term and preterm newborn infant. In: Harel S, Anastolsiow N Y (eds) The at-risk infant: psycho/social/medical aspects. Paul H. Brooks, Baltimore, pp 185–196

Dubowitz L M S, Dubowitz V 1977 Gestational age of the newborn: a clinical manual. Addison-Wesley, California

Dubowitz L, Dubowitz V 1981 The neurological assessment of the preterm and full-term newborn infant. Clinics in Developmental Medicine, No 79. SIMP/Heinemann, London

Dubowitz V, Whittaker G F, Brown B H, Robinson A 1968 Nerve conduction velocity: an index of neurological maturity of the newborn infant. Developmental Medicine and Child Neurology 10: 741–749

Dubowitz L M S, Dubowitz V, Goldberg C 1970 Clinical assessment of gestational age in the newborn infant. Journal of Pediatrics 77: 1–10

Dubowitz L M S, Dubowitz V, Morante A, Verghote M 1980 Visual function in the premature and full-term newborn infant. Developmental Medicine and Child Neurology 22: 465–475

Dubowitz L M S, Levene M I, Morante A, Palmer P, Dubowitz V 1981 Neurological signs in neonatal intraventricular hemorrhage: correlation with real-time ultrasound. Journal of Pediatrics 99: 127–133

Dubowitz L M S, Dubowitz V, Goldberg C 1983 Comparison of neurological function in growth-retarded and appropriate sized full-term newborn infants in two ethnic groups. South African Medical Journal 61: 1003–1007

Dubowitz L M S, Dubowitz V, Palmer P G, Miller G, Fawer C-L, Levene M I 1984 Correlation of neurologic assessment in the preterm newborn infant with outcome at one year. Journal of Pediatrics 105: 452–456

Dubowitz L M S, Mushin J, de Vries L, Arden G B 1986 Visual function in the newborn infant: is it cortically mediated? Lancet i: 1139–1140

Graham F K 1956 Behavioural differences between normal and traumatized newborns: I. The test procedures. Psychological Monographs 70: 1–16

Graham F K, Matarazzo R G, Caldwell B M 1956 Behavioural differences between normal and traumatized newborns: II. Standardization, reliability and validity. Psychological Monographs 70: 127–28

Hittner H M, Hirsh N J, Rudolph A J 1977 The lens in the assessment of gestational age. Journal of Pediatrics 91: 455–460

Howard J, Parmelee A H, Kopp C B, Littman B 1976 A neurological comparison of preterm and fullterm infants at term conceptual age. Journal of Pediatrics 88: 995–1002

Koenigsberger M R 1966 Judgment of foetal age. I. Neurological evaluation. Pediatric Clinics of North America 13: 822–833

Lacey J L, Henderson-Smart D J, Edwards D A, Storcy B 1985 The early development of head control in preterm infants. Early Human Development 11: 199–212

Leijon I, Finnstrom O 1982 Correlation between neurological examination and behavioural assessment of the newborn infant. Early Human Development 7: 119–130

Miller G, Heckmatt J Z, Dubowitz L M S, Dubowitz V 1983 Use of nerve conduction velocity to determine gestational age in infants at risk and in very low birth weight infants. Journal of Pediatrics 103: 109–112

Miranda S B, Hack M 1979 The predictive value of neonatal visual perceptual behaviours. In: Field T M (ed) Infants born at risk. SP Medical and Scientific Books, London

Mitchell R G, Farr V 1965 The meaning of maturity and the assessment of maturity at birth. In: Dawkins M, MacGregor B (eds) Gestational age, size and maturity. Clinics in Developmental Medicine, No 19. SSMEIU/Heinemann, London, pp 83–99

Moosa A, Dubowitz V 1971 Postnatal maturation of peripheral nerves in preterm and full term infants. Journal of Pediatrics 79: 915–922

Ounsted M K, Chalmers C A, Yudkin P L 1978 Clinical assessment of gestational age at birth: the effect of sex, birthweight and weight for length of gestation. Early Human Development 2: 73–80

Palmer P G, Dubowitz L M S, Verghote M, Dubowitz V 1982 Neurological and neurobehavioural differences between preterm infants and term and full term newborn infants. Neuropediatrics 13: 183–189

Papile L, Burnstein J, Burnstein R, Koffler H 1978 Incidence and evolution of subependymal and intraventricular haemorrhage: a study of infants with birthweight less than 1500 g. Journal of Pediatrics 92: 529–534

Parmelee A H, Michaelis M D 1971 Neurological examination of the newborn. In: Hellmuth J (ed) The exceptional infant, Vol 2. Brunner Mazel, New York, pp 3–23

Peiper A 1928 Die Hirntatigkeit des Sauglings. Julius Springer, Berlin

Peiper A 1963 Cerebral function in infancy and childhood (translation of the 3rd revised German edition by Nagler B and Nagler H). Consultants Bureau, New York

Piper M C, Kunos I, Willis D M, Mazer B 1985 Effect of gestational age on neurological functioning of the very low birthweight infant at 40 weeks. Developmental Medicine and Child Neurology 27: 596–605

Prechtl H F R 1972 Pattern of reflex behaviour related to sleep in the human infant. In: Clements C D, Purpura D P, Mayer F E (eds) Sleep and the maturing nervous system. Academic Press, New York, pp 287–301

Prechtl H F R 1977 The neurological examination of the full term newborn infant, 2nd edn. Clinics in Developmental Medicine, No 63. SIMP/Heinemann, London

Prechtl H F R, Beintema D 1964 The neurological examination of the full term newborn infant. Clinics in Developmental Medicine, No 12. SIMP/Heinemann, London

Prechtl H F R, Fargel J W, Weinmann H M, Bakker H H 1979 Postures, motility and respiration of low-risk preterm infants. Developmental Medicine and Child Neurology 21: 3–27

Robinson H P, Fleming J E E 1975 A critical evaluation of sonar 'crown–rump length' measurements. British Journal of Obstetrics and Gynaecology 82: 702–710

Robinson R J 1966 Assessment of gestational age by neurological examination. Archives of Disease in Childhood 41: 437–447

Saint-Anne Dargassies S 1955 Methode d'examen neurologique du nouveau-ne. Etudes Neonatales 3: 101–123

Saint-Anne Dargassies S 1966 Neurological maturation of the premature infant of 28 to 41 weeks gestational age. In: Falkner F (ed) Human development. Saunders, Philadelphia, pp 306–325

Saint-Anne Dargassies S 1977 Neurological development in full term and premature neonate. Elsevier/North Holland/Excerpta Medica, Amsterdam

Sarnat H B, Sarnat M S 1976 Neonatal encephalopathy following fetal distress. Archives of Neurology 33: 696–705

Schulte F J, Michaelis R, Linke I, Nolter R 1968 Motor nerve conduction velocity in term, preterm and small for date infants. Pediatrics 42: 17–21

Schulte F J, Schrempf G, Hinze G 1971 Maternal toxemia, fetal malnutrition and motor behaviour of the newborn. Pediatrics 48: 871–882

Smith D W 1982 Recognizable patterns of human malformation, 3rd edn. Saunders, Philadelphia

Touwen B C L, Bierman van Eendenburg M E C, Jurgens-van der Zee A D 1977 Neurological screening in full term newborn infants. Developmental Medicine and Child Neurology 19: 739–747

Usher R, McLean F, Scott K E 1966 Judgment of fetal age. II. Clinical significance of gestational age and an objective method for its assessment. Pediatric Clinics of North America 13: 835–848

Volpe J J 1978 Neonatal periventricular hemorrhage, past, present and future. Pediatrics 92: 693–696

Volpe J J 1981 Neurology of the newborn. Major Problems in Clinical Pediatrics, No 22. Saunders, Philadelphia

4. Fetal habituation

Dr L. R. Leader and Prof M. J. Bennett

The assessment of the quality of life in utero presents considerable methodological difficulties. Present measures, such as cardiotocography and fetal movement observation or ultrasound evaluation assess general well-being which only has an indirect relationship with cortical function, the ultimate arbitor of excellence in man. An ideal method of monitoring fetal well-being would be the measurement of fetal cortical function but no such test is currently available. Antenatal cardiotocography uses the fetal heart to assess the integrity of the autonomic nervous system pathways. In contrast, a test which elicits a behavioural response provides more information about the central nervous system because it involves both sensory and motor responses which require a high degree of neuronal involvement.

Habituation is a decrease leading to cessation of a behavioural response that occurs when an initially novel stimulus is presented repeatedly (Thompson & Glansman 1966). Although habituation is remarkably simple, it is one of the most widespread forms of learning (Buchwald & Humphrey 1973, Kandel 1979, Stevenson & Siddle, 1983) and there is good evidence that a normal habituation pattern reflects an intact central nervous system (Jeffrey & Cohen 1971, Wyers et al 1973). Overt activity reflects only a minor part of the information processed by the central nervous system. In an environment of constant sensory stimulation this ability to ignore meaningless stimuli is essential for the efficient functioning and survival of the organism. Unresponsiveness is one of the most prominent sustained behavioural patterns of mammalian life (Buchwald & Humphrey 1973).

RESPONSE TO STIMULATION

When a novel stimulus is presented to an organism it may evoke and activate almost any of the response systems of the organism. These include psychological, motor and autonomic phenomena. With repeated stimulation the organism learns to recognize the stimulus and if innocuous or unrewarding will reduce and ultimately suppress its response.

TYPES OF RESPONSE TO STIMULATION

Three reflexes in response to stimulation have been described:

1. Startle reflex
2. Orienting reflex
3. Defensive reflex

Although all three reflexes are generalized reactions, they have distinguishable components and characteristics. They also differ with respect to the stimuli that elicit them (Graham 1979).

Temporal relationships

Gogan (1970) studied the temporal relationship of two components of the response to stimulation and suggested that the startle response has a latency of 20–40 ms and a duration of about 160 ms. This is followed by the orienting response (OR) which lasts from 3 s to 10 s or longer. The OR may be present when the startle falls to zero and similarly a startle is not always followed by an OR. Although the startle and OR correspond to two different psychomotor activities, they appear to be engendered by a common neural pathway.

Startle reflex

If the stimulus is intense enough it will initially provoke a startle reflex, which occurs within milliseconds of the stimulus. It is associated with a unique skeletal muscle pattern of widespread flexor contraction. It is also associated with an increase in heart rate.

Although the whole-body startle habituates very rapidly in human subjects, some aspects of the response, such as the blink, decrease relatively slowly (Landis & Hunt 1939, Graham et al 1975). Heart rate acceleration seen with the startle reflex habituates rapidly.

Startle can be dissociated from the other reflexes through brain lesions and drugs. Lower brainstem lesions that abolished the startle response left orienting movements to sound stimulations intact (Szabo & Hazafi 1965). Others have shown that the startle response was not affected by pain-reducing drugs but the defensive reflex was (Evans 1961, 1962).

Orienting reflex

This follows the startle (Gogan 1970) and is by definition a non-specific generalized reaction to the presentation of a novel stimulus (Pakula & Sokolov 1973). It has behavioural components (e.g. movements of parts of the body) and physiological components (e.g. changes in heart rate, galvanic skin response (GSR) and electro-encephalographic changes (Brackbill 1971)). Orienting reflexes usually habituate rapidly.

The orienting response was first described by Pavlov in 1927 who referred to it as the investigatory or 'what is it' reflex. According to Sokolov (1963), orienting is the first phase of information processing and sets in motion the appropriate response. The appropriateness of continued responding is related to the importance of the stimulus to the continued functioning of the organism.

Orienting reflexes may be measured objectively as a behavioural response (Brackbill 1971, Brackbill et al 1974), electrodermal response (Goldwater & Lewis 1978), direct electro-encephalographic measurement (Rust 1977) or by heart rate changes (Holloway & Parsons 1971, Graham 1979). According to Graham (1979) the orienting reflex results in a decrease in the heart rate.

Defensive reflex

This response serves to protect the organism from harmful or noxious stimuli by the reduction of stimulus effect. It usually follows a much stronger stimulus and takes much longer to habituate or may not habituate at all (Brackbill et al 1974). The orienting reflex (OR) is associated with a decrease in heart rate whereas defensive reflex (DR) is associated with an increase (Graham & Clifton 1966, Graham 1979).

The OR is a system responsive to stimulus information whereas the DR is a system responsive to stimulus intensity.

HABITUATION THEORIES

Stimulus-model comparator

Sokolov (1963) suggested that a stimulus model is formed in the sensory cortex. The sensory input is compared with the neuronal model of the expected stimulus. If a repetitive stimulus matches the model, then the system which normally subserves a behavioural output amplification function, i.e. the reticular formation, is inhibited. If a new or altered stimulus occurs which does not match the model,

then inhibition is released and response strength recovers accordingly.

Dual-process theory

This has been suggested by Groves & Thompson (1970). Two hypothetical processes, one decremental, which is habituation, and the other incremental, which is sensitization, are assumed to develop independently in the central nervous system and the response elicited by a repeated stimulus is the net outcome of these two independent processes. Dishabituation is said to be a special case of sensitization which is produced by a temporary masking of habituation by the independent transient sensitization process.

Priming theory

Two recent theories of habituation (Ohman 1979, Wagner 1976, 1979) also focus on the matching of afferent stimulation with elements of an internal representation of stimulation. Both suggest interaction between long- and short-term memory in determining response decrement to repeated stimulation. They propose that there will be no response to the stimulus if it is prepresented or primed in a limited-capacity short-term store (STS). There are thought to be two ways in which elements of the stimulus may be primed into the STS. It may be by means of self-priming in which representation is activated in STS through a recent presentation of the stimulus. The second is retrieval-generated or associated priming in which activation of the stimulus representation in STS is produced by the presence of contextual cues which have been associated with the stimulus in the past.

Afferent neuronal inhibition

Hernandez-Peon (1960) suggested that habituation results from inhibition of sensory input which can occur as far peripherally as the first sensory relay nucleus (e.g. the cochlear nucleus).

Limbic forebrain theory

Pribam (1967) has suggested that the limbic system is involved and that there are two forms of afferent inhibition which normally oppose one another in the regulation of orienting and other aspects of complex information processing.

HABITUATION CRITERIA

In the experimental situation, the criteria that have been used to define habituation are:

1. a response decrement to some percentage of the subjects initial response level (Ferguson et al 1978);
2. the same arbitrary amount of response decrement in all subjects (Buckwald & Humphrey 1973);
3. a specified number of consecutive non-response trials (Brackbill et al 1974).

We have defined habituation as a failure to respond to five consecutive stimuli. These criteria are similar to those used by Brackbill et al (1974).

CENTRAL NERVOUS PATHWAYS

It is not known with any certainty which part of the central nervous system controls habituation. Both Brackbill (1971) and Sokolov (1963) proposed that the cortex is essential for normal habituation and this is widely supported by other data (Buchwald & Humphrey 1972, Gulbrandsen et al 1972, Davis & Gendelman 1977). However, the cerebral cortex may not be essential for all aspects of response habituation in that the electro-encephalographic response in decerebrate cats shows habituation (Sharpless & Jasper 1956, Buchwald & Humphrey 1972). In these experiments the response decrements were larger and occurred more rapidly than in the intact animal. Davis & Gendelman (1977) studying the startle response in rats, found that they failed to habituate after decerebration. There is also some evidence that short- and long-term habituation may have different neural pathways (Davis & File 1984). Depending on the response measured and the criteria used, habituation can be demonstrated at all levels of the central nervous system and on all scales of phylogenetic development (Buchwald & Humphrey 1973, Kandel 1979).

The cerebral cortex is essential for dishabituation as it is readily demonstrated in intact but not in decerebrate cats (Buchwald & Humphrey 1972). Dishabituation classically refers to the recovery of an habituated response to the original stimulus following presentation of an extraneous or differing stimulus. Some authors, however, have used the term dishabituation to refer to the elicitation of a previously habituated response by the introduction of a different or new stimulus into the sequence (Jeffrey & Cohen 1971, Eisenstein & Peretz 1973). This process is very important as it differentiates between neural fatigue and habituation.

METHODS OF ASSESSING FETAL HABITUATION

Peiper (1925) noted cessation of the fright response in the human fetus to repetitive sound stimuli using an automobile horn. Ray (1932) attempted to establish the conditioned response in the human fetus but his results were inconclusive. Sontag & Wallace (1935) also observed a fetal startle reaction and habituation in response to a vibrotactile stimulus but were unable to establish a conditioned response in the fetus. Spelt (1948) claimed to have established a conditioned response in the last two months of pregnancy. Further attempts have been made to establish a conditioned response in the unborn fetus (Goodlin 1979).

Fleischer (1955) noted habituation of fetal movements to repeated strong sound stimuli. Habituation of the fetal heart rate response has also been described (Goodlin & Lowe 1974), and human fetal habituation has been reported to a repeated vibro-acoustic stimulus (Leader et al 1982a,b, Birnholz & Benacerraf 1983, Bennett 1984, Hills et al 1985). Madison et al (1986) in a study of human fetuses using two different vibro-acoustic stimuli in a randomized format have confirmed that the response decrement seen is habituation and not response fatigue.

We have found the most suitable stimulus to be a 9 V battery-powered toothbrush and this produced a greater response than a pure-tone stimulus of frequencies varying from 50 to 3000 Hz. The toothbrush produces a complex waveform of frequencies with the energy peak at 2.4 kHz (68 dB referred to 20 μPa) and consisting largely of a fundamental of 98 Hz and third harmonics thereof. The highest frequency present was 6 kHz; the overall sound level was 74 dB.

Responses were measured by a combination of a modified cardiotocographic method (Leader & Baillie 1979), real-time ultrasound or maternal observation of fetal movements. Spontaneous fetal movement must be distinguished from response to stimulation and we have considered only movement that occurs during the 5 seconds stimulus or within 2.5 seconds of its cessation to be a response. Lack of response to five consecutive stimuli is taken to indicate short-term habituation and the duration to habituation is recorded by the number of responses required to produce extinction of the response (Brackbill et al 1974). Habituations to between 10 and 50 stimuli are regarded as showing a normal pattern (Leader et al 1982b). Those fetuses who show no response at all to stimulation are referred to as non-responders. Those who habituate 1–9 stimuli are fast habituators and those still responding after 50 stimuli are slow habituators. These abnormal patterns have also been described in schizophrenics (Gruzelier & Venables 1972, Patterson & Venables 1978, Gruzelier & Connolly 1979).

Dishabituation

This term refers to breaking the habituated behaviour by a counter-stimulus. Dishabituation is achieved by applying two new vibro-acoustic stimuli 5 seconds apart and lasting 5 seconds to the maternal abdomen (Leader et al 1982a), followed by gently balotting the uterus from side to side in a further attempt to deliver a completely different stimulus. The original stimulus can then be applied to reassess habituation.

FACTORS INFLUENCING HABITUATION

State effect

It is believed that fetal responsiveness to varying stimuli is dependent in part on the fetal behavioural state at the time of stimulation (Prechtl 1985, Schmidt et al 1985). We are highly critical of published stimulation studies which have not taken account of fetal state at the time of stimulation. Most studies which have examined the effect of fetal state on the response to stimulation have unfortunately paid little attention to the type and intensity of the stimulus, how it is delivered, or the experimental design, particularly when repetitive stimuli are used.

The stimulus strength may be an important factor in the effect of state on responsiveness. For example, in fetal sheep, responses to varying mild stimuli (i.e. percussion of the ewe's abdomen or the sounding of a bell, Ruckebusch 1972, Ruckebusch et al 1977, and hindlimb nerve stimulation, Rigatto et al 1982) have been found during high-voltage state (HVS) but not during low-voltage state (LVS). In contrast, Leader et al (1988), using a broad-spectrum intense vibro-acoustic stimulus, showed that in fetal sheep, responsiveness and the rate of habituation were not significantly influenced by the electrocortical state of the fetus. Furthermore, studies using a similar vibro-acoustic stimulus (Leader et al 1982b, Divon et al 1985, Hills et al 1985, Ohel et al 1985, 1986, Madison et al 1986) all report reliable responses to stimulation in uncomplicated human pregnancies. Timor-Tritsch (1986) supports the importance of the intensity of the stimulus in evoking a response. Using an auditory stimulus, he was unable to show consistently a fetal heart rate (FHR) response. However, when using injections of cold saline through the cervix of patients in labour as a stimulus, more than 75% of cases showed a fetal heart rate response even during the quiet state. Similarly Lamper & Eisdorfer (1971) found that in neonates, responses to a mild stimulus were state-dependent whilst responses to strong stimuli were not. Hutt et al (1968) found that responses in neonates were dependent on the type of stimulus used.

In a further study in fetal sheep using an injection of saline against the fetal skin as a stimulus, fetal responses were found to be independent of fetal electrocortical activity. In this study significant increases in fetal heart rate and blood pressure after stimulation were demonstrated (Leader et al 1986b). Natale & Nasello-Paterson (1986) used multiple rapid stimulations at 0.01 or 0.05 pulses per second to show that in fetal sheep the response was not only influenced by the state but also by the frequency of the stimulus. A more frequent stimulus resulted in a greater response. They unfortunately did not take the effect of stimulus repetition into account and did up to eight experiments per day on sheep.

A study by Schmidt et al (1985) used two different auditory stimuli and found that in contrast to the animal data (e.g. Ruckebusch 1972), fetal responses occurred more commonly during state 2F (similar to low-voltage state). Only 1 of 28 fetuses in stage 1F (similar to high-voltage state) showed a response. This is in contrast to Divon et al (1985) who demonstrated a startle response to all 100 stimuli in 28 full-term fetuses tested using a vibro-acoustic stimulus and Ohel et al (1986) using a similar stimulus who showed consistent heart rate and movement responses in 10 full-term fetuses during periods of low heart reactivity. Recently Gagnon et al (1986), using a similar stimulus but a randomized format, were able to show changes in the fetal heart rate and fetal body movements in all patients who had the stimulus applied to their abdominal walls but no responses in patients who received the stimulus on the hand, confirming that the response is due to the stimulus and not the result of maternal catecholamine release from anxiety.

Madison et al (1986) have also demonstrated reliable responses to vibro-acoustic stimulation and habituation in human fetuses. In a study of human fetal habituation (Leader et al 1982a,b, Leader 1986) failure to obtain a response was only observed in 14 of 750 tests in 350 patients. Eight infants were found to be small for gestational age and in four, the mother had clinical abnormalities such as hypertension, decreased fetal movements or antepartum haemorrhage. The remaining two infants were only at 29 and 30 weeks of gestation when tested and both responded when tested two weeks later. Of fetuses who failed to show an increase in heart rate in response to a vibro-acoustic stimulus, 80% were found to be small for gestational age (Leader et al 1984). Earlier studies using fetal cardiotocography to determine state found habituation to be independent of fetal state (Goodlin & Schmidt 1972). Most human fetuses will respond to vibro-acoustic stimulation after 30 weeks of gestation (Leader et al 1982a, Birnholz & Benacerraf 1983, Hills et al 1985). As neither the responsiveness nor the rate of habituation alters significantly with gestational age (Leader et al 1986, Madison et al 1986), and since fetal behavioural states as described by Nijhius et al (1982) have only been consistently described after 36 weeks of gestation in multiparous and after 38 weeks in nulliparous patients (Van Vliet et al 1985), it is most unlikely that fetal state is a major factor in determining the response to a vibro-acoustic stimulus. Unquestionably it is a major factor in responsiveness with mild stimulation but not to more intense broad-spectrum stimuli.

Gestational age

A total of 27 non-smoking subjects were studied prospectively from 20 weeks of gestation at two-weekly intervals. The gestational age at which a fetal response was first obtained is shown in Figure 4.1. Only two (7%) responded at 23–24 weeks of gestation but by 27–28 weeks 89% responded. By 30 weeks of gestation all fetuses responded. The onset of the response occurred earlier in female than in

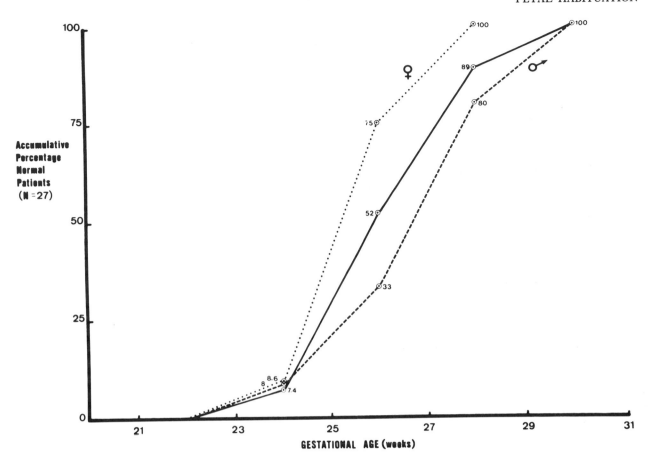

Fig. 4.1 Accumulative percentage of normal fetuses responding for the first time: females ...... ; males ----- ; mean —. (Reproduced with permission from Leader et al 1982.)

male fetuses. Of the 12 females, 75% responded by 25–26 weeks compared with only 33% of the 15 males ($P<0.05$ Fisher exact test). All the females responded by the 28th week whilst 80% of the males responded at this gestational age (Leader et al 1982a).

Birnholz & Benacerraf (1983), using a similar stimulus to elicit the blink-startle response found that the response was first noted at 24–25 weeks and was consistently present after 28 weeks. The finding that the onset of habituation was earlier in females is in keeping with established physiological data that females have advanced neuromuscular development compared with males of the same age (Singer et al 1968, Robinson 1969).

Long-term habituation

The fetuses of 40 subjects who were more than 36 weeks pregnant and did not smoke were tested for habituation. In 15 the test was repeated the following day, while in 12 the test was repeated after three days. The remaining 13 fetuses were tested after four days. The numbers of stimuli required for habituation in the two tests in each group were compared by means of the Sign test.

In the group retested the following day, the Sign test was significantly negative ($P = 0.035$), in that all but one of the 15 fetuses showed a decrease in the number of stimuli required for habituation. In the other two groups, the sign test was not significant and there was no consistent pattern of habituation. A previous study (Keen et al 1965) found that neonates who habituated to an auditory stimulus returned the habituation effect for 24 hours. This result is consistent with those mentioned above.

Sedative drugs

Drugs known to affect the central nervous system have also been shown to alter the rate of habituation. These include barbiturates and chlordiazepoxide (Lader & Wing 1965), amphetamines (Davis et al 1975), chlorpromazine and lysergic acid diethylamide (Key 1961).

Newborn babies whose mothers are given pethidine in labour (Brackbill et al 1971) or have a general anaesthetic (Moreau & Birch 1974) take significantly longer to habituate to an acoustic stimulus when tested in the neonatal period.

We have tested the habituation of fetuses of seven patients, who were prescribed either phenobarbitone or diazepam for specific medical indications. In eight tests, the habituation patterns were in the abnormal range (0–9 or >50). In two patients the habituation pattern returned to normal (10–50) when the drug was withdrawn. In a third patient, the fetus initially did not respond to stimulation but two days after the diazepam was stopped, the fetus habituated after nine stimuli.

We further tested fetuses of nine consenting volunteers who had normal uncomplicated pregnancies and who did not smoke and were more than 36 weeks pregnant for habituation (Day 0). They took 30 mg phenobarbitone 8 hourly for three days. The subjects took their last phenobarbitone tablet on the morning of the second test (Day 4). Where possible, the test was repeated the following day. They were tested for the fourth time three to five days later.

A group of 14 subjects with similar characteristics acted as controls. They were tested at approximately the same time intervals but did not receive any phenobarbitone. None of the fetuses of the 14 subjects in the control group failed to habituate on Day 4 or 5, compared with 7 of the 9 in the patients taking phenobarbitone. This was significantly different comparing Day 4 alone or together with Day 5 ($P<0.05$, Wilcoxon matched-pairs signed-ranks test). Sedative drugs affect the rate of fetal habituation. The most common change is an increase in the number of stimuli needed for habituation. The varying habituation patterns seen after the withdrawal of the drug may reflect a fetus's ability to metabolize the drug or the dosages used.

Maternal smoking

Cigarette smoking during pregnancy is associated with an increase in complications of pregnancy (Andrews & McGarry 1972) and in perinatal mortality and morbidity (Meyer et al 1976). We found the fetuses of eight subjects who smoked to have normal habituation patterns (10–50) when the time elasped from their last cigarette was 1.5 or more hours. The test was repeated three to seven days later. When tested within one hour of their last cigarette, seven had an abnormal habituation pattern (<9 or >50). One subject who smoked 40 cigarettes/day required 6 hours before the fetal habituation pattern returned to normal. In an individual such as this, the effects of smoking would take longer to wear off as there is a correlation between the number of cigarettes smoked and the levels of carboxyhaemoglobin, plasma thiocyanate (Vesey et al 1982) and nicotine (Russell et al 1976, Feyerabend et al 1982).

An additional study involved 13 subjects who did not smoke and 9 smokers who were at more than 36 weeks of gestation. Smokers were tested for habituation after they had refrained from smoking for 6 hours. They were retested after a 30 minute break. They were then asked to smoke two consecutive cigarettes in 20 minutes and the habituation test was repeated. Non-smoking controls were similarly tested

but the smoking omitted. The difference in habituation rates between smokers and non-smokers was significant ($P<0.01$, Mann–Whitney U-test).

These findings are consistent with those of Manning & Feyeraband (1976) who showed a decrease in fetal breathing which lasted for 75 minutes after subjects had smoked two cigarettes. The maternal plasma nicotine levels remained significantly raised for one hour after a cigarette. Thaler et al (1980) found a decrease in spontaneous movement activity after smoking. Lehtovirta & Forss (1978) using ^{133}Xe showed a decrease in the intervillous blood flow for an hour after a cigarette and Quigley et al (1979) have shown a rise in maternal catecholamines after smoking a cigarette, starting after 2.5 minutes and lasting for 20 minutes. This was followed by a smaller secondary peak at 60 minutes. The peak of carbon monoxide was also found to occur at about 60 minutes. Longo (1976) has found that the partial pressure of oxygen in the fetal blood decreases in proportion to the carboxyhaemoglobin concentrations in the fetal and maternal blood and results in a shift to the left of the oxygen dissociation curve. Socol et al (1982) found that the fall in fetal arterial oxygen was greatest an hour after pregnant rhesus monkeys were exposed to cigarette smoke.

Maternal smoking appears to result in a greater likelihood of a non-reactive antenatal cardiotocograph (Phelan 1980). In addition Eriksen & Gennser (1984) have shown changes following maternal smoking in the arterial flow velocity waveforms in human fetuses.

Smoking appears to result in decreased fetal perfusion and hypoxia. The effects of smoking a cigarette on the fetus appear to last 60–90 minutes and there is an accumulation of metabolic products with an increase in the number of cigarettes smoked. This would explain why the fetal complications associated with smoking are more marked in mothers who smoke more than 10 cigarettes per day; these fetuses live under an almost constant tobacco siege.

Maternal hypoxia

Studies have examined the fetal cardiovascular responses to alterations in the maternal inspired oxygen (O_2) concentrations between 8 and 20% (Hellman et al 1961, John 1965, Copher & Huber 1967). Wood et al (1971) reported severe late decelerations and acidosis in fetuses whose mothers were breathing 10% O_2. Baillie (1974) described the hypoxic stress test using an inspired maternal O_2 concentration of 11.6%. Breathing 12% O_2 is the equivalent of living at 13 000 feet above sea-level and this reduces the maternal P_aO_2 from 99 (±4.3) to 44 (±2.8) mmHg. The arterial saturation falls to 86% and has been shown in over 600 tests to be quite safe for both mother and fetus.

The fetuses of 23 (5 control) non-smoking volunteers who had had an uncomplicated antenatal course and were 36 or more weeks pregnant were tested for habituation on two successive days, whilst exposed to air or a specially prepared mixture of 12% (±0.5%) oxygen in nitrogen, and breathed by the mother using the delivery system described by Baillie (1974). The order of the test was reversed the second day.

This study showed quite clearly that reducing the O_2 concentration inspired by the mother to 12%, alters the fetal habituation pattern. Of 18 fetuses, 17 had a normal pattern when tested in air. Only 2 of the 18 had a normal pattern when tested whilst their mothers breathed 12% O_2 (Fig. 4.2). The most common abnormal pattern seen in 13 fetuses was the failure to habituate by 51 stimuli. Three of four fetuses whose habituation patterns were at variance with the rest of the group were found to have meconium-stained amniotic fluid when labour commenced 3–5 days later. The remaining fetus, who had an abnormal pattern when tested in air, was found to have an arterial base deficit of 17 mmol at caesarian section and was small for gestational age (SGA). There is a high incidence of abnormal fetal habituation patterns in infants who are SGA (Leader et al 1982b). Studies in fetal sheep (Natale et al 1981, Leader et al 1986) have shown decreased fetal forelimb activity during periods of fetal hypoxia produced by reducing the inspired O_2 concentration to 9%. In addition, fetal lambs failed to show fetal movement, blood pressure or heart rate responses to cutaneous stimulation using cold saline during periods of hypoxia (Leader et al 1986).

It is unlikely that catecholamine release due to anxiety in mothers tested is the reason for the changes in habituation

patterns seen as four of the five fetuses in the control group had a normal habituation pattern when tested the following day, while their mothers breathed air through the same apparatus used to deliver the 12% O_2.

The alterations in habituation patterns may be due either to the direct effects of reduced O_2 tension in the fetus or to the changes in catecholamines due to hypoxia (Jones & Robinson 1975, Rosen et al 1984). The differences in response noted between the sheep and human studies are probably due to the greater degree of hypoxia induced in sheep.

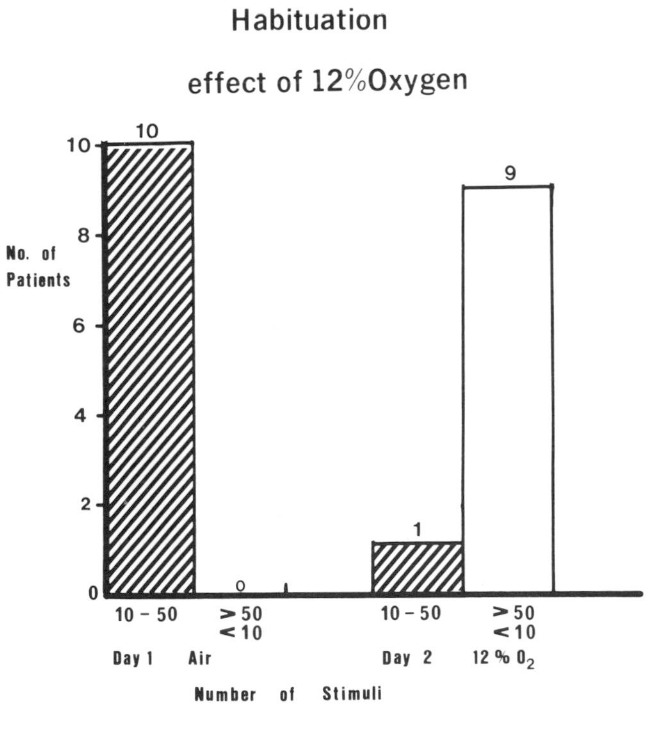

HABITUATION IN PATHOLOGICAL STATES

A normal habituation pattern reflects an intact central nervous system (Lewis 1971). In animal studies failure to habituate to repeated stimuli has been found in decerebrate rats (Davis & Gendelman 1977) and those with septal lesions (Sagvolden & Webster 1974), and with drugs such as barbiturates (Webster 1969), amphetamines (Davis et al 1975) and lysergic acid diethylamide (Key 1961).

In human studies, impaired habituation to repeated stimuli has been reported in high-risk (Eisenberg et al 1966) and traumatized newborn infants (Bronstein et al 1968), hyperkinetic (Hutt & Hutt 1964, Tizard 1968) and autistic children (Hutt et al 1965), Down's syndrome (Dustman & Callner 1979), brain damage (Thompson & Spencer 1966, Holloway & Parsons 1971), schizophrenics (Gruzelier & Venables 1972) and anxiety states (Lader & Wing 1965).

In animal studies, faster habituation has been found after decerebration (Buchwald & Humphrey 1972), lesions of the dorsal raphe nucleus and with drugs such as clonidine (Davis et al 1977), low doses of p-chlorphenylalanine (Pearson et al 1974) and during a noradrenaline infusion (Leader et al 1986).

Failure to respond or accelerated habituation has also been reported in adults with such abnormalities as unconsciousness (Gulbrandsen et al 1972), schizophrenia (Gruzelier & Venables 1972, Pattern & Venables 1978) and severe depression (Lader & Wing 1969). Chlordiazepoxide and amylobarbitone increase the rate of habituation in patients with anxiety states (Lader & Wing 1965) whereas propranolol improves habituation in schizophrenics (Gruzelier & Connolly 1979).

Few studies of habituation of the abnormal fetus have been described. To assess abnormal responses a normal control group must be established. We included patients with normal pregnancies who fulfilled all of the antenatal criteria required in an optimal group (Leader et al 1982b). Their final inclusion depended on the course of labour and neonatal outcome and therefore could only be determined retrospectively.

Habituation

effect of 12%Oxygen

Fig. 4.2 The effect of breathing 12% O_2 on habituation patterns in 10 subjects. On Day 1 they were tested breathing room air; on Day 2 they were tested breathing 12% O_2 mixture.

This control group (Group 1) was compared with five other groups of high-risk pregnancies, complicated by factors known to be associated with increased perinatal mortality and morbidity. All patients were tested within 10 days of delivery.

Group 1. Forty patients who had a normal uncomplicated antenatal, intrapartum and neonatal course and were delivered of infants thought to be in an optimal condition (Michaelis et al 1980) were used as control subjects.

Group 2 comprised five patients whose infants had major central nervous system abnormalities. Four infants were anencephalic and one was microcephalic. One of these patients had twins: one anencephalic and the other normal.

Group 3 comprised 46 patients whose infants had birth-weights below the 10th centile for the local population (Jaroszewicz et al 1975) and were classified as small for gestational age (SGA).

Group 4 comprised 28 patients with meconium-stained amniotic fluid. In 16 patients this was detected by amniocentesis before labour.

Group 5 comprised 38 patients in whom serial ultrasound measurements of the fetal biparietal diameter (BPD) showed a lag in the expected rate of growth (Campbell & Newman 1971).

Group 6 comprised 28 patients in whom serial ultrasound fetal BPD estimations showed a normal growth pattern (Campbell & Newman 1971) with the last measurement being made within 10 days before delivery. This was a mixed group and consisted of some normal pregnancies and others complicated by hypertension, antepartum haemorrhage and decreased fetal movements. Only one infant was small for gestational age.

Fetuses in Group 2 (major central nervous system abnormalities) showed no response to stimulation. In the twin pregnancy the anencephalic infant showed no response while the normal twin showed a normal response. Figure 4.3 shows the distribution of the habituation results in the different groups.

Five infants had 5 minute Apgar scores of less than 6. All of these infants had abnormal habituation patterns.

There were very highly significant differences between the normal control group (Group 1) and the high-risk groups (Groups 3–5, $P<0.0005$) but not among the high-risk groups. There were no significant differences in habituation patterns in Group 4, whether the meconium-staining of the amniotic fluid was detected antenatally or intrapartum.

Dishabituation

Of the 24 patients tested, 19 (79%) in Group 1 responded when the second vibrator was applied while 18 (75%) responded again to the re-introduction of the original stimulus.

CONCLUSIONS

The finding of highly significant differences in fetal short-term habituation patterns between normal and high-risk pregnancies, complicated by conditions that are often associated with an increased incidence of neurological damage, suggests that it may be possible to identify individual fetuses within an abnormal group that are at a particular risk as suggested by Goodlin & Lowe (1974). Early delivery of these infants may reduce the risks of long-term neurological damage.

This is supported by the finding that one-year-old infants who had a normal habituation pattern during intra-uterine life rated more highly on a Griffiths Mental Developmental Scale (Griffiths 1954) than those infants who had had abnormal habituation patterns during intra-uterine life (Leader et al 1984). In addition, Lewis (1971) has shown a significant relationship between visual habituation at one year of age, learning tasks such as two choice discrimination, concept formation and the IQ as measured by a full Stanford Binet test at 44 months.

It is not known why the bimodal patterns of abnormal habituation rates occur. The suggested hypothesis is that in an event such as intra-uterine hypoxaemia or inadequate placental function, the fetus progresses through three stages of behavioural responsiveness.

1. In the initial stages or when the 'stress' is not too severe, the fetus habituates rapidly due to effects of endogenously induced hormones such as catecholamines.
2. This is followed by generalized depression of the central nervous system as the 'stress' or hypoxia becomes more severe. At this stage, the fetus will still respond to the sensory stimulus but will fail to habituate at a normal rate.
3. Finally as fetal compromise becomes more extreme, the fetus will fail to respond at all to sensory stimulation.

It remains to be established how long an abnormal habituation pattern must be present before long-term neurological sequelae occur and whether the patterns of faster or slower habituation have different prognostic implications. It may also be possible to use an animal model of fetal habituation to study fetal ability to metabolize and excrete sedative drugs.

As most physiological systems have well-developed reserve mechanisms, testing under basal conditions can only provide limited information. It is likely that future tests for fetal well-being will incorporate some form of stimulation. Tests such as habituation, using different response systems may offer more information about central nervous system integrity because of the complexity of the information processing required.

As with all tests of fetal well-being, the difficulty of assessing neonatal outcome still remains with there being no clear-cut 'gold standard' (Grant & Mohide 1982). This is

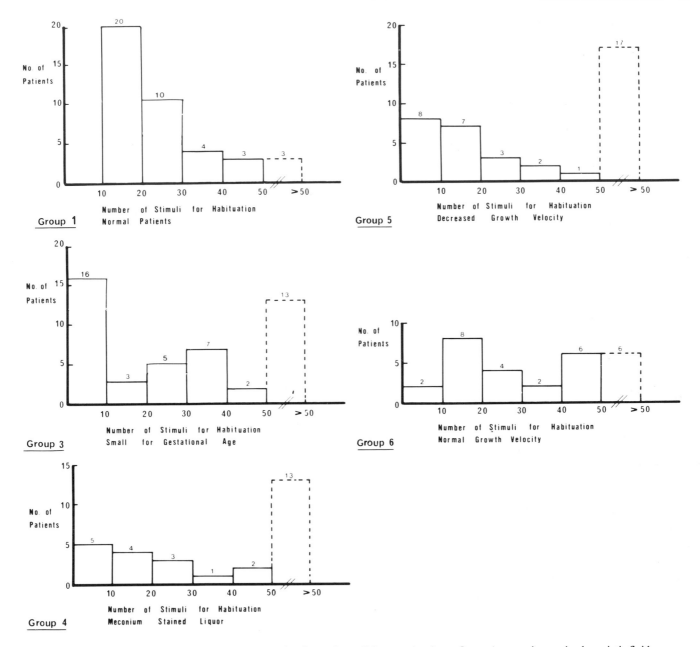

Fig. 4.3 Habituation patterns in: Group 1, normal pregnancies; Group 3, small for gestational age; Group 4, meconium-stained amniotic fluid; Group 5, decreased growth velocity; Group 6, normal growth velocity. Dashed columns are fetuses that failed to habituate by 50 stimuli.

compounded by the plasticity of the infant's central nervous system which allows undamaged brain areas to take over the function of damaged areas. This makes detection of abnormal function even more difficult.

One solution to the problem of fetal outcome may lie in a change in attitude by investigators. Because of the difficulties involved in measuring poor outcome perhaps the time has come to try and measure optimal or quality outcome. This may be easier to define and antenatal tests should not only be used to see what their sensitivity, specificity and predictive values are at detecting poor outcome but also optimal outcome.

REFERENCES

Andrews J, McGarry J M 1972 A community study of smoking in pregnancy. Journal of Obstetrics and Gynaecology of the British Commonwealth 79: 1057–1073

Baillie P 1974 Non hormonal methods of antenatal monitoring. In: Beard R W (ed) Clinics in obstetrics and gynaecology, Vol 1, No 1. Saunders, London, pp 103–122

Bennett M J 1984 The assessment of fetal-wellbeing. In: Bennett M J (ed) Ultrasound in perinatal care. John Wiley, London, pp 117–126

Birnholz J C, Benacerraf B R 1983 The development of human fetal hearing. Science 222: 516–518

Brackbill Y 1971 The role of the cortex in orienting. Orienting reflex in an anencephalic human infant. Developmental Psychobiology 5: 195–201

Brackbill Y, Kane J, Manniello R L, Adamson D 1974 Obstetric premedication and infant outcome. American Journal of Obstetrics and Gynecology 118: 377–384

Bronstein A I, Itina N A, Kamenetsaia A G 1968 The orienting reaction in newborn children. In: Varonin L G, Leontiev A N, Luris A R, Sokolov E N, Vinogradova O S (eds) Orienting reflex and exploratory behaviour. Moscow Academy of Pedagogical Sciences of RSFSR

Buchwald J A, Humphrey G L 1972 Response plasticity in cochlear nucleus of decerebrate cats during acoustic habituation procedures. Journal of Neurophysiology 35: 864–878

Buchwald J S, Humphrey G L 1973 An analysis of habituation in specific sensory systems. In: Steller E, Sprague J (eds) Progress in physiological psychology, Vol 5. Academic Press, New York, pp 1–75

Campbell S, Newman G B 1971 Growth of the fetal biparietal diameter during normal pregnancy. Journal of Obstetrics and Gynaecology of the British Commonwealth 78: 513–519

Copher D E, Huber C P 1967 Heart rate response of the human fetus to induced maternal hypoxia. American Journal of Obstetrics and Gynecology 98: 320–335

Davis M, File S E 1984 Intrinsic and extrinsic mechanisms of habituation and sensitization. In: Peek H V S, Petrinovich L (eds) Habituation, sensitization and behaviour. Academic Press, Florida

Davis M, Gendelman P M 1977 Plasticity of the acoustic startle response in the acutely decerebrate rat. Journal of Comparative Physiological Psychology 91: 549–563

Davis M, Svensson T H, Aghajanian G K 1975 Effects of D- and L-amphetamine on habituation and sensitization of the acoustic startle response in rats. Psychopharmacology 43: 1–11

Divon M Y, Platt L D, Cantrell C J, Smith C V, Yeh S, Paul R H 1985 Evoked fetal startle response: a possible intrauterine neurological examination. American Journal of Obstetrics and Gynecology 153: 454–456

Dustman R E, Callner D A 1979 Cortical evoked responses and response decrement in non-retarded and Down's syndrome individuals. American Journal of Mental Deficiency 83: 391–397

Eisenberg R, Coursin D B, Rupp N R 1966 Habituation to an acoustic pattern as an index of differences among human neonates. Journal of Auditory Research 6: 239–248

Eisenstein E M, Peretz B 1973 Comparative aspects of habituation in invertebrates. In: Peeke H V S, Herz M V (eds) Habituation. Physiological substrates, Vol 2. Academic Press, New York, pp 1–34

Erikson P, Gennser G 1984 Acute responses to maternal smoking of the pulsatile movements in fetal aorta. Acta Obstetricia et Gynecologica Scandinavica 63: 647–654

Evans W O 1961 A new technique for the investigation of some analgesic drugs on a reflex behaviour in the rat. Psychopharmacologia 2: 318–325

Evans W O 1962 A comparison of the analgesic potency of some analgesics as measured by the 'flinch-jump' procedure. Psychopharmacologia 3: 51–54

Ferguson I T, Lenman J A R, Johnston B B 1978 Habituation of the orbicularis oculi reflex in dementia and dyskinetic states. Journal of Neurology, Neurosurgery and Psychiatry 41: 824–828

Feyerabend C, Higenbottam T, Russel M A 1982 Nicotine concentrations in urine and saliva of smokers and non-smokers. British Medical Journal 2841: 1002–1004

Fleischer K 1955 Untersuchungen zur Entwicklung der Innenohrfunktion (interuterine Kindsbewegungen nag Schallreizen). Zeitschrift fur Laryngologie, Rhinologie, Otologie und ihre Grenzgebiete 34: 733–740

Gagnon R, Patrick J, Hunse C, Carmichael L 1986 Vibroacoustic stimulus causes changes in human fetal heart and movement pattern near term. Presented at the 13th Conference of the Society for the Study of Fetal Physiology, Banff

Gogan P 1970 The startle and orienting reactions in man. A study of their characteristics and habituation. Brain Research 18: 117–135

Goldwater B C, Lewis J 1978 Effects of arousal on the electrodermal orienting reflex. Psychophysiology 15: 221–225

Goodlin R C 1979 History of fetal monitoring. American Journal of Obstetrics and Gynecology 133: 323–352

Goodlin R C, Lowe E W 1974 Multiphasic fetal monitoring. A preliminary evaluation. American Journal of Obstetrics and Gynecology 119: 341–357

Goodlin R C, Schmidt R 1972 Human fetal arousal levels as indicated by heart rate recordings. American Journal of Obstetrics and Gynecology 114: 613–621

Graham F K 1979 Distinguishing among orienting, defense, and startle reflexes. In: Kimmel H D, van Olst E H, Orlebeke J F (eds) The orienting reflex in humans (An international conference sponsored by the Scientific Affairs Division of the North Atlantic Treaty Organization). Lawrence Erlbaum Associates, New York, pp 137–167

Graham F K, Clifton R K 1966 Heart rate change as a component of the orienting response. Psychological Bulletin 65: 305–320

Graham F K, Putnam L E, Leavitt L A 1975 Lead stimulation effects on human cardiac orienting and blink reflexes. Journal of Experimental Psychology: Human Perception and Performance 1: 161–169

Grant A, Mohide P 1982 Screening and diagnostic tests in antenatal care. In: Enkin M, Chalmers I (eds) Effectiveness and satisfaction in antenatal care. Clinics in Developmental Medicine. Heinemann Medical, London

Griffiths R 1954 The abilities of babies. University of London Press, London

Groves P M, Thompson R F 1970 Habituation: a dual process theory. Psychological Reviews 77: 419–450

Gruzelier J H, Connolly J F 1979 Differential drug action of electrodermal orienting responses as distinct from non-specific responses and electrodermal levels. In: Kimmel H D (ed) The orienting reflex in humans. Erlbaum, New York

Gruzelier J H, Venables P H 1972 Skin conductance orienting activity in a heterogenous sample of schizophrenics. Journal of Nervous and Mental Disease 155: 277–287

Gulbrandsen G B, Kristiansen K, Ursin H 1972 Response habituation in unconscious patients. Neuropsychologia 10: 313–320

Hellman L M, Johnston H L, Tolks W E, Jones E H 1961 Some factors effecting the fetal heart rate. American Journal of Obstetrics and Gynecology 82: 1055–1063

Hernandez-Peon R 1960 Neurophysiological correlates of habituation and other manifestations of plastic inhibition (internal inhibition). Electroencephalography and Clinical Neurophysiology 3 (suppl): 101–114

Hills D, Rodriquez P, Lawson W, Baim R 1985 Habituation testing in utero: its relation to fetal outcome. Presented at the meeting of the American Institute of Ultrasound in Medicine, Dallas

Holloway F A, Parsons O A 1971 Habituation of the orienting response in brain damaged patients. Psychophysiology 8: 623–634

Hutt S J, Hutt C 1964 Hyperactivity in a group of epileptic (and some non-epileptic) brain damaged children. Epilepsia 5: 334–351

Hutt S J, Hutt C, Lee D, Dunstead C 1965 A behavioural and electroencephalographic study of autistic children. Journal of Psychiatric Research 3: 181–197

Hutt C, von Bernuth H, Lenard H G, Hutt S J, Prechtl H F R 1968 Habituation in relation to state in the human neonate. Nature 220: 618–620

Jaroszewicz A M, Schuman D E W, Keet M P 1975 Intrauterine growth standards in Cape coloured infants. South African Medical Journal 49: 568–572

Jeffrey W E, Cohen L B 1971 Habituation in the human infant. In: Reese H W (ed) Advances in child development and behaviour, Vol 6. Academic Press, New York, pp 63–97

John A H 1965 The effect of maternal hypoxia on the heart rate of the foetus in utero. British Journal of Anaesthesia 37: 515–519

Jones C T, Robinson R O 1975 Plasma catecholamines in foetal and adult sheep. Journal of Physiology (London) 248(1): 15–33

Kandel E R 1979 Small system of neurones. Scientific American 241: 67–76

Keen R E, Chase H H, Graham F K 1965 Twenty-four low retention by neonates of an habituated heart rate response. Psychonomic Science 2: 265–266

Key B J 1961 Effects of chlorpromazine and lysergic acid diethylamide on the role of habituation of the arousal response. Nature (London) 190: 275–277

Lader M H, Wing L 1965 Comparative bioassay of chlordiazepoxide and amylobarbitone sodium therapies in patients with anxiety states using physiological and clinical measures. Journal of Neurology, Neurosurgery and Psychiatry 28: 414–424

Lader M H, Wing L 1969 Physiological measures in agitated and retarded depressed patients. Journal of Psychiatric Research 7: 89–100

Lamper C, Eisdorfer C 1971 Prestimulus activity level and responsivity in the neonate. Child Development 42: 465–473

Landis C, Hunt W A 1939 The startle pattern. Farrar & Rinehart, New York (Reprinted in 1968 by Johnson Reprint Corp., New York

Leader L R 1986 Unpublished data

Leader L, Baillie P 1979 The accuracy of maternal assessment of fetal movements. South African Medical Journal 55: 836–837

Leader L R, Baillie P, Martin B, Vermeulen E 1982a The assessment and significance of habituation to a repeated stimulus by the human fetus. Early Human Development 7: 211–219

Leader L R, Baillie P, Martin B, Vermeulin E 1982b Fetal habituation in high risk pregnancies. British Journal of Obstetrics and Gynaecology 89: 441–446

Leader L R, Baillie P, Martin B, Molteno C, Wynchank S 1984 Fetal responses to vibrotactile stimulation: a possible predictor of fetal and neonatal outcome. Australian and New Zealand Journal of Obstetrics and Gynaecology 24: 251–256

Leader L R, Lumbers E R, Stevens A D 1986 The effect of hypoxia and catecholamines on cardiovascular, forelimb and habituation responses to repeated tactile stimulation in fetal sheep. Presented at the 4th Annual Meeting of the Australian Perinatal Society, Brisbane

Leader L R, Stevens A D, Lumbers E R 1988 Biology of the Neonate 53: 73–85

Lehtovirta P, Forss P 1978 The acute effect of smoking on intervillous blood flow in the placenta. Journal of Obstetrics and Gynaecology of the British Commonwealth 85: 729–731

Lewis M 1971 Individual differences in the measurement of early cognitive growth. Exceptional infant 2. In: Hellmuth J (ed) Studies in abnormalities. Brunner Mazel, New York, pp 172–210

Longo L D 1976 Carbon monoxide: effects on oxygenation of the fetus in utero. Science 194: 523–525

Madison L S, Adubato S A, Madison J K et al 1986 Fetal response decrement: true habituation? Journal of Developmental and Behavioral Pediatrics 7(1): 14–20

Manning F A, Feyerabend C 1976 Cigarette smoking and fetal breathing movements. British Journal of Obstetrics and Gynaecology 83: 262–270

Meyer M B, Jonas B S, Tonascia J A 1976 Perinatal events associated with maternal smoking during pregnancy. American Journal of Epidemiology 103: 464–476

Michaelis R, Rooschuz B, Dopfer R 1980 Prenatal origin of spastic hemiparesis. Early Human Development 4: 243–255

Moreau T, Birch H G 1974 Relationship between obstetrical general anaesthesia and rate of neonatal habituation to repeated stimulation. Developmental Medicine and Child Neurology 16: 612–619

Natale R, Clewlow F, Dawes G S 1981 Measurement of fetal forelimb movements in the lamb in utero. American Journal of Obstetrics and Gynecology 140: 545–551

Natale R, Nasello-Paterson C 1986 The effect of electrical stimulation on behavioural states in the fetal lamb. American Journal of Obstetrics and Gynecology 154: 321–328

Nijhuis J G, Prechtl H F R, Martin C B Jr, Bots R S G M 1982 Are there behavioural states in the human fetus? Early Human Development 6: 177–195

Ohel G, Rabinovitz R, Sadovsky E 1985 Fetal response to vibroacoustic stimulation in periods of low activity, low variability. Presented at the 12th Annual Meeting of the Society for the Study of Fetal Physiology, Haifa

Ohel G, Birkenfeld A, Rabinowitz R, Sadovsky E 1986 Fetal response to vibratory acoustic stimulation in periods of low heart rate reactivity and low activity. American Journal of Obstetrics and Gynecology 154: 619–621

Ohman A 1979 The orienting response, attention and learning: an information-processing perspective. In: Kimmel H D, van Olst E H, Orlebeke J F (eds) Orienting reflex in humans. Erlbaum, Hillsdale, pp 443–471

Pakula A, Sokolov E N 1973 Habituation in gastropoda: behavioural, interneuronal and endoneural aspects. In: Peeke H V S, Herz M J (eds) Habituation. Physiological substrates, Vol 2. Academic Press, New York, pp 35–107

Patterson T, Venables P H 1978 Bilateral skin conductance and skin potential in schizophrenic and normal subjects. The identification of the fast habituator group of schizophrenics. Psychophysiology 15: 556–560

Pavlov I P 1927 Conditioned reflexes. An investigation of the physiological activity of the cerebral cortex. Oxford University Press, London

Pearson J A, Wills L, MacDonald J F 1974 The effect of PCPA and lesions of the dorsal raphe nucleus on habituation of the flexor withdrawal reflex. Brain Research 77: 515–520

Peiper A 1925 Sinnesempfindungen des Kindes vor seiner Geburt. Monatsschrift fur Kinderheilkunde 29: 236–241

Phelan J P 1980 Dimished fetal reactivity with smoking. American Journal of Obstetrics and Gynecology 136: 230–233

Prechtl H F R 1985 Ultrasound studies of human fetal behaviour. Early Human Development 12: 91–98

Pribam K H 1967 The limbic systems, efferent control of neural inhibition and behaviour. In: Adey W R, Tokizane T (eds) Progress in brain research. Structure and function of the limbic system, Vol 2. Elsevier, Amsterdam

Quigley M E, Sheehan K L, Wilkes M M, Yen S S C 1979 Effects of maternal smoking on circulating catecholamine levels and fetal heart rates. American Journal of Obstetrics and Gynecology 133: 685–690

Ray W S 1932 A preliminary study of fetal conditioning. Child Development 3: 173–177

Rigatto H, Blanco C E, Walker D W 1982 The response of stimulation of hindlimb nerves in fetal sheep, in utero, during different phases of electrocortical activity. Journal of Developmental Physiology 4: 175–185

Robinson A 1969 Sex differences in development. Developmental Medicine and Child Neurology 11: 245–246

Rosen K G, Dagbjartsson A, Henriksson B A, Lagercrantz H 1984 Kjellmer I: The relationship between circulating catecholamines and ST waveform in the fetal lamb electrocardiogram during hypoxia. American Journal of Obstetrics and Gynecology 149: 190–195

Ruckebusch Y 1972 Development of sleep and wakefulness in the foetal lamb. Electroencephalography and Clinical Neurophysiology 32: 119–128

Ruckebusch Y, Gaujoux M, Eghbali B 1977 Sleep cycles and kinesis in the foetal lamb. Electroencephalography and Clinical Neurophysiology 42: 226–237

Russell M A, Feyeraband C, Cole P V 1976 Plasma nicotine levels after cigarette smoking and chewing nicotine gum. British Medical Journal 1: 1043–1046

Rust J 1977 Habituation and the orienting response in the auditory cortical evoked potential. Psychophysiology 14(2): 123–126

Sagvolden T, Webster K 1974 Habituation of the startle reflex in rats with septal lesions. Behavioral Biology 12: 413–418

Schmidt W, Boos R, Gnirs J, Auer L, Schulze S 1985 Fetal behavioural states and controlled sound stimulation. Early Human Development 12: 145–153

Sharpless S, Jasper J 1956 Habituation of the arousal reaction. Brain 79: 655–680

Singer J E, Westphal M, Niswander K R 1968 Sex differences in the incidence of neonatal abnormalities and abnormal performance in early childhood. Child Development 39: 103–112

Socol M L, Manning F A, Murata Y, Druzin M L 1982 Maternal smoking causes fetal hypoxia: experimental evidence. American Journal of Obstetrics and Gynecology 142: 214–218

Sokolov Y N 1963 Perception and the conditioned reflex (trans. by S. W. Waydenfeld). Pergamon Press, Oxford

Sontag L W, Wallace R F 1935 Preliminary report of the Fels Fund. American Journal of Diseases of Children 48: 1050–1057

Spelt D K 1948 The conditioning of the human fetus in utero. Journal of Experimental Psychology 38: 338–346

Stevenson D, Siddle D 1983 Theories of habituation. In: Siddle D (ed) Orienting and habituation: perspectives in human research. John Wiley, New York, pp 183–236

Szabo I, Hazafi K 1965 Elicitability of the acoustic startle reaction after brain stem lesions. Acta Physiologica, Academy of Science, Hungary 27: 155–165

Thaler I, Goodman J D S, Dawes G S 1980 Effects of maternal cigarette smoking on fetal breathing and fetal movements. American Journal of Obstetrics and Gynecology 138: 282–287

Thompson R F, Glansman D L 1966 Neural and behavioural mechanisms of habituation and sensitization. In: Tighe T J, Leaton R N (eds) Habituation. Lawrence Earlbaum Associates, Hillsdale, NJ, p 49

Thompson R F, Spencer W A 1966 Habituation: a model for the study of neuronal subtrates of behaviour. Psychological Review 73: 16–43

Timor-Tritsch I E 1986 The effect of external stimuli on fetal behaviour. European Journal of Obstetrics and Gynaecology 6: 321–331

Tizard B 1968 Habituation of EEG and skin potential changes in normal and severely sub-normal children. American Journal of Mental Deficiency 73: 16–43

Van Vliet M A T, Martin C B Jr, Nijhuis J G, Prechtl H F R 1985 Behavioural states in the fetuses of nulliparous women. Early Human Development 12: 121–135

Vesey C J, Saloojee Y, Cole P V, Russell M A H 1982 Blood carboxyhaemoglobin, plasma thiocyanate, and cigarette consumption: implications for epidemiological studies in smokers. British Medical Journal 284: 1516–1518

Wagner A R 1976 Priming in STM: an information-processing mechanism for self-generated or retrieval-generated depression in performance. In: Tighe T G, Leaton R N (eds) Habituation: perspectives from child development, animal behaviour and neurophysiology. Erlbaum, Hillsdale, pp 95–128

Wagner A R 1979 Habituation and memory. In: Dickenson A, Boakes R A (eds) Mechanisms of learning and motivation: a memorial volume to Jerzy Konorski. Erlbaum, Hillsdale, pp 53–82

Webster W 1969 Auditory habituation and barbiturate induced neurological activity. Science 164: 970–971

Wood C, Hammond J, Lumley J et al 1971 Effect of maternal inhalation of 10% oxygen upon the human fetus. Australian and New Zealand Journal of Obstetrics and Gynaecology 11: 85–90

Wyers E J, Peek H V S, Herz M J 1973 Behavioural habituation in invertebrates. In: Peek H V S, Herz M J (eds) Habituation. Physiological Substrates, Vol 2. Academic Press, New York, pp 1–57

5. Assessment of neurodevelopmental outcome

Dr C-L. Fawer and Prof A. Calame

During the last 25 years, there has been a growing interest in perinatal medicine. Better knowledge of fetal and neonatal physiology, improvements in both obstetrics and neonatal intensive care together with progress in technology and better health organization have accounted for a reduction in perinatal mortality (Calame et al 1972, 1977, Hack et al 1979, Stanley & Hobbs 1980, Pharoah & Alberman 1981, Stewart et al 1981, Falkner 1984, Tenovuo et al 1986). Regionally organized programmes for prenatal care (involving genetic counselling, fetal screening, identification of high-risk pregnancies, maternal education) and for perinatal care (involving resuscitation, examination and management of infants at high risk, introduction of new technology) as well as research studies have been introduced and rapidly implemented in varying degrees of development. Therefore, financial investment to support such programmes rapidly became very important (Pomerance et al 1978, Sinclair et al 1981, Boyle et al 1983, Newns et al 1984).

As there is no definite and unique approach to evaluate the relationship between the high cost and the expected benefits in terms of health improvement and in the needs of a particular community or society that is served, the effectiveness of neonatal intensive care has been regularly questioned (McCarthy et al 1979, Kiely et al 1981a,b, Sinclair et al 1981, Boyle et al 1983, Swyer 1984, Walker et al 1984).

If perinatal mortality is easily recorded and provides useful parameters for evaluation and comparison — when registration data at a regional or national level are available — perinatal morbidity and long-term outcome are much more difficult to define and assess (Bax 1986, Dunn 1986). With the introduction of neonatal intensive care and the concomitant decline in mortality, the quality of survival became a major concern for all neonatologists. This has been summarized by the World Health Organization (1978) 'Improved survival is not sufficient. If the reduction of perinatal mortality rates were accompanied by increased numbers of surviving infants who subsequently endured short, miserable lives, then the gain from the reduced level of perinatal mortality would be illusory.'

Because of numerous problems associated with medical progress, i.e. economical, ethical and human, there were solid and rational grounds for creating follow-up programmes to measure short- and long-term effects of neonatal intensive care.

Technological development, changes in resuscitation criteria and management of the newborn, modification in defining viability and limits of survival of critically ill infants implied a need for monitoring the validity of such financial investment and human engagement. This is the justification for follow-up studies. Health services, at least in industrialized nations, have to face explosive increases in medical demands and at the same time have to distribute resources equally.

Since 1960, the efficacy of perinatal medicine has been analysed and assessed in various ways, depending mainly on changing concepts of risk over periods of time, on local and environmental conditions, and on the background of medical and scientific observers. Follow-up studies have thus been performed with reference to a variety of points:

1. Epidemiological analyses which provided useful figures at regional or national levels for health organization, the utilization of services and distribution of wealth (Douglas & Gear 1976, Stanley 1979, Hagberg et al 1982, Eksmyr 1985, 1986).
2. The cost-effectiveness evaluation of neonatal intensive care (Boyle et al 1983, Newns et al 1984, Walker et al 1984).
3. Perinatology and neonatology with regard to advances in technology, to newborn management regimes, potential hazards and their subsequent effects on mortality and morbidity (Davies 1976, Fitzhardinge et al 1976, 1978, Stewart et al 1978, Ruiz et al 1981, Horwood et al 1982, Nelson & Ellenberg 1984, Paneth 1986).
4. Neurodevelopmental paediatrics and neurology with analyses of changing patterns of clinical conditions and neurological abnormalities (Calame et al 1972, Calame 1983, Hagberg et al 1984, Largo et al 1986). These last

two approaches have specific targets and can be assessed by appropriate data collection.

In the early 1980s, the validity of follow-up studies was also questioned in a debate involving many neonatologists, neurologists, epidemiologists and health services (Jones et al 1979, Lancet 1980, Department of Health and Social Security 1980, Medical Research Council 1980, Social Services Committee 1980, Stewart et al 1981).

Surveys of infants born too soon, too small, extremely ill, exposed to hazardous treatment and with confounding risk factors provided controversial results leading to scepticism, if not confusion.

There are indeed, meticulous and meaningful follow-up studies which answer the relevant and essential questions but there are other reports without rigorous methodology and asking inadequate questions. Minimal requirements, however, can be defined to properly design a study, describe the population, report and interpret results, whatever the purpose and particular conditions of the study.

One of the major aims of medicine is to find the right 'marker' for evaluating not only gains that it is hoped will be achieved but also subsequent disadvantages and even harmful effects. Only an objective and critical control of the quality of care will provide ethical guidelines and the basis for a rational health policy. This demands regular reappraisal of intended aims.

FOLLOW-UP STUDIES

The Neonatal Unit of Lausanne (Switzerland) opened in 1966 and the need for neurodevelopmental surveillance became obvious very rapidly. Since 1970, high-risk infants have been selected and prospectively included in a longitudinal follow-up study. During these 15 years of experience, numerous problems have been encountered; some of these could be overcome, others were unavoidable and remain so. They are related 1. to study design including methodology, population factors, results analysis, staff and financial organization; and 2. to the consequences of rapid changes in neonatology and their possible effects on analysis and interpretation of the results.

STUDY DESIGN

Aim of the study

The aim of the study should be reasonable, properly defined and should reflect true needs and demands. To do this, the relevant question must be chosen with regard to the local working conditions. It will also depend on the clear-sightedness of the observers. The following prerequisites ought to be taken into consideration:

1. A precise evaluation of the health care system in order to define the geographical region and the population being served by the hospital.
2. A definition of the level of care provided by the unit.
3. A careful selection of the sample.
4. An evaluation of the feasibility of the study and the effectiveness of data collection.

Based on these preliminary evaluations, the framework of the follow-up programme will be delineated in terms of a hospital-based or area-based study. Hospital-based evaluation is used to assess the current activity of the Neonatal Unit, to control the quality of care and establish the prognosis of a particular risk factor. Area-based studies refer to a county or a health region and assess the value and effectiveness of neonatal intensive care, as well as determining the overall outcome of a representative population of high-risk newborn infants.

Population

Selection criteria of the sample, period of recruitment, nationality, race and sex distribution, should be described. Various biases, such as socio-economic class, perinatal risk factors and loss to follow-up should be controlled for.

Socio-economic class

The concept of socio-economic class and its impact on later outcome has been much debated. Definition and classification vary from one country to another (Cougalton 1963, Blishen 1965, Hollingshead 1975). Most classifications are based mainly on the occupation of the child's father. Others have included variables such as income, housing and parents' education and provide a more comprehensive and appropriate, although time-consuming profile (Graffar 1961).

Low socio-economic status has been shown to be associated with complications of pregnancy including increased incidence of low-birth-weight infants, perinatal complications and child morbidity (Butler & Bonham 1963, Butler & Alberman 1969, Davie et al 1972, Chamberlain et al 1975, 1978, Butler et al in press). If one wishes to assess the outcome of neonatal intensive care, not only in relation to perinatal mortality and morbidity but also in relation to later social and academic achievement, the social class distribution of the population, based on a detailed evaluation, should be included in each investigation.

Perinatal factors

Although social status is a very important determinant of health outcome (Egbuonu & Starfield 1982, Rumeau-Rouquette 1984, Papiernik et al 1985) several surveys show that other social factors such as maternal height, age, nutrition, parity, smoking history, drug abuse, and attitudes towards health have additional adverse effects.

Mothers in the lower social classes are more likely to have a complicated pregnancy with a compromised fetus leading to a newborn infant with perinatal complications and subsequent major sequelae. Perinatal factors and birth represent the end-point of a 'continuum of casualties'.

Pre-, peri- and postnatal injuries are interdependent and the difficulty in interpreting the immediate and long-term impact of each risk factor on a child's outcome is confounding.

In each follow-up investigation, the concept of risk has to be clearly defined and described. Its potential role should be considered in a multifactorial approach and weighed in a covariance analysis, as performed in the study of Nelson & Ellenberg (1986).

Loss to follow-up

When defining a study group, it implies not only a description of the overall population, the selection criteria, perinatal mortality, postneonatal mortality, but also the loss to follow-up. This last factor causes inaccuracy in data collection and misleading interpretation, either by underestimating or overestimating the incidence of both healthy and handicapped children. To ensure an optimal follow-up, clinic attendance, time, money, staff organization and co-ordination with other health professionals are required. Reasons for incorporating a newborn in a follow-up programme should be clearly explained to parents, community paediatricians and family doctors before discharge from hospital. Appointments to the clinic must be scheduled and not only based on the goodwill of the parents. Neurodevelopmental assessment should be performed in a quiet and comfortable atmosphere where parents feel free to ask questions. Psychometric testings should be described, interpreted to the family, and if any abnormality is detected, appropriate management should be planned with them.

Control group

There are major hazards in reporting, analysing and interpreting 'raw' data, without any attempt at comparison. A control group is of critical importance and has a number of functions including minimizing bias or extraneous factors, avoiding misleading inferences about outcome, as well as recognizing iatrogenic hazards.

The choice of the control group depends on the aim of the study, the factor being evaluated and the global hypothesis being tested. The control group should reflect race, sex and the socio-economic class distribution of the population under study.

The relevance of a control group has been stressed in follow-up studies of low-birth-weight infants (Kitchen et al 1980, Kiely & Paneth 1981, Lloyd 1984, Calame et al 1986). Their purpose was to establish either the prognosis in terms of mortality or morbidity and to recognize changes over periods of time. In addition the control group serves to monitor the effects of neonatal intensive care and of specific neonatal management techniques. The constitution of a control group and its selection therefore varies, according to the hypothesis formulated by the investigators.

Methods

The accurate identification of abnormalities depends on a wide spectrum of tests. These, however, vary considerably from one country to another, from one culture to another, and depend on the level of care and technology available. Furthermore, the choice of the method of neurological assessment and of adequate psychometric tests, and their use, require a qualified and well-trained developmental team. Knowledge of normative data, variations and individual fluctuations in development are essential, as the detection of neurological abnormalities in infancy and early childhood and a neurodevelopmental diagnosis involve measurements of specific abilities.

There is an important distinction to be made between developmental assessment and developmental screening. The latter is the procedure of checking the development of a general population of presumed healthy children. Various methods have been developed which rely on a brief developmental history and a precise but simple method of testing to detect abnormalities at optimal ages (Wilson & Jungner 1968, Hart et al 1978, Baird & Hall 1985, Hall & Baird 1986). Developmental assessment is a far more complex approach requiring a Developmental Unit and an experienced team. It encompasses an exhaustive developmental history, an evaluation of development with appropriate psychometric tests, a physical and neurological examination (including vision and hearing) and medical investigations, if necessary.

As far as assessment of survivors of neonatal intensive care or outcome of neonatal intensive care is concerned, recruitment of study groups of children, fulfilling specific selection criteria is needed, and assessment must be performed according to a rigorous methodology.

Assessment tests

Brain growth and development of the neonate is a continuous process involving various sequences of structures and functional changes and any assessment has to take into account the subjects maturation. To ensure diagnostic accuracy, a psychometric test should be standardized, reproducible, reliable and have a predictive value.

With advances in neonatology and the growing interest in the neurology of the newborn infant and young child, several methods of both neurological and developmental assessment have been reported.

Neurological assessment in infancy. The various methods for neurological assessment of the newborn and infant are discussed in detail in Chapter 3.

Neurological examination in childhood (2–8 years). A conventional neurological examination encompasses evaluation of the cranial nerves, motor system (tone, muscle power and motility), co-ordination, sensory system and tendon reflexes (Paine & Oppé 1966, Touwen 1982). At 5 and 8 years, fine and gross motor ability can be evaluated by specific methods described by Ozeretski (1936) and Grant et al (1973) for example.

In both infancy and childhood, the visual examination includes reflected light test and cover test, optokinetic nystagmus in response to a rotating drum, fixation and following of a moving object. Visual acuity is tested with the stycar graded balls up to 2–2.5 years, the Stycar Miniature Toys Test from 2 to 3 years and the Stycar Letter Cards from 2.5 to 5 years (Sheridan 1969). From 5 to 8 years colour vision and binocular vision are also evaluated. A good estimate of visual acuity can often be obtained by watching a child at play.

Testing visual fields can be performed by eliciting the response of head and eye turning to a stimulus presented from behind the patient in one or other visual field (4–5 months to 8 years).

Assessment of hearing in infancy involves free field testing as described by Sheridan (1968). This involves a variety of general sounds (spoon on cup, rattle, bell, paper, voice). More sophisticated investigations are recommended between 6 and 9 months, if hearing loss is suspected. These include auditory brainstem responses, audiometry and ears, nose and throat (ENT) examination.

Developmental testing. The primary aim of a developmental scale is to produce a measure of the current general and intellectual ability of the child, expressed as a Developmental Quotient (DQ) or Intelligence Quotient (IQ). It consists of an inventory of performances and milestones.

Many developmental tests have been devised. Some of them are more analytical and explore both general and specific abilities.

The Bayley scale (Bayley 1969) is well standardized and widely used. The Denver developmental scale (Frankenberg & Dodds 1968) is more a screening test. The Griffiths scale (Griffiths 1970a,b) and the McCarthy scales of children's abilities (McCarthy 1972) are attractive because of their developmental emphasis. The Standford Binet (Terman & Merrill 1961) is a well-known intelligence test, but with a verbal bias, therefore unsuitable for children with language disorders. Gesell development schedules (Gesell & Amatruda 1969) and Sheridan's assessment (Sheridan 1973) have a clinical diagnosis orientation and are applicable to handicapped children. Wechsler Intelligence Scale for Children (Wechsler 1944) and Wechsler Preschool and Primary Scale of Intelligence (Wechsler 1967) distinguish verbal and performance intelligence. The Reynell developmental language scales (Reynell 1969) separately assess verbal comprehension and expressive language.

Specific problems may need more sophisticated and appropriate tests to investigate a particular ability. For example the 'Raven's progressive matrix' is applied for testing non-verbal performance in a child with a language disorder (Raven 1948).

Developmental scales are usually divided into five main subscales: gross and fine motor abilities; hearing and speech; vision-manipulation; performance (or quantitative subscale); and personal and social.

Developmental Quotient and Intelligence Quotient and their distributions are useful for interstudy-group comparisons.

The most comprehensive development scale is no substitute for a neurological examination, although there is much overlap between these two approaches. A neurological examination is a standardized technique for eliciting neural function, detecting abnormal signs and evaluating the quality of a response eventually leading to a diagnosis. The developmental tests, however, measure the level of achievement, whatever the child's condition.

It is noteworthy that one of the most serious problems encountered by the investigators, is the lack of appropriate and standardized tests and methods for examination. For example in the French-speaking countries, there is no language scale available. Reviewers therefore may have difficulty in understanding study design and choice of testings — more particularly at school age.

Efforts are needed to adapt, revise, translate and standardize neurological examinations and testings.

Definitions and classification

Most follow-up studies refer to major and minor sequelae but they do not always agree on the definition. The terms of impairment or defect, disability and handicap are extensively used to express, report and analyse data. In a recent article, Baird & Hall (1985) reviewed diagnosis definition and stressed once again the 'important philosophical distinction between them'.

According to these authors and many others (World Health Organisation 1980), an impairment is an anatomical or physiological abnormality; a disability refers to the functional effect of the impairment; and handicap implies that the disability prevents or hinders attainment of socially desirable role and behaviour.

For clinical description of the various types of neurodevelopmental problem, the same authors proposed the following classification, already in use by several investigators.

Major handicaps include conditions that almost inevitably have a major effect on the child's life — that is severe mental handicap with Intelligence Quotient (IQ) less than 50, cerebral palsy, sensory–neural hearing loss, and partial or total blindness.

Minor defects involve important organic conditions,

although they are less severe. They include minor hearing losses, squint, refractive errors and amblyopia.

Developmental disorders include global delay, speech and language problems, clumsiness, learning disabilities, hyperactivity and transient behavioural disturbances. They are more difficult to define and identify as they are often close to normality. Their detection depends on the choice of specific testing and the observer's expertise.

Cerebral palsy. The classification of cerebral palsy has varied from study to study, depending mainly on the author's background. Cerebral palsy has been defined as a non-progressive, chronic disability, characterized by aberrant control of movement and posture, and appearing in early life. Although clinical experience has shown that the distinction between a mild cerebral palsy and minor abnormal neurological signs may be difficult, five main categories of cerebral palsy are usually proposed aiming at neurological description and comparison of results (Ingram 1964, Hagsberg et al 1972, 1975, Drillien & Drummond 1977, Holt 1977, Ellison 1984).

1. Hemiplegia: a unilateral spastic paresis affecting the arm more than the leg.
2. Spastic quadriplegia or tetraplegia (bilateral hemiplegia): affecting all four limbs with more marked involvement of arms than legs.
3. Diplegia: paresis affecting all four limbs but much more marked in the legs than in the arms.
4. Ataxic cerebral palsies: characterized by hypotonia, lack of co-ordination of voluntary movements and impairment of balance.
5. Dyskinetic cerebral palsy: characterized by involuntary movements and disorderly changes of tone affecting the bulbar musculature, the face, trunk and all four limbs.
6. Other cerebral palsies: mixed and unclassifiable conditions.

The severity of the cerebral palsy should also be reported on the basis of functional impairment and described as mild, moderate, or severe (Ingram 1964).

Mental retardation. The following categories of IQ are recommended: DQ or IQ 71–85 borderline; 51–70 mild mental retardation; and <50 severe mental retardation (Grossmann et al 1973).

Transient tone and posture abnormalities of infancy. Description of the clinical picture varies with different authors. Amiel-Tison (1976) reported an early appearance of abnormalities within weeks or months, disappearing by late infancy. Drillien (1972) described various 'dystonic' conditions as well as their possible significance. Two studies (Matile et al 1984, Furrer et al 1984) described the long-term prognosis of these abnormalities. The hypertonic patterns, affecting mainly pre-term infants, had a better prognosis compared with the hypotonic patterns occurring most commonly in asphyxiated full-term infants.

Age at testing; age at diagnosis

The concept of 'key ages' has been developed to improve the understanding of developmental problems and to facilitate clinical documentation and interpretation. 'Key age' defined by Gesell & Amatruda (1969) is an empirical age at which a characteristic developmental and behavioural feature can be specified. The 'initial age' gives a minimal developmental age level of a particular ability (Gessell & Amatruda 1969, Holt 1977) and the 'limit age' or 'upper limit age' (Neligan & Prudham 1969) is the latest age for acceptable appearance of the ability. The absence of a permanent ability requires further investigations. The 'mean age' is the age at which 50% of the population of normal children achieve a particular milestone.

On the basis of these concepts and the use of standard deviations (initial age corresponding to 2 SD below the mean age and limit age to 2 SD above), optimal age at testings as well as optimal age at diagnosis of specific disorders are established within rational and empirical ranges.

Throughout the last 15 years of follow-up investigations in Lausanne, the following scheme has been adopted with regular updating to include new techniques and tests (Table 5.1). In our experience, this proposed programme has proved to be reasonable, efficient and accurate for the detection of abnormalities.

Assessment in the neonatal period, at 6 and 18 months and 3.5, 5 and 8 years is mandatory and is the minimal requirement for longitudinal surveillance. The 3, 9, 12, 24-months and 4-years assessments are performed, either on request or if a particular ability has not been evaluated, or if intervention, specific management and parental guidance are necessary. If for example the hearing of a 6-month-old child is not properly assessed, a further test will be planned at 9 months.

There is an overall agreement to examine babies up to 24-months (age corrected for prematurity). At the age of testing, the corrected age of the child is the chronological age minus the number of weeks that the infant had been born before full-term.

Major handicap (severe cerebral palsy, severe sensory–neural hearing loss and severe visual impairment) should be detected as early as possible and within the first few months of life. The diagnosis of transient abnormalities in tone and posture is ascertained only by sequential assessment; they should have disappeared by 18 months. Minor defects such as squint, myopia and amblyopia are frequent and should be detected within the first 18 months of life. Other refractive errors (hypermetropia and astigmatism) as well as partial hearing loss, behavioural problems and language and speech disorders should be diagnosed in preschool children because early intervention may be beneficial.

Furthermore, it has been demonstrated that developmental problems identified at preschool age persisted into school

Table 5.1 Scheme for neurodevelopmental follow-up programme

Age at testing	Methods of testing	Age at diagnosis	Further specialized investigations
Birth 40th postmenstrual week	Standardized neonatal neurological examination (Dubowitz & Dubowitz)	Chromosomal anomalies Congenital anomalies Congenital infections Infants at high risk	EEG ABR Fundi Ultrasound
3 months	Systematic development history Standardized neurological examination (Amiel–Tison, St-Anne Dargassies)	Major handicaps (Severe CP, severe visual and auditory impairment) Transient abnormalities	EEG ABR Fundi Ultrasound
6 months	Vision-audition (Sheridan)	Development delay	
9 months 12 months	Developmental assessment (DQ, Griffiths)	Major handicaps (moderate, mild CP partial deafness) Minor defects* Development delay	EEG Audiometry Ophthalmology Orthopaedics
18 months 3.5 years	Systematic developmental history Conventional neurological examination Developmental assessment (DQ, Griffiths) Systematic developmental history Conventional neurological assessment Developmental assessment (DQ, McCarthy)	Major handicaps (moderate, mild CP) Minor defects* Developmental delay Mental retardation Minor defects* Developmental disorders†	Neuropaediatrics ENT investigations Speech evaluation Ophthalmology Specific psychometric testings
5 years 8 years	Systematic developmental history Conventional neurological assessment Developmental assessment (DQ, McCarthy) Evaluation of school performances	Minor defects* Developmental disorders† School problems	Specific psychometric testings

*Minor defects: minor hearing losses, squint, refractive errors, amblyopia
†Developmental disorders: global delay, speech and language disorders, clumsiness, learning disabilities, behavioural disorders

age and were frequently associated with early school failure (Francis-Williams 1976, Camp et al 1977, Michelsson 1982, Gillberg & Gillberg 1983a,b, Claeys et al 1984). This is likely to result in lower school attainment, modifying social and professional success. Only follow-up studies of longer duration will aid the assignment of a precise prognosis of high-risk newborn infants.

Reporting and analysis

From our own experience and from the literature, the following recommendations are made:

1. Data on the overall population, neonatal and post-neonatal mortality, loss to follow-up, sex, race and socio-economic class distributions should all be provided.
2. Birth weight and gestational age (mean, standard deviation, ranges) as well as birth weight and gestational age categories should be reported.
3. Age at testing (mean, standard deviation, ranges) and choice of tests should be specified.
4. A conventional classification of major handicaps, minor defects and developmental disorders should be adopted.

5. The incidence of major handicaps should be reported. This should be expressed as percentages of the total live-born population (for epidemiological purposes) and percentages of the survivors (for appraisal of quality of survival).
6. A comprehensive table of handicapped children should be included, specifying the type of handicap (cerebral palsy, multiple handicap, i.e. cerebral palsy ± visual impairment ± hearing loss ± mental retardation), its severity (mild, moderate and severe) and individual DQ or IQ scores.
7. The incidence of minor defects, developmental disorders and their type should be reported.
8. DQs and IQs (mean, standard deviation, ranges) as well as their distributions should be reported separately for each study group.

RAPID CHANGES IN NEONATOLOGY: THEIR POSSIBLE EFFECTS ON REPORTING AND ANALYSIS

Some problems are difficult to overcome when carrying out follow-up studies. A perennial difficulty is the argument that, as modifications in neonatal intensive care occur over relatively few years, long-term data could become outdated. Furthermore, because of the ongoing assessment, subtle changes in care may influence results and thus alter interpretation.

Constant improvements in neonatology should in any case not discourage paediatricians from setting up follow-up programmes. On the contrary, there are sound reasons to justify such studies. These include:

1. the control of the quality of intensive care;
2. the establishment of the true long-term prognosis of high-risk newborn infants in terms not only of mortality, morbidity and major handicaps but also minor defects and school achievement;
3. the evaluation of changing patterns in outcome of neonatal intensive care, in relation to periods of time and changes in neonatology. A new technique or a new treatment ought to be assessed in randomized trials, with rigorous methodology.

Figure 5.1 summarizes our current concepts on follow-up investigations. If Health Services can afford neonatal intensive care, they should also afford follow-up programmes. The Neonatal Unit is defined as either hospital-based or area-based. Newborn infants are selected into follow-up on the basis of concept of risk and allocated to the study group or control group with regards to the hypothesis being tested. Prerequisites of such projects are adequate choice of methods and diagnosis classification. Longitudinal examination at various ages allows the early detection of major handicaps, minor defects, developmental disorders and school problems.

Consequences of such follow-up programmes are handicap detection, involving precise definition of the extent of handicap and its management, parental guidance, co-ordination with other specialists and health professionals.

Finally, inferences about outcome, prognosis of a particular risk and treatment, will provide reappraisal of the quality of care and perspective for a rational health policy.

OUTCOME OF NEONATAL INTENSIVE CARE

Neonatology started in 1907 when the French obstetrician Pierre Budin claimed in an 'historical' statement: 'de nos jours, grâce à l'antisepsie et aux progrès techniques, l'accoucheur libéré de son anxiété quant du destin maternel, peut porter son attention sur les besoins de l'enfant'*

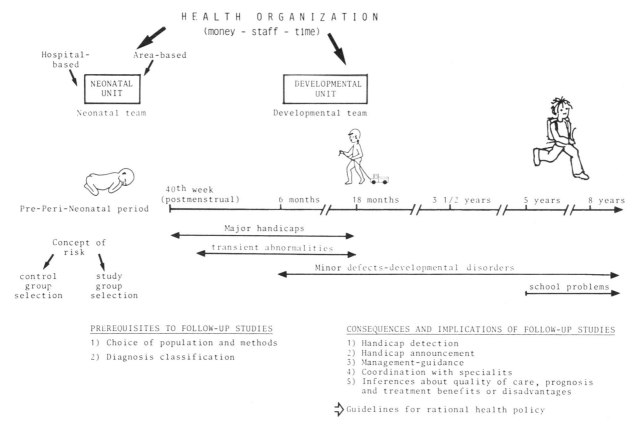

Fig. 5.1 Follow-up programme in the health organization.

*'Now, thanks to the discovery of disinfection and technical progress, the obstetrician freed of his anxiety concerning the mother's fate, can attend to the needs of the newborn infant.'

(Budin 1907). Thereafter, management of the newborn and fetus can be reported in several phases as described by some authors (Davies 1976, Silverman 1977, Hack et al 1979, Stewart et al 1981, Calame 1983). These phases are represented on the upper part of Figure 5.2. Results of follow-up studies, summarized in the lower part of the figure, reflect true gains due to successive improvements in neonatology and perinatology, as well as hazards, mistakes and iatrogenic complications. Neonatal history went through alternating periods of success and optimism, misadventures and scepticism, with economic and political involvement.

Up to 1940, neonatal care was confined to the control of environmental temperature and avoidance of infections. Mortality rate remained high. Long-term outcome was nevertheless fairly good, although numbers of survivors were very small (Hess 1953, Douglas & Gear 1976).

From 1940 to 1960, specific treatments were introduced, such as oxygen administration, exchange-transfusion and antibiotics. Methodology of follow-up studies of this second phase was mainly retrospective, entailing numerous biases in population selection and data collection. They nevertheless, showed alarming results and highlighted iatrogenic complications (Lubchenco et al 1963, Drillien 1964). Retrolental fibroplasia provided an invaluable lesson for all neonatologists. Its late diagnosis and the discovery of its aetiological mechanism is an example of an empirical treatment in neonatal care, without any control trial, resulting in long-term sequelae (McDonald 1963, Bolton & Gross 1974, Silverman 1977).

The third and fourth phases were marked by advances in obstetrics, fetal monitoring, neonatal management (mechanical ventilation, phototherapy, nutrition and drugs), better understanding in pathophysiology and improved health organization. The concept of risk was developed, categories of risk defined, as well as pre-, peri- and postnatal complications identified as being potentially responsible for later sequelae.

From 1970 onwards, methodology of follow-up studies changed. Authors adopted a prospective approach with greater rigour in methodology, data collection and study design. Follow-up investigations were set up to determine the short- and long-term prognoses of particular risk factors, such as very low birthweight, intra-uterine growth retardation and mechanical ventilation.

These studies showed that with concomitant improvement in both obstetrics and neonatology, decline in mortality rate and better quality of survival were observed (Rawlings et al 1971, Calame & Prod'hom 1972, Stewart et al 1978, 1981).

However, because of the lack of appropriate techniques, it was difficult at that time to establish a direct relationship between adverse events and a subsequent cerebral injury. The approach to the central nervous system was restricted to indirect methods (electro-encephalography, pneumo-encephalography, lumbar puncture) or to postmortem findings.

The fifth phase is characterized by the advent of brain imaging. Computerized tomography in 1977 and cerebral ultrasonography in 1979, made it possible for the first

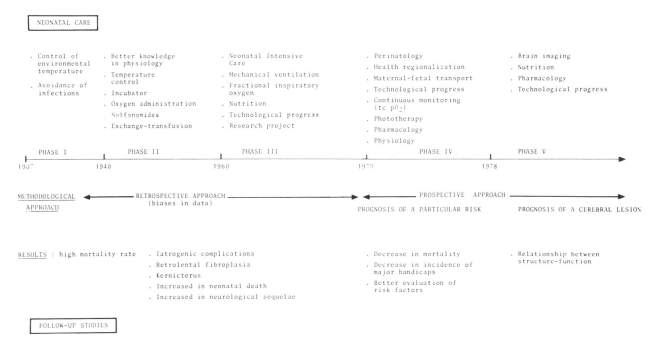

Fig. 5.2 Evolving phases of neonatal care and follow-up studies (1900–1986).

time to diagnose accurately cerebral lesions. The concept of risk changed entirely and was based on the absence or presence of a particular cerebral lesion. This implied again profound modifications in follow-up programmes, with new questions, new hypotheses and therefore new study design.

REVIEW OF THE LITERATURE

In an attempt to summarize the vast literature, the most recently published studies were selected and compiled in tables. The choice might appear arbitrary but data comparison is difficult and inferences about outcome perilous. There is indeed in all these studies wide disparity in methodology and in population selection and characteristics.

Neurodevelopmental outcome of infants weighing 1500 g or less at birth (VLBW infants)

In 1979, Jones et al reported that, despite increasing complexity of care, the neonatal mortality and the prevalence of major handicaps in VLBW babies did not significantly decrease over 15 years at Hammersmith Hospital in London. However, in the subsequent correspondence, several centres from both the UK and USA reported much improved neonatal mortality rates over corresponding periods of time (Lancet 1979, 1980).

In 1981, Stewart et al, in a survey of the world literature showed again that there was a decrease in mortality of VLBW infants between the years 1946 and 1977, with however, a stable and low handicap rate of 6–8% of VLBW live births since 1960. This paper again opened a passionate debate in the Lancet, illustrating the real difficulties in establishing the long-term prognosis of VLBW infants and in assessing the 'true' impact of neonatal intensive care on outcome (Lancet 1981a,b, 1982).

Hagberg et al (1984) in an epidemiological panorama of cerebral palsy over the 20-year-period 1959–78, reported that the incidence of cerebral palsy among VLBW infants surviving the first week of life did not change between 1963 and 1978.

The Neonatal Unit of Lausanne opened in 1966 and is the only reference centre for a geographically well-defined population of 600 000 inhabitants and 5000 deliveries per year. As most VLBW neonates are admitted to the unit, our conditions are very close to those of an area-based study. The outcome of VLBW babies from 1961 to 1985 is shown in Figures 5.3 and 5.4. Data are shown for different periods of time, corresponding to successive studies.

The overall incidence of major handicaps expressed as percentage of total VLBW live-born infants is shown in Figure 5.3. Results of periods 1961–5 and 1966–8 were retrospectively collected in 1970 after the opening of the Neonatal Intensive Care Unit. A marked decrease in the incidence of major handicaps was observed, although this

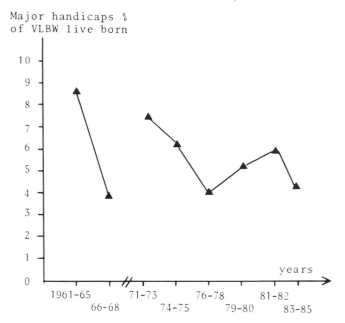

Fig. 5.3 Incidence of major handicaps among live-born VLBW infants between 1961 and 1985.

type of study is likely to be biased. Since 1971, VLBW infants have been prospectively followed-up. Over the years, there was a progressive reduction in major handicaps from 7.6% in 1971–3 to 4.2% in 1983–5.

Survival rate and evolving patterns of handicaps are shown in Figure 5.4.

Survival rate remained stable between 1961 and 1965. With the introduction of neonatal intensive care, survival

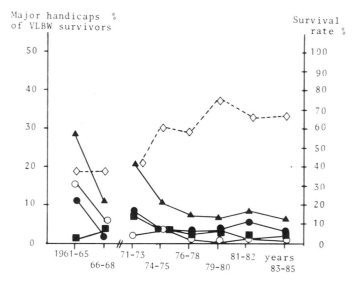

Fig. 5.4 Survival rate and incidence of major handicaps among surviving VLBW infants between 1961 and 1985. ▲ Major handicaps include cerebral palsy, mental retardation, severe visual impairment, severe sensory–neural hearing loss and are divided into the following subgroups: ● cerebral palsy, ○ cerebral palsy + mental retardation ± other major handicaps, ■ other major handicaps without cerebral palsy (i.e. blindness, deafness, mental retardation).

steadily increased to reach in the early 1980s a rate of about 70%.

The incidence of major handicaps, expressed as percentage of VLBW survivors (including neonatal and postnatal survivors) decreased from 21.9% in 1971–3 to 6.1% in 1983–5. Furthermore, the handicaps were found to be less severe over the years, as shown by the fall in the incidence of cerebral palsy and mental retardation and the incidence of other handicaps. Contrary to recently published data (Phelps 1980, Shohat et al 1983, Purohit et al 1985), severe and moderate retrolental fibroplasia have not been detected in our Unit by ophthalmologists since 1977, despite systematic examination in the neonatal period and in the first year of life.

As we are working in a privileged situation, close to a population study, our data strongly suggest that with increasingly sophisticated neonatal intensive care, there is a concomitant decrease in both mortality rate and incidence of major handicaps among VLBW infants over years.

Many centres from UK, USA and Australia have recently published their long-term outcome of VLBW infants. These studies are summarized in Table 5.2 (Stewart et al 1978, Jones et al 1979, Kitchen et al 1980, Steiner et al 1980, Peacock & Hirata 1981, Saigal et al 1982, Lloyd 1984, Ross et al 1985, Calame et al 1986b). Although there are wide variations in the periods of selection from the 1960s to the 1970s, in duration of follow-up and in survival rate (expressed in some studies as the neonatal survival rate or in others as the survival at discharge), the reported incidence of major handicaps, nevertheless, is relatively constant from one study to another and varies between 8.5 and 16.8%.

If there is general agreement to describe major handicaps, minor handicaps are subjected to variability in definition and methodology for their detection and age at testings. Their incidence ranges from 8.5 to 47%.

We assessed at 8 years of age the neurodevelopmental outcome and school performances of 50 AGA (appropriate for gestational age) and 33 SGA (small for gestational age)/VLBW infants, compared with a control group of 41 full-term neonates. Our results stressed the following points:

1. The overall incidence of major handicaps was similar to other reports (Stewart & Reynolds 1974, Kitchen et al 1980, Stewart et al 1981, Lloyd 1984), but the incidence and type of major handicaps were found to differ among SGA and AGA/VLBW. The latter group comprised more cerebral palsy and retrolental fibroplasia. Thus, gestational age and postnatal complications appeared to be predisposing risk factors to sequelae. It is therefore essential to specify gestational age and intra-uterine growth retardation when reporting outcome in VLBW studies.

2. As VLBW babies often come from disadvantaged backgrounds and are likely to present a high incidence of minor handicaps and poor school performances, a matched control group is of critical value in long-term follow-up, to minimize the influence of environmental

Table 5.2   Survival rate and neurodevelopmental outcome of very-low-birth-weight (VLBW) infants ≤1500 g

Reference and centre	Year of birth	No. VLBW (≤1500 g)	Survival rate (%)	Age at follow-up (months, years)	Survivors with neurodevelopmental handicaps Major/moderate (%)	Minor (%)
Stewart et al (1978) UCH London	1966–76	259	54	18 months–8 years	8.5	18
Jones et al (1979) Hammersmith	1961–75	357	41.5	2–17 years	13	14
Steiner et al (1980) King's Mill	1963–71	236	50.4	6–16 years	14	24
Kitchen et al (1980) Melbourne	1966–70	456	37	8 years	16	40
Peacock & Hirata (1981) San Francisco	1972–75	164	62	1–8 years	8.5	8.5
Saigal et al (1982) Hamilton	1973–78	294	62.6	2–5 years	16.8	17
Lloyd (1984) Wolverhampton	1975–79	159	58	3–7 years	14	22
Ross et al (1985) New York	1978–79	148	81	1–3 years	13	23
Calame (1986b) Lausanne	1972–76	179	58	8 years	12	47

and socio-economic factors. Our study demonstrated that VLBW infants and more particularly AGA/VLBW infants had more developmental disorders and more school failure compared with the control group. (Developmental disorders included fine and gross motor disorders, language, visuomotor disorders, and behavioural disturbances). School failure was most often related to the presence of several developmental disorders and also to isolated language disorders.

As developmental disorders and early school problems are likely to persist in young adulthood, resulting in lower academic attainment, lower social and professional status, only follow-up studies of longer duration will ascertain the long-term prognosis of VLBW infants.

Neurodevelopmental outcome of infants weighing less than 1001 g at birth

Over the last few years, a marked increase in the survival rate among the very-low-birth-weight and extremely-low-birth-weight infants has been reported (Cohen et al 1982, Bennett et al 1983, Hack & Fanaroff 1986). With such increasing survival capability, neonatologists became very concerned about the long-term outcome of these tiny babies. Few centres had, until recently, published their data, reporting a relatively high incidence of major handicaps. This has raised the ethical questions of justification of neonatal intensive care and limits of viability for intact survival (Schechner 1980, Britton et al 1981, Ruiz et al 1981, Yu et al 1985). Selected follow-up data are summarized in Table 5.3 (Stewart et al 1977, Yu & Hollingsworth 1979, Driscoll et al 1982, Buckwald et al 1984, Skouteli et al 1985, Calame et al 1986a).

As Dubowitz score (Dubowitz et al 1970) assessment has been established on a population of pre-term infants of a gestation greater than 27 weeks, a clinical evaluation

of gestation of very immature infants based on these criteria may therefore not be accurate. This could account for the disparity in results when comparing SGA and AGA immature infants and could also explain why most data are presented in relation to birth weight rather than gestation.

The overall reported mortality rate remained very high, particularly among infants weighing less than 800 g (Bennett et al 1983). Results of neurodevelopmental outcome are variable, the incidence of major handicaps varying between 0% and 35%. A poor outcome was strongly associated with sepsis (Driscoll et al 1982), asphyxia (Britton et al 1981, Driscoll et al 1982), the infant's condition on arrival at the Neonatal Unit (Britton et al 1981), acidosis (Skouteli et al 1985), mode of delivery (Stewart et al 1977) and intra-uterine growth retardation (Worthington et al 1983).

Our own experience was marked by major changes in both fetal and neonatal management occurring in 1982, with the introduction of sequential cerebral ultrasonography. This technique has enabled us to assess regularly 'brain status' and thus to decide upon engaging or continuing intensive care (Calame et al 1986a). Characteristics of our population with regard to the periods 1978–81 and 1982–4 are given in Table 5.4. Birth weight, gestation, sex, race and AGA, SGA distributions are similar in both groups. Changes in care are illustrated by the increase in both percentage of infants born by caesarean section and percentage of ventilated infants. The neonatal mortality of inborn infants fell from 61.9 to 34.8%, whereas the mortality of outborns remains stable. There is also an impressive fall from 67 to 18% in the mortality among SGA infants between 1978–81 and 1982–4.

The neurodevelopmental outcome of the 32 survivors expressed by the Developmental Quotient (Griffiths) and Intellectual Quotient (Terman–Merrill) is good (Fig. 5.5). No infant had major handicap and quotients are all above 80. Eight (25%) children were found to have

Table 5.3   Survival rate and neurodevelopmental outcome of very-low-birth-weight (VLBW) infants <1001 g

Reference and centre	Year of birth	No. VLBW (<1001 g)	Survival rate (%)	Age at follow-up (months, years)	Survivors with neurodevelopmental handicaps	
					Major (%)	Minor (%)
Stewart et al (1977) UCH London	1966–75	148	32	15 months–8 years	7	15
Yu & Hollingsworth (1979) QVMC, Melbourne	1977–78	55	60	3–24 months	6	not reported
Driscoll et al (1982) Columbia, NY	1977–78	54	48	8–36 months	17	19
Buckwald et al (1984) Buffalo, NY	1977–81	145 (VLBW <800 g)	44	>1 year	35	22
Skouteli et al (1985) Hammersmith	1979–81	67	43	≤3 years	8	13
Calame (1986a) CHUV, Lausanne	1978–84	84	42	12 months–7 years	0	25

Table 5.4 Neonatal data and mortality in very-low-birth-weight (VLBW) infants <1001 g in the Neonatal Unit of Lausanne (1978–1984)

Patients	1978–1981 (n=42)	1982–1984 (n=42)	Total (n=84)
Birth weight (g) (x̄ ± 1SD)	869 ± 104	877 ± 99	873 ± 101
Gestational age (weeks) (x̄ ± 1SD)	28.2 ± 2.3	28 ± 2.4	28 ± 2.4
Birth weight ≤750 g	5 (11.9%)	6 (14.3%)	11 (13.1%)
SGA infants	9 (21.4%)	11 (26.2%)	20 (23.8%)
Boys/girls	22/20	25/17	47/37
Caesarian section	9 (21.4%)	16 (38.1%)	25/84
Ventilated (IPPV)	6 (14%)	19 (45%)	25/84
Neonatal mortality	27 (64.3%)	22 (52.4%)	49 (58.3%)
Death (BW ≤750 g)	3/5	6/6	9/11
Death (25–27 weeks)	16/21 (76.2%)	15/22 (68.2%)	34/43 (72.1%)
Death (SGA)	6/9 (66.7%)	2/11 (18.2%)	8/20 (40%)

minor handicaps and developmental disorders. Most of them presented the association of clumsiness, language disorders and myopia. It is important to detect these developmental problems as they were found to be associated in very-low-birth-weight infants with early school failure.

Most interesting are the ultrasound findings among survivors. Of the 17 survivors of the period 1982–4, 11 developed only small cerebral lesions (grade I and II haemorrhages with or without small lesions of periventricular leukomalacia). On the contrary, death was always associated

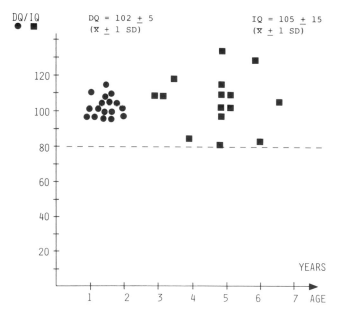

Fig. 5.5 DQ (Griffiths) and IQ (Terman-Merrill) distributions of children weighing less than 1001 g.

with extensive cerebral lesions (see p. 141 for the definitions of ultrasound abnormalities).

In summary, mortality rate is still very high among extremely-low-birth-weight and immature infants. The prognosis in our study is rather good, as no major handicap is diagnosed, the number of survivors being nevertheless small. However, the incidence of neurodevelopmental disorders is high.

Since 1982, the following recommendations have been adopted in our Perinatal Unit and they define our current policy towards these immature infants:

1. early identification of high-risk pregnancies;
2. early maternal transfer;
3. choice of optimal timing and mode of delivery;
4. continuity in the management of the fetus and newborn in the Perinatal Unit;
5. immediate and vigorous resuscitation and neonatal intensive care involvement;
6. early and regular neurological assessment.

This last encompasses clinical examination, sequential ultrasonography and electro-encephalography. If the assessment demonstrates strong evidence of extensive brain damage, together with iso-electric or paroxysmal EEG, intensive care will be withdrawn after a reappraisal of the risk factors and the infant's conditions in a multidisciplinary discussion involving medical and nursing staff. Gestational age, course of pregnancy, the state of the infant at birth, the timing and presence of complications, the ultrasound and EEG findings and the family circumstances are reviewed with the greatest care. Doctors and nurses should be convinced that the option of withdrawing intensive care is in the best interest of the infant and the family. Such a decision should not be hasty nor arbitrary and should leave time for reflection and to prepare parents for bereavement.

Neurodevelopmental outcome of small-for-gestational-age infant

The population of small-for-gestational-age infants is a heterogeneous one, with multiple causes. The diagnosis of small-for-gestational-age (SGA) is usually made at birth on the basis of birth weight charts (Lubchenco et al 1966, Gruenwald 1966, Usher & McLean 1969, Tanner & Thomson 1970). Most follow-up studies distinguish between full-term and pre-term SGA infants. They also exclude chromosomal disorders, congenital infections and anomalies, conditions that are known to account for long-term sequelae as well as growth retardation. Throughout the last two decades, major surveys and careful studies have been performed, with regular reappraisal of SGA outcome (Drillien 1970, Neligan et al 1976, Allen 1984). An extensive review of the literature would be illusory. A few studies are presented in Table 5.5 (Fitzhardinge & Steven 1972, Francis-Williams & Davies 1974, Neligan et al 1976,

Table 5.5 Survival rate and neurodevelopmental outcome of small-for-gestational age (SGA) infants

Reference and centre	Year of birth	No. SGA pre-term	No. SGA full-term	Survival rate (%)	Age at follow-up (years)	Survivors with neurodevelopmental handicaps		
						Major (%)	Minor (%)	Low IQ (%)
Fitzhardinge & Steven (1972) Montréal	1960–66	–	96	98.5	4–8	7.3	17	25 (SGA Boys IQ<90)
Francis-Williams & Davies (1974) Hammersmith	1961–68	–	+33§	nr	5–8	?	21.9*	15 (IQ<70)
Neligan et al (1976) Newcastle	1960–62	–	337	nr	5–7	0.6		
Commey & Fitzhardinge (1979) Toronto	1974–75	109	–	75	2	21	28	–
Hack et al (1979) Cleveland	1975–76	43	–	nr	2	21	–	–
Calame et al (1981) Lausanne	1971–75	–	25	nr	5	0	16	5 (IQ<80)
Low et al (1982) Kingston	–	–	76	nr	1–5	0	25	6.6 (IQ<85)
Winer et al (1982) New York	1973–76	–	+55§	nr	4–7	9	20	–
Calame (1983) Lausanne	1971–75	110	–	88	5	8.5	28.2	5.6 (IQ<80)
Vohr & Oh (1983) Providence	1975–76	21	–	nr	5	14	26	5 (IQ<80)
Westwood et al (1983) Montréal	1960–66	–	33	nr	13–19	0	†	

*Performance IQ <verbal IQ
†Verbal arithmetic scale lower compared with control children
nr = not reported
§No distinction between pre-term and full-term infants

Commey & Fitzhardinge 1979, Hack et al 1979, Calame et al 1981, 1983, Winer et al 1982, Low et al 1982, Vohr & Oh 1983, Westwood et al 1983). Again methodologies differ, classifications of handicaps, IQs, minor defects and neurodevelopmental disorders are not uniform or even not reported.

The following conclusions can nevertheless be drawn:

1. There is general agreement in most studies to describe a very low incidence of major handicaps in SGA full-term infants, with however, an increased risk of minor handicaps including minor defects, neurodevelopmental disorders and school failure.
2. The prognosis of SGA pre-term infants is far less clear and results are controversial; pathogenesis of sequelae is not yet fully understood as both prematurity and growth retardation can account for these.
3. SGA pre-term infants appear to have a higher incidence of major and minor handicaps compared with SGA full-term infants.
4. School performances and comparison with AGA pre-term infants are rarely reported.

In the Lausanne study, the incidence of major handicaps was lower (6%) in the SGA pre-term infants compared with the AGAs (16%) of similar birth weight. The types of handicap were different. Neurodevelopmental disorders were frequent in both groups, whereas school failure occurred less commonly in the SGA infants. As AGA pre-term infants were less mature (mean gestational age ± 1 SD: 29.9 weeks ± 1.4) than the SGA pre-term infants (mean gestational age ± 1 SD: 34.6 weeks ± 1.9), the poorer outcome of the AGA pre-term infants ought to be ascribed to gestational age and postnatal complications. In the SGA infants, the degree of prematurity is certainly an additional adverse risk factor, which should not be neglected when assessing outcome of small-for-gestational-age infants.

Asphyxia

Over the years, the clinical concept of asphyxia has varied in its definition, classification and incidence, as have inferences about its outcome. Most of our knowledge has been based on experimental data. However, a wide variety of techniques and assessments have been developed to establish in the neonatal period reliable criteria for the prediction of neurological sequelae. Outcome is discussed in detail in Chapter 34.

Neurodevelopmental outcome in relation to ultrasonographic appearances

Haemorrhage, ventricular dilatation and periventricular leukomalacia

Since 1979, real-time ultrasonography has been used in many Units as a research tool. It has now become an invaluable routine procedure. If its validity for the diagnosis of intracerebral haemorrhage has been rapidly recognized by most centres, its use for the detection of periventricular leukomalacia (PVL) has been much more controversial. However, with careful correlation studies between ultrasound appearances consistent with PVL and postmortem observations, the accurate diagnosis of PVL has recently been achieved (Levene et al 1985a). To evaluate the effect of cerebral lesions on neurodevelopmental outcome, numerous follow-up studies have been set up and some of them reported (Table 5.6) (Palmer et al 1982, Shankaran et al 1982, Stewart et al 1983, Bowerman et al 1984, McMenamin et al 1984, Catto-Smith et al 1985, De Vries et al 1985, Dubowitz et al 1985, Fawer et al 1985, 1986b, Weindling et al 1985, Calvert et al 1986).

Table 5.6   Neurodevelopmental outcome of infants with cerebral lesions diagnosed by ultrasonography

Reference and centre	Year of birth	Population*	Followed-up (n)	Age at testings (months)	MHz	Ultrasound diagnosis	Outcome (%)		Predictor for poor outcome
Palmer et al (1982) London	1979–80	<34 w	39	12	5	Normal IVH IVH + dilatation	0 0 60	Major handicaps	Ventricular dilatation
Shankaran et al (1982) Detroit	1979–80		32	6–18	5	Mild PVH + IVH Moderate PVH + IVH Severe PVH + IVH	0 53 90	Abnormalities	Parenchymal haemorrhage
Stewart et al (1983) London	1979–80	<33 w ≤1250 g ventilated	109	16–23	5 7	Normal Uncomplicated PVH Enlarged ventricles	8 8 71	Abnormalities	Cerebral ischaemia and infarction
McMenamin et al (1984) St Louis		460–2250 g	56	8–24	5	Small IPE Large IPE	30 100	Major handicaps	Large IPE
Bowerman et al (1984) Michigan			6		5	PVL	100	Major handicaps	PVL
Fawer et al (1985) Lausanne	1982–83	≤34 w	54	12	7.5	Normal Isolated PVH Associated lesions	0 0 33		PVL
Catto-Smith et al (1985) Melbourne	1981	23–28 w	31	24	5	Normal GLH IVH ICH	9 25 67 100	Major handicaps	Extensive periventricular haemorrhage
Dubowitz et al (1985) London		30–31 w	3	18	5 7	PVL	100	Major handicaps	PVL
Weindling et al (1985) Oxford	1982–83	<1500 g <34 w	8	12–18	7.5	PVL	100	Major handicaps	Periventricular cysts
De Vries et al (1985) London	1982–85	≤34 w	25	6–18	5 7.5	Large PVH PVL	11 100	Major handicaps	Severe cystic PVL
Calvert et al (1986) Toronto	1981–84	<1500 g	8	12–18	7.5	PVL	100	Major handicaps	Periventricular cysts
Fawer et al (1986) Lausanne	1982–83	≤34 w	82	18	7.5	Normal Isolated PVH Posthaemorrhagic hydrocephalus PVL	0 0 0 33	Major handicaps	Echogenic and cystic lesions of PVL

*w = gestational weeks
IVH, intra-ventricular haemorrhage; PVH, periventricular haemorrhage; IPE, intraparenchymal echodensity; GLH, germinal layer haemorrhage; PVL, periventricular leukomalacia, ICH, intracerebral haemorrhage

Conflicting conclusions have been drawn on the predictive value of cerebral ultrasound. Such disparity and controversy in results may be explained by differences in populations studied and variations in classifications of ultrasound abnormalities. Ultrasonographic definitions have been regularly modified, together with technological advances, the availability of high-frequency transducer, timing of scannings and investigators' experience.

Ventricular dilatation was firstly incriminated for poor outcome (Pape et al 1979, Palmer et al 1982). Then, with improved descriptions of periventricular haemorrhage, subsequent studies showed that small haemorrhages tended to have a good prognosis, while parenchymal or massive intraventricular haemorrhages were likely to be associated with major handicaps (Shankaran et al 1982, Stewart et al 1983, McMenamin et al 1984, Catto-Smith et al 1985). The identification of PVL among survivors has prompted several authors to publish case-reports (Hill et al 1982, Dolfin et al 1984, Dubowitz et al 1985, Weindling et al 1985, Calvert et al 1986). Periventricular leukomalacia and more particularly the cystic lesions appeared to be the best predictors for later major handicap.

The Lausanne study suggested that a better prediction of neurodevelopmental outcome can be based on a careful description of ultrasonographic changes consistent with PVL (Fawer et al 1986a). Emphasis is given to regular scanning and reports of both echogenic appearances of PVL as well as cystic formations. Both of these could be associated with major handicaps. A clear relationship between site and extent of the lesion and type and severity of the handicap can be demonstrated. Parietal involvement is likely to lead to motor dysfunction, occipital involvement to visual impairment and extensive lesions in the frontal, parietal and occipital regions to multiple handicap. These conditions are discussed in detail in Section 8.

ACKNOWLEDGEMENTS

We wish to thank Prof E. Gautier for his advice and support. We also thank P. Bernoulli, M. Marion and M. Michel for their help in preparing the manuscript. We are grateful to all the doctors, nurses and psychologists of the Neonatal and Development Units, who have been involved in this long drawn-out study; 15 years of hard work!

This work was supported by the Swiss National Science Foundation Nos 3.703-0.82 and 3.895-0.83 and by the Stanley Thomas Johnson Foundation, Berne, Switzerland.

REFERENCES

Allen M C 1984 Developmental outcome and follow-up of the small for gestational age infant. Seminars in Perinatology 8: 123–154

Amiel-Tison C 1976 A method for neurologic evaluation within the first year of life. Current problems in pediatrics, Vol III. Year Book Medical Publishers, Chicago, pp 1–50

Amiel-Tison C, Grenier A 1985 La surveillance neurologique au cours de la première année de vie. Masson, Paris

Baird G, Hall D M B 1985 Developmental paediatrics in primary care: what should we teach? British Medical Journal 291: 583–586

Bax M 1986 Perinatal care — success or failure? Editorial. Developmental Medicine and Child Neurology 28: 277–278

Bayley N 1969 Bayley scales of infant development. Psychological Corporation, New York

Bennett F C, Robinson N M, Sells C J 1983 Growth and development of infants weighing less than 800 grams at birth. Pediatrics 71: 319–323

Blishen B R 1965 The construction and use of an occupational class scale. In: Blishen B R, Jones S E, Neagele K D, Porter J C (eds) Canadian Society: Sociological perspectives. Macmillan, Toronto

Bolton D P G, Gross K W 1974 Further observations on cost of preventing retrolental fibroplasia. Lancet i: 445–448

Bowerman R A, Donn S M, DiPietro M A, D'Amato C J, Hicks S P 1984 Periventricular leukomalacia in the pre-term newborn infant: sonographic and clinical features. Radiology 51: 383–388

Boyle M H, Torrance G W, Sinclair J C, Horwood S P 1983 Economic evaluation of neonatal intensive care of very-low-birth-weight infants. New England Journal of Medicine 308: 1330–1337

Britton B S, Chir B, Fitzhardinge P M, Ashby S 1981 Is intensive care justified for infants weighing less than 801 gm at birth? Journal of Pediatrics 99: 937–943

Brown J K, Purvis R J, Forfar J O, Cockburn F 1974 Neurological aspects of perinatal asphyxia. Developmental Medicine and Child Neurology 16: 567–580

Buckwald S, Zorn W A, Egan E A 1984 Mortality and follow-up data for neonates weighing 500 to 800 g at birth. American Journal of Diseases of Children 138: 779–782

Budin P 1907 The nursling. Caxton Publishing Company, London

Butler N R, Alberman E D 1969 Perinatal problems: the second report of the 1958 British perinatal mortality survey. Churchill-Livingstone, Edinburgh

Butler N R, Bonham D G 1963 Perinatal mortality: the first report of the 1958 British perinatal mortality survey. Churchill-Livingstone, Edinburgh

Butler N R, Golding J, Dowling S, Howlett B From birth to five. Clinics in Developmental Medicine. Spastics Society, London (in press)

Calame A 1983 Etre prématuré: hier, aujourd'hui, demain. Revue Médicale de la Suisse Romande 103: 319–332

Calame A, Prod'hom L S 1972 Pronostic vital et qualité de survie des prématurés pesant 1500 gm et moins à la naissance soignés en 1966–1968. Schweizerische Medizinische Wochenschrift 102: 65–70

Calame A, Prod'hom L S, Van Melle G 1977 Outcome of infants of very low birthweight treated in neonatal intensive care unit. Revue d'Épidémiologie et de Santé Publique 25: 21–32

Calame A, Plancherel B, Jaunin L, Ducret S 1981 Les grandes hypotrophies foetales: devenir à moyen terme. XXVIe Congrès de Pédiatrie, Toulouse

Calame A, Ducret S, Jaunin L, Plancherel B 1983 High risk appropriate for gestational age (AGA) and small for gestational age (SGA) preterm infants. Helvetica Paediatrica Acta 38: 39–50

Calame A, Fawer C L, Anderegg A, Perentes E 1985 Interaction between perinatal brain damage and processes of normal brain development. Developmental Neuroscience 7: 1–11

Calame A, Fawer C L, Charpié-Dubrit M, Micheli J L, Arrazola L 1986a Devenir neuropsychologique à long terme des enfants avec un poids de naissance (PN) <1000 g. Progrès en Néonatologie 6. S. Karger, Bâle, pp 189–193

Calame A, Fawer C L, Claeys V, Arrazola L, Ducret S, Jaunin L 1986b Neurodevelopmental outcome and school performance of very-low-birth-weight infants at 8 years of age. European Journal of Pediatrics 145: 461–466

Calvert S A, Hoskins E M, Fong K W, Forsyth S C 1986 Periventricular leukomalacia: ultrasonic diagnosis and neurological outcome. Acta Paediatrica Scandinavica 75: 489–496

Camp B W, van Doorninck W J, Frankenburg W K, Lampe J M 1977 Preschool developmental testing in prediction of school problems. Clinical Pediatrics 16: 257–263

Casaer P 1979 Postural behaviour in newborn infants. Clinics in Developmental Medicine, No 72. SIMP/Heinemann, London

Catto-Smith A G, Yu V Y H, Bajuk B, Orgill A A, Astbury J 1985 Effect of neonatal periventricular haemorrhage on neurodevelopmental outcome. Archives of Disease in Childhood 60: 8–11

Chamberlain R, Chamberlain G, Howlett B, Claireaux A 1975 British births 1970: The first week of life, Vol 1. Heinemann, London

Chamberlain G, Philipp E, Howlett B, Masters K 1978 British births 1970: Obstetric care, Vol 2. Heinemann, London

Claeys V, Calame A, Fawer C L, Ducret S, Arrazola L, Jaunin L 1984 Neurodevelopmental abnormalities in preschool children with high perinatal risk. Helvetica Paediatrica Acta 39: 293–306

Cohen R S, Stevenson D K, Malachowski N et al 1982 Favorable results of Neonatal Intensive Care for very low-birth-weight infants. Pediatrics 69: 621–625

Commey J O O, Fitzhardinge P M 1979 Handicap in the preterm small-for-gestational age infant. Journal of Pediatrics 94: 779–786

Congalton A A 1963 Occupational status in Australia. Studies in Sociology, No 3. University of New South Wales, Sydney

Davie R, Butler N R, Goldstein H 1972 From birth to seven. Longman, London

Davies P A 1976 Infants of very low birth weight: an appraisal of some aspects of their present neonatal care and of their later prognosis. In: Hull D (ed) Recent advances in pediatrics. Churchill-Livingstone, London, pp 89–128

Department of Health and Social Security 1980 Arrangements for research and development. Written and oral evidence to Social Service Committee of House of Commons. In: Second report from the Social Services Committee. Perinatal and Neonatal Mortality, Vols IV, V. HMSO, London

De Vries L S, Dubowitz L M S, Dubowitz V et al 1985 Predictive value of cranial ultrasound in the newborn baby: a reappraisal. Lancet i: 137–140

Dolfin T, Skidmore M B, Fong K W, Hoskins E M, Shennan A T, Hill A 1984 Diagnosis and evolution of periventricular leukomalacia: a study with real time ultrasound. Early Human Development 9: 105–109

Douglas J W B, Gear R 1976 Children of low birth weight in the 1946 national cohort: behaviour and educational achievement in adolescence. Archives of Disease in Childhood 51: 820–827

Drillien C M 1964 The growth and development of the prematurely born infant. Churchill-Livingstone, Edinburgh

Drillien C M 1970 The small-for-date infant: etiology and prognosis. Pediatric Clinics of North America 17: 9–24

Drillien C M 1972 Abnormal neurologic signs in the first year of life in low-birthweight infants: possible prognostic significance. Developmental Medicine and Child Neurology 14: 575–584

Drillien C M, Drummond M B 1977 Neurodevelopmental problems in early childhood. Assessment and management. Blackwell, Oxford

Driscoll J M, Driscoll Y T, Steir M E et al 1982 Mortality and morbidity in infants less than 1,001 grams birth weight. Pediatrics 69: 21–26

Dubowitz L, Dubowitz V 1981 The neurological assessment of the preterm and full-term newborn infant. Clinics in Developmental Medicine, No 79. SIMP/Heinemann, London

Dubowitz L M, Dubowitz V, Goldberg C 1970 Clinical assessment of gestational age in the newborn infant. Journal of Pediatrics 77: 1–10

Dubowitz L M S, Bydder G M, Mushin J 1985 Developmental sequence of periventricular leukomalacia. Archives of Disease in Childhood 60: 349–355

Dunn H G 1986 Sequelae of low birthweight: the Vancouver Study. Clinics in Developmental Medicine, Nos 95/96. MacKeith Press, London with Blackwell Scientific, Philadelphia

Egbuonu L, Starfield B 1982 Child health and social status. Pediatrics 69: 550–557

Eksmyr R 1985 Two geographically defined populations with different organization of medical care. Comparison of perinatal risks. Acta Paediatrica Scandinavica 74: 855–860

Eksmyr R 1986 Two geographically defined populations with different organization of medical care. Cause-specific analysis of early neonatal deaths. Acta Paediatrica Scandinavica 75: 10–16

Eksmyr R, Eklund G 1985 Early neonatal deaths in geographically defined populations with different organization of medical care. Acta Paediatrica Scandinavica 74: 848–854

Ellison P H 1984 Neurologic development of the high-risk infant. Clinics in Perinatology, 11(1): 41–58

Falkner F 1984 Prevention of perinatal mortality and morbidity. In: Manciaux M (ed) Child health and development. Karger, Paris, p 1–8

Fawer C L, Calame A, Furrer M T 1985 Neurodevelopmental outcome at 12 months of age related to cerebral ultrasound appearances of high risk preterm infants. Early Human Development 11: 123–132

Fawer C L, Calame A, Vaudaux B, Bammatter C 1986 Brain ultrasasonographic study in neonatal sepsis: new concepts of pathophysiology of cerebral damages and early developmental outcome. Pediatric Research 20: 1057

Fawer C L, Diebold P, Calame A 1986 Periventricular leukomalacia and neurodevelopmental outcome in preterm infants. Archives of Disease in Childhood 62: 30–36

Fitzhardinge P M, Steven E M 1972 The small-for-date infant. II. Neurological and intellectual sequelae. Pediatrics 50: 50–57

Fitzhardinge P M, Pape K, Arstikaitis M et al 1976 Mechanical ventilation of infants less than 1501 grams birth weight: health, growth and neurologic sequelae. Journal of Pediatrics 88: 531–541

Fitzhardinge P M, Kalman E, Ashby S et al 1978 Present status of the infant of very low birth weight treated in a referral neonatal intensive care unit in 1974. Ciba Foundation Symposium 59: 139–144

Francis-Williams J 1976 Early identification of children likely to have specific learning difficulties: report of a follow-up. Developmental Medicine and Child Neurology 18: 71–77

Francis-Williams J, Davies P A 1974 Very low birthweight and later intelligence. Developmental Medicine and Child Neurology 16: 709–728

Frankenberg W K, Dodds J B 1968 The Denver developmental screening test. University of Colorado Press, Denver

Furrer M T, Calame A, Ducret S, Jaunin L, Arrazola L 1984 Anomalies transitoires du tonus et de la posture durant la première année de vie: devenir en âge scolaire. Helvetica Paediatrica Acta 50 (suppl): 27

Gesell A, Amatruda C S 1947 Developmental diagnosis. Harper & Row, New York

Gesell A, Amatruda C S 1969 Developmental diagnosis. Harper & Row, New York

Gillberg C, Gillberg Ch 1983 Three-year follow-up at age 10 of children with minor neurodevelopmental disorders. I: Behavioral problems. Developmental Medicine and Child Neurology 25: 438–449

Gillberg C, Gillberg Ch 1983 Three-year follow-up at age 10 of children with minor neurodevelopmental disorders. II: School achievement problems. Developmental Medicine and Child Neurology 25: 566–573

Graffar M 1961 Etude sociale des échantillons en croissance et développement de l'enfant normal. In: F Falkner (ed) 28. Masson, Paris

Grant W M, Boelsche A R, Zin D 1973 Developmental patterns of two motor functions. Developmental Medicine and Child Neurology 15: 171–177

Griffiths R 1970a The abilities of babies. University of London Press, London

Griffiths R 1970b The abilities of young children. Young, Chard, Somerset

Grossman H J et al 1973 Manual on terminology and classification. American Association on Mental Deficiency, Washington

Gruenwald P 1966 Growth of the human fetus. I. Normal growth and its variation. American Journal of Obstetrics and Gynecology 94: 1112–1119

Hack M, Fanaroff A A 1986 Changes in the delivery room care of the extremely small infant (<750 g) Effects on morbidity and outcome. New England Journal of Medicine 314: 660–664

Hack M, Fanaroff A A, Merkatz I R 1979 The low-birth-weight infant: evolution of a changing outlook. New England Journal of Medicine 301: 1162–1165

Hagberg B, Scanner G, Steen M 1972 The dysequilibrium syndrome in cerebral palsy. Acta Paediatrica Scandinavica 226 (suppl)

Hagberg B, Hagberg G, Olow I 1975 The changing panorama of cerebral palsy in Sweden 1954–1970. II. Analyis of various syndromes. Acta Paediatrica Scandinavica 64: 193–200

Hagberg B, Hagberg G, Olow I 1982 Gains and hazards of intensive neonatal care: an analysis from Swedish cerebral palsy epidemiology. Developmental Medicine and Child Neurology 24: 13–19

Hagberg B, Hagberg G, Olow I 1984 The changing panorama of cerebral palsy in Sweden. IV. Epidemiological trends 1959–78. Acta Paediatrica Scandinavica 73: 433–440

Hall D M B, Baird G 1986 Developmental tests and scales. Archives of Disease in Childhood 61: 213–215

Hart H, Bax M, Jenkins S 1978 The value of a developmental history. Developmental Medicine and Child Neurology 20: 442–452

Hess J H 1953 Experiences gained in a thirty year study of prematurely born infants. Pediatrics 11: 425–434

Hill A, Melson G L, Clark H B, Volpe J J 1982 Hemorrhagic periventricular leukomalacia: diagnosis by real time ultrasound and correlation with autopsy findings. Pediatrics 69: 282–284

Hollingshead A B 1975 Four factor index of social status, working paper. Yale University, New Haven

Holmes G, Rowe J, Hafford J, Schmidt R, Testa M, Zimmerman A 1982 Prognostic value of the electroencephalogram in neonatal asphyxia. Electroencephalography and Clinical Neurophysiology 53: 60–72

Holt K S 1977 Developmental paediatrics: perspectives and practice. Postgraduate Paediatrics Series. Butterworths, London

Horwood S P, Boyle M H, Torrance G W, Sinclair J C 1982 Mortality and morbidity of 500- to 1,499-gram birth weight infants live-born to residents of a defined geographic region before and after neonatal intensive care. Pediatrics 69: 613–620

Illingworth R S 1975 The development of the infant and young child, normal and abnormal, 6th edn. Churchill-Livingstone, Edinburgh

Ingram T T S 1964 Definition and classification of cerebral palsy. In: Paediatric aspect of cerebral palsy. Churchill-Livingstone, Edinburgh

Jones R A K, Cummins M, Davies P A 1979 Infants of very low birthweight: a 15-year analysis. Lancet i: 1332–1335

Kiely J L, Paneth N 1981 Follow-up studies of low-birthweight infants: suggestions for design, analysis and reporting. Developmental Medicine and Child Neurology 23: 96–99

Kiely J L, Paneth N, Stein Z, Susser M 1981 Cerebral palsy and newborn care. I. Secular trends in cerebral palsy. Developmental Medicine and Child Neurology 23: 533–537

Kiely J L, Paneth N, Stein Z, Susser M 1981 Cerebral palsy and newborn care. II. Mortality and Neurological impairment in low-birthweight infants. Developmental Medicine and Child Neurology 23: 650–659

Kitchen W H, Ryan M M, Rickards A et al 1980 A longitudinal study of very low birthweight infants. IV. An overview of performance at eight years of age. Developmental Medicine and Child Neurology 22: 172–188

Knobloch H, Pasamanick B, Sherard E S 1966 A developmental screening inventory for infants. Pediatrics 38: 1095–1108

Lancet 1979 ii: 36, 254, 255, 362, 523

Lancet Editorial 1980 The fate of the baby under 1501 g at birth 1: 461–463

Lancet 1981a i: 1415

Lancet 1981b ii: 194, 527, 1052, 1162

Lancet 1982 i: 281

Largo R H et al 1986 Language development of term and preterm children during the first five years of life. Developmental Medicine and Child Neurology 28: 333–350

Levene M I, Williams J L, Fawer C L 1985 Ultrasound of the infant brain. Chap 6 Clinics in Developmental Medicine, No 92. SIMP/Blackwell (UK)/Lippincott (US), London, pp 76–92

Levene M I, Williams J L, Fawer C L 1985 Ultrasound of the infant brain. Clinics in Developmental Medicine, No 92. SIMP/Blackwell (UK)/Lippincott (US), London, pp 110–117

Lipp-Zwahlen A E, Deonna T, Micheli J L, Calame A, Chrzanowski R, Cêtre E 1985 Prognostic value of neonatal CT scans in asphyxiated term babies: low density score compared with neonatal neurological signs. Neuropediatrics 16: 209–217

Lloyd B W 1984 Outcome of very-low-birthweight babies from Wolverhampton. Lancet ii: 739–741

Low J A, Galbraith R S, Muir D, Killen H, Pater B, Karchmar J 1982 Intrauterine growth retardation: a study of long-term morbidity. American Journal of Obstetrics and Gynecology 142: 670–677

Lubchenco L O, Horner F A, Reed L H et al 1963 Sequelae of premature birth: evaluation of premature infants of low birth weights at ten years of age. American Journal of Disease of Children 106: 101–115

Lubchenco L O, Hansman C, Boyds E 1966 Intrauterine growth in length and head circumference as estimated from live births at gestational ages from 26–42 weeks. Pediatrics 37: 403–408

McCarthy D 1972 Manual for the McCarthy scales of children's abilities. Psychological Corporation, New York

McCarthy J, Koops B, Honeyfield P et al 1979 Who pays the bill for neonatal intensive care? Journal of Pediatrics 95: 755–761

McDonald A D 1963 Cerebral palsy in children of very low birth weight. Archives of Disease in Childhood 38: 579–588

McMenamin J B, Shackelford G D, Volpe J J 1984 Outcome of neonatal intraventricular hemorrhage with periventricular echodense lesions. Annals of Neurology 15: 285–290

Matile P A, Calame A, Plancherel B 1984 Valeur pronostique du status neuro-développemental durant la première année de vie chez les enfants à risque périnatal élevé. Helvetica Paediatrica Acta 39: 449–462

Medical Research Council 1980 Written and oral evidence to Social Services Committee of House of Commons. In: Second report from the Social Services Committee. Perinatal and Neonatal Mortality, Vol IV. HMSO, London

Michelsson K 1982 Un examen de dépistage du développement neurologique des enfants de 5 ans. Médecine et Hygiène 40: 3657–3664

Neligan G, Prudham D 1969 Potential value of four early developmental milestones in screening children for increased risk of later retardation. Developmental Medicine and Child Neurology 11: 423

Neligan G A, Kolvin I, Scott D M et al 1976 Born too soon or born too small. A follow-up study to seven years of age. Clinics in Developmental Medicine, No 61. JB Lippincott, Philadelphia

Nelson K B, Ellenberg J H 1984 Obstetric complications as risk factors for cerebral palsy or seizure disorders. Journal of the American Medical Association 251: 1843–1848

Nelson K B, Ellenberg J H 1986 Antecedents of cerebral palsy. Multivariate analysis of risk. New England Journal of Medicine 315: 81–86

Newns B, Drummond M F, Durbin G M, Culley P 1984 Costs and outcomes in a regional neonatal intensive care unit. Archives of Disease in Childhood 59: 1064–1067

Ozeretski N 1936 L'échelle métrique du développement de la motricité chez l'enfant et chez l'adolescent. Hygiène Mentale 3: 3–75

Paine R S, Oppé T E 1966 Neurological examination of children. Clinics in Developmental Medicine, Nos 20/21. Spastics Society/Heinemann, London

Palmer P, Dubowitz L M S, Levene M I, Dubowitz V 1982 Developmental and neurological progress of preterm infants with intraventricular haemorrhage and ventricular dilatation. Archives of Disease in Childhood 57: 748–753

Paneth N 1986 Birth and the origins of cerebral palsy. New England Journal of Medicine 315: 124–126

Paneth N, Kiely J L, Stein Z, Susser M 1981 Cerebral palsy and newborn care. III. Estimated prevalence rates of cerebral palsy under differing rates of mortality and impairment of low birthweight infants. Developmental Medicine and Child Neurology 23: 801–807

Pape K E, Blackwell R J, Cusick G et al 1979 Ultrasound detection of brain damage in preterm infants. Lancet i: 1261–1264

Papiernik E, Bouyer J, Dreyfus J et al 1985 Prevention of preterm births: a perinatal study in Haguenau, France. Pediatrics 76(2): 154–158

Peacock W G, Hirata T 1981 Outcome in low-birth-weight infants (750 to 1,500 grams): a report on 164 cases managed at Children's Hospital, San Francisco, California. American Journal of Obstetrics and Gynecology 140: 165–172

Peiper A 1928 Die Hirntätigkeit des Säuglings. Julius Springer, Berlin

Peiper A 1963 Cerebral function in infancy and Childhood. Springer, New York

Pharoah P O D, Alberman E D 1981 Mortality of low birthweight infants in England and Wales 1953 to 1979. Archives of Disease in Childhood 56: 86–89

Phelps D L 1980 Retinopathy of prematurity: an estimate of vision loss in the United States — 1979. Pediatrics 67: 924–926

Pomerance J, Ukrainski C, Ukra T et al 1978 Cost of living for infants weighing 1000 grams or less at birth. Pediatrics 61: 908–910

Purohit D M, Ellison R C, Zierler S, Miettinen O S, Nadans A S 1985 Risk factors for retrolental fibroplasia: experience with 3,025 premature infants. Pediatrics 76: 339–344

Raven J C 1948 The comparative assessment of intellectual ability. British Journal of Psychology 39: 12–19

Rawlings G, Reynolds E O R, Stewart A et al 1971 Changing prognosis for infants of very low birth weight. Lancet i: 516–519

Reynell J 1969 Reynell developmental language scales. National Foundation for Educational Research, Windsor

Ross G, Lipper E G, Auld P A M 1985 Consistency and change in the development of premature infants weighing less than 1,501 grams at birth. Pediatrics 76: 885–891

Ruiz M P, LeFever J A, Hakanson D O, Clark D A, Williams M L 1981 Early development of infants of birth weight less than 1,000 grams with reference to mechanical ventilation in newborn period. Pediatrics 68: 330–335

Rumeau-Rouquette C 1984 The French perinatal program: 'Born in France'. In: Manciaux M (ed) Child Health, Vol 3. Karger, Paris, pp 137–163

Saigal S, Rosenbaum P, Stoskopf B, Milner R 1982 Follow-up of infants 501 to 1,500 gm birth weight delivered to residents of a geographically defined region with perinatal intensive care facilities. Journal of Pediatrics 100: 606–613

Sainte-Anne Dargassies S 1966 Neurological maturation of the premature infant of 28 to 41 weeks' gestational age. In: Falkner F (ed) Human development. Saunders, Philadelphia, pp 306–325

Sainte-Anne Dargassies S 1972 Neurodevelopmental symptoms during the first year of life. I. Essential landmarks for each key age. Developmental Medicine and Child Neurology 14: 235–246

Saint-Anne Dargassies S 1972 Neurodevelopmental symptoms during the first year of life. II. Practical examples and the application of this assessment method to the abnormal infant. Developmental Medicine and Child Neurology 14: 247–264

Sainte-Anne Dargassies S 1977 Neurological development in full term and premature neonate. Elsevier/North-Holland/Excerpta Medica, Amsterdam

Schechner S 1980 For the 1980s: how small is too small? (Symposium on Neonatal Intensive Care). Clinics in Perinatology 7: 135–143

Shankaran S, Slovis T L, Bedard M P, Poland R L 1982 Sonographic classification of intracranial hemorrhage. A prognostic indicator of mortality, morbidity, and short-term neurologic outcome. Journal of Pediatrics 100: 469–475

Sheridan M 1968 Manual for the STYCAR hearing test. NFER, UK

Sheridan M 1969 Manual for the STYCAR vision test. NFER, UK

Sheridan M D 1973 Children's developmental progress. National Foundation for Educational Research, Windsor

Shohat M, Reisner S H, Krikler R, Nissenhorn I, Yassur Y, Ben-Sira I 1983 Retinopathy of prematurity: incidence and risk factors. Pediatrics 72: 159–163

Silverman W A 1977 The lesson of retrolental fibroplasia. Scientific American 236(6): 100–107

Sinclair J C, Torrance G W, Boyle M H, Horwood S P, Saigal S, Sackett D L 1981 Evaluation of neonatal intensive care programs. New England Journal of Medicine 305: 489–494

Skouteli H N, Dubowitz L M S, Levene M I, Miller G 1985 Predictors for survival and normal neurodevelopmental outcome of infants weighing less than 1001 grams at birth. Developmental Medicine and Child Neurology 27: 588–595

Social Services Committee 1980 Research, innovation and equipment. In: Second report from the Social Services Committee. Perinatal and Neonatal Mortality, Vol I. HMSO, London

Stanley F J 1979 An epidemiological study of cerebral palsy in Western Australia, 1956–1975. I. Changes in total incidence of cerebral palsy and associated factors. Developmental Medicine and Child Neurology 21: 701–713

Stanley F J, Hobbs M S T 1980 Neonatal mortality and cerebral palsy: the impact of neonatal intensive care. Australian Paediatric Journal 16: 35–39

Steiner E S, Sanders E M, Philipps E C K, Maddok C R 1980 Very low birthweight children at school age: comparison of neonatal management methods. British Medical Journal 281: 1237–1240

Stewart A L, Reynolds E O R 1974 Improved prognosis for infants of very low birth weight. Pediatrics 54: 724–735

Stewart A L, Turcan D M, Rawlings G, Reynolds E O R 1977 Prognosis for infants weighing 1000 g or less at birth. Archives of Disease in Childhood 52: 97–104

Stewart A, Turcan D, Rawlings G, Hart S, Gregory S 1978 Outcome for infants at high risk of major handicap. Ciba Foundation Symposium 59: 151–171

Stewart A L, Reynolds E O R, Lipscomb A P 1981 Outcome for infants of very low birthweight: survey of world literature. Lancet i: 1038–1041

Stewart A L, Thorburn R J, Hope P L, Goldsmith M, Lipscomb A P, Reynolds E O R 1983 Ultrasound appearance of the brain in very preterm infants and neurodevelopmental outcome at 18 months of age. Archives of Disease in Childhood 58: 598–604

Swyer P R 1984 Regionalization of perinatal care. In: Manciaux (ed) Prevention of perinatal mortality and morbidity. Child Health and Development. Karger, Paris, pp 90–109

Tanner J M, Thomson A M 1970 Standards for birthweight at gestational period from 32 to 42 weeks, allowing for maternal height and weight. Archives of Disease in Childhood 45: 566–569

Tenovuo A, Kero P, Piekkala P, Sillpanpää M, Erkkola R 1986 Advances in perinatal care and declining regional neonatal mortality in Finland, 1968–82. Acta Paediatrica Scandinavica 75: 362–369

Terman L M, Merrill M A 1961 Stanford Binet intelligence scale, 3rd edn. Harrap, London

Touwen B C L 1982 Die Untersuchung von Kindern mit geringen neurologischen Funktionsstörungen. Georg Thieme Verlag, Stuttgart

Usher R, McLean F 1969 Intrauterine growth of live born caucasian infants at sea level: standards obtained from measurements in 7 dimensions of infants born between 25 and 44 weeks of gestation. Journal of Pediatrics 74: 901–910

Vohr B R, Oh W 1983 Growth and development in preterm infants small for gestational age. Journal of Pediatrics 103: 941–945

Walker D J B, Feldman A, Vohr B R, Oh W 1984 Cost-benefit analysis of neonatal intensive care for infants weighing less than 1,000 grams at birth. Pediatrics 74: 20–25

Wechsler D 1944 The measurement of adult intelligence, 3rd edn. Williams & Wilkins, Baltimore

Wechsler D 1967 Manual for the Wechsler preschool and primary scale of intelligence. Psychological Corporation, New York

Weindling A M, Rochefort M J, Calvert S A, Fok T F, Wilkinson A 1985 Development of cerebral palsy after ultrasonographic detection of periventricular cysts in the newborn. Developmental Medicine and Child Neurology 27: 800–806

Westwood M, Kramer M S, Munz D, Lovett J M, Watters G V 1983 Growth and development of full-term nonasphyxiated small-for-gestational age newborns: follow-up through adolescence. Pediatrics 71: 376–382

Wilson J, Jungner G 1968 Principles and practice of screening for disease. Public Health Papers, No 34. WHO, Geneva

Winer E K, Tejani N A, Atluru V L, DiGiuseppe R, Borofsky L G 1982 Four-to-seven-year evaluation in two groups of small-for-gestational age infants. American Journal of Obstetrics and Gynecology 143: 425–429

World Health Organization 1978 Main findings of a comparative study of social and biological effects on perinatal mortality. World Health Statistic Quarterly 31: 74–83

World Health Organization 1980 International classification of impairments, disabilities and handicaps: a manual of classification relating to the consequences of disease. WHO, Geneva

Worthington D, Lowell D E, Grausaz P, Sobocinski K 1983 Factors influencing survival and morbidity with very low birth weight delivery. Obstetrics and Gynecology 62: 550–555

Yu V Y H, Hollingsworth E 1979 Improving prognosis for infants weighing 1000 g or less at birth. Archives of Disease in Childhood 55: 422–426

Yu V Y H, Bajuk B, Orgill A A, Astbury J 1985 Viability of infants born at 24 to 26 weeks gestation. Annals of the Academy of Medicine 14: 563–571

Imaging

Probably the greatest advance this century in neurology was the introduction of imaging techniques for visualization of the brain. Parallel advances in the field of obstetric imaging with ultrasound gave rise to serious study of both the structural and pathological anatomy of the developing brain. Ultrasound, computerized X-ray tomography and most recently magnetic resonance imaging provide the clinician and researcher with a powerful range of tools with which to assess the fetal or neonatal brain. This section reviews the role of these methods in providing information on both the normal and abnormal brain in terms of structure and function. It is clearly important for the clinician to choose the imaging modality best suited to the cerebral pathology he or she considers most likely and Chapters 8 and 9 discuss both the advantages and disadvantages of these techniques. Table 9.1 (p. 139) summarizes the most appropriate imaging technique for a variety of important pathological conditions occurring in the neonatal brain. This table must be read in conjunction with the discussions in Chapters 8 and 9.

6. Ultrasound evaluation of fetal neurology

Prof J. C. Birnholz

Ultrasonic studies of a human fetal nervous system have become progressively more sophisticated during the past decade. Initial clinical interest in detecting structural abnormalities has been refined and there is current work concerning normal developmental processes. Four types of ultrasound-derived information contribute to these studies:

1. detailed morphology of the skull, brain, spine and cord;
2. detailed morphology of the remainder of the fetus;
3. Doppler flow profiles of the carotid arteries, jugular veins and various intracranial vessels; and
4. neurobehavioural information from the type, incidence, and association of spontaneous and provoked movements.

These areas are also discussed elsewhere in this book. Although these topics are distinct from a didactic standpoint, they are pursued conjointly in the prospective evaluation. This chapter will emphasize composite results for normal development and for the specific problems of neural tube defect, hydrocephalus and dysmorphic brain development.

Instrumentation for evaluation of the fetal central nervous system must have contrast resolution that will, at least, discriminate cerebral cortex and cerebrospinal fluid in the second trimester (Fig. 6.1), despite the water content of the brain at that time (Wladimiroff et al 1975). Spatial resolution (for high-contrast targets) should be in the 0.5 to 1 mm range or better. The focal depth must be adjustable to suit the target, either with a range of single focus transducers or, optimally, a system with dynamic focusing capabilities. Performance is dependent principally upon the effective transducer aperture. For our own studies, we prefer an 80 to 100 wavelength (or longer) aperture with rectilinear scan format, although we will defer to smaller aperture sector scanning options in the later third trimester whenever fetal cranial position requires a physically small probe for positioning over a fontanelle or the foramen magnum. For dynamic studies, the scanning rate should be at least 24 Hz. Finally, it is quite important that there is a 'write' form of image magnification. The region of interest should be extended to fill the display surface, with the resultant increase in number of display pixels per tissue millimetre pertinent to both spatial and temporal resolution performance.

Ultrasonic images are two-dimensional. They are rich in data, which is acquired and updated at high speeds. There is a wide choice of scan planes and, as transducer orientation is changed and different path lengths, materials and target shapes are encountered, the instrument must be readjusted for optimal performance. Instrument operation and image interpretation are not yet separable functions. Consequently, the operator remains the crucial part of the system, particularly since the scope of the study is changed as imaging proceeds, observations are made and clinical, pathological, or pathophysiological possibilities are defined or excluded (Birnholz & Hayes 1987).

A final preliminary consideration is the 'philosophical' foundation for human fetal studies. It is easy to dismiss the fetus as an immature organism without neuromotor integrity or more than random activity. This has been the prevailing notion until the last few years. Preyer (1885) and Ahlfeld's (1905) attribution of movements transmitted through the maternal abdominal wall as fetal 'breathing' was thought a fantastic notion. Similarly, there was persistent controversy over whether it is hours, days or weeks after delivery that an infant hears (Peiper 1961), dismissing entirely the possibility that hearing and other sensory factors develop long before birth. Fetal studies, particularly those of the nervous system, which involve organizational considerations require an appreciation of the complexity and, perhaps, directivity of fetal development (see Ch. 2). As an organism, the fetus is adapted for an environment that is different from that of the postnatal world (Liley 1972). Human development includes many relatively abrupt transition phases, one of which is delivery from the uterine environment; however, there are minimal developmental differences between a fetus and an infant at the same age. Saint-Anne Dargassies (1979) refers to 'the fetus living in the incubator' versus 'the fetus observed in utero'. All of the central nervous system capabilities of the newborn infant appear and function prenatally. Fetal and

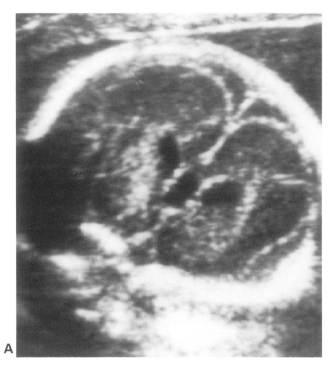

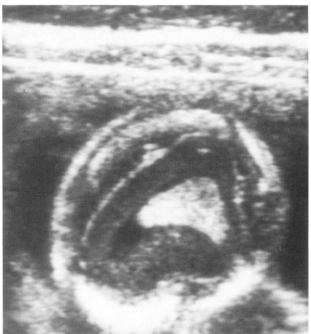

Fig. 6.1 (a) Coronal midcranial section at 20 weeks gestational age. The lateral ventricles and cavum septi pellucidi form the 'face' centrally. The mantle is thick but uniform in reflectivity, and the smoothness of the convexities is marred only by prominent surface vessels. (b) The mantle, cerebrospinal fluid and highly reflective choroid glomus are distinct. The choroid is situated posteriorly.

neonatal studies are fully complementary. The continuity of fetal and infant development was emphasized by Preyer (1885) long before survival of the small premature infant provided the direct observation making this concept axiomatic.

ASSESSMENT OF CNS DEVELOPMENT

The early ultrasound units showed the outline of the fetal skull and, consequently, observations of brain growth were limited to inferences from the size, shape and mineralization of the calvarium. When it became possible to visualize some intracranial structures, like the interhemispheric fissure, the brainstem or the thalamus, these were applied to refining the definition of cranial scan planes (Shepard & Filly 1982) so that measurements of the skull could be made with greater assurance and repeatability. The emphasis now has shifted to the brain itself (Fig. 6.1). We study the calvarium when the clinical problem appears to involve an abnormality of ossification. The same sequence of events has occurred with the spine. Initially, attention was limited to skeletal appearance (Fig. 6.2), while now we pursue examination of the membranes, cord and nerve roots (Fig. 6.3). Measurement standards more easily obtained for infants (Kawahara et al 1987) can be transposed to the fetal realm.

The transverse diameter of the skull is the 'classic' fetal ultrasound measurement, following some 40 years after radiographic determination and a hundred or more years after its use in pathology (Scammon & Calkins 1929). The transverse diameter (referred to universally as the biparietal diameter (BPD) but in practice usually representing a bitemporal path) was used for many years for staging fetal development. BPD charts are available for large, often ethnically defined or mixed, populations (Sabbagha 1979). We improve upon the use of a single diameter by taking an orthogonal measurement, e.g. the occipitofrontal diameter, or by working with the skull perimeter or cross-sectional area, to correct for moulding (Birnholz 1986b). Even so, the general experience is that these correlations with age are quite reasonable in the first half of pregnancy but become much less accurate in the third trimester. We assume that cranial growth is largely but not exclusively driven by cerebral development later in pregnancy. We surmise that timing of growth phases of the brain bears a direct relation to gestational age throughout pregnancy. Transcranial diameters provide information about the volumetric growth of the skull and its contents. The brain increases its volume monotonically in the first half of pregnancy, hence the observed correlation between gestational age and transcranial diameter during that part of development. Later, however, it is the increase in surface area with sulcation that becomes the predominant growth factor. Cranial diameters are insensitive to changes in brain surface area, hence the failure of that morphological clue for staging later in pregnancy.

One of the practical consequences of instrumentation advances in ultrasound has been the ability to visualize directly anatomical features of the developing brain (Birnholz 1986c). At all ages, the cortical mantle is distinguished from cerebrospinal fluid. The arachnoid boundary of the cerebral convexities and the margins of

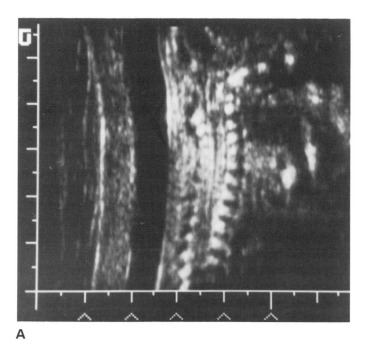
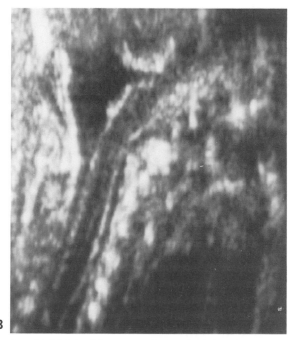

A

B

Fig. 6.2 (a) Sagittal view of the posterior neck emphasizes the skin border and the spine. (b) Slightly oblique, magnified sagittal view shows the cervical cord and medulla.

the lateral ventricles are distinct and the vascular choroid glomi are highly reflective internal landmarks.

Between 10 and 12 weeks gestational age the unossified cranial boundary is well defined, the mantle is small, the ventricles are relatively large, and they are filled almost entirely by choroid (Fig. 6.4). As the mantle grows after 12 weeks, the relative size of the ventricles becomes small. A slit-like cross-section in coronal views, typical of the full-term infant, is evident from 16 to 17 weeks (Fig. 6.1). There is some residual fullness of the frontal horns to around 18 weeks; while the occipital horns remain prominent to 26 weeks. These changes represent regional cortical growth differences.

We observed a linear increase in motor strip thickness from about 12 to 16 weeks gestational age; continued increase but with lesser velocity between 16 and 20 weeks; and an abrupt increase in thickness after 20 weeks (Birnholz & Farrell in preparation, Fig. 6.5). We believe that these phases correspond to neuronal proliferation, neuronal migration and glial proliferation (Sidman & Rakic 1973, Lou 1982).

We expect that growth disturbances affecting the brain during any of these second trimester phases will result in profound, probably unrecoverable, deficits. Low-dose radiation, possibly only deleting a single cell line, is associated with learning or behavioural disabilities, unmasked at three or more years of age (Gaulden & Murry 1980). We have identified two types of case with delayed cortical growth early in the second trimester. The first were cases of trisomy 21, with relative ventriculomegaly at 16 weeks gestational age due to a lag in the primary spurt of the cortex, no longer evident by 26 weeks. Necropsy studies

of infants with trisomy 21 have tended to show low brain weight with normal thickness of cortex but with regional decreases in neurone density (Wisniewski et al 1986). Decreased neuroblast proliferation and cortical thinning are also features of murine trisomy 16 (Oster-Granite et al 1986). The other form of deficit involved discordant-sized twins, one having severe placental vascular insufficiency due to velamentous insertion of a cord.

Concerning overall cortical thickness, it is important to consider that there is an initial 'over-production' of neurones and neural connections and that selective cell

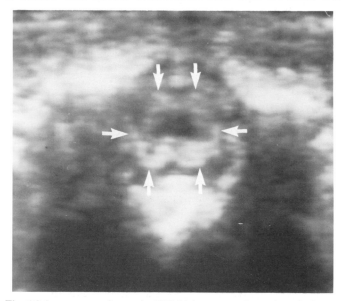

Fig. 6.3 A transverse view at the T10–11 interspace shows the spinal cord (arrows). Note the shape of the cord and the relative size of the central canal.

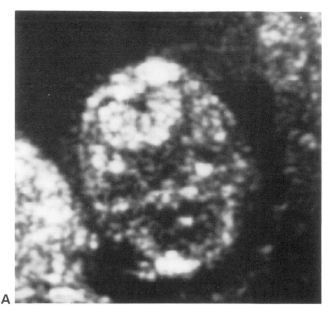

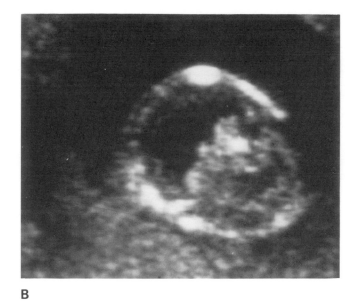

A **B**

Fig. 6.4 (a) Coronal view of a 14 mm wide cranium. The ventricles are filled with highly reflective choroid. This appearance can be seen from 9 weeks gestational age. (b) Holoprosencephaly with single, wide, fluid-filled ventricle; there is no choroid glomus anteriorly.

death is necessary for appropriate 'wiring' (Shatz & Kirkwood 1984). Cortical thickness may be maintained adventitiously with trisomy 21 by associated failures in this stage (Huttenlocher 1984). We have also seen cases of microcephaly with growth deficit beginning after 20 weeks gestational age, presumably reflecting decreased glial proliferation. The observations of Goldman-Rakic (1980) that localized prefrontal surgical lesions in fetal monkeys during a 'critical period' result in widespread distortion of gyration are particularly interesting. As Lewis & Patel (1979) have emphasized, there is an 'inflexible chronology of neurogenesis. A given nerve cell population is produced at a certain period of development, and if an adverse influence on acquisition were to be present on its 'birthday', its number might be permanently deleted with repercussion on the cellular make-up and functional capabilities of the brain regions inhabited.'

The corpus callosum (CC) is readily visualized in midline sagittal views (Fig. 6.6). It completes its structural formation as late as 20 to 21 weeks gestational age (Rakic & Yakovlev 1968). The overall length appears to increase linearly with fetal age after 17 weeks in a relationship described by CC – 1.568 GA – 12.32 (mm, weeks) (Birnholz in preparation). After formation, the ratio of corpus callosal length of cranial occipitofrontal diameter is about 0.45 (Davidson et al 1985). De Lacoste et al (1986) have shown a sex-related influence on callosal development.

Midline sagittal views also reveal either cingulate sulcus. These are short, faint and difficult to visualize at 24 weeks gestational age, penetrating less than a millimetre into cortex at that stage. Depth is best evaluated in coronal planes (Fig. 6.7). There is rapid increase in length and definition during the next 2 weeks and afterwards, there is progressive complexity in shape and branching (Fig. 6.8). Gyral patterning

has been related to fetal age (Larroche 1962, Chi et al 1977, Dorovini-Zis & Dolam 1977). Time standards of sulcation can be applied prognostically for cases sustaining perinatal asphyxial injury.

Hypo-echoic rims surround the major anterior sulci from about 30 weeks (Fig. 6.7). This is an additional developmental marker that probably represents changing cortical vascularity before myelination. This feature is also delayed with asphyxial injuries sustained in the first half of the third trimester and appears to predict the delayed myelination found in long-term follow-up of these infants when studied with nuclear magnetic resonance imaging (Johnson et al 1983).

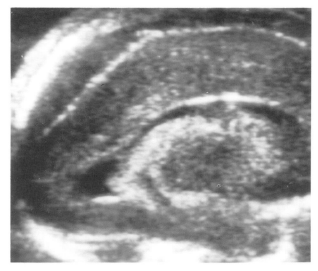

Fig. 6.5 Parasagittal view of cortex along the course of the right lateral ventricle at 20 weeks gestational age. While we prefer measurements of cortical thickness in coronal views, this plane permits direct comparison of different portions of the cortex.

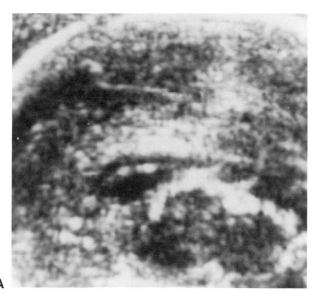

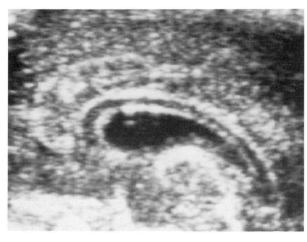

Fig. 6.6 Compare the incomplete corpus callosum at 18 weeks gestational age (a) with the fully formed structure at 24 weeks (b).

The issue of laterality is now amenable to further study. We have not observed any left–right differences in anterior coronal views in our studies of motor strip thickness but about 4% of cases at 26 weeks gestational age will have slight degrees of ventricular asymmetry, usually left slightly larger than right. The temporal gyri appear asymmetrically in a substantial portion of third trimester cases (Chi et al 1977). This may be difficult to utilize clinically with ultrasound because of ipsilateral image degradation when pulses traverse the meniscus-lens like temporal bone with typical base plane viewing. In two cases of identical twins, with comparable intra-uterine growth rates and uncomplicated neonatal courses, we observed differences in gyral pattern and in behavioural characteristics, chiefly in their social interactions (Birnholz 1986c). Sulcal thickening is also the earliest finding in infants with asphyxial injury progressing to atrophy.

The choroid glomi have not received a great deal of attention. They are a site of glycogen deposition and small glomi and poor outcome have been associated (Crade et al 1981). Small- to medium-sized cysts are seen in about 1 to 2% of early second trimester cases and usually regress spontaneously well before full-term. Small cysts, apparently with no developmental or clinical significance, are found occasionally elsewhere in ependymal tissue, typically at a boundary of the germinal matrix. These are to be distinguished from (solid) subependymal nodules that may be seen with tuberous sclerosis (Volpe 1986). The prenatal appearance of the choroid glomi is discussed in detail on p. 109.

Gestational age standards are available for transverse width of the cerebellum (McLeary et al 1984, and see p. 292), and for cross-sectional area of the mid-portion of the vermis (Birnholz 1982). Surface ridging of the cerebellum is seen earlier and it progresses more rapidly than sulcation of the cerebral hemispheres.

The ability to visualize the cord is new (Fig. 6.3), and detailed study of this portion of the nervous system remains to be undertaken. The reflectivity of the cervical cord is low, like that of the hemispheres. The cauda equina has a quite high reflectivity because of the composite backscattering of numerous braided nerve roots. Lack of tapering of the cauda equina predicts tethering (Fig. 6.9). The central canal at the thoracic level is large with the bulk of thickness growth at this level occurring postnatally.

We have been interested in morphological development of the eye as an indicator of overall cerebral development

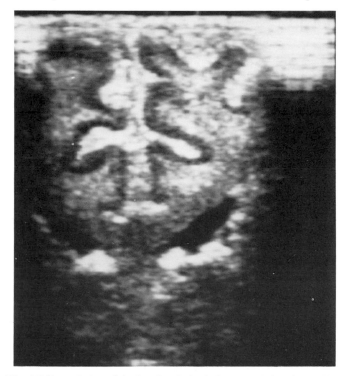

Fig. 6.7 Coronal view of the interhemispheric fissure and cingulate sulci. Each sulcus extends about 10 mm (into cortex) from the midline.

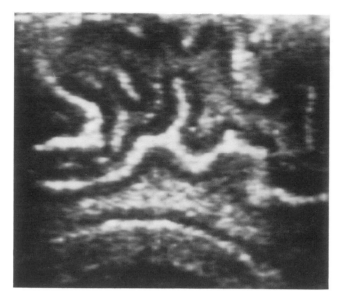

Fig. 6.8 The right cingulate sulcus is seen along its length; note the hypo-echoic border in this view and in Figure 6.7.

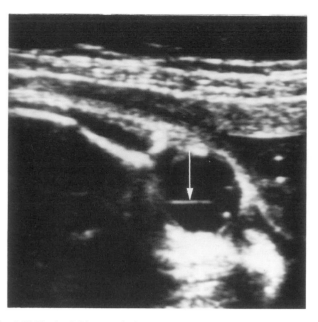

Fig. 6.10 The hyaloid artery is the central intra-ocular structure (arrow) bridging the retina (left) and lens (right).

(Birnholz 1985). Embryologically the eye derives from the forebrain. Its fluid content provides high acoustic contrast and the near-spherical shape facilitates measurement, which can be compared with infant standards (Scammon & Armstrong 1925, O'Rahilly & Bossy 1982). The lens can be seen from the early second trimester. The pupil is seen in some selected cases in the third trimester but is uniformly miotic because of absence of functioning sympathetic innervation (Lind et al 1971). An interesting feature of the mammalian eye is the presence of the hyaloid artery, (Fig. 6.10) which vascularizes the posterior lens early in development but which regresses spontaneously at about the time of potential extra-uterine viability (Ozaniks & Jakobiec 1982). Since the hyaloid artery is occasionally

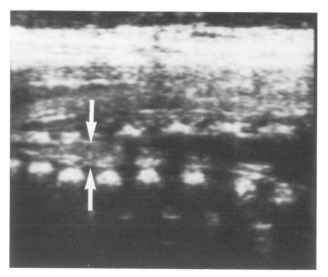

Fig. 6.9 Note how the filum terminale (arrows) expands to fill the distal canal. The proximal part of the cauda equina is unusually narrow in this case also.

found in healthy, full-term infants, persistence of this vessel can be a normal variation. We wonder, however, if delayed regression can be a marker of more general developmental retardation and we await eagerly correlations with long-term developmental and neurological assessment of infants with this antenatal finding. Persistence of a hyaloid artery to the mid-third trimester appears to be associated typically with trisomy 21. Vitreous diameter of volume measurements in the second and third trimesters increases with spurts and plateaux mirroring the cortical growth pattern. Clinical associations between relative microphthalmia and mental retardation are reiterated (Warburg 1971).

Pulsations of larger arteries are obvious during ultrasonic inspection when frame rates are 20 Hz or faster. The cerebellar arteries, the basilar and circle of Willis branch arteries and lateral portions of the middle cerebral arteries are all evident in base plane views of the cranium and coronal and sagittal views permit observation of the pericallosal, callosomarginal and other anterior cerebral branches. Visualization will, of course, depend upon cranial position and ossification. It is relatively easy to visualize the common carotid arteries and jugular veins within the neck at and below the level of the larynx. It is almost always possible to gain access to one side of the neck and in the majority of instances the two sides can be compared. Blood flow itself can be quantitated to some degree by using Doppler methods which acquire target velocity from measurement of the frequency shift that occurs when an acoustic pulse interacts with a moving structure (Figs. 6.11, 6.12). In this case, the 'moving targets' are the vessel wall and an ensemble average of intraluminal blood (see Ch. 11).

We determine volume flow within the umbilical vein routinely during our third trimester fetal examinations;

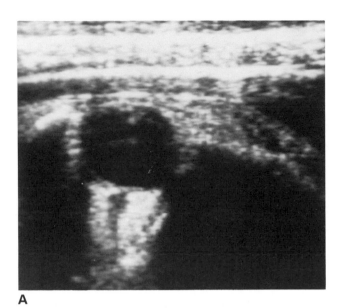
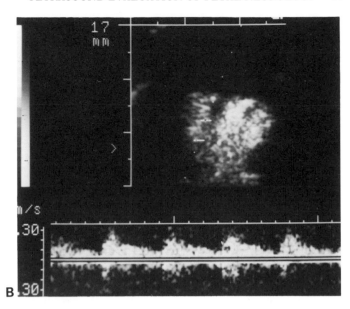

Fig. 6.11 (a) The optic nerve is less reflective than surrounding retro-orbital fat. (b) The Doppler window (upper panel) is aligned with the nerve, the tracing shows ophthalmic artery pulsations in a 2.6 second time interval.

however, this technique has not been exploited for quantitative cerebrovascular flow studies. These calculations can be performed for the jugular vein because of the size of the vessel and capability for achieving a 60 degree or less angle of incidence in most cases. However they may not be appropriate for the carotid arteries because of the smaller size and because of relatively large changes in the size of the lumen of these very flexible vessels during each pressure pulse cycle. An alternate stratagem is employed when angle of incidence of lumen area cannot be determined within a preset error level, which is to extract information from the shape, rather than the magnitude, of an arterial waveform (Griffin et al 1984). In many instances, the up-stroke of an arterial waveform relates to the pump properties of the heart; the width of the systolic peak may be related to blood viscosity, which in the fetus translates to the hematocrit; and the level of diastolic flow conveys information about the resistance downstream from the sampling site. A low-resistance vascular net, like the full-term infant brain after ductal closure, is associated with continued diastolic flow; moderately high resistance by absence of any diastolic flow; and a very high resistance by diastolic flow reversal. Such qualitative flow profiles can be obtained from most of the major intracranial arteries. This approach is used in detecting or grading asphyxial injury in newborn infants but it remains to be exploited as a research tool in the fetal realm, when diastolic components are relatively low. Dynamic survey of vascular anatomy refines antenatal (and neonatal) diagnoses of malformations, such as vein of Galen aneurysm.

FUNCTIONAL DEVELOPMENT

We infer functional information from motor behaviour.

This includes overt movements and covert mechanisms of control, co-ordination and rhythm. We will need to define activity norms for each gestational age and learn through experience which departures convey prognostically significant information. In later pregnancy, we are concerned additionally with recognizing the acute brain syndrome that occurs with fetal hypoxia, which requires prompt delivery.

Conventional ultrasound imaging is cross-sectional with depth. We can characterize movements that occur within a plane but not those that are three-dimensional. For example, we can describe fully movements of a lens

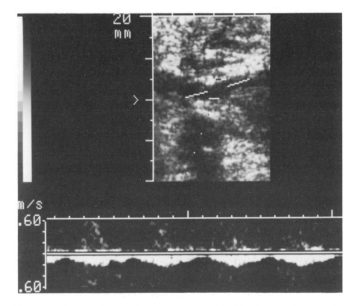

Fig. 6.12 The Doppler window traverses the right jugular vein, intersecting it at 55 degrees. Venous flow is intermittent (not continuous). Peak velocity here is about 0.12 m/s.

in coronal scan planes (Fig. 6.13), but we cannot be equally thorough in looking at the hands (Fig. 6.14). Motion-sensing fidelity varies greatly among different types of instrument. Important technical concerns are

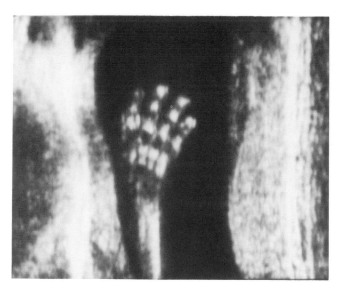

Fig. 6.14 The hands and their movements are not characterized fully with thin-section two-dimensional scan planes.

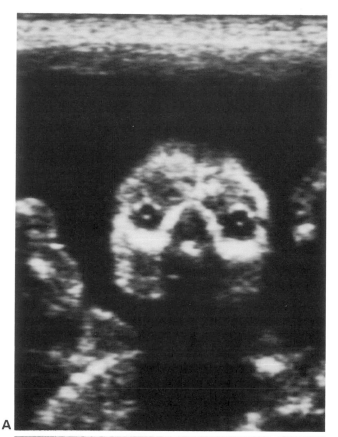

A

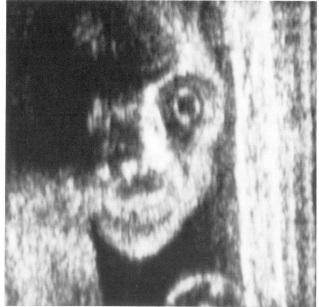

B

Fig. 6.13 (a) Both lenses are seen in this supra-orbital coronal view, which is usually only obtained in the second trimester with single fetuses. (b) A typical lateral coronal view shows one lens and permits complete description of lens movements.

the magnification factor (namely the number of display pixels per tissue millimetre), the beam focal pattern and the frame rate. For example, recent observations with large-aperture, dynamically focused equipment shows that diaphragm excursions are prevalent in the third trimester (Birnholz 1986a) with only brief phases of 'apnoea', while earlier studies concluded erroneously that fetal breathing movements were relatively infrequent (Patrick et al 1978).

Prior concepts of fetal activity tended to assume that fetal movements were 'reflex' patterns, while we now regard most activity as having intrinsic, central origin. The first body movements we observe are simple extensions of the trunk which are seen by the seventh postmenstrual week. The movement repertory at 8 to 10 weeks is quite limited, again being an active extension followed by slower return to rest position, usually elevating the fetus within its membranous bubble. Isolated movements of one limb are seen by 11 weeks, with arm movements recognized a week or more before those of a leg. These movements appear to be spontaneous, more or less random in timing. Normal fetuses do not exhibit a movement preference for right side or left. Chronologies of second trimester movement patterns are now becoming available (de Vries et al 1982).

Tonic–clonic seizure activity is an important observation. We have seen a few instances of such repetitive movements of one or both arms at 19 to 20 weeks gestational age which were absent later. We do not know yet if these children will show any predilection for seizure activity later. Ianniruberto & Tajani (1981) have observed these movements in a few cases of elective late second trimester termination after maternal diazepam (Valium) administration. Seizure-type movements occurring later in pregnancy are pathological. Seizure movements should, of course, be distinguished from repetitive forceful hiccups which are misinterpreted by some prospective mothers as 'seizures'. A particular type of seizure activity with poor long-term prognosis is small-amplitude, high-frequency pericentral eye movement. Coarse, large-amplitude bursts of eye movements, 'REM storms' also convey a poor prognosis (Beckert & Thomas 1981).

We have been concerned with the technical aspects of studying eye movements (Birnholz 1981). The majority of eye movements are transverse, occurring in an arc from the centre between 3 o'clock and 5 o'clock. Relatively slow, isolated eye movements are observed occasionally, as early as 14 weeks gestational age. During the mid-second trimester the eyes will often remain deviated before shifting to another location but by 19 to 20 weeks a more or less central rest position is typical. By 20 weeks, also, eye movement velocities increase. By 23 to 24 weeks, high-velocity movements frequently occur in pairs and triplets and may be classified as a rapid eye movement (REM). These movements increase in incidence and duration between 24 and 35 weeks. REMs are conjugate. They are abolished by maternal sedation. We have seen a number of cases of Rh iso-immunization in which absent or rare REM activity became frequent a few hours after fetal transfusion. Correspondingly, auditory brainstem responses improve promptly after (infant) exchange transfusion (Nwaesei et al 1984). In some late third trimester examinations (especially after auditory startle) there may be slow, drifting eye movements, associated with lid opening (Fig. 6.15). It is during this last 'state', presumably arousal, that we can demonstrate an orienting response to a bright light source applied to the maternal lower abdomen (Birnholz 1985). Phototropism is thought to develop around 34 weeks gestational age (Robinson 1966, Brandt 1979).

Even the simple movements we observe ultrasonically follow a complicated time-course of development. It is as if a movement appears as a primary capability, followed

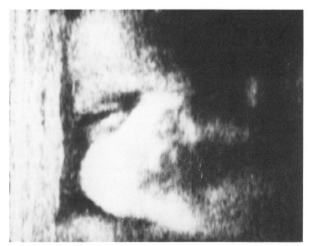

Fig. 6.15 A 'frontal' (lateral coronal) view of the right side of the face anterior to the plane of the lens (Fig. 6.13b) shows the lids. They are open here. Note the fullness of the cheek in this well-nourished late third trimester male fetus.

by a mechanism for its inhibition. Later, the movement reappears, usually having a smoother more co-ordinated quality, after which it becomes integrated with other movement patterns, themselves having individual phases of activation, suppression or reinforcement. Consequently, we can derive a great deal of information from the association between movements, trying to infer, thereby, some of the control and integrative functions of the central nervous system. Recognition of stable associations between activity patterns, i.e. 'behavioural states' was a landmark concept in newborn evaluation (Prechtl 1974, Prechtl & O'Brien 1982); antenatal extension is discussed in detail in Chapter 2.

State analysis involves, specifically, combined observations. Conceptually, this can include simultaneous activities of different parts and also the presence of one movement and the absence of another, when reciprocal inhibition is operative. This area has not been pursued in detail, probably because of technical difficulties. Usually, observations are obtained by a single observer viewing a single screen. Two or more instruments (and multiple observers) are possible when steps are taken to avoid radiofrequency interference between the devices. Second, with conventional cross-sectional imaging, observations are confined to excursions that are constrained to occur within a plane, or which can be characterized from sampling two-dimensional movement components, e.g. dynamics of the eye, mouth, tongue, heart, diaphragm and torso. Simultaneous observations are facilitated in those few cases in which one scan-plane suffices, as with movement of eyes and lips. One can make near-simultaneous observations for some regions by shifting probe position. Volumetric movements may eventually be described as forms of three-dimensional sampling.

There has been a great deal of technical attention to breathing movements, particularly with the expectation of their conveying information about fetal condition. Regular diaphragm excursions can be seen at 12 to 13 weeks gestational age. Their already low incidence at that stage declines after the mid-second trimester, suggesting some type of inhibition. They are seen more often after 23 weeks gestational age, when they increase progressively in incidence throughout the rest of the pregnancy. There are also pattern changes in the third trimester, with definition of periodic, high-frequency excursions, usually associated with REM sleep, the slow, deep and regular movements seen in deep sleep and various intermediate conditions as noted in foundation studies of fetal lambs (Dawes et al 1972). Early studies inferred diaphragm activity from in and out movements of the chest wall. Later works concentrated upon more readily observed (but still incompletely representative) movements of the abdominal wall or viscera. As mentioned earlier, magnification ultrasonic imaging reveals near-continuous, though subtle, diaphragmatic activity. This indicates that the third trimester fetus, like the equivalent premature infant, does spend most of this time 'breathing'. Phases of apnoea do occur and there is compelling evidence in sheep that these are due to central inhibition (Harding 1980). The incidence of breathing movements declines greatly with chronic hypoxia. More-over, all body movements decrease under those conditions and there is an average slowing of heart rate, which may be considered as energy conservation. Blanco et al (1983) have shown in sheep that decreased reflex response of the hindlimb during hypoxia is also mediated centrally.

Movements of the larynx are an integral part of breathing (Harding 1984). The entire glottic region can be visualized and developing integration between excursions of the dia-phragm and movement of the larynx are now amenable to physiological dissection in situ. Laryngeal movements are isolated, apparently independent of diaphragm excursions, at 16 to 17 weeks, but integration is achieved by 22 to 23 weeks. One can also study fluid flow within the trachea (Fig. 6.16), which depends upon the valve action of the larynx and the piston-like effect of the diaphragm. Early in the third trimester, fluid movement is back and forth, with little net efflux. Periods of exaggerated, unidirectional flow occur later when the larynx tends to open just during inspiration. Intermediate phases of considerable variability in flow direction and timing are associated with rapid eye movement phases. Hypoxia involves laryngospasm, which is distinguished electrophysiologically from laryngeal closure (Suzuki & Sasaki 1977). Viewing the neck also permits observation of the hypopharynx and epiglottis.

The previous activity patterns are observed passively and, correspondingly, their characterizations will involve

sampling for a sufficiently long time under fixed conditions for statistical significance (Campbell et al 1981). It is, however, possible to make active observations, i.e. stimulus response behaviour (see also Ch. 4). Prodding a late third trimester fetus over the legs to provoke a kick was one of the earliest tests of fetal well-being (Cazeau 1871). Tactile 'reflexes' were studied by Hooker (1952) and by Humphrey (1964) in prematurely delivered but non-viable second trimester cases, and there has been some progress in understanding the development of olfactory and gustatory sensitivity (Pedersen & Blass 1982). That the third trimester fetuses will have a motor response to loud sounds has been reported since the 1920s (Peiper 1961) and sound-induced change in heart rate was investigated during the 1940s (Bernard & Sontag 1947). Functional development of the auditory system has been reviewed thoroughly by Rubel (1978). Ando & Hattori (1970) have shown behavioural differences in infants subdivided by prenatal environmental noise level. There are developmental changes in auditory response (Bench & Parker 1971), probably coinciding with behavioural state differentiation, further influenced by perfusion (Pettigrew et al 1985). Leider et al (1982), Gelman et al (1982) and others have evaluated general fetal body movements after intentional sound stimulation. We have studied the time-course of auditory responsiveness using ultrasound for monitoring blink–startle behaviour (Birnholz & Benacerraf 1983) and to demonstrate the presence of decremental behaviour to repetitive stimulation (Birnholz 1984). Failure to habituate is a feature of trisomy 21 (Barnet & Lodge 1967, Barnet et al 1971). We distinguish a motor response to a noise stimulus from the sensation of 'hearing', with the assumption that the sensorium can itself be tested eventually, with the correct choice of stimulus and observational response. Finally, it is technically difficult but not impossible to measure response time, as is done with evoked potentials (Hrbek et al 1973). We would expect from nerve conduction time studies in infants that the response interval would convey specific information about functional maturation (Dubowitz et al 1968). In the context of testing, peripheral nerve conduction findings relate to age, while central auditory markers tend to be stable over time but are influenced more readily by hypoxia (Miller et al 1984).

PATHOLOGY

The ultrasound diagnosis of specific congenital abnormal-ities of the fetal central nervous system is discussed in the next chapter. This section will discuss these abnormalities in a more general way.

NEURAL TUBE DEFECTS

A great deal of attention has been directed towards neural tube defects, particularly in the United Kingdom

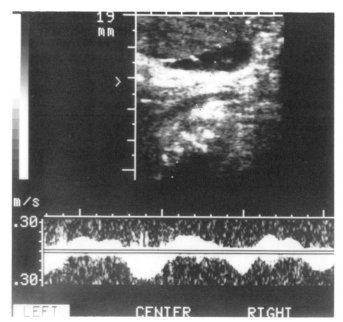

Fig. 6.16 The Doppler window is placed over the trachea (chin right, thorax left). Lung fluid flow is biphasic, uneven in timing during coincident rapid eye movements.

and British Commonwealth. This group includes exencephaly (anencephaly), spinal rachisis, and myeloceles or meningo-myeloceles at any level. This group is aetiologically hetero-geneous (Holmes et al 1976) with probable causes including a true genetic factor, thermal stress (Smith et al 1978), dietary deficiency (Lawrence 1982), or other toxic agent exposure at the 6 to 8 week stage. Neural tube defects may accompany any of the trisomies but are particularly common with trisomy 13. Subtle skeletal abnormalities of the lumbar spine (with intact membranes and normal-appearing cord) can be seen with most trisomies and with triploidy (Fig. 6.17), and rounding of the anterior margins of the lumbar bodies, well away from the canal, has been noted (Kramer & Scheers 1987). Statistically, the recurrence risk is about 1.5%, although this may be misleading because it probably averages some few families with high risk of recurrence and those at no greater risk than the remainder of the general population.

Diagnostically, this group of disorders should pose little problem, assuming that the cranium and spine are inspected carefully using satisfactory equipment. For the spine, attention is directed to the membranes and not just bony appearance. A small lumbar or sacral lesion may be missed as a sampling error but these lesions should be visible from the mid-second trimester onwards if sought specifically.

The relative uses of ultrasound and α-fetoprotein (AFP) for screening (Wald et al 1977) will need to be redefined and

this is discussed in detail in Ch. 24. Serum AFP testing is sensitive but not specific with the result that relatively few women with mildly elevated AFP levels will be carrying a child with a neural tube defect. We have not yet seen a case in which ultrasound survey at the time of amniocentesis for amniotic fluid AFP had any errors in detecting or excluding a significant neural tube abnormality, although we recognize that these errors can occur in a subjectively interpreted procedure.

At this time, there are relatively few unidentified cases of anencephaly presenting for the first time in the third trimester or at delivery (Fig. 6.18). These cases invariably have adrenal hypoplasia and somatic growth retardation, usually mild. One early anthropometric study suggested that arm length is greater than leg length in anencephalics (Nanagas 1925), mimicking the simian norm, although this has not been our experience in relatively few cases. Late anencephalics tend to exhibit exaggerated motor response to auditory stimuli. Occasionally, a decremental auditory reponse will be observed (Amiel-Tison 1985), although true 'habituation' is believed to be mediated cortically. Muscle tone and primitive reflexes are usually intact (Turkewitz & Birch 1971).

Cases with lumbar or sacral neural tube defects discovered in the second trimester are usually not continued in our patient population, so that we have not developed material for relating second trimester anatomical observations to functional outcome later. We know that some of these cases will have minimal deficits, while in others, with or without lower extremity paralysis and incontinence, slowly progress-ive communicating hydrocephalus and impaired cerebral mantle growth will eventuate (Fig. 6.19). In this context it is well to remember that (later asymptomatic) filum terminale lipoma and variations in membrane appearance are relatively common and can be visualized ultrasonically. These findings are significant when associated with signs of delayed cerebral cortical development (i.e. hydrocephalus, microphthalmia, thick sulci) but can be found, incidentally, in otherwise normal fetuses. It is to be hoped that further observations bearing upon functional development will

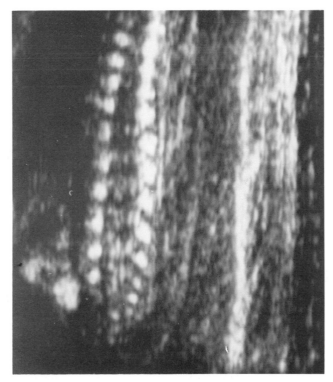

Fig. 6.17 There is subtle widening of the lumbar canal with intact membranes and normal appearing cord in this case of triploidy.

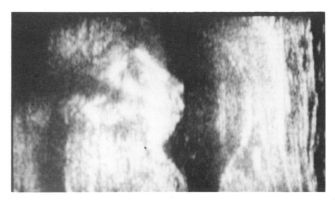

Fig. 6.18 Typical profile facial appearance with anencephaly.

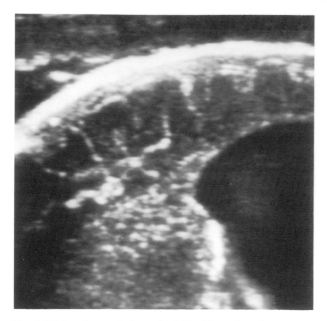

Fig. 6.19 Note the poorly formed sulci in this section of parietal cortex adjacent to a distended ventricle (L2 meningomyelocele case).

refine counselling of prospective parents faced with this difficult problem.

HYDROCEPHALUS

Hydrocephalus is a general term for dilatation of some or all of the ventricular system without particular reference to extra-axial fluid. Cerebrospinal fluid over-production from a choroid papilloma is one of the least common causes but one with a clear-cut pathophysiology. All other cases are obstructive with the block occurring either intracranially (at the level of the aqueduct or one of the anterior foramina) or as an impairment of CSF resorption at the level of subarachnoid granulation tissue. Fetal hydrocephalus is due rarely to germinal matrix haemorrhage (Birnholz 1984, Hill & Rozdilsky 1984), which is usually a postnatal event.

The conventional thinking about newborn infants has focused upon the size and configuration of the ventricles but in fetal evaluation our primary concern is the appearance of the cortex. Features of normal mantle growth are described in the next chapter. The mantle is thin and the ventricles correspondingly large at 12 to 14 weeks gestational age. The ventricles are filled by choroid. Cortical growth is such that by 17 weeks gestational age, the mid and anterior portions of the lateral ventricles have already reached the small convex–concave shape in coronal section that they will maintain for most of the remainder of gestation. Apparent ventricular dilatation recognized between 17 and 22 weeks gestational age is associated with limited cortical growth. There is also increased extra-axial fluid. The cortical growth deficiency is usually primary but it may be secondary. In any case,

ventricular dilatation can be recognized definitively during this part of development and the neurological prognosis is uniformly dismal. Evaluation is aided by short-term serial observation, by exacting study of other morphological features of development and by chromosome analysis (by amniocyte culture before 20 weeks gestational age or with percutaneous fetal blood sampling (Hobbins et al 1985) when more rapid diagnosis is required). We have found ear length helpful in identifying or excluding aneuploidy (Birnholz in press). Parenthetically, there has been considerable progress in recognizing other morphological features of the trisomies antenatally (Fig. 6.20), including redundant suboccipital skin folds, middle phalanx abnormalities of the fifth finger and relative decrease in femur length (trisomy 21) (Benacerraf, in preparation).

Percutaneous placement of indwelling stent catheters is a well-established capability in several different adult interventional applications, such as drainage of obstructed biliary or urinary tracts. Percutaneous, transuterine placement of a catheter between the ventricle and amniotic fluid (Clewell et al 1982) is identical conceptually but there are few situations in which this will be helpful clinically. This is discussed in detail in Chapter 42.

Another situation in which cranial decompression might be considered is multiple pregnancy with one affected fetus. Presumably, the procedure might lessen the risk of premature labour occurring with unconstrained craniomegaly. Contractions will be provoked by percutaneous instrumentation, although this effect can be lessened by tocolytic

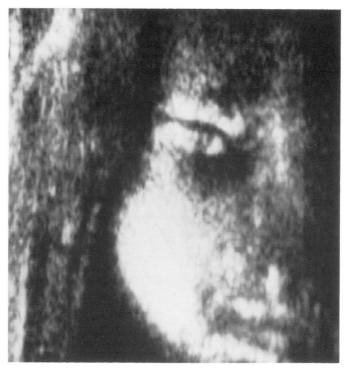

Fig. 6.20 Aneuploid facies with epicanthal fold and lax cheek. This was trisomy 18, although the appearance is initially suggestive of trisomy 21.

pretreatment. Finally, the procedure does involve cerebral mantle injury and carries a risk of intracranial haemorrhage, both of which are acceptable if the hydrocephalus is progressive and delivery is not possible or practical. The septum cavum pellucidi is almost always fenestrated with longstanding congenital hydrocephalus (Birnholz 1983), so that drainage of one side is generally adequate. Finally, needle decompression has been used in late third trimester cases of extreme hydrocephalus to permit vaginal delivery when there is no likelihood of infant survival (Osathanondh et al 1980).

The established prognostic imaging sign for infant hydrocephalus is mantle thickness, as originally defined for frontal cortex by pneumo-encephalography (Yashon et al 1965, Young et al 1973). Extreme thinning probably implies an early onset hydrocephalus with cortical growth arrest, although some element of mantle compression can occur if the calvarium is stiff enough to result in raised intracranial pressure. In most cases, the thinning will be uneven with some regional sparing perhaps of portions of the frontal or occipital lobes. Free movement of the falx with gentle ballottment over the head implies low intracranial pressure, as is usually the case with longstanding, late cases with marked dilatation, splaying of the sutures, thinning of the calvarium and a thin cortical rind. Many of these cases will have associated microphthalmia. We have also found that absence of motor response with auditory stimulation (i.e. deafness) also implies a limited developmental prognosis.

OTHER MAJOR ABNORMALITIES

Other problems, besides dysraphia, hydrocephalus and, perhaps, encephalocele, sought (and encountered) in routine practice involve either regional or global underdevelopment or an abnormal fluid collection. Vascular malformation and neoplasms are quite uncommon but have specific and predictable signs. Chronic viral infections usually have most obvious findings in the liver or skeleton, although microcephaly and basal ganglia calcifications are characteristic late findings. There is evidence that prenatal viral or protozoal infections induce cerebral abnormalities via a vasculitis rather than through intracellular infection per se (Marques et al 1984). Cystic encephalomalacia prompts particular consideration of herpes infection. Cranial findings of tuberous sclerosis tend to appear postnatally, as do skin changes, although intracardiac rhabdomyomas occur and can be found prenatally and subependymal nodules have been found in affected infants (Volpe 1987).

In our own examples of primary microcephaly, ventricular appearance has been normal and cranial and cerebral dimensions did not begin to depart from the norm until the start of the fifth month. This suggests that some component of the process involves failure of glial proliferation and further that early second trimester diag-

nosis, or prediction, may not be possible. Grossly evident microcephaly in the early and mid second trimester implies an underlying, systemic condition, such as neural tube defect and triploidy (Fig. 6.21). Microcephaly is usually accompanied (paradoxically) by a large anterior fontanelle. I have also seen one case in which mild microcephaly in the mid-second trimester was associated with absence of the cerebellum. Additional findings in that case were vault asymmetry, frontal pointing and a flat occiput (Fig. 6.22), an appearance also frequent with neural tube defects. In some cases of global underdevelopment associated with chromosome abnormalities we have seen an excessively large extra-axial fluid component within the head and a 'shaggy' cerebral boundary (Fig. 6.23). Mild microcephaly is typical with maternal alcohol and marijuana syndromes and will also be associated with delayed fetal, neuromotor milestones. Affected cases will have mandibular hypoplasia. Polymicrogyria is another form of global underdevelop-

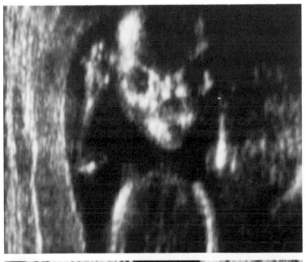

A

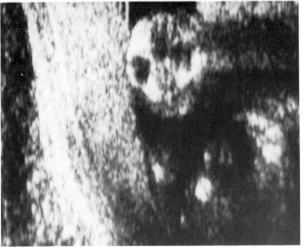

B

Fig. 6.21 (a) The normal bony facial configuration in the early second trimester. (b) The orbits appear large because of maxillary (and mandibular) hypoplasia. The frontal bones narrow conically towards the skull apex. In cases of triploidy, growth deficits are even evident as delayed body length in the first trimester.

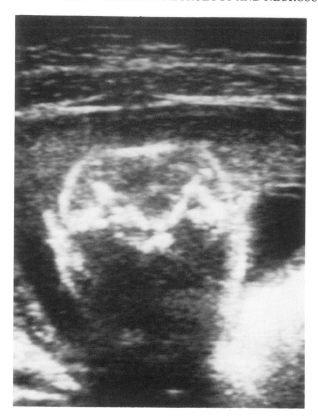

Fig. 6.22 Microcephaly with flattening of the occiput. The foramen magnum is large and the cerebellum absent.

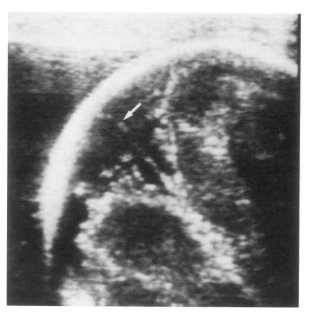

Fig. 6.23 Microcephaly with 'shaggy' boundary of the occipital lobes. The extra-axial fluid is increased (arrow identifies the falx).

ment which can be recognized ultrasonically (see p. 145), although (for the cerebrum) not until the 24 to 26 and 28 to 30 week phases of rapid sulcation fail to appear.

Holoprosencephaly has graphic intracranial findings due to cleavage failure of the prosencephalon early in development (i.e. a dorsal midline dysgenesis) and is described in detail in Chapter 19. We have detected two cases at 12 weeks gestational age (Fig. 6.4b): one associated with fetal triploidy and the other with first trimester maternal use of cocaine and 'angel dust'. Some authorities consider agenesis of the corpus callosum a forme fruste of this same condition (Loeser & Alford 1968). Most of our own cases of agenesis of the corpus callosum have had slit-like frontal and dilated occipital horns (i.e. colpocephaly, Herkewitz et al 1985) thought to be related to failure or deficiency of formation of the forceps major (Loeser & Alford 1968, Kendall 1983). At least 80% of cases of agenesis of the corpus callosum have other malformations (Parrish et al 1979, Atlas et al 1986). We have now seen two cases of typical holoprosencephaly, in whom there were multiple amniotic bands causing finger and toe amputations, and in whom a partially swallowed band had caused palato–facial clefting. Because of the obvious structural anomaly and the early origin, these cases can be recognized in utero by the mid-second trimester.

An infarct will evolve to liquefaction necrosis in the

compromised arterial distribution followed by fluid clearing and cyst formation. When the infarct is peripheral, porencephaly results; with carotid occlusion, there is hydrancephaly. Infants surviving with hydrancephaly should have extreme neurological deficits, although one case diagnosed as pneumo-encephalography was said to have a satisfactory outcome (Lorber 1965). Marked ventricular asymmetry identified late in pregnancy (Fig. 6.24) is due to global undergrowth of one hemisphere. This is a non-genetic event, probably also due to a unilateral vascular process and perhaps compromise of venous drainage. As with postasphyxial atrophy in the infant, there will be growth delay and the sulci will be thick. Large intracranial haemorrhages, though quite rare, are a complication of twin–twin transfusion states (Fig. 6.25), and cystic encephalomalacia has been reported following death of one mono-amniotic twin (Yoshioka et al 1979).

Gross motor deficits are evident from the mid-second trimester with Werdnig–Hoffman disease, Prader–Willi syndrome and central nuclear palsy. Polyhydramnios can be seen with these conditions and with myotonic dystrophy, presumably due to impaired swallowing. Experience with muscle disorders in infants remains to be extended antenatally with comparable precision. Periodic fetal motor deficits are also seen with maternal myasthenia (Lefvert & Osterman 1983), although diaphragmatic activity is usually present and lung hypoplasia is not anticipated.

PROSPECTS

Recent technical advances in ultrasonic imaging have increased our observational capabilities for fetal nervous sys-

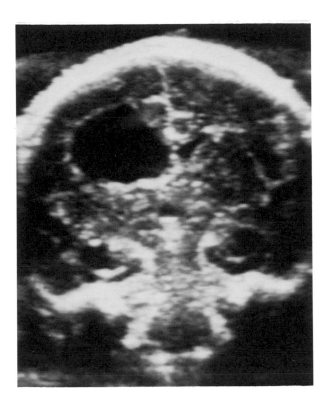

Fig. 6.24 Coronal view with normal left lateral ventricle and distended right ventricle due to focal undergrowth of the frontoparietal cortex.

tem. The most important of these has been large-aperture, dynamically focused instrumentation with its extended spatial contrast and temporal resolution performances, which also minimize the extraneous effects of maternal habitus, fluid volume and fetal position on our ability to study individual cases thoroughly.

Antenatal studies of the central nervous system have a dual emphasis on primary developmental abnormalities and on acquired damage from asphyxial injury. Brief decreases in cerebral blood flow in the neonate result in significant functional deficits later (Skov et al 1984). Similar concerns arise any time in the third trimester if placental inadequacy ensues or umbilical venous flow is compromised mechanically.

Ultrasonic image quality appears to have reached the level that the next group of advances will be analytical, following careful, unbiased and exacting observations of many cases and, where possible, of individual subjects followed serially. What are normal neurodevelopmental horizons? What are their intrinsic biological variations? How are these events influenced by changes in the uterine environment occurring naturally, intentionally, or as a result of disease such as pre-eclampsia, growth retardation, premature labour, maternal diabetes or from drugs used in treating those conditions. Most important will be long-term follow-up, for which careful second and third trimester (as well as perinatal) events are compared

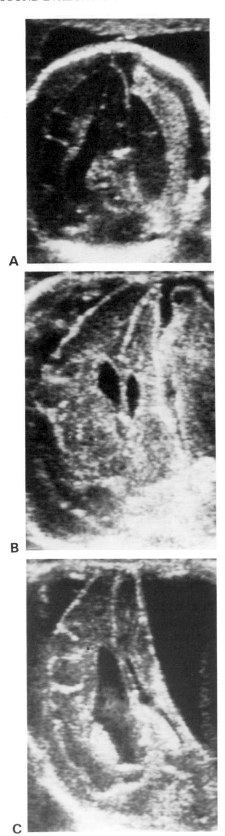

Fig. 6.25 The brain is compressed by a large subdural blood dissection, echodense on the left in utero (a) and shortly after delivery (b). Two weeks after birth (c) the clot has lysed leaving echo-free fluid (bilaterally). The brain is atrophic, especially the left.

with later motor and intellectual performance. Such work might also address conditions for stimulatory regimes which may enhance development.

Further technical developments may also be antici-pated, leading to better prenatal anatomical display, to quantitative measures of reflectivity and to quantitation of dynamic events related to spontaneous and provoked fetal movements.

REFERENCES

Ahlfeld F 1905 Die intrauterine tatigkeit der Thorax und Zwerchfellmuskulatur, intrauterine at mung. Mschr Geburtsch Gynaek 21: 143–163

Amiel-Tison C 1985 Pediatric contribution to the present knowledge on the neurobehavioral status for infants at birth in neonatal cognition. In: Mehler J, Fox R (eds). Erlbaum, Hillsdale, Ch 18

Ando Y, Hattori H 1970 Effects of intense noise during fetal life upon postnatal adaptability (statistical study of the reactions of babies to aircraft noise). Journal of the Acoustical Society of America 47: 1128–1130

Atlas S W, Zimmerman R A, Bilaniuk L T et al 1986 Corpus callosum and limbic system: neuroanatomic MR evaluation of developmental anomalies. Radiology 160: 355–362

Barnet A B, Lodge A 1967 Click evoked EEG responses in normal and developmentally retarded infants. Nature 214: 252–255

Barnet A B, Ohlrich E S, Shanks B L 1971 EEG evoked responses to repetitive auditory stimulation in normal and Down's syndrome in infants. Developmental Medicine and Child Neurology 13: 321–329

Beckert P T, Thomas E B 1981 Rapid eye movement storms in infants: rate of occurrence at 6 months predicts mental development at 1 year. Science 212: 1415–1416

Bench J, Parker A 1971 Hyper-responsivity to sounds in the short-gestation baby. Developmental Medicine and Child Neurology 13: 15–19

Bernard J, Sontag L W 1947 Fetal reactivity to tonal stimulation. Journal of Genetic Psychology 70: 205–210

Birnholz J C (in press) Fetal ear length. Pediatrics

Birnholz J C 1981 The development of fetal eye movement patterns. Science 213: 679–681

Birnholz J C 1982 Newborn cerebellar size. Pediatrics 70: 284–288

Birnholz J C 1983 Septum pellucidum fenestration. Radiology 149: 122

Birnholz J C 1984 Fetal neurology. In: Sanders R, Hill M (eds) Ultrasound annual. Raven Press, New York, pp 139–160

Birnholz J C 1985 Ultrasonic fetal opthalmology. Early Human Development 12: 199–209

Birnholz J C 1986a Studies of fetal dynamics. In: Deter R, Harris R B, Birnholz J C, Hadlock F P (eds) Qualitative obstetrical ultrasonography. Wiley, New York, Ch 8

Birnholz J C 1986b Techniques and observations for ultrasonic charac-terization of fetal growth. In: Greenleaf J (ed) Tissue characterization with ultrasound, Vol II. CRC, Boca Raton, Ch 12

Birnholz J C 1986c Ultrasonic studies of human fetal brain development. Trends for Neuroscience 9: 329–333

Birnholz J C, Benacerraf B R 1983 The development of fetal hearing. Science 222: 516–518

Birnholz J C, Frigoletto F D 1981 Antenatal treatment of hydrocephalus. New England Journal of Medicine 304: 1021–1023

Birnholz J C, Hayes T 1987 The effect of instrumentation and examination. In: McGaham J P (ed) Controversies in ultrasound. Churchill Livingstone, New York, pp 143–153

Blanco C E, Dawes G S, Walker D W 1983 Effect of hypoxia on polysynaptic hind-limb reflexes of unanaesthetized fetal and new-born lambs. Journal of Physiology 339: 453–466

Brandt I 1979 In: Falkner F, Tanner J M (eds) Patterns of early neurological development in human growth, Vol 3. Plenum, New York, Ch 8

Campbell K, MacNeill I, Patrick J 1980 Time series analysis of human fetal breathing activity at 30–39 weeks gestation. Journal of Biomedical Engineering 2: 108–112

Campbell K, MacNeill I, Patrick J 1981 Time series analysis of ultrasonic observations of gross fetal body movements during the last 10 weeks of pregnancy. Ultrasonic Imaging 4: 330–341

Cazeau P 1871 In: Bullock W R (ed) A theoretic and practical treatise on midwifery, American edn. Linday & Balkison, Philadelphia

Chi J G, Dooling E C, Gilles F H 1977 Gyral development of the human brain. Annals of Neurology 1: 86–93

Clewell W H, Johnson M L, Meier P R et al 1982 A surgical approach to hydrocephalus. New England Journal of Medicine 306: 1320–1325

Crade M, Patel J, McQuown D 1981 Sonographic imaging of the glycogen stage of the fetal choroid plexus. American Journal of Roentgenology 137: 489–491

Davidson H D, Abraham R, Skinner R E 1985 Agenesis of the corpus callosum: magnetic resonance imaging. Radiology 155: 371–373

Dawes G S, Fox H E, Leduc B M et al 1972 Respiratory movements and rapid eye movement sleep in the foetal lamb. Journal of Physiology (London) 220: 119–143

de Lacoste M-C, Holloway R I, Woodward D J 1986 Sex differences in the fetal human corpus callosum. Human Neurobiology 5: 93–96

Demayer W 1971 Classification of cerebral malformations. Birth Defects (original article series) 7: 78–93

de Vries J I P, Vissir G H A, Prechtl H F R 1982 The emergence of fetal behavior. I. Qualitative aspects. Early Human Development 7: 301–322

Dorovini-Zis K, Dolman C L 1977 Gestational development of the brain. Archives of Pathology and Laboratory Medicine 101: 192–195

Dubowitz V, Whitaker G F, Brown B H et al 1968 Nerve conduction velocity: an index of neurological maturity of the newborn infant. Developmental Medicine and Child Neurology 10: 741–746

Gaulden M E, Murry R C 1980 Medical radiation and possible adverse effects on the human embryo. In: Meyn R E, Withers H R (eds) Radiation biology in cancer research. Raven Press, New York, pp 277–294

Gelman S R, Wood S, Spellacy W N et al 1982 Fetal movement in response to sound stimulation. American Journal of Obstetrics and Gynecology 143: 484–485

Goldman-Rakic P C 1980 Morphological consequences of prenatal injury to the primate brain. Progress in Brain Research 53: 3–19

Griffin D, Bilardo K, Masini L et al 1984 Doppler blood flow intravenous in the descending thoracic aorta of the human fetus. British Journal of Obstetrics and Gynaecology 91: 997–1006

Harding R 1980 State related and developmental changes in laryngeal function. Sleep 3: 307–322

Harding R 1984 Perinatal development of laryngeal function. Journal of Developmental Physiology 6: 249–258

Herskewitz J, Roeman P, Wheeler C B 1985 Colpocephaly: Clinical radiologic, and pathogenetic aspects. Neurology 35: 1594–1598

Hill A, Rozdilsky 1984 Congenital hydrocephalus secondary to intrauterine germinal matrix/intraventricular hemorrhage. Developmental Medicine in Child Neurology 26: 524–527

Hobbins J C, Grannum P A, Romero R et al 1985 Percutaneous umbilical blood sampling. American Journal of Obstetrics and Gynecology 152: 1–6

Holmes L B, Driscoll S G, Atkins L 1976 Etiologic heterogeneity of neural tube defects. New England Journal of Medicine 294: 365–369

Hooker D 1952 The prenatal origin of behavior. University of Kansas Press, Lawrence

Hrbek A, Karlberg P, Olsson T 1973 Development of visual and somatosensory evoked responses in preterm newborn infants. Electroencephalographical Clinical Neurophysiology 34: 225–232

Humphrey J 1964 Some correlations between the appearance of human fetal reflexes and the development of the nervous system. Progress in Brain Research 4: 93–135

Huttenlocher P R 1984 Synapse elimination and plasticity in developing human cerebral cortex. American Journal of Mental Defects 88: 488–496

Ianniruberto A, Tajani E 1981 Ultrasonic study of fetal movement. Seminars in Perinatology 5: 175–181

Kawahara H, Andon Y, Takashima S et al 1987 Normal development of the spinal cord in neonates and infants seen on ultrasonography. Neuroradiology 29: 50–52

Kendall B E 1983 Dysgenesis of the corpus callosum. Neuroradiology 25: 239–256

Kramer P P G, Scheers I M 1987 Round anterior margin of lumbar bodies in children with a meningomyelocele. Pediatric Radiology 17: 263

Larroche J C L 1962 Quelques aspects anatomiques du developpment cerebral. Biology of the Neonate 4: 126–153

Lawrence K M 1982 Prevention and prenatal diagnosis of neural tube defects. In: Persand T V N (ed) Central nervous system and craniofacial malformations, Vol 7. Liss, New York

Lefvert A K, Osterman P O 1983 Newborn infants to myasthenic mothers: a clinical study and an investigation of acetylcholine receptor antibodies in 17 children. Neurology 33: 133–138

Leider L R, Baillie P, Martin B et al 1982 Fetal habituation in high risk pregnancies. British Journal of Obstetrics and Gynaecology 89: 441–446

Lewis P D, Patel A 1979 Psychotropic drugs and brain development effects on all acquisition. In: Di Benedetta C, Balazs R, Combos G, Purcellate G (eds) Multidisciplinary approach to brain development. Elsevier, Amsterdam, pp 509–517

Liley A W 1972 The foetus as a personality. Australian and New Zealand Journal of Psychiatry 6: 99–105

Lind N, Shinebourne E, Turner P, Cotton D 1971 Adrenergic neurone and receptor activity in the iris of the neonate. Pediatrics 47: 105–112

Lockwood G, Benacerraf B, Krinsky A et al 1987 A sonographic screening method for Down's syndrome. American Journal of Obstetrics and Gynecology 157: 803–808

Loeser J D, Alford E C Jr 1968 Agenesis of the corpus callosum. Brain 91: 553–568

Lorber J 1965 Hydrancephaly with normal development. Developmental Medicine and Child Neurology 7: 628–633

Lou H C 1982 Developmental neurology. Raven Press, New York, Ch 1

McLeary R D, Kuhns R R, Barr M 1984 Ultrasonography of the fetal cerebellum. Radiology 151: 439–442

Marques M J, Harmant-Van Rijckevorse L, Landrieu P, Lyon G 1984 Prenatal cytomegalovirus disease and cerebral microgyria: evidence for perfusion failure, not disturbance of histogenesis, as the major cause of fetal cytomegalovirus encephalopathy. Neuropediatrics 15: 18–24

Miller G, Skouteli H, Dubowitz M S, Lary S 1984 The maturation of the auditory brainstem response compared to peripheral nerve conduction velocity in preterm and full term infants. Neuropediatrics 15: 25–27

Nanages J J C 1925 A comparison of the growth of the body dimensions of anencephalic human fetuses with normal fetal growth as determined by graphic analysis and empirical formulae. American Journal of Anatomy 35: 455–495

Nicolaides K H, Gabbe S G, Guidetti R et al 1986 Ultrasound screening for spina bifida: cranial and cerebellar signs. Lancet i: 72–73

Nwaesei C G, Van Aerde J, Boyden M, Perlman Y 1984 Changes in auditory brainstem respones in hyperbilirubinemic infants before and after exchange transfusion. Pediatrics 74: 800–803

O'Rahilly R, Bossy J 1982 The growth of the eye. I. In utero. Anal Desarrollo 16: 31–51

Osathanondh R, Birnholz J C, Altman A M et al 1980 Ultrasonically guided transabdominal encephalocentesis. Journal of Reproductive Medicine 25: 125–128

Oster-Granite M L, Gaerhart J D, Reeves R H 1986 Neurobiological consequences of trisomy 16 in mice. In: Epstein C J (ed) The neurobiology of Down's syndrome. Raven Press, New York, pp 137–151

Ozanics V, Jakobiec F A 1982 Prenatal development of the eye and its adnexa. In: Ocular anatomy, embryology and teratology. Harper & Row, Philadelphia, Ch 2

Parrish M L, Roessman U, Levinsohn M W 1979 Agenesis of the corpus callosum: a study of the frequency of associated malformations. Annals of Neurology 6: 349–354

Patrick J, Natale R, Richardson B 1978 Patterns of human fetal breathing activity at 34 to 35 weeks gestational age. American Journal of Obstetrics and Gynecology 132: 507–511

Pedersen P E, Blass E M 1982 Prenatal and postnatal determination of the 1st suckling episode in albino rats. Developmental Psychobiology 15: 349–355

Peiper A 1961 Die Eigenart der Kindlichen Hirntatigkeit. Georg Verlag, Leipsig, Ch 2

Pettigrew A G, Edwards D A, Henderson-Smart D J 1985 The influence of intrauterine growth retardation on brainstem in development of preterm infants. Developmental Medicine and Child Neurology 26: 467–471

Prechtl H F R, O'Brien M J 1982 Behavioral states of the full-term newborn: emergence of a concept. In: Psychobiology of the human newborn. Wiley, New York, Ch 3

Prechtl H F R 1974 The behavioral states of the newborn infant (a review). Brain 76: 1304–1311

Preyer W 1885 Die spezielle physiologie des embryo. Grieben, Liepsig, p 161

Rakic P, Yakovlev P E 1968 Development of the corpus callosum and the cavum septi in man. Journal of Comparative Neurology 132: 45–72

Robinson R J 1966 Assessment of gestational age by neurological examination. Archives of Diseases in Childhood 41: 437–447

Rubel E W 1978 Ontogeny of structure and function in the vertebrates auditory system. In: Jacobson M (ed) Development of sensory systems. Springer Verlag, Berlin, Ch 5

Sabbagha R E 1979 The use of ultrasound in defining gestational age. In: Hobbins J C (ed) Diagnostic ultrasound in obstetrics. Churchill Livingstone, New York, Ch 3

Saint-Anne Dargassies S 1979 Normal and pathological fetal behavior as seen through neurological study of the premature newborn. Controversies in Gynecology and Obstetrics 6: 42–56

Scammon R E, Armstrong 1925 On the growth of the human eyeball and optic nerve. Journal of Comparative Neurology 38: 165–219

Scammon R E, Calkins K A 1929 The development and growth of external dimensions of human body in the fetal period. University of Minnesota, Minneapolis

Shatz C, Kirkwood P A 1984 Prenatal development of functional connections in the cat's retinogeniculate pathway. Journal of Neuroscience 4: 1378–1379

Shepard M, Fily R A 1982 A standardized plane for biparietal diameter measurement. Journal of Ultrasound in Medicine 1: 145–150

Sidman R L, Rakic P 1973 Neuronal migration. Brain Research 62: 1–35

Skov H, Lou H, Pederson H 1984 Perinatal brain ischaemia: impact at four years of age. Developmental Medicine and Child Neurology 26: 353–357

Smith D W, Clarren S K, Harvey M A 1978 Hyperthermia as a possible teratogenic agent. Journal of Pediatrics 92: 878–883

Sulik K, Lauder J M, Dehart D B 1984 Brain malformations in prenatal mice following acute maternal ethanol administration. International Journal of Developmental Neuroscience 2: 203–214

Suzuki M, Sasaki C T 1977 Laryngeal spasm: a neurophysiologic redefinition. Annals of Neurology 86: 100–157

Turkewitz G, Birch H G 1971 Neurobehavioral organization of the human newborn. In: Hobbins J C (ed) Ultrasound in Obstetrics. Churchill Livingstone, New York, Ch 3

Volpe J J 1987 Neurology of the newborn. Saunders, Philadelphia, Ch 2

Wald N J, Cuckle H S 1977 Antenatal screening for neural tube defects. In: Weitzel H K, Schneider J (eds) Alpha-fetoprotein in clinical medicine. Georg Thieme, Stuttgart, pp 29–34

Warburg M 1971 The heterogeneity of microphthalmia in the mentally retarded. Birth Defects (original article series) 7: 136–141

Wisniewski K E, Laure-Kamionowska M, Connell F, Wen G Y 1986 Neuronal density and synaptogenesis in the postnatal stage of brain maturation in Down's syndrome. In: Epstein C J (ed) The neurobiology of Down's syndrome. Raven Press, New York, pp 29–44

Wladimiroff J W, Craft I L, Talbert D G 1975 In vitro measurements of sound velocity in human fetal brain tissue. Ultrasound in Medicine and Biology 1: 377–381

Yashon P, Jane J A, Sugar O 1965 The course of severe untreated infantile hydrocephalus: prognostic significance of the cerebral mantle. Journal of Neurosurgery 23: 509–516

Young H F, Nulsen F E, Weiss M H, Thomas P 1973 The relationship of intelligence and cerebral mantle in treated infantile hydrocephalus. Pediatrics 52: 38–44

Yoshioka J, Icadomoto Y, Mino M et al 1979 Multicystic encephalomalacia in live born twin with a stillborn macerated co-twin. Journal of Pediatrics 91: 798–799

7. The ultrasound appearances of normal and abnormal anatomy of the fetal central nervous system

Dr G. Pilu and Prof J. C. Hobbins

In the early 1970s prenatal diagnosis was possible for only a small group of catastrophic lesions, namely anencephaly (Campbell et al 1972) and gross hydrocephalus (Freeman et al 1977) but in more recent years Johnson et al (1980) Fiske & Filly (1982) and Hidalgo et al (1982) must all be given credit for providing considerable insight into the sonographic interpretation of ventricular and vascular anatomy of the brain before birth. Johnson et al (1980) and Jeanty et al (1981) first established nomograms for ventricular size thus addressing the important issue of early recognition of hydrocephalus. Chervenak et al (1983, 1984a,b,c) have considered on several occasions the problems of prenatal diagnosis and rational clinical management of fetal central nervous system anomalies.

The purpose of this chapter is to review the principles of embryogenesis and gestational development of the brain and to provide guidelines for both sonographic identification and management of fetal abnormalities.

DEVELOPMENTAL ANATOMY OF THE NERVOUS SYSTEM

The embryological development of the central nervous system is described in detail in Part 1 of this book and will only be briefly reiterated here for the purposes of appreciating the corresponding sonographic appearances that are relevant for the understanding of congenital abnormalities amenable to prenatal diagnosis. We will also consider the morphological modifications normally occurring during the first half of pregnancy that can be recognized with ultrasound.

The nervous system is originally derived from a dorsal thickening of the ectoderm (the neural plate) which can be recognized as early as the 14th day of development. The faster growth rate of the lateral portions of the plate results in the formation of two longitudinal folds demarcating an internal groove. The folds fuse with each other in the midline, starting the transformation of the groove into a tube at about the midportion of the embryonic disk. Closure proceeds then cephalad and caudad. From 20 to 24 days the neural tube is almost entirely closed with the exception of two openings at the extremities — the anterior and posterior neuropores. The anterior neuropore first undergoes obliteration, followed by the posterior neuropore at about 24 to 26 days.

At this time, the rostral portion of the neural tube is cleaved along two horizontal planes, giving rise to the three primary vesicles of the brain: the prosencephalon, mesencephalon and rhombencephalon. Two further cleavages occur in the following weeks, leading to the subdivision of the prosencephalon into telencephalon and diencephalon, and of the rhombencephalon into metencephalon and myelencephalon.

The cerebral hemispheres originate from two paired diverticula ballooning out of the telencephalon. At the same time, the diencephalon (the primordium of the optic thalami) gives rise to two anterior paired diverticula, the optic bulbs, and two unpaired buds on the median plane, the anterior neurohypophysis and posterior pineal body. The mesencephalon will form the cerebral penduncles and quadrigeminal plate. The metencephalon will develop into the pons, cerebellum and rostral portion of the fourth ventricle, while the myelencephalon will give rise to the medulla oblongata and caudal portion of the fourth ventricle.

Cleavage of the primitive cerebrum along four horizontal planes leading to the formation of the five primary cerebral vesicles results in constrictions and secondary enlargements of the cavity of the neural tube which will develop eventually into the ventricular system. The cavity contained within the telencephalon (telocele) undergoes paired symmetrical division and diverticulation along the sagittal plane with formation of two distinct cavities that will give rise to the lateral ventricles. The cavities contained within the diencephalon (diocele), mesencephalon (mesocele) and metencephalon–myelencephalon (metacele, myelocele) will form the third ventricle, aqueduct of Sylvius and fourth ventricle respectively. The remaining portion of the neural tube cavity will develop into the ependymal canal which runs within the spinal cord.

The rapidly growing hemispheres rotate inwardly thus enfolding the thin membranous roof of the telocele (the tela choroidea) deep into the brain. The hemispheres are now separated by a thin mesenchymal layer which is the primordium of the falx cerebrii. The cerebral cortex is quite thin at this point in gestation, most of the hemispheres being occupied by the primitive ventricular cavities. At about the sixth week of gestation, the medial wall of the lateral ventricles is seen bulging within the cavity, thus forming a fold which is rapidly covered by pseudostratified epithelium and moulded by the proliferation of the underlying blood vessels into a villous structure — the choroid plexus. Both anatomical studies on animal models (Tennyson & Pappas 1964) and sonographic investigation of the human fetus in utero (Crade et al 1981) have outlined the generous size of the choroid plexus, which fills almost entirely the lateral ventricles from about 8 to 16 weeks. The peculiar echogenicity of this structure in vivo (Fig. 7.1) has been attributed to a high glycogenic content,

which is thought to represent a major energy supply for the rapidly growing cerebrum.

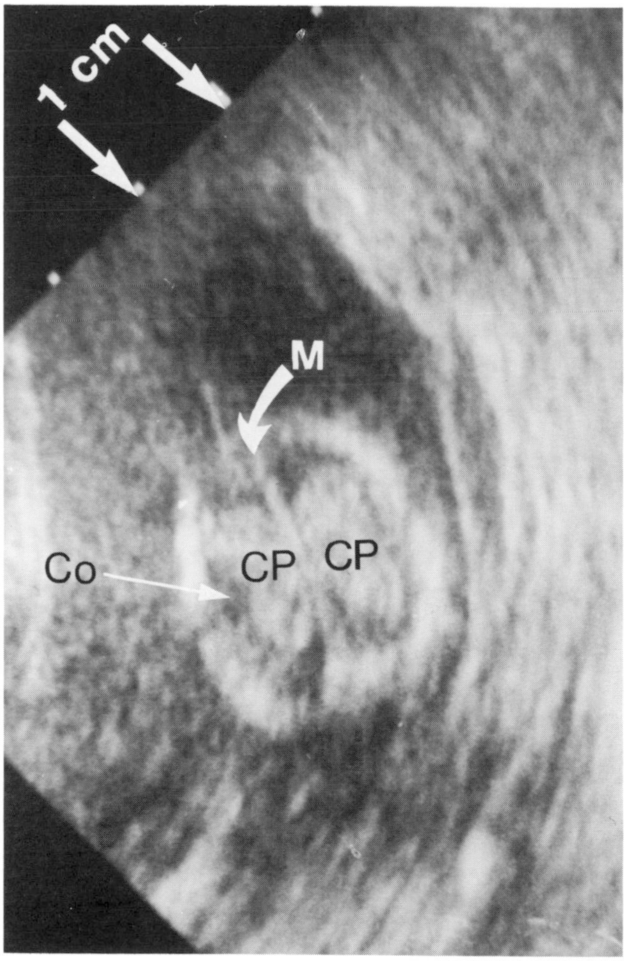

While the choroid plexus decreases in size relative to both brain mass and ventricular volume, the lateral ventricles are stretched and moulded by the many developing processes occurring within the forebrain (growth of cerebral lobes, basal ganglia and thalami, formation and deepening of the cerebral sulci). Assessment of the developmental anatomy of the ventricular system in the fetus has depended mainly upon complex dissection procedures and barium casting techniques (Kier 1977). More recently, real-time high-resolution ultrasound equipment has allowed documentation from a large number of living fetuses the observations originally made on abortion specimens (Fig. 7.2). By the fourth month of gestation, the lateral ventricles are large in size when compared to the cortex and intracranial cavity. At this time, the bodies and frontal horns are short, the atrium being by far the most prominent portion. Both ontogenetically and phylogenetically, the last modification in the shape of the lateral ventricles to occur is the formation of the occipital horns, as only higher mammals and mature fetuses have an occipital lobe large enough to allow a well-defined internal cavity. The lateral ventricles are fully developed at about the 30th week of gestation. As the fetus usually lies on one side inside the amniotic cavity, ultrasound examination of the intracranial contents mainly relies on axial scans.

The obstetric sonographer should be familiar with the tomographic anatomy of the brain. Figure 7.3 displays three views that can be easily obtained in the vast majority of fetuses and enable a proper assessment of all the different portions of the lateral ventricles. Another axial view, obtained at a slightly lower level than the previous ones, and slightly angled towards the posterior fossa permits the simultaneous visualization of the third and fourth ventricles (Fig. 7.4).

A few other anatomical structures will be considered in this section. The cavum septi pellucidi is a fluid-filled

Fig. 7.1 Axial scan of the fetal head at 10 weeks. Most of the intracranial cavity is occupied by the large echogenic choroid plexuses (CP). The thin cerebral cortex (Co) is seen as an hypo-echoic crescent interposed between the prominent choroid plexus and the calvarium. (M: midline).

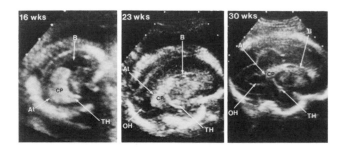

Fig. 7.2 Parasagittal scans of the fetal head in three normal fetuses at 16, 23 and 30 weeks. Note the modifications in size and shape of the body (B), atrium (At) and temporal horn (TH) of lateral ventricles throughout gestation. At 16 weeks the atrium is prominent and it ends blindly posteriorly, the occipital horn (OH) appearing only at about mid-gestation. At any gestational interval, the choroid plexus (CP) is seen filling entirely the atrium. (Reproduced with permission from Romero et al 1987.)

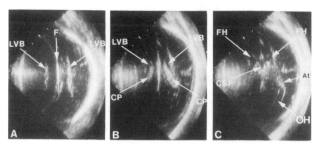

Fig. 7.3 Tomographic evaluation of the mature fetal ventricular system (32 weeks). (a) At the higher level, the bodies of lateral ventricles (LVB) are seen as two single lines running parallel on both sides of the falx cerebrii (F). (b) At a slightly lower level the echogenic choroid plexus (CP) is seen coursing along the floor of the body; (c) A lower scan demonstrating the frontal horns (FH), separated by a cavum septi pellucidi (CSP), the atria (At) filled by the choroid plexuses and the well-developed occipital horns (OH).

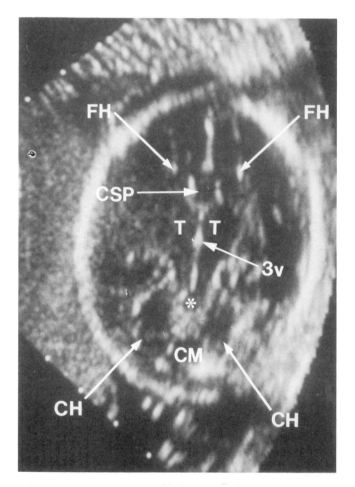

Fig. 7.4 Suboccipito–bregmatic scan of the head of a 25-week-old fetus. The frontal horns of the lateral ventricles (FH), separated by a large cavum septi pellucidi (CSP), the thalami (T) and the third ventricle (3v) are well demonstrated. At the level of the posterior fossa the fourth ventricle (*) is seen as a small anechoic quadrangular area, delineated inferiorly by the echogenic cerebellar vermis (unlabelled) and laterally by the hypoechoic cerebellar hemispheres (CH). Between the cerebellar vermis and the echogenic calvarium, the sonolucent cisterna magna (CM) is seen. (Reproduced with permission from Pilu et al in press a.)

cavity which is formed between the leaves of the septum pellucidum. The cavum is largely patent in the fetus and it decreases progressively in size during gestation, being sonographically recognizable in 40 to 60% (Farruggia & Babcock 1981, Cerisoli et al 1984) of normal newborn infants. A caudal prolongation of the cavum septi pellucidum, the cavum Vergae, can be seen at times (Fig. 7.5).

The development of cerebral fissure and sulci has been extensively reviewed by Dorovini-Zis & Dolman (1977). The distinct feature of the human brain before the 22nd week of gestation is a peculiar smoothness. Only the calcarine and parieto–occipital fissures are discernible. In the following 8 weeks the rapid growth of the cerebral cortex leads to the formation of the rolandic fissure and of the cingulate, frontal and parietal sulci. The formation of cortical convolutions proceeds steadily up to the 40th week, when tertiary sulci can finally be seen. Evaluation of the convolutional pattern is a well-established method to assess maturity both in pathological (Dorovini-Zis & Dolman 1977) and neonatal ultrasound studies (Worthen et al 1986). Cerebral sulci can be appreciated sonographically in utero as well (Figs 7.6, 7.7 and 7.8) but adequate visualization requires the use of transfontanellar coronal and sagittal scans. As these views can be obtained only in a minority of cases, such an otherwise promising approach to the intra-uterine estimation of fetal maturity has important limitations.

Development of the brain results in conspicuous modifications of the subarachnoid cisterns. This issue has been the subject of both anatomical (Lanman et al 1958) and sonographic studies (Pilu et al 1986a). Knowledge of the normal sonographic anatomy of the subarachnoid space is useful both in avoiding misinterpretation of normal sonograms and in the differential diagnosis of congenital anomalies. The main features of the cisterns that are particularly relevant for the obstetric sonographer will be

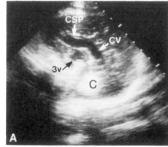
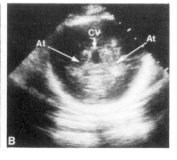

Fig. 7.5 (a) midsagittal scan of the head of a normal 29-week-old fetus demonstrating a prominent cavum septi pellucidi (CSP) prolonging posteriorly into a patent cavum Vergae (CV). The third ventricle (3v) and cerebellar vermis (C) are seen in the same scanning plane. (b) Transfontanellar posterior coronal scan in the same fetus. The patent cavum Vergae (CV) is seen as an oval-shaped sonolucent area between the atria of lateral ventricles (At).

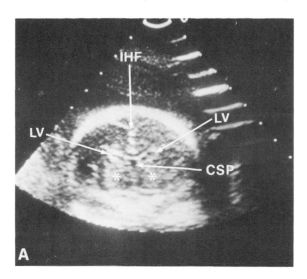

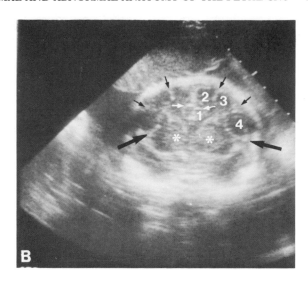

Fig. 7.6 Anterior coronal scans of the fetal head passing through the bodies of lateral ventricles (LV), cavum septi pellucidi (CSP) and basal ganglia (*). (a) At 21 weeks, the surface of the cerebral hemispheres appears smooth; (b) At 31 weeks, a well-developed convolutional pattern can be seen. The cingulate (1), superior frontal (2), middle frontal (3) and inferior frontal (4) gyri can be recognized. The large black arrows indicate the Sylvian fissure. In these scans, the corpus callosum can be seen as a thin sonolucent area interposed between the interhemispheric fissure (IHF) and the cavum septi pellucidi.

briefly considered, the interested reader being referred to the specific works on this subject (Mahony et al 1984, Pilu et al 1986a).

The extracortical space overlying the cerebral convexities is very prominent early in gestation and decreases steadily starting from about 20 weeks until it becomes of minimal dimensions in the adult (Fig. 7.9). Before 24 weeks of gestation, the frontal and temporal lobes adjacent to the insula (the opercula) are separated by an ample space the base of which is the insula (Fig. 7.10). The opercula progressively converge until they meet to form the Sylvian fissure. The beginning of the Sylvian fissure demarcation

is already visible by 22 weeks of gestation but it is not until 32 to 34 weeks of gestation that opercularization is complete (Fig. 7.11). The cistern of the vein of Galen (or

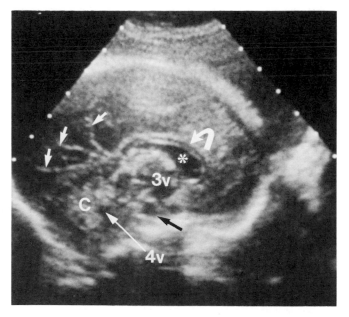

Fig. 7.8 Midsagittal scan of the fetal head at 29 weeks. The corpus callosum is seen as a thin sonolucent crescent interposed between the echogenic pericallosal cistern (curved arrow) and the patent cavum septi pellucidi (*). Anteriorly to the third ventricle (3v) the chiasmatic cistern is seen (black arrow). The cerebellar vermis (C) is indented by the fourth ventricle (4v). Note the well-developed cerebral sulci (parieto–occipital, calcarine and collateral) on the medial surface of the hemisphere (white arrows).

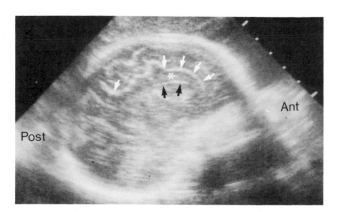

Fig. 7.7 Midsagittal scan of the fetal head at 30 weeks. The cingulate (white arrows) and callosal (black arrows) sulci demarcating the cingulate gyrus (*) are demonstrated. (Ant denotes anterior, Post posterior.)

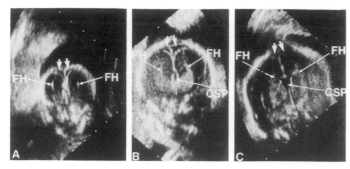

Fig. 7.9 Coronal scans of the fetal head at 16 (a), 24 (b) and 30 weeks of gestation (c), demonstrating the progressive reduction in size of the subarachnoid space overlying the cerebral convexities (arrows). A patent cavum septi pellucidi (CSP) separating the frontal horns of lateral ventricles (FH) is seen in b and c. (Reproduced with permission from Pilu et al 1986a.)

quadrigeminal cistern), which lies in the angle between the superior surfaces of the cerebellum and mesencephalon, can be seen on sonographic studies as early as the 15th week (Fig. 7.10). It can be seen extending laterally on both sides in the ambient cisterns, which separate the thalami from the hippocampal and parahippocampal gyri (Fig. 7.11). Neither the ambient cistern nor the vein of Galen cistern undergoes significant modification in shape or relative size throughout gestation. The cisterna magna, which is situated between the inferior surface of the cerebellum and the posterior aspect

of the medulla oblongata can be consistently visualized with ultrasound, and it is quite generous in size up to the third trimester (Mahony et al 1984, Pilu et al 1986a).

CONGENITAL ANOMALIES OF THE NERVOUS SYSTEM

HYDROCEPHALUS

Congenital hydrocephalus arises in most cases from an obstruction along the normal pathway of the cerebrospinal fluid. The incidence ranges between 0.3 and 1.5 in 1000 births in different series (Myrianthopoulos 1977). In a series of 205 infants with congenital isolated hydrocephalus, aqueductal stenosis was found in 43%, communicating hydrocephalus in 38% and Dandy–Walker malformation in 13% (Burton 1979).

Congenital infections and genetic factors are both involved in the pathogenesis of aqueductal stenosis. Infectious

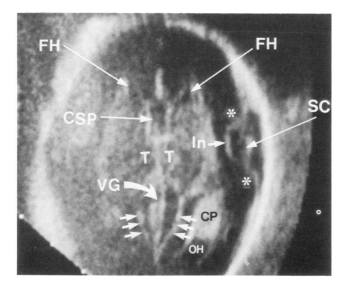

Fig. 7.10 Axial scan of the fetal head at 25 weeks passing through the frontal horns of lateral ventricles (FH), cavum septi pellucidi (CSP), atria (unlabelled) and occipital horns (OH). The opercula (*) are widely separated and the Sylvian cistern (SC) appears as an ample square-shaped area extending from the base of the insula (In) to the inner calvarium. The vein of Galen cistern is seen as a triangular sonolucent space demarcated anteriorly by the thalami (T) and posteriorly by the medial surface of the occipital lobes (triple arrowhead). Within this cistern, the great cerebral vein of Galen (VG) is clearly seen. Note that the echogenic choroid plexus (CP) fills entirely the atrium, being closely apposed to both the medial and lateral walls (unlabelled). (Reproduced with permission from Pilu et al 1986a.)

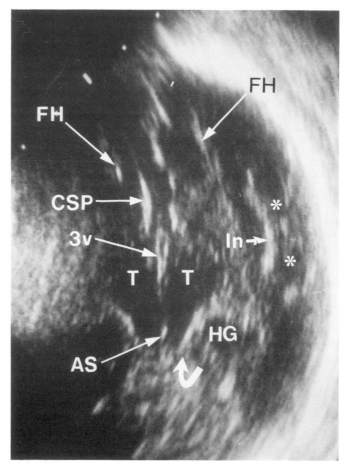

Fig. 7.11 Axial scan of the fetal head passing through the frontal horns of lateral ventricles (FH), cavum septi pellucidi (CSP), thalami (T) and third ventricle (3v) and aqueduct of Sylvius (AS). The opercularization is almost complete. The Sylvian cistern is now only seen as an echogenic line interposed between the base of the insula (In) and the closely apposed opercula (*). The curved arrow indicates the ambient cistern, which is interposed between the thalamus and the hippocampal gyrus (HG).

agents include toxoplasmosis, syphilis, cytomegalovirus, mumps and influenza virus (Salam 1977).

Infections result in gliotic stenosis of the aqueduct. True malformations include narrowing and forking (multicanalization), and less frequently a transverse septum obstructing the lumen. In an autopsy series, 50% of cases of aqueductal stenosis were due to gliosis, 46% to forking and 4% to simple narrowing (Milhorat 1972). Congenital tumours such as gliomas, pinealomas and meningiomas cause aqueductal stenosis by external compression. Outlet obstruction of the third ventricle results in enlargement of the third and lateral ventricles. The degree of ventriculomegaly, even if variable, is severe in the vast majority of cases.

Communicating hydrocephalus usually results from failure of reabsorption of cerebrospinal fluid. It has been found in cases of agenesis (Gutierrez et al 1975) or blockage of arachnoid granulation due to subarachnoid haemorrhage (Ellington & Margolis 1969), venous occlusion of the superior sagittal sinus, torcular Herophilii or lateral sinuses (Kalbag & Woolf 1967) and over-production of cerebrospinal fluid by a choroid plexus papilloma (Gradin et al 1983). Communicating hydrocephalus in its most typical manifestation is characterized by a variable degree of enlargement of the entire ventricular system associated with dilatation of the subarachnoid spaces. A radiological study has outlined the natural history of this lesion demonstrating that in the earliest stage enlargement is confined to the subarachnoid channels overlying the cerebral hemispheres (Robertson & Gomez 1978). At a further stage simultaneous dilatation of both the subarachnoid spaces and the ventricular system is seen. Eventually, only ventriculomegaly can be demonstrated.

According to recent experience, isolated communicating hydrocephalus carries a good prognosis. In a series of 13 treated infants no deaths occurred and the intelligence was normal in all cases (McCullough & Balzer-Martin 1982).

It should be stressed that the traditional view that considers stenosis of the aqueduct and communicating hydrocephalus as two separate entities has been challenged, when it has been postulated that ventriculomegaly may be the cause instead of the consequence of aqueductal stenosis (Williams 1973).

DANDY–WALKER MALFORMATION

Dandy–Walker malformation is frequently associated with other central nervous system abnormalities such as agenesis of the corpus callosum, hetertopia, polymicrogyria, agyria and macrogyria, systemic anomalies such as congenital heart disease (mainly ventricular septal defects), polydactyly–syndactyly, cleft palate and polycystic kidneys (Brown 1977, Hirsch et al 1984, Murray et al 1985) and it may be a part of a number of genetic and non-genetic syndromes that are reviewed Chapter 20.

In spite of the classical definition of Dandy–Walker malformation, it has been demonstrated that in 80% of cases, hydrocephalus is absent at birth and it develops only after several months or years (Hirsch et al 1984). This observation is relevant for the obstetric sonographer as it indicates that Dandy–Walker malformation cannot be excluded on the pure basis of the absence of ventriculomegaly. Recent paediatric series indicate that treated infants have an overall mortality rate ranging between 12 and 26% and an IQ above 80 in 30 to 40% of cases (Sawaja & McLaurin 1981, Hirsch et al 1984).

The issue of prenatal diagnosis of hydrocephalus by sonography has been addressed by many investigators. As macrocrania usually does not develop until late in gestation, head measurements are unreliable and the identification of hydrocephalus should depend upon the direct demonstration of the enlargement of the ventricular system. Nomograms of the normal size of frontal horns (Denkhaus & Winsberg 1979, Pearce et al 1985), bodies (Denkhaus & Winsberg 1979, Johnson et al 1980, Jeanty et al 1981), temporal horns (Denkhaus & Winsberg 1979) and atria (Pearce et al 1985) of the lateral ventricles throughout gestation are now available. Measurement of the bodies is by far the most widely used. This determination easily allows the immediate recognition of moderate and severe ventriculomegaly as early as mid-gestation (Fig. 7.12). However, in the experience of other investigators (Fiske et al 1980, Pearce et al 1985) as well as in our own, the size of both bodies and frontal horns of lateral ventricles is often within the normal range in cases of early or mild hydrocephalus. Measurement of the atria probably yields a greater accuracy, as these portions of the ventricles usually undergo the earliest and maximal enlargement (Pearce et al 1985). Several authors have demonstrated that a qualitative evaluation of the intracranial structures is most useful in cases of mild hydrocephalus. Fiske et al (1980) have pointed out that, in the third trimester, axial scans of the normal fetal head only reveal the lateral wall of the body of the lateral ventricle (Fig. 7.3), while in cases of mild hydrocephalus, due to the enlargement of the ventricular lumen, the medial wall can be demonstrated. Chinn et al (1983) have observed that the large fetal choroid plexus entirely fills the cavity of the lateral ventricle at the level of the atria, being closely apposed to both the medial and lateral walls (Fig. 7.10). In early hydrocephalus, the choroid plexus is shrunken and anteriorly displaced, thus being clearly detached from the medial wall (Fig. 7.13). In our experience, the latter criterion is both simple to apply, as it eliminates the need for a quantitative evaluation, and highly effective in screening for fetal hydrocephalus early in the second trimester. We have never had any false positive or negative diagnoses and we could successfully identify many lesions in which biometry was within normal range.

Once hydrocephalus has been recognized, the site of the obstruction may be inferred by identifying the enlarged portion of the ventricular system. Dilatation of the lateral

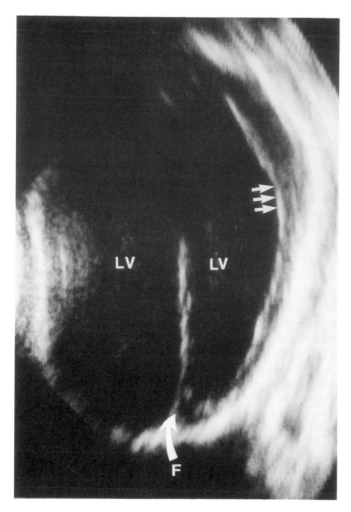

Fig. 7.12 Severe fetal hydrocephalus at 28 weeks of gestation. An axial scan at the level of the bodies of lateral ventricles (LV) clearly demonstrates gross ventriculomegaly. The thin cortex is indicated by arrows. F: falx.

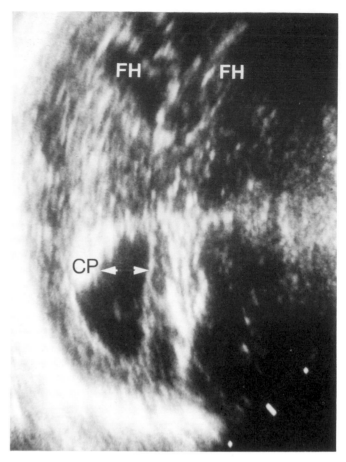

Fig. 7.13 Mild hydrocephalus. In this third trimester fetus with spina bifida, an axial scan reveals slightly prominent frontal horns of lateral ventricles (FH) and atria (unlabelled). The detachment of the choroid plexus (CP) from the medial wall of the atrium (double-pointed arrow) is evident.

and third ventricles suggests aqueductal stenosis (Fig. 7.14). Tetraventricular enlargement in the presence of a normal cerebellar vermis associated with distension of the subarachnoid cisterns (Fig. 7.15) suggests communicating hydrocephalus (Pilu et al 1986a,b). A defect in the cerebellar vermis through which the fourth ventricle communicates with a posterior fossa cyst indicates Dandy–Walker malformation (Fig. 7.16) (Pilu et al in press a). An attempt to differentiate the anatomical type of hydrocephalus should always be made, as each form carries a different prognosis (see Ch. 46). Unfortunately, the previously described sonographic approach to differential diagnosis is of limited accuracy. Non-contrast computed tomographic studies in infants have clearly demonstrated that communicating hydrocephalus often mimics aqueductal stenosis (Raybaud et al 1978, Naidich et al 1982). In our prenatal series, in only 22% of cases of communicating hydrocephalus could the enlarged subarachnoid spaces be demonstrated clearly (Pilu et al 1986b). A certain diagnosis can probably be made only

in cases of Dandy–Walker malformation (Pilu et al 1987a) and in cases with spina bifida, in which communicating hydrocephalus is almost always the rule.

Much work has been done trying to correlate the outcome of ventriculomegalic infants with the extent of ventricular enlargement. Measurements such as the frontal cerebral mantle thickness (Lorber 1970, Young et al 1973), average cerebral mantle thickness (Yashon et al 1965) and the brain mass, calculated on the basis of the frontal cerebral mantle thickness and occipito–frontal diameter (Cochrane & Myles 1982, McCullough & Balzer-Martin 1982) have been used. All these studies uniformly indicate that the prognosis is rather unpredictable on the basis of a quantitative evaluation of the spared cerebral cortex. Many reports indicate that even infants with a cerebral mantle thickness of a few millimetres have sometimes developed a normal or superior intelligence following treatment. At present, the outcome of affected infants seems to depend more upon the nature of the underlying lesion than upon the degree of ventriculomegaly.

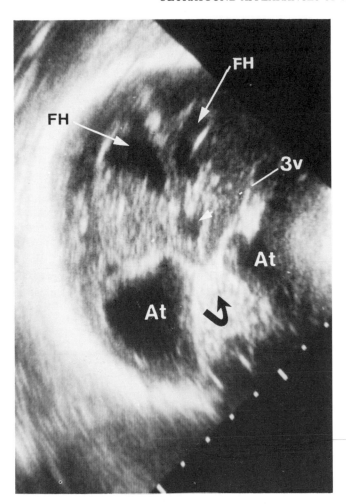

Fig. 7.14 Axial scan demonstrating enlargement of the lateral and third ventricles (3v) in a fetus with aqueductal stenosis. The fourth ventricle (curved arrow) is small. FH: frontal horns and At: atria of lateral ventricles.

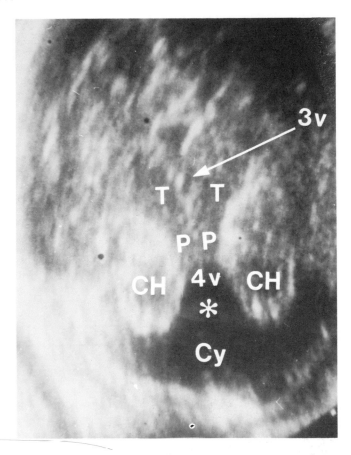

Fig. 7.16 Dandy–Walker syndrome in a 25-week-old fetus. A suboccipito–bregmatic scan reveals a wide defect in the cerebellar vermis (★) through which the fourth ventricle (4v) directly communicates with a retrocerebellar cyst (Cy). The cerebellar hemispheres (CH) are widely separated. Compare this figure with the normal appearance of the suboccipito–bregmatic view of the fetal head which is shown in Figure 7.4. T: thalami; 3v: third ventricle; P: cerebral peduncles.

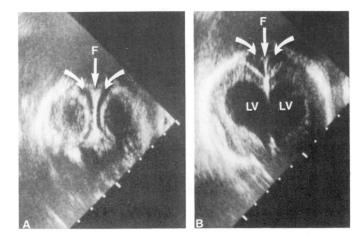

Fig. 7.15 Coronal scans of the head of a 30-week-old fetus with communicating hydrocephalus. (a) Prominent interhemispheric fissure (curved arrows). (b) Enlarged lateral ventricles (LV) and subarachnoid spaces overlying the cerebral convexities (curved arrows). F. falx. (Reproduced with permission from Pilu et al 1986a.)

Difficulties in establishing a reliable prognosis in utero are reflected in uncertainties in deciding upon proper obstetric management. When the diagnosis of hydrocephalus is made before viability, many parents would probably request termination of pregnancy. When this option is not accepted, and in those cases recognized later on in pregnancy, a thorough discussion of the possible choices with the couple is recommended. The management of fetal ventriculomegaly is fully discussed in Chapter 45.

It should be stressed that one of the main factors influencing the outcome of hydrocephalic fetuses is the possible association with other important life-threatening anomalies. In the experience of Yale–New Haven Hospital, in which the association of hydrocephalus–spina bifida was also considered, 60% of fetuses have associated anomalies (Chervenak et al 1984a). In the experience of the Bologna Unit, in which only isolated hydrocephalus was considered, the incidence was 30% (Pilu et al 1986b). Associated anomalies included chromosomal abnormalities and malformations involving virtually all fetal systems. In view of these figures, an effort to identify associated anomalies should always be made before considering aggressive obstetric management. Detailed examination of the entire fetal anatomy by high-resolution ultrasound, echocardiography and karyotyping are strongly recommended. If severe anomalies are found suggesting that postnatal survival is unlikely, vaginal delivery might be strongly considered.

HOLOPROSENCEPHALY

Holoprosencephaly is a complex developmental anomaly of the telencephalic and diencephalic structures (see Ch. 19). The incidence is unknown as milder forms are probably unrecognized. Two subtypes of this anomaly, cyclopia and cebocephaly, have been reported to occur in 1:40 000 and 1:16 000 births respectively (DeMyer 1977). An incidence of 4:1000 abortions has also been reported (Matsunaga & Shiota 1977) suggesting a high intra-uterine fatality rate from this defect. The ætiology is discussed fully in Chapter 19.

Several cases of sonographic antenatal diagnosis of holoprosencephaly have been reported in the literature. A variety of findings has been described, including microcephaly and absence of the midline (Kurtz et al 1980), absence of the midline and intracranial cyst (Hill et al 1982), absence of the midline and cyclopia (Blackwell et al 1982), absence of the midline and enlarged holoventricle (Hidalgo et al 1982), microcephaly, intracranial fluid collection and proboscis (Lev-Gur et al 1983), holoventricle, hypothelorism (Chervenak 1984d), cyclopia and unspecified intracranial anomalies (Benacerraf et al 1984), holoventricle, uncleft thalami dorsal sac and cyclopia (Filly et al 1984). In our own series of 8 cases (Pilu et al in press b), the most valuable finding was the demonstration of the single primitive ventricle, which was possible in all cases (Fig. 7.17). We were also able to recognize the dorsal sac, when present, and to predict facial anomalies such as hypotelorism, anophthalmia, arhinia, proboscis and median cleft lip (Pilu et al in press b,c). Recognition of facial anomalies strengthens the diagnosis of holoprosencephaly based upon central nervous system findings. Conversely, should any of the mentioned facial features be serendipitously encountered, a careful examination of the intracranial contents is recommended.

Only one case of antenatal diagnosis of semilobar holoprosencephaly has been reported thus far (Cayea 1984). The ultrasonic findings were very similar to the ones described in cases of alobar holoprosencephaly. In newborns, semilobar holoprosencephaly can be identified for sure by visualizing well-developed occipital horns in either computed tomographic or ultrasound studies (see Ch. 8 and 9).

It is yet to be demonstrated that this is possible in the fetus. To our knowledge, the lobar variety has never been identified in utero. However, fusion of the frontal horns of lateral ventricles and absence of the cavum septi can probably be recognized by a careful sonographic examination.

When either alobar or semilobar holoprosencephaly are identified in utero, termination of pregnancy should be offered before viability and conservative management is strongly recommended in continuing pregnancies.

AGENESIS OF THE CORPUS CALLOSUM

Agenesis may be complete or partial. In the latter case aplasia affects the posterior portion, which is ontogenically the first one to be formed. The incidence of agenesis of the corpus callosum is highly controversial. Figures ranging from 1 in 100 to 1 in 19 000 have been reported (Ettlinger 1977). The ætiology is unknown. Agenesis of the corpus callosum can be found in association with chromosomal

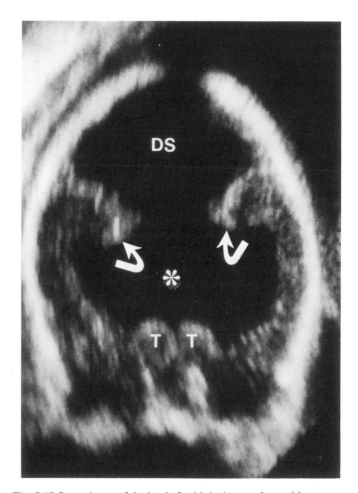

Fig. 7.17 Coronal scan of the head of a third trimester fetus with holoprosencephaly. There is a single enlarged ventricular cavity (*). The cortex is only partially enfolded above the ventricular lumen (curved arrows), which thus amply communicates with a large dorsal sac (DS). The hypoplastic bulb-like thalami (T) can be seen on the floor of the ventricle. (Reproduced with permission from Pilu et al in press a.)

aberrations (trisomy 13 and 18), mostly as a part of the holoprosencephalic malformative sequence. The familial cases reported in the literature have been reviewed recently by Young et al (1985). A marked genetic heterogeneity was found, with evidence supporting autosomal dominant, autosomal recessive and X-linked inheritance as well.

The high frequency of associated malformations suggests that agenesis of the corpus callosum may be a part of a widespread developmental disturbance. In a review of the literature (Parrish et al 1979), associated central nervous system abnormalities, including microcephaly, abnormal convolutional patterns, neural tube defects, Dandy–Walker malformation, aplasia or hypoplasia of the pyramidal tracts were found in 85% of cases. Systemic anomalies including a variety of musculo–skeletal, cardiovascular, genito-urinary and gastrointestinal malformations were found in 62% of cases.

The criteria for the postnatal diagnosis of agenesis of the corpus callosum by diagnostic imaging techniques are well established and are discussed in Section 2 of this book. They mainly depend upon the demonstration of the typical alterations of the cerebral architecture which are found in this condition. The bodies of the lateral ventricles are invariably widely separated and the atria and occipital horns are enlarged (colpocephaly). The third ventricle is frequently enlarged and dorsally extended, being found at the same level or higher than the bodies of lateral ventricles.

Two cases of prenatal sonographic diagnosis of agenesis of the corpus callosum have been reported by Comstock et al (1985). In both cases, colpocepahly and upward displacement of the third ventricle were observed. In our own series of 9 cases, a prenatal diagnosis was possible in 7 (Sandri et al 1987). The most valuable sonographic antenatal finding was the demonstration of colpocephaly. The wide separation of the bodies of lateral ventricles and the enlargement of the atria resulted in a very typical image that was found in all cases, and was not similar to any of the other congenital brain anomalies we have seen (Fig. 7.18). Dorsal extension of the third ventricle (Fig. 7.19) appears to be an inconsistent finding, as it was present in only 45% of our cases.

Establishing a reliable prognosis for agenesis of the corpus callosum is extremely difficult. Many patients suffer from mental retardation, neurological abnormalities, including increased muscle tone and seizures, and are psychologically abnormal (Ettlinger 1977) but in some cases the condition is totally asymptomatic. It is likely that disabilities depend more upon the amount and extent of associated anomalies than upon agenesis of the corpus callosum per se. No specific figures are available at present. Difficulties in assessing the prognosis are reflected in uncertainties as to

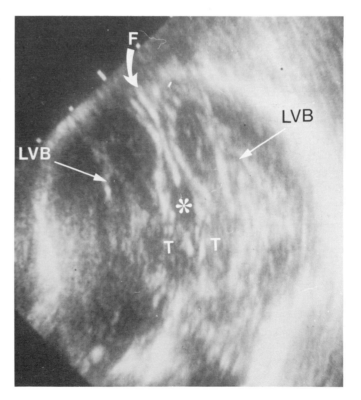

Fig. 7.19 Coronal scan of the head of a second trimester fetus with agenesis of the corpus callosum. The third ventricle (★) is enlarged and displaced upward in the position normally occupied by the corpus callosum. The bodies of lateral ventricles (LVB) are widely separated. The interhemispheric fissure (unlabelled) is prominent. The falx cerebri (F) is closely apposed to the third ventricle. Compare this figure with the normal appearance of the fetal head in this sonographic view, as it is shown in Figure **7.9a**.

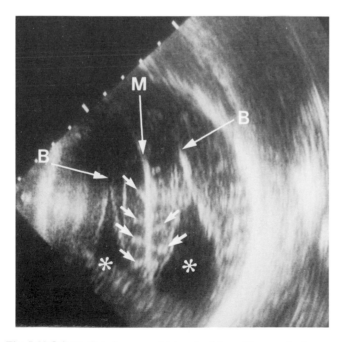

Fig. 7.18 Colpocephaly in a second trimester fetus with agenesis of the corpus callosum. The bodies of lateral ventricles (B) are widely separated and diverge anteriorly. The atria (★) are typically enlarged. An abnormal convolutional pattern of the medial cerebral sulci is seen (arrows). M: midline.

prenatal counselling and obstetric management. A careful search for associated anomalies, including echocardiography and karyotyping is mandatory but it should be stressed that the ability of prenatal ultrasound to identify several of the anomalies classically associated with agenesis of the corpus callosum, such as abnormal convolutional patterns, has not been tested yet. Abnormalities of the pyramidal tracts, which may cause significant disability are obviously unpredictable. Termination of pregnancy can be offered before viability but the parents should be informed that there is a chance of an entirely normal intellectual and neurological development. In continuing pregnancies no specific obstetric management is required. Agenesis of the corpus callosum may be associated with macrocephaly. In these cases, a caesarean delivery is indicated. (See also Ch. 19.)

PORENCEPHALY

The term porencephaly refers to a condition in which cystic cavities are found within the brain matter. It may be either the consequence of a morphogenetic disorder (true porencephaly or schizencephaly) or the result of an intra-uterine or postnatal destructive process (pseudoporencephaly or encephaloclastic porencephaly) — see Chapters 19 and 30. The cavities usually communicate with the ventricular system, the subarachnoid space or both. The developmental form is often bilateral and symmetrical. In pseudoporencephaly a unilateral lesion is usually found. In both cases, there is a wide variability in the size of the lesion. Hydrocephalus is frequently associated.

Both true porencephaly and congenital pseudoporencephaly are severe anomalies with a dismal prognosis. The vast majority of patients are affected by severe mental retardation and important neurological sequelae such as blindness and tetraplegia.

Prenatal sonographic identification of intracerebral cystic cavities is easy (Pilu et al 1986b) (Fig. 7.20) but the differential diagnosis with intracranial cysts of different nature, such as arachnoid cysts and congenital tumours (Sauerbrei & Cooperberg 1983) may be impossible.

When a confident diagnosis of porencephaly is made before viability, termination of pregnancy should be offered to the parents. In continuing pregnancies, conservative obstetric management is recommended.

HYDRANENCEPHALY

Hydranencephaly is thought to result from an intra-uterine destructive process and may be considered as an extreme form of pseudoporencephaly. Most of the cerebral hemispheres are absent and the intracranial cavity is filled with fluid. Remnants of the temporal and occipital lobes can be

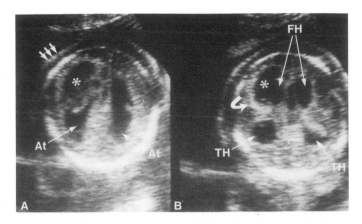

Fig. 7.20 Coronal scans of the head of a second trimester fetus with non-immune hydrops and multiple congenital anomalies. (a) A posterior coronal scan reveals a large porencephalic cyst (*). The atria of lateral ventricles (At) are enlarged. Prominent oedema of the scalp is seen (triple arrow). (b) An anterior coronal scan demonstrates an ample communication between the porencephalic cyst and the corresponding frontal horn (FH). The cyst is lined by an irregular and hyperechogenic wall (curved arrow). TH: temporal horns of lateral ventricles.

found. The brainstem and rhombencephalic structures are usually spared. The head may be small, of normal size or extremely enlarged (Halsey et al 1977). The aetiology is heterogeneous and is discussed in Chapter 20. Prognosis is very poor but long survival has been reported (Halsey et al 1968). These infants are obviously incapable of any intellectual achievement.

Even if replacement of intracranial structures with fluid is easily detected by antenatal sonography, certain identification of hydranencephaly may be difficult. The differential diagnosis includes severe hydrocephalus and holoprosencephaly. However, even in the most devastating forms of ventriculomegaly, it is possible to demonstrate the falx cerebrii and some spared cortex. In alobar holoprosencephaly, the falx is absent but a crescent-shaped frontal cortex can usually be seen. In hydranencephaly the falx is in the vast majority of cases absent or incomplete. In our experience, the most valuable finding for a specific diagnosis is the demonstration of the bulb-like brainstem, which, in the absence of the surrounding cortex, bulges inside the fluid-filled intracranial cavity (Pilu et al 1986b) (Fig. 7.21). The sonographic appearance is somewhat similar to that of hypoplastic thalami which can be seen in cases of alobar or similobar holoprosencephaly (Fig. 7.17). Obviously, confusion between holoprosencephaly and hydranencephaly is inevitable as both conditions share a dismal prognosis and the obstetric management is the same.

MICROCEPHALY

The definition of microcephaly is a highly controversial issue. Some authors suggest the diagnostic criterion of

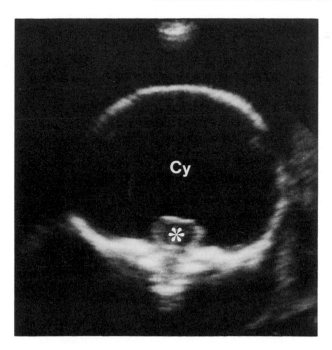

Fig. 7.21 Coronal scan of the head of a third trimester fetus with hydrancephaly. Note the brain stem (*) typically protruding inside the cystic intracranial cavity (Cy). (Reproduced with permission from Pilu et al 1986b.)

a head circumference two standard deviations below the mean (O'Connell et al 1965). Others believe that a threshold of minus three standard deviations should be used (Book et al 1953). Differences in diagnostic modalities probably account for the wide variability of the incidence of this condition reported in different studies. Figures ranging from 1.6 in 1000 births (Myrianthopoulos 1977) to 1 in 25 000–50 000 (Book et al 1953) can be found in the literature. The ætiology is extremely heterogeneous. Microcephaly should not be considered as a separate entity but rather as a symptom of many ætiological disturbances. Genetic and environmental causative factors are both well accepted and are fully discussed in Chapter 20. The widely accepted classification suggested by Book et al (1953) includes two main categories. Microcephaly resulting from non-genetic insults such as infections, anoxia, radiations, etc.; and genetic microcephaly, which includes all those cases in which microcephaly is a part of an inherited syndrome.

Microcephalic individuals have in common a typical disproportion in size between the splanchnocranium and neurocranium. The forehead is sloping. The correlation between a small head circumference and reduced brain mass and total cell number is well established (Winnick & Rosso 1969). The cerebral hemispheres are affected to a greater extent than the diencephalic and rhombencephalic structures. Abnormal convolutional patterns (macrogyria, microgyria, agyria) are frequently found. The ventricles

may be enlarged. Microcephaly is frequently found in cases of porencephaly, lissencephaly and holoprosencephaly.

Establishing a reliable prognosis for infants affected by microcephaly is difficult. Associated anomalies obviously have a major influence on the outcome. Controversial clinical data exist with regard to isolated microcephaly. In one series of 134 infants with head circumference two standard deviations below the mean, only one had a normal intelligence (O'Connell et al 1965). More recent studies are in disagreement with these observations. Avery et al (1972) reported a group of 28 infants with head circumference below two standard deviations from the mean and found either a normal intellectual development or mild retardation in 50%. Martin (1970) found normal intellectual development in 82% and 28% of infants with a head circumference between minus two and minus three standard deviations and below minus three standard deviations respectively. Even if it is hard to derive precise prognostic figures from these studies, there is evidence indicating that a small head size does not necessarily imply mental retardation.

Many difficulties arise in attempting to identify fetal microcephaly. The utility of head measurements alone is limited, as these can be markedly biased by factors such as incorrect dating or intra-uterine growth retardation. Furthermore, the natural history of fetal microcephaly is largely unknown. Campbell et al (1983) have described a progressive intra-uterine development of the lesion, thus making early diagnosis impossible in some cases. This observation is in agreement with our own experience. Nevertheless, recognition before viability is of paramount importance as microcephaly has genetic implications and many couples with a positive familial history demand prenatal diagnosis. A comparison of biometric parameters such as the head circumference:abdominal circumference ratio (Kurtz et al 1980, Campbell et al 1983) and the femur length:biparietal diameter ratio (Hohler & Quetal 1981) has been suggested. With this regard, Chervenak et al (1984e) have provided nomograms that are extremely useful for diagnostic practice. Nevertheless, both false positive and false negative diagnoses have been reported (Chervenak et al 1984e). It is clear that the predictive value of ultrasound has some limitations at present and that further investigations are required. A qualitative evaluation of the intracranial structures is a very useful adjunct to biometry. All cases of fetal microcephaly seen at the Bologna Unit had some degree of morphological derangement. It is obvious that our observations may be biased by the probably higher detection rate of those cases associated with cerebral anomalies recognizable by prenatal ultrasound.

CONCLUSIONS

Modern ultrasound equipment yields a unique potential for the evaluation of the normal and abnormal fetal central nervous system from very early in pregnancy. The bulk of the experience accumulated in the last 10 years indicates that a large number of congenital anomalies can be consistently recognized. Even if criteria for identification of nervous malformations are well established, it should be stressed that many uncertainties exist as to the parental counselling and obstetric management. At present, the prognostic figures derived by paediatric studies are used. It is important to realize that there is no evidence indicating that these figures can be applied to the fetus. The natural history of many congenital anomalies is still unknown. It is possible that pediatric series are biased by high perinatal mortality rates and failure of referral. The first large series of nervous malformations recognized in utero seems to indicate a much worse outcome that expected from postnatal series (Chervenak et al 1984a). Establishing reliable prognostic figures to be applied to affected fetuses and drawing precise guidelines for obstetric management seems to be the priority for the next decade.

REFERENCES

Avery G B, Meneses L, Lodge A 1972 The clinical significance of 'measurement microcephaly'. American Journal of Diseases of Children 123: 214

Benacerraf B R, Frigoletto F D, Bieber F R 1984 The fetal face. Ultrasound examination. Radiology 153: 495

Blackwell D E, Spinnato J A, Hirsch G, Giles H R, Sackler J 1982 Prenatal diagnosis of cyclopia. American Journal of Obstetrics and Gynecology 143: 848

Book J A, Schut J W, Reed S C 1953 A clinical and genetical study of microcephaly. American Journal of Mental Deficiency 57: 637

Brown J R 1977 The Dandy–Walker syndrome. In: Vinken P J, Bruyn G W (eds) Handbook of clinical neurology, Vol 30. Elsevier, Amsterdam, pp 623–646

Burton B K 1979 Recurrence risks for congenital hydrocephalus. Clinical Genetics 16: 47

Campbell S, Johnstone F D, Holt E M, May P 1972 Anencephaly: early ultrasonic diagnosis and active management. Lancet ii: 1226

Campbell S, Allan L, Griffin D, Little D 1983 The early diagnosis of fetal structural abnormalities. In: Lerski R A, Morley P (eds) Ultrasound 82. Pergamon Press, Oxford, pp 547–563

Cayea P D, Balcar I, Alberti O et al 1984 Prenatal diagnosis of semilobar holoprosencephaly. American Journal of Roentgenology 142: 455

Cerisoli M et al 1984 Ultrasound recognition of the cavum septi pellucidi and the cavum Vergae in the newborn. Journal of Nuclear Medicine and Allied Sciences 28: 163

Chervenak F A et al 1984a Outcome of fetal ventriculomegaly. Lancet ii: 179

Chervenak F A et al 1984b Diagnosis and management of fetal cephalocele. Obstetrics and Gynecology 64: 86

Chervenak F A et al 1984c Perinatal management of myelomeningocele. Obstetrics and Gynecology 63: 376–380

Chervenak F A, Farley M A, Walters L, Hobbins J C, Mahoney M J 1984d When is termination of pregnancy during the third trimester morally justifiable? New England Journal of Medicine 310: 501

Chervenak F A, Isaacson G, Mahoney M J et al 1984e The obstetric significance of holoprosencephaly. Obstetrics and Gynecology 63: 114

Chervenak F A, Jeanty P L, Cantraine F et al 1984f The diagnosis of fetal microcephaly. American Journal of Obstetrics and Gynecology 149: 512

Chinn D H, Callen P W, Filly R A 1983 The lateral cerebral ventricle in early second trimester. Radiology 148: 529

Cochrane D D, Myles S T 1982 Management of intrauterine hydro-cephalus. Journal of Neurosurgery 57: 590

Comstock C H, Culop D, Gonzalez J et al 1985 Agenesis of the corpus callosum in the fetus: its evolution and significance. Journal of Ultrasound in Medicine 4: 613

Crade M, Patel J, McQuown D 1981 Sonographic imaging of the glycogen state of the fetal choroid plexus. American Journal of Neuroradiology 2: 345

DeMyer W 1977 Holoprosencephaly. In: Vinken P J, Bruyn G W (eds) Handbook of clinical neurology, Vol 30. Elsevier, Amsterdam, pp 431–478

Denkhaus H, Winsberg F 1979 Ultrasonic measurement of the fetal ventricular system. Radiology 131: 781

Dorovini-Zis K, Dolman C L 1977 Gestational development of the brain. Archives of Pathology and Laboratory Medicine 101: 192

Ellington G, Margolis G 1969 Block of arachnoid villus by subarachnoid hemorrhage. Journal of Neurosurgery 30: 651

Ettlinger G 1977 Agenesis of the corpus callosum. In: Vinken P J, Bruyn G W (eds) Handbook of clinical neurology, Vol 30. Elsevier, Amsterdam, pp 285–297

Farruggia S, Babcock D S 1981 The cavum septi pellucidi: its appearance and incidence with cranial ultrasonography in infancy. Radiology 139: 147

Filly R A, Chinn D H, Callen P W 1984 Alobar holoprosencephaly. Ultrasonographic prenatal diagnosis. Radiology 151: 455

Fiske C E, Filly R A, Callen P W 1980 Sonographic measurement of lateral ventricular width in early ventricular dilation. Journal of Clinical Ultrasound 9: 303

Fiske C E, Filly R A 1982 Ultrasound evaluation of the normal and abnormal fetal neural axis. Radiologic Clinics of North America 20: 285

Freeman R K, McQuown D S, Secrist L J, Larson E 1977 The diagnosis of fetal hydrocephalus before viability. Obstetrics and Gynecology 49: 109

Gradin W C, Taylor C, Fruin A H 1983 Choroid plexus papilloma: case report and review of the literature. Neurosurgery 12: 217

Gutierrez Y, Friede R L, Kaliney A J 1975 Agenesis of arachnoid granulations and its relationship to communicating hydrocephalus. Journal of Neurosurgery 43: 553

Halsey J H, Allen N, Chamberlin H R 1968 The chronic decerebrate state of infancy. Archives of Neurology 19: 339

Halsey J H, Allen N, Chamberlin H R 1977 Hydranencephaly. In: Vinken P J, Bruyn J W (eds) Handbook of clinical neurology, Vol 30. Elsevier, Amsterdam, pp 661–680

Hidalgo H et al 1982 In utero sonographic diagnosis of fetal cerebral anomalies. American Journal of Roentgenology 139: 143

Hill L M, Breckle R, Bonebrake R 1982 Ultrasonic findings with holoprosencephaly. Journal of Reproductive Medicine 27: 172

Hirsch J F, Pierre, Kahn A, Reiner D et al 1984 The Dandy–Walker malformation: a review of 40 cases. Journal of Neurosurgery 61: 515

Hohler C W, Quetal T A 1981 Comparison of ultrasound femur length and biparietal diameter in late pregnancy. American Journal of Obstetrics and Gynecology 141: 759

Jeanty P, Dramaix-Wilmet M, Delbeke D, Rodesch F, Struyven J 1981 Ultrasonic evaluation of fetal ventricular growth. Neuroradiology 21: 127

Johnson M L, Dunne M G, Mack L A et al 1980 Evaluation of fetal intracranial anatomy by static and real-time ultrasound. Journal of Clinical Ultrasound 8: 311

Kalbag R M, Woolf A L 1967 Cerebral venous thrombosis. Oxford University Press, London

Kier E L 1977 The cerebral ventricles: aphylogenetic and ontogenetic study. In: Newton T H, Potts D G (eds) Radiology of the skull and brain: anatomy and pathology. C V Mosby, St Louis, pp 2787–2914

Kurtz A B, Wagner R J, Rubin C S et al 1980 Ultrasound criteria for in utero diagnosis of microcephaly. Journal of Clinical Ultrasound 8: 11

Lanman J T, Partanen Y, Ullberg S et al 1958 Extracortical cerebrospinal fluid in normal human fetuses. Pediatrics 21: 403

Lev-Gur M, Maklad N F, Patel S 1983 Ultrasonic findings in fetal cyclopia. A case report. Journal of Reproductive Medicine 28: 554

Lorber J 1970 Medical and surgical aspects in the treatment of congenital hydrocephalus. Neuropaediatrie 2: 239

McCullough D C, Balzer-Martin L A 1982 Current prognosis in overt neonatal hydrocephalus. Journal of Neurosurgery 57: 378

Mahony B S, Callen P W, Filly R A et al 1984 The fetal cisterna magna. Radiology 153: 773

Martin H P 1970 Microcephaly and mental retardation. American Journal of Diseases of Children 119: 128

Matsunaga E, Shiota Y 1977 Holoprosencephaly in human embryos: epidemiological studies of 150 cases. Teratology 16: 261

Milhorat T H 1972 Hydrocephalus and the cerebrospinal fluid. Williams & Wilkins, Baltimore

Murray J C, Johnson J A, Bird T D 1985 Dandy–Walker malformation: etiologic heterogeneity and empiric recurrence risks. Clinical Genetics 28: 272

Myrianthopoulos N C 1977 Epidemiology of central nervous system malformations. In: Vinken P J, Bruyn G W (eds) Handbook of clinical neurology. Elsevier, Amsterdam, pp 139–171

Naidich T P, Schott L H, Baron R L 1982 Computed tomography in evaluation of hydrocephalus. Radiologic Clinics of North America 20: 143

O'Connell E J, Feldt R H, Stickler G B 1965 Head circumference, mental retardation and growth failure. Pediatrics 36: 62

Parrish M, Roessman U, Levinsohn M 1979 Agenesis of the corpus callosum: a study of the frequency of associated malformations. Annals of Neurology 6: 349

Pearce J M, Little D, Campbell S 1985 The diagnosis of abnormalities of the fetal central nervous system. In: Sanders R C, James A E (eds) The principles and practice of ultrasound in obstetrics and gynecology. Appleton Century-Crofts, Norwalk, pp 243–256

Pilu G, DePalma L, Romero R et al 1986a The fetal subarachnoid cisterns: an ultrasound study with report of a case of congenital communicating hydrocephalus. Journal of Ultrasound Medicine 5: 365

Pilu G, Rizzo N, Orsini L F, Bovicelli L 1986b Antenatal recognition of cerebral anomalies. Ultrasound in Medicine and Biology 12: 319

Pilu G, Romero R, DePalma L a Antenatal diagnosis and obstetrical management of Dandy–Walker syndrome. Journal of Reproductive Medicine (in press)

Pilu G, Romero R, Rizzo N b Criteria for the antenatal diagnosis of holoprosencephaly. American Journal of Perinatology (in press)

Pilu G, Reece E A, Romero R c Prenatal diagnosis of cranio-facial malformations by sonography. American Journal of Obstetrics and Gynecology (in press)

Raybaud C, Bamberger Bozo C, Laffont J et al 1978 Investigations of nontumoral hydrocephalus in children. Neuroradiology 16: 24

Robertson W C, Gomez M R 1978 External hydrocephalus: early finding in congenital communicating hydrocephalus. Archives of Neurology 35: 541

Salam M Z 1977 Stenosis of the aqueduct of Sylvius. In: Vinken P J, Bruyn G W (eds) Handbook of clinical neurology, Vol 30. Elsevier, Amsterdam, pp 609–622

Sandri F, Pilu G, Cerisoli M Sonographic diagnosis of agenesis of the corpus callosum in the fetus and newborn infant (submitted)

Sauerbrei E E, Cooperberg P L 1983 Cystic tumors of the fetal and neonatal cerebrum: ultrasound and computed tomographic evaluation. Radiology 147: 689

Sawaja R, McLaurin R L 1981 Dandy–Walker syndrome: clinical analysis of 23 cases. Journal of Neurosurgery 55: 89

Tennyson V M, Pappas G D 1964 The fine structure of the developing telencephalic and myelencephalic choroid plexus in the rabbit. Journal of Comparative Neurology 123: 379

Williams B 1973 Is aqueduct stenosis a result of hydrocephalus? Brain 96: 399

Winick M, Rosso P 1969 Head circumference and cellular growth of the brain in normal and marasmic children. Journal of Pediatrics 74: 7744

Worthen N J, Gilberton V, Lau C 1986 Cortical sulcal development seen on sonography: relationship to gestational parameters. Journal of Ultrasound Medicine 5: 153

Yashon D, Jane J A, Sugar O 1965 The course of severe untreated infantile hydrocephalus: prognostic significance of the cerebral mantle. Journal of Neurosurgery 23: 509

Young H F, Nulsen F E, Weiss M H, Thomas P 1973 The relationship of intelligence and cerebral mantle in treated infantile hydrocephalus. Pediatrics 52: 38

Young I D, Trounce J Q, Levene M I et al 1985 Agenesis of the corpus callosum and macrocephaly in siblings. Clinical Genetics 28: 225

8. Computed tomography and magnetic resonance imaging of the neonatal central nervous system

Prof O. Flodmark

The clinical examination of the central nervous system in the neonate is often difficult with complex pathology. Diagnostic imaging of the neonatal brain has become extremely useful and has developed during the last decade along two main directions: computed tomography (CT) and ultrasonography (US). Ultrasonography has several obvious advantages over CT including portability and relative low cost but using the fontanelles and sutures as acoustic windows limits the use of US to the first few months of life. Furthermore some areas of the brain are less well-visualized by US, e.g. extracerebral and posterior fossa lesions. The role of CT scanning in the neonate is to provide additional information when US is unsatisfactory and when unusual pathology is encountered (Harwood-Nash & Flodmark 1982). Ultrasonography is discussed in detail in the next chapter. A new technique, magnetic resonance imaging (MRI), has been used recently with varying success in the diagnosis of pathology in the neonatal brain (Johnson et al 1983). Despite technical difficulties, this imaging method is likely to become increasingly important in the neonate.

TECHNIQUES

The fragile physiology of the neonate and the distressed newborn in particular, must be protected at all times. This becomes particularly important whenever the neonate leaves the nursery, i.e. for a diagnostic test in the Radiology Department. The transport must be carried out in such a way that all ongoing treatment can continue, the infant's temperature can be maintained and the handling of the neonate, particularly if premature, is kept to a minimum (Harwood-Nash & Flodmark 1981).

COMPUTED TOMOGRAPHY (CT)

Infants in the intensive care nursery should be moved to the CT scanner in a fully equipped transport incubator. All ongoing treatment and monitoring must be maintained, including intravenous infusions and assisted ventilation.

The temperature in the CT gantry room must be between 24° and 26°C. The body temperature is maintained by a heating lamp, so equipped that overheating of the infant is impossible, or a rubber blanket, with circulating warm water, wrapped around the neonate. A medical attendant or nurse skilled in resuscitation of neonates must be suitably protected and present in the CT gantry room at all times (Harwood-Nash & Flodmark 1981, 1982).

CT imaging of a small object, such as the neonatal brain, is difficult. Every precaution must be taken to avoid artefacts caused by improper radiographic technique. The neonate must be placed in the centre of the gantry in a proper head rest. Scanning with the infant directly on the table usually creates severe artefacts in the image. The CT scanner must be programmed correctly including proper X-ray technique as well as correct reconstruction algorithm used by the computer.

The detectors in the CT scanner record the amount of transmitted radiation. This amount is dependent on the initial energy of the X-ray beam and the amount of radiation absorbed and scattered in the patient. Thus a small object such as an infant's head will absorb and scatter a smaller amount of radiation. The output of the X-ray tube must therefore be reduced to prevent overload of the detectors. Although some CT scan systems indicate to the operator that such over-ranges have occurred, overload may only be detected as artefacts in the image. The artefact caused by over-ranges is an error in calculation of the image attenuation which usually will be assigned a lower value than the actual attenuation. Although the artefact will influence the entire image it will be more obvious in parts of the image if the object is placed asymmetrically in the scanner. The combination of excessive X-ray technique and asymmetrical positioning of the head is most devastating for the quality of the image (Fig. 8.1). This is known as 'shading' in which a gradient is seen over the entire image. Correct tension (voltage, kV) and current (amperage, mAs) applied to the X-ray tube in each case will depend on the equipment used but must always be reduced since a small object such as an infant's head is being imaged (Lassen 1986).

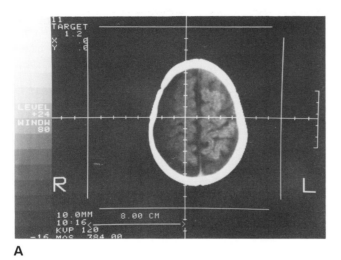
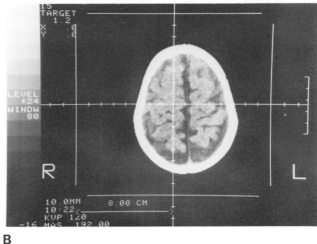

A   B

Fig. 8.1 Image artefact. (a) Decreased brain tissue attenuation caused by improper centring of the patient and excessive radiation dose. Note that the midline of the head is just 1 cm from the gantry centre. The mAs was too high at 384. (b) Correction of the artefact was achieved by reduction in radiation dose to 192 mAs, thereby eliminating over-range. The improper position of the head is now less critical. Note that both images have been recorded at identical 'level' and 'window' values.

Most CT scanners allow a small image or part of an image to be reconstructed to take advantage of the entire image matrix. Thus the picture element, pixel, remains the same size, as opposed to electronic magnification of the image in which each pixel is magnified, leading to a magnified image with poor spatial resolution. Thus the spatial resolution can be improved without compromising density resolution if a correct algorithm is used to reconstruct the image of a small neonate's head. However, spatial resolution is also dependent on slice thickness. The most commonly used image thickness, 10 mm, is generally too thick in neonates leading to significant volume-averaging. An image thickness of 5 mm is usually sufficient. It may not be necessary to obtain contiguous slices. An image interval of 10 mm will significantly reduce the radiation dose and if necessary interjacent images can be obtained at the end of the procedure. It is, however, important to include the entire brain in the study, to properly evaluate the posterior fossa.

The radiation dose involved in a CT scan is not insignificant. The actual dose depends mostly on equipment used, X-ray technique (kVp and mAs) and slice thickness. Contiguous slices always involve some overlap of radiation, thus increasing the skin dose approximately 50% from that of a single slice. The dose is also increased in a small subject (Lassen 1986, Wagner et al 1986). The most radiosensitive organs that may be included in the radiation field is the lens of the eye and the thyroid. Thus every precaution should be taken to avoid inclusion of the orbits in the scan, i.e. the scanning plane should be 20° over the cantho–meatal line. The X-ray beam in the CT scanner is extremely well collimated, thus radiation of the rest of the body, e.g. gonads, is usually not detectable. Radiation dose to staff in the CT room is therefore also minimal. Reliable values for radiation delivered by different scanners are not readily available and may even be difficult to calculate (Lassen 1986). As a rule of thumb, the dose to the head in each complete CT scan can be compared to a series of skull films including three views. However, due to scatter the gonadal dose is much higher with the skull films.

The use of intravenously administered contrast material is rarely necessary. In particular, contrast enhancement is not indicated in the asphyxiated neonate but may be necessary in a rare case of a congenital tumour (Harwood-Nash & Flodmark 1981). The less toxic non-ionic contrast materials (iohexol or iopamidol) should then be used in a dose of 2 to 3 ml per kg body weight.

Sedation is rarely necessary in neonates. Feeding immediately before the study is usually sufficient. Seizures may require additional medication to avoid motion artefacts.

There are several pitfalls that must be avoided in interpretation of CT images. It is important to assess and measure the brain tissue attentuation when the images are viewed and the hard copies being produced from the video image. Images of the neonatal brain should be viewed and documented using a narrow window of 60–80 Hounsfield units. The 'level' must be properly selected at about 25–30 and not based on the visual appearance only. Brain tissue with abnormally low attenuation can easily be made to appear 'normal' by decreasing the 'level' on the video display. Areas of normal brain tissue may then appear abnormally dense and may mimic fresh haemorrhage or calcifications causing misinterpretation of the image (Fig. 8.2) (Shewmon et al 1981, Masdeu et al 1982, Voorhies et al 1984, Aicardi & Goutieres 1984). Accurate interpretation is also dependent on a correct and complete history and good knowledge of the normal appearance of the brain in premature and full-term neonates respectively.

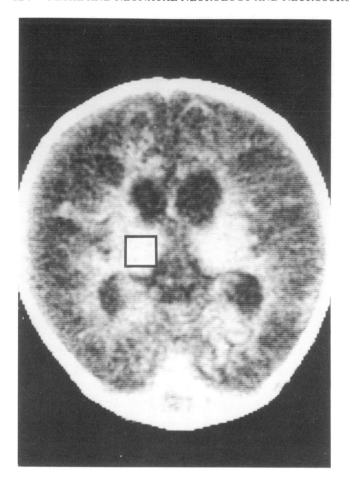

Fig. 8.2 'Attenuation artefact'. This image from a three-month-old infant born at full-term shows an apparent increase in attenuation within the basal ganglia (square box). However, the attenuation within the cursor box is 35 and consistent with normal brain tissue. The infant suffered severe asphyxia at birth with abnormally low cortical tissue attenuation indicating damage to these structures.

MAGNETIC RESONANCE IMAGING (MRI)

A magnetic resonance imaging system is centred around a magnet which is capable of generating a strong homogeneous magnetic field. This field generates a stable net magnetization of the protons within a patient located in the core of the magnet. Weak radiofrequency (RF) pulses are used to temporarily influence this net magnetization in a plane perpendicular to the long axis of the magnetic field. A relaxation process follows RF excitation by which the magnetization of the individual proton returns to its original magnitude and orientation. A weak electromagnetic signal is generated during the relaxation process and this signal can be detected by a receiver coil applied around the infant's head. The proton relaxation is dependent on and can be described by two time constants $T1$ and $T2$. Both constants are in turn dependent on the chemical environment in which the protons are found. This chemical environment can be affected by pathological and developmental factors. The

electromagnetic signal is furthermore dependent on the amount of excitable protons available (proton density). The MRI computer generates a video image that is a two-dimensional representation of the signal received and contains spatial as well as signal intensity information, which in turn depends on $T1$ and $T2$ constants as well as the RF characteristics (pulse-sequence) used in the specific application (Bradley et al 1983).

Many practical problems associated with neonatal MR imaging are similar to those of CT scanning. However, MRI poses additional problems unique to the environment in and around the magnet. The strong magnetic field prohibits the use of ferromagnetic life-support equipment in or close to the scanner (Johnson et al 1983, Nixon et al 1986). Electronic equipment is likely to malfunction in the rapidly changing magnetic field making the task of monitoring vital signs in the neonate difficult (Roth et al 1985, McArdle et al 1986). These problems must be solved for each type of magnet and field strength and are currently being addressed by manufacturers of most MR equipment. In general MRI is a safe imaging method approved for imaging during pregnancy after the first trimester (National Radiological Protection Board 1983).

The water content in the neonatal brain is high with little difference between white and grey matter (Larroche 1977). Because MR images are dependent in part on the presence of protons, i.e. water, the tissue characteristics in the neonatal brain become difficult. Therefore pulse-sequences appropriate for adults may not yield useful information in the newborn (Lee et al 1986). At the present time $T1$-weighted images have proved more informative in neonatal brain imaging than $T2$-weighted images but further development of software may change this in the future (Johnson et al 1983, Dubowitz et al 1985, Dubowitz & Bydder 1985, Lee et al 1986). The introduction of close fitting, helmet-like RF coils has significantly improved image quality in small infants as shown in Figs 8.3 and 8.4 (Dubowitz et al 1986). MRI will almost certainly provide important information regarding normal and abnormal brain development currently not possible by other imaging techniques.

INDICATIONS

COMPUTED TOMOGRAPHY

The indications for CT scanning of the neonatal brain are twofold. Firstly where the result of the study will have an immediate impact on the acute care for the neonate and secondly where the CT scan is used as an adjunct in establishing a diagnosis and hence prognosis for the neonate.

Perinatal asphyxia is the most common indication for CT scanning of the neonatal brain but the indications differ

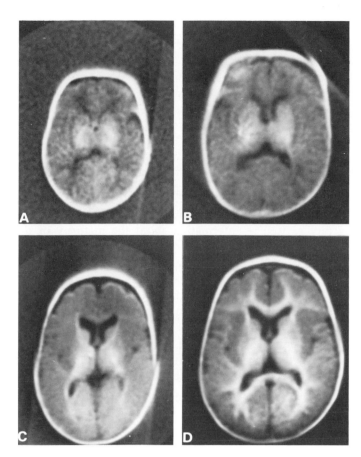

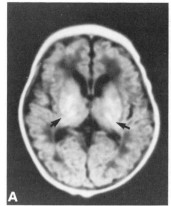

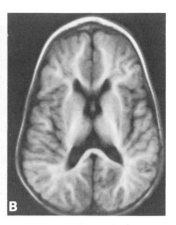

Fig. 8.4 High-resolution MRI scans using closely applied spherical receiver coils. (a) Normal scan (IR 2400/800/44) from a 9 day old infant. Early myelination can be seen in the thalami (arrowed) much earlier than the older image shown in Fig. 8.3a. (b) The same infant scanned at 12 months. Note the greatly improved resolution in both unmyelinated periventricular white matter in scan (a), and the myelinated white matter in scan (b). (Reproduced with permission from Johnson et al 1987.)

Fig. 8.3 Progression of myelination. Four IR scans (IR 1800/600/13f) from the same normal child at full-term (a), 3 months (b), 6 months (c) and 10 months (d). (Reproduced with permission from Johnson et al 1987.)

depending on the maturity of the neonate. Ultrasonography is the primary imaging method for the pre-term neonate (see Ch. 9). Intracerebral haemorrhage, a common lesion in pre-term infants, is delineated well by this method and the ventricular size can readily be assessed (Bejar et al 1980). The role of CT scanning in such patients is limited to situations in which ultrasound findings are inconsistent with the clinical impression of the patient (Harwood-Nash & Flodmark 1982, Kirks & Bowie 1986). In this instance, investigation should focus on possible pathology located in areas not well visualized by ultrasonography, i.e. the posterior fossa (Perlman et al 1983) and the extracerebral space (Cremin et al 1984). Early diagnosis of periventricular leukomalacia is difficult and unreliable but is more amenable to ultrasound imaging which shows periventricular increased echogenicity and later cysts. These findings may not be possible to confirm by CT scanning in the neonatal period (Flodmark 1981) but a characteristic reduction of periventricular white matter can be shown by CT scanning later in life (Schellinger et al 1986, Flodmark et al 1987).

The asphyxiated full-term neonate is subject to different mechanisms of brain injury and thus develops specific pathology (Volpe 1976, Brann & Dykes 1977, Hill &

Volpe 1985). The presence of cerebral œdema, extra- or intracerebral haemorrhage, posterior fossa pathology or subarachnoid blood, may be difficult to assess with ultrasonography alone (Wilson-Davis et al 1983, Siegel et al 1983, 1984). CT scanning may therefore have significant and immediate impact on the acute care and is usually considered the primary imaging method for the asphyxiated full-term infant (Harwood-Nash & Flodmark 1982). Furthermore the appearance of the brain tissue has proved to be an useful adjunct in determining the long-term prognosis for these neonates (see p. 390).

Seizures in the neonate may be secondary to asphyxia (Hill & Volpe 1981) but other causes may be identified by CT scanning, including cerebral artery infarction which is discussed in detail on p. 335 (Mannino & Trauner 1983, Trauner & Mannino 1986). A significant proportion of young infants with infantile spasm have organic pathology (Cavazzuti et al 1984) that can be diagnosed radiographically, including congenital malformations, phakomatoses, intra-uterine infections or rarely tumours. However, accurate diagnosis depends on correct timing of the CT scan. Although indication exists early in life for a scan, it may be important to delay the study. The pathology may be easier to define in a more mature brain, hence, if possible, the CT scan should be delayed until about six months of age to improve the diagnostic accuracy. This may be even more important in neonates with dysmorphic features, in whom genetic counselling may be the main indication for investigation.

The investigation of the neonate with raised intracranial pressure must focus on two issues. Firstly, to confirm the clinically suspected presence of hydrocephalus, i.e. an imbalance between production and absorption of cerebrospinal fluid (CSF). Secondly, hydrocephalus must be considered a symptom and the aetiology must therefore be identified. The most common reason for hydrocephalus in neonates is intraventricular haemorrhage (see p. 347). Thus ultrasonography is the best modality to evaluate the aetiology as well as ventriculomegaly (Horbar et al 1980, Levene 1981, Fleischer et al 1983) but if the aetiology remains obscure, the investigation must include CT scanning. Rarely tumour or congenital malformations may cause hydrocephalus in the neonatal period.

The indications for CT scanning in the neonate with meningitis are relative. Ultrasonography is a better method for monitoring ventricular size in hydrocephalus arising as a complication of meningitis. However, the incidence of complicating abscess formation is particularly high with some infectious agents, e.g. enterobacteria such as *Citrobacter* and other nosocomial infections, thus making it important to obtain a CT scan under certain circumstances (Enzmann 1984). Furthermore, atrophic lesions following meningitis are shown well by CT scanning and may be helpful in establishing the long-term prognosis.

MAGNETIC RESONANCE IMAGING

The absence of ionizing radiation will make MRI the preferred imaging modality in neonates and infants in the future. Specific indications for MR imaging of the neonatal brain are not yet established but the method has proven useful to follow the myelination of the brain (Dubowitz & Bydder 1985) (Fig. 8.3) and the flow of CSF in various compartments (Bradley et al 1986). The capability of direct sagittal imaging (Fig. 8.5) is an advantage for defining the pathology in congenital malformations (Johnson et al 1983).

RADIOGRAPHIC PATHOLOGY

The pattern of hypoxic–ischaemic cerebral injury in the newborn infant is dependent on the maturity of the brain at the time of injury (see Ch. 33). Thus, the findings on the CT scan must be interpreted in the light of the history as well as information about the maturity of the neonate. In fact, the neuroradiologist must have in-depth knowledge of the normal development of the brain as well as neonatal pathology, to properly understand sonographic and radiographic findings in the neonatal brain.

The CT scan in a pre-term neonate without significant pathology will demonstrate a smooth brain without more than a few wide gyri. The Sylvian fissures are open, exposing the insula. The cortex is thin and most of the hemisphere consists of rather homogeneous tissue with low attenuation (Fig. 8.6) (Picard et al 1980, Harwood-Nash & Flodmark 1982). The normal mature neonate will demonstrate a more prominent cortex with a more complex pattern of gyri. The Sylvian fissures are closed. The brain tissue attenuation shows clear differentiation between white and grey matter. Central white matter may be prominent and have a strikingly low attenuation; however, cortex with a higher attenuation will still be seen around the periphery (Fig. 8.7) (Picard et al 1980).

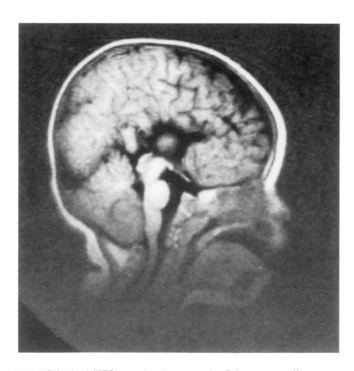

Fig. 8.5 Sagittal MRI scan showing agenesis of the corpus callosum. IR scan in a 14-month-old infant showing total absence of the corpus callosum with an abnormally high roof to the third ventricle. (Reproduced with permission from Fielder et al 1986.)

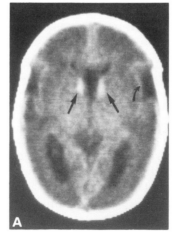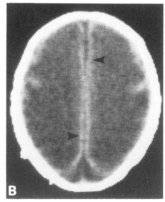

Fig. 8.6 Normal appearances in severe prematurity (27 weeks gestation, birth-weight 1070 g). (a) Image at the level of the foramen of Monro showing the normal hypervascularity of the germinal matrix (arrows) and the wide-open Sylvian fissures with the insula exposed (curved arrow). (b) Image at the level of the centrum semiovale showing the extensive homogeneous white matter with low attenuation. The cortex is a thin structure best seen outlining the interhemispheric fissure (arrows). (Also note the paucity of cortical convolutions in both **a** and **b**.)

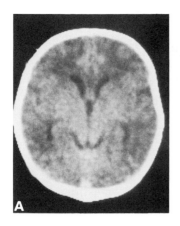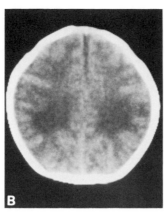

Fig. 8.7 Normal scans from a full-term, appropriately grown infant. (a) Image at the level of the foramen of Monro demonstrates normal Sylvian fissures and a higher attenuation throughout the brain and a good differentiation between white and grey matter. Note prominent white matter in both frontal lobes. (b) Image at the level of the centrum semiovale showing normal amounts of grey matter but prominent white matter. However, note that grey matter surrounds the white matter and has maintained normal attenuation.

PRE-TERM NEONATES

Intracranial haemorrhage

The detection of the haemorrhagic components of hypoxic–ischaemic brain damage, germinal matrix and intraventricular haemorrhage (GMH–IVH), may be accomplished accurately with CT scanning (Burstein et al 1977, Rumack et al 1978, Burstein et al 1979, Lee et al 1979, Ahmann et al 1980, Flodmark et al 1980a, Flodmark et al 1980b, Leblanc & O'Gorman 1980, Albright & Fellows 1981). As the attenuation of a haemorrhage is decreasing with time, the timing of the CT scan is important for correct diagnosis. Thus a haemorrhage 10–14 days old may be of the same attenuation as brain-tissue and difficult to delineate or may even totally escape detection. High-resolution CT scanners are capable of detecting the normal hypervascularity of the normal germinal matrix (Harwood-Nash & Flodmark 1982), an image that may be confused with a haemorrhage in this location (Fig. 8.6a). More recently neurosonography has proven to have a comparable sensitivity and specificity for diagnosis of GMH–IVH (Grant et al 1980, Dewbury & Bates 1981, Grant et al 1981, Sauerbrei et al 1981, Babcock et al 1982, Shankaran et al 1982, Pape et al 1983, Quisling et al 1983, Slovis & Shankaran 1984, Szymonowicz et al 1984) but not necessarily other forms of haemorrhagic or non-haemorrhagic injury (Grant et al 1983, Bowerman et al 1984, Nwaesei et al 1984, Szymonowicz et al 1984, Delaporte et al 1985, DiPietro et al 1986, Laub & Ingrisch 1986). Subarachnoid haemorrhage is common secondarily to GMH–IVH (Flodmark et al 1980a). The radiographic diagnosis is uncertain with CT scanning (Fig. 8.8) (Flodmark et al 1980b, Ludwig et al 1983)

and virtually impossible with ultrasonography (Babcock et al 1982, Quisling et al 1983).

The different forms of GMH–IVH have been assumed to represent lesions with the same ætiology but with an increasing severity (Burstein et al 1979, Flodmark et al 1980b). Defining a grading system should therefore be useful for prognostic purposes (Krishnamoorthy et al 1979, Papile et al 1983, Krishnamoorthy et al 1984, TeKolste et al 1985) but the usefulness has been difficult to confirm (Bada et al 1982, Fitzhardinge et al 1982, Palmer et al 1982, Stewart et al 1983, Dubowitz et al 1984, de Vries et al 1985, Ment et al 1985). Although several grading systems for germinal matrix–intraventricular haemorrhage have been suggested (Burstein et al 1979, Flodmark et al 1980b, Shankaran et al 1982, Slovis & Shankaran 1984) the most widely used system (Papile et al 1978) includes four grades: grade 1, isolated haemorrhage into the germinal matrix; grade 2, IVH with normal ventricular size; grade 3, IVH with ventriculomegaly; grade 4, IVH associated with intraparenchymal haemorrhage (Fig. 8.9). The grade assigned to a specific case depends on the most severe grade diagnosed and may be different in each hemisphere.

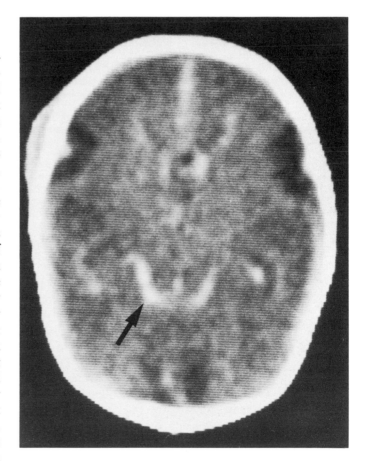

Fig. 8.8 An image from a CT scan of a prematurely born neonate in whom higher sections showed a significant IVH. The quadrigeminal cistern (arrow) is full of fluid with a high attenuation indicating fresh subarachnoid haemorrhage.

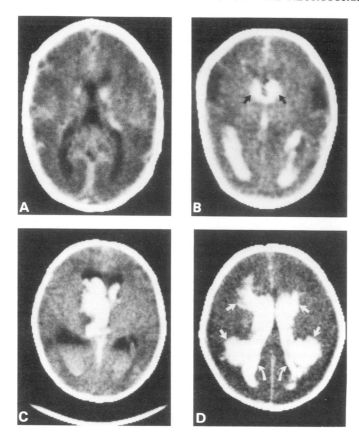

Fig. 8.9 Intraventricular haemorrhage. (a) IVH grade 1. This image, at the level of the lateral ventricles, shows a haemorrhage confined to the germinal matrix on the left side. The germinal matrix with the haemorrhage extends posteriorly along the body of the caudate nucleus in this immature neonate of 27 weeks gestation. No haemorrhage is seen in the ventricles. (b) IVH grade 2. Note bilateral germinal matrix haemorrhage (arrows) with evidence of haemorrhage in the occipital horns of the lateral ventricles bilaterally. (c) IVH grade 3. Extensive germinal matrix haemorrhage on the right side associated with ventricular dilatation, primarily caused by the haemorrhage itself but there is also ventriculomegaly due to hydrocephalus. (d) IVH grade 4. This image is obtained in the plane of the lateral ventricles and show non-dilated ventricles full of fresh haemorrhage (curved white arrows) as well as extensive areas of poorly demarcated haemorrhage in the periventricular brain substance (white arrows).

The application of this grading system is associated with some difficulties. The intention of the grading system is to grade the amount of haemorrhage (Papile et al 1978, Burstein et al 1979). Introducing the ventricular size is a source of some confusion (Fleischer et al 1983). An IVH large enough to fill the entire lateral ventricle and dilate the ventricle is a grade 3 haemorrhage. However, every patient with even a small IVH subsequently develops some degree of ventriculomegaly (Fig. 8.9c) (Flodmark et al 1980b). This is probably due to a disturbed CSF circulation and should thus be recognized as an early sign of hydrocephalus and not be confused with a progression to a higher degree of IVH.

Grade 4 intraventricular haemorrhage was defined as IVH associated with intraparenchymal haemorrhage (Papile et al 1978) without any provisions for varying severity of the lesion. The general assumption was that the haemorrhage broke through the ventricular wall and extended into the brain tissue. However, pathology studies have not been able to confirm this (Flodmark et al 1980a) and the aetiology for intraparenchymal haemorrhage in pre-term neonates is presently thought to be a secondary haemorrhage into an area of periventricular leukomalacia or venous infarction (see p. 317). Although parenchymal haemorrhage usually is combined with IVH, the lesion can occur isolated or associated with only a very small amount of IVH (Fig. 8.10) (Bowerman et al 1984, Sauerbrei 1984). Furthermore, the extent and location of the intraparenchymal haemorrhage can vary greatly. Thus lesions of different severity can all be classified as a grade 4 IVH. The findings of a grade 4 IVH must therefore be carefully described by the radiologist to allow a qualified assessment of the prognosis in each individual case.

The ability to detect intracerebral haemorrhage with MRI depends on the age of the haemorrhage. The presence in the haematoma of various paramagnetic substances, deoxyhaemoglobin, methaemoglobin free or within red blood cells and haemosiderin, influence the signal. The relaxation times and thus signal intensities of paramagnetic substances are also dependent on the magnetic field strength. Imaging of fresh haematomas (<7 days) appears at present to be only possible at high magnetic field strength, 1.5 T or more (Gomori et al 1985). Thus, MRI may not be as useful as US or CT in the early diagnosis of neonatal intracranial haemorrhage.

Periventricular leukomalacia (PVL)

The diagnosis of PVL in the newborn is difficult. Prompt detection is possible when a haemorrhage has complicated

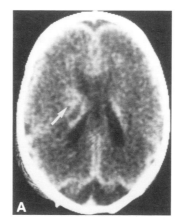
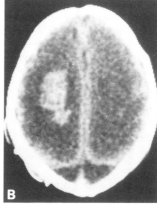

Fig. 8.10 Periventricular haemorrhage in a premature infant. (a) This image is obtained in the plane of the lateral ventricles and shows evidence of a haemorrhage into the germinal matrix on the right side (white arrow). Note the absence of haemorrhage in the ventricles. (b) An image of the same patient as in (a) at a level just above the lateral ventricles showing an intraparenchymal haemorrhage which appears to be an extension of the germinal matrix haemorrhage seen in (a).

the ischaemic infarct (Pasternak et al 1980, Sauerbrei 1984) and this lesion is commonly known, somewhat misleadingly, as grade 4 GMH–IVH. Despite early reports (Di Chiro et al 1978, Albright & Fellows 1981) non-haemorrhagic PVL cannot be diagnosed by CT scanning in the neonatal period (see p. 328) (Flodmark et al 1980a). High water content in the brain (Larroche 1977) does not allow sufficient contrast between the hypoxic–ischaemic lesions and surrounding normal brain tissue. Thus low attenuation is a normal finding in an immature brain (Estrada et al 1980, Flodmark et al 1980b, Picard et al 1980, Quencer et al 1980, Schrumpf et al 1980, Brant-Zawadzki & Enzmann 1981). Late stages of PVL when atrophy has developed can be recognized on CT scanning (Chow et al 1985) as a specific type of decrease in the amount of white matter with prominent deep sulci, secondary ventricular dilataton and in severe cases large cystic spaces adjacent to the ventricles (Fig. 8.11) (Levene et al 1983, Schellinger et al 1984, 1985, 1986, Flodmark et al 1987). These findings have been present in patients with cerebral palsy of a type compatible with the pathological diagnosis of PVL (Koch et al 1980, Kulakowski & Larroche 1980, Kotlarek et al 1981, Taudorf et al 1984). Recent experience with MRI confirms these observations and in addition shows evidence of delayed myelination in the affected periventricular white matter (for example, see Ch. 29) (Johnson et al 1983, Dubowitz et al 1985, Dubowitz & Bydder 1985, Wilson & Steiner 1986). No attempts have yet been made to assess possible damage to the periventricular white matter during the first week of life. The diagnosis of PVL is more fully discussed in Chapter 29.

FULL-TERM NEONATES

The value of CT scanning in hypoxic–ischaemic brain injury has been clearly demonstrated (Ludwig et al 1980, Schrumpf et al 1980, Hill et al 1983, Lipper et al 1986). An association has been demonstrated between general or focal decrease in brain tissue attenuation in early CT scans and adverse neurological outcome (Fitzhardinge et al 1981, Adsett et al 1985). High-resolution CT scanning of the full-term neonate, as described above, should permit identification of white and grey matter, respectively, in a normal full-term infant. However, the brain tissue attenuation will decrease as the interstitial or intracellular amount of water increases with developing cerebral œdema. The attenuation of grey matter will then approach that of white matter and the discrimination between these two tissue-types will become difficult. The attenuation is truly decreased to values around 20 units or lower in severe œdema and the brain becomes featureless (Fig. 8.12). These findings of generalized œdema are most prominent at one to three days of age and may disappear after five days. Regional cerebral blood flow changes with gradual onset of asphyxia, common in birth asphyxia, with preservation of perfusion

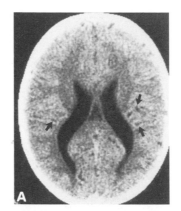
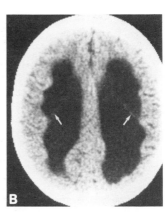
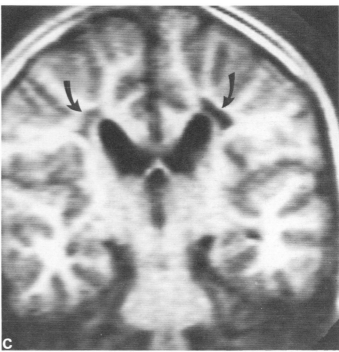

Fig. 8.11 Periventricular leukomalacia (PVL). (**a**) Mild changes with specific reduction of white matter in the periventricular region at the trigone. Note the dilated deep cortical sulci (arrows) associated with this focal form of atrophy. (**b**) Severe changes of PVL demonstrate complete absence of periventricular white matter. This has been replaced by cystic spaces. A thin remnant of the ependyma (white arrows) may separate the ventricles from these cysts. (**c**) Anterior coronal T1-weighted images (TE 400 ms, TR 1650 ms) from an MR scan of an 8-year-old patient with moderate PVL. Note that the bilateral periventricular cysts in the white matter (curved arrows) are separate from the lateral ventricle and the ependyma is intact. These cysts are located in the corona radiata and would interrupt the cortico–spinal tract.

to basal ganglia and cerebellum (Volpe et al 1985). As a result these structures maintain more normal attenuation and become clearly visible against the darker background formed by the oedematous cerebrum.

Focal areas of brain damage and less severe generalized changes may be more difficult to evaluate in CT scans during the first days of life. Prominence of white matter is common but this correlates poorly with adverse outcome as

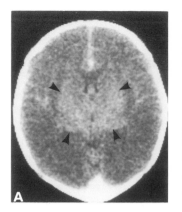
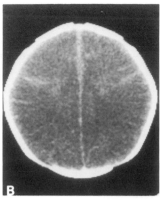

Fig. 8.12 Severe asphyxia in a full-term neonate. (**a**) Generalized decrease in attenuation of the brain tissue (21 Hounsfield units). The discrimination between white and grey matter is lost except in the basal ganglia (arrowhead) which have maintained a more normal attenuation contrasting against the darker background. (**b**) A more cephalad image of the same neonate showing an homogeneous decrease in attenuation with only a few strands of tissue frontally with preservation in attenuation. Grey matter cannot be distinguished from white matter (compare with Fig. 8.7).

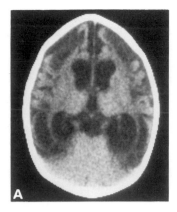
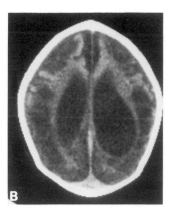

Fig. 8.13 Multicystic encephalomalacia in the same patient as shown in Fig. 8.12 when scanned at 4 months of age. (**a**) There is preservation of the basal ganglia and cerebellum but almost complete destruction of the frontal cortex. (**b**) Image at the level of the lateral ventricles showing marked ventriculomegaly secondary to almost complete cystic destruction of the entire cortex. Note how strands of preserved tissue correspond to structures seen with a more normal attenuation in Fig. 8.12**b**.

long as the grey matter has maintained normal attenuation. Modern high-resolution CT scanners are capable of better tissue discrimination and should permit better accuracy than earlier reports (Adsett et al 1985). Furthermore, elaborate scoring systems have been developed (Lipp-Zwahlen et al 1985, Lipper et al 1986) in an attempt to improve the prognostic accuracy. This is discussed in detail on p. 390.

Severe asphyxia in the full-term neonate leads to extensive destruction of brain tissue. The final stage is usually named multicystic encephalomalacia in which large portions of cortical tissue are replaced by cystic lesions (Fig. 8.13) (Babcock & Ball 1983, Raybaud 1983, Stannard & Jimenez 1983, Naidich & Chakera 1984, Slovis et al 1984). The ventricles dilate as the atrophy progresses. Confident CT diagnosis in this stage of the disease depends on careful assessment of brain tissue attenuation (Schellinger et al 1985). As described above under CT technique, the bright contrast between the relatively normal tissue attenuation in the basal ganglia and the low attenuation throughout the rest of the cerebrum may been mistaken for haemorrhage or even calcifications in the basal ganglia. This mistake must be avoided. Lesser degrees of atrophy are seen after less severe hypoxic–ischaemic brain damage. The loss of brain tissue is diffuse and mainly cortical, although axonal degeneration will cause secondary white matter atrophy.

Increased attenuation along the tentorium and straight sinus is very common in the full-term neonate (Fig. 8.14). Sometimes this increased attenuation extends forward and includes the internal cerebral veins. The cause for this is unclear and its significance is unknown. This finding may represent subarachnoid haemorrhage (Flodmark et al 1980a) which is a common finding in full-term neonates with seizures. Other possibilities include sinus thrombosis

(Wendling 1978, Eick et al 1981, Lee et al 1984, Voorhies et at 1984) or high haematocrit.

Intracerebral, subdural (Flodmark et al 1980a) or epidural (Gama & Fenichel 1985) haematoma and haemorrhage in the posterior fossa are not uncommon (Towbin 1970, Rom et al 1978, Ravenel 1979, Scotti et al 1981, Koch et al 1985, Williamson et al 1985) and it is quite important to correctly diagnose haemorrhage as extracerebral since surgery may be indicated. Tentorial tearing due to birth trauma is a more common lesion than previously thought and even large haematomas may be found in neonates with minimal symptoms (Fig. 8.15) (Schrumpf et al 1980). Correct localization of this lesion is much easier on coronal CT images of the posterior fossa (Fig. 8.15**b**), a technique that should be used whenever posterior fossa pathology is encountered. CT scanning should be the primary imaging

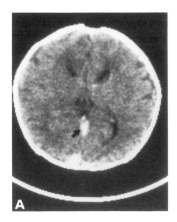
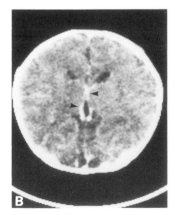

Fig. 8.14 Severe asphyxia in a full-term infant (non-enhanced). (**a**) Increased attenuation in a location compatible with the straight sinus (arrow). (**b**) A lower image of the same CT scan showing the internal cerebral veins outlined in a similar manner (arrowhead).

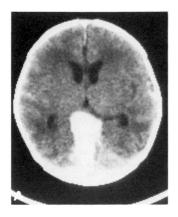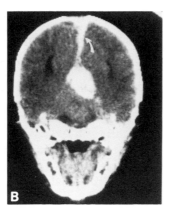

Fig. 8.15 Subdural haemorrhage. (a) Axial CT scan showing fresh haemorrhage in the region of the tentorium. (b) Coronal CT scan delineates the haemorrhage well localized within the tentorium, presumably between the two dural leaflets. Haemorrhage (probably subdural) is seen in the interhemispheric fissure (curved white arrow). A follow-up scan was normal and the infant recovered completely.

method in the full-term neonate with suspected intracranial pathology (Harwood-Nash & Flodmark 1982). The value of ultrasound for the recognition of cerebral hypoxic brain damage in full-term infants has been demonstrated in a few cases (Babcock & Ball 1983, Martin et al 1983, Wilson-Davis et al 1983, Siegal et al 1983, 1984). Unfortunately, no long-term follow-up studies have been performed and the general usefulness of this technique has yet to be established (Winchester et al 1986). Furthermore, surgically important lesions such as extracerebral haemorrhage and posterior fossa haematomas may be very difficult to diagnose by ultrasonography.

The impact of MRI in the asphyxiated full-term neonate is not known. Pure cortical pathology in adults has proven less suitable for MR imaging (Weinstein et al 1986) and this may prove true in the full-term neonate as well.

Raised intracranial pressure — cerebral atrophy

Raised intracranial pressure is a clinical diagnosis (see Ch. 34) but neuroradiological investigation is indicated. No imaging method can at the present time assess the intracranial pressure and the diagnosis of hydrocephalus may be difficult and depend entirely on clinical correlation with the imaging results. Ultrasonography is the ideal method to detect ventriculomegaly and to follow the effect of treatment on ventricular size (Horbar et al 1980, Levene 1981, Fleischer et al 1983). However, dilated ventricles are not synonymous with hydrocephalus and must be viewed with suspicion as this may be due to other causes such as congenital malformation or loss of brain tissue, atrophy. The distinction between cerebral atrophy and hydrocephalus can be very difficult, as communicating hydrocephalus in a neonate is characterized by ventriculomegaly as well as prominent subarachnoid

spaces. In fact, the distinction may be impossible unless clinical data about head circumference and head growth are available. Although the patterns of cerebral atrophy may vary greatly, two patterns are more common as sequelae to perinatal injury. A central form of atrophy with loss of periventricular white matter and secondarily ventricular dilatation (PVL), is most common in infants who were born prematurely (Fig. 8.11b) (Flodmark et al 1987). Cortical or peripheral atrophy, either generalized or focal is usually the result of hypoxic–ischaemic brain damage in the full-term neonate. Ventricular dilatation can be secondary and quite marked and associated with prominence of cortical sulci (Fig. 8.16) (Martin et al 1983, Schellinger et al 1985). Both these patterns can, for different reasons, be difficult to distinguish from hydrocephalus on CT scanning alone (Flodmark et al 1981). Thus, clinical correlation and knowledge of the patients history is imperative. As the finding of cerebral atrophy in an infant would have far-reaching consequences, the diagnosis should be made with great reluctance and only in cases when the diagnosis is clearly confirmed by clinical evidence of a small head or abnormally slow head growth and absence of intracranial hypertension.

Hydrocephalus, on the other hand, may be suspected but cannot be diagnosed by ventriculomegaly alone (Flodmark

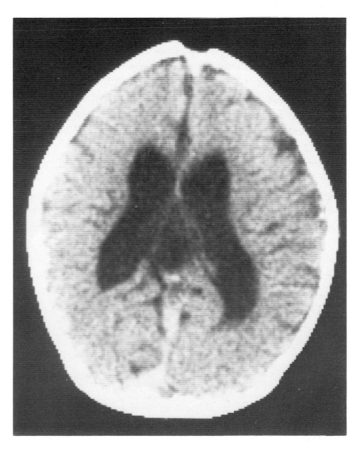

Fig. 8.16 Cerebral atrophy. The lateral ventricles are dilated subsequent to loss of brain tissue. The cortical sulci are prominent.

et al 1981). The diagnosis can only be made if large ventricles are associated with clinical evidence of raised intracranial pressure (Allan et al 1982). This is an extremely important limitation as almost all neonates, whether they have suffered IVH or not, will develop some degree of usually transient ventriculomegaly (Flodmark et al 1980b, Flodmark et al 1981, Levene & Starte 1981, Shinnar et al 1982, Szymonowicz & Yu 1984). The word hydrocephalus has a high emotional value and is generally considered synonymous with poor prognosis and life-long treatment (Boynton et al 1986). Thus, the diagnosis 'hydrocephalus' must be used with as much care as 'atrophy' and only be made if radiological findings are supported by clinical symptoms. It must also be remembered that hydrocephalus may be superimposed on atrophy, although this is extremely rare in neonates.

MRI may be of value in detecting raised intracranial pressure due to hydrocephalus and thus confirming the diagnosis as there is evidence that $T2$-weighted images can detect increased signal in the periventricular white matter, indicating transependymal CSF absorption (Johnson et al 1983, Bradley et al 1986, Sherman et al 1986). However, this has not yet been confirmed in small neonates. MRI may therefore prove to be the investigation of choice in this group.

The primary role of CT scanning in the context of raised intracranial pressure is to establish an ætiology if this is not already known. For example, the diagnosis of aqueduct stenosis is a diagnosis by exclusion and should only be made if other causes are excluded by careful imaging using CT scanning (Fig. 8.17). Small tumours in and around the third ventricle can obstruct the aqueduct and cause obstructive hydrocephalus. These are best diagnosed by CT.

Infection

Intra-uterine infection by various viruses may have devastating effects on the brain. Neuroradiological imaging may aid in the investigation of prenatal infection by detecting calcification in neonates exposed to toxoplasmosis and cytomegalovirus (CMV) in utero (see Ch. 36). The calcifications in toxoplasmosis are usually in the immediate ventricular wall and tend to form dense plaques (Fig. 8.18). Small specks of calcification scattered deeper into the white matter are usually an indication of intra-uterine CMV infection (Bale et al 1985). Both diseases can be associated with loss of brain tissue which can be extensive and cause microcephaly with or without associated ventriculomegaly (Enzmann 1984).

Postnatal infection with a virus from the herpes group can result in necrotizing encephalitis with extensive destructive lesions. This form of encephalitis is commonly more extensive in neonates than in adults or older children and may have a non-characteristic appearance with large areas of decreased brain tissue attenuation, sometimes associated with diffuse haemorrhage (Sage et al 1981).

Abscess formation and ventriculitis may occur in neonates with Gram-negative meningo-encephalitis, particularly if

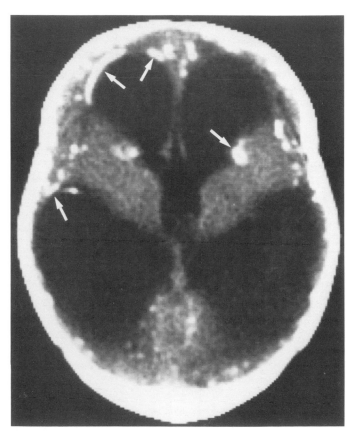

Fig. 8.18 Intra-uterine infection caused by toxoplasmosis. Densely calcified plaques are seen to outline dilated ventricles (white arrows). The infant was microcephalic.

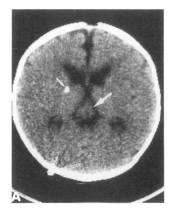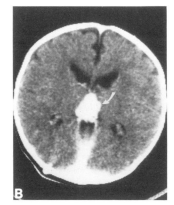

Fig. 8.17 Choroid plexus papilloma in an infant presenting with hydrocephalus. (a) Unenhanced CT scan showing v–p shunt (small white arrow) and a mass in the region of the third ventricle (white arrow). (b) Following injection of contrast, enhancement is seen in the mass. A choroid plexus papilloma was removed surgically from the third ventricle.

the infectious agent is uncommon, e.g. *Citrobacter* or other nosocomial infections (Fig. 8.19). It appears as if abscess formation in neonates is quite rapid and usually extensive. Ventriculitis is diagnosed on CT by the presence of debris in the ventricles that tend to sediment in dependent parts of the ventricular system. Neurosonography will show an increased echogenicity of the CSF mimicking a snow-storm (Hill et al 1981, Reeder & Sanders 1983). Contrast injection will show dense enhancement of the ependymal lining and other parts of the brain surrounding the abscess.

Congenital malformations of the brain

Congenital malformations are fully discussed in Chapter 19. Diagnosis during life may be made by either CT or ultrasonography (Edwards et al 1980, Raybaud 1983) but distinction between various types may be difficult. The differential diagnosis between extreme hydrocephalus and hydranencephaly (Dublin & French 1980, Sutton et al 1980) may be impossible with either imaging method and angiography may be necessary to show the presence of branches from the internal carotid artery and thus prove the diagnosis of hydrocephalus.

With the ability of MRI to directly image in the sagittal plane, this modality is well suited to provide a better understanding of the pathology of most malformations (Fig. 8.5), particularly of the limbic system which is difficult or impossible to delineate well on CT or US (Davidson et al 1985, Atlas et al 1986, Lee et al 1986).

Failure of migration of nerve cells from the germinal matrix to the cortex is usually not diagnosed until later in childhood. However, complete failure of migration,

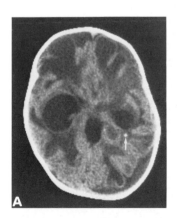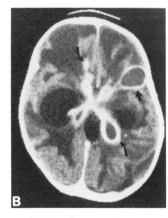

Fig. 8.19 Meningo-encephalitis caused by *Citrobacter* in a neonate. (a) Unenhanced CT image showing cystic structures in the brain associated with widespread areas of decreased brain tissue attenuation. The ventricular system cannot be clearly seen. Calcification (white arrow) in brain tissue is commonly associated with infection. (b) After contrast enhancement the ependymal surfaces are seen and the ventricular system can now be identified (curved arrows). This indicates ventriculitis. Note the high density of CSF in the ventricles in (a) compared with other CSF-containing cysts in the brain. An abscess with rim enhancement is seen in the left hemisphere (arrow).

lissencephaly, may be recognized in early infancy. The cortex is found to be smooth without formation of sulci or gyri (Norman et al 1976). The white matter is abnormally arranged in a featureless lump centrally in the hemisphere. Normal interdigitations extending into the cortex are absent. The corpus callosum is usually absent (Zimmerman et al 1983). However, the poor development of cerebral convolutions in the immature brain precludes this diagnosis to be made radiographically in a pre-term neonate. US may also be useful in this diagnosis (p. 145).

Phakomatosis

This group of disorders includes a number of hereditary entities characterized by presence of tumour-like malformations within the central nervous system (Gardeur et al 1983). Entities usually included in this group include tuberous sclerosis (Bourneville's disease), Sturge–Weber angiomatosis, neurofibromatosis (von Recklinghausen's disease) and von Hippel–Lindau disease. Only the first two may be of interest in the neonatal period.

The diagnosis of tuberous sclerosis can be made if a number of different diagnostic criteria are met. One of these is the detection of cerebral tubers and calcifications by CT scanning (Kingsley et al 1986, McLaurin & Towbin 1986). Tubers may be found in cortical grey matter but the typical calcifications are usually found in the subependymal region, most commonly in the region of foramen of Monro and trigone (Fig. 8.20). In contrast to calcifications due to toxoplasmosis, the lesions in tuberous sclerosis tend to protrude into the ventricles and are usually calcified. The natural history of these calcifications is poorly understood but it is reasonable to suggest that they develop slowly over the first years of life and may therefore not be detected if a CT scan is performed early in postnatal life (Kingsley et al 1986). Genetic counselling to parents is the main indication to confirm the diagnosis, hence the CT scan should, if possible, be delayed until at least six months of age and then performed using thin-slice thickness (5 mm) of relevant areas to minimize volume-averaging.

Seizures that are difficult to control is the usual presenting symptom in Sturge–Weber angiomatosis. Angiomatosis of the meninges causes secondary atrophy with mineralization of the underlying cortex. The calcifications are in the beginning quite diffuse and may therefore be difficult to see. Intravenous contrast injection will, however, show the meningeal angiomatosis as enhancement (Fig. 8.21). The calcifications progress with time, and atrophy becomes more pronounced (Gardeur et al 1983).

Spinal dysraphism

The need for initial radiographic imaging of neonates with open meningo–myelocele is usually quite limited. Neurosonography is capable of assessing the degree of

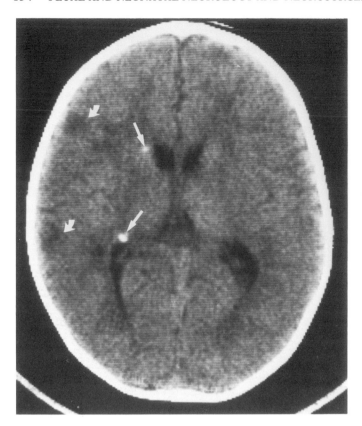

Fig. 8.20 Tuberous sclerosis. Subependymal calcifications (white arrows) may be associated with focal hemispheric lesions with decreased attenuation (curved white arrows) representing cortical tubers.

associated hydrocephalus and thus the need for ventriculo–peritoneal shunting. Diagnostic imaging is, however, important in the evaluation of neonates with lipo–meningoceles. Early corrective surgery is the indication for radiographic evaluation in the neonatal period. Plain films have a limited value and should not be performed as

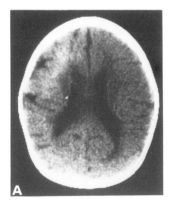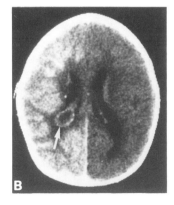

Fig. 8.21 Sturge–Weber angiomatosis. (a) An unenhanced CT image shows evidence of widespread diffuse calcifications throughout the entire right hemisphere associated with loss of brain tissue. (b) Dense enhancement is seen throughout the entire hemisphere following contrast administration. Note the cyst in the choroid plexus (white arrow), a not uncommon association with this affliction.

dysraphism, unless gross, is impossible to evaluate becase of absent ossification of the posterior elements in the spine.

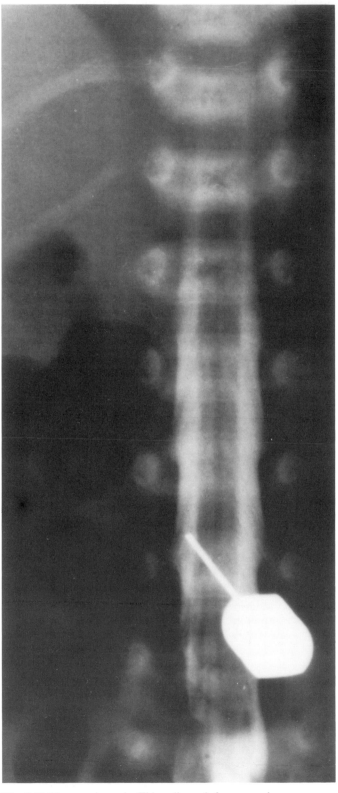

Fig. 8.22 Lipo–meningocele. This radiograph from a myelogram performed with water-soluble contrast material demonstrates how the spinal cord extends farther caudal than normally and is attached to a distal lipoma. Note the position of the spinal needle, deliberately off the midline.

Spinal neurosonography in experienced hands may provide all the information necessary to plan corrective surgery (Raghavendra et al 1983, Kangarloo et al 1984, Naidich et al 1984), however myelography combined with CT scanning will probably remain the standard procedure (Pettersson & Harwood-Nash 1982) until MRI can achieve comparable spatial resolution (Pojunas et al 1984, Roos et al 1986).

Myelography should be performed with care. The aim of the study is to establish a complete evaluation of anatomy before surgery. The lumbar puncture has to be performed at the level of the spinal cord. Thus, the puncture should be off the midline (Fig. 8.22). A preliminary film of the lumbar spine may indicate a spinal curve. The spinal cord usually follows the inner curve of the spine, thus the lumbar puncture should be done on the convex side to avoid damage to neural tissue. Two or three millilitres of isotonic non-ionic contrast material is usually sufficient to opacify the thecal sac. A small number of films provide the overview of the entire spinal canal. Associated hydromyelia is common and can be found at more rostral levels of the spinal cord and is seen as an expansion of the cord. CT scanning can confirm the diagnosis by showing the presence of a cystic structure within the cord. CT scanning is usually necessary to diagnose commonly associated diastematomyelia with a split cord and to allow detailed evaluation of the lipo–meningocele. The small size of the patient necessitates CT images not thicker than 5 mm. These slices can be non-contiguous to allow CT imaging of longer sections of the spinal cord without exposing the neonate to unnecessarily large doses of radiation.

Vascular malformations

The diagnosis of ectasia (or aneurysm) of the vein of Galen may be confirmed by ultrasonography or CT scanning. Angiography is required to assess the malformation in detail (Fig. 8.23) (Martelli et al 1980, Hoffman et al 1982, Brunelle et al 1983). These neonates are usually very unstable and suffer from cardiac failure. Contrast material must be used with care so as not to preclude possible urgent treatment with endovascular embolization.

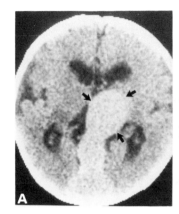
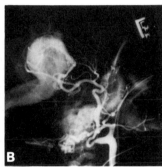

Fig. 8.23 Arterio–venous malformation with ectasia of the vein of Galen. (**a**) This image from a CT scan obtained without prior contrast injection demonstrates the ectatic vein of Galen (arrows). (**b**) Cerebral angiogram of the same patient delineates the arterio-venous malformation in detail. Feeding vessels were found from all major cerebral vessels.

REFERENCES

Adsett D B, Fitz C R, Hill A 1985 Hypoxic–ischaemic cerebral injury in the term newborn: correlation of CT findings with neurological outcome. Developmental Medicine and Child Neurology 27: 155–160

Ahamnn P A, Lazzara A, Dykes F D, Brann A W, Schwartz J F 1980 Intraventricular hemorrhage in the high-risk preterm infant: incidence and outcome. Annals of Neurology 7: 118–124

Aicardi J, Goutieres F 1984 A progressive familial encephalopathy in infancy with calcifications of the basal ganglia and chronic cerebrospinal fluid lymphocytosis. Annals of Neurology 15: 49–54

Albright L, Fellows R 1981 Sequential CT scanning after neonatal intracerebral hemorrhage. American Journal of Neuroradiology 2: 133–137

Allan W C, Holt P J, Sawyer L R, Tito A M, Meade S K 1982 Ventricular dilation after neonatal periventricular–intraventricular hemorrhage: natural history and therapeutic implications. American Journal of Diseases in Childhood 136: 589–593

Atlas S W, Zimmerman R A, Bilaniuk L T et al 1986 Corpus callosum and limbic system: neuroanatomic MR evaluation of developmental anomalies. Radiology 160: 355–362

Babcock D S, Ball W Jr 1983 Postasphyaxial encephalopathy in full-term infants: ultrasound diagnosis. Radiology 148: 417–423

Babcock D S, Bove K E, Han B K 1982 Intracranial hemorrhage in premature infants: sonographic–pathologic correlation. American Journal of Neuroradiology 3: 309–317

Bada H S, Miller J E, Menke J A et al 1982 Intracranial pressure and cerebral arterial pulsatile flow measurements in neonatal intraventricular hemorrhage. Journal of Pediatrics 100: 291–296

Bale J F, Bray P F, Bell W E 1985 Neuroradiographic abnormalities in congenital cytomegalovirus infection. Pediatric Neurology 1: 42–47

Bejar R, Curbelo V, Coen R W, Leopold G, James H, Gluck L 1980 Diagnosis and follow-up of intraventricular and intracerebral hemorrhages by ultrasound studies of infant's brain through the fontanelles and sutures. Pediatrics 66: 661–673

Bowerman R A, Donn S M, DiPietro M A, D'Amato C J, Hicks S P 1984 Periventricular leukomalacia in the pre-term newborn infant: sonographic and clinical features. Radiology 151: 383–388

Boynton B R, Boynton C A, Merritt T A, Vaucher Y E, James H E, Bejar R F 1986 Ventriculoperitoneal shunts in low birth weight infants with intracranial hemorrhage: neurodevelopmental outcome. Neurosurgery 18: 141–145

Bradley W G, Newton T H, Crooks L 1983 Physical principles of nuclear magnetic resonance. In: Newton T H, Potts D G (eds) Advanced imaging techniques. Clavadel Press, San Anselmo, CA

Bradley W G, Kortman K E, Burgoyne B 1986 Flowing cerebrospinal fluid in normal and hydrocephalic states: appearance on MR images. Radiology 159: 611–616

Brann A W, Dykes F D 1977 The effects of intrauterine asphyxia on the full-term neonate. Clinics of Perinatology 4: 149–161

Brant-Zawadzki M, Enzmann D R 1981 Using computed tomography of the brain to correlate low white-matter attenuation with early gestational age in neonates. Radiology 139: 105–108

Brunelle F O S, Harwood-Nash D C, Fitz C R, Chuang S H 1983 Intracranial vascular malformations in children: computed tomographic and angiographic evaluation. Radiology 149: 455–461

Burstein J, Papile L A, Burstein R 1977 Subependymal germinal matrix and intraventricular hemorrhage in premature infants: diagnosis by CT. American Journal of Roentgenology 128: 971–976

Burstein J, Papile L A, Burstein R 1979 Intraventricular hemorrhage and hydrocephalus in premature newborns: a prospective study with CT. American Journal of Roentgenology 132: 631–635

Cavazzuti G B, Ferrari P, Lalla M 1984 Follow-up study of 482 cases with convulsive disorders in the first year of life. Developmental Medicine and Child Neurology 26: 425–437

Chow P P, Horgan J G, Taylor K J W 1985 Neonatal periventricular leukomalacia: real-time sonographic diagnosis with CT correlation. American Journal of Neuroradiology 6: 383–388

Cremin B J, Lipinski K J, Sharp J A, Peacock W J 1984 Ultrasonic detection of subdural collections. Pediatric Radiology 14: 191–194

Davidson H D, Abraham R, Steiner R E 1985 Agenesis of the corpus callosum: magnetic resonance imaging. Radiology 155: 371–373

Delaporte B, Labrune M, Imbert M C, Dehan M 1985 Early echographic findings in non-hemorrhagic periventricular leukomalacia of the premature infant. Pediatric Radiology 15: 82–84

De Vries L S, Dubowitz L M S, Dubowitz V et al 1985 Predictive value of cranial ultrasound in the newborn baby: a reappraisal. Lancet ii: 137–140

Dewbury K C, Bates R I 1981 The value of transfontanellar ultrasound in infants. British Journal of Radiology 54: 1044–1052

Di Chiro G, Arimitsu T, Pellock J M, Landes R D 1978 Periventricular leukomalacia related to neonatal anoxia: recognition by computed tomography. Journal of Computer Assisted Tomography 2: 352–355

DiPietro M A, Brody B A, Teele R L 1986 Peritrigonal echogenic 'blush' on cranial sonography: pathologic correlates. American Journal of Neuroradiology 7: 305–310

Dublin A B, French B N 1980 Diagnostic image evaluation of hydranencephaly and pictorially similar entities, with emphasis on computed tomography. Radiology 137: 81–91

Dubowitz L M S, Bydder G M 1985 Nuclear magnetic resonance imaging in the diagnosis and follow-up of neonatal cerebral injury. Clinics of Perinatology 12(1): 243–260

Dubowitz L M S, Dubowitz V, Palmer P G, Miller G, Fawer C L, Levene M I 1984 Correlation of neurologic assessment in the preterm newborn infant with outcome at 1 year. Journal of Pediatrics 105: 452–456

Dubowitz L M S, Bydder G M, Mushin J 1985 Developmental sequence of periventricular leukomalacia: correlation of ultrasound, clinical, and nuclear magnetic resonance functions. Archives of Disease in Childhood 60: 349–355

Dubowitz L M S, Pennock J M, Johnson M A, Bydder G M 1986 High-resolution magnetic resonance imaging of the brain of children. Clinical Radiology 37: 113–117

Edwards M K, Brown D L, Muller J, Grossman C B, Chua G T 1980 Cribside neurosonography: real-time sonography for intracranial investigation of the neonate. American Journal of Neuroradiology 1: 501–505

Eick J J, Miller K D, Bell K A, Tutton R H 1981 Computed tomography of deep cerebral venous thrombosis in children. Radiology 140: 399–402

Enzmann D R 1984 Imaging of infections and inflammations of the central nervous system: computed tomography, ultrasound, and nuclear magnetic resonance. Raven Press, New York

Estrada M, El Gammal T, Dyken P R 1980 Periventricular low attenuations: a normal finding in computerized tomographic scans of neonates? Archives of Neurology 37: 754–756

Fielder A R, Gresty M A, Dodd K L, Mellor D H, Levene M I 1986 Congenital oculomotor apraxia. Transactions of the Ophthalmological Societies of the United Kingdom 105: 589–598

Fitzhardinge P M, Flodmark O, Fitz C R, Ashby S 1981 The prognostic value of computed tomography as an adjunct to assessment of the full-term neonate with post-asphyxial encephalopathy. Journal of Pediatrics 99: 777–781

Fitzhardinge P M, Flodmark O, Fitz C R, Ashby S 1982 The prognostic value of computed tomography of the brain in asphyxiated premature infants. Journal of Pediatrics 100: 476–481

Fleischer A C, Hutchinson A A, Bundy A L et al 1983 Serial sonography of posthemorrhagic ventricular dilatation and porencephaly

after intracranial hemorrhage in the preterm neonate. American Journal of Neuroradiology 4: 971–975

Flodmark O 1981 Diagnosis by computed tomography of intracranial hemorrhage and hypoxic/ischemic brain damage in neonates. Thesis, Karolinska Institutet, Stockholm

Flodmark O, Becker L E, Harwood-Nash D C, Fitzhardinge P M, Fitz C R, Chuang S H 1980a Correlation between computed tomography and autopsy in premature and full-term neonates that have suffered perinatal asphyxia. Radiology 137: 93–103

Flodmark O, Fitz C R, Harwood-Nash D C 1980b CT diagnosis and short term prognosis of intracranial hemorrhage and hypoxic/ischemic brain damage in neonates. Journal of Computer Assisted Tomography 4: 775–787

Flodmark O, Scotti G, Harwood-Nash D C 1981 Clinical significance of ventriculomegaly in children who suffered asphyxia with or without intracranial hemorrhage. Journal of Computer Assisted Tomography 5: 663–673

Flodmark O, Roland E H, Hill A, Whitfield M F 1987 Radiologic diagnosis of periventricular leukomalacia (PVL). Radiology 162: 119–124

Gama C H, Fenichel G M 1985 Epidural hematoma of the newborn due to birth trauma. Pediatric Neurology 1: 52–53

Gardeur D, Palmieri A, Mashaly R 1983 Cranial computed tomography in the phakomatoses. Neuroradiology 25: 293–304

Gomori J M, Grossman R I, Goldberg H I, Zimmerman R A, Bilaniuk L T 1985 Intracranial hematomas: imaging by high-field MR. Radiology 157: 87–93

Grant E G, Schellinger D, Borts F T et al 1980 Real-time sonography of the neonatal and infant head. American Journal of Neuroradiology 1: 487–492

Grant E G, Borts F T, Schellinger D, McCullough D C, Sivasubramanian K N, Smith Y 1981 Real-time ultrasonography of neonatal intraventricular hemorrhage and comparison with computed tomography. Radiology 139: 687–691

Grant E G, Schellinger D, Richardson J D, Coffey M L, Smirniotopoulous J G 1983 Echogenic periventricular halo: normal sonographic finding or neonatal cerebral hemorrhage. American Journal of Neuroradiology 4: 43–46

Harwood-Nash D C, Flodmark O 1981 CT of the neonate. In: Moss A A, Goldberg H I (eds) Interventional radiographic techniques: computed tomography and ultrasonography. University of California, pp 157–165

Harwood-Nash D C, Flodmark O 1982 Diagnostic imaging of the neonatal brain: review and protocol. American Journal of Neuroradiology 3: 103–115

Hill A, Volpe J J 1981 Seizures, hypoxic–ischemic brain injury, and intraventricular hemorrhage in the newborn. Annals of Neurology 10: 109–121

Hill A, Volpe J J 1985 Pathogenesis and management of hypoxic–ischemic encephalopathy in the term newborn. Neurologic Clinics 3: 31–34

Hill A, Shackelford G D, Volpe J J 1981 Ventriculitis with neonatal bacterial meningitis: identification by real-time ultrasound. The Journal of Pediatrics 99: 133–136

Hill A, Martin D J, Daneman A, Fitz C R 1983 Focal ischemic cerebral injury in the newborn: diagnosis of ultrasound and correlation with computed tomographic scan. Pediatrics 71: 790–793

Hoffman H J, Chuang S, Hendrick E B, Humphreys R P 1982 Aneurysms of the vein of Galen. Journal of Neurosurgery 57: 316–322

Horbar J D, Walters C L, Philip A G S, Lucey J F 1980 Ultrasound detection of changing ventricular size in posthemorrhagic hydrocephalus. Pediatrics 66: 674–678

Johnson M A, Pennock J M, Bydder G M et al 1983 Clinical NMR imaging of the brain in children: normal and neurologic disease. American Journal of Neuroradiology 4: 1013–1026

Johnson M A, Pennock J M, Bydder G M, Dubowitz L M S, Thomas D J, Young I R 1987 Serial MR imaging in neonatal cerebral injury. American Journal of Neuroradiology 8: 83–92

Kangarloo H, Gold R H, Diament M J, Boechat M I, Barrett C 1984 High resolution spinal sonography in infants. American Journal of Roentgenology 142: 1243–1247

Kingsley D P E, Kendall B E, Fitz C R 1986 Tuberous sclerosis: a clinicoradiological evaluation of 110 cases with particular reference to atypical presentations. Neuroradiology 28: 38–46

Kirks D R, Bowie J D 1986 Cranial ultrasonography of neonatal periventricular/intraventricular hemorrhage: who, how, why and when Pediatric Radiology 16: 114–119

Koch B, Braillier D, Eng G, Binder H 1980 Computerized tomography in cerebral-palsied children. Developmental Medicine and Child Neurology 22: 595–607

Koch T K, Jahnke S E, Edwards M S B, Davis S L 1985 Posterior fossa hemorrhage in term newborns. Pediatric Neurology 1: 96–99

Kotlarek F, Rodewig R, Brull D, Zeumer H 1981 Computed tomographic findings in congenital hemiparesis in childhood and their relation to etiology and prognosis. Neuropediatrics 12: 101–109

Krishnamoorthy K S, Shannon D C, DeLong G R, Todres I D, Davis K R 1979 Neurologic sequelae in the survivors of neonatal intraventricular hemorrhage. Pediatrics 64: 233–237

Krishnamoorthy K S, Kuehnle K J, Todres I D, DeLong G R 1984 Neurodevelopmental outcome of survivors with posthemorrhagic hydrocephalus following grade II neonatal intraventricular hemorrhage. Annals of Neurology 15: 201–204

Kulakowski S, Larroche J C 1980 Cranial computerized tomography in cerebral palsy. An attempt at anatomo–clinical and radiological correlations. Neuropediatrics 11: 339–353

Larroche J C 1977 Developmental pathology of the neonate. Excerpta Medica, Amsterdam, p. 320

Lassen M N 1986 Dedicated CT technique for scanning neonates. Radiology 161: 363–366

Laub M C, Ingrisch H 1986 Increased periventricular echogenicity (periventricular halos) in neonatal brain: a sonographic study. Neuropediatrics 17: 39–43

Leblanc R, O'Gorman A M 1980 Neonatal intracranial hemorrhage: a clinical and serial computerized tomographic study. Journal of Neurosurgery 53: 642–651

Lee B C P, Grassi A E, Schechner S, Auld P A M 1979 Neonatal intraventricular hemorrhage: a serial computed tomography study. Journal of Computer Assisted Tomography 3: 483–490

Lee B C P, Voorhies T M, Ehrlich M E, Lipper E, Auld P A M, Vannucci R C 1984 Digital intravenous cerebral angiography in neonates. American Journal of Neuroradiology 5: 281–286

Lee B C P, Lipper E, Nass R, Ehrlich M E, de Ciccio-Bloom E, Auld P A M 1986 MRI of the central nervous system in neonates and young children. American Journal of Neuroradiology 7: 605–616

Levene M I 1981 Measurement of the growth of the lateral ventricles in preterm infants with real-time ultrasound. Archives of Disease in Childhood 56: 900–904

Levene M I, Starte D R 1981 A longitudinal study of post-haemorrhagic ventricular dilatation in the newborn. Archives of Disease in Childhood 56: 905–910

Levene M I, Wigglesworth J S, Dubowitz V 1983 Hemorrhagic periventricular leukomalacia in the neonate: a real-time ultrasound study. Pediatrics 71: 794–797

Lipper E G, Voorhies T M, Ross G, Vannucci R C, Auld P A M 1986 Early predictors of one-year outcome for infants asphyxiated at birth. Developmental Medicine and Child Neurology 28: 303–309

Lipp-Zwahlen A E, Deonna T, Micheli J L, Calame A, Chrzanowski R, Cetre E 1985 Prognostic value of neonatal CT scans in asphyxiated term babies: low density score compared with neonatal neurological signs. Neuropediatrics 16: 209–217

Ludwig B, Brand M, Brockerhoff P 1980 Postpartum CT examination of the heads of full term infants. Neuroradiology 20: 145–154

Ludwig B, Becker K, Rutter G, Bohl J, Brand M 1983 Postmortem CT and autopsy in perinatal intracranial hemorrhage. American Journal of Neuroradiology 4: 27–36

McArdle C B, Nicholas D A, Richardson C J, Amparo E G 1986 Monitoring of the neonate undergoing MR imaging: technical considerations. Radiology 159: 223–226

McLaurin R L, Towbin R B 1986 Tuberous sclerosis: diagnostic and surgical considerations. Pediatric Neurosciences 12: 43–48

Mannino F L, Trauner D A 1983 Stroke in neonates. Journal of Pediatrics 102: 605–610

Martelli A, Scotti G, Harwood-Nash D C, Fitz C R, Chuang S H 1980 Aneurysms of the vein of Galen in children: CT and angiographic correlations. Neuroradiology 20: 123–133

Martin D J, Hill A, Fitz C R, Daneman A, Havill D A, Becker L E 1983 Hypoxic/ischaemic cerebral injury in the neonatal brain: a

report of sonographic features with computed tomographic correlation. Pediatric Radiology 13: 307–331

Masdeu J C, Fine M, Shewmon D A, Palacios E, Naidu S 1982 Postischemic hypervascularity of the infant brain: differential diagnosis on computed tomography. American Journal of Neuroradiology 3: 501–504

Ment L R, Scott D T, Ehrenkranz R A, Duncan C C 1985 Neurodevelopmental assessment of very low birth weight neonates: effect of germinal matrix and intraventricular hemorrhage. Pediatric Neurology 1: 164–168

Naidich T P, Chakera T M H 1984 Multicystic encephalomalacia: CT appearance and pathological correlation. Journal of Computer Assisted Tomography 8: 631–636

Naidich T P, Fernbach S K, McLone D G, Shkolnik A 1984 Sonography of the caudal spine and back: congenital anomalies in children. American Journal of Roentgenology 142: 1229–1242

National Radiological Protection Board ad hoc Advisory Group on Nuclear Magnetic Resonance Clinical Imaging: 1983 Revised guidance on acceptable limits of exposure during nuclear magnetic resonance clinical imaging. British Journal of Radiology 56: 974–977

Nixon C, Hirsch N P, Ormerod I E C, Johnson G 1986 Nuclear magnetic resonance: Its implications for the anaesthetist. Anaesthesia 41: 131–137

Norman M G, Roberts M, Sirois J, Trembaly L J M 1976 Lissencephaly. Canadian Journal of Neurological Sciences 3: 39–46

Nwaesei C G, Pape K E, Martin D J, Becker L E, Fitz C R 1984 Periventricular infarction diagnosed by ultrasound: a postmortem correlation. Journal of Pediatrics 105: 106–110

Palmer P, Dubowitz L M S, Levene M I, Dubowitz V 1982 Developmental and neurological progress of preterm infants with intraventricular haemorrhage and ventricular dilatation. Archives of Disease in Childhood 57: 748–753

Pape K E, Bennett-Britton S, Szymonowicz W, Martin D J, Fitz C R, Becker L E 1983 Diagnostic accuracy of neonatal brain imaging: a postmortem correlation of computed tomography and ultrasound scans. Journal of Pediatrics 102: 275–280

Papile L A, Burstein J, Burstein R, Koffler H 1978 Incidence and evolution of subependymal and intraventricular hemorrhage: a study of infants with birth weights less than 1500 gm. Journal of Pediatrics 92: 529–534

Papile L A, Munsick-Bruno G, Schaefer A 1983 Relationship of cerebral intraventricular hemorrhage and early childhood neurologic handicap. Journal of Pediatrics 103: 273–277

Pasternak J F, Mantovani J F, Volpe J J 1980 Porencephaly from periventricular intracerebral hemorrhage in a premature infant. American Journal of Diseases in Childhood 134: 673–675

Perlman J M, Nelson J S, McAlister W H, Volpe J J 1983 Intracerebellar hemorrhage in a premature newborn: diagnosis by real-time ultrasound and correlations with autopsy findings. Pediatrics 71: 159–162

Pettersson H, Harwood-Nash D C 1982 CT and myelography of the spine and cord: techniques, anatomy and pathology in children. Springer-Verlag, Berlin, pp. 39–56

Picard L, Claudon M, Roland J et al 1980 Cerebral computed tomography in premature infants, with an attempt at staging developmental features. Journal of Computer Assisted Tomography 4: 435–444

Pojunas K, Williams A L, Daniels D L, Haughton V M 1984 Syringomyelia and hydromyelia: magnetic resonance evaluation. Radiology 153: 679–683

Quencer R M, Parker J C, Hinkle D K 1980 Maturation of normal primate cerebral tissue: preliminary results of a computed tomographic–anatomic correlation. Journal of Computer Assisted Tomography 4: 464–465

Quisling R G, Reeder J D, Setzer E S, Kaude J V 1983 Temporal comparative analysis of computed tomography with ultrasound for intracranial hemorrhage in premature infants. Neuroradiology 24: 205–211

Raghavendra B N, Epstein F J, Pinto R S, Subramanyam B R, Greenberg J, Mitnick J S 1983 The tethered spinal cord: diagnosis by high-resolution real-time ultrasound. Radiology 149: 123–128

Ravenel S D B 1979 Posterior fossa hemorrhages in the term newborn: report of two cases. Pediatrics 64: 39–42

Raybaud C 1983 Destructive lesions of the brain. Neuroradiology 25: 265–291

Reeder J D, Sanders R C 1983 Ventriculitis in the neonate: recognition by sonography. American Journal of Neuroradiology 4: 37–41

Rom S, Serfontein G L, Humphreys R P 1978 Intracerebellar hematoma in the neonate. Journal of Pediatrics 93: 486–488

Roos R A C, Vielvoye G J, Voormolen J H C, Peters A C B 1986 Magnetic resonance imaging in occult spinal dysraphism. Pediatric Radiology 16: 412–416

Roth J L, Nugent M, Gray J E et al 1985 Patient monitoring during magnetic resonance imaging. Anesthesiology 62: 80–83

Rumack C M, McDonald M M, O'Meara O, Sanders B B, Rudikoff J C 1978 CT detection and course of intracranial hemorrhage in premature infants. American Journal of Roentgenology 131: 493–497

Sage M R, Dubois P J, Oakes J, Rothman S, Heinz E R, Drayer B 1981 Rapid development of cerebral atrophy due to perinatal herpes simplex encephalitis: a case report. Journal of Computer Assisted Tomography 5: 763–766

Sauerbrei E E 1984 Serial brain sonography in two children with leukomalacia and cerebral palsy. Journal of the Canadian Association of Radiologists 35: 164–167

Sauerbrei E E, Digney M, Harrison P B, Cooperberg P L 1981 Ultrasonic evaluation of neonatal hemorrhage and its complications. Radiology 139: 677–685

Schellinger D, Grant E G, Richardson J D 1984 Cystic periventricular leukomalacia: sonographic and CT findings. American Journal of Neuroradiology 5: 439–445

Schellinger D, Grant E G, Richardson J D 1985 Neonatal leukoencephalopathy: a common form of cerebral ischemia. Radiographics 5: 221–242

Schellinger D, Grant E G, Manz H J, Lavenstein B L, Patronas N 1986 Ventricular shapes, distortions, and deformities: mirrors of past cerebral insults. A study based on early sonographic follow-up studies. Pediatric Neurology 2: 193–201

Schrumpf J D, Sehring S, Killpack S, Brady J P, Hirata T, Mednick J P 1980 Correlation of early neurologic outcome and CT findings in neonatal brain hypoxia and injury. Journal of Computer Assisted Tomography 4: 445–450

Scotti G, Flodmark O, Harwood-Nash D C, Humphries R P 1981 Posterior fossa hemorrhages in the newborn. Journal of Computer Assisted Tomography 5: 68–72

Shankaran S, Slovis T L, Bedard M P, Poland R L 1982 Sonographic classification of intracranial hemorrhage. A prognostic indicator of mortality, morbidity, and short-term neurologic outcome. Journal of Pediatrics 100: 469–475

Sherman J L, Citrin C M, Bowen B J, Gangarosa R E 1986 MR demonstration of altered cerebrospinal fluid flow by obstructive lesions. American Journal of Neuroradiology 7: 571–579

Shewmon D A, Fine M, Masdeu J C, Palacios E 1981 Postischemic hypervascularity of infancy: a stage in the evolution of ischemic brain damage with characteristic CT scan. Annals of Neurology 9: 358–365

Shinnar S, Molteni R A, Gammon K, D'Souza B J, Altman J, Freeman J M 1982 Intraventricular hemorrhage in the premature infant: a changing outlook. New England Journal of Medicine 306: 1464–1468

Siegel M J, Patel J, Gado M H, Shackelford G D 1983 Cranial computed tomography and real-time sonography in full-term neonates and infants. Radiology 149: 111–116

Siegel M J, Shackelford G D, Perlman G M, Fulling K H 1984 Hypoxic–ischemic encephalopathy in term infants: diagnosis and prognosis evaluated by ultrasound. Radiology 152: 395–399

Slovis T L, Shankaran S 1984 Ultrasound in the evaluation of hypoxic–ischemic injury and intracranial hemorrhage in neonates: the state of the art. Pediatric Radiology 14: 67–75

Slovis T L, Shankaran S, Bedard M P, Poland R L 1984 Intracranial hemorrhage in the hypoxic–ischemic infant: ultrasound demonstration of unusual complications. Radiology 151: 163–169

Stannard M W, Jimenez J F 1983 Sonographic recognition of multiple cystic encephalomalacia. American Journal of Neuroradiology 4: 1111–1114

Stewart A L, Thorburn R J, Hope P L, Goldsmith M, Lipscomb A P, Reynolds E O R 1983 Ultrasound appearance of the brain in very preterm infants and neurodevelopmental outcome at 18 months of age. Archives of Disease in Childhood 58: 598–604

Sutton L N, Bruce D A, Schut L 1980 Hydranencephaly versus maximal hydrocephalus: an important clinical distinction. Neurosurgery 6: 35–38

Szymonowicz W, Yu V Y H 1984 Timing and evolution of periventricular haemorrhage in infants weighing 1250 g or less at birth. Archives of Disease in Childhood 59: 7–12

Szymonowicz W, Schafler K, Cussen L J, Yu V Y H 1984 Ultrasound and necropsy study of periventricular haemorrhage in preterm infants. Archives of Disease in Childhood 59: 637–642

Taudorf K, Mechior J C, Pedersen H 1984 CT findings in spastic cerebral palsy: clinical, aetiological and prognostic aspects. Neuropediatrics 15: 120–124

TeKolste K A, Bennett F C, Mack L A 1985 Follow-up of infants receiving cranial ultrasound for intracranial hemorrhage. American Journal of Diseases in Childhood 139: 299–303

Towbin A 1970 Central nervous system damage in the human fetus and newborn infant. American Journal of Diseases in Childhood 119: 529–542

Trauner D A, Mannino F L 1986 Neurodevelopmental outcome after neonatal cerebrovascular accident. Journal of Pediatrics 108: 459–461

Volpe J J 1976 Perinatal Hypoxic–Ischemic brain injury. Pediatric Clinics of North America 23(3): 383–397

Volpe J J, Herscovitch P, Perlman J M, Kreusser K L, Raichle M 1985 Positron emission tomography in the asphyxiated term newborn: parasagittal impairment of cerebral blood flow. Annals of Neurology 17: 287–296

Voorhies T M, Lipper E G, Lee B C P, Vannucci R C, Auld P A M 1984 Occlusive vascular disease in asphyxiated newborn infants. Journal of Pediatrics 105: 92–96

Wagner L K, Archer B R, Zeck O F 1986 Conceptus dose from two state-of-the-art CT scanners. Radiology 159: 787–792

Weinstein M A, LaValley A, Rosenbloom S A, Duchesnan P M 1986 Limitations of MRI for the detection of gray matter lesions. Presented at 24th Annual Meeting of The American Society of Neuroradiology, San Diego, CA, 19–23 January

Wendling L R 1978 Intracranial venous sinus thrombosis: diagnosis suggested by computed tomography. American Journal of Roentgenology 130: 978–980

Williamson W D, Percy A K, Fishman M A et al 1985 Cerebellar hemorrhage in the term neonate: developmental and neurologic outcome. Pediatric Neurology 1: 356–360

Wilson D A, Steiner R E 1986 Periventricular leukomalacia: evaluation with MR imaging. Radiology 160: 507–511

Wilson-Davis S L, Lo W, Filly R A 1983 Limitations of ultrasound in detecting cerebral ischemic lesions in the neonate. Annals of Neurology 14: 249–251

Winchester P, Brill P W, Cooper R, Krauss A N, Peterson H 1986 Prevalence of 'compressed' and asymmetric lateral ventricles in healthy full-term neonates: sonographic study. American Journal of Neuroradiology 7: 149–153

Zimmerman R A, Bilaniuk L T, Grossman R I 1983 Computed tomography in migratory disorders of human brain development. Neuroradiology 25: 257–263

9. Ultrasound imaging of the neonatal brain

Dr J. Q. Trounce and Dr M. I. Levene

The first reports of ultrasound to image pathology in the neonatal brain appeared in the late 1970s (Heimburger et al 1978, Johnson et al 1979, Pape et al 1979) and it has rapidly become the most widely used imaging technique in the neonatal period. The ubiquity of ultrasound is due to its safety, portability and ease of use and it has been widely adopted as a clinical tool by neonatologists. The value of ultrasound in evaluating cardiac and abdominal pathology contributes to its importance as a dedicated instrument on a neonatal intensive care unit. Whilst it remains the first-line method for screening all intracranial problems in early infancy, the most appropriate imaging technique to use depends on the pathology or condition to be detected as shown in Table 9.1.

BASIC PHYSICS

The application of a short electrical pulse to a thin piezo-electric crystal causes it to vibrate at ultrasonic frequencies and to transmit a longitudinal sound wave into the tissues. Originally quartz crystals were used but more recently ferro-electric materials such as lead zirconate and lead titanate have been preferred. On passage through the tissue, ultrasound waves are affected by the acoustic properties of the tissue. Reflection of the sound waves back to the transducer occurs from interfaces between tissues with different acoustic properties. The reflected signal is detected by the transducer, extraneous electronic noise is filtered out, and the time of flight of the pulse is measured. The distance of the object from the transducer can then be calculated and an image displayed on the screen.

The frequencies of the ultrasound waves used for medical imaging usually lie between about 2 to 10 million cycles per second (MHz). A higher frequency is associated with a proportionally shorter wavelength. Sound waves of lower frequency experience less attenuation as they travel through the tissues and thus allow greater penetration. The longer wavelength, however, decreases the resolution of the image and makes it more difficult to differentiate closely adjacent structures.

The width and focusing of the ultrasound beam is also important in the quality of image production. Axial resolution refers to the minimum distance between two objects in the axial direction which can be resolved by the ultrasound beam. Lateral resolution refers to the minimum distance between objects at right angles to the axis of the ultrasound beam and is dependent on the degree of focusing of the beam and whether the reflecting object lies in the near or far field.

Table 9.1 The relative value of computerized tomography (CT), magnetic resonance imaging (MRI), and ultrasound (US) in the diagnosis of various forms of intracranial pathology

	CT	MRI	US
GMH–IVH	++		++
Parenchymal haemorrhage	++	++	++
Subdural haemorrhage	++		+
Subarachnoid haemorrhage	++		+
Leukomalacia	+	+	++
Cerebral artery infarction	++		+
Cerebral oedema	++		
Intracranial calcification	+		++
Ventriculomegaly	++	+	++
Congenital abnormalities	++	++	++
Vein of Galen aneurysm			++
Tumour	++	++	
Meningitis (complications)	++		+
Abnormal myelination		++	

++represents the best method; +gives some useful, but less than definitive information

INSTRUMENTATION

Real-time ultrasound images may be produced by the sequential firing of a linear array of crystals. This type of transducer is relatively large and makes relatively poor contact with the anterior fontanelle. The original scanners used for imaging of the infant's head were of this type and were mainly applied against the flatter temporoparietal bone, producing a scan in axial plane.

An alternative method is to use a single oscillating

or rotating crystal to produce a wedge or sector image. Transducers of this type are smaller and may be used over the open anterior fontanelle, which has been referred to as an 'acoustic window' (Volpe 1982), to give a much wider range of view.

More recently, electronic phased array transducers have been used to steer the ultrasound beam to produce angled or sectored views from non-mobile crystals. The imaging crystals may also be used to produce a pulsed wave Doppler beam, allowing simultaneous imaging and haemodynamic assessment of the brain and these machines are referred to as duplex Doppler instruments (see Ch. 11).

TECHNIQUE

Scanning can be performed in the incubator or cot and no sedation is required. Scans should be performed in both the coronal plane (sweeping from anterior to posterior) and sagittally (from the midline as far laterally as possible on both sides). Transaxial scans performed through the temporoparietal bones are seldom of value except for the following situations:

1. to measure the size of dilated lateral ventricles which cannot be seen clearly through the anterior fontanelle or if this has closed;
2. to demonstrate small extracerebral collections such as a small subdural haemorrhage.

A 5 MHz scan-head will usually serve to demonstrate most abnormalities and carries sufficient penetration to allow good imaging in the larger infant. In the pre-term brain (<32 weeks gestation) more precise definition can be achieved with 7.5 MHz scan-heads which utilize shorter wavelengths (see above); these scan-heads, however, generally have insufficient penetration for the larger infant. Modern ultrasound machines often produce excellent and high-resolution images even in the smallest infants with a 5 MHz transducer. There is little, if any, place for lower frequencies in neonatal practice.

BIOLOGICAL EFFECT

Parents will frequently ask if there are any dangers associated with ultrasound scanning. The major areas to be considered are as follows:

Heat production. This occurs largely as a result of the absorption of ultrasound energy causing vibration at the molecular level with heat generation. However, the pulsed waves of low intensity used in diagnostic ultrasound produce very little heat.

Cavitation. This depends on the property of all normal liquids in containing a population of submicroscopic gas bubbles. The vibration induced by the ultrasound causes the microbubbles to grow by a process of rectified diffusion (i.e. transfer of gas to the bubble from solution in the surrounding liquid). The larger bubbles may then induce sequelae including shearing effects, which may in turn lead to DNA degradation, and the release of free radicals. It appears that the pulsed waves used in clinical imaging are free of this effect (Hill & ter Haer 1982).

Genetic risks. Liebeskind et al (1979) found an increase in sister chromatid exchange in human lymphocytes and lymphoblasts but this effect has not been reproduced (Stewart & Stratmeyer 1982) and it is thought that current diagnostic ultrasound procedures are very unlikely to result in a genetic hazard (Thacker 1973).

Neural effects. A follow-up study has found no behavioural or developmental sequelae in children previously exposed to ultrasound in utero (Carstensen & Gates 1983). Although further work is needed on the possible hazards the WHO report (Hill & ter Haer 1982) is a reasonable statement of our present understanding:

> There is at present no clearly established evidence to indicate that the ultrasonic exposures involved (in diagnostic medicine) constitute a hazard to the patient.

Ultrasound exposure should, however, be kept to an essential minimum.

PATHOLOGY

To fully appreciate minor degrees of abnormality a clear understanding of the normal appearances is essential. These are illustrated elsewhere (Cremin et al 1983, Levene et al 1984, Rumack & Johnson 1984) and will not be reproduced here. It is of note that the brain shows a sequence of changes from 26 weeks to full-term which are apparent on sequential ultrasound scans. Initially the brain appears smooth with a wide cleft in the region of the developing insula. The relative proportions of the basal ganglia and other structures change as the fetus develops up to full-term.

INTRACRANIAL HAEMORRHAGE

Ultrasound imaging is of particular value in the detection of intracranial haemorrhage. All the important varieties of haemorrhage occurring in the neonatal head have been described by real-time ultrasound but this method is considerably more sensitive to some forms compared with others. Enzmann et al (1981), using a canine model, proposed that the echogenicity of haemorrhages related to the tightly packed red cell mass. Dewbury & Bates (1983) have suggested from in-vitro studies that the three-dimensional fibrin polymer is a strongly reflective substance and is responsible for the echodense appearance of intracranial haemorrhage.

Germinal matrix and intraventricular haemorrhage (GMH–IVH)

Haemorrhage in the germinal matrix appears echogenic and will be detected if the lesion exceeds 1–2 mm in size. The haemorrhage is identified in two planes (coronal and sagittal) as an echogenic area in the region of the head of the caudate nucleus, usually in front of the caudothalamic notch when viewed in the parasagittal plane (Fig. 9.1). Although GMH may occur behind the notch this is uncommon and occurs particularly in the most immature infants. Confusion between the GMH and normal choroid plexus may also occur but the choroid does not extend anterior to the caudothalamic notch and lies in the curve of the thalamus within the lateral ventricle. Liquid blood in the ventricles is not echogenic and minor degrees of IVH will be missed on ultrasound. More extensive liquid-phase IVH will cause some anechoic distension of the lateral ventricles. Once clot develops then these appear as echogenic structures. Occasionally, bright symmetrical echoes will be seen in the region of the germinal matrix which show no change with time. At autopsy no haemorrhage is present and this probably represents unusually echogenic but otherwise normal fornices (Levene et al 1984). Echoes from the floor of the lateral ventricle may also occasionally cause confusion with minor degrees of GMH. Even with repeated scanning a minor proportion of 'small haemorrhages' must remain equivocal. The accuracy of real-time ultrasound in recognizing autopsy proven GMH–IVH is about 90% (Babcock et al 1982, Thorburn et al 1982, Pape et al 1983, Szymonowicz et al 1984, Trounce et al 1986a).

Intraparenchymal extension of ventricular haemorrhage and its differentiation from periventricular leukomalacia (PVL) is discussed fully in Chapter 29. Trounce et al (1986b) have recently described the sonographic distinction between these two conditions (Figs 9.2 and 9.3).

Parenchymal haemorrhage is seen as an echodense area involving the ventricle and the parenchyma. The apex of the echoes lies near the midline with its base extending into

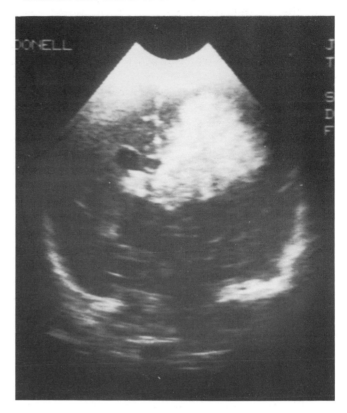

Fig. 9.2 Parenchymal haemorrhage. There is an extensive echodense area involving the ventricle and parenchyma with complete loss of the outline of ventricular structures. (Reproduced with permission from Trounce et al 1986b.)

the parenchyma and there is complete loss of the outline of ventricular structures (Fig. 9.2). In surviving infants a porencephalic cyst develops within 7 to 10 days, with loss of the ependyma of the lateral part of the lateral ventricle.

Cerebral artery infarction (see Ch. 29) is often echogenic and may be due to bleeding into infarcted tissue. This may easily be confused with spontaneous parenchymal haemorrhage. If this is considered, computerized tomographic (CT) scanning is of much more value and will show a characteristic wedge-shaped area of low attenuation. Just such an appearance was seen in the middle cerebral artery distribution in four of the five babies reported by Mannino & Trauner (1983) and they all had normal ultrasound scans. The fifth had a haemorrhagic infarct in the posterior cerebral artery distribution and this was seen on both ultrasound and CT.

Grading of GMH–IVH is controversial. Many adopt the method of Papile et al (1978) first described for haemorrhage diagnosed by CT scan (see p. 128). For the reasons discussed by Flodmark in Chapter 8 we chose to describe ventricular size separately from haemorrhage and a suitable grading system to describe the extent of GMH–IVH is shown in Table 9.2.

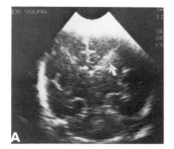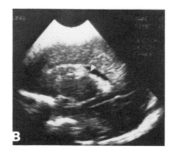

Fig. 9.1 Small haemorrhage in the region of the germinal matrix. Coronal scan (a) showing increased echos on the left (arrow) and parasagittal view (b) showing an echodense region in front of the caudothalamic notch (arrow).

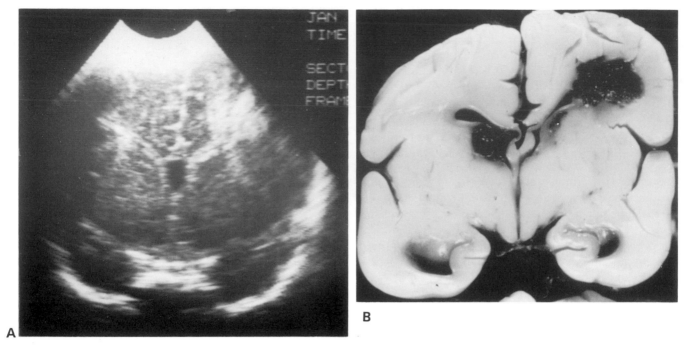

Fig. 9.3 Early periventricular leukomalacia. Coronal ultrasound scan (**a**) showing a triangular echodense flare in the right hemisphere with its apex at the external angle of the lateral ventricle. Pathological specimen (**b**) showing the haemorrhagic nature of this lesion. There is also germinal matrix haemorrhage (GMH) on the left side. (Reproduced with permission from Trounce et al 1986a and 1986b.)

Subdural subarachnoid haemorrhage

These appearances are well described on ultrasound imaging but confident exclusion of these lesions by this modality is difficult. Convexity haemorrhages (Morgan et al 1983) are easier to detect with ultrasound than those related to the tentorium or those high in the parietal region. An axial scan with either linear or sector imaging transducers is probably the best method to detect small lesions in this position (Fig. 9.4). The problem with the sonographic diagnosis of subarachnoid haemorrhage (SAH) is the close proximity of the subarachnoid space to the bone echo. It is extremely unlikely that small volumes of blood will be detected but it is possible that thrombus within the Sylvian fissure may be recognized. In addition we believe it is probably impossible to distinguish between subarachnoid and subdural haemorrhage ultrasonographically. Clinically significant lesions are likely to be associated with some

Table 9.2 Classification system for grading germinal matrix and intraventricular haemorrhage (GMH–IVH). (Modified from Levene & De Crespigny 1983)

Haemorrhage
- 0 — No haemorrhage
- 1 — Localized haemorrhage <1 cm in its largest measurement
- 2 — Haemorrhage >1 cm in its largest measurement but not extending beyond the atrium
- 3 — Blood clot forming a cast of the lateral ventricle and extending beyond the atrium
- 4 — Intraparenchymal haemorrhage

Ventricular dilatation
- 0 — No dilatation
- 1 — Transient dilatation
- 2 — Persistent but stable dilatation
- 3 — Progressive ventricular dilatation requiring treatment
- 4 — Persistent asymmetrical ventricular dilatation

Parenchymal
- 1 — Porencephalic cyst in communication with the ventricle
- 2 — Intraparenchymal cyst separated from the ventricle by ependyma

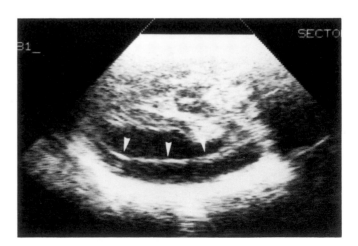

Fig. 9.4 Subarachnoid haemorrhage. Axial scan through the temporoparietal bone showing haemorrhage lying between the dense echo of the contralateral skull and the edge of brain (arrows). (Reproduced with permission from Levene et al 1984.)

midline shift and if present on ultrasound examination, CT scanning should be performed as this is more reliable in the diagnosis of these conditions.

Other patterns of haemorrhage

Although parenchymal haemorrhage usually occurs in association with intraventricular haemorrhage, it may occasionally occur as a primary condition. Intracerebellar haemorrhage producing an echodensity in the cerebellar region associated with loss of the normal appearance of brainstem structures has been reported as a rare finding in the pre-term infant (Peterson et al 1984). Primary thalamic haemorrhage (see p. 307) has a characteristic ultrasound appearance with unilateral echodensity of the thalamus well seen on both coronal and parasagittal views and usually with spread of haemorrhage into the ventricular system (Trounce et al 1985). Extensive GMH–IVH in the pre-term infant may also involve the basal ganglia.

Thrombus may adhere to the choroid plexus in the occipital horn as a sequel to germinal matrix haemorrhage, so the choroid is enlarged with an irregular outline and of increased echogenicity. Rarely these appearances are seen in the absence of GMH and represent a choroid plexus bleed (Veyrac & Couture 1985). This should be readily identifiable with real-time ultrasound and an example is shown on p. 307.

PERIVENTRICULAR LEUKOMALACIA (PVL)

This condition is discussed in detail in Chapter 29. Trounce et al (1986a) have recently defined the sonographic appearances of PVL.

The early appearance is an echodense triangle with its apex at the lateral border of the lateral ventricle (Fig. 9.3). In surviving infants the echodensity resolves to discrete echo-free cavities representing cyst formation. The ependyma of the lateral ventricles remains intact in most cases (see p. 327). Some infants die in the echodense, precystic phase; this is referred to as precystic PVL.

Prolonged flare refers to an appearance of relatively increased echodensity in the periventricular region seen in both coronal and parasagittal views and persisting for at least two weeks but not undergoing cystic degeneration (Fig. 9.5). Subjectively these lesions are less echogenic than either parenchymal haemorrhage or precystic PVL despite standardized gain and energy output settings.

The accuracy of the real-time ultrasound diagnosis of PVL subsequently identified at autopsy has been reported to range from 78% (Nwasei et al 1984) to 90% (Trounce et al 1986a). The improved accuracy in the latter study is probably due to the use of a 7.5 MHz transducer. We found that in the few autopsy specimens examined, the appearance of prolonged flare correlated with histological

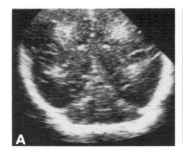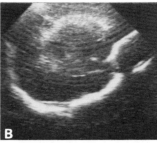

Fig. 9.5 Prolonged flare. Bilateral echogenic areas (arrows) in the periventricular white matter lasting for more than two weeks. Coronal (a) and parasagittal (b) sections. (Reproduced with permission from Levene et al 1983.)

evidence of gliosis and microcalcification. This represents the less severe end of the PVL spectrum.

HYPOXIC–ISCHAEMIC INJURY

A variety of abnormalities seen on ultrasound examination have been reported in full-term infants who have suffered birth asphyxia. These may be focal or generalized. Subdural and subarachnoid haemorrhage, or cerebral artery infarction, are discussed elsewhere.

Kreusser et al (1984) described a full-term infant who suffered severe perinatal asphyxia. Ultrasound scanning at 24 hours of age showed bilateral echodensity of the thalamus and putamen, which correlated with the autopsy findings of haemorrhagic necrosis of the thalamus and basal ganglia. We have seen similar changes in severely asphyxiated infants born at full-term (Fig. 9.6), who survived with significant neurodevelopmental sequelae.

More generalized echodensity throughout the brain has been described as 'bright brain' by Skeffington and

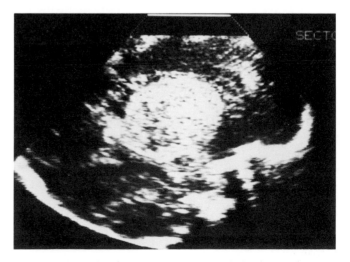

Fig. 9.6 Bright thalamic echoes seen on parasagittal scan in a severely asphyxiated full-term infant.

Pearse (1983). There is partial or complete obliteration of anatomical structures which are normally seen clearly. This condition is probably due to cerebral oedema but does not necessarily correlate with raised intracranial pressure. It is our impression that CT scanning is a much better modality for assessing cerebral structure in asphyxiated infants than ultrasound and CT gives remarkably accurate prognostic information (see p. 390). A normal ultrasound scan may be seen in infants with areas of low attenuation on CT due to cerebral oedema. Hill et al (1983) described four full-term infants with focal echodensity on ultrasound corresponding to areas of low attenuation on the CT scan: in two of the four there was absence of arterial pulsation on ultrasound within the areas of echodensity. It is believed that the changes represent non-haemorrhagic ischaemic cerebral injury.

Leukomalacia is a well-recognized complication of asphyxia. In full-term infants with hypoxic–ischaemic cerebral injury subcortical leukomalacia (SCL) is readily diagnosed by ultrasound (Trounce & Levene 1985, De Vries & Dubowitz 1985). This is also rarely seen in more immature infants. The sequence of appearances comprises an initial echodense phase in the region of the subcortical structures, particularly around the interhemispheric fissure. This gives way to multiple echofree cavities over the course of 7–10 days in the region of the cortex and these appearances are illustrated on p. 352. The greater resolution of modern ultrasound machines for small echofree cavities makes this the best method for diagnosing cystic SCL.

VENTRICULAR DILATATION

Ultrasound is of particular value in this condition as the safety of the procedure and portability allows repeated assessment to determine whether ventricular dilatation is progressive or static. To detect ventricular dilatation, a normal range for ventricular size must be established. Unfortunately there is no consensus view as to the best measurement to make. The width of the lateral ventricles may be expressed as a ratio of the total width of the cranium; the ventricles may be measured directly, or an estimate of cerebrospinal fluid (CSF) volume attempted. Levene (1981) measured the ventricular size from midline to the lateral-most point of the lateral ventricle (referred to as the ventricular index — VI) in 273 infants from 26 to 42 weeks gestation. This measurement can be made in either coronal or axial planes. In coronal section the measurement was made at the level of the hippocampal gyrus, just posterior to the foramen of Monro. A centile chart expressing the 3rd, 50th and 97th centiles from 26 to 42 weeks gestation was produced (Fig. 9.7). Sauerbrei et al (1981) in addition to using a measurement similar to the ventricular index, recorded the depth of the lateral ventricle, defined as the widest measurement taken perpendicular to the longest axis of the lateral ventricle on coronal section. Good correlation

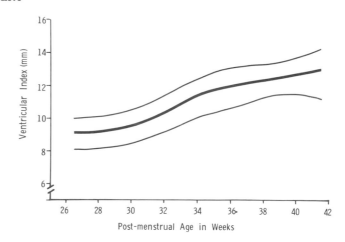

Fig. 9.7 Chart to show ventricular index from 26 to 42 postmenstrual weeks. The lines represent 97th (upper), 50th and 3rd (lower) centiles. (Reproduced with permission from Levene 1981.)

has been found between various ultrasound measurements and similar estimates made on CT imaging (Skolnick et al 1979, London et al 1980, Sauerbrei et al 1981). When dilatation occurs it is often the occipital horns of the lateral ventricles that dilate first and dilatation of the body of the lateral ventricle often lags behind this. For this reason we also recommend measurement of the depth of the lateral ventricles. Dilated third and fourth ventricles can also be recognized on a coronal ultrasound scan. The cavum septi pellucidi, present in almost all premature infants, should not be confused with an enlarged third ventricle. A normal third ventricle should never be seen clearly on coronal scan but is often apparent in the sagittal plane.

Therapeutic manoeuvres can also be performed under ultrasound guidance — either ventricular tap (Levene 1982) or shunt insertion. Alternatively the position of a ventricular shunt can be clearly demonstrated postoperatively.

ATROPHY

The differentiation of the ultrasound appearance of ventricular enlargement representing either pressure-driven dilatation or cerebral atrophy ('hydrocephalus ex vacuo') has been debated for several years. It is likely that in many very-low-birth-weight (VLBW) infants, both conditions can co-exist as a sequel to haemorrhagic or ischaemic insult. Distinction between the two may be very difficult but the following guidelines may prove helpful:

1. the enlargement associated with pressure related dilatation tends to produce ballooning of the ventricles whereas with atrophy the outline is more irregular;
2. pressure-driven dilatation is often bilateral, especially if progressive, whereas atrophy may produce asymmetrical ventricular enlargement;

3. there may be other clues to loss of brain tissue, such as widening of the interhemispheric fissure.

In our experience one of the most common precursors to atrophy is cystic PVL. In the majority of cases the cysts resorb after weeks or months leaving irregular ventricular enlargement (see p. 328).

CONGENITAL ABNORMALITIES

The central nervous system is second only to the heart in the frequency of major congenital abnormalities. The ventricular dilatation associated with myelomeningocele is readily diagnosed and infants with Arnold–Chiari malformation and hydrocephalus often have a characteristic shape to the lateral ventricles (Fig. 9.8).

Agenesis of the corpus callosum has a characteristic appearance with widely spaced lateral ventricles and the corpus callosum is absent in both coronal and midline sagittal views (Skeffington 1982). We have seen this abnormality in otherwise healthy babies being scanned for other reasons and the follow-up of these infants is awaited with interest to ascertain its exact significance. The low echogenicity of cerebrospinal fluid (CSF) allows easy detection of many abnormalities containing fluid. In its most extreme form hydranencephaly is revealed by a large volume of CSF with, perhaps, residual basal ganglia, a rim of cortex and the falx. It may be impossible to distinguish this from severe hydrocephalus by ultrasound. Holoprosencephaly, a disorder of ventral induction in early embryonic life, consists of a single ventricular cavity and absence of the interhemispheric fissure. Septo-optic dysplasia, a condition characterized by agenesis of the septum pellucidum and optic nerve hypoplasia, is also represented by a single ventricular cavity although the interhemispheric fissure is present. Fluid-filled cystic masses such as Dandy–Walker malformation may also be diagnosed as reported by Chilton & Cremin (1983). A vein of Galen aneurysm produces an echofree area in the midline just posterior to the third ventricle in both coronal and sagittal planes; final confirmation is achieved by demonstrating filling of this defect by microbubbles following the intravenous injection of 1 ml of normal saline (Jones et al 1982). We have recently reported the diagnosis of lissencephaly (p. 242) in a neonate who demonstrated a smooth cerebral surface and very wide interhemispheric and Sylvian fissures on scanning; he had agenesis of the corpus callosum as an associated defect (Trounce et al 1986c). This must be distinguished from the smooth brain normally seen in extremely premature infants.

Most congenital abnormalities of the brain seen in the perinatal period can be diagnosed accurately by real-time ultrasound. Confusion may arise between a number of disorders where midline structures may be absent and it is possible that magnetic resonance imaging (MRI) or CT may clarify the precise nature of the abnormality. Ultrasound should be the first-line technique used to image the brain of any infant with suspected congenital abnormality.

INFECTION

Prenatal viral infection is well known for causing intracranial calcification and this is readily detected by ultrasound. This characteristically occurs as small highly echodense lesions, typically in the periventricular region or basal ganglia. Other sequelae to early intra-uterine infection which are also readily recognized on ultrasound are subependymal pseudocysts (Shackelford et al 1983), ventricular dilatation and an echodense ependymal reaction.

Bacterial meningitis in the neonate is associated with various complications, some of which may be recognized on ultrasound. In our experience, scans in the acute stage are often normal although an increase in cortical echodensity has been reported (Edwards et al 1982). The development of ventricular dilatation is recognized on serial scans. Hill et al (1981) described the changes seen in bacterial ventriculitis and these included diffuse intraventricular echoes (probably representing exudate), echogenic strands attached to the ependymal surface and progressive ventricular dilatation. A recent report has shown that veins normally present in the septum pellucidum can give a very similar appearance and must be distinguished from intraventricular adhesions (Goldstein et al 1986).

Abscess formation gives a characteristic appearance of

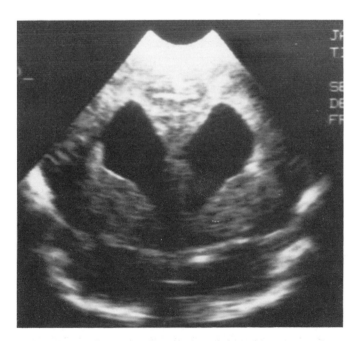

Fig. 9.8 Marked ventricular dilatation in an infant with open neural tube defect and Arnold–Chiari malformation. Note the angular peak to the roof of the lateral ventricles.

localized increase in echodensity within the parenchyma. Subsequently, cavity formation may develop (Edwards et al 1982) and this may be associated with shift of the midline structures. Infarction of the periventricular white matter may occur, leading to widespread cyst formation. The development of significant subdural effusion complicating *Haemophilus influenzae* meningitis can also be monitored by serial scans. CT is probably a better modality for the detection of severe complications that occur following infection.

DISCRETE AREAS OF ECHOGENICITY

As mentioned above echoes are produced from tissue interfaces and are dependent on the acoustic properties of the brain. Brightly echogenic lesions are produced by a number of conditions and interpretation may be difficult. Calcification occurs commonly in the developing brain and a number of disease processes may lead to deposition of discrete areas of calcium and in some cases calcification may be massive (Fig. 9.9). Ultrasound is particularly sensitive to intracranial calcification, more so than CT, and routine MRI will not detect calcification. Haemorrhage and gliosis give echogenic appearances as described above and fat cells (lipomata) within the corpus callosum are also strongly echogenic (Fig. 9.10). Air or oxygen embolus affecting the brain will also produce echogenic lesions within the distribution of the blood vessels. The diagnosis of tumour has been reported by ultrasound (Babcock & Han 1981) and usually has the appearance of an echodense mass which may be associated with ventricular dilatation. Some reports comment on the cystic changes seen within the tumourous mass and we have seen just such an appearance in a primitive neuronal tumour which also showed calcification. We have also seen calcification in association with neurofibromatosis and tuberose sclerosis. Choroid plexus papilloma appear as a strongly echogenic mass in association with ventricular dilatation.

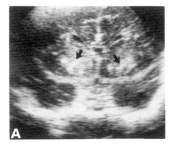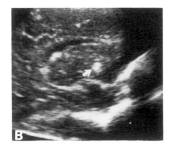

Fig. 9.9 Extensive calcification (arrows) in the basal ganglia seen on coronal (**a**) and parasagittal (**b**) sections. This was not seen on plain skull X-Ray. (Reproduced with permission from Levene et al 1984.)

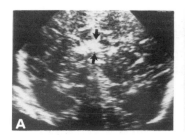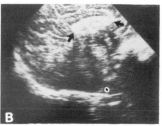

Fig. 9.10 Lipoma of the corpus callosum. This appears as an echodense region (arrows) on coronal (**a**) and sagittal (**b**) scan.

ROUTINE CEREBRAL ULTRASOUND SCANS

To detect the majority of important intracranial lesions in the infant brain we recommend routine scanning of the following infants:

1. All infants less than 32 weeks gestation and/or <1500 g birth-weight. They should be scanned at least once at the end of the first week and again on discharge from the neonatal unit.
2. All infants with neurological abnormality (e.g. seizures, cranial bruit, meningitis) should be scanned at the time the problem is observed.
3. Dysmorphic infants, especially those with craniofacial abnormalities, should be scanned at birth.
4. All infants with a rapidly increasing occipitofrontal circumference. If ventriculomegaly is recognized then the infant should be scanned at least once weekly until stable.

THE SPINE

The unossified spinous process and dorsal arches of the young infant make the spinal cord amenable to ultrasound examination and this is proving to be a valuable method of investigating the child with actual or suspected neural tube disorder. High-frequency transducers are required, up to 10 MHz, to give good visualization in the near field. A water-path or stand-off device may be particularly useful in this respect.

Scans are obtained with the infant in the prone position and the head turned to one side. The sagittal (longitudinal) plane is most valuable for routine scanning. The normal appearances have been well described (Raghavendra & Epstein 1985, Levene et al 1984). The spinal cord appears as a tubular structure superficial to the dense echoes of the vertebral bodies. The cord produces an appearance of relatively low echodensity and on longitudinal view three parallel echoes are seen (Fig. 9.11). These are produced by the anterior and posterior borders of the cord with the central canal providing the echogenic midline. At the caudal end the conus medullaris can be seen to taper at the

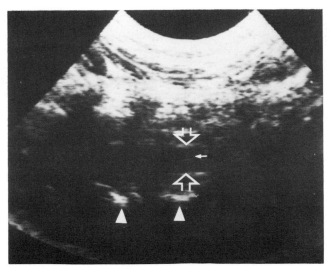

Fig. 9.11 Longitudinal section through a normal spine. Vertebral bodies (arrowheads). The anterior and posterior surfaces of the spinal cord are shown by the open arrows with the central canal (small arrow). The spinal cord is of relatively low echodensity.

level of L3 in infants. The filum terminale is of relatively higher echogenicity and the nerve roots of the cauda equina

combine to form a diffuse echogenic mass extending from the conus. On real-time scanning, vascular pulsations are seen in the region of the cauda equina and the whole cord moves up and down on respiration.

Ultrasound may be of value in the assessment of infants with spina bifida cystica or occulta (see Section 7). A meningocele produces an echofree appearance corresponding to the fluid-filled sac. Septae are often seen within it and may be difficult to distinguish from nerve roots (Raghavendra & Epstein 1985). Nerve roots pulsate when scanned in real-time in distinction to septae which do not. Lipomata, a well-recognized feature in association with neural tube defects, appear as more echogenic lesions and may be followed into the spinal canal to infiltrate the conus medullaris or cauda equina.

Ultrasound may be useful in screening infants with cutaneous lesions suggestive of spina bifida occulta. The most important abnormality seen on ultrasound examination in infants with this condition is tethering of the cord and absence of the normal rhythmical up and down movements. In addition, thickened filum terminale may be evident as an increase in the echogenicity of the structures extending caudally from the conus (Scheible et al 1983).

REFERENCES

Babcock D S, Han B K 1981 The accuracy of high resolution, real-time ultrasonography of the head in infancy. Radiology 139: 665–676

Babcock D S, Bove K E, Han B K 1982 Intracranial hemorrhage in premature infants: sonographic–pathologic correlation. American Journal of Neuroradiology 3: 309–317

Carstensen E L, Gates A H 1983 University of Rochester New York Electrical Engineering Technical Report, No GM09933-21R

Chilton S J, Cremin B J 1983 Ultrasound diagnosis of CSF cystic lesions in the neonatal brain. British Journal of Radiology 56: 613–620

Cremin B J, Chilton S J, Peacock W J 1983 Anatomical landmarks in anterior fontanelle ultrasonography. British Journal of Radiology 56: 517–526

De Vries L S, Dubowitz L M S 1985 Cystic leukomalacia in preterm infants: site of lesion in relation to prognosis. Lancet ii: 1075–1076

Dewbury K C, Bates R I 1983 Neonatal intracranial haemorrhage: the cause of the ultrasound appearances. British Journal of Radiology 56: 783–789

Edwards M K, Brown D L, Chua G T 1982 Complicated infantile meningitis: evaluation by real-time sonography. American Journal of Neuroradiology 3: 431–434

Enzmann D R, Britt R H, Lyons B E, Buxton J L, Wilson D A 1981 Natural history of experimental intracerebral hemorrhage: sonography, computer tomography and neuropathology. American Journal of Neuroradiology 2: 517–526

Goldstein R B, Filly R A, Toi A 1986 Septal veins: a normal finding on neonatal cranial sonography. Radiology 161: 623–624

Heimburger R, Fry F, Patrick J T, Gardner G, Gresham E 1978 Ultrasound brain tomography for infants and young children. Perinatology Neonatology 2: 27–31

Hill C R, ter Haer G 1982 Ultrasound. In: Suess M J (ed) Nonionizing radiation protection. WHO Regional Publications, European Series 10. Copenhagen.

Hill A, Shackelford G D, Volpe J J 1981 Ventriculitis with neonatal bacterial meningitis: identification by real-time ultrasound. Journal of Pediatrics 99: 133–136

Hill A, Martin D J, Daneman A, Fitz C R 1983 Focal ischaemic cerebral injury in the newborn: diagnosis by ultrasound and correlation with computed tomographic scan. Pediatrics 71: 790–793

Johnson M L, Mack L A, Rumack C M, Frost M, Rashbaum C 1979 B-mode echoencephalography in the normal and high risk infant. American Journal of Roentgenology 133: 375–381

Jones R W A, Allan L D, Tynan M J, Joseph M C 1982 Ultrasound diagnosis of cerebral arteriovenous malformations in the newborn. Lancet i: 102–103

Kreusser K L, Schmidt R E, Shackelford G D, Volpe J J 1984 Value of ultrasound for identification of acute hemorrhagic necrosis of thalamus and basal ganglia in an asphyxiated term infant. Annals of Neurology 16: 361–363

Levene M I 1981 Measurement of the growth of the lateral ventricles in preterm infants with real-time ultrasound. Archives of Disease in Childhood 56: 900–904

Levene M I 1982 Ventricular tap under direct ultrasound control. Archives of Disease in Childhood 57: 873–875

Levene M I, de Crespigny L Ch 1983 Classification of intraventricular haemorrhage. Lancet i: 643

Levene M I, Wigglesworth J S, Dubowitz V 1983 Hemorrhagic periventricular leukomalacia in the neonate: a real-time ultrasound study. Pediatrics 71: 794–797

Levene M I, Williams J L, Fawer C-L 1984 Ultrasound of the Infant Brain. SIMP Blackwell Scientific Publications, Oxford.

Liebeskind D, Bases R, Eleguin F et al 1979 Diagnostic ultrasound: effects on the DNA and growth patterns of animal cells. Radiology 131: 177–184

London D A, Carroll B A, Enzmann D R 1980 Sonography of ventricular size and germinal matrix hemorrhage in premature infants. American Journal of Neuroradiology 1: 295–300

Mannino F L, Trauner D A 1983 Stroke in neonates. Journal of Pediatrics 102: 605–610

Morgan M E I, Hensey O J, Cooke R W I 1983 Convexity cerebral haemorrhage in the neonate: in vivo ultrasound diagnosis. Archives of Disease in Childhood 58: 814–818

Nwaesei C G, Pape K E, Martin D J, Becker L E, Fitz C R 1984 Periventricular infarction diagnosed by ultrasound: a postmortem correlation. Journal of Pediatrics 105: 106–110

Pape K E, Blackwell R J, Cusick G et al 1979 Ultrasound detection of brain damage in preterm infants. Lancet ii: 1261–1264

Pape K E, Bennett-Britton S, Szymonowicz W et al 1983 Diagnostic accuracy of neonatal brain imaging: a postmortem correlation of computed tomography and ultrasound scans. Journal of Pediatrics 102: 275–280

Papile L A, Burstein J, Burstein R, Koffler H 1978 Incidence and evolution of subependymal and intraventricular hemorrhage: a study of infants with birth weights less than 1500 gm. Journal of Pediatrics 92: 529–534

Peterson C M, Smith W L, Franken E A 1984 Neonatal intracerebellar hemorrhage: detection by real-time ultrasound. Radiology 150: 391–392

Raghavendra B N, Epstein F J 1985 Sonography of the spine and spinal cord. Radiologic Clinics of North America 23: 91–105

Rumack C M, Johnson M L 1984 Perinatal and infant brain imaging. Year Book Medical, New York.

Sauerbrei E E, Digney M, Harrison P B, Cooperberg P L 1981 Ultrasonic evaluation of neonatal intracranial hemorrhage and its complications. Radiology 139: 677–685

Scheible W, James H E, Leopold G R, Hilton S 1983 Occult spinal dysraphism in infants: screening with high-resolution real-time ultrasound. Radiology 146: 743–746

Shackelford G D, Fulling K H, Glasier C M 1983 Cysts of the subependymal germinal matrix. Sonographic demonstration with pathologic correlation. Radiology 149: 117–121

Skeffington F S 1982 Agenesis of the corpus callosum: neonatal ultrasound appearances. Archives of Disease in Childhood 57: 713–714

Skeffington F S, Pearse R G 1983 The bright brain. Archives of Disease in Childhood 58: 509–511

Skolnick M L, Rosenbaum A E, Matzuk T, Guthkelch A N, Heinz E R 1979 Detection of dilated cerebral ventricles in infants: a correlative study between ultrasound and computed tomography. Radiology 131: 447–452

Stewart H F, Stratmeyer M E 1982 US Department of Health and Human Services (Food and Drug Administration)

Szymonowicz W, Schafer K, Cussen L J, Yu V Y H 1984 Ultrasound and necropsy study of periventricular haemorrhage in preterm infants. Archives of Disease in Childhood 59: 637–642

Thacker J 1973 The possibility of genetic hazard from ultrasonic radiation. Current Topics in Radiation Research Quarterly 8: 235–258

Thorburn R J, Reynolds E O R, Blackwell R J et al 1982 Accuracy of imaging of the brains of newborn infants by linear-array real-time ultrasound. Early Human Development 6: 31–46

Trounce J Q, Levene M I 1985 Diagnosis and outcome of subcortical cystic leucomalacia. Archives of Disease in Childhood 60: 1041–1044

Trounce J Q, Fawer C-L, Punt J, Dodd K L, Fielder A R, Levene M I 1985 Primary thalamic haemorrhage in the newborn: a new clinical entity. Lancet i: 190–192

Trounce J Q, Fagan D, Levene M I 1986a Intraventricular haemorrhage and periventricular leucomalacia: ultrasound and autopsy correlation. Archives of Disease in Childhood 61: 1203–1207

Trounce J Q, Rutter N, Levene M I 1986b Periventricular leucomalacia and intraventricular haemorrhage in the preterm neonate. Archives of Disease in Childhood 61: 1196–1202

Trounce J Q, Fagan D G, Young I D, Levene M I 1986c Disorders of neuronal migration: sonographic features. Developmental Medicine and Child Neurology 28: 467–471

Veyrac C, Couture A 1985 Normal and pathological choroid plexus ultrasound. Annals of Radiology 28: 215–223

Volpe J J 1982 Anterior fontanel: window to the neonatal brain. Journal of Pediatrics 100: 395–398

Cerebral haemodynamics

Cerebral blood flow is the key to understanding many perinatally acquired cerebral insults. A variety of methods exist to measure volume flow to the brain but few are acceptable either methodologically or ethically for routine use in the newborn and these are discussed in Chapter 10. For this reason, indirect methods have been applied to assess cerebral haemodynamics, of which Doppler ultrasound has been most widely used. It is important to understand the limitations of these techniques and Doppler ultrasound is reviewed in some detail in Chapters 11 and 12. Because Doppler ultrasound has not yet been widely used to assess directly the fetal brain, we have put the chapter on the neonatal brain before that of the fetus. This reflects the relative importance of these techniques in assessing brain function at present.

10. Methods for assessing cerebral blood flow

Dr G. Greisen

Cerebral perfusion may be quantitated as blood flow in millilitres per 100 grams brain weight per minute (ml/100 g^{-1}/min^{-1}). This quantity is commonly termed cerebral blood flow (CBF) and relates to the brain as a whole or to a specified region, depending on the methods of measurements.

CBF was first estimated in a few newborn infants by Garfunkel et al in 1954. However, only recently did the interest in neonatal CBF increase, when it was hypothesized that some important types of perinatal brain damage may be caused by perturbation of CBF. Observing proportionality between arterial blood pressure and CBF in eight distressed infants shortly after birth (Fig. 10.1), Lou et al (1977) proposed that abolishment of the normal pressure–flow autoregulation after asphyxia may allow moderate arterial hypotension to cause ischaemia as well as moderate hypertension to be transmitted to the capillary bed and cause rupture and cerebral haemorrhage.

Whereas the main problem for experimental animal studies is the differences among species in cerebrovascular anatomy and physiology, the main problem in clinical research is the lack of reliable and applicable methods for measurement of CBF. Therefore, this chapter describes the clinical research methods in some detail, to allow critical interpretation of the available data. Furthermore, a brief outline of the regulation of CBF is given along with a review of the available data concerning human neonatal CBF.

CLINICAL RESEARCH METHODS

CBF is a complex variable. It may change within seconds in hypoxia, epileptic seizures, or with abrupt changes in blood pressure. CBF varies from one part of the brain to the other and between brain structures. During functional activation, or during stress, the flow distribution may change markedly. The methods available for estimation of CBF in human newborns provide only crude measures of those complexities.

THE KETY–SCHMIDT METHOD

This method is based on Fick's principle for metabolically inert tracers, stating that the change of the mean tracer concentration in a tissue equals the perfusion rate multiplied by the arterio–venous concentration difference. Nitrous oxide, a freely diffusible inert gas, is administered by inhalation. The tracer concentration in arterial and jugular venous blood is followed by taking six to eight samples over 10 minutes after the start of inhalation of 15% nitrous oxide.

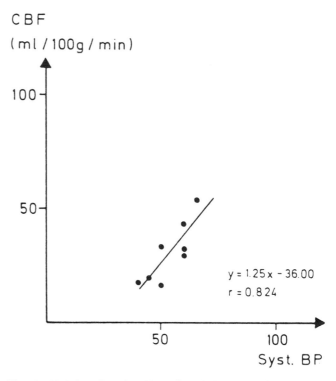

Fig. 10.1 Relation of cerebral blood flow (CBF) to systolic blood pressure in eight stressed newborn infants, a few hours after birth. CBF was estimated by the intra-arterial ^{133}Xe clearance method, using an early slope index, reflecting mainly flow to grey matter. (Reproduced with permission from Lou et al 1977.)

The calculation of CBF depends on the brain–blood partition coefficient and on the assumption of equilibrium between brain tissue and jugular venous blood by 10 minutes. This assumption may not hold good if parts of the brain are perfused at low rates and therefore remain unsaturated. If counter-current exchange of nitrous oxide from artery to vein takes place, the difference between venous concentration and tissue concentration will be even greater. The result is overestimation of CBF. The error is, however, not likely to be large and the method is generally accepted as a kind of gold standard.

The value of CBF obtained by the Kety–Schmidt method is a mean over a period of 10 minutes and relates to the part of the brain drained by the jugular vein at the sampling site; even at the jugular bulb there may be a small admixture of extracerebral blood.

The Kety–Schmidt method was used by Garfunkel et al in 1954. It was made possible by the development of a micromethod for analysis of nitrous oxide but the application is strictly limited by the need for arterial and jugular venous blood sampling.

[11]CO-LABELLED ERYTHROCYTES

Erythrocytes are non-diffusible tracers and may be used to estimate cerebral blood volume and the mean transit time within this volume. Arnot et al (1970) labelled erythrocytes in vitro by [11]CO and reinjected them through an umbilical artery catheter placed in the aortic arch near the origin of the left carotid artery.

The gamma emissions from the infant's head were monitored. The mode transit time was measured as the time between the inflections of the increasing and decreasing count rate. The cranial blood volume was measured as the equilibrium count rate over the head related to the count rate over a one millilitre blood sample obtained from the superior sagittal sinus by direct puncture. When calculating cranial blood flow, it is assumed that the mode transit time approximates the mean transit time. Furthermore, the calculation depends on the accuracy of the calibration of the scintillation detectors for the measurement of cerebral blood volume. The method is invasive, whereas the whole-body radiation dose due to the [11]CO is only about 5 mrad (0.05 mGy). Furthermore, the high radiation energy requires heavy shielding and transport of the infant to the stationary equipment.

[133]Xe CLEARANCE

Xenon clearance methods have become widely used for measuring CBF in adult humans. The results are comparable to those obtained by the Kety–Schmidt method. Xenon is a freely diffusible inert tracer like nitrous oxide

and the methods are also based on Fick's principle. The methods differ in that xenon is detected not in venous blood but in the tissue by means of the gamma emissions. It is assumed that the tissue concentration at any time is proportional to the concentration in venous blood, the relationship being expressed by the brain–blood coefficient. The assumption may not hold good at high perfusion rates where equilibration may be incomplete. The result is underestimation of CBF. Xenon is highly lipophilic and the brain–blood partition coefficient is therefore dependent on brain myelination. Not until recently (Greisen 1986) has the brain–blood partition coefficient been known for newborn infants.

Lou et al (1977) have described the use of ^{133}Xe clearance. During umbilical artery catheterization the catheter was advanced to the root of the left carotid artery or into the common carotid artery where a one millilitre bolus of [133]Xe (0.5 mCi = 20 MBq) dissolved in normal saline was injected over 5 seconds. Gamma emissions were monitored over the head from 15 to 60 seconds after the injection and recorded on a semilogarithmic recorder. The mean clearance rate was estimated by fitting a straight line, as it may be assumed the arterial xenon concentration drops to zero shortly after the bolus injection. The brain–blood partition coefficient of cerebral cortex for adults was used and this is valid for newborn grey and white matter. The measure of CBF relates to the best perfused parts of a poorly defined, rather large (100–200 g), mass of brain tissue under the scintillation detector.

Owing to the injection at a level below the origin of the external carotid artery, the flow to the scalp and skull is included and there is a certain recirculation of xenon. Neither of these factors, however, is likely to significantly affect the clearance of xenon during the first minute after injection. The application of this method is limited by the need for umbilical artery catheterization. The radiation dose to the brain is about 50 mrad (0.5 mGy) and about 5 mrad (0.06 mGy) to the whole body. There may be a theoretical risk associated with the injection of saline into the cerebral circulation because of a transient decrease in oxygen delivery.

Modifications of the intra-arterial ^{133}Xe clearance method have been worked out for adults and xenon may be injected intravenously or administered by inhalation. The CBF values obtained by these non-invasive methods compare favourably with the results obtained by the intra-arterial method.

The inhalation method has been applied to newborn infants using a portable gamma-camera (Ment et al 1981). An air–oxygen mixture containing 5 mCi (200 MBq) of ^{133}Xe is administered for two minutes and then abruptly stopped and the patient returned to the ventilator using the same air–oxygen mixture. The clearance rate of xenon is calculated in a two-minute period, starting 30 seconds after the end of ^{133}Xe inhalation. The clearance rate in this time interval relates to the highly perfused parts of the brain, cortical as well as subcortical structures. Owing to the large amount of xenon used and the take-up in all tissues, the arterial xenon concentration does not drop to zero after stopping inhalation. An estimate of arterial xenon concentration may, however, be obtained from monitoring gamma emissions over the chest, since it may be assumed that the alveolar air equilibrates with pulmonary capillary blood. The calculation of the clearance rate requires the deconvolution of the cranial clearance curve from the estimated arterial concentration curve by a computer.

This method is non-invasive, is applied within the incubator, and the whole-body radiation of 11 mrad (0.11 mGy) is comparable to a plain chest X-ray.

The method, however, has several sources of error in addition to those discussed for the intra-arterial ^{133}Xe method. Since a larger amount of ^{133}Xe is used, the gamma emissions over the head will include a certain amount of Compton scatter from xenon in the airways, resulting in an overestimation of the clearance rate. Since the gamma emissions detected over the chest include emissions from the chest wall, the arterial concentration will be overestimated during the last part of the clearance also resulting in an overestimation of the clearance rate. Finally, the calculated CBF is overestimated by a third since the mean brain–blood partition coefficient for grey and white matter in adults is one-third higher than that in newborns.

The intravenous injection ^{133}Xe clearance technique was first applied to newborns by Younkin et al (1982), 0.5 to 1 mCi (20–40 MBq) per kilogram body weight is injected as a bolus dissolved in 1–2 millilitres of normal saline in a peripheral vein. The arterial xenon concentration is estimated from the gamma emissions detected over the chest. The clearance is followed for 15 minutes and a correction for the chest wall contribution is applied to the gamma emissions from the chest.

Valid estimation of the arterial concentration of xenon may, however, be affected by two factors particular to intravenous administration. In the presence of significant right-to-left shunting of blood past the lungs through the foramen ovale or through intrapulmonary shunts, the arterial concentration will exceed the alveolar concentration especially during the passage of the bolus and during the late part of the study. Uptake of ^{133}Xe in the vein and perivenous tissues and later slow release will result in an elevated tail in the arterial concentration curve and underestimation of CBF.

A two-compartment cranial clearance curve is deconvoluted from the arterial concentration curve to obtain an estimate of the flow to a fast compartment 'grey matter' and a slow compartment 'white matter' with some contribution from extracranial tissue. The estimation of the fast compartment flow rate by the intravenous injection technique is uncertain in newborn infants due to the sources of error discussed above (Greisen et al 1984). The slow compartment

flow rate is overestimated if the adult brain–blood partition coefficient for xenon in white matter is used, being nearly twice that in newborns.

A weighted mean flow rate to the two compartments is calculated to estimate mean (global) CBF relating to the poorly defined mass of tissue seen by the detector (180–200 g). If the weighting is done for the 15 minute study period, the results are about 10% higher than the value obtained when the weighting is carried out to infinity by extrapolation. This estimate of global CBF is reproducible (Greisen & Trojaborg 1987).

The whole-body radiation is comparable to the inhalation method, whereas the radiation to the lungs is somewhat less. The method requires venepuncture but the fitting of a tight mask is not required, provided that the exhaled xenon is removed from the field by adequate suctioning.

JUGULAR VENOUS OCCLUSION PLETHYSMOGRAPHY

Venous occlusion plethysmography is a standard method for measurement of limb blood flow. It is based on measurement of the rate of increase in limb volume when the venous drainage is effectively occluded. It estimates mean blood flow to all tissues within the limb.

When the jugular veins are compressed bilaterally in the newborn infant by two fingers, the cranial circumference increases stepwise with each heartbeat. Owing to patency of non-jugular venous return, the increase in circumference gradually slows down and reaches a plateau when the increased intracranial pressure allows venous outflow to equal arterial inflow (Fig. 10.2). On the release of compression, the decrease of the cranial circumference to the baseline is faster when compared to the increase following onset of compression. The changes in circumference may be recorded by a mercury in silastic strain gauge.

Two methods of quantitative analysis, resulting in estimates of cranial blood flow have been developed. One method is based on the fitting of an exponential term to the end-diastolic circumference of heartbeats two to six after the onset of compression. The rate of increase in cranial circumference at the onset of compression may then be calculated by extrapolation (Cross et al 1976). The other method depends on measurement of the actual increase of circumference during the first heatbeat (Cooke 1978). The latter method, however, is open to a compression artefact since a small amount of jugular blood is pressed back into the head when compression is induced. Actually this method does result in higher estimates of cranial blood flow at flow rates below average when compared to the method of exponential fitting (Dear 1980). At flow rates about average, the estimates are lower than those of the exponential method, possibly due to an

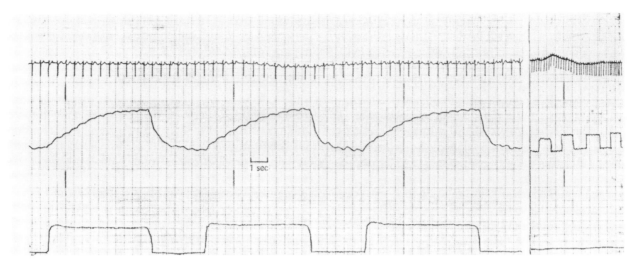

Fig. 10.2 Venous occlusion plethysmography trace showing a set of waves obtained by bilateral jugular compression. From above downwards the traces are: electrocardiogram, strain-gauge measurement of occipito–frontal circumference, and balloon pressure showing the period of compression. (Reproduced with permission from Cross et al 1979.)

increased non-jugular outflow present during the very first heartbeat. This may be particularly marked in infants with low cranial compliance. The calculation of flow rate depends on estimation of increase in cranial volume from the increase in cranial circumference (occipital–frontal circumference). Provided there is no change in shape, the factor relating small changes of volume to small changes in distance is three. The base of the skull, however, is unlikely to expand during jugular venous compression and the factor may be somewhat less.

Cross et al (1979) carried the analysis further to a qualified estimate of cerebral blood flow. The circumference increase following compression (impeding jugular outflow) and the circumference decrease following decompression (reflecting jugular as well as non-jugular outflow) have different rate constants. Assuming that the resistances to the flow in the jugular veins and in the non-jugular 'vertebral' veins are constant, the sum of the flow in these systems may be estimated from the two rate constants. It is, however, likely that the veins dilate when the flow through them increases and thereby the resistance is reduced. Finally, from estimates of cranial volume and brain weight, 'total' cranial blood flow may be converted into CBF expressed in ml/100 g^{-1}/min^{-1}. As well as the introduction of another source of variation, a systematic overestimation is caused by assigning extracerebral blood flow to the brain.

The jugular venous occlusion plethysmographic methods have the virtue of technical simplicity. The risk to the infant is unlikely to exceed that of ordinary handling. An estimate of global blood flow is obtained within a few seconds although the average of results from several jugular compressions is required to obtain adequate precision. The coefficient of variation of the flow variable obtained from a simple compression is 15 to 35%. The infant must be quiet and the head unrestrained. Unfortunately the method has

not been validated against other methods as described above and the results may show error on either side.

ELECTRICAL IMPEDANCE PLETHYSMOGRAPHY

The transcephalic impedance, as measured by applying a small alternating electrical current, is slightly pulsatile. The pulsatility is related to pulse-synchronous changes in cerebral blood volume, cranial volume, and displacement of cerebrospinal fluid. Several different flow indices can be calculated from the impedance waveform. In newborns there have been no attempts to estimate absolute values of CBF (Costeloe et al 1984). This method has theoretical risks only and appears to be well-suited for long-term monitoring.

POSITRON EMISSION TOMOGRAPHY

For a short period of observation, water may be considered as an inert, freely diffusible tracer. Using [^{15}O]water, the spatial resolution of positron emission tomography is $14 \times 12 \times 12$ mm in tiny pre-term infants. This is sufficient to separate the left and right hemispheres and the frontal, temporal, parietal and occipital regions (see Frontispiece I). Owing to the volume-averaging effect within the individual image element, the cortex cannot be separated from subcortical white matter.

For the first 40 seconds after intravenous injection the local brain concentration of the tracer will be higher, the higher the local perfusion rate (the bolus distribution principle). The area under the local tissue indicator concentration curve is measured by integration of the emissions detected from the time of injection for 40 seconds. The calculation of perfusion rate in ml/100 g^{-1}/min^{-1} depends on measurement of indicator concentration in frequent samples of arterial blood and on the brain–blood coefficient for water. Underestimation of flow rate will result from local perfusion heterogeneity, and high flow rates will be underestimated due to the diffusion limitation, more important for water than for xenon. Furthermore, the absolute value depends on the accuracy of the attenuation calibration and on an accurate assumption of the artery-to-brain delay.

The method was first applied to newborn infants by Volpe et al (1983). The radiation exposure is 90 mrad (0.9 mGy), a venepuncture is required, and the infant has to be transported to the stationary equipment.

DOPPLER ULTRASOUND

The use of Doppler ultrasound for estimation of cerebral blood flow in ml.100 g^{-1}.min^{-1} has not yet been reported. The major problem is related to estimation of vessel diameter (see Ch. 11).

STABLE XENON-ENHANCED COMPUTED TOMOGRAPHY

The use of this method in newborn infants with posthaemorrhagic hydrocephalus was recently reported (Manwarring et al 1984). The method is based on the high density of xenon to X-rays. By repeated CT scans during inhalation of 35% stable (non-radio-active) xenon, brain saturation can be followed. In principle the spatial resolution is as good as for conventional CT-scanning, unfortunately, the low brain–blood partition coefficient of xenon in newborn brain results in a low signal-to-noise ratio and imprecise estimates of CBF. The repeated CT-scans result in a greater patient radiation dose, compared with the use of ^{133}Xe.

THE PHYSIOLOGICAL REGULATION OF CBF

COUPLING OF CBF TO CEREBRAL ENERGY METABOLISM

Through a wide range of metabolic rates, from deep hypothermia to electrical seizures, CBF increases in proportion to the increase in metabolism. The precise mechanism of this coupling is not known, nor is it known when in fetal life it develops. Proportionality between local CBF and local glucose metabolism is present in newborn puppies which are rather immature at birth. In newborn

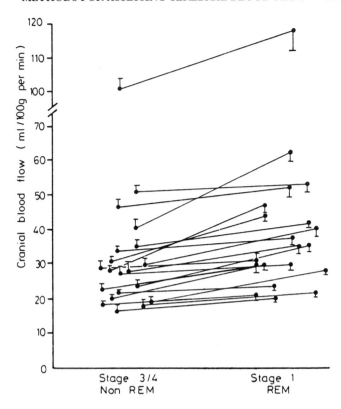

Fig. 10.3 Changes in cerebral blood flow (CBF) estimated by venous occlusion plethysmography, in 20 healthy full-term infants in different sleep states (the bars show SE of the mean of 10 compressions in each infant and sleep state). (Reproduced with permission from Rahilly 1980a.)

full-term infants, indirect evidence of the flow–metabolism coupling was obtained by the demonstration of increased CBF, as estimated by venous occlusion plethysmography, during active sleep as compared to quiet sleep (Fig. 10.3) (Milligan 1979, Rahilly 1980a, Mukhtar et al 1982). Using ^{133}Xe clearance after intravenous injection in pre-term infants of 32 to 35 weeks postconceptional age, Greisen et al (1985) found CBF increased in the awake state when compared to quiet or active sleep.

The clinical relevance of the flow–metabolism coupling is most clearly appreciated by considering focal electrical seizures. If the flow–metabolism coupling is insufficient, the highly increased local metabolic demands may not be met and local tissue injury may ensue. A 50% increase in local CBF was demonstrated by positron emission tomography in a postasphyxiated full-term newborn infant with unilateral tonic–clonic seizures (Perlmann et al 1982). This is less than the increase seen during seizures in adult experimental animals but the difference may be due to the volume-averaging effect of PET-scanning.

From the above observations it appears that cerebral circulation reacts to changes in cerebral metabolism in newborn infants in a way comparable to that of older patients.

PERFUSION PRESSURE–FLOW AUTOREGULATION

Cerebral perfusion rate is haemodynamically determined by the perfusion pressure (the arterial blood pressure minus the intracranial pressure) and by the cerebrovascular resistance. The cerebrovascular resistance in adults is mainly determined by the degree of contraction of the precapillary arterioles. In adults only about 20% of the cerebrovascular resistance is located in the pre-arteriolar arteries. In newborn infants and in particularly in pre-term infants, the arterial tree is smaller. Since the resistance varies with the inverse of the radius in the fourth power it may be estimated that these arteries may contribute as much as 50% of the cerebrovascular resistance.

Normally cerebral perfusion pressure may vary considerably while the cerebral metabolic rate remains stable. The ability of the brain to keep its perfusion constant in view of a varying perfusion pressure is termed the cerebral autoregulation. The precise mechanism of the autoregulation is not known, although both rapid myogenic reflexes and slower acting mediators relating to metabolism seem to be involved.

Autoregulation has been demonstrated in a range of fetal and newborn experimental animals. The range of perfusion pressures over which CBF is kept constant is lower when compared with adult animals and is adapted to the prevailing low normal perfusion pressure. Furthermore, the range appears to be narrower.

The autoregulation is easily disrupted in pre-term lambs. Moderate hypoxia (arterial oxygen saturation less than 50% for 20 minutes) results in disruption of the autoregulation lasting for 4 to 7 hours. Using the intra-arterial ^{133}Xe clearance method in 19 stressed newborn infants a few hours after birth, Lou et al (1979) found CBF to vary in direct proportion to the systolic blood pressure, the correlation between CBF and systolic blood pressure being independent of birth-weight and Apgar scores. Furthermore, in two infants the measurements were repeated, and in these infants CBF varied over time in proportion to systolic blood pressure.

Similar results were reported by Milligan (1980), who estimated CBF by venous occlusion plethysmography in five very pre-term, ventilated infants before and after blood transfusion (Fig. 10.4). In all the infants blood pressure and CBF increased significantly. In several other studies of CBF in newborn infants the relationship to arterial blood pressure has been examined and found insignificant. None of them, however, has been directly concerned with the demonstration or quantification of the pressure–flow autoregulation. Meanwhile it may be reasonably assumed that autoregulation is present in normocapnic newborn infants unless interrupted by recent hypoxic or asphyxic insults. The range of perfusion pressures covered in

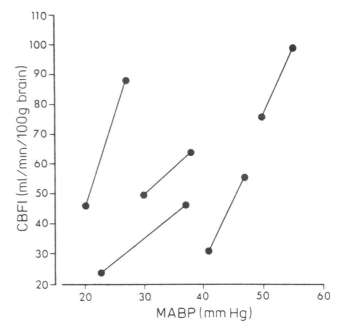

Fig. 10.4 The relationship between changes in cerebral blood flow (CBF), estimated by venous occlusion plethysmography, and changes in mean arterial blood pressure (MABP), following blood transfusions in five ill, pre-term infants. (Reproduced with permission from Milligan 1980.)

newborn infants and the gestational age at which it develops can only be guessed at.

As described in other chapters in this book, it has been hypothesized that abolition of the pressure–flow autoregulation is a crucial pathogenetic element of cerebral haemorrhage as well as of ischaemia. Until now, however, there is little direct evidence in at-risk infants to support this hypothesis.

CARBON DIOXIDE–CBF REACTIVITY

Carbon dioxide is a strong cerebral vasodilator. In normocapnic adults small changes in arterial carbon dioxide tension (P_{a,CO_2}) result in a change in CBF by 4%/mmHg (30%/kPa). At extreme hypocapnia no further decrease in CBF occurs, the limit being around 50% of normal resting CBF values. Adaptation, with return of CBF to normal values, occurs within 24 hours after a chronic change of P_{a,CO_2}. A similar or even higher CO_2–CBF reactivity has been demonstrated in pre-term and full-term infants by venous occlusion plethysmography (Leahy et al 1980, Rahilly 1980b). This has also been shown in full-term infants by venous occlusion plethysmography and electrical impedance plethysmography (Costeloe et al 1984) and in pre-term ventilated infants by ^{133}Xe after intravenous injection (Fig. 10.5) (Greisen & Trojaborg 1987).

The clinical importance of the CO_2–CBF reactivity is related to three major issues. Firstly, severe hypercarbia will decrease cerebrovascular resistance, increase the transmural

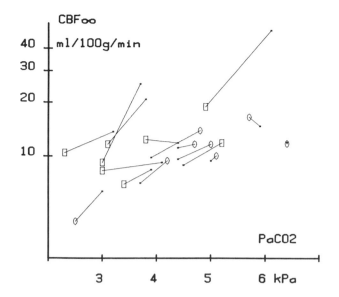

Fig. 10.5 The relationship between changes in cerebral blood flow (CBF), estimated by intravenous ^{133}Xe clearance, and changes in arterial carbon dioxide tension in 16 mechanically ventilated, pre-term infants. In eight infants the change occured spontaneously (○), whereas in the other eight infants the carbon dioxide tension changed after a change in the ventilator settings (□). (Reproduced with permission from Greisen & Trojaborg 1987.)

pressure in the capillary bed and increase the risk of germinal matrix haemorrhage. Furthermore, at high P_{a,CO_2} the range of pressure–flow autoregulation is narrowed, potentiating the cerebral effects of arterial hypertensive peaks. Secondly, moderate hyperventilation has been proposed in the postasphyxic period to decrease the flow to the undamaged parts of the brain and thereby to induce an inverse steal to the more severely affected parts of the brain. Moderate hyperventilation has also been proposed to restore pressure–flow autoregulation. Thirdly, it is possible that severe hyperventilation, to very low levels of P_{a,CO_2} may induce frank cerebral ischaemia in pre-term infants.

NEUROGENIC REGULATION OF CBF

This is a complex area of physiology where small differences in the conditions of experimentation may produce contradictory results.

It now seems clear that increased sympathetic tone may shift the pressure–flow autoregulatory plateau towards the right, allowing the brain to withstand the extraordinary perfusion pressures related to physical or emotional stress. The mechanism is in part a contraction of larger cerebral arteries and the effect may be more marked in newborn infants.

In two studies of full-term newborn infants using venous occlusion plethysmography (Dear 1980, Rahilly 1980a), a consistent decrease in CBF by 25–35% was found within the first 30–60 minutes after a feed (Fig. 10.6). In one of the

studies sleep state was controlled for, and it seems unlikely that postprandial decrease in P_{a,CO_2} or blood pressure could be responsible for the marked decrease in CBF. The results suggest a redistribution of cardiac output from the brain to the gastrointestinal tract, possibly by neurogenic mediation.

ABSOLUTE VALUES OF CBF IN NEWBORN INFANTS

Nearly all of the methods discussed above may be used to obtain estimates of CBF expressed in ml/100 g brain weight^{-1}/min^{-1} but it must be appreciated that all of them are based on a number of assumptions and may be subject to error. When comparing the results obtained by different methods it should furthermore be appreciated that the values may refer to different flow compartments or different anatomical parts of the brain. The Kety–Schmidt

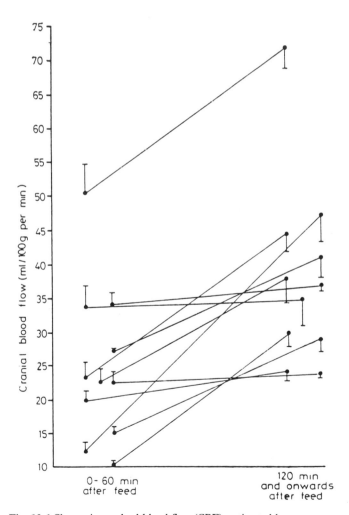

Fig. 10.6 Change in cerebral blood flow (CBF), estimated by venous occlusion plethysmography, after feeding in 11 healthy full-term infants. Each baby was in a constant sleep state. (Reproduced with permission from Rahilly 1980a.)

method, the venous occlusion plethysmographic method, the ^{11}CO-labelled erythrocyte method, and the ^{133}Xe method estimating CBF extrapolated to infinity, all provide estimates of global CBF, still there are small differences concerning the precise volume of brain represented. These differences, however, are likely to be of minor importance when compared to the other sources of error. Very different estimates, on the other hand, are obtained by the ^{133}Xe clearance technique when initial slopes from 15–60 seconds or from 0.5–2.0 minutes are used. In these slopes the most richly perfused parts of the brain are over represented; in adults the initial slopes are considered to represent mainly 'grey matter' and are by nature 50 to 150% higher than estimates of global CBF.

Apart from the methodological problems, it is clear from the discussion earlier that several biological factors may contribute to variations between reported CBF values in newborn infants including gestational age, postnatal age, state of sleep, timing of feed and possible immobilization stress — all likely to influence resting CBF in healthy infants during the first days of life. Haematocrit is usually high and haemoglobin dissociation curve shifted to the left. Rapid changes in P_{a,CO_2} associated with handling of the infants before and during CBF measurement may further contribute to the variation.

The three infants studied by Garfunkel et al (1954) were all abnormal (one with myelomeningocele, one with microcephaly and one with hydrocephalus) — CBF ranged from 15 to 23 ml.100 g^{-1}.min^{-1}, as estimated by the Kety–Schmidt method. These values were surprisingly low and this has been assumed to be due to the brain pathologies. Since then, many more attempts to estimate CBF in healthy and apparently normal newborn infants have been made and are summarized in Table 10.1. For comparison the available values for older infants, children and reference values for adults are also given. The available data suggest that CBF is low in newborn infants and that it increases with gestational age and postnatal age. In animal species, as immature at birth as man, neonatal CBF is also low when compared to adults. Whereas little is known of the energy metabolism of brain growth, in the immature brain there is a balance between the low CBF and the low metabolic rate. The rapid increase in anatomical, electrophysiological and behavioural complexity during the last part of fetal life and the first few months of human life would also suggest a rapid increase in metabolic rate and CBF.

PATHOPHYSIOLOGY

ISCHAEMIA

Decrease of CBF below a threshold, when oxygen supply is no longer sufficient, is termed ischaemia. In animal

Table 10.1 Values of cerebral blood flow (CBF) obtained in healthy, apparently normal, infants, children and adults

Author	Method	n	Gestational age	Age	CBF (ml/100g^{-1}/min^{-1})
Leahy et al 1980	Venous occlusion plethysmography (one pulse)	24	34 weeks	2–24 days	33 (16–50)
Younkin et al 1982	Intravenous ^{133}Xe	15	31 weeks	3–57 days	28 ± 8[a]
Greisen 1986	Intravenous ^{133}Xe	11	31 weeks	0–5 days	20 ± 5
Arnot et al 1970	^{11}Co-labelled erythrocytes	5	35–42 weeks	1–2 days	66 (30–106)[b]
Cross et al 1979	Venous occlusion plethysmography (exponential)	16	full-term	2–8 days	40 (22–59)
Cooke et al 1979	Venous occlusion plethysmography (one pulse)	13	full-term	3–24 hours	31 (23–48)
Milligan 1979	Venous occlusion plethysmography (one pulse)	12	full-term	3–4 days	37 (31–44)[c] 30 (24–37)[d]
Rahilly 1980a	Venous occlusion plethysmography (exponential)	20	full-term	1–7 days	40 (21–118)[c] 32 (18–102)[d]
Mukhtar et al 1982	Venous occlusion plethysmography (exponential)	29	full-term	2–9 days	40 ± 16[c] 31 ± 13[d]
Costeloe et al 1984	Venous occlusion plethysmography (one pulse)	8	full-term	3–8 days	28 ± 7
Settergren et al 1976	Kety–Schmidt, N$_2$O	12	–	11 days–12 months	69 ± 27[e]
Kennedy & Sokoloff 1957	–	9	–	3–11 years	106 ± 10[f]
Lou et al 1984	Inhalation ^{133}Xe tomography	9	–	7–15 years	71 ± 10
Meyer et al 1978	Inhalation ^{133}Xe	15	–	23–62 years	45 ± 8

[a]Recalculated using the neonatal brain–blood partition coefficient and extrapolated to infinity.
[b]The infants had recovered from asphyxia, respiratory distress and hypoglycaemia.
[c]Active sleep.
[d]Quiet sleep.
[e]Under N$_2$O-anaesthesia.
[f]Distribution by moving pictures.

experiments, in which ischaemia was induced by middle cerebral artery occlusion potentiated by systemic arterial hypotension, it has been demonstrated that there are at least two ischaemic thresholds. In adult brain cortex, electrical function ceases at about 18 ml/100 g^{-1}/min^{-1}. In subcortical grey matter and the brainstem the values reach down to 12 ml/100 g^{-1}/min^{-1}. When the other threshold is passed there is rapid neuronal depolarization, potassium efflux, calcium influx, and a series of autodigestive processes are initiated, which ultimately cause cell death.

The threshold values for newborn infants are not known but in view of the low resting levels of CBF and the comparatively much longer survival in total ischaemia or anoxia, the thresholds are likely to be considerably below 10 ml/100 g^{-1}/min^{-1}. Thus, in ventilated pre-term infants visual evoked responses were unaffected at flow levels below 10 ml/100 g^{-1}/min^{-1} as estimated by ^{133}Xe clearance after intravenous injection (Greisen & Trojaborg 1987). (See also Chapter 29.)

ASPHYXIA

Perinatal and postnatal asphyxia result in complex disturbances of blood gases and tissue perfusion. Some degree of hypoxia and hypercarbia is always present and in long-lasting asphyxia, acidosis and arterial hypotension supervene. During the early phases of asphyxia, an increased cardiac output combined with diminished oxygen supply put a particular stress on the myocardium, which is the 'target' organ of asphyxia. Arterial blood pressure is kept up by severe systemic and visceral vasoconstriction to the benefit of the brain, adrenal glands and kidneys.

Experimental asphyxia in perinatal animals has been produced by hypobaric oxygen, occlusion of the maternal aorta, occlusion of the umbilical cord, suffocation and rebreathing techniques — all producing a different combination of hypoxia, hypercarbia, acidosis and arterial hypotension. Accordingly, during experimental asphyxia global CBF may be increased. Neuronal damage may occur even with increased CBF, if the increase is insufficient in providing the oxygen required. Severe glial cell oedema may result from excessive accumulation of lactate, resulting in brain oedema, increased intracranial pressure and subsequent ischaemia. During longer lasting asphyxia, global CBF tends to be decreased. It is of greater interest, however, that very significant local inhomogeneities in CBF changes may occur. Firstly, when the arterial blood pressure drops, great local differences in perfusion pressure may result and the terminal arterial branches supplying the watershed territories between the anterior, middle and posterior cerebral arteries suffer most. Secondly, flow may be redistributed from the hemispheres to the brainstem and cerebellum. In newborn puppies this redistribution is mediated by the sympathetic system. Thirdly, in newborn puppies, which are rather immature at birth, the subcortical white matter suffers more than the cortex. Finally, at the end of prolonged partial asphyxia in near-term monkey fetuses, patchy areas of severe ischaemia in the cerebral hemispheres and central nuclei were observed. This corresponds well to the finding of rather circumscript cerebral infarcts in asphyxiated full-term infants. The mechanisms are unknown, although emboli, thrombosis or local arterial compression have been implicated.

At recovery, CBF increases dramatically when arterial blood pressure increases. At first the increase is probably mediated by tissue acidosis and the increased extracellular concentrations of potassium and adenosine and makes good the energy deficit.

After ischaemic insults, insufficient reperfusion may aggravate the resulting brain injury. This is likely to be true also after asphyxia, in particular when the metabolic needs are increased by paroxysmal electric discharges. The reactive hyperaemia may last only 5 to 10 minutes but a disturbance of the regulation of CBF may, however, last for hours after asphyxia. The perfusion pressure-autoregulation appears to be most easily disturbed, the CO_2-flow reactivity less easily, whereas the ability for vasodilatation in response to hypoxia appears most resistant. Owing to these complexities it may be difficult to interpret values of global CBF after asphyxia. Sankaran et al (1981) used venous occlusion plethysmography and found CBF to be low in the first days of life in moderately asphyxiated full-term infants whereas Friis-Hansen (1985) reported increased CBF, as estimated by the intravenous ^{133}Xe method, in a few severely asphyxiated full-term infants. Volpe et al (1985) reported local decrease in CBF, as estimated by positron emission tomography, in the parasagittal regions 3 to 20 days after the insult in a large proportion of asphyxiated infants.

The important aspects of CBF regulation after asphyxia have as yet not been studied in newborn infants. In particular, the effect of increased P_{a,CO_2} on a cerebral vasculature with inhomogeneous reactivity may be complex. It is possible, as has been demonstrated in adult patients with focal ischaemia, that a steal phenomenon may develop, when blood flow to the least damaged areas improves at the cost of the flow to the most damaged areas.

Finally, there are no data on the relationship between CBF in the reperfused asphyxiated brain with cerebral oedema and intracranial hypertension. The benefit of hyperventilation on the relationship between CBF and energy requirements following cerebral oedema in these infants has not yet been documented.

(See also Chapters 32 and 33.)

INTRACRANIAL HAEMORRHAGE

When pressure–flow autoregulation is abolished, arterial blood pressure peaks may reach the capillary bed in the germinal matrix. When the capillary wall is weak by constitution or by preceding ischaemia the increased transmural pressure may cause rupture and haemorrhage. The lack of autoregulation will be witnessed by increased CBF when arterial blood pressure is high. The importance of the loss of autoregulation for the development of germinal matrix haemorrhage has been widely accepted but the evidence is still only circumstantial (see Ch. 28).

After germinal matrix haemorrhage and in particular when blood spreads to the ventricular fluid or into surrounding tissue, vasoconstriction may ensue, as has been demonstrated after subarachnoid haemorrhage in adults. The vasoconstriction causes ischaemia which may, if severe, result in tissue injury. On the other hand, haemorrhage is often associated with electrical seizures and as long as the flow metabolism coupling is present, seizures will cause increased CBF.

The expected complexity of the relationship between intracranial haemorrhage and CBF is matched by the contradictory results obtained from the study of newborn infants. High CBF preceding haemorrhage (Cooke et al 1979, Milligan 1980, Ment et al 1981) and low CBF following haemorrhage (Cooke et al 1979, Ment et al 1981, Volpe et al 1983, Ment et al 1984) has been well documented. But even the opposite situation of low CBF preceding haemorrhage (Ment et al 1984) and high CBF following haemorrhage (Greisen 1986) has been reported. The clinical implications of these findings are unclear.

RESPIRATORY DISTRESS AND ARTIFICIAL VENTILATION

Respiratory distress may affect CBF through hypercarbia or hypoxia (Cooke et al 1979) or through decreasing perfusion pressure due to systemic hypotension or increased intrathoracic pressure. A decrease in perfusion pressure may only change CBF when the lower threshold of pressure–flow autoregulation is passed, or when autoregulation has been abolished altogether. During artificial ventilation there is a particular risk of increased intrathoracic pressure. Respiratory distress syndrome is characterized by several circulatory features of which decreased visceral blood flow is one. It is possible that brain blood flow is affected similarly. Thus, among 42 pre-term infants (Fig. 10.7) artificial ventilation was associated with a significant decrease in CBF which could not be explained by differences in P_{a,CO_2}, arterial blood pressure, or gestational age (Greisen 1986).

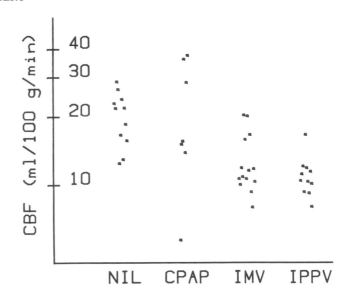

Fig. 10.7 Cerebral blood flow (CBF) in 42 pre-term infants less than 5 days of age, estimated by the intravenous ^{133}Xe method. Of these infants 11 required no respiratory assistance (NIL), 6 had continuous positive airway pressure (CPAP), 14 were mechanically ventilated at a rate <20/min (IMV), whereas 11 required a faster rate (IPPV). (Reproduced with permission from Greisen 1986.)

MEASUREMENT OF CBF IN CLINICAL PRACTICE

At present there is no place for CBF measurements in the intensive care of newborn infants. We do not know with any precision the lower limit of acceptable CBF at which it will be appropriate to intervene by increasing the perfusion pressure and/or P_{a,CO_2}. On the other hand, while it is likely that increased CBF may be a forerunner of intracranial haemorrhage, it has not been demonstrated that haemorrhage may be prevented by decreasing CBF.

Very low CBF as estimated by ^{133}Xe clearance after intra-arterial injection or inhalation a few hours after birth carried a significant risk of later death, cerebral atrophy or neurodevelopmental deficit (Lou & Skov 1979, Ment et al 1983). It is, however, uncertain if the outcome could have been improved by management to increase CBF.

The avoidance of perinatal brain damage will, however, be a principal task for those caring for newborn infants in the near future. Cerebral perfusion seems to be a most important variable. Future research will hopefully help in improving our understanding of this complex field. Efficient use of the available methods, as well as development of new and more applicable and reliable methods, with less patient risk is needed. The combination of measurement of CBF with estimation of cerebral function and cerebral metabolism may open the door to a soundly based clinical practice of brain-oriented intensive care.

REFERENCES

Arnot R N, Glass H I, Clark J C, Davis J A, Schiff D, Picton-Warlow C G 1970 Methods of measurement of cerebral blood flow in the newborn infant using cyclotron produced isotopes. Radioaktive Isotope in Klinik und Forschung 9: 60–74

Cooke R W I 1978 Cerebral blood flow measurement using venous occlusion plethysmography in the human newborn infant. In: Rolfe P (ed) Non-invasive physiological measurements. Academic Press, London

Cooke R W I, Rolfe P, Howat P 1979 Apparent cerebral blood flow in newborns with respiratory disease. Developmental Medicine and Child Neurology 21: 154–160

Costeloe K, Smyth D P L, Myrdoch N, Rolfe P, Tizard J P M 1984 A comparison between electrical impedance and strain gauge plethysmography for the study of cerebral blood flow in the newborn. Pediatric Research 18: 290–295

Cross K W, Dear P R F, Warner R M, Watling G B 1976 An attempt to measure cerebral blood flow in the newborn infant. Journal of Physiology 260: 42–43

Cross K W, Dear P R F, Hathorn M K S, Hyams A, Kerslake D McK, Milligan D W A, Rahilly P M, Stothers J K 1979 An estimation of intracranial blood flow in the newborn infant. Journal of Physiology 289: 329–345

Dear P R F 1980 Effect of feeding on jugular venous blood flow in the normal infant. Archives of Diseases in Childhood 55: 365–370

Friis-Hansen B 1985 Perinatal brain injury and cerebral blood flow in newborn infants. Acta Paediatrica Scandinavica 74: 323–331

Garfunkel J M, Baird H W, Siegler J 1954 The relationship of oxygen consumption to cerebral functional activity. Journal of Pediatrics 44: 64–72

Greisen G 1986 Cerebral blood flow in preterm infants during the first week of life. Acta Paediatrica Scandinavica 75: 43–51

Greisen G, Trojaborg W 1987 Cerebral blood flow, $PaCO_2$ changes, and visual evoked potentials in mechanically ventilated, preterm infants. Acta Paediatrica Scandinavica 76: 394–400

Greisen G, Frederiksen P S, Mali J, Friis-Hansen B 1984 Analysis of cranial 133-clearance in the newborn by the two-compartment model. Scandinavian Journal of Clinical and Laboratory Investigation 44: 239–250

Greisen G, Hellstrom-Westas L, Lou H, Rosen I, Svenningsen N 1985 Sleep-waking shifts and cerebral blood flow in stable preterm infants. Pediatric Research 19: 1156–1159

Kennedy C, Sokoloff L 1957 An adaptation of the nitrous oxide method to the study of the cerebral circulation in children: normal values for cerebral blood flow and cerebral metabolic rate in childhood. Journal of Clinical Investigation 36: 1130–1137

Leahy F A N, Cates D, MacCallum M, Rigatto H 1980 Effect of CO_2 and 100% O_2 on cerebral blood flow in preterm infants. Journal of Applied Physiology 48: 468–472

Lou H C, Skov H 1979 Low cerebral blood flow: a risk factor in the neonate. Journal of Pediatrics 95: 606–609

Lou H C, Lassen N A, Friis-Hansen B 1977 Low cerebral blood flow in hypotensive perinatal distress. Acta Neurologica Scandinavica 56: 343–352

Lou H C, Lassen N A, Friis-Hansen B 1979 Impaired autoregulation of cerebral blood flow in the distressed newborn infant. Journal of Pediatrics 94: 118–121

Lou H C, Henriksen L, Bruhn P 1984 Focal cerebral hypoperfusion in children with dysphasia and/or attention deficit disorder. Archives of Neurology 41: 825–829

Manwarring K H, Kodak J A, Tarby T J, Johnson S D, Suess D M 1984 Stable xenon computed tomography in the assessment of neonatal intraventricular haemorrhage and posthaemorrhagic hydrocephalus. Annals of Neurology 16: 411

Ment L R, Ehrenkrantz R A, Lange R C, Rothstein P T, Duncan C C 1981 Alterations in cerebral blood flow in preterm infants with intraventricular hemorrhage. Pediatrics 68: 763–769

Ment R L, Scott D T, Lange R C, Ehrenkrantz R A, Duncan C C, Warshaw J B 1983 Postpartum perfusion of the preterm brain: relationship to neurodevelopmental outcome. Childs Brain 10: 266–272

Ment L R, Duncan C C, Ehrenkranz R A et al 1984 Intraventricular hemorrhage in the preterm neonate: timing and cerebral blood flow changes. Journal of Pediatrics 104: 419–425

Meyer J S, Isihara N, Deshmukh V D et al 1978 Improved method for measurement of regional cerebral blood flow by 133-xenon inhalation. I. Description of method and normal values obtained in healthy volunteers. Stroke 9: 195–205

Milligan D W A 1979 Cerebral blood flow and sleep state in the normal newborn infant. Early Human Development 3/4: 321–328

Milligan D W A 1980 Failure of autoregulation and intraventricular haemorrhage in preterm infants. Lancet i: 896–899

Mukhtar A I, Cowan F M, Stothers J K 1982 Cranial blood flow and blood pressure changes during sleep in the human neonate. Early Human Development 6: 59–64

Perlman J M, Herscovitch P, Kreusser K, Raichle M, Volpe J J 1982 Positron emission tomography in the newborn: effect of seizure on regional cerebral blood flow in an asphyxiated infant. Annals of Neurology 12: 403

Rahilly P M 1980a Effects of sleep state and feeding on cranial blood flow of the human neonate. Archives of Diseases in Childhood 55: 265–270

Rahilly P M 1980b Effects of 2% carbon dioxide, 0.5% carbon dioxide and 100% oxygen on cranial blood flow of the human neonate. Pediatrics 66: 685–689

Sankaran K, Peters K, Finer N 1981 Estimated cerebral blood flow in term infants with hypoxic–ischemic encephalopathy. Pediatric Research 15: 1415–1418

Settergren G, Lindblad B S, Persson B 1976 Cerebral blood flow and exchange of oxygen, glucose, ketone bodies, lactate, pyruvate and amino acids in infants. Acta Paediatrica Scandinavica 65: 343–353

Volpe J J, Herscovitch P, Perlman J M, Raichle M E 1983 Positron emission tomography in the newborn. Extensive impairment of regional cerebral blood flow with intraventricular hemorrhage and hemorrhagic cerebral involvement. Pediatrics 72: 589–601

Volpe J J, Herscovitch P, Perlman J M, Kreusser K L, Raichle M E 1985 Positron emission tomography in the asphyxiated term newborn: parasagittal impairment of cerebral blood flow. Annals of Neurology 17: 287–296

Younkin D P, Reivich M, Jaggi J, Obrist W, Delivoria-Papadopoulos M 1982 Noninvasive method of estimating newborn regional cerebral blood flow. Journal of Cerebral Blood Flow Metabolism 2: 415–420

11. Doppler assessment of the neonatal cerebral circulation

Dr L. N. J. Archer and Dr D. H. Evans

The use of Doppler ultrasound for the assessment of blood flow in the fetal and neonatal brain is comparatively recent, the first report of its use in the neonatal brain being that of Bada et al (1979). It has great potential since it is non-invasive and can be carried out at the cot-side of even severely ill infants and may be repeated at will. It has been used to research into many pathological conditions in the neonate but many studies have been carried out using inadequate equipment and have drawn unjustifiable conclusions from the results obtained. It is important for the long-term credibility of the method that the limitations of the technique are appreciated so that extravagant claims are not made for it. As yet little work has been carried out on the fetal cerebral circulation.

A brief review of the principles and some practical aspects of the technique is followed by a discussion of its validity and of its clinical applications.

INSTRUMENTATION AND SIGNAL PROCESSING

The ultrasonic Doppler velocimeter works by sensing the change in frequency imposed on an ultrasonic wave as it is reflected or scattered from a moving target. That change in frequency is given by the Doppler equation:

$$f_d = 2\, v\, f_t \cos \theta\, /\, c \tag{1}$$

where v is the velocity of the target, f_t the transmitted frequency, θ the angle between the ultrasound beam and the direction of flow, and c the velocity of ultrasound in tissue.

There are two distinct types of Doppler velocimeter, continuous wave (CW) and pulsed wave (PW). CW Dopplers employ a transducer containing two piezo-electric crystals, one of which is used to transmit continuously a beam of ultrasound into the tissue, whilst the second is used for receiving. These devices have no depth resolution except in the sense that the signals from targets close to the transducer experience less attentuation than those at a distance.

PW Dopplers usually contain only a single crystal which serves both as a transmitter and a receiver. They emit short bursts of ultrasound several thousand times every second, usually at regular intervals. After each pulse has been transmitted there is a delay before a gate in the receiving circuit is opened for a short period of time to admit returning signals from a small volume of tissue. The delay between transmission and opening the gate may be altered by the operator to determine the depth from which signals are gathered, whilst the time for which the gate is left open (also operator adjustable) taken together with the length of the transmitted pulse determines the length of the sample volume. As with CW the width of the sample volume is determined by transducer geometry and ultrasound frequency. PW Doppler has the obvious advantage that it makes it possible to select signals from a particular depth but it can cause misleading results, due to a phenomenon known as aliasing, if high velocity flow is present in the sample volume. To avoid this problem (where spectral power corresponding to high frequencies is incorrectly interpreted as being of lower frequency) it is essential that the sampling rate, determined by the pulse repetition frequency (PRF), is at least twice the highest Doppler shift frequency. High PRFs bring their own problems as they introduce multiple gates (and hence range ambiguity) and also increase the ultrasonic dose to the tissue. Despite these problems PW Doppler is generally to be preferred in regions, such as the fetal or neonatal brain, where there is a high risk of insonating the wrong vessel if range gating is not used.

Once the returning ultrasound signal (continuous or pulsed) has been received by the transducer it is necessary to process it in order to obtain a Doppler signal. This may be achieved in many ways but in essence all methods compare the transmitted signal with the received signal and derive a difference signal, the frequency of which is proportional to the velocity of the target. In practice there will be many targets in the ultrasound field and they will be travelling with a variety of velocities. The Doppler signal therefore contains many frequencies (which will vary with time). This makes it necessary to apply further processing to the signal before it can be displayed and recorded in a meaningful manner. It is possible either to extract a frequency envelope from the signal, or to perform a spectral analysis on the signal and display the results as a sonogram. The former method has the advantage of simplicity but is prone to error, whilst the latter requires more sophisticated equipment both for analysis and display. Envelope detectors may extract the instantaneous mean, maximum or root mean square (rms) frequency of the signal and the outputs are normally written to a chart recorder. Each of these methods is prone to errors (Evans 1985a) but the rms detector (the zero-crossing detector) which is used in many commercial instruments is particularly bad in this respect (Lunt 1975) and should be avoided. The preferred method of processing Doppler signals is to perform a full spectral analysis using a real-time spectrum analyser, and to display the results in the form of a sonogram. In this type of display (Fig. 11.1), time is represented along the abscissa (x-axis), Doppler shift frequency along the ordinate (y-axis), and the power of the signal at a given frequency and time by the intensity of the corresponding pixel. A maximum frequency envelope may be derived by following the outline of the sonogram either automatically or by hand using a digitizer. The spectral information may also be used to calculate a mean frequency envelope but this is susceptible to many of the same problems as the mean frequency follower.

Both CW and PW Dopplers may be used in isolation and this may be appropriate in some monitoring situations. However, it is generally much better to define the direction of the beam and the position of the sample volume with the help of anatomical information. Duplex scanners combine a Doppler unit with an ultrasound imaging device and superimpose cursors on the image which depict the position of the sample volume (Fig. 11.2). This has the additional

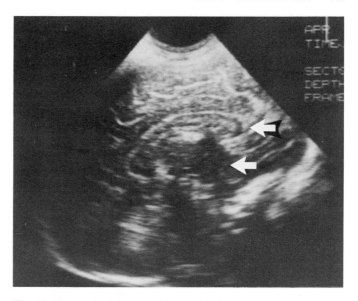

Fig. 11.2 Parasagittal ultrasound B-scan of a baby's brain showing the position of two sites at which the anterior cerebral artery can be insonated with a low value for θ.

advantage that it allows the angle between the Doppler beam and the blood vessel (θ in Eqn 1) to be measured, and thus allows Doppler shift frequencies to be converted to velocities.

Having obtained a good signal from a known point in the head, some interpretation is necessary. There are several options available which include waveform analysis, velocity measurement and flow measurement. At this stage of the application of Doppler techniques to the fetal and neonatal brain, waveform analysis techniques are by far the most widely used. These techniques are aimed at correlating changes in the shape of the velocity waveforms with different physiological and pathological states. The method that has been used almost exclusively to date is to calculate a 'Resistance Index' defined as $(S–D)/S$ (Fig. 11.3) where S and D are the maximum and minimum values of the Doppler shift frequency envelope during the cardiac cycle (Pourcelot 1976). This index does correlate with changes in vascular resistance distal to the recording site but it is also

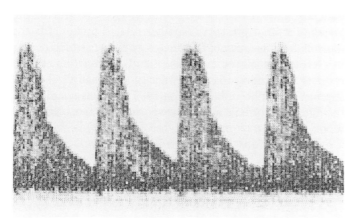

Fig. 11.1 A sonogram of the Doppler signal from a normal baby. In this type of display time is represented along the abscissa, Doppler frequency shift along the ordinate, and the power of the signal at a given frequency and time by the intensity of the corresponding pixel.

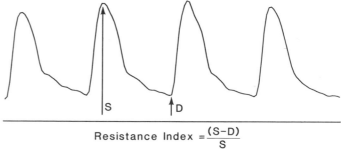

$$\text{Resistance Index} = \frac{(S-D)}{S}$$

Fig. 11.3 Definition of resistance index (RI).

Table 11.1 Current uses for neonatal cerebral Doppler examination

Condition	Use
Postasphyxial encephalopathy	Waveform shape a reliable prognostic tool
Hydrocephalus/ventricular dilatation	Waveform pulsatility may help in management
Brain death	May help with diagnosis
Cerebral AV malformation	Value unclear
Haemorrhagic/ischaemic lesions	True blood velocities may be of value in research

influenced by many other factors. Therefore, although it is a useful and simple objective statement about the waveform shape, care is necessary with its interpretation. Principal component analysis, a sophisticated pattern recognition technique has also been tried with some success (Evans et al 1985). Waveform analysis techniques have much to offer because they do not require the angle θ to be measured and it is probable that waveform shape is altered by lesser degrees of circulatory perturbation than are either mean blood velocity or mean blood flow.

Measurements of mean blood velocity are relatively easy to make with duplex Doppler scanners. They can be used to measure proportional changes in blood flow, provided that the diameter of the vessel under study does not alter significantly. There is some evidence, as yet unconfirmed, that it may not always be possible to assume a constant vessel cross-section (Drayton & Skidmore 1987). The mean velocity may be obtained directly from the temporal average of the mean frequency envelope or may, if the flow is unidirectional and the velocity profiles fully established, be estimated from half the temporal average of the maximum frequency envelope (Evans 1985b). Frequently investigators report the value of, and changes in the 'Area Under The Curve' (AUTC), which may represent either the temporal average of the mean, rms or maximum Doppler shift frequency depending on the type of processing in use. Volumetric flow is given by the product of mean velocity and cross-sectional area. Unfortunately it is at present impossible to measure the size of cerebral vessels in the fetus or neonate in vivo and therefore absolute blood flow measurements must await further technological advances.

METHODOLOGY

In the newborn the usual way to obtain Doppler signals from the cerebral vessels is to use the anterior fontanelle as an acoustic window through which the anterior cerebral arteries can be insonated. Using this approach the angle of incidence is not greatly different from 0 degrees (Archer et al 1985) (Fig. 11.2). However, without concomitant imaging the angle is not known and cannot be assumed to be constant on different occasions or between babies.

Indeed it is possible that at times a pericallosal branch rather than the anterior cerebral artery itself will be insonated. With a Duplex system it is possible to obtain signals from two positions on the anterior cerebral arteries with a small angle of insonation, one being shortly above the origin of the anterior communicating artery and the other being at the most anterior point before the vessel turns backwards above the corpus callosum (Fig. 11.2). We do not consider it possible to distinguish reliably between right and left sides because the vessels run virtually adjacent to each other. Access to the middle cerebral artery via the fontanelle is unsatisfactory and this vessel is better insonated through the temporal bone, a technique first used in adults (Aaslid et al 1982, Padayachee et al 1986). There is little information on examination of posterior cerebral artery velocities although Padayachee and colleagues (1986) have reported findings in adults.

The clinical situations in which cranial Doppler ultrasound waveforms have been reported are many and have recently been reviewed by Perlman (1985). The question of exactly what information the technique provides about underlying haemodynamic processes is a vexed one (Bejar et al 1982, Volpe et al 1982, Ahmann et al 1983a, Batton et al 1983a, Bada & Sumner 1984). A different consideration is whether or not cranial Doppler ultrasound can be used as a clinical tool even if the reasons for waveform shape changes are not understood.

FACTORS AFFECTING THE DOPPLER WAVEFORM

Cerebral Doppler waveform shape is affected by a large number of variables acting both proximal and distal to the site of recording. The blood pressure waveform will affect the shape of cerebral blood velocity waveforms and this has been well demonstrated by Perlman et al (1983) who recorded fluctuating cerebral blood velocities from babies with respiratory distress syndrome (RDS) and fluctuating systemic arterial pressure. Another related proximal factor in neonates is patency of the ductus arteriosus which results in a left to right shunt and consequently a reduction or even reversal of cerebral diastolic velocity (Perlman et al 1981, Lipman et al 1982, Martin et al 1982). Resistance distal to the site of recording affects waveform and the commonly reported resistance index (RI, see Fig. 11.3) is said to be a reflection of distal vascular resistance (Pourcelot 1976). There is some evidence for this in the effect of carbon dioxide (Hauge et al 1980) and other vasodilating agents (Pourcelot 1976) on reducing RI in adults. In animal experiments cerebral vasodilation induced by hypercapnia increased velocities as expected but showed a weak negative association with RI in puppies (Batton et al 1983b) and no association with RI in piglets (Hansen et al 1983). In human newborn babies there are two reported studies specifically designed to examine the effect of changes in inspired carbon dioxide concentration on Doppler signals. Costeloe et al (1984) were unable to show correlation between changes in any Doppler parameter and a stepwise increase in inspired carbon dioxide from air to 2–3%. Archer et al (1986a), however, showed a correlation between end-tidal carbon dioxide concentration with both RI and area under the velocity curve. In a clinical setting Daven et al (1983) and Jorch & Menge (1985) have similarly shown a low RI and increased velocities in hypercapnia or hypoxia. Drayton & Skidmore (1986) also report a fall in RI with hypercapnia but point out that there are in addition major changes in the aortic velocity waveform. Viscosity of blood also affects RI in newborn infants (Rosenkrantz & Oh 1982). It is not clear whether this is a result of altered rheological properties of the blood or whether it reflects a physiological response of the cerebral vasculature to oxygen delivery but there is some reason to believe the latter explanation from lamb experimental work involving altering oxygen content but not viscosity of blood (Rosenkrantz et al 1984).

It is unclear to what extent changes in RI reflect changes in cerebral vascular resistance (CVR) but it appears that it relates poorly or not at all to cerebral blood flow (CBF) (Batton et al 1983b, Hansen et al 1983, Greison et al 1984). Greison et al (1984) using a xenon clearance technique did, however, find a significant correlation between Doppler measured velocities and CBF in newborn infants as did Batton et al (1983b) with puppies and Hansen et al (1983) with piglets. It seems likely that actual velocities when reliably obtained may prove of more value in following blood flow changes but RI may also have a clinical role (see later).

EFFECT OF PHYSIOLOGICAL VARIABLES ON WAVEFORM

The effects of postnatal age (Gray et al 1983, Archer et al 1985) and sleep state (Cowan 1985, Archer et al 1986b) on cerebral Doppler signals have been reported. RI falls over the first few postnatal days in normal full-term infants and this is probably due to a combination of cerebrovascular as well as central cardiovascular changes. Sleep state shows a variable effect on RI and velocity but probably one that does not matter in clinical practice, the important point being to have a quiet settled infant for examination. There is little information on the effect of head position on cerebral arterial RI (Emery & Peabody 1983) and none on the effect on velocity but the expected marked changes in venous velocity (Cowan & Thoresen 1985) brought about by posture and pressure have been described. It is advisable whenever possible to avoid excessive rotation of the baby's head to prevent venous obstruction and also to avoid abnormal pressure being applied to the skull during

Doppler examination. In studying healthy infants a mild degree of fluctuation in maximum frequency in time with respiration is often seen. A more exaggerated fluctuation has been reported in ventilated babies with respiratory distress syndrome (Perlman et al 1983). Cowan & Thoresen (1984) have reported a critical peak ventilator pressure above which the Doppler waveform shows a reduction in velocity coinciding with peak inspiration.

CLINICAL STUDIES

Fetal cranial vessel Doppler examination has only recently been reported (Wladimiroff et al 1986) and further work is needed before assessment of its worth is possible. The newborn's cerebral circulation has been examined with Doppler ultrasound in many clinical conditions. In some, the abnormalities detected clearly represent major disturbances in cardiac output or blood pressure. Thus changes seen in apnoea and bradycardia (Perlman & Volpe 1985), seizures (Perlman & Volpe 1983a), endotracheal tube suction (Perlman & Volpe 1983b) and pneumothorax (Peabody 1981a, Hill et al 1982, Batton et al 1984) are only to be expected. These are all events known to influence the cardiovascular system and Doppler demonstration of changes in the cerebral circulation only serves to underline the potentially damaging effect they may have. Marked fluctuations in cerebral blood flow velocity seen in respiratory distress syndrome (Perlman et al 1983) are a marker for increased risk of germinal matrix haemorrhage–intraventricular haemorrhage (GMH–IVH). Abolition of fluctuation by neuromuscular paralysis (Perlman et al 1985) reduces the incidence of severe GMH–IVH. These fluctuations appear to be transmission of fluctuations in systemic arterial pressure and may be a cardiovascular manifestation of the respiratory lack of co-ordination described by Greenough et al (1984). In any case it is unnecessary to use Doppler to detect them if direct continuous arterial pressure monitoring is performed. The changes in cranial Doppler waveform in infants with patent ductus arteriosus (PDA) have already been referred to (Perlman et al 1981, Lipman et al 1982, Martin et al 1982) and are not a recommended way of diagnosing PDA (although aortic and pulmonary artery Doppler examination is to be recommended). They do, however, warn of possible deleterious effects on cerebral perfusion of a large shunt through the ductus arteriosus. Furthermore, attempted closure of the DA by indomethacin (Cowan 1986, Archer et al 1987, Lundell & Sonesson 1987) is also associated with dramatic changes in cerebral haemodynamics, probably reflecting reduced CBF induced by the drug. Surgical ligation of the ductus arteriosus is also accompanied by dramatic changes in cerebral blood flow velocity (Lundell & Sonesson 1986, Sonesson et al

1986) but in the opposite direction. Diminution or reversal of diastolic flow velocity in cranial vessels has also been reported in other cardiovascular abnormalities with a large systemic to pulmonary connection (Snider 1985). The effect of drugs other than indomethacin on the cerebral circulation assessed by Doppler ultrasound has only been reported for aminophylline (Rosenkrantz & Oh 1984) which reduced peak systolic velocity and AUTC acutely, and pancuronium (Peabody 1981b) which caused RI to fall although detailed information on direct blood pressure values is not given in either case. Neonatal meningitis did not have a major effect on Doppler waveforms in the four cases reported by McMenamin & Volpe (1984), nor indeed was intracranial pressure or blood pressure significantly abnormal.

In the original description of neonatal cerebral Doppler ultrasound Bada et al (1979) reported a high RI in GMH–IVH. The haemorrhage was preceded by a lower RI in infants who bled compared with those who did not. Ando et al (1985) have recently described similar results. For reasons already given it is not possible to interpret these observations and Perlman & Volpe (1982) did not find any consistent association. Bada et al (1982) also found a high RI to indicate worse outcome in GMH–IVH but at present Doppler ultrasound is not clinically useful in assessing babies with haemorrhage nor has it provided information about disturbed haemodynamics causing or following haemorrhagic or ischaemic lesions in the neonatal brain. Attempts to assess the efficiency of cerebral autoregulation using Doppler are premature (Ahmann et al 1983b) with the current state of development of the method.

Doppler changes in cranial vessels in vein of Galen aneurysm have been described in two cases (Perlman 1985, McCord et al 1987). It is not clear whether Doppler ultrasound will have a role in the management of these cases.

There are three conditions in which characteristic changes in the Doppler waveform have been described with the suggestion that clinical management may be aided thereby. Neonatal brain death is not a diagnosis commonly made in Europe, but McMenamin & Volpe (1983) describe a gradual diminution in and eventual disappearance of Doppler signals which they consider helpful in making this diagnosis rather than progressing to more invasive evaluation. In perinatal asphyxia low values of RI have been described by several groups (Bada et al 1979, van Bel & Grimberg 1982, Archer et al 1986c). In a series of patients with all grades of severity of postasphyxial encephalopathy (PAE) we have found a normal RI to be a very sensitive and specific marker for good outcome regardless of severity of PAE (Archer et al 1986c). An abnormally high RI has been described in hydrocephalus (Hill & Volpe 1982, Ando et al 1985, Saliba et al 1985) with return to more normal values after drainage. Clear guidelines as to whether this will serve as a useful tool in planning intervention or monitoring progress in hydrocephalus are not available yet.

SAFETY OF DOPPLER ULTRASOUND

Recently concern has been expressed about the power levels produced by some ultrasound machines and much has been written about potential hazards. That ultrasound of sufficient power may have deleterious effects is not in question (Nyborg & Ziskin 1985) but 'there have been no independently confirmed significant biological effects in mammalian tissue exposed to intensities below 100mW/cm² (SPTA)' (American Institute of Ultrasound in Medicine 1984). It is important that operators of ultrasound machines are aware of potential hazards and of the output powers their machines are capable of producing. Prudence dictates that wherever possible the ultrasonic dose to the fetal or neonatal brain should be kept to a minimum compatible with obtaining relevant clinical information and that the spatial peak temporal average power should at all times be kept below 100mW/cm².

CONCLUSIONS

There are many theoretical and methodological issues to be clarified before neonatal cerebral Doppler ultrasound examination can be used with confidence as a basic research tool to provide information on CBF and CVR. Use of PW and Duplex scanning is likely to be of value in resolving these problems. Abnormalities in Doppler waveforms seen in pathological conditions are only very loosely interpretable with equipment and analysis techniques used to date and in many cases provide no more information than knowledge of heart rate, blood pressure or systemic arterial waveforms. Table 11.1 summarizes the uses of neonatal cerebral Doppler examination. In PAE, Doppler is a reliable prognostic indicator. Doppler ultrasound may possibly be of value in assessing the significance of ventricular dilatation and planning appropriate intervention.

REFERENCES

Aaslid R, Markwalder T M, Nornes H 1982 Non-invasive transcranial Doppler ultrasound recording of flow velocity in basal cerebral arteries. Journal of Neurosurgery 57: 769–774
Ahmann P A, Dykes F D, Lazzara A, Wilcox W D, Carrigan T 1983a Cerebral blood flow. Pediatrics 71: 296–298

Ahmann P A, Dykes F D, Lazzara A, Holt P J, Giddens D P, Carrigan T A 1983b Relationship between pressure passivity and subependymal/intraventricular hemorrhage as assessed by pulsed Doppler ultrasound. Pediatrics 72: 665–669
American Institute of Ultrasound in Medicine, Bioeffects Committee 1984

Safety considerations for diagnostic ultrasound. AIUM Publication 316

Ando Y, Takashima S, Takeshita K 1985 Cerebral blood flow velocity in pre-term neonates. Brain and Development 7: 385–391

Archer L N J, Evans D H, Levene M I 1985 Doppler ultrasound examination of the anterior cerebral arteries of normal newborn infants: the effect of post-natal age. Early Human Development 10: 255–260

Archer L N J, Evans D H, Levene M I 1986a The effect of controlled hypercapnia on anterior cerebral artery Doppler waveforms in healthy newborn infants. Pediatric Research 20: 218–221

Archer L N J, Evans D H, Levene M I, Paton S Y, Hall H S 1986b The effect of some physiological variables on the Doppler ultrasound waveform in healthy newborn infants. In: Rolfe P (ed) Fetal and neonatal physiological measurements, Vol 2. Butterworths, London, pp. 111–116

Archer L N J, Evans D H, Levene M I 1986c Cerebral artery Doppler ultrasonography predicts outcome in perinatal asphyxia. Archives of Disease in Childhood 61: 632 (abstract)

Archer L N J, Evans D H, Levene M I 1987 The effects of indomethacin on cerebral blood velocity in premature infants. In: Sheldon C D, Evans D H, Salvage J R (eds) Obstetric and neonatal blood flow. Biological Engineering Society, London

Bada H S, Sumner D S 1984 Transcutaneous Doppler ultrasound: pulsatility index, mean flow velocity, end diastolic flow velocity and cerebral bloodflow. Journal of Pediatrics 104: 395–397

Bada H S, Hajjar W, Chua C, Sumner D S 1979 Non-invasive diagnosis of neonatal asphyxia and intraventricular hemorrhage by Doppler ultrasound. Journal of Pediatrics 95: 775–779

Bada H S, Miller J E, Meuke J A et al 1982 Intracranial pressure and cerebral arterial pulsatile flow measurements in neonatal intraventricular hemorrhage. Journal of Pediatrics 100: 291–296

Batton D G, Hellmann J, Maisels M J 1983a Doppler pulsatility index. Pediatrics 71: 298

Batton D G, Hellmann J, Hernandez M J, Maisels M J 1983b Regional cerebral blood flow, cerebral blood velocity and pulsatility index in newborn dogs. Pediatric Research 17: 908–912

Batton D G, Hellmann J, Nardis E E 1984 Effect of pneumothorax induced systemic blood pressure alterations on the cerebral circulation in newborn dogs. Pediatrics 74: 350–353

Bejar R, Merritt T A, Coen R W 1982 Pulsatility index, patent ductus arteriosus and brain damage. Pediatrics 69: 818–822

Costeloe K, Weindling A M, Tarressenko L, Murphy D, Wollner J C, Rolfe P 1984 An attempt to validate the use of pulsatility index in the study of the newborn cerebral circulation. Biology of the Neonate 45: 300 (abstract)

Cowan F 1985 Cerebral blood velocities and their variability in different sleep states in the newborn infant. Pediatric Research 19: 1084 (abstract)

Cowan F 1986 Acute effects of indomethacin on neonatal cerebral blood velocities. Early Human Development 13: 343 (abstract)

Cowan F, Thoresen M 1984 Effect of differing ventilation rates and pressures on cranial blood flow velocities in the newborn infant. Biology of the Neonate 45: 151 (abstract)

Cowan F, Thoresen M 1985 Changes in superior sagittal sinus blood velocities due to postural alterations and pressure on the head of the newborn infant. Pediatrics 75: 1038–1047

Daven J R, Milstein J M, Guthrie R D 1983 Cerebral vascular resistance in premature infants. American Journal of Diseases of Children 137: 328–331

Drayton M R, Skidmore R 1986 Doppler studies of the neonatal cerebral circulation. In: Kurjak A (ed) Recent advances in ultrasound diagnosis, Vol. 6. Excerpta Medica, Amsterdam, pp. 113–127

Drayton M R, Skidmore R 1987 A volumetric approach to the Doppler assessment of neonatal cerebral perfusion. In: Sheldon C D, Evans D H, Salvage J R (eds) Obstetric and neonatal blood flow. Biological Engineering Society, London, pp. 95–99

Emery J R, Peabody J L 1983 Head position affects intracranial pressure in newborn infants. Journal of Pediatrics 103: 950–953

Evans D H 1985a Doppler signal processing. In: Altobelli A, Voyles W F, Green E R (eds) Cardiovascular ultrasonic flowmetry. Elsevier, New York, pp. 239–261

Evans D H 1985b On the measurement of the mean velocity of blood flow over the cardiac cycle using Doppler ultrasound. Ultrasound in Medicine and Biology 11: 735–741

Evans D H, Archer L N J, Levene M I 1985 The detection of abnormal cerebral haemodynamics using principal component analysis of the Doppler ultrasound waveform. Ultrasound in Medicine and Biology 11: 441–449

Gray P H, Griffin E A, Drumm J E, Fitzgerald D E, Duignan N M 1983 Continuous wave Doppler ultrasound in evaluation of cerebral blood flow in neonates. Archives of Disease in Childhood 58: 677–681

Greenough A, Wood S, Morley C J, Davis J A 1984 Pancuronium prevents pneumothoraces in ventilated premature babies who actively expire against positive pressure inflation. Lancet i: 1–3

Greisen G, Johansen K, Ellison P H, Fredenksen P S, Mali J, Friis-Hansen B 1984 Cerebral blood flow in the newborn infant: comparison of Doppler ultrasound and 133-Xenon clearance. Journal of Pediatrics 104: 411–418

Hansen N B, Stonestreet B S, Rosenkrantz T S, Oh W 1983 Validity of Doppler measurements of anterior cerebral artery blood flow velocity: correlation with brain blood flow in piglets. Pediatrics 72: 526–531

Hauge A, Thoresen M, Walloe L 1980 Changes in cerebral blood flow during hyperventilation and CO_2-breathing measured transcutaneously in humans by a bi-directional, pulsed, ultrasound Doppler velocity meter. Acta Physiologica Scandinavica 110: 167–173

Hill A, Volpe J J 1982 Decrease in pulsatile flow in the anterior cerebral arteries in infantile hydrocephalus. Pediatrics 69: 4–7

Hill A, Perlman J M, Volpe J J 1982 Relationship of pneumothorax to occurrence of intraventricular hemorrhage in the premature newborn. Pediatrics 69: 144–149

Jorch G, Menge V 1985 Die Bedeutung des pCO_2 fur die Hirndurchblutung in der Neonatologie. Monatsschrift fur Kinderheilkunde 133: 38–42

Lipman B, Serwer G, Brazy J E 1982 Abnormal cerebral haemodynamics in preterm infants with patent ductus arteriosus. Pediatrics 69: 778–781

Lundell B P W, Sonesson S E 1987 Surgery or indomethacin? Ductus closure and cerebral blood flow. Early Human Development 14(2): 141 (abstract)

Lunt M J 1975 Accuracy and limitations of the ultrasonic Doppler blood velocimeter and zero-crossing detector. Ultrasound in Medicine and Biology 2: 1–10

McCord F B, McNeil A, Shields M D, McClure B G, Halliday H L, Reid M McC 1987 Pulsed Doppler in cerebral arteriovenous malformation. In: Sheldon C D, Evans D H, Salvage J R (eds) Obstetric and Neonatal Blood Flow. Biological Engineering Society, London, pp. 109–112

McMenamin J B, Volpe J J 1983 Doppler ultrasonography in the determination of neonatal brain death. Annals of Neurology 14: 302–307

McMenamin J B, Volpe J J 1984 Bacterial meningitis in infancy: effects on intracranial pressure and cerebral blood flow velocity. Neurology 34: 500–504

Martin C G, Snider A R, Katz S M, Peabody J L, Brady J P 1982 Abnormal cerebral blood flow patterns in preterm infants with a large patent ductus arteriosus. Journal of Pediatrics 101: 587–593

Nyborg W L, Ziskin M C 1985 Biological effects of ultrasound. Clinics in Diagnostic Ultrasound, No. 16. Churchill Livingstone, Edinburgh

Padayachee T S, Kirkham F J, Lewis R R, Gillard J, Hutchinson M C E, Gosling R G 1986 Transcranial measurement of blood velocities in the basal cerebral arteries using pulsed Doppler ultrasound: a method of assessing the circle of Willis. Ultrasound in Medicine and Biology 12: 5–14

Peabody J L 1981a Mechanical ventilation of the newborn: good news ... bad news. Critical Care Medicine 9: 710–713

Peabody J L 1981b Muscle relaxants — a potential danger to infants at risk for intraventricular hemorrhage. Pediatric Research 15: 709 (abstract)

Perlman J M 1985 Neonatal cerebral blood flow velocity measurement. Clinics in Perinatology 12: 179–193

Perlman J M, Volpe J J 1982 Cerebral blood flow velocity in relation to intraventricular hemorrhage in the premature newborn infant. Journal of Pediatrics 100: 956–958

Perlman J M, Volpe J J 1983a Seizures in the pre-term infant: effects on cerebral blood flow velocity, intracranial pressure and arterial blood pressure. Journal of Pediatrics 102: 288–293

Perlman J M, Volpe J J 1983b Suctioning in the pre-term infant: effects on cerebral blood flow velocity, intracranial pressure and arterial blood pressure. Pediatrics 72: 329–334

Perlman J M, Volpe J J 1985 Episodes of apnea and bradycardia in the preterm newborn: impact on cerebral circulation. Pediatrics 76: 333–338

Perlman J M, Hill A, Volpe J J 1981 The effect of patent ductus arteriosus on flow velocity in the anterior cerebral arteries: ductal steal in the premature newborn infant. Journal of Pediatrics 99: 767–771

Perlman J M, McMenamin J B, Volpe J J 1983 Fluctuating cerebral blood flow velocity in respiratory distress syndrome. New England Journal of Medicine 309: 204–209

Perlman J M, Goodman S, Kreusser K L, Volpe J J 1985 Reduction in intraventricular hemorrhage by elimination of fluctuating cerebral blood flow velocity in preterm infants with respiratory distress syndrome. New England Journal of Medicine 312: 1353–1357

Pourcelot L 1976 Diagnostic ultrasound for cerebral vascular diseases. In: Donald I Levis (ed) Present and future of diagnostic ultrasound. Kooyker, Rotterdam, pp. 141–147

Rosenkrantz T S, Oh W 1982 Cerebral blood flow velocity in infants with polycythemia and hyperviscosity: effects of partial exchange transfusion with plasmanate. Journal of Pediatrics 101: 94–98

Rosenkrantz T S, Oh W 1984 Aminophylline reduces cerebral blood flow velocity in low birth weight infants. American Journal of Diseases of Children 138: 489–491

Rosenkrantz T S, Stonestreet B S, Hansen N B, Nowicki P, Oh W 1984 Cerebral blood flow in the newborn lamb with polycythemia and hyperviscosity. Journal of Pediatrics 104: 276–280

Saliba E, Santini J J, Arbeille Ph et al 1985 Mesure non invasive du flux sanguin cerebral chez le nourisson hydrocephale. Archives Francaises de Pediatrie 42: 97–102

Snider A R 1985 The use of Doppler ultrasonography for the evaluation of cerebral artery flow patterns in infants with congenital heart disease. Ultrasound in Medicine and Biology 11: 503–514

Sonesson S E, Lundell B P W, Herin P 1986 Changes in intracranial arterial blood flow velocities during surgical ligation of the patent ductus arteriosus. Acta Paediatrica Scandinavica 75: 36–42

van Bel F, Grimberg M Th Th 1982 Intracraniele bloedingen en asfyxic bij de pasgeborene nadep onderzocht met de Doppler ultrasonoor methode. Tijdschrift Kindergeneeskd 50: 1–10

Volpe J J, Perlman J M, Hill A, McMenamin J 1982 Cerebral blood flow velocity in the human newborn: the value of its determination. Pediatrics 70: 147–152

Wladimiroff J M, Tonge H M, Stewart P A 1986 Doppler ultrasound assessment of cerebral blood flow in the human fetus. British Journal of Obstetrics and Gynaecology 93: 471–475

12. Doppler assessment of fetal blood flow

*Dr P. S. Warren, Dr R. W. Gill and
Dr W. J. Garrett*

The main aim of ultrasonic examination in the second half of pregnancy is to identify and monitor those babies who are at risk of perinatal death or morbidity so that an optimal time for delivery can be determined. The traditional approach has been to devise ultrasonic techniques to establish criteria for the recognition of those clinical entities which are known to be associated with increased perinatal morbidity and mortality, such as pre-eclampsia, antepartum haemorrhage, premature rupture of membranes, maternal diabetes, Rhesus iso-immunization, and the fetus being small-for-dates. Although some impact has been made, the results fall short of ideal. In particular, when a baby has been deemed on ultrasound grounds to be associated with a high-risk entity, there is difficulty in ascertaining whether or not that particular baby is in fact at risk. The usual morphological approach involves an assessment of the overall size of the baby, its nourishment and gross anatomy, the umbilical cord, placental texture and liquor volume. There remains, however, the problem of identifying which specific babies are in strife because firstly there is a time lag between the functional onset of a problem and its morphological expression and secondly the degree of compromise cannot be quantified morphologically.

These limitations in detecting not only overt fetal morbidity but also suboptimality have resulted in an increasing interest in the assessment of fetal function and well-being using ultrasonic techniques. Much attention has been directed recently at the use of Doppler ultrasound to assess the umbilical circulation, which is a low-resistance, high-flow circulation between the placenta and the fetus, and vessels within the fetus, notably the fetal descending aorta and vessels supplying the fetal brain.

DOPPLER ULTRASOUND

The physics of Doppler ultrasound is discussed in detail in Chapter 11.

Ultrasound is scattered by the large number of red cells in the fetal blood but as the scattering is very weak the Doppler instrumentation must be extremely sensitive to produce worthwhile signals. Generally the red cells within the sample volume in the blood vessel under study do not all travel at the same velocity and, furthermore, the distribution of velocities across the diameter of the vessel may be quite complex (O'Rourke 1982). This range of velocities produces a spectrum of Doppler shifts.

From the spectrum of shifts information can be obtained, including the maximum velocity of flow in the vessel and its variation with time (i.e. the flow-velocity waveform). Alternatively, the technique devised by Gill (1979) can be used to estimate the volume flow rate in the vessel. Here the ultrasound beam geometry is such that Doppler-shifted signals are received approximately equally from all points across the vessel lumen. Under these circumstances, processing of the detected Doppler signal by a mean frequency demodulator produces an output proportional to the average blood velocity over the vessel's cross-section, regardless of the particular velocity distribution within the vessel. With knowledge of the angle θ between the line of sight and the long axis of the vessel, the average velocity can be computed from the standard Doppler equation. The blood flow rate in millilitres per minute (Q) can then be calculated by multiplying the average velocity by the cross-sectional area of the vessel:

$$Q = V (\pi d^2)/4$$

where d = vessel diameter.

Continuous-wave Doppler uses relatively simple equipment, generally consisting of two transducers housed in a pencil probe — one to transmit continuously at a fixed frequency and the other to receive the echoes. Although the sample volume is relatively large, and hence the spatial selectivity poor, it does enable the equipment to be used for some applications without imaging guidance, as positioning is less critical.

With pulsed Doppler equipment the transducer transmits a few cycles at a fixed frequency and then switches to reception to pick up the returning echoes. The use of a Doppler range-gate allows detection of only those echoes returning after a given time. This enables the signals from scatterers at a predetermined depth to be studied, as distance is the product of the speed of sound and time and the sound speed is known.

APPLICATIONS

There are two main ways in which Doppler techniques are applied to the study of the fetus. The most widely used and easiest technique involves using either continuous-wave or pulsed Doppler ultrasound to study arterial flow velocity waveforms, there being no significant difference between the two methods for recording the waveforms (Giles et al 1986). With the use of various measurements and indices (Table 12.1) these waveforms can provide dynamic information about the circulation, particularly downstream

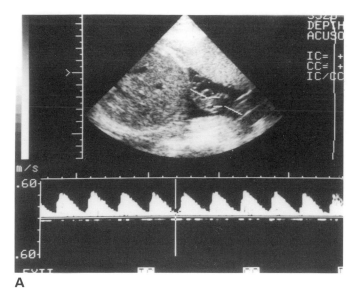

A

Table 12.1 Waveform indices

S/D ratio (A/B ratio)	$= \dfrac{\text{Peak systolic velocity}}{\text{Least diastolic velocity}}$
Pourcelot resistance index	$= \dfrac{\text{Peak systolic velocity} - \text{least diastolic velocity}}{\text{Peak systolic velocity}}$
Pulsatility index	$= \dfrac{\text{Peak systolic velocity} - \text{least diastolic velocity}}{\text{Mean velocity}}$

resistance (see Fig. 11.3, p. 163). The rate of acceleration of the arterial pressure wave depends on the pressure gradient, vessel elasticity and blood density. During systole the work of the myocardium is stored in part as potential energy in the vessel wall, so that in diastole continued forward flow of blood occurs. The flow at the end of diastole is thought to reflect vascular resistance peripheral to the point of measurement in the target circulation (Stuart et al 1980). In the case of the umbilical arteries and fetal descending thoracic aorta, this reflects the resistance in the placental bed, while in the carotid arteries it reflects the resistance in the intracranial circulation.

A commonly used index obtained from the waveform is the systolic/diastolic ratio (S/D) (Table 12.1). Being a ratio, it is independent of the angle between the vessel and the ultrasound beam. The S/D ratio in the umbilical cord has been shown to diminish progressively throughout the third trimester of pregnancy (Stuart et al 1980) (Fig. 12.1), reflecting a steady decrease in the placental vascular resistance. Van Eyck et al (1985) have shown that the behavioural state of the fetus (Table 12.2) influences the waveform in the fetal aorta in later weeks of pregnancy (37–38 weeks). They found that the Pourcelot index (Table 12.1), which is also an indicator of vascular resistance, was significantly lower in state 2F than in 1F, suggesting increased perfusion of fetal skeletal muscle to meet energy demands. They also found a significant inverse relationship

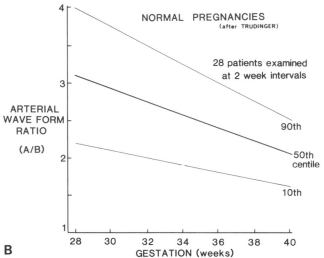

B

Fig. 12.1 (**a**) Section through umbilical cord showing sample volume encompassing the artery, and the waveform obtained. (**b**) In normal pregnancies the S/D ratio steadily diminishes throughout the third trimester.

between the Pourcelot resistance index and fetal heart rate in state 2F, mainly due to a significant increase in the velocity at end-diastole.

A more demanding and less widely available technique requires the use of pulsed Doppler for the quantitative assessment of flow in vessels (Gill 1979). In-vivo and in-vitro tests have shown that such methods can be applied with

Table 12.2 Fetal behavioural states

1F:	Quiescence, which may be regularly interrupted by brief gross body movements, mainly startles. Stable heart rate pattern.
2F:	Frequent and periodic gross body movements which are mainly stretches and retroflexions, and movements of the extremities. Greater heart rate variation than 1F.

From Van Eyck et al 1985.
For further details see Chapter 2.

good absolute accuracy (±10%) when the measurement is repeated several times and the results averaged (Gill 1985). Studies were initially aimed at the umbilical vein (Gill et al 1981) (Fig. 12.2) and more recently the fetal descending aorta (Jouppila et al 1982). The rate of umbilical venous blood flow steadily increases with gestational age, reaching a maximum at around 37 weeks of amenorrhoea followed by a slight fall-off to full-term (Fig. 12.3). The flow per kilogram remains essentially constant until 35 weeks amenorrhoea with an average value of around 120 ml.min^{-1}.kg^{-1} but there is a gradual decrease to an average value of around 90 ml.min^{-1}.kg^{-1} at 40 weeks amenorrhoea (Gill et al 1984).

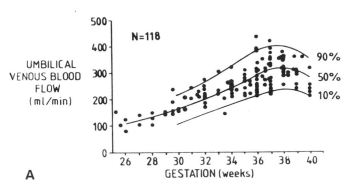

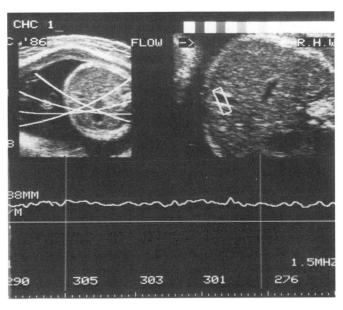

Fig. 12.2 Section through intra-abdominal portion of umbilical vein showing sample volume encompassing the vessel (rectangular box) and the computed flow tracing (in ml/min).

ABNORMALITIES

The recognition of the baby at risk of perinatal death or morbidity is the cornerstone of modern antenatal care. Those babies who are known to be small for gestational age (SGA) constitute a high-risk group which has been extensively studied by Doppler ultrasound (Gill et al 1984, Giles et al 1986, Warren et al). Low values of flow (i.e. below the tenth percentile) correlate strongly with fetal growth retardation, and an increased risk of perinatal hypoxia, morbidity and death (Gill et al 1984) (Fig. 12.3). Recently Jouppila et al (1986) demonstrated a significant negative correlation between umbilical venous blood flow and blood viscosity in 'chronic fetal distress' and in hypertensive pregnancies but not in normal or diabetic pregnancies. They postulated that haemoconcentration leading to increased fetal blood viscosity might act as a cause of the reduced flow in developing fetal distress. Recently the risk of morbidity and mortality in SFD babies

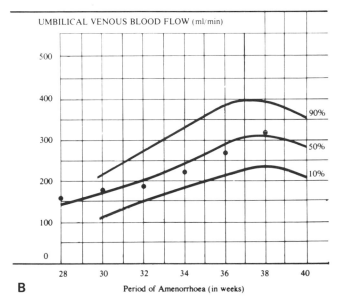

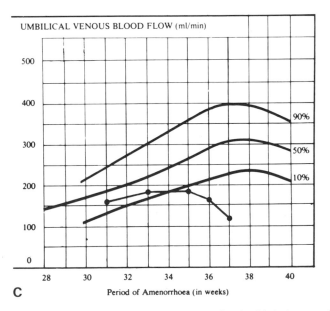

Fig. 12.3 Umbilical venous blood flow changes during the third trimester of pregnancy. (a) 10th to 90th centile range. (b) Normal serial measurements in a woman who had a previous unexplained stillbirth near full-term. (c) Progressive falling of flow rates in a very growth-retarded baby.

(i.e. babies whose birthweights are below the fifth centile for gestational age) has been studied (Gill et al 1984) using both the umbilical venous blood flow rate and the S/D ratio in the umbilical artery. Morbidity was defined as occurring when the baby required admission to the Neonatal Intensive Care Unit for seven or more days. Of 277 high-risk patients who were delivered within two weeks of their last Doppler study, 50 were SGA. Flow rate measurements were performed in all of these patients and the S/D ratio was assessed in 44. Of the 50 SGA babies, 37 recorded one or more low flows and 13 had normal flows, while 24 recorded a high S/D ratio and 20 recorded normal ratios. The results for those SGA babies who died or experienced 'morbidity' is shown in Table 12.3. Table 12.4 shows that assessment of the umbilical venous blood flow rate offers the possibility of classifying an SGA fetus as high-risk or low-risk with reasonable accuracy. The results also suggest that in this group the assessment of the umbilical venous blood flow rate is a more accurate predictor of risk than assessment of the umbilical artery S/D ratio.

Intra-uterine growth retardation and perinatal hypoxia (low five minute Apgar score) are associated with an increase in the placental vascular resistance, which manifests itself in a high S/D ratio in the umbilical arterial waveform (Trudinger et al 1985). It would appear that this high S/D ratio is due to a reduction in the diastolic flow velocity, rather than to an increase in systolic flow velocity. Trudinger & Cook (1982) have shown that serial studies in growth-retarded fetuses reveal a rise in the S/D ratio with gestational age rather than the normal reduction. In their study 20 SGA babies who were delivered after 34 weeks of amenorrhoea showed increased resistance to placental blood flow with high S/D ratios. In the same series, 11 grossly malnourished babies actually had reversed flow in diastole and they were delivered electively before 32 weeks of amenorrhoea.

Jouppila & Kirkinen (1984), and Kirkinen & Jouppila (1986) have described nine patients, all with hypertensive complications of pregnancy, in whom there was absent end-diastolic flow in the fetal descending thoracic aorta. All fetuses were 'growth retarded', and most had an abnormal cardiotocograph and low Apgar scores at birth. The umbilical venous blood flow was unmeasurable in one,

abnormally low in five and normal in three. Some studies in sheep have suggested that the reduction in the umbilical venous blood flow rate in acute and chronic hypoxia is a late phenomenon (Berman et al 1976, Clapp et al 1980, Parer 1980, Peeters et al 1980) which occurs after reduction in flow to other tissues. Jouppila & Kirkinen (1984) found three patients with a normal umbilical venous blood flow pattern who at the same time had absent end-diastolic flow in the fetal descending aorta suggesting that the same might occur in humans. Fetuses with absent end-diastolic flow have also been shown to have a significantly increased risk of perinatal death, necrotizing enterocolitis and haemorrhage (Hackett et al 1987).

REDISTRIBUTION TO BRAIN

Using radionuclide techniques and catheters Cohn et al (1974) studied the circulatory responses to induced hypoxaemia (6% oxygen) and acidaemia (3% carbon dioxide) in 10 fetal lambs. In all fetuses there was a two- to three-fold increase in blood flow to the brain, heart and adrenals, and a reduction in flow to the lungs, kidneys, spleen, gut and carcass. These changes were greater during combined hypoxaemia and acidaemia. They also noted that the umbilical blood flow was maintained in all fetuses during hypoxaemia. A similar redistribution of the cardiac output during hypoxaemia was reported by Reuss et al (1982).

Lingman et al (1986) using Doppler ultrasound, studied five exteriorized fetal lambs during acute asphyxia induced by cord clamping. They found typical changes in the time velocity waveforms, with an increase in the pulsatility index (Table 12.1) in the aorta reflecting the marked resistance to flow in the clamped cord, and a significant reduction in the pulsatility index in the common carotid artery suggesting reduced resistance in the cranial circulation. This, together with a large increase in the diameter of the common carotid artery, demonstrated increased blood flow to the head during the insult.

Similar observations are now being made in the human

Table 12.3 The incidence of mortality and morbidity in small-for-gestational age fetuses who had flow measurements (50 cases) and S/D ratios (44 cases)

	Mortality	Morbidity	Mortality and morbidity
Flow <10th centile	4/37 (11)*	26/33 (79)	30/37 (81)
Flow >10th centile	0/13 (0)	3/13 (23)	3/13 (23)
S/D ratio >90th centile	2/24 (8)	16/22 (73)	18/24 (75)
S/D ratio <90th centile	1/20 (5)	9/19 (47)	10/20 (50)

*Figures in brackets are percentages.

Table 12.4 Prediction of morbidity and mortality in small-for-gestational-age babies

	Flow	S/D ratio
True positive	30	18
True negative	10	10
False positive	7	6
False negative	3	10
	50	44
Sensitivity	91%	64%
Specificity	59%	63%
Positive predictive value	81%	75%
Negative predictive value	77%	50%
Accuracy	80%	64%

fetus using Doppler ultrasound. Marsal et al (1985) recorded waveforms from the umbilical artery, fetal descending aorta and common carotid artery in 87 'high-risk' pregnancies. Five fetuses with growth retardation, when compared with 15 non-growth retarded fetuses, showed an increased pulsatility index in the umbilical artery and descending aorta (indicating raised placental vascular resistance) and a lower pulsatility index in the common carotid artery (suggesting that the head was receiving at least some of the redistributed blood). These findings have been supported by Wladimiroff et al (1986) who studied the internal carotid artery in 42 normal pregnancies and nine growth-retarded babies between 26 and 41 weeks.

CONCLUSIONS

With appropriate instrumentation and experience, Doppler ultrasound allows accurate, non-invasive studies of the fetal and umbilical circulations. Estimation of the rate of flow in the umbilical vein has been shown to be a sensitive indicator of fetal and perinatal risk. When the flow rate is shown to lie outside the 10th to 90th centile range, the risk of perinatal morbidity or mortality is significantly raised irrespective of the cause (Gill et al 1985). This risk is increased further when serial flow measurements are shown to lie outside the normal range and when there is progressive deviation away from normal.

Waveform analysis can also provide useful information on fetal compromise, particularly in relatively small fetal vessels where the narrow diameter of the lumen may compromise the accuracy of volume flow estimations. Information acquired from waveforms not only enables us to recognize increasing placental vascular resistance but also indicates the redistribution of blood flow to the fetal head when asphyxia is imminent.

Flow and waveform abnormalities are known to precede other signs of fetal distress, such as cardiotocograph abnormalities, but the appropriate management reaction has yet to be determined, particularly in regard to that perennial problem for the obstetrician, the timing of delivery.

REFERENCES

Berman W, Goodlin R C, Heymann M A, Rudolph A M 1976 Relationships between pressure and flow in the umbilical and uterine circulations of the sheep. Circulation Research 38: 262–266

Clapp J F, Szeto H H, Larrow R, Hewitt J, Mann L I 1980 Umbilical blood flow response to embolization of the uterine circulation. American Journal of Obstetrics and Gynecology 138: 60–67

Cohn H E, Sacks E J, Heymann M A, Rudolph A M 1974 Cardiovascular responses to hypoxemia and acidemia in fetal lambs. American Journal of Obstetrics and Gynecology 120: 817–824

Giles W B, Lingman G, Marsal K, Trudinger B J 1986 Fetal volume blood flow and umbilical artery flow velocity waveform analysis: a comparison. British Journal of Obstetrics and Gynaecology 93: 461–465

Gill R W 1979 Pulsed Doppler with B-mode imaging for quantitative blood flow measurement. Ultrasound in Medicine and Biology 5: 223–235

Gill R W 1985 Measurement of blood flow by ultrasound: accuracy and sources of error. Ultrasound in Medicine and Biology 11: 625–641

Gill R W, Trudinger B J, Garrett W J, Kossoff G, Warren P S 1981 Fetal umbilical venous flow measured in utero by pulsed Doppler and B-mode ultrasound. I. Normal pregnancies. American Journal of Obstetrics and Gynecology 139: 720–725

Gill R W, Warren P S, Kossoff G, Garrett W J 1984 Umbilical venous flow in normal and complicated pregnancy. Ultrasound in Medicine and Biology 10: 349–363

Gill R W, Warren P S, Stewart A, Garrett W J, Kossoff G 1985 Blood flow measurement in the umbilical vein — current status. In: Gill R W, Dadd M J (eds) Proc. 4th Meeting WFUMB. Pergamon Press, Sydney

Hackett G A, Campbell S, Gamsu H, Cohen-Overbeek T, Pearce J M F 1987 Doppler studies in the growth-retarded fetus and prediction of neonatal necrotising enterocolitis, haemorrhage, and neonatal morbidity. British Medical Journal 294: 13–16

Jouppila P, Kirkinen P 1984 Increased vascular resistance in the descending aorta of the human fetus in hypoxia. British Journal of Obstetrics and Gynaecology 91: 853–856

Jouppila P, Kirkenen P, Koivula A, Jouppila R 1982 The effect of maternal oxygen inhalation on blood flow in the intervillous space and fetal umbilical vein and descending aorta. WFUMB '82 Abstract Book

Jouppila P, Kirkinen P, Puukka R 1986 Correlation between umbilical vein blood flow and umbilical blood velocity in normal and complicated pregnancies. Archives of Gynecology 237: 191–197

Kirkinen P, Jouppila P 1986 Prognostical significance of the analysis of blood velocity waveforms in fetal descending aorta. In: Jung H, Fendel H (eds) Doppler techniques in obstetrics. Georg Thieme, New York

Lingman G, Marsal K, Rosen K G, Kjellmer I 1986 Blood flow measurements in exteriorised lamb fetuses during asphyxia. In: Jung H, Fendel J (eds) Doppler techniques in obstetrics. Georg Thieme, New York

Marsal K, Lingman G, Laurin J, Giles W 1985 Fetal circulatory changes in imminent intrauterine asphyxia. In: Gill R W, Dadd M J (eds) Proc. 4th meeting WFUMB. Pergamon Press, Sydney

O'Rourke M F 1982 Arterial function in health and disease. Churchill Livingstone, New York

Parer J T 1980 The effect of acute material hypoxia on fetal oxygenation and the umbilical circulation in the sheep. European Journal of Obstetrics, Gynecology, and Reproductive Biology 10: 125–136

Peeters L L H, Sheldon R E, Jones M D, Makowski E L, Meschai G 1980 Blood flow to fetal organs as a function of arterial oxygen content. American Journal of Obstetrics and Gynecology 135: 638–646

Reuss M L, Parer J T, Harris J L, Krueger T R 1982 Hemodynamic effects of alpha-adrenergic blockade during hypoxia in fetal sheep. American Journal of Obstetrics and Gynecology 142: 410–415

Stuart B, Drumm J, Fitzgerald D E, Duignan N M 1980 Fetal blood velocity waveforms in normal pregnancy. British Journal of Obstetrics and Gynaecology 87: 780–785

Trudinger G J, Cook C M 1982 Fetal umbilical artery velocity waveforms. WFUMB '82 Abstract Book

Trudinger B J, Giles W B, Cook C M, Bombardieri J, Collins L 1985 Fetal umbilical artery flow waveforms and placental resistance: clinical significance. British Journal of Obstetrics and Gynaecology 92: 23–30

Van Eyck J, Wladimiroff J W, Noordam M J, Tonge H M, Prechtl H F R 1985 The blood velocity waveform in the fetal descending aorta: its relationship to fetal behavioural states in normal pregnancy at 37–38 weeks. Early Human Development 12: 137–143

Warren P S, Gill R W, Stewart A Identification of the at-risk small-for-dates baby. Submitted for publication

Wladimiroff J W, Tonge H M, Stewart P A 1986 Doppler ultrasound assessment of cerebral blood flow in the human fetus. British Journal of Obstetrics and Gynaecology 93: 471–475

Neurophysiology

Recording of cerebral electrical activity from the scalp has been widely used for a number of years as the only method for continuously monitoring cerebral function. The majority of cortical neurones discharge asynchronously and are therefore 'silent' to scalp recording. It is probably only postsynaptic discharges from specific neurones that under normal conditions are detectable using clinical electro-encephalographic (EEG) techniques. The role of EEG monitoring in the newborn has expanded recently with the introduction of imaging techniques used to document intracranial pathology and EEG signals could then be correlated with a variety of brain insults. The development of portable and reliable techniques for continuously recording EEG activity, or a function of it (referred to as cerebral function monitoring), in the newborn has recently broadened the role for this method in the management of the critically ill neonate. The clinical value of the neonatal EEG is in the detection of occult seizures and in providing accurate prognostic information. EEG abnormalities relate well to the functional severity of a lesion but are aetiologically non-specific. There may also be a role for cerebral function monitoring in the detection of cerebral compromise during labour.

The integrity of neural pathways within the brain has more recently been assessed by evoked potentials. These involve a specific sensory stimulus with recording of ensuing electrical potentials from scalp electrodes. The stimulus produces a potential of a few microvolts with a characteristic waveform pattern. A large number of these responses to repeated stimuli can be computer-averaged and displayed to give a clear record of the response. A regular sequence of maturational changes is seen in infants with advancing postconceptual age. Visual, auditory and sensory stimuli have all been used in the assessment of cerebral integrity in the newborn infant. Using these techniques it is possible to localize specific components of the evoked potential to anatomical generators within the central nervous system. This allows for more precise assessment of neural function and can relate focal pathology to specific abnormalities with a better understanding of the developing nervous system. These techniques may soon be applied to the fetus but as yet there are no clinical data.

13. Neonatal electro-encephalography

Dr J. Connell and Mrs R. Oozeer

This chapter reviews the current status of electro-encephalographic (EEG) monitoring in the assessment of normal and abnormal neonates, with particular reference to seizure disorders, intraventricular haemorrhage, cystic leukomalacia and birth asphyxia. Also reviewed are currently available methods of recording the neonatal EEG, with particular reference to newer techniques of continuous monitoring.

METHODS FOR MONITORING THE NEONATAL EEG

CONVENTIONAL MULTICHANNEL RECORDING

This remains the classical method against which all others should be compared. The main technical details of its application are beyond the scope of this review but have been well covered by Werner et al (1977).

Its main asset is the ability to provide simultaneous recording from multiple cerebral foci, detecting amplitude and frequency of discharges together with their symmetry and synchrony. These may be related to behavioural states and other physiological parameters by polygraphic recording and direct observation. Normal and abnormal intermittent discharges may be distinguished and ictal activity occurring during a recording can be detected. Important insights into cerebral function in both normal and abnormal states have been gained with this method.

Despite its acknowledged value it is, however, an investigation which has found relatively limited application in 'high-risk' neonates undergoing intensive care. Its propensity to electrical interference may be aggravated by the multiple electronic devices with which it must compete for space at the bedside, and its relative bulk may also impede access if applied over a long period. The main technical artefacts to which it may be liable are also summarized in the atlas of Werner et al (1977) and have more recently been reviewed by Scher (1985). It requires the application of multiple electrodes to the small area of scalp that may be available in very-low-birth-weight

(VLBW) infants, which are least likely to tolerate handling. It may also be harder to reconcile this electrode placement with the maintenance of scalp vein infusions and the need to leave the fontanelle area free for other monitoring such as ultrasound scanning.

In view of these limitations, it has not usually been possible to obtain extended EEG monitoring on these most unstable infants. Thus, potentially valuable information on cerebral function at a most critical period of neurological vulnerability regularly goes by default on many occasions.

CONTINUOUS MONITORING SYSTEMS

In view of the limitations of conventional recording, great interest has developed in the application of continuous EEG monitoring systems to the newborn. These are the Continuous Ambulatory EEG Monitor (Medilog) and the Cerebral Function Monitor (CFM) which have the outstanding advantage of providing ready access to EEG activity as an index of cerebral function throughout the most critical parts of the neonatal period.

The Medilog was designed for continuous EEG monitoring of adults and older children and was first reported as applicable to neonates by Eyre et al (1983). It is a light, compact, battery-driven recorder which can record four channels of data, providing simultaneous monitoring of the 'raw' EEG with other variables such as ECG and respiration (Fig. 13.1). The Cerebral Function Monitor was also first designed for use in adults (Maynard et al 1969) and reported as applicable to neonates by Bjerre et al (1983). In contrast with the Medilog, it provides a processed EEG signal displayed in terms of amplitude and, with some models, frequency. The application of both systems is much simpler than that of the standard EEG and both are compatible with prolonged use for several days in even the most unstable infants. Both are compact and do not interfere with other intensive care procedures. With the Medilog, the short distance between electrodes and pre-amplifiers, which are both attached to the scalp with

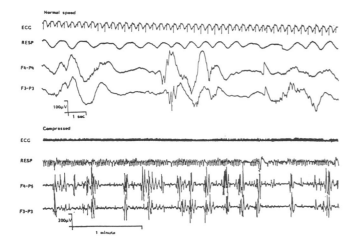

Fig. 13.1 Four-channel Medilog recording of continuous ECG, respiration and right- and left-sided EEG traces from the fronto–parietal regions, shown at standard speed (above) as seen on visual display unit and on compressed transcription (below), demonstrating the characteristic discontinuity of the pre-term EEG.

collodion, minimizes electrical interference and movement artefact. In our experience, no adverse effects of such fixatives have been noted, although care must be taken not to produce excessive abrasion of the scalp. The CFM has also been regarded as relatively free of interference. Nevertheless, it is very important that impedance should be constantly monitored, preferably with an alarm system attached, as the CFM will analyse all artefacts in the same way as true EEG activity and display this as a change in amplitude. Since the CFM provides only a processed signal, access to raw EEG data is advisable when interpretation is in doubt.

Storage and display of data are handled differently by these systems. Medilog data is stored for 24 hour periods on an ordinary C-120 cassette tape. The tape can then be displayed visually by a rapid playback system, on which a 24 hour tape can be reviewed in 24 minutes and the data can also be printed out via a standard EEG machine. The Medilog is not marketed with a bedside display facility, although it is possible to provide this by connecting the output signal from the recorder to a monitor, while the tape recording is in progress. The CFM can be viewed immediately at the bedside since it is printed out constantly at a slow paper speed, usually 6 cm/h.

The systems differ also in the type of EEG information which they provide. The detection of changes in amplitude is the particular strong point of the CFM, which provides a constant analysis of this most important EEG feature. Amplitude changes are also easily detectable by the Medilog. Thus both monitors can also distinguish the intermittent periods of low-amplitude discontinuous activity that are a common feature of the neonatal EEG. The systems also share the capacity to detect frequency changes, although the more basic CFM is not provided with this.

The Medilog has additional capabilities in that it allows recording from at least two channels of EEG, so that it can assess interhemispheric symmetry and synchrony (Fig. 13.2). The CFM usually carries only one channel of EEG and thus cannot detect lateralized abnormalities. Furthermore, since the Medilog permits visualization of the raw EEG on a time-scale comparable with conventional recording, it allows more detailed inspection of other types of activity, especially short-duration transients such as spikes and sharp waves, which would not be detectable by the CFM (Fig. 13.3).

Seizures have been reported as detectable by both systems. In the Medilog system seizures are displayed in exactly the same way as on conventional recording (Fig. 13.4). In the CFM, seizures are distinguished only by their amplitude characteristics, having a characteristic profile against that of the background activity and are perhaps seen most clearly when prolonged with a distinctive onset and termination (Fig. 13.5). It is not yet clear, however, whether the CFM will be equally successful in detecting the shorter, less organized seizures seen in pre-term infants and reliable in distinguishing them from short bursts of high-voltage slow waves which are a normal feature of their background activity. Furthermore, many neonatal seizures are of very slow frequency (1 Hz or less) and may not be detected by CFM recorders which have a low frequency filter of 2 Hz.

Both systems are limited in the number of channels from which they record, although the eight-channel Medilog is likely to improve on this. The information they provide is still most valuable, however, and is sufficient to permit meaningful analysis. They may still of course be used in conjunction with conventional recording and further study

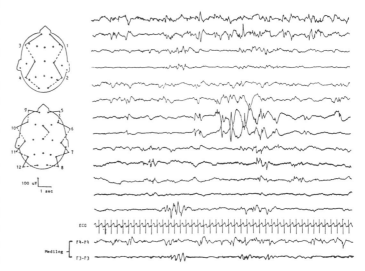

Fig. 13.2 Simultaneous standard and Medilog EEG recordings. Asymmetrical, asynchronous and discontinuous trace shown on Medilog (lower trace) as well as standard EEG.

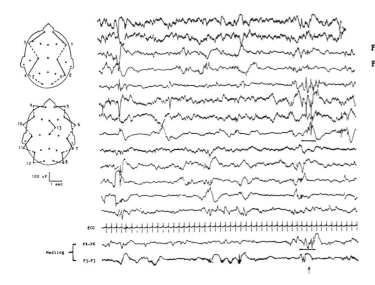

Fig. 13.3 Simultaneous standard and Medilog EEG. The asymmetrical right-sided spikes (underlined) are seen on the Medilog (lower trace) as well as the standard EEG.

is needed to determine the optimal combination of these methods. Overall, they represent a most exciting development in neonatal electro-encephalography with considerable potential for making this most valuable investigation much more available to the neonatal neurologist.

THE NORMAL AND ABNORMAL NEONATAL EEG: GENERAL CONSIDERATIONS

THE NORMAL NEONATAL EEG: MATURATION

The neurophysiological basis of the maturing neonatal EEG is not precisely defined but is generally held to be related to the extensive concomitant cellular, synaptic and neurochemical development of the neonatal brain, which has recently been reviewed by Sarnat (1984).

There is no standardized system of interpretation applied uniformly throughout the literature although terminology has been classified by Anders et al (1971) and a helpful

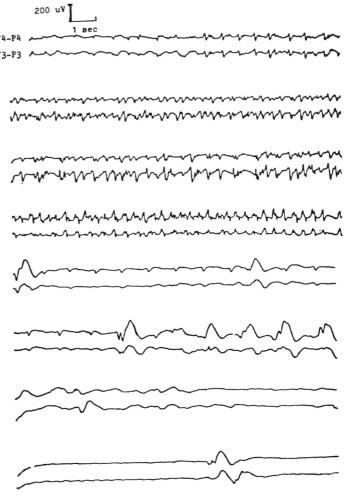

Fig. 13.4 Medilog recording throughout a seizure showing a gradual buildup and termination of bilateral, asymmetrical sharp waves, followed by a period of discontinuous activity. The continuous trace runs from top left to bottom right.

recent clarification is provided in the review of Lombroso (1985). Analysis should include description of the amplitude and frequency, continuity, symmetry and synchrony, and spatiotemporal organization of background, transient and ictal activity. It should be related to behavioural state and to gestational age.

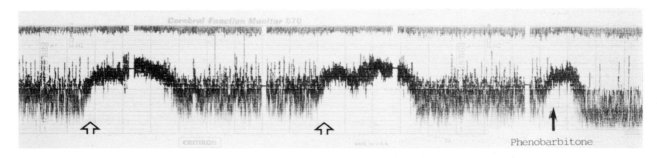

Fig. 13.5 Cerebral function monitor trace showing two seizures of approximately 6 minutes duration (onset marked by an open arrow). On the third occasion phenobarbitone was given intravenously (thin arrow) with termination of the electroconvulsive seizure and reduction in overall voltage.

Using standard techniques, well-defined criteria of EEG maturation have been established, in both full-term and pre-term infants (Parmelee et al 1968, Graziani et al 1974, Werner et al 1977, Lombroso 1978, Dreyfus-Brisac 1979, Dehkharghan 1984, Anderson et al 1985, Lombroso 1985, Torres & Anderson 1985). These may be summarized as follows. (See Figs 13.6 and 13.7.)

Frequency and amplitude

In extreme prematurity, the dominant activity consists of very high-amplitude slow waves around 400 μV and 1 Hz, with few faster frequencies. As the infant matures, this is gradually replaced by faster activity of more moderate amplitude of around 100 μV, with high-voltage slow activity being found only in some phases of quiet sleep.

Continuity of activity

The early pre-term EEG is characterized by short bursts of high voltage slow activity, interspersed with longer low-amplitude intervals. The upper limit of normal of these inactive periods is uncertain but intervals of at least 60 seconds may be found below 30 weeks. With increasing maturity, these intervals gradually shorten until, at full-term, the EEG is entirely continuous except in some phases of quiet sleep when it is known as 'tracé alternans'. Quantitative parameters of this increasing continuity can be used as an index of maturation.

Focal organization

Particular stages of maturation are characterized by the predominance of activity in particular areas. An example of this is the occipital predominance found mainly between 29 and 34 weeks.

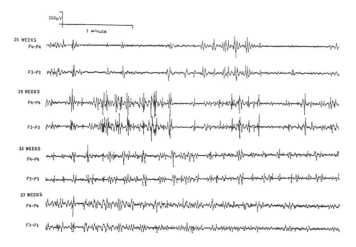

Fig. 13.6 EEG maturation. The characteristic increase in continuity between 25 and 37 weeks gestation is readily appreciated on compressed Medilog recordings.

Transient activity

Certain stages of maturation are marked by the temporary appearance of characteristic types of transient activity which should be recognized as normal phenomena, e.g: bursts of spindle-like fast waves superimposed on high-amplitude slow activity (delta brush) seen mainly between 28 and 34 weeks; bursts of temporal theta activity mainly between 27 and 32 weeks (temporal sawtooth); frontal sharp transients (encoches frontales), maximal between 35 and 36 weeks; and high voltage frontal slow waves, most evident between 28 and 32 weeks (slow anterior dysrhythmia).

Emergence of stages

These have particularly been studied by Dreyfus-Brisac et al (1957), Parmelee et al (1968), Prechtl et al (1969), Shirataki & Prechtl (1977), Ellingson & Peters (1980). Sleep states do not emerge fully until 36 weeks, although their origins may probably be discerned earlier. At full-term, four well-defined EEG states have been described with behavioural correlates. These are as follows (see also Fig. 13.8).

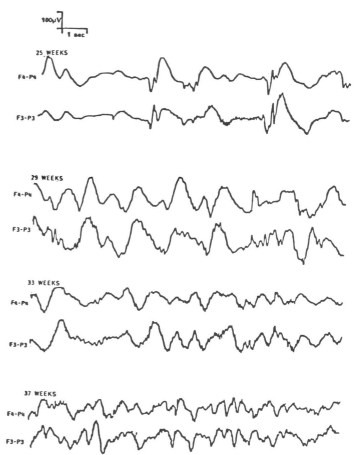

Fig. 13.7 EEG maturation. The gradual replacement of high-voltage slow activity by mixed frequencies of more moderate amplitude is shown by the Medilog recordings between 25 and 37 weeks of gestation.

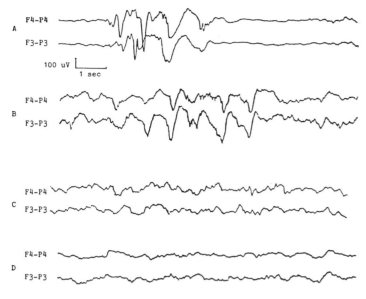

F4-P4
A
F3-P3

100 uV
1 sec

F4-P4
B
F3-P3

F4-P4
C F3-P3

F4-P4
D
F3-P3

Fig. 13.8 EEG sleep states at full-term: (**a**) tracé alternans; (**b**) high-voltage slow activity; (**c**) mixed activity; (**d**) low-voltage irregular activity.

Low-voltage irregular activity. Continuous mixed frequencies in theta, alpha and even beta ranges between 15 and 30 μV found in wakefulness and active sleep.

Mixed activity. Continuous mainly delta and slower theta activity of intermediate amplitude found in wakefulness and active sleep.

High-voltage slow activity. Continuous delta actvity at 50–150 μV or higher found in quiet sleep.

Tracé alternans. Discontinuous bursts of high-voltage slow activity, including some faster frequencies, interspersed with short intervals of low-voltage irregular activity, lasting up to 8 seconds and found in quiet sleep. This may persist till up to 6 weeks after full-term, following which the EEG is normally continuous in all states.

The relative proportions of different sleep states also vary with gestational age. A feature of particular note is the decrease in active sleep from 60% at 34 weeks gestation to 25% by 8 months of age. Recordings should, when possible, be sufficiently prolonged to encompass all states of sleep and wakefulness and interpreted in relation to these.

These maturational features of the normal neonatal EEG have mainly been derived from a rather different population than that now encountered in many neonatal intensive care units. They may require further refinement in view of recent advances in neonatal care which permit the survival of larger numbers of VLBW infants who have been maintained in optimal condition by advanced intensive care techniques. The use of ultrasound to identify clinically silent haemorrhagic lesions that may adversely affect the EEG has further aided the definition of a normal group for study. In addition to standard recording, developments in continuous monitoring allow study of 'low-risk' infants

over longer periods. Use of the Medilog monitor in a group of optimal pre-term infants has allowed us to quantify and establish normal values for variations in continuity of activity and interburst interval duration within a 24 hour period in relation to gestational age (Fig. 13.9). This has allowed us to establish that such 'optimal' infants may have considerably better EEG function than has previously been generally appreciated. We have been able to demonstrate that, even in infants of 26 weeks gestation, runs of completely continuous activity lasting more than 15 minutes may be found, while interburst intervals rarely exceed 60 seconds at most and are usually no more than 20 seconds mean (Connell et al 1987b). This is of particular interest in relation to earlier reports of normal interburst intervals of 2–3 minutes in such infants or statements such as those of Lombroso (1985) that at less than 29 weeks 'the EEG patterns are invariantly discontinuous'. Further integrated studies taking advantage of advances in neonatal care, such as that of Anderson et al (1985) may continue to improve appreciation of optimal cerebral function in the VLBW infant and refine the detection of abnormal EEG features which are considered below.

THE ABNORMAL NEONATAL EEG

EEG abnormalities relate closely in their extent, duration and rate of resolution to the functional severity of a given lesion and its clinical outcome although they are aetiologically non-specific. They have been reviewed by Monod et al (1972), Engel (1975), Werner et al (1977), Dreyfus-Brisac (1979), Tharp et al (1981), Dehkharghan (1984), and Lombroso (1985).

Seizures (Fig. 13.10)

These are considered first as they are often regarded as the most dramatic of all EEG abnormalities, although other features may be of equal or greater significance. Seizures are defined as repetitive discharges with gradual buildup and termination and characteristic pattern of evolution lasting several seconds. The waveforms are generally rhythmic and frequently display increasing amplitude and decreasing frequencies during the same episode. With particular reference to neonates, these waveforms were described by Harris & Tizard (1960) as including the following: rhythmic slow wave discharges at 1–2 Hz and 50–200 μV; repeated stereotyped sharp waves or spikes at frequencies from 2–3/s to ½–3/s, often of high amplitude and lasting for several minutes; persistent focal sharp waves and spikes; short bursts of rhythmic fast activity at up to 20 Hz. They also reported that in some convulsing infants the EEG showed only flattening during fits (see also Ch. 41).

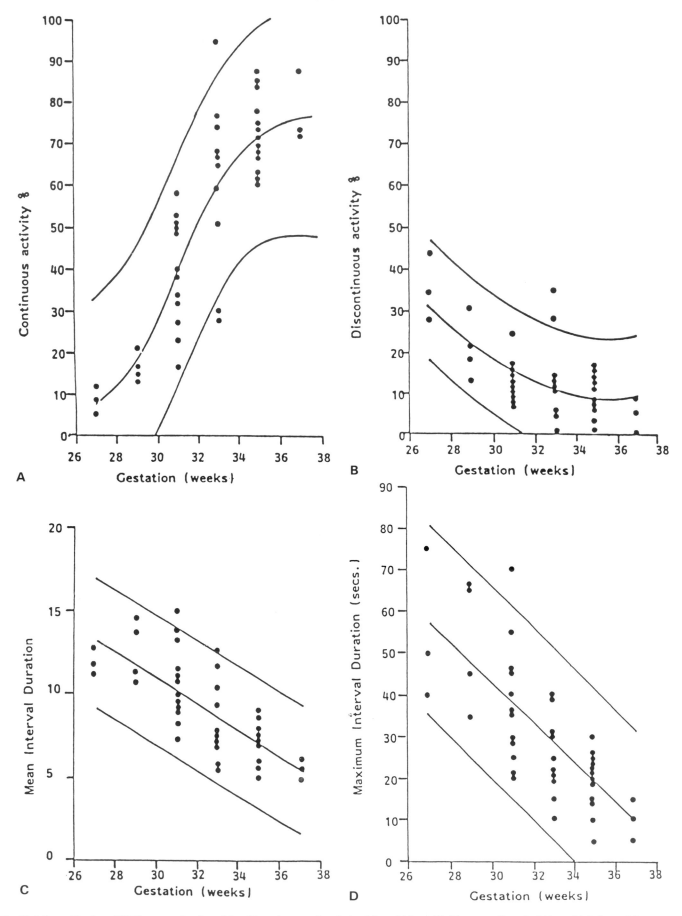

Fig. 13.9 Quantification of EEG maturation from 26 to 38 weeks gestation derived from 24 hour Medilog recordings in 44 low-risk infants: (a) increase in total continuous activity; (b) decrease in total discontinuous activity; (c) decrease in mean interburst interval duration; (d) decrease in maximum interburst interval duration (mean ±2SD).

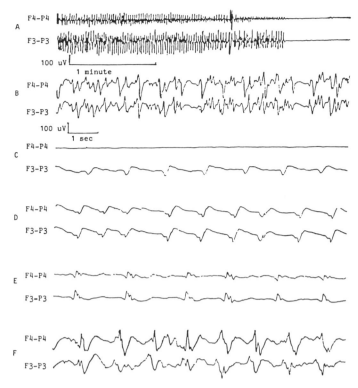

Fig. 13.10 Varieties of EEG seizure activity recorded on Medilog at compressed and standard speeds: (**a**) Compressed version. Bilateral, synchronous seizures on low-amplitude background. Details of individual complexes cannot be distinguished at this speed and must be confirmed as seizure by review at standard time-scale (see below). (**b**) Standard time-scale. Bilateral, irregular spike and slow wave complexes. (**c**) Standard time-scale. Asymmetrical seizure activity with unilateral long-duration sharp waves and low-amplitude background. (**d**) Standard time-scale. Synchronous, bilateral, long-duration sharp and slow wave complexes. (**e**) Standard time-scale. Synchronous, bilateral, long-duration sharp waves. (**f**) Standard time-scale. Irregular bilateral spike and slow wave complexes.

Disturbance of amplitude and frequency

Amplitudes persistently less than 10 μV are abnormal irrespective of gestation and state. Amplitudes of less than 2–5 μV may be difficult to differentiate from background 'noise' and a completely iso-electric recording may not be completely distinguishable from this. Other abnormalities of amplitude should be interpreted in relation to gestation and state. Abnormalities of frequency should also be interpreted in this context, e.g. persistence of excessive slow activity at full-term.

Interhemispheric asymmetry and asynchrony

The extent to which these are normal is ill-defined. Asynchrony of bursts (burst precedence greater than two seconds) is abnormal if severe but there is no clear point of demarcation from the normal, although an incidence greater than 50% is probably excessive. The limits of normal asymmetry are also unclear but an amplitude difference greater than 50% would seem to be abnormal.

Disturbance of continuity

This should be interpreted with caution in relation to established quantitative normal values for gestation and sleep state since such activity may be physiological in pre-term infants or in full-term infants during quiet sleep (tracé alternans). Terminology may also be confusing. 'Burst suppression' is used also in adult recording and implies an abnormal, persistent discontinuity, although it has also been applied to the normal discontinuity of prematurity. The full-term 'tracé paroxystique' has been used for records wherein short bursts of high amplitude sharp activity were interspersed with longer low-amplitude intervals. This may be translated as 'paroxysmal' or 'periodic' in English language literature.

Abnormal transients

Persistent focal spikes and sharp waves are generally regarded as abnormal features although their significance is controversial. Particular interest has focused on their occurrence in the Rolandic area, especially in view of a suggested relationship with intraventricular haemorrhage, which is discussed further below.

Sleep state disturbance

Abnormalities of sleep state have been thoroughly investigated (Prechtl et al 1969, Dreyfus-Brisac & Monod 1970, Theorell et al 1974, Thoman et al 1981). They may be completely absent and such lack of reactivity is a significant abnormality. Other abnormalities include the presence of immature or insufficiently defined states, or the exhibition of an EEG pattern inappropriate to the behavioural state of the infant.

CLINICAL APPLICATIONS OF THE NEONATAL EEG

GENERAL CONSIDERATIONS

The overall significance of the normal and abnormal neonatal EEG has been established in long-term follow-up studies. As well as those dealing with specific conditions, some important general reviews should be considered. Monod et al (1972) reported the outcome in 270 infants of more than 36 weeks gestation followed up until 3–14 years of age. A normal EEG was strongly associated with a normal outcome. Conversely, a severe prognosis was attached to patterns such as inactive or paroxysmal recordings, low voltage with theta rhythm, absence of lability, or persistent absence of occipital activity. Tharp et al (1981) reported essentially similar conclusions in 81 pre-term infants of 30–36 weeks gestation, and followed up at 2–7 years of age. In this study, while moderate abnormalities were not prognostically significant, normal records were usually associated with good outcome but no infant with a severely abnormal EEG survived without neurological sequelae. Further detailed analyses have been provided in authoritative reviews such as those of Engel (1975), Werner et al (1977), Dreyfus-Brisac (1979) and Lombroso (1985). These studies refer to EEGs initially recorded at various times within the first weeks of life but similar prognostic associations for EEGs recorded as early as within the first 24 hours after birth have recently been asserted by Pezzani et al (1986).

SPECIFIC APPLICATIONS

Seizure disorders

Although seizures are also discussed in other sections in relation to some specific associated conditions, it is necessary to consider some more general features of the EEG in neonatal convulsions, with reference to clinically relevant aspects of diagnosis and prognosis. Neurophysiological aspects of the origins of neonatal seizure activity have been reviewed by Purpura (1969).

Diagnosis

The EEG is of particular value both in primary diagnosis of seizures, and in monitoring their response to therapy in view of the clinical subtlety of many neonatal seizures. A good example of this is provided by the problem of diagnosis of apnoea, which may be a feature of convulsions. However, Watanabe (1982) found that the overall incidence of apnoeic seizures was relatively low. Most infants in this study who had apnoeic seizures also had other clinical manifestations at different phases of their illness, while most apnoeic episodes witnessed during polygraphic recording were not associated with seizures. A point of diagnostic importance in this study was that the most common type of ictal discharge seen in apnoeic seizures took the form of fast rhythmic activity in the alpha range. This association of periodic alpha seizures and apnoea has also been noted by Willis & Gould (1980).

The situation in which the EEG is of greatest diagnostic value is that of the infant paralysed for mechanical ventilation. Monod et al (1969) found it to be a reliable guide to seizure activity in such infants. This has been confirmed by Staudt et al (1981). In this context, continuous monitoring has been found to be of great value. Coen et al (1982), using a conventional EEG technique, detected seizures in 13 out of 16 paralysed infants, some of whom had more than 200 fits. Continuous monitoring has been made more feasible by the use of the Medilog Continuous Ambulatory Monitor described above. Eyre et al (1983) reported EEG seizures in 20 of 25 infants only 11 of whom had clinical manifestations, suggesting an important role for this investigation in the detection of subclinical seizures. Bridges et al (1986) found

the method less useful, detecting EEG seizure activity in only 7 out of 37 infants. In this study, however, infants were only monitored with the Medilog if a standard EEG failed to detect seizures. Such differences may reflect the selection of the study groups and make it difficult at present to make firm recommendations as to the indications for use of continuous monitoring systems. Our own experience of continuous EEG monitoring with the Medilog in a regional referral unit suggests a seizure incidence of 25% in high-risk infants, 42% of whom have subclinical episodes. More selective and early use of continuous monitoring may thus be of value in these high-risk cases, when the chance of detecting seizures is sufficient to justify its application.

The specific indications for the optimal use of continuous EEG monitoring and in particular its role in monitoring response to therapy require further evaluation (Fig. 13.11). This is especially important when EEG seizure activity persists after clinical seizures have apparently ceased in response to therapy, as reported by Eyre et al (1983). There are no clear published guidelines at present as to how far clinical management should be determined by the EEG in this situation, and particularly whether continuing anticonvulsant therapy is warranted on this basis.

Prognosis

The degree of abnormality of the background EEG has been found to be a most important factor in prognosis (Fig. 13.12). Monod et al (1969) stressed this point in a review of outcome in 150 cases of neonatal convulsion. A paroxysmal or inactive EEG was prognostically catastrophic; only 1 out of 42 such infants had a normal outcome. Conversely, intermediate abnormalities were associated with a 31% outcome and this rose to 77% in infants with normal interictal EEGs. They recommended that, for prognostic purposes, the initial EEG should be performed no later than 10 days, since most abnormalities had resolved by then. Rose & Lombroso (1970) also emphasized the

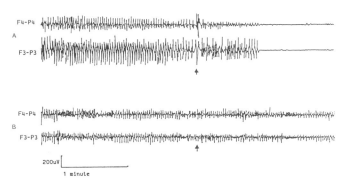

Fig. 13.11 Monitoring of phenobarbitone response on compressed Medilog recording in two full-term infants: (**a**) rapid termination of seizures; (**b**) no response. Arrow indicates i.v. injection.

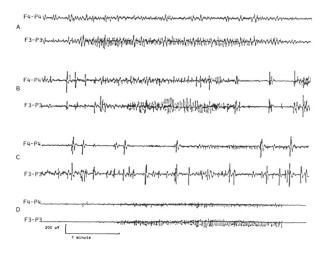

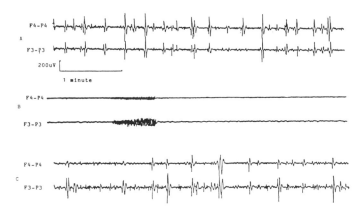

Fig. 13.12 Varieties of EEG background activity during seizures (compressed Medilog recording): (**a**) normal background; (**b**) burst suppression; (**c**) asynchronous and asymmetrical background; (**d**) low-amplitude background.

Fig. 13.13 Medilog recording of rapid changes in EEG background and seizure activity during acute insult (pneumothorax) in a 26-week-gestation infant. (**a**) Normal discontinuous EEG immediately before insult. (**b**) Bilateral seizures on low-amplitude background during the episode. (**c**) Thirty minutes later. Successful drainage of the pneumothorax has produced rapid recovery of the EEG. This infant survived with only minor neurological abnormalities at one year.

value of background EEG in prognosis. Infants with a normal background EEG had an 86% chance of normal development at 4 years but this fell to 7% if the EEG was either periodic or very low amplitude. The review of Engel (1975) also asserted the significance of the interictal EEG and reported the author's own finding that no infant out of 16 with a severely depressed background had a normal outcome. In contrast with the general consensus, the study of Harris & Tizard (1960) failed to find any general prognostic function for the EEG. However, its value in the prognosis of seizures has been reasserted and shown to apply also to pre-term infants by Rowe et al (1985), who found that burst suppression, low voltage or electrically inactive recordings had an equal prognostic gravity in this group. Our own experience using the Medilog continous monitor also supports the significance of such abnormalities in both full-term and pre-term infants with seizures. No infant with such severe background abnormalities has yet had a normal outcome.

Continuous EEG monitoring, which has already been discussed in its diagnostic capacity, also has considerable potential in providing extra prognostic definition. Indeed it has several potential advantages over conventional monitoring in this respect, although insufficient time has passed for the full significance of initial findings to be assessed by long-term follow-up studies. It can easily be applied very early in an acute illness during periods of the greatest physiological instability when abnormalities are most likely to be present (Fig. 13.13). This is particularly important in view of the tendency of all but the most severe abnormalities to resolve. It can then be maintained throughout the illness until resolution has occurred. It thus permits more detailed assessment of the persistence of the abnormality and the rate of its resolution. The overall integration of the prognostic function of continuous

EEG monitoring with that of the conventional technique requires further assessment. Persistent, severe, generalized abnormalities with their acknowledged poor outcome are detectable by either method. The greatest contribution of continuous monitoring may therefore lie in refining the prognostic capacity of the EEG for early detection, in acutely ill infants, of lesser, though still significant, abnormalities that may have improved or resolved before a conventional EEG is feasible.

In the determination of the EEG features of prognostic importance for the development of later epilepsy, the most extensive recent survey has been that of Watanabe et al (1982). In this study of 264 full-term infants with neonatal seizures, particular comparison was made of infants with cerebral dysgenesis and perinatal hypoxia. Although subsequent epilepsy was commoner in those with dysgenesis, the EEG was only predictive of its development in the hypoxic group. The degree of background depression was most important, e.g. later epilepsy developed in 9 of 10 with maximal depression and 22 of 37 with marked depression, whereas none of 52 with mildly depressed or normal records had further fits. A further point of interest in this study was the connection between certain EEG features and the type of seizure that subsequently developed. Infantile spasms and myoclonic seizures occurred only in those infants with maximal or markedly depressed neonatal EEGs. Of 9 with maximal depression, 5 developed infantile spasms and 4 myoclonic seizures, while of the 22 with marked depression 11 developed infantile spasms and 1 myoclonic seizures.

Anticonvulsants are not generally thought to interfere significantly with the prognostic function of the EEG. Concern regarding this arises from observations of the EEG depressant effects of very high barbiturate levels found in anaesthesia or poisoning. These EEG effects have actually been used as a guide to therapy in thiopentone-induced coma in asphyxiated infants by Eyre & Wilkinson (1986) but have not been found to occur to any significant extent within the therapeutic range of phenobarbitone. Staudt et al (1982) compared the degree of background EEG depression, plasma phenobarbitone levels, and clinical outcome in 26 neonates with seizures. The EEG abnormalities correlated well with outcome, as in other studies, but bore no relation to the phenobarbitone level. They concluded that in the range of 1.3–5.9 mg/dl phenobarbitone, EEG suppression was related to brain pathology and not to therapy, so that the EEG could still be used as a guide to prognosis even in infants treated with phenobarbitone. These findings have been supported in other studies. In the CFM study of Bjerre et al (1983) high phenobarbitone concentrations were deliberately aimed for so as to produce brain protection in asphyxiated infants. Even at concentrations as high as 130 μmol/dl, CFM traces did not change from continuous to discontinuous. Couto-Sales et al (1979) have also reported no prolonged effect of anticonvulsant on the EEG. Radvanyi-Bouvet et al (1985) described 19 infants given phenobarbitone (20 mg/kg) or diazepam (1 mg/kg) intravenously during EEG recordings. Some increase in discontinuity was noted and in two cases there was complete suppression of EEG activity, but this effect lasted for only 15 minutes. They never found longer periods of inactivity to be related to overdosage of anticonvulsant.

Since many neonates with seizures are already treated with anticonvulsants at the time of recording, these studies are therefore particularly important in establishing that such therapy does not restrict the prognostic function of the EEG.

Germinal matrix haemorrhage–intraventricular haemorrhage (GMH–IVH)

The role of the EEG in both the diagnosis and prognosis of this condition has been investigated. In terms of diagnosis, most interest has been concentrated on the importance of positive Rolandic sharp waves (PRS) as a specific marker of GMH–IVH which were first reported by Cukier et al (1972). Blume & Dreyfus-Brisac (1982) described two types, according to whether they appeared in isolation or in bursts, finding a poorer clinical outcome in those with isolated PRS. That PRS are neither specific nor sensitive for GMH–IVH, however, is apparent from this and other studies (Clancy & Tharp 1984, Lombroso 1985). In any case, the recent advances in imaging, particularly cranial ultrasound scanning, have revolutionized the diagnosis of GMH–IVH to the point where the EEG is no longer necessary primarily for this purpose but is of most value in the assessment of functional severity and clinical prognosis of the lesion.

There are relatively few reports of the value of the EEG in comparison with assessment based on scanning. Such as do exist mainly suggest an important role for the EEG in this respect. Watanabe et al (1983) found, in a comparative study of 19 infants in which GMH–IVH was diagnosed by CT scan or at postmortem, that the grade of severity of haemorrhage as assessed by these methods generally correlated well with the EEG assessment. Where discrepancies were found, the EEG proved the more reliable predictor. Infants with a severely abnormal EEG had the worst outcome, even with milder grades of GMH–IVH, while infants with larger lesions had a better outcome if their EEG was well preserved. Similar conclusions were reached by Clancy et al (1984) in a larger, retrospective study of EEG in relation to CT scan in 44 infants with GMH–IVH. Neither of these studies found any particular EEG features to be diagnostic but important adverse prognostic features were severe background depression, discontinuity and seizures. However, Lacey et al (1986) correlated standard EEG with GMH–IVH diagnosed by CT scan and clinical outcome in 102 VLBW infants but were unable to find any significant correlations with either of these although infants with the type of severe background abnormalities noted in other studies also had poor outcomes.

Abnormal EEG activity in infants with GMH–IVH may also be detected using the Medilog recorder. Several of the infants in whom Eyre et al (1983) detected seizures had GMH–IVH. Continuous EEG monitoring is likely to be of particular value as it can be applied throughout the first 72 hours of life when haemorrhage is most likely to occur. When combined with serial cranial ultrasound, as in our own study (Connell et al 1988), it is able not only to confirm the prognostic importance of the EEG found in conventional EEG studies but also to determine the relative timing of the appearance of the abnormalities. In our own series, when precedence can be established, the EEG deterioration has always anticipated the ultrasound changes (Fig. 13.14). This suggests that the EEG change relates mainly to the fundamental insult that precipitates the haemorrhage rather than to the effects of the bleed itself, although these may, of course, also affect cerebral function. This study also confirmed the significance of some particular EEG abnormalities. Major amplitude depression, asymmetry and asynchrony were all adverse prognostic features. Seizures were found mainly in infants with parenchymal extension and were a constant adverse feature when occurring on an abnormal background.

The ultimate role of EEG monitoring in infants with GMH–IVH remains to be determined, but serial correlative studies may well contribute further to understanding of this problem.

Echodense lesions and cystic leukomalacia

Recent advances in ultrasound scanning, using the 7.5 MHz probe, have facilitated appreciation of areas of increased echogenicity, particularly in the periventricular and subcortical regions, which may either resolve or proceed to cystic

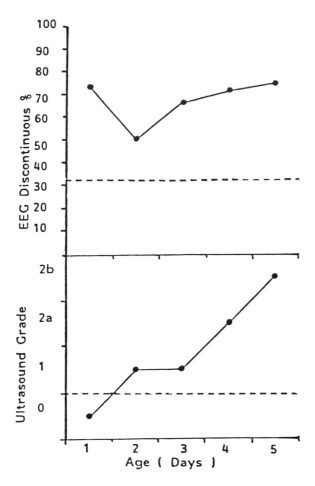

Fig. 13.14 Continuous EEG monitoring in GMH–IVH at 28 weeks of gestation, illustrating the precedence of EEG abnormality. Discontinuous activity exceeds upper limit of normal (dotted line) on day 1 when ultrasound is still normal. Further EEG deterioration is seen from day 3 as haemorrhage progresses. The infant died on day 5.

contributory in the 19 infants who did not develop cysts, since the presence of marked EEG abnormalities such as low amplitude and excessively discontinuous recordings together with seizures, identified the three who had neurological sequelae at follow-up.

Birth asphyxia

Extensive studies of the role of the EEG in this problem have established the important general principle that the degree of abnormality of the EEG and the rate at which it recovers are reliable indicators of the functional severity of

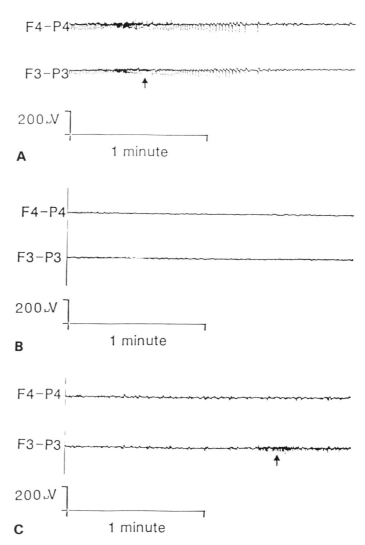

Fig. 13.15 Continuous EEG monitoring in subcortical leukomalacia at 35 weeks postmenstrual age illustrating the precedence of EEG abnormalities. (a) Day 1. Bilateral seizures (arrow) on low-amplitude background with a normal ultrasound scan. (b) Day 5. Very low amplitude EEG. Ultrasound at this time showed echodense lesions in the subcortical region. (c) Week 5. Low amplitude, discontinuous EEG with unilateral seizure (arrow). Ultrasound scan at this time showed extensive subcortical leukomalacia. The poor outcome suggested by the first day EEG was confirmed as this infant showed severe mental retardation and spastic quadriplegia at 1 year of age.

leukomalacia during the next 2–4 weeks (DeVries et al 1987) (see Ch. 29). The EEG may provide an earlier guide to those infants liable to develop cystic leukomalacia. Positive Rolandic sharp waves, discussed previously in relation to GMH–IVH, were found by Marret et al (1986) to provide an early indication of periventricular leukomalacia in four infants studied within the first week of life. These findings were transitory and a relationship with periventricular ischaemia was suggested.

Our own study (Connell et al 1987a) of 31 infants with densities established that EEG abnormalities, which usually preceded the appearance of the cysts and sometimes even the densities, were related in grade of severity to the degree of ultrasound abnormality. The EEGs of the four infants with subcortical leukomalacia all showed maximal background depression while the eight with periventricular cysts showed lesser degrees of abnormality. EEG abnormalities were of particular value in leukomalacia since they preceded by several weeks the appearance of the prognostically significant cystic changes on ultrasound (Fig. 13.15). They were also the asphyxial insult and the prognosis for the neurological outcome of the infant suffering it.

A normal EEG usually carries a good prognosis. Dreyfus-Brisac (1979) stated that a normal EEG between the first and third days of life was associated with a good prognosis in the great majority of cases, even if a severe clinical state was present. Several other authors, including Sarnat & Sarnat (1976), Watanabe et al (1980), and Holmes et al (1982) have also reported the essentially good prognostic significance of a normal EEG in asphyxiated infants.

The poor prognosis associated with a severely abnormal EEG in asphyxia is also generally agreed (Engel 1975, Sarnat & Sarnat 1976, Werner et al 1977, Dreyfus-Brisac 1979, Watanabe et al 1980, Holmes et al 1982). Persistently low-amplitude, discontinuous, or unreactive traces are particularly associated with a poor outcome. While seizures are also a significant abnormality, the degree of background EEG abnormality is a more important factor in determining prognosis. Particular points of note may be illustrated by specific reference to some of the studies cited above.

Correlations with clinical state are most important. In a study of 21 asphyxiated full-term infants, Sarnat & Sarnat (1976) described three clinical stages and their EEG correlates, emphasizing the importance of serial examinations to determine the relative duration of each stage (see p. 390). Stage 1 was essentially one of clinical hyperactivity, during which time the EEG was normal. In stage 2, depressed consciousness and hypotonia were accompanied by seizures and a discontinuous EEG pattern. Stage 3 was characterized by severe neurological depression clinically, with an iso-electric or extremely discontinous EEG. Infants who remained in stage 1 had a good prognosis, and those in stage 3 a poor prognosis. For infants in stage 2 the most important factor was the duration of the abnormality. The outcome was good if it persisted for less than 5 days and poor thereafter. They therefore recommended EEG examinations on the second and sixth days, with further studies every 3–4 days till two weeks in those infants whose sixth day EEG was still abnormal.

In a retrospective study of 38 asphyxiatcd full-term infants, Holmes et al (1982) found that a single EEG recorded in the first two weeks had a higher predictive efficiency for outcome than neurological examination performed by a paediatric neurologist or neonatologist.

The importance of serial studies was also stressed by Watanabe et al (1980) as being of particular value in clarifying prognosis in intermediate grades of EEG abnormality in a study of 132 asphyxiated full-term infants. Normal EEGs carried a good prognosis and severely abnormal EEGs a poor prognosis, at all times. The most important factor in assessing the prognosis of intermediate abnormalities was their duration. Mild depression was associated with good outcome in most infants if present in weeks 1 and 2 but if it persisted by week 3 the outcome was always poor. Moderate depression was still associated with normal outcome in 36% of infants in week 1 but if it persisted in weeks 2 and 3 outcome was always poor.

The prognostic sensitivity of the EEG has been reported not only in conventional recording studies but also more recently with the cerebral function monitor. Bjerre et al (1983) found that a persistently discontinuous CFM trace was always associated with abnormal outcome. Of 18 infants with such traces, 15 died and the 3 survivors all had serious neurological abnormalities. In this particular study, however, a continuous trace was not constantly related to a good outcome. Of 8 such infants, 2 died, 2 were neurologically abnormal, and only 4 were normal. In the complementary studies of Verma et al (1984) and Archbald et al (1984) of the CFM in normal and asphyxiated infants those with a normal CFM trace had a better outcome. Eighteen surviving infants out of 20 with normal traces were normal at follow-up, whereas all 8 infants with low-voltage pattern died and all 3 survivors with lesser CFM abnormalities were neurologically abnormal. Our own experience with continuous monitoring using the Medilog system also supports the significance of EEG appearances in birth asphyxia that has been found in other studies. This system is most likely to be of value in view of the ease with which it can monitor infants throughout their acute illness, as is discussed in the section on seizures.

Considerable evidence thus exists that the EEG, whatever the method of recording used, is of major significance in determining prognosis in the asphyxiated neonate. Low amplitude and very discontinuous records are especially significant but some caution is needed in interpreting moderately discontinuous traces so as to avoid confusing persistent discontinuity, which is abnormal (burst suppression), from the normal discontinuous activity seen in quiet sleep at full-term (tracé alternans) or more generally in pre-term infants. This may be relevant in assessing the significance of the prospective correlative EEG-clinical study of Torres & Blaw (1968), in which a normal outcome at 4 years was found in 6 out of 10 children whose neonatal EEGs were interpreted as showing burst suppression. This study has been criticised by Watanabe et al (1980) on the grounds that insufficient attention may have been paid to sleep states. This does at least emphasize the importance of recording for long enough to study all sleep states that may be present, which may require more than an hour of recording, especially for the interpretation of discontinuous traces.

The balance of specific factors that may contribute to the EEG changes in asphyxia is not fully understood, but some interesting, if conflicting, findings have emerged from studies of postnatal hypoxia. Roberton (1969) reported significant, though reversible, EEG depression in pre-term infants who became hypoxic and acidotic during attempted weaning from mechanical ventilation. Intra-arterial monitoring of blood pressure was performed simultaneously but was not found to correlate significantly with the EEG changes. However, these findings have been challenged by Radvanyi et al (1973), who found no significant effect on the EEG at P_{O_2} and pH levels as low as 20 mmHg and 7.02 respectively. Roberton suggested that cerebral blood flow and factors affecting this might be significant in determining the variable EEG response to hypoxia. Correlative studies of EEG and cerebral blood flow may further elucidate EEG changes in this and other conditions.

Existing evidence demonstrates that the standard EEG is one of the most sensitive indices of the severity of the asphyxial insult and the prognosis of the affected infant.

It should always be serially monitored as part of the comprehensive neurological assessment of the asphyxiated infant in whom it is an essential non-invasive investigation.

REFERENCES

Anders T, Emde R, Parmelee A H (eds) 1971 A manual of standardised terminology, techniques, and criteria for scoring of states of sleep and wakefulness in newborn infants. UCLA Brain Information Service/BRI Publications Office, Los Angeles

Anderson C M, Torres F, Faoro A 1985 The EEG of the early premature. Electroencephalography and Clinical Neurophysiology 60: 95–105

Archbald F, Verma U L, Tejani N A, Handwerker S M 1984 Cerebral function monitor in the neonate: birth asphyxia. Developmental Medicine and Child Neurology 26: 162–168

Bjerre I, Hellstrom-Westas L, Rosen I, Svenningsen N 1983 Monitoring of cerebral function after severe asphyxia in infancy. Archives of Disease in Childhood 58: 997–1002

Blume W T, Dreyfus-Brisac C 1982 Positive Rolandic sharp waves in neonatal EEG: types and significance. Electroencephalography and Clinical Neurophysiology 53: 277–282

Bridges S L, Ebersole J S, Ment L R, Ehrenkranz R A, Silva C G 1986 Cassette electroencephalography in the evaluation of neonatal seizures. Archives of Neurology 43: 49–51

Clancy R R, Tharp B R 1984 Positive Rolandic sharp waves in the electroencephalograms of premature neonates with intraventricular hemorrhage. Electroencephalography and Clinical Neurophysiology 57: 395–404

Clancy R R, Tharp B R, Enzman D 1984 EEG in premature infants with intraventricular hemorrhage. Neurology 34: 583–590

Coen R W, McCutcheon C B, Werner D, Snyder J 1982 Continuous monitoring of the electroencephalogram following perinatal asphyxia. Journal of Pediatrics 100: 628–630

Connell J A, Oozeer R, Regev R, de Vries L S, Dubowitz L M S, Dubowitz V 1987a Continuous 4-channel EEG monitoring in the evaluation of echodense ultrasound lesions and cystic leukomalacia. Archives of Diseases of Childhood 62: 1019–1026

Connell J A, Oozeer R, Dubowitz V 1987b Continuous 4-channel EEG monitoring: a guide to interpretation, with normal values, in preterm infants. Neuropediatrics 18: 138–145

Connell J, de Vries L, Oozeer R, Reger R, Dubowitz L M S, Dubowitz V 1988 Predictive value of early continuous EEG monitoring in ventilated preterm infants with intraventricular hemorrhage. Pediatrics (in press)

Couto-Sales S, Rey E, Radvanyi M-F, Dreyfus-Brisac C 1979 Essai d'evaluation des therapeutiques (Diazepam–Phenobarbital) sur l'EEG neonatal pendant les premieres 24 heures de traitement. Revue EEG Neurophysiologie Clinique 9: 26–34

Cukier F, Andre M, Dreyfus-Brisac C 1972 Apport de l'EEG au diagnostic des hemorragies intra-ventriculaires du premature. Revue EEG Neurophysiologie Clinique 2: 318–322

Dehkharghan F 1984 Application of electroencephalographical and evoked potential studies in the neonatal period. In: Topics in neonatal neurology. Grune & Stratton, New York, pp 257–287

de Vries L S, Connell J A, Pennock J M, Dubowitz L M S, Dubowitz V 1987 Neurological, electrophysiological and MRI abnormalities in infants with extensive cystic leukomalacia. Neuropediatrics 18: 61–66

Dreyfus-Brisac C 1979 Neonatal electroencephalography. Reviews in Perinatal Medicine 3: 397–471

Dreyfus-Brisac C, Monod N 1970 Sleeping behaviour in abnormal newborn infants. Neuropediatrie 11: 101–129

Dreyfus-Brisac C, Fischgold H, Samson-Dollfus D, Saint-Anne Dargassies S, Monod N, Blanc C 1957 Veille, sommeil, reactivite sensorielle chez le premature, le nouveau-ne, et le nourisson. Electroencephalography and Clinical Neurophysiology 6 (suppl): 417–440

Ellingson R J, Peters J F 1980 Development of EEG and daytime sleep patterns in normal fullterm infants during the first three months of life: longitudinal observations. Electroencephalography and Clinical Neurophysiology 49: 112–124

Engel R 1975 Abnormal electroencephalogram in the neonatal period. Charles C Thomas, Springfield

Eyre J A, Wilkinson A R 1986 Thiopentone induced coma after severe birth asphyxia. Archives of Disease in Childhood 61: 1084–1089

Eyre J A, Oozeer R C, Wilkinson A R 1983 Diagnosis of neonatal seizure by continuous recording and rapid analysis of the electroencephalogram. Archives of Disease in Childhood 58: 785–790

Graziani L, Katz L, Cracco R, Cracco J, Weitzman E 1974 The maturation and inter-relationship of EEG pattern and auditory evoked responses in premature infants. Electroencephalography and Clinical Neurophysiology 36: 367–375

Harris R, Tizard J P M 1960 The electroencephalogram in neonatal convulsions. Journal of Pediatrics 57: 501–521

Holmes G, Rowe J, Hafford J, Schmidt R, Testa M, Zimmerman A 1982 Prognostic value of the electroencephalogram in neonatal asphyxia. Electroencephalography and Clinical Neurophysiology 53: 60–72

Lacey D J, Topper W H, Buckwald S, Zorn W A, Berger P E 1986 Preterm and very low birth weight neonates: relationship of EEG to intracranial haemorrhage, perinatal complications, and developmental outcome. Neurology 34: 1084–1087

Lombroso C T 1978 Quantified electrographic scales on 10 preterm healthy newborns followed up to 40–43 weeks of conceptional age by serial polygraphic recording. Electroencephalography and Clinical Neurophysiology 46: 460–474

Lombroso C T 1985 Neonatal polygraphy in full-term and premature infants: a review of normal and abnormal findings. Journal of Clinical Neurophysiology 2: 105–155

Marret S, Parain D, Samson-Dollfus D, Jeannot E, Fessard C 1986 Positive Rolandic sharp waves and periventricular leukomalacia in the newborn. Neuropediatrics 17: 199–202

Maynard D, Prior F, Scott F D 1969 Device for continuous monitoring of cerebral activity in resuscitated patients. British Medical Journal 4: 545–546

Monod N, Dreyfus-Brisac C, Sfaello Z 1969 Depistage et pronostic de l'etat de mal neo-natal d'apres l'etude de 150 cas. Archives Francais de Pediatrie 26: 1085–1102

Monod N, Pajot N, Guidasci S 1972 The neonatal EEG: statistical studies and prognostic value in full-term and pre-term babies. Electroencephalography and Clinical Neurophysiology 32: 529–544

Parmelee A H, Schulte F J, Akiyama Y, Wenner W H, Stern E 1968 The maturation of EEG activity during sleep in premature infants. Electroencephalography and Clinical Neurophysiology 24: 319–329

Pezzani C, Radvanyi-Bouvet M-F, Relier J P, Monod N 1986 Neonatal electroencephalography during the first twenty-four hours of life in full-term newborn infants. Neuropediatrics 17: 11–18

Prechtl H F R, Weinmann H, Akiyama Y 1969 Organisation of physiological parameters in normal and neurologically abnormal infants. Neuropaediatrie 1: 101–129

Purpure D P 1969 Stability and seizure susceptibility. In: Jasper H H, Ward A, Pope A (eds) Basic mechanisms of the epilepsies. Little Brown, Boston, pp 481–505

Radvanyi M-F, Monod N, Dreyfus-Brisac C 1973 Electroencephalogramme et sommeil chez le nouveau-ne en detresse respiratoire: etude de l'influence des variations de la PaO₂ et de l'equilibre acido–basique. Bulletin de Physio-Pathologique Respiratoire 9: 1569–1585

Radvanyi-Bouvet M-F, Vallecalle M H, Morel-Kahn F, Rellier J P, Dreyfus-Brisac C 1985 Seizures and electrical discharges in premature infants. Neuropediatrics 16: 143–148

Roberton N R C 1969 Effect of acute hypoxia on blood pressure and electroencephalogram of newborn babies. Archives of Disease in Childhood 44: 719–725

Rose A L, Lombroso C T 1970 A study of clinical, pathological, and electroencephalographical features in 137 full-term babies with a long-term follow-up. Pediatrics 45: 404–425

Rowe J C, Holmes G L, Hafford J et al 1985 Prognostic value of the electroencephalogram in term and preterm infants following neonatal seizures. Electroencephalography and Clinical Neurophysiology 60: 183–196

Sarnat H B 1984 Anatomic and physiologic correlates of neurologic development in prematurity. Topics in Neonatal Neurology. Grune & Stratton, New York, pp 1–25

Sarnat H B, Sarnat M S 1976 Neonatal encephalopathy following foetal distress. Archives of Neurology 33: 696–705

Scher M S 1985 Physiological artefacts in neonatal electroencephalography: the importance of technical comments. American Journal of EEG Technology 25: 257–277

Shirataki S, Prechtl H F R 1977 Sleep state transitions in newborn infants: preliminary study. Developmental Medicine and Child Neurology 19: 316–325

Staudt F, Roth J G, Engel R C 1981 The usefulness of electroencephalography in curarised newborns. Electroencephalography and Clinical Neurophysiology 51: 205–208

Staudt F, Scholl M L, Coen R W, Bickford R W 1982 Phenobarbital therapy in neonatal seizures and the prognostic value of the EEG. Neuropediatrics 13: 24–33

Tharp B R, Cukier F, Monod N 1981 The prognostic value of the electroencephalogram in premature infants. Electroencephalography and Clinical Neurophysiology 51: 219–236

Theorell K, Prechtl H F R, Vos J E 1974 A polygraphic study of normal and abnormal newborn infants. Neuropaediatrie 5: 279–317

Thoman E B, Denenberg V H, Sievel J 1981 State organisation in neonates: developmental inconsistency indicates risk for developmental dysfunction. Neuropediatrics 12: 45–54

Torres F, Anderson C 1985 The normal EEG of the human newborn. Journal of Clinical Neurophysiology 2: 89–103

Torres F, Blaw M E 1968 Longitudinal EEG-clinical correlations in children from birth to 4 years of age. Pediatrics 41: 945–954

Verma U L, Archbald F, Tejani N A, Handwerker S M 1984 Cerebral function monitor in the neonate. 1. Normal Patterns. Developmental Medicine and Child Neurology 26: 154–161

Wasterlain C G 1978 Neonatal seizures and brain growth. Neuropediatrics 9: 213–228

Watanabe K, Miyazaki S, Hara K, Hakamada A 1980 Behavioural state cycles, background EEGs, and prognosis of newborns with perinatal hypoxia. Electroencephalography and Clinical Neurophysiology 49: 618–625

Watanabe K, Kuroyanagi M, Hara K, Miyazaki S 1981 Neonatal seizures and subsequent epilepsy. Brain and Development 4: 342–346

Watanabe K, Hara K, Miyazaki S, Hakamada S, Kuroyanagi M 1984 Apneic seizures in the newborn. American Journal of Diseases of Children 136: 980–984

Watanabe K, Hakamada S, Kuroyanagi M, Yamazaki T, Takeuchi T 1983 Electroencephalographic study of intraventricular hemorrhage in the preterm newborn. Neuropediatrics 14: 225–230

Werner S S, Stockard J E, Bickford R G 1977 Atlas of neonatal electroencephalography. Raven Press, New York

Willis J, Gould J B 1980 Periodic alpha seizures with apnea in a newborn. Developmental Medicine and Child Neurology 22: 214–222

14. Fetal intrapartum electro-encephalography

Dr D. A. Viniker

Obstetricians have been able to increasingly concentrate their attention towards the prevention of fetal morbidity as perinatal mortality has steadily declined. With each contraction during labour, the oxygen supply to the placenta is reduced and the resulting oxygen deprivation may occasionally lead to fetal mortality and morbidity. Brain damage is the morbidity of greatest concern. The aim of intrapartum fetal monitoring is to detect evidence of fetal compromise early so that, when indicated, the delivery of the fetus can be expedited before disaster strikes.

Continuous fetal heart rate recording combined with intermittent fetal blood sampling for pH estimation may reflect evidence of oxygen deprivation, but their place in the prevention of brain damage will remain debatable until the relationship between oxygen deprivation in labour and brain damage is established. The fetal electro-encephalogram (EEG) directly reflects the functional state of the brain and provides a sensitive indicator of cerebral metabolic disturbance (Rosen & Scibetta 1970, Chachava 1976).

THE FETAL EEG SIGNAL

Electro-encephalography is the study of the minute, constantly varying potentials originating from the brain that are recorded from electrodes attached to the scalp. The scalp averages out localized random rhythms generated by millions of neurones and transmits those rhythms which are synchronous and common to relatively large areas. Only cortical activity is recorded by an EEG but deeper structures influence the behaviour of the cortex.

The shape of the waveforms of an EEG trace will be influenced by the characteristics of the recording system and in particular by the physical composition of the electrodes, quality of the signal amplifiers, filter settings and paper speed. The waveforms of an EEG are described in terms of their amplitude and frequency. The fetal EEG has an amplitude of less than 100 μV and most of the activity is at a frequency of less than 15 Hz.

RECORDING TECHNIQUES

The earliest attempts at recording the fetal EEG were described by Lindsley (1942) who attached electrodes over the lower abdomen of his pregnant wife. The first useful recordings were obtained with clips attached to the fetal scalp (Rosen & Satran 1965).

As the EEG signal is of small amplitude, successful fetal EEG recording requires the incorporation of techniques that provide a high signal to noise ratio. The noise content of a recording is dependent upon the quality of the signal amplifiers and the composition of the electrodes. Artefacts may also arise from fetal and maternal movement and fetal ECG.

The introduction of suction to maintain electrode-to-skin apposition (Rosen & Scibetta 1969) provided electrode isolation and mechanical stability. Rosen and his team, who have been pioneers in the field of fetal EEG research, have, for several years been using platinum pin electrodes (Sokol et al 1976). After the membranes have been ruptured, two electrodes, each housed in a 2.5 cm diameter suction cup, are introduced through the cervix and applied to the fetal scalp with at least 4 cm separation. A negative pressure of 250 mmHg, maintained through a suction line, keeps the electrodes firmly in position. Fetal ECG contamination tends to disappear as the suction is applied (Zorn et al 1974) but if the ECG contamination persists, the electrodes may have to be repositioned.

Researchers trying to record the fetal EEG have developed a variety of electrodes. Barden et al (1968) followed Rosen's early example and used FHR type clips but later used a screw electrode (Peltzman et al 1973). Garcia-Austt (1969) applied a number of hook-shaped platinum needles during advanced labour. The majority have used modifications of the Rosen suction pin electrode (Feldman et al 1970, Hopp et al 1972, Wilson et al 1979, Fig. 14.1). Mann et al (1972) were happy with recordings from suction disc electrodes.

Contamination of the fetal EEG by fetal ECG has been a major problem (Rosen et al 1973, Zorn et al

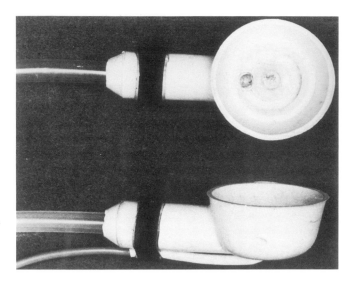

Fig. 14.1 A pair of suction fetal EEG electrodes.

1974, Spies 1976, Maynard et al 1979, Weller et al 1981). This problem is almost certainly related to the liquor. It is imperative that the ECG be removed before any processing of the EEG (Fig. 14.2).

Maynard (1979) found that a tripolar suction electrode assembly, with the three electrodes just 1 cm apart, seemed to provide a satisfactory answer to the ECG problem. The EEG signal from each of the three possible pairs was observed in turn and the pair with the least ECG contamination chosen. Any residual ECG was removed by electronic balancing with the signal from the third electrode. Some acceptable recordings were obtained (Maynard et al 1979). Despite a variety of modifications, the close proximity of the electrodes usually resulted in signals that were too weak for interpretation (Viniker 1986). A modification of the tripolar electrode with the electrode separation at 2.5 cm (Viniker 1986) has proved to be rather unwieldy (Viniker 1988).

More recently, two techniques for removing the ECG have been described. In the first each QRS complex is removed (Viniker 1986a). In practice, other ECG complexes

such as the T wave may remain to contaminate the EEG. A more successful method involves averaging the ECG complex which can be computed by a microprocessor and this can be subtracted from the ECG contaminated fetal EEG (Viniker 1984).

In the latest development in fetal cerebral activity technology Blum et al (1985) have applied the neuromagnetometer to the maternal abdomen to obtain recordings antenatally. Fetal ECG contamination is also a problem with this technique.

FETAL EEG ANALYSIS

The difficulties of using the fetal EEG may be divided into the problems of obtaining a good quality signal and the problems of reading and interpreting the voluminous unprocessed trace produced by conventional recorders (108 m/h).

The need for techniques that can reduce the fetal EEG into simplified and comprehensible format have been well recognized (Peltzman et al 1973, Chik et al 1975, Sureau 1977, Maynard et al 1979, Viniker 1979).

The simplest method of reducing the voluminous paper trace is to set the paper write-out to a very slow paper speed resulting in a 'compressed EEG' (Fig. 14.3). Hundreds of methods have been described for automatic processing of the EEG into comprehensible format and the advance in computer technology is rapidly adding to these. One instrument, the Cerebral Function Monitor (CFM — Maynard et al 1969) has found useful applications in a variety of clinical and research situations (Prior 1979). It is compact, easy to operate and produces a simple, on-line, write-out with a paper speed at 30 cm/h. The write-out

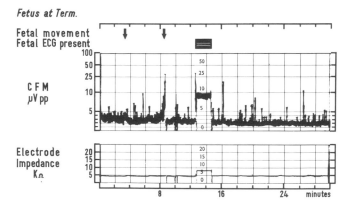

Fig. 14.2 CFM record showing artificially elevated activity due to fetal ECG contamination.

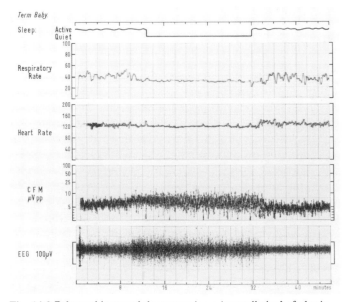

Fig. 14.3 Polygraphic record demonstrating a 'constellation' of physiological alterations in association with altered behavioural state.

appears as a band (Figs 14.2 and 14.3) the upper and lower borders representing the maximum and minimum levels of cerebral electrical activity respectively. A simple method of quantifying cerebral electrical activity in the perinatal period from CFM recordings has been described (Viniker et al 1984).

THE NORMAL FETAL EEG

The characteristics of cerebral electrical activity of the fetus and neonate of similar conceptional age are the same (Lindsley 1942, Rosen & Satran 1965, Mann et al 1972, Fargier et al 1974, Zorn et al 1974, Viniker 1983). In the perinatal period there are cycles of higher voltage and lower voltage activities and with polygraphic recordings it is possible to demonstrate that these cycles correspond to quiet sleep (non-rapid eye movement) and active sleep (rapid eye movement) respectively (Jost et al 1972, Ruckebusch 1972, Viniker et al 1980, Viniker 1988, Fig. 14.3). In the human fetus, the mean duration of quiet sleep is 20 minutes and the mean duration of the sleep cycles is 68 minutes (Viniker 1988).

The maturation of the normal EEG is described in Chapter 13 (p. 179). Differentiation between quiet sleep and active sleep develops at about 32 weeks gestational age (Dreyfus-Brisac 1975).

Cycles of cerebral electrical EEG patterns consistent with active and quiet sleep have been demonstrated during labour in the presence of uterine contractions and maternal pushing (Zorn et al 1974). Challamel et al (1975) consider that the presence of these fetal EEG sleep cycles is indicative of fetal well-being.

ABNORMALITIES OF THE FETAL EEG

STUDIES IN ANIMALS

In a pilot study, we have assessed the feasibility of using the CFM to determine whether factors such as acidosis alter the response of the fetal brain to hypoxia in the fetal guinea pig. Sibling fetal animal models were employed to reduce the number of variables. The sow was anaesthetized and the head and thorax of the fetuses exteriorized whilst taking care not to disturb the placental circulation.

Multistranded steel wire electrodes were introduced through tiny burr holes and held in place with a rubber disc and 'superglue' (Viniker 1983). Similar electrodes were attached to the fetal thorax to record the fetal ECG.

The fetal CFM outputs and fetal heart rates were recorded during hypoxia induced by reducing the maternal oxygen supply. There was no difference in the rate of fall or recovery of cerebral electrical activity of the siblings in five preparations (Fig. 14.4).

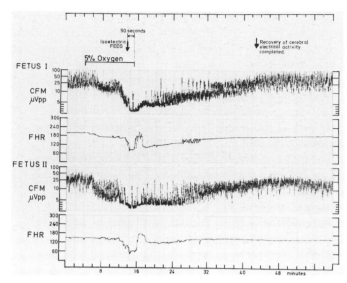

Fig. 14.4 The effect of oxygen deprivation on heart rate and cerebral electrical activity (CFM) of two sibling fetal guinea pigs.

In 17 preparations one fetus was rendered relatively acidotic by administering lactic acid and saline or sodium bicarbonate to the control. It was found that the brain of the fetus that had been intended to be more acidotic was the most sensitive in the majority of recordings (Fig. 14.5) and this was statistically significant.

In the majority of our fetal guinea pig recordings, following the onset of hypoxia, cerebral electricity activity (as indicated by the CFM) tended to fall before the fetal heart rate. The fetal heart rate recovered before cerebral electrical activity with re-oxygenation.

It has previously been observed that during hypoxia the fetal heart rate falls before alteration of the conventional EEG (Mann et al 1970, Scibetta et al 1973, Myers 1977). Other researchers, comparing the CFM and conventional EEG in anaesthetic studies have observed that the CFM can clearly detect alterations of cerebral electrical activity when these are not apparent on the conventional EEG (Schwartz et al 1974).

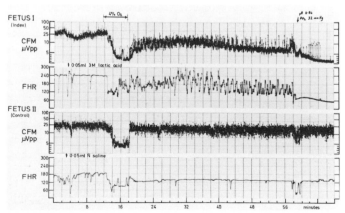

fig. 14.5 Effect of hypoxia on cerebral function of an acidotic fetal guinea pig compared with sibling control.

Rosen (1967), who observed that the fetal heart rate of the guinea pig returns to prehypoxia levels before cerebral electrical activity following re-oxygenation, commented that it was disturbing to note that the normal fetal heart rate could be present despite the continuing cerebral dysfunction indicated by an abnormal fetal EEG. Mann et al (1970) who made similar observations in the fetal lamb believed that their results indicated that cerebral function could not be dependent on oxygen supply alone.

The effect of oxygen deprivation on the fetal brain may be influenced by a variety of factors. The serum glucose level has been shown to influence the neuropathological results of oxygen deprivation in the rhesus monkey to a greater extent than the degree or duration of hypoxia (Myers 1977). The tolerance to hypoxia of the brain of newborn animals decreases with increasing maturation (Glass et al 1944) and the site of brain damage due to perinatal asphyxia depends on gestational age (Towbin 1970). Swedish workers have demonstrated that the evoked somatosensory response to moderate oxygen deprivation is reduced or completely abolished by the presence of acidosis in the fetal lamb (Hrbek et al 1974).

STUDIES IN THE HUMAN

Rosen et al (1973) have classified abnormalities of the fetal EEG into transient and non-transient changes. The transient changes are associated with alterations of fetal heart rate, medication and application of obstetric forceps.

The most common type of non-transient fetal EEG change is prolonged voltage suppression which has been associated with low Apgar score and the need for resuscitation at delivery (Borgstedt et al 1978). In an analysis of recordings from the last hour of labour or the hour immediately preceding the decision to deliver by caesarean section, the percentage time of iso-electrical fetal EEG was used as the only criterion of fetal EEG abnormality (Wilson et al 1979). There was a significant increase of iso-electrical fetal EEG in association with fetal heart rate decelerations and fetal acidosis. Iso-electrical fetal EEG was present for more than 20% of the hour in the presence of moderate acidosis (pH 7.25–7.30).

In the neonate, sleep cycles are present only when there is normal oxygenation and acid–base balance (Radvanyi et al 1973). Absence of fetal EEG sleep cycles over prolonged recordings has been considered to be a specific sign of fetal cerebral distress (Fargier et al 1974, Challamel et al 1975).

Rosen and his team (Chik et al 1976) wrote a computer program which recognized normal fetal EEG patterns and also depressed and iso-electrical activities. The tape-recorded fetal EEGs of nine babies with known neurological impairment at one year were analysed by their computer and the number of 10 second epochs of each EEG pattern was summated. The results were compared with the analysis of the fetal EEGs of 11 babies known to be normal at one year. There was a highly significant difference between the two groups.

By combining factors including fetal EEG frequencies and trends at onset and end of uterine contractions, uterine pressure record area and fetal heart rate derivations, sensitivity (defined as correct prediction rate for low Apgar score) and specificity (defined as correct prediction for high Apgar score), each in the order of 90% were obtained (Chik et al 1979).

By simultaneous visual observation of fetal EEG and cardiotocograph recordings, Rosen et al (1973) found no fetal EEG changes with early fetal heart rate decelerations. With some late and variable decelerations the EEG falls to an iso-electrical state and recovers with the recovery of the fetal heart rate. Occasionally, the recovery of the fetal EEG is slower than that of the fetal heart rate and they considered that this might indicate cerebral compromise. Polygraphic recordings of CFM, compressed EEG, fetal heart rate and uterine contractions facilitate comparison of alterations of cerebral electrical activity and fetal heart rate (Viniker 1986, Viniker 1988).

The pattern of acute fall and slow recovery of fetal cerebral electrical activity described by Rosen et al (1973) with the conventional EEG may be compared to a similar pattern demonstrated by the CFM in patients undergoing open-heart surgery who subsequently developed neurological impairment (Branthwaite 1972). In a retrospective analysis of the case notes of 417 patients submitted to open-heart surgery during 1970, Branthwaite found that brain damage had occurred in 20% of the patients. The timing of the cerebral insult was unknown. CFM recordings demonstrated an acute fall and slow recovery of cerebral electrical activity which occurred with the onset of cardio–pulmonary bypass in the majority of patients with subsequent brain damage. With the timing of the cerebral insult defined by the CFM, appropriate technical improvements were rapidly introduced leading to a highly significant reduction in the incidence of neurological complications to 7% in 1973 (Branthwaite 1975).

FUTURE DEVELOPMENTS

The role of current methods of intrapartum fetal monitoring in the prevention of brain damage has become the subject of current debate. This debate is unlikely to be resolved before the exact relationship between oxygen deprivation in labour and brain damage is determined. Acute fall and slow recovery of fetal cerebral electrical activity may be an important clue to the timing of fetal cerebral compromise and subsequent impaired cerebral function. Comparison of this pattern as it relates to fetal monitoring and open-heart surgery indicates that further studies are needed before the exact significance of acute fall and slow recovery of fetal cerebral electrical activity is elucidated (Viniker 1988).

The majority of advances in medical investigations have been achieved by the application of technology borrowed from other disciplines, ultrasound being a typical example. By contrast, the theoretical advantages of fetal electro-encephalography are apparent in advance of satisfactory technology. Despite the many excellent techniques for analysing a good quality EEG signal, the perfect fetal EEG electrode remains to be described.

Many fetal electrodes have been designed and produced. These have been attached to the fetus during labour and tested. It may be that the particular problems of recording cerebral electrical activity from the fetus should be investigated initially with models in the laboratory.

REFERENCES

Barden T P, Peltzman P, Graham J T 1968 Human fetal electroencephalographic response to intrauterine acoustic signals. American Journal of Obstetrics and Gynecology 100: 1128–1134

Blum T, Saling E, Bauer R 1985 First magnetoencephalographic recordings of the brain activity of a human fetus. British Journal of Obstetrics and Gynaecology 92: 1224–1229

Borgstedt A D, Heriot J T, Rosen M G, Laurence R A, Sokol R J 1978 Fetal electroencephalography and one minute and five minute Apgar scores. Journal of the American Medical Women's Assocation 33: 220–222

Branthwaite M A 1972 Neurological damage related to open-heart surgery: a clinical survey. Thorax 27: 248–253

Branthwaite M A 1975 Prevention of neurological damage during open-heart surgery. Thorax 30: 258–261

Chachava K V 1976 Fetal EEG. Fifth European Congress of Perinatal Medicine, Uppsala, Sweden, p 116

Challamel M J, Revol M, Bremond A, Fargier P 1975 Electroencephalogramme foetal au cours du travail. Revue Francaise de Gynecologie et d'Obstetrique 70: 235–239

Chik L, Rosen M G, Sokol R J 1975 An interactive computer program for studying fetal electroencephalograms. Journal of Reproductive Medicine 14: 154–158

Chik L, Sokol R J, Rosen M G, Borgstedt A D 1976 Computer interpreted fetal electroencephalogram. II. Patterns in infants who were neurologically abnormal at one year of age. American Journal of Obstetrics and Gynecology 125: 541–544

Chik L, Sokol R J, Rosen M G, Pillay S K, Jarrell S E 1979 Trend analysis of intrapartum monitoring data: a basis for a computerized fetal monitor. Clinical Obstetrics and Gynecology 22: 665–679

Dreyfus-Brisac C 1975 Neurophysiological studies in human premature and full-term newborns. Biological Psychiatry 10: 485–496

Fargier P, Bremond A, Challamel M J et al 1974 Electroencephalogram of the fetus during delivery. Journal de Gynecologie, Obstetrique et Biologie de la Reproduction 3: 1023–1033

Feldman J P, Le Houzec R, Sureau C 1970 Electro-encephalographie. Mise au point d'une electrode permettant l'enregistrement permenent au cours du travail. Gynecologie et Obstetrique 69: 491–493

Garcia-Austt E 1969 Effect of uterine contractions on the EEG of the human fetus during labour. In: Perinatal factors affecting human development. Pan American Health Organization, Scientific Publications, p 127

Glass H G, Snyder F F, Webster E 1944 The rate of decline in resistance to anoxia of rabbits, dogs and guinea-pigs from onset of viability to adult life. American Journal of Physiology 140: 609–615

Hopp H, Heinrich J, Seidenschnur G, Beier R, Schultz H 1972 Fetale electroenzephalographie und kardiotokographie. Geburtshilfe und Frauenheilkunde 32: 629–634

Hrbek A, Karlsson K, Kjellmer I, Olsson T, Riha M 1974 Cerebral reactions during intrauterine asphyxia in the sheep. II. Evoked electroencephalogram responses. Pediatric Research 8: 58–63

Jost R G, Quilligan E J, Sze-Ya Yeh, Anderson G G 1972 Intrauterine electroencephalogram of the sheep fetus. American Journal of Obstetrics and Gynecology 114: 535–539

Lindsley D B 1942 Heart and brain potentials of human fetuses in utero. American Journal of Psychology 55: 412–416

Mann L I, Prichard J W, Symmes S 1970 EEG, ECG, and acid base observations during acute hypoxia. American Journal of Obstetrics and Gynecology 106: 39–51

Mann L I, Zwies A, Duchin S, Newman M 1972 Human fetal electroencephalography: application of a vacuum electrode. American Journal of Obstetrics and Gynecology 114: 898–903

Maynard D E 1979 Removal of EKG from fetal CFM recordings. Annales de l'Anesthesiologie Francaise 20: 243–246

Maynard D, Prior P F, Scott D F 1969 Device for continuous monitoring of cerebral activity in resuscitated patients. British Medical Journal 4: 545–546

Maynard D E, Cohen R J, Viniker D A 1979 Intrapartum fetal monitoring with the Cerebral Function Monitor. British Journal of Obstetrics and Gynaecology 86: 941–947

Myers R E 1977 Experimental models of perinatal brain damage: relevance to human pathology. In: Gluck L (ed) Intrauterine asphyxia and the developing brain. Year Book Medical, Chicago, p 37

Peltzman P, Goldstein P J, Battagin R 1973 Quantitative analysis of fetal electrophysiologic data. American Journal of Obstetrics and Gynecology 115: 1117–1124

Prior P F 1979 Monitoring cerebral function. Elsevier, Amsterdam

Radvanyi M F, Monod N, Dreyfus-Brisac C 1973 Electroencephalogramme et sommeil chez le nouveau-ne en detresse respiratoire. Bulletin de Physio-Pathologique Respiratoire 9: 1569–1585

Rosen M G 1967 Effects of asphyxia on the fetal brain. Obstetrics and Gynecology 29: 687–693

Rosen M G, Satran R 1965 Fetal electroencephalography during birth. Obstetrics and Gynecology 26: 740–745

Rosen M G, Scibetta J J 1969 The human fetal electroencephalogram. I. An electrode for continuous recording during labour. American Journal of Obstetrics and Gynecology 104: 1057–1060

Rosen M G, Scibetta J J 1970 The human fetal electroencephalogram. II. Characterizing the EEG during labour. Neuropediatrie 2: 17–26

Rosen M G, Scibetta J J, Chik L, Borgstedt A D 1973 An approach to the study of brain damage: the principles of fetal electroencephalography. American Journal of Obstetrics and Gynecology 115: 37–47

Ruckebusch Y 1972 Development of sleep and wakefulness in the fetal lamb. Electroencephalography and Clinical Neurophysiology 32: 119–128

Schwartz M S, Virden S, Scott D F 1974 Effects of ketamine on the electroencephalograph. Anaesthesia 29: 135–140

Scibetta J J, Fox H E, Chik L, Rosen M G, Steinbrecher M, Braun L 1973 On correlating the fetal heart rate and brain in the sheep. American Journal of Obstetrics and Gynecology 115: 946–952

Sokol R J, Rosen M G, Chik L 1976 Fetal electroencephalography. In: Beard R W, Nathanielsz P W (eds) Fetal physiology and medicine. Saunders, London, p 476

Spies S 1976 A preliminary report on foetal EEG monitoring. Journal of the Electrophysiological Technology Association 2: 251–260

Sureau C 1977 Electronics and Clinical Measurement. In: Phillip E E, Barnes J, Newton M (eds) Scientific foundations of obstetrics and gynaecology. Heinemann, London, p 882

Towbin A 1970 Central nervous system damage in the human fetus and newborn infant. American Journal of Diseases of Children 119: 529–542

Viniker D A 1979 The fetal EEG (detection of oxygen deprivation). British Journal of Hospital Medicine 22: 504–510

Viniker D A 1983 Perinatal Cerebral Function Monitoring. MD Thesis, University of London

Viniker D A 1984 Intrapartum fetal electroencephalography, so near and yet so far. William Blair Bell Memorial Lecture. Royal College of Obstetricians and Gynaecologists, 11 May 1984

Viniker D A 1986 Human fetal electroencephalography. In: Di Renzo

G C, Hawkins D F (eds) Perinatal medicine: problems and controversies. Raven Press, New York, pp 37-43

Viniker D A 1988 Fetal electroencephalography. In: Chamberlain G, Cockburn F (eds) Perinatal practice. Wiley, Chichester (in press)

Viniker D A, Bromley I E, Maynard D E 1980 Monitoring the neonate with the Cerebral Function Monitor. In: Rolfe P (ed) Fetal and neonatal physiological measurements. Pitman Medical, London, pp 297–306

Viniker D A, Maynard D E, Scott D F 1984 Cerebral Function Monitor studies in neonates. Clinical Electroencephalography 15: 185–192

Weller C, Dyson R J, McFadyen I R, Green H L, Arias E 1981 Fetal electroencephalography using a flexible electrode. British Journal of Obstetrics and Gynaecology 88: 983–986

Wilson P C, Philpott R H, Spies S, Ahmed Y, Kadichza M 1979 The effect of fetal head compression and fetal acidaemia during labour on human fetal cerebral function as measured by the fetal electroencephalogram. British Journal of Obstetrics and Gynaecology 86: 269–277

Zorn J R, Monod N, Le Houezec R, Dreyfus-Brisac C, Sureau C 1974 Electroecencephalographie foetale. Journal de Gynecologie, Obstetrique et Biologie de la Reproduction 3: 1035–1055

15. Brainstem evoked potentials

Dr S. Lary

The auditory brainstem responses (ABR) are measures of electrical events generated within the auditory brainstem pathway. These responses provide an objective method for the assessment of function in the peripheral auditory apparatus (middle ear and cochlea) and the central auditory pathways through the brainstem. The role of the ABR is better assessed in the newborn than either visual or somatosensory evoked responses. The responses are independent of level of arousal or attention and thus provide an advantage over other neurophysiological tests in infancy. The ABR is, however, significantly affected by changes in stimulus input and disease processes of the primary sensory organs, therefore attention to methodological detail is important in its interpretation.

THE RESPONSE

The auditory brainstem responses are the far-field potentials recorded from scalp electrodes and consist of seven small vertex positive waves designated by the Roman numerals I to VII (Jewitt & Williston 1971). They occur in the first 10 ms from the acoustical stimulus (Fig. 15.1). Modern

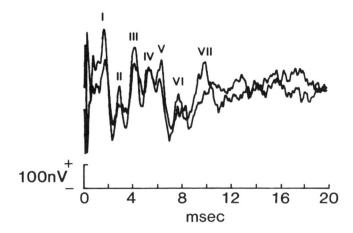

Fig. 15.1 Normal auditory brain responses (ABR) in a full-term infant. There are seven waves, designated by Roman numerals I–VII and elicited by 60 dB, 10/s click stimuli.

computer equipment averages the responses and typically over 1000 are collected and displayed as a representative pattern. Because these waves have short latencies they cannot represent either neural events at the level of the cerebral cortex or myogenic responses mediated through a cerebral reflex arc.

Animal studies have elucidated the origin of the seven positive waves and this is illustrated in Fig. 15.2. Hashimoto et al (1981) have confirmed the animal data in humans. Component I is dependent on the auditory nerve and occurs simultaneously with the compound action potential of the nerve recorded at the round window. Component II arises from the cochlear nuclei especially their ventral parts, and component III arises from generators in the region of the superior olivary nuclei complex. Component IV represents the ventral nucleus of the lateral lemniscus and depends on both crossed and uncrossed fibres. Midline lesions reduce its amplitude but do not abolish it. Component V probably arises from the inferior colliculi and also represents the result of crossed pathways. Components VI and VII are still controversial in their origin. It has been suggested that they arise from the medial geniculate body and auditory cortical radiations, respectively, but there is little experimental evidence for this.

ANALYSIS

The relationship between any response and the stimulus eliciting that response is called the latency. Latency may be further subdivided into absolute latencies and interpeak intervals (Fig. 15.3). Interpeak interval (IPI) refers to the interval between two component waves. IPI I–V for instance is the interval between the peaks of waves I and V. Both the absolute latency and interpeak intervals are measured in milliseconds. The amplitude of a wave is determined by the difference between the highest peak and the subsequent negative trough (assuming that vertex positive waves are displayed as upward deflections). Amplitude is measured in nanovolts (nV). Waves I, III and V are most prominent

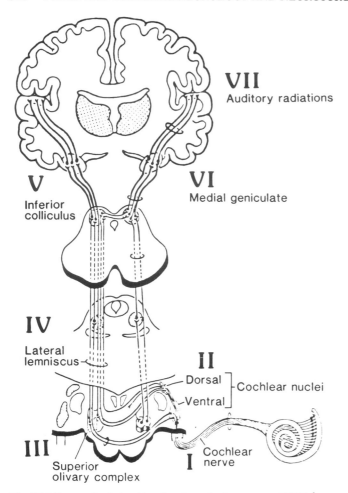

VII
Auditory radiations

V
Inferior colliculus

VI
Medial geniculate

IV
Lateral lemniscus

II
Dorsal ⎱ Cochlear nuclei
Ventral ⎰

III
Superior olivary complex

I
Cochlear nerve

Fig. 15.2 Proposed relationship of auditory brain response (ABR) waves to various structures of the auditory pathway. The input from each nerve ascends both ipsilaterally and contralaterally and there are crossing fibres at each level as far rostrally as the colliculi. (Adapted from Pansky & Delmas 1980.)

and waves II, IV and VI are not commonly used in clinical interpretation. By decreasing stimulus intensity the last group of waves tends to diminish markedly, thus greatly facilitating identification of waves I, III and V.

FACTORS AFFECTING ABR

The ABR is a dependent variable. It has certain measurable properties and is influenced by a host of technical and instrumental factors including the nature of the stimulus, recording procedures and the subject.

Stimulus

An ideal stimulus should have a sharp onset (for good synchronization) and be timed accurately so that response latencies are unequivocal. It must also be frequency-specific so that a chosen section of the cochlea may be selectively

stimulated. Threshold assessment should be of precisely known latency. A click stimulus meets the first requirement but has no frequency-specificity. It nevertheless evokes an excellent 'whole nerve' action potential. A frequency-specific stimulus is a pure tone, devoid of any click artefacts. Such a stimulus must have a gradual rise and fall to avoid high-frequency transients. This slow rise-time prevents the stimulus from meeting the first requirement. Moreover, it does not allow for close synchrony of firing of the individual hair cells within the basal turn of the cochlea. In practice clicks are most commonly used. They tend to produce larger and consequently better-defined evoked potentials than other more frequency-specific stimuli such as tone bursts or pips (Picton & Devrieux-Smith 1978). Clicks generated at a rate of 10 per second are generally accepted as the most suitable frequency for neurological diagnosis. There is controversy as to the effects of click stimulation rates on ABR in the neonate. Hecox (1975) compared infants aged from 3 weeks to 16 months, stimulating them at 10 and 30 clicks/second. He found no age-dependent differences in ABR in relation to the frequency of stimulation. Stockard et al (1979, 1983) on the other hand reported greater rate-dependent changes in absolute latencies and interpeak interval measurements in newborns. Standardization of click repetition of 10/second is important for comparison

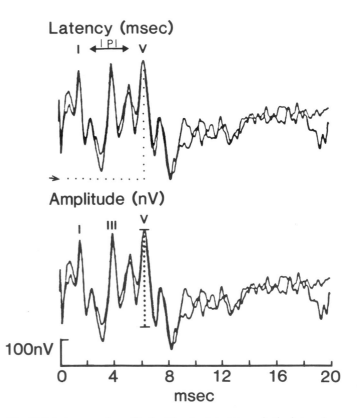

Fig. 15.3 Latency and amplitude. The absolute latency is the interval between the onset of the stimulus and the response it evokes. Interpeak interval is the distance between two peaks. Amplitudes are measured from the peak of a wave to the next trough.

between studies. In the newborn there is no evidence that repeated stimuli (up to 100 000 cause 'fatigue' in the neural pathways (Schulman-Galambos & Galambos 1975, Salamy & McKean 1977).

The ABR wave components (latencies and amplitudes) change in an orderly manner as a function of signal intensity (Hecox & Galambos 1974, Starr & Achor 1975). The wave components are best observed in response to high-intensity stimuli. In general, a decrease in stimulus intensity is associated with increase in wave latencies and decrease in amplitude. At lower intensities the ABR waves lose many of their peaks but wave V persists long after other waves have receded and is often the only remaining wave in response to stimulus intensities that approximate threshold levels.

The stimulus is presented to the infant by a small earphone which is held gently over the ear when the infant lies prone and with the other ear on the mattress. Care is taken not to occlude or collapse the external auditory canal which may result in appearances simulating a conductive lesion. Each ear is tested separately. Binaural stimulation should be avoided because monaural abnormalities are common with brainstem lesions and may be masked by the responses from the normal ear (Stockard et al 1978).

Electrode placement

Three scalp electrodes are usually used. One is attached to the vertex (Cz) just behind the anterior fontanelle, one relative to the stimulated ear on the ipsilateral mastoid (M1), and the ground electrode on the contralateral mastoid process (M2). The vertex and mastoid electrodes are called the 'active' and 'reference' electrodes respectively. A fourth electrode is sometimes applied to the forehead and used for grounding while M2 records from the contralateral ear in a second channel.

Bandpass filters

To achieve a successful ABR recording, a favourable signal-to-noise ratio is necessary, as the response must be extracted from a background of myogenic and neurogenic noise. Computer-averaging results in considerable noise reduction but the use of filters before averaging can make a further contribution to successful recording. The filters eliminate unwanted low- and high-frequency information; only those frequencies between the selected low- and high-frequency cut-off settings being allowed through the 'bandpass'. In neonatal ABR recordings, the filters are usually set between 100 and 3000 Hz.

Effects of maturation

Maturation has a significant influence on ABR measurements (Hecox & Galambos 1974, Salamy et al 1975, 1978, 1979, Salamy & McKean 1976, Starr et al 1977, Stockard

et al 1983). Age affects ABR variables such as latency and amplitude (Fig. 15.4). Latencies are greatly prolonged in premature infants and neonates and become progressively shorter in the first two years of life (Mokotoff et al 1977).

A decrease in absolute latency with increasing age has been observed throughout the second year of life (Hecox & Galambos 1974, Salamy et al 1975, Salamy & McKean 1976). Hecox & Galambos (1974) found that the latency of wave V decreased systematically in infants whose ages ranged from three weeks to 32 months. Salamy & McKean (1976) reported that in infants aged from 20 hours to 12 months the latencies of the first five waves were reduced as the child grew older. The changes in mean latency were greater for wave V (1.12 ms) than for wave I (0.41 ms). In addition, after six to eight weeks there was a slight decrease of the latencies throughout the first 12 months of life. The interpeak intervals were also prolonged for infants under 2 years of age compared with adult values and varied inversely with age. During the first year of life the I–V IPIs have been shown to decrease from 5.12 ms in full-term newborns to 4.2 ms in 12-month-old infants (Hecox 1975, Salamy et al 1975, Salamy & McKean 1976). Salamy & McKean (1976) found an abrupt decrease in I–V interval by 6 weeks of age, a fairly stable value through the next 6 months, and then another abrupt decrease between the ages of 6 and 12 months.

Latency shifts occurring with advancing age are due to changes in neural structure including increases in fibre diameter, progressive myelination and increased dendritic arborization (Hecox 1975). Myelination and the shortening of latency with age have been described (Hecox 1975, Salamy & McKean 1976, Salamy 1984). Myelination of the eighth cranial nerve is said to be complete by

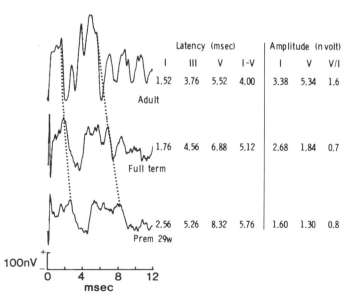

Fig. 15.4 Changes in latency (decrease) and amplitude (increase) with maturation in three subjects (29 weeks gestation, full-term and adult).

birth. Myelination proceeds caudo–rostrally and the lower brainstem structures are well myelinated before birth (Flechsig 1920, Langworthy 1933, Yakovlev & Lecours 1967) but Rorke & Riggs (1969) have suggested that myelination of the inferior colliculus and medial geniculate bodies is not complete at birth.

A high correlation has been found between gestational age and nerve conduction velocity (Dubowitz et al 1968, Moosa & Dubowitz 1972, Miller et al 1983). Increases in nerve conduction velocity (NCV) depend on myelination brought about by Schwann cells which are also responsible for the myelination of the auditory nerve. Miller et al (1984) compared NCV with wave I latency and conduction velocity through the auditory brainstem pathways as reflected by the interpeak latency (IPI I–V) in pre-term and full-term infants. Although they found a linear relationship between wave I latency and NCV, they found a poor correlation between IPI I–V and NCV. This suggests that the factors governing normal maturation of central transmission were not related to myelination of the peripheral nerves. Central transmission is easily affected by many of the risk factors often present in this age group.

The ABR is not affected by the infant's sex, the presence of most CNS depressants (Stockard et al 1980) and state of alertness. Sohmer et al (1978) studied the effects of sedation-induced sleep on the ABRs of six normal children (aged 5 to 10 years) and found no significant latency differences.

NORMAL RANGE FOR GESTATIONAL AGE

Data for normal ABR values have been reported from gestational age of 28 weeks and upwards (Starr et al 1977, Goldstein et al 1979, Despland & Galambos 1980, Cox et al 1982, Stockard et al 1983, Salamy 1984). Unfortunately inconsistencies in the selection of the 'normal' population have led to wide variations in the reported normal values for different components of the ABR at various gestational ages.

Two studies from the Hammersmith Hospital have carefully defined a normal group of infants of varying gestational ages (Fawer & Dubowitz 1982, Lary 1986). They selected infants with a low postnatal complication score (Drillien et al 1980) and those found to be repeatedly normal on sequential neurological examination. In addition none of the infants had intracranial ultrasound abnormalities. Charts have been produced from these data to show the normal ranges for the wave I and V latencies and the I–V interpeak interval (Fig. 15.5). The latencies showed a regular and consistent decrease with age but amplitude ratios did not vary with maturation.

Caution is necessary in comparing normal data from different laboratories. Published norms can be used for comparison but must not be taken as exact values against which to test data obtained in quite different settings with non-comparable equipment (Weber 1982, Stockard et al 1983, Cox 1984).

CLINICAL APPLICATIONS

The two main clinical applications for ABR are assessment of hearing impairment (audiological disorders) and abnormalities of brainstem function (neurological disorders). ABR appears to be of particular value in view of its reproducibility and consistency of responses from patient to patient. In addition it is not affected by the level of alertness, muscle artefact or ongoing activity and provides valuable objective assessment of brainstem function.

AUDIOLOGICAL DISORDERS

ABRs may be used to predict the degree and type of hearing impairment. When infants with such disorders are screened by ABR an audiological diagnosis can usually be made provided one takes into account:

1. the threshold
2. the latency and amplitudes of wave I
3. the latency of wave V
4. the I–V interval
5. the latency–intensity curve.

The ABR is the only reliable method for estimating threshold sensitivity in infants (Schulman-Galambos & Galambos 1975, Galambos & Hecox 1978, Lary et al 1985). The most commonly used criterion for threshold estimation is the minimum intensity required to detect wave V in the response.

Several investigators have compared electrical response audiometry (particularly the ABR) with behaviourally determined thresholds. Mokotoff et al (1977) compared ABR results with impedance thresholds in 81 infants and children and established the ABR as a highly reliable test. Pratt & Sohmer (1978) found that ABR thresholds differed by +6 dB from behavioural thresholds in adults. Jerger et al (1980) reported a threshold agreement between electrical and behavioural tests in 94% of the 141 children tested. Ruth et al (1983) compared behavioural observation, audiometry and the ABR in 63 infants with normal hearing whose ages ranged from 1 to 12 months. They concluded that the ABR provided the most consistent threshold for all subjects tested, regardless of age.

ABR has been shown to quantify hearing deficits in full-term and prematurely born infants (Galambos & Despland 1980, Marshall et al 1980, Roberts et al 1982, Stein et al 1983, Lary et al 1985). The deficits can be classified as mild, moderate or severe. In full-term babies a mild hearing deficit will range from 20 to 40 dB and a moderate deficit from 40 to 60 dB. Severe deficits will

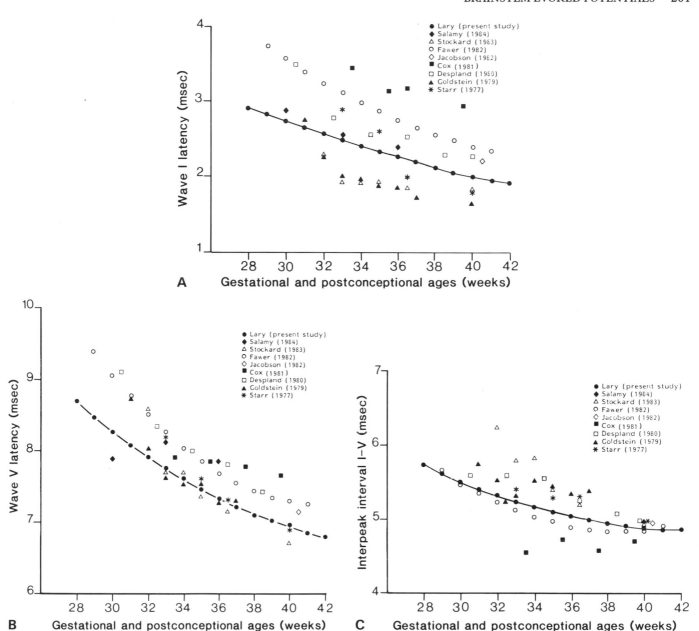

Fig. 15.5 Absolute latencies as a function of gestational age of waves I (**a**) and V (**b**). The results from nine studies are shown. Interpeak interval I–V as reported in nine studies is shown in (**c**). By 40 weeks of gestational age most studies report similar data.

exceed 70 dB. Lary et al (1985) found hearing threshold to be at 40 dB in pre-term infants between 28 and 34 weeks gestational age, at 30 dB in infants between 35 and 38 weeks and below 20 dB in full-term infants.

Stein et al (1983) reported follow-up data on infants with abnormal ABRs identified in the neonatal unit and found four infants to have apparently normal hearing who had failed their initial ABR assessment. Two of these four infants continued to show neurologically abnormal ABR results. ABR appears to be a highly sensitive test for subsequent deafness but is not very specific.

Diagnostic information in identifying the type of hearing impairment comes from determining the curves of latency–

intensity function (LIF). LIF curves represent the relationship of wave V latency and its changes with intensity of the stimulus. Curves obtained from patients with impaired hearing differ from normal curves, and it is the analysis of these differences that identifies the type of hearing deficits. In conductive deafness, the effective stimulus reaching the cochlea is reduced. When a patient with a conductive deficit of 40 dB is tested with a 60 dB click, only 20 dB reach the cochlea. The response will correspond to a stimulus of 20 dB only. When the latency–intensity function for wave V is plotted, the slope is normal but the latency is abnormally prolonged. The pathological curve is parallel but above the normal curve. In sensorineural hearing impairment, latency–

intensity curves show a rapid decrease in wave V latency from an elevated threshold at low intensities of stimulation to near-normal latencies at higher intensities (Yamada et al 1975, Galambos & Hecox 1977, 1978). These two patterns are shown in Fig. 15.6.

In conclusion, judgement about hearing deficits is not always conclusive when based solely on ABR data obtained before discharge. Subsequent ABR re-testing at follow-up improves the diagnostic accuracy considerably. Decisions regarding hearing impairment based solely on ABRs elicited in the neonatal unit should be guarded. Behavioural and audiological testing must also be performed before a diagnosis of hearing loss is made. ABR abnormalities may reflect transient disturbances.

NEUROLOGICAL DISORDERS

Certain laboratories use ABR techniques solely for audiological purposes, while others are interested primarily in the neurological information which the ABR can provide.

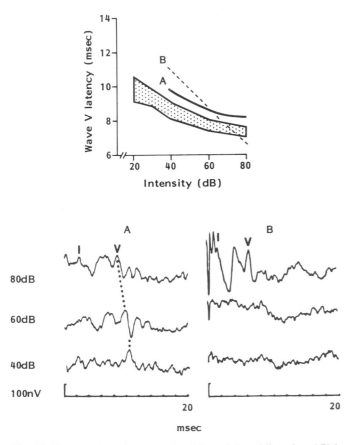

Fig. 15.6 Latency–intensity curves (straight and dotted lines A and B) in two infants with hearing deficits plotted against a background of normal data (hatched area) for ages 33–37 weeks. Curves A and B relate to traces A and B below. Curve A suggests conductive deafness in an infant aged 33 weeks. Curve B suggests hearing deficit of sensorineural type in an infant aged 34 weeks.

The two approaches should not be separated; the exact hearing status may influence the neurological diagnosis and vice versa.

The application of ABR results to neurological diagnosis is based on certain factors known to reflect the activity of neural structures in the eighth nerve and brainstem pathways. When these pathways are involved by lesions or disease, certain ABR parameters will be affected. The effect may involve the disappearance of waves, increases in latencies, decreases in amplitude, morphological changes, or any combination of these.

The most common changes in ABR seen with lesions in the central nervous system are of three types. The first is a prolongation in latency between various ABR components (mainly an increase in the I–V interval). This measure of 'central conduction time' was developed for neurological evaluation because the absolute latency of all the various waves might be affected by middle ear or cochlear disturbances, whereas the interpeak intervals are relatively independent of both click intensity and hearing loss (Starr et al 1977, Stockard & Rossiter 1977, Rowe 1978). The second type of abnormality is a change in the amplitude ratio of waves V to I (Starr & Achor 1975, Rowe 1978, Chiappa 1983). An amplitude ratio of 0.1 at 60 dB hearing level is considered normal. The third is a loss or marked attenuation of certain ABR components. Complete absence or marked attenuation of all waves may be seen in pre-term infants which may resolve within a few weeks. Such abnormality may indicate hearing or neurological disturbances or both and therefore, a separate category may be advisable. This classification may prove later to have a predictive value when compared with audiological or neurological outcome.

Researchers have shown a relationship between abnormal ABR and such neonatal risk factors as low birth-weight (Benitez et al 1979, Barden & Peltzman 1980, Galambos & Despland 1980), asphyxia (Goldstein et al 1979, Barden & Peltzman 1980, Kilney et al 1980), acidosis (Galambos & Despland 1980), hyperbilirubinaemia (Benitez et al 1979, Chisin et al 1979, Kotagal et al 1981), intracranial haemorrhage (Hazell et al 1980, Galambos & Despland 1980, Marshall et al 1980), respiratory disorders (Benitez et al 1979), apnoea (Abramovich et al 1979) and aminoglycoside therapy (Bernard et al 1980, Cox et al 1982, Cox 1984). Unfortunately many of these studies did not perform ABRs early enough to establish the precise temporal relationship between the insult and the ABR findings.

Lary (1986) studied prospectively 67 sick infants with gestational ages of 34 weeks or less admitted to a neonatal intensive care unit. ABRs were assessed at the end of the first week of life, at discharge from the unit and again at follow-up assessment (2–24 months). Those factors that reached statistical significance in relation to abnormal ABR at follow-up were hypoxia, hypercapnia and acidosis exceeding one week and an abnormal ABR at discharge. Risk factors with transient effect included germinal matrix–intraventricular haemorrhage, early abnormal clinic-al neurological findings, apnoea and gentamicin therapy.

Hyperbilirubinaemia and the ototoxic aminoglycosides have been suggested to alter the ABR in some infants (Benitez et al 1979, Chisin et al 1979, Kotagel et al 1981, Mjoen et al 1982). Others have reported that hyperbilirubinaemia causes only transient and reversible changes (Perlman et al 1983, Lenhardt et al 1984, Nakamura et al 1985). Wennberg et al (1982) reported improvement of the ABR following exchange transfusion but other groups found no significant relationship between hyperbilirubinaemia and abnormal ABR (Marshall et al 1980, Streletz et al 1986, Lary 1986). It is possible that additional risk factors are necessary to alter the background which increases the affinity of neural tissue to the effects of bilirubin or which enhances the vulnerability of neurones, thus precipitating damage.

Only one study has suggested a direct association between the use of aminoglycoside antibiotics and abnormal ABR results (Bernard et al 1980). Others found the drug effect to be transient and to normalize on follow-up (Cox et al 1982, 1984, Lary 1986). Finitzo-Hieber et al (1985) found that testing with ABR revealed early hearing impairment in some infants treated with netilmicin or amikacin but that this had preceded antibiotic treatment. This reinforces the difficulty in allocating a single cause to ABR abnormalities. Others have reported that aminoglycosides have no effect on the ABR (Galambos & Despland 1980, Marshall et al 1980).

Abnormalities of the ABR have been associated with intracranial haemorrhage (Schulmann-Galambos & Galam-bos 1975, Marshall et al 1980, Despland & Galambos 1980, Galambos & Despland 1980, Roberts et al 1982, Mjoen et al 1982, Fawer et al 1983). Lary (1986) found that all 28 infants with germinal matrix haemorrhage and/or intraventricular haemorrhage (GMH–IVH) in whom ABRs were performed had abnormal evoked potentials. In the non-GMH–IVH group only half had abnormal ABRs. Interestingly in 10 at-risk infants tested soon after birth, ABR abnormalities were present before GMH–IVH was diagnosed and in infants with definite haemorrhage all had ABR abnormalities including absent responses and prolonged interpeak intervals. Lary (1986) reported the presence of fusion between waves V and VI in infants with GMH–IVH. This was usually associated with abnormal morphology of wave V. These changes together with the finding of prolonged IPI and abnormal V:I ratio can be considered as evidence of a compromised brainstem. There was no consistent correlation between ABR abnormalities and the site of the haemorrhage or whether it was unilateral or bilateral.

Ventricular dilatation is an important and common sequel to GMH–IVH and disturbances in ABRs have been reported in association with this complication in infants and children (De Vlieger et al 1981, Starr & Amlie 1981, Stockard & Stockard 1981, Kraus et al 1984). It has been shown that in the presence of ventricular dilatation there were increased I–V interpeak intervals attributed to increased intracranial pressure (De Vlieger et al 1981, Starr & Amlie 1981). Lary (1986) found that in pre-term infants ABR abnormalities did not necessarily develop simultaneously with, or evolve in parallel with, the development of posthaemorrhagic ventricular dilatation (see Ch. 31). Initially abnormal ABRs all reverted to normal despite variable persistence of ventricular dilatation. Intermittent drainage of CSF in two infants was followed by an increase of amplitude of the ABR waves after 24 hours but not earlier. In pre-term infants there was no correlation between CSF pressure and I–V interpeak intervals.

In conclusion, any attempt to analyse factors predisposing to ABR abnormalities must take into account both anatomical and physiological variables which may alter the distribution or regulation of the cerebral blood flow, and in particular the effect of such changes upon the auditory brainstem pathway. It is against this background of haemodynamic disturbances and associated risks that the neonatal ABR has to be studied.

REFERENCES

Abramovich S, Gregory S, Slemick M, Stewart A 1979 Hearing loss in very low birthweight infants treated with neonatal intensive care. Archives of Disease in Childhood 54: 421–426

Barden T P, Peltzman P 1980 Newborn brainstem auditory evoked response and perinatal clinical events. American Journal of Obstetrics and Gynecology 136: 912–919

Benitez L D, Salomon R, Martinez A 1979 Longterm follow-up of deaf ICU babies detected by BSER. Paper presented at the International Evoked Response Auditory Study Group Symposium. Santa Barbara (abstract)

Bernard Ph A, Pechere J C, Hebert R 1980 Altered objective audiometry in aminoglycoside-treated human neonates. Arch fur Ahoren Nasen Kehl Heilk 228: 205–210

Chiappa K H 1983 Brainstem auditory evoked potentials: methodology. In: Chiappa K (ed) Evoked potentials in clinical medicine. Raven Press, New York, pp 105–143

Chisin R, Perlman M, Sohmer H 1979 Cochlear and brainstem responses in hearing loss following neonatal hyperbilirubinaemia. Annals of Otology, Rhinology and Laryngology 88: 352–357

Cox L C, Hack M, Metz D 1982 Longitudinal ABR in the NICU infant. International Journal of Pediatric Otorhinolaryngology 4: 225–231

Cox L C 1984 Auditory brainstem response abnormalities in the very low birthweight infant: incidence and risk factors. Ear and Hearing 5: 47–51

Despland P A, Galambos R 1980 The auditory brainstem response (ABR) is a useful diagnostic tool in the intensive care nursery. Pediatric Research 14: 154–158

De Vlieger M, Sadikoglu S, Van Eijndhoven J H M, Atac M 1981 Visual evoked potentials, auditory evoked potentials and EEG in shunted hydrocephalic children. Neuropediatrics 12(1): 55–61

Drillien C M, Thompson A J M, Burgoyne K 1980 Low birthweight children at early school age: a longitudinal study. Developmental Medicine and Child Neurology 22: 26–47

Dubowitz V, Whittaker G F, Brown B H, Robinson A 1968 Nerve conduction velocity: an index of neurological maturity of the newborn infant. Developmental Medicine and Child Neurology 10: 741–749

Fawer C, Dubowitz L M S 1982 Auditory brainstem response in neurologically normal preterm and fullterm newborn infants. Neuropediatrics 13: 200–206

Fawer C, Dubowitz L M S, Levene M, Dubowitz V 1983 Auditory brainstem responses in neurologically abnormal infants. Neuropediatrics 14: 88–92

Finitzo-Hieber T, McCracken G H, Brown K C 1985 Prospective controlled evaluation of auditory function in neonates given netilmicin or amikacin. Journal of Pediatrics 106: 129–136

Flechsig P 1920 Anatomie des Menschlichen Gehirns und Ruckenmarks auf Myelogenetischer Grundlage, Vol. 1 Georg Thieme, Leipzig

Galambos R, Despland P A 1980 The auditory brainstem response (ABR) evaluates risk factors for hearing loss in the newborn. Pediatric Research 14: 159–163

Galambos R, Hecox K 1977 Clinical applications of the brainstem evoked potentials. In: Desmedt J E (ed) Auditory evoked potential in man. Karger, Basel, pp 1–19

Galambos R, Hecox K E 1978 Clinical applications of the auditory brainstem response. Otolaryngologic Clinics of North America II 3: 709–722

Goldstein P J, Krumholz A, Felix J K, Dhannon D, Carr R 1979 Brainstem evoked response in neonates. American Journal of Obstetrics and Gynecology 135: 622–628

Hashimoto I, Ishiyama Y, Yoshimoto T, Nemoto S 1981 Brainstem auditory evoked potentials recorded directly from human brainstem and thalamus. Brain 104: 841–859

Hazell J W P, Sheldrake L B, Reynolds E O R 1980 Auditory evoked potentials in the newborn. In: Rolfe P (ed) Fetal and neonatal physiological measurements. Pitman Medical, Tunbridge Wells, pp 198–205

Hecox K 1975 Electrophysiological correlates of human auditory development. In: Cohen L B, Salapatek P (eds) Infant perception; from sensation to cognition, Vol. II. Academic Press, New York, pp 151–191

Hecox K, Galambos R 1974 Brainstem auditory evoked responses in human infants and adults. Archives of Otolaryngology 99: 30–33

Jerger J, Hayes D, Jordan C 1980 Clinical experience with auditory brainstem response audiometry in pediatric assessment. Ear and Hearing 1: 19–25

Jewitt D L, Williston J S 1971 Auditory-evoked far-fields averaged from scalp of humans. Brain 94: 681–696

Kilney P, Connelly C, Robertson C 1980 Auditory brainstem responses in perinatal asphyxia. International Journal of Pediatric Otorhinolaryngology 2: 147–159

Kotagal S, Rudd D, Rosenberg C, Horenstein S 1981 Brainstem auditory evoked potentials in neonatal hyperbilirubinaemia. Neurology 31: 48 (abstract)

Kraus N, Ozdamar O, Stein L, Reed N 1984 Absent auditory brainstem dysfunction. Laryngoscope 94: 400–406

Langworthy O R 1933 Development of behaviour patterns and myelination of the nervous system in the human fetus and infant. Carnegie Contributions to Embryology 443: 1–57

Lary S 1986 Auditory brainstem responses in normal and abnormal preterm and fullterm infants. PhD Thesis. London University, pp 112–188

Lary S, Briassoulis G, De Vries L, Dubowitz L M S, Dubowitz V 1985 Hearing threshold in preterm and term infants by auditory brainstem response. Journal of Pediatrics 107: 593–599

Lenhardt M L, McArtor R, Bryant B 1984 Effects of neonatal hyperbilirubinaemia on the brainstem electric response. Journal of Pediatrics 104: 281–284

Marshall R E, Reichert T J, Kerley S M, Davis H 1980 Auditory function in newborn intensive care unit patients revealed by auditory brainstem potentials. Journal of Pediatrics 96: 731–735

Miller G, Skouteli H, Dubowitz L M S, Dubowitz V 1983 The use of nerve conduction velocity to determine gestational age in at risk and very low birthweight neonates. Journal of Pediatrics 103: 109–112

Miller G, Skouteli H, Dubowitz L M S, Lary S 1984 The maturation of the auditory brainstem response compared to peripheral nerve conduction velocity in preterm and fullterm infants. Neuropediatrics 15: 25–27

Mjoen S, Langslet A, Tangsrub S E, Sundby A 1982 Auditory brainstem responses (ABR) in high-risk neonates. Acta Paediatrica Scandinavica 71: 711–715

Mokotoff B, Schulman-Galambos C, Galambos R 1977 Brainstem auditory evoked responses in children. Archives of Otolaryngology 103: 38–43

Moosa A, Dubowitz V 1972 Assessment of gestational age in newborn infants: nerve conduction velocity versus maturity score. Developmental Medicine and Child Neurology 14: 290–295

Nakamura H, Takada S, Shimabuku R, Matsuo M, Matsuo T, Negishi H 1985 Auditory nerve and brainstem responses in newborn infants with hyperbilirubinaemia. Pediatrics 75: 703–708

Pansky B, Delmas J A 1980 Cochlear (VIII) nerve: auditory system. In: Review of neuroscience. Macmillan, USA, pp 238–239

Perlman M, Fainmesser P, Sohmer H, Tamari H, Wax Y, Pevsner B 1983 Auditory nerve-brainstem evoked responses in hyperbilirubinemic neonates. Pediatrics 72: 658–664

Picton T W, Devrieux-Smith A D 1978 The practice of evoked potential audiometry. Otolaryngologic Clinics of North America 11: 263–282

Pratt H R, Sohmer H 1978 Comparison of hearing threshold determined by auditory pathway electric responses and by behavioural responses. Audiology 17: 285–292

Roberts J L, Davis H, Phon G L, Reichert T J, Sturtevant E M, Marshall R E 1982 Auditory brainstem responses in preterm neonates: maturation and follow-up. Journal of Pediatrics 101: 257–263

Rorke L B, Riggs H E 1969 Myelination of the brain in the newborn. Lippincott, Philadelphia

Rowe J 1978 Normal variability of the brainstem auditory evoked response in young and old adult subjects. Electroencephalography and Clinical Neurophysiology 44: 459–470

Ruth R, Horner J S, McCoy G S, Chandler C R 1983 Comparison of auditory brainstem response and behavioural audiometry in infants. Scandinavian Audiology 17 (suppl.): 94–98

Salamy A 1984 Maturation of the auditory brainstem response from birth through early childhood. Journal of Clinical Neurophysiology 1: 293–329

Salamy A, McKean C M 1976 Postnatal development of human brainstem potentials during the first year of life. Electroencephalography and Clinical Neurophysiology 40: 418–426

Salamy A, McKean C M 1977 Habituation and dishabituation of cortical and brainstem evoked potentials. International Journal of Neuroscience 7: 175–182

Salamy A, McKean C M, Buda F 1975 Maturational changes in auditory transmission as reflected in human brainstem potentials. Brain Research 96: 361–366

Salamy A, McKean C M, Pettett G, Mendelson T 1978 Auditory brainstem recovery processes from birth to adulthood. Psychophysiology 15(3): 214–221

Salamy A, Birtley-Fenn C, Bronshvag M 1979 Ontogenesis of human brainstem evoked potential amplitude. Developmental Psychobiology 12(5): 519–526

Schulman-Galambos C, Galambos R 1975 Brainstem auditory evoked responses in premature infants. Journal of Speech and Hearing Research 18: 456–465

Sohmer H, Gafni M, Chisin R 1978 Auditory nerve and brainstem responses: comparison in awake and unconscious subjects. Archives of Neurology 35: 228–230

Starr A, Achor J 1975 Auditory brainstem responses in neurological diseases. Archives of Neurology 32: 761–768

Starr A, Amilie R N, Martin W J, Sanders S 1977 Development of auditory function in newborn infants revealed by auditory brainstem potentials. Pediatrics 60: 831–839

Starr A, Amilie R N 1981 The evaluation of newborn brainstem and cochlear functions by auditory brainstem potentials. In: Korobkin R, Guilleminault C (eds) Progress in perinatal neurology. Williams & Wilkins, Baltimore, pp 65–83

Stein L et al 1983 Follow-up of infants screened by auditory brainstem response in the neonatal intensive care unit. Journal of Pediatrics 103: 447–453

Stockard J E, Stockard J J 1981 Brainstem auditory evoked potentials in normal and otoneurologically impaired newborns and infants. In: Henry C E (ed) Current clinical neurophysiology: update on EEG and evoked potentials. Elsevier, Amsterdam, pp 9–71

Stockard J J, Rossiter V S 1977 Clinical and pathologic correlates of brainstem auditory response abnormalities. Neurology 27: 316–325

Stockard J J, Stockard J E, Sharbrough F W 1978 Non-pathologic factors influencing brainstem auditory evoked potentials, II. American Journal of EEG Technology 18: 265–286

Stockard J E, Stockard J J, Westmoreland B F, Corfits J 1979 Brainstem auditory-evoked responses: normal variation as a function of stimulus and subject characteristics. Archives of Neurology 36: 823–831

Stockard J J, Stockard J E, Sharbrough F W 1980 Brainstem auditory evoked potentials in neurology: methodology; interpretation; clinical application. In: Aminoff M J (ed) Electrodiagnosis in clinical neurology. Churchill Livingstone, Edinburgh, pp 370–413

Stockard J E, Stockard J J, Coen R W, Gluck L 1983 Auditory brainstem response variability in infants. Ear and Hearing 4: 11–23

Streletz L, Graziani L, Branca P, Desai H, Travis S, Mikaelian D 1986 Brainstem auditory evoked potentials in fullterm and preterm newborns with hyperbilirubinaemia and hypoxaemia. Neuropediatrics 17: 66–71

Weber B A 1982 Comparison of auditory brainstem response latency for premature infants. Ear and Hearing 3: 257

Wennberg R, Ahlfors C, Bickers R, McMurtry C, Shetter J 1982 Abnormal auditory brainstem response in a newborn infant with hyperbilirubinaemia: improvement with exchange transfusion. Journal of Pediatrics 100: 624–626

Yakovlev P I, Lecours A R 1967 The myelogenetic cycles of regional maturation of the brain. In: Minkowski A (ed) Regional development of the brain in early life. Blackwell Scientific, Oxford, pp 3–70

Yamada O, Yagi T, Yamane H, Suzuki J 1975 Clinical evaluation of auditory evoked brainstem response. Auris, Nasus, Larynx 2: 97–105

16. Visual evoked potentials

Dr J. Mushin

The visual evoked potential (VEP) is a gross electrical signal generated by the occipital region of the brain in response to visual stimulation. It is a more specific response than the electro-encephalogram (EEG) and more sensitive to changes in the type of visual stimulus used. The VEP can provide information both on the normal development of vision and on the integrity of the visual pathways. Unlike behavioural testing and pattern preference techniques, the VEP does not require the co-operation of the infant. The electroretinogram is discussed in Chapter 42.

RECORDING VEP

Two types of visual stimuli can be used to elicit the VEP — diffuse unpatterned flashes of light and patterned stimuli. The xenon-discharge stroboscope used to produce unpatterned stimuli gives a very high-intensity, brief duration flash, and has other disadvantages particularly when used in a neonatal intensive care unit. The bulky light-housing makes precise positioning of the light difficult and the high-voltage discharge generated is undesirable if the incubator contains raised oxygen levels. Most strobo-scopes produce an audible click which might cause cortical activity confusible with the VEP. These disadvantages can be overcome with the use of photostimulators designed using light-emitting diodes (LED). The LEDs can be incorporated in a small box which can be hand-held inside the incubator in front of the infant's face (Mushin et al 1984) or in goggles (Chin et al 1985). The red light produced by the LEDs is less attenuated by closed eyelids, an advantage when recording from newborn infants.

Since one of the primary functions of the human visual system is to analyse contours and edges, pattern stimulation in which a spatial dimension is present would seem to provide a much more sensitive test of visual function than the flash. A flash-elicited pattern VEP can be obtained by placing a checkerboard (or grating) pattern in front of a stroboscope (Harter et al 1977). However, the most usual form of pattern stimulation, which may be generated using a

television screen, is the reversing checkerboard in which the VEP is evoked by movement of the checkerboard through one square at constant mean luminance. The waveform of the pattern reversal VEP shows less interindividual variability than the flash VEP, and by altering the size of the checkerboard squares and the black/white contrast, a measure of visual acuity can be obtained (Sokol 1976). To record accurate pattern VEPs, however, it is necessary for the subject to maintain fixation on a central spot during the one minute or so of recording time, thus the technique is clearly not applicable to very young infants.

A minimum of three scalp electrodes is required to record the VEP, an active electrode placed on the midline at or just above the level of the inion is referenced to a midfrontal electrode and a ground electrode is placed on the mastoid or the earlobe. Two-channel recording from electrodes placed on either side of the midline allows hemispheric asymmetries in the VEP to be investigated. VEPs have also been recorded using multiple electrode locations to map the electrical field distribution of the occipital cortex (Halliday & Michael 1970), but this is time consuming to do in a clinical situation. More recently, computer-based electrodiagnostic topographic brain mapping techniques (VEPM) have been developed (Duffy et al 1979) which allow responses to be studied simultaneously over large areas of the brain in a dynamic manner. This technique has been used in children (Whiting et al 1985) and is potentially applicable to newborn infants.

MATURATION OF VEP IN THE NORMAL INFANT

VEPs have been recorded in infants from 25 weeks gesta-tional age (Hrbek et al 1973). The first response is a slow surface negative wave with a peak between 300 and 400 ms following the stimulus flash (Fig. 16.1). Between 32 and 35 weeks gestational age a positive wave precedes the negativity occurring at a peak time of around 200 ms (Umezaki & Morrell 1970). By 40 weeks postmenstrual age (PMA) the positive wave has increased in amplitude and an early

Maturation of the VER

Post menstrual age (weeks)

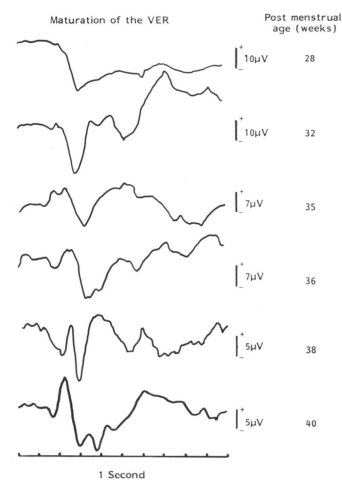

Fig. 16.1 VEPs at different postmenstrual ages. Negative wave only before 30 weeks postmenstrual age. Small positivity appears preceding the negativity between 32 and 35 weeks which increases in amplitude. By 40 weeks an early negative wave is present before the positive wave. Positivity at midline occipital electrode recorded upwards.

been found between the positive peak latency and stages of the wakefulness–sleep cycle in infants (Ellingson 1986, Watanabe et al 1972).

VEP IN NEUROLOGICALLY ABNORMAL NEWBORN INFANTS

Abnormalities in the waveform of the VEP have been reported in 85% of newborn infants with perinatal asphyxia as judged by low Apgar scores, the most characteristic features being an abnormal response pattern, an increase in latency and poor photic driving (Hrbek et al 1977). In infants suffering from severe idiopathic respiratory distress (Hrbek et al 1978, Gambi et al 1980), the VEP amplitude was decreased and the latency prolonged in the initial period. A reduction in the number of VEP components present was reported in premature infants at risk for CNS damage (Weiss et al 1982).

In a study of the evolutionary changes occurring in the VEP from the neonatal period to the age of one year in infants with various perinatal disorders (Hakamada et al 1981), the VEP was classified as atypical if there was:

1. abnormal waveform including low amplitude,
2. prolonged latency, or
3. asymmetry in the responses from the two hemispheres.

Absent responses and abnormal waveforms persisting beyond the age of 2 months were associated with later brain dysfunction. Kurtzberg (1982) recorded the VEP in a group of 79 very-low-birth-weight infants: 49% demonstrated abnormal flash VEPs at 40 weeks PMA and these tended to be the infants with a poorer neurological outcome at the age of one year.

The introduction of imaging techniques such as cranial ultrasonography, CT scanning and magnetic resonance imaging in the neonatal unit has made possible the early diagnosis of ischaemic–hypoxic lesions such as germinal matrix haemorrhage–intraventricular haemorrhage (GMH–IVH), periventricular leukomalacia (PVL), porencephalic cysts and ventricular dilatation. This has allowed the correlation of the VEP with the evolution of well-defined pathological lesions (Placzek et al 1985), and with behavioural tests of visual function (Dubowitz et al 1986).

Placzek et al (1985) recorded the VEP in a series of 70 premature infants, 26 of whom had evidence of GMH–IVH on ultrasound examination. The appearance of the positive wave immediately preceding the negative deflection was taken to indicate maturation of the VEP (Fig. 16.2). This positive wave was present in over 90% of records from neurologically normal infants by 35–36 weeks postmenstrual age but a high incidence of immature VEPs was found in infants suffering from GMH–IVH. The delay in maturation was not found to be related to the presence of ventricular enlargement but tended to be more marked in cases where

negativity has appeared giving a negative–positive–negative complex (Ellingson 1960, Watanabe et al 1972, Mushin et al 1984, Chin et al 1985). Placzek et al (1985) report little change in component latencies in the neonatal period, in contrast to Watanabe et al (1972) who observed a steady decrease in peak latency with gestational age, although it must be pointed out that components labelled N1, P2, etc cannot be assumed to be the same component across ages.

The component latencies subsequently shorten and the waveform becomes more complex, so that by the age of 6 months the response has a nearly adult waveform with the prominent surface positive component occurring at 100–150 ms after the flash. Ellingson (1960, 1986) has described a steep reduction in the latency of the positivity occurring in the first two months post-term. The sequence of development of the VEP, and in particular the appearance of the positive wave, appears to be a more reliable indicator of maturation than either latency or amplitude measurements (Watanabe et al 1972). No relationship has

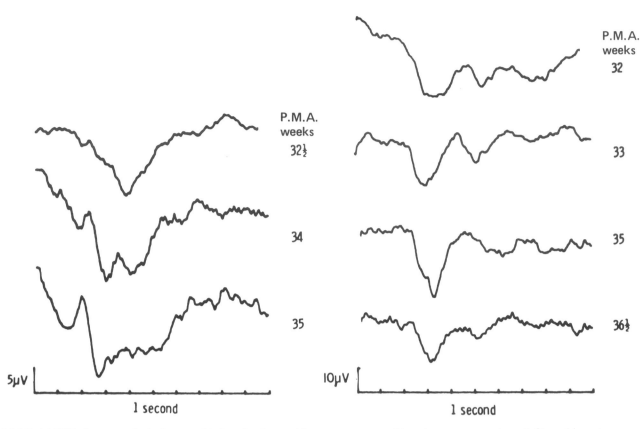

Fig. 16.2 Serial VEPs from neurologically normal infant showing positive wave present at 34 weeks postmenstrual age (left), and immature VEPs from an infant with severe periventricular haemorrhage with parenchymal extension showing small positivity at 36 ½ weeks PMA only (right). Positivity recorded upwards.

the haemorrhage extended down towards the thalamus. In infants in whom asymmetrical ventricular dilatation was associated with cyst formation, bilateral VEP recording demonstrated no difference in the VEP waveform between the two hemispheres in infants under 40 weeks PMA. Later recordings in the same infants obtained after the age of 2 months post-term showed asymmetrical responses (Fig. 16.3), even though the lesion had not progressed (however one cannot exclude the possibility that this may have been due to slight differences in electrode placement).

Abnormalities in the VEP in infants with cystic leukomalacia appear to depend on the site of the lesions. In infants with periventricular leukomalacia, in whom the cysts were most prominent around the occipital horn in the region of the trigone, the VEP was normal or became normal, despite in some cases, widespread involvement of the occipital cortex (Fig. 16.4A,B). In contrast, atypical responses were recorded from infants with cysts predominantly in the subcortical white matter (Fig. 16.4C). Infants in whom the VEP was persistently absent during the neonatal period were later usually found to have gross visual impairment. It is also interesting to note that a VEP, although abnormal,

was obtained in the first 2 days of life in an infant with complete absence of the occipital cortex (Dubowitz et al 1986).

VEP AS AN INDICATOR OF VISUAL FUNCTION

FLASH VEP

The clinical usefulness of the flash VEP in the neonatal period is limited, partly because of the high degree of interindividual variability in response amplitude and waveform at this age (Ellingson 1986) and partly because of the non-specificity of the VEP abnormalities for diagnosis and prognosis. In general, an absent VEP in the neonatal period indicates a poor prognosis for vision but we have examined one infant with cystic leukomalacia in whom the VEP was persistently absent between 30 and 36 weeks PMA. This infant later developed cerebral palsy but by the age of 3 years had apparently normal vision although a squint was present. Immature VEPs recorded in premature infants with neurological abnormalities tend to normalize soon after full-term and the infants appear to have no visual

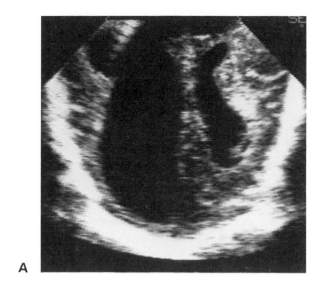

K.T. Gestational age 27 weeks

age 40 days

R

L

5uV

age 6 months

R

L

15uV

age 9 months

R

L

20uV

1 second

A

B

Fig. 16.3 Posterior coronal ultrasound scan showing asymmetrical ventricular dilatation in an infant born at 27 weeks gestational age examined at the age of 40 days (**a**). Serial VEPs performed in the same infant (**b**). The first VEP recorded at the time of the scan appears symmetrical but later VEPs show an asymmetry between the two hemispheres. R = right; L = left.

deficit although many have squints. Longitudinal studies are currently in progress to determine if such delays in VEP maturation are associated with later visual or learning difficulties. Serial VEPs together with electroretinograms have been helpful in the investigation of children under the age of six months with delayed visual maturation (Mellor & Fielder 1980). This is discussed in detail in Chapter 42.

It is important to point out that the VEPs do not always agree with psychophysical or behavioural tests of visual acuity. In particular, in the neonatal period infants may appear to be able to fix and follow a moving target, yet may have completely absent VEPs (Dubowitz et al 1986). The VEP cannot determine visual function accurately in children with grossly abnormal EEGs, critically ill infants with electrolyte abnormalities, sedated or anaesthetized infants, and children with nystagmus. In a study of over 70 children who experienced hypoxic insults to the visual cortex during infancy, Hoyt (1984) concluded that VEPs were of no value in the diagnosis of the original insult nor in establishing the prognosis for long-term visual recovery. It has recently been reported that VEP mapping studies in a group of children suffering from permanent cortical visual impairment gave more information than VEP data; the VEP mapping being abnormal in all 23 cases tested while the VEP was only abnormal in 10 (Whiting et al 1985).

PATTERN VEP

Although Harter et al (1977) claimed that it is possible to use flashed checkerboard pattern VEPs to estimate the visual acuity in newborn infants, the small changes presented in their amplitude versus check size function make clear inferences of acuity difficult. On the other hand, there seems to be general agreement that a true VEP cannot be elicited to pattern reversal stimulation in the newborn period. Marcus (1977) found no difference in the waveform to flash and pattern stimulation in early infancy, whereas a clear difference was noted in a 12-week-old infant. Below the age of about 8 weeks post-term the VEP can only be elicited by checkerboard patterns containing large checks or gratings (Porciatti 1984). Hoffman (1978) compared the VEP evoked by different check sizes in two groups of subjects, one group aged 4–6 weeks, the other 10–12 weeks. The younger subjects had longer latency responses which showed relatively little change in amplitude with check size

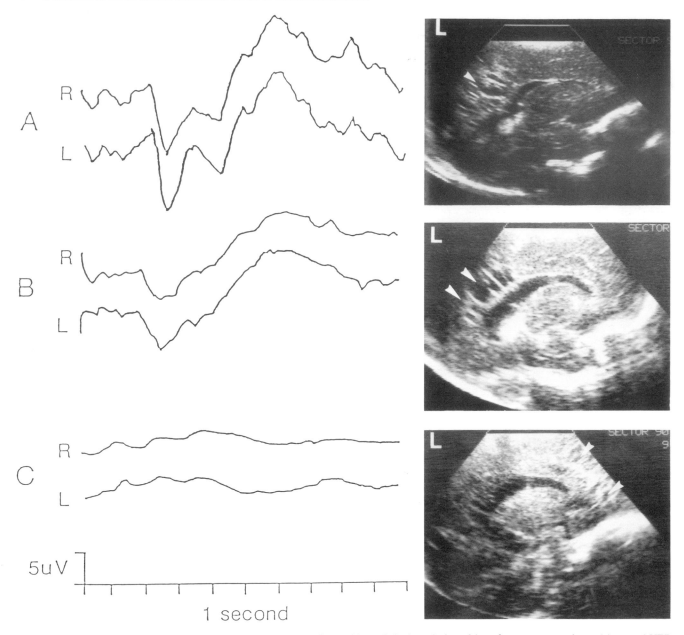

Fig. 16.4 VEPs and parasagittal ultrasound scans recorded in three infants with cystic leukomalacia at 36 weeks postmenstrual age. (a) normal VEP from right and left hemispheres in an infant showing cysts mainly in the occipital area, (b) immature VEP in an infant with periventricular lesions, (c) absent VEP in an infant with subcortical leukomalacia (arrows).

compared to the older subjects who showed an increase in amplitude as check size decreased from 5 degrees to 40 min arc. No recordable signals were obtained for small checks for infants under 2 months (Moscovitz & Sokol 1983) and even larger checks (60 min arc) produced only a very small simple waveform at this age.

The form of the visual stimulus used to elicit the VEP can be manipulated to study particular mechanisms within the visual system that respond to specific stimuli. In this way, Braddick et al (1986) have used dynamic random dot correlograms to elicit VEPs that indicate cortical binocularity, and a moving grating display which

elicits VEPs specific to orientation-selective mechanisms in the visual cortex. Normal infants showed no evidence of binocularity at birth, the first positive results on the VEP test of binocularity occurring at a median age of 13 weeks. In the second study, no response to orientation change occurred in the newborn and the first orientation-specific response was found to be present at around 6 weeks of age.

IS NEONATAL VEP CORTICAL IN ORIGIN?

In adults, the VEP is considered to be for the most

part cortical in origin and is composed of activity from two sources, a primary source originating from activity of the retinal receptors which reaches the occipital lobe via the lateral geniculate nucleus, and secondary activity which arises initially from the retina but then travels to the cortex via the superior colliculus and the diffuse thalamic projection system (Ciganek 1961). There is some evidence to support the hypothesis that these two systems mature at different rates in the neonatal period (Bronson 1974).

Only one study has attempted to show the correlation between the morphological development of the VEP and neuronal maturation of the neonatal visual cortex in the human infant (Purpura 1977). This study suggested that the characteristic negative wave of the VEP which occurs before 30 weeks PMA probably reflects the activity of grossly immature pyramidal and non-pyramidal neurones, while the appearance of the positive wave in the VEP at around 32 weeks PMA is associated with extensive dendritic differentiation and the development of dendritic spines in pyramidal neurones.

However, studies on neurologically abnormal infants suggest that in the newborn period the VEP, as well as behavioural tests of visual function, are more affected by lesions involving the midbrain and subcortical areas than by those affecting the occipital cortex (Placzek et al 1985). It has been suggested that visual function in the neonatal period, both behavioural and electrophysiological, is not dependent on the visual cortex but is mediated through subcortical pathways (Dubowitz et al 1986).

There are known to be a number of changes which occur in the visual system at around two months post-term. It is at this time that the latency of the flash VEP shortens markedly (Ellingson 1960), it becomes possible to elicit evidence of binocular stereopsis which is known to be a cortical function (Braddick et al 1986), a pattern reversal VEP can be elicited (Marcus 1977) and visual acuity determined by the pattern VEP begins to improve (Moskowitz & Sokol 1983). These changes support the hypothesis that there is a developmental shift in the physiological locus of control of infant visual function from a subcortical to a cortical locus at around 2 months of age (Hoffman 1978).

SUMMARY

The pattern VEP can provide a measure of visual function but only in infants over the age of 2 months. The flash VEP, although giving limited information on visual and general cerebral functioning, is simple to perform in the neonate, can be elicited even in quite premature infants, and has a waveshape which changes systematically with age in the neonatal period. Persistently absent or abnormal VEPs in the first few weeks of life generally indicate a poor neurological outcome, which may or may not be associated with visual impairment. Newer techniques which record not only from the primary visual cortex but also from the association areas may eventually give a better guide to diagnosis and prognosis of visual pathway lesions in the young infant.

REFERENCES

Braddick O, Atkinson J, Wattam-Bell J 1986 VER testing of cortical binocularity and pattern detection in infancy. In: Jay B (ed) Detection and measurement of visual impairment in pre-verbal children. Documenta Ophthalmologica Proceedings, No. 45. Dr W Junk, Dordrecht, pp 107–115

Bronson G 1974 The postnatal growth of visual capacity. Child Development 45: 873–890

Chin K C, Taylor M J, Menzies R, Whyte H 1985 Development of visual evoked potentials in neonates. Archives of Diseases of Childhood 60: 1166–1168

Ciganek L 1961 The EEG response (evoked potential) to light stimulus in man. Electroencephalography & Clinical Neurophysiology 13: 165–172

Dubowitz L M S, Mushin J, De Vries L, Arden G B 1986 Visual function in the newborn infant: is it cortically mediated? Lancet i: 1139–1141

Duffy F H, Burchfield J L, Lombroso C T 1979 Brain electrical activity mapping: a new method for extending the clinical utility of EEG and evoked potential data. Annals of Neurology 5: 309–321

Ellingson R J 1960 Cortical electrical responses to visual stimulation in the human infant. Electroencephalography and Clinical Neurophysiology 12: 663–677

Ellingson R J 1986 Development of visual evoked potentials and photic driving responses in normal full term, low risk premature, and trisomy-21 infants during the first year of life. Electroencephalography and Clinical Neurophysiology 63: 309–316

Gambi D, Rossini P M, Albertini G, Sollazzo D, Torrioli M G, Polidori G C 1980 Follow-up of visual evoked potential in full-term and pre-term control newborns and in subjects who suffered from perinatal respiratory distress. Electroencephalography and Clinical Neurophysiology 48: 509–516

Hakamada S, Watanabe K, Hara K, Miyazaki S 1981 The evolution of visual and auditory potentials in infants with perinatal disorder. Brain Development 3: 339–344

Halliday A M, Michael W F 1970 Changes in pattern evoked responses in man associated with the vertical and horizontal meridians of the visual field. Journal of Physiology 208: 499–513

Harter M R, Deaton F K, Odom J V 1977 Pattern visual evoked potentials in infants. In: Desmedt J E (ed) Visual evoked potentials in man: new developments. Clarendon, Oxford, pp 332–352

Hoffmann R F 1978 Developmental changes in human infant visual evoked potentials to patterned stimuli recorded at different scalp locations. Child Development 49: 110–118

Hoyt C S 1984 The clinical usefulness of the visual evoked response. Paediatric Ophthalmology and Strabismus 21: 231–234

Hrbek A, Karlberg P, Olsson T 1973 Development of visual and somatosensory evoked responses in preterm newborn infants. Electro-encephalography and Clinical Neurophysiology 34: 225–232

Hrbek A, Karlberg P, Kjellmer I, Olsson T, Riha M 1977 Clinical application of evoked encephalographic responses in newborn infants. I. Perinatal asphyxia. Developmental Medicine and Child Neurology 19: 34–44

Hrbek A, Karlberg P, Kjellmer I, Olsson T, Riha M 1978 Clinical application of evoked EEG responses in newborn infants. II. Idiopathic respiratory distress syndrome. Developmental Medicine and Child Neurology 20: 619–626

Kurtzberg D 1982 Event-related potentials in the evaluation of high-risk infants. In: Bodis Wollner I (ed) Evoked potentials. Annals of the New York Academy of Sciences 388: 557–571

Marcus M M 1977 Visual evoked potentials to flash and pattern in normal and high-risk infants. In: Desmedt J E (ed) Visual evoked potentials in man: new developments. Clarendon, Oxford, pp 490–499

Mellor D H, Fielder A R 1980 Dissociated visual development: electrodiagnostic studies in infants who are 'slow to see'. Developmental Medicine and Child Neurology 22: 327–335

Moskowitz A, Sokol S 1983 Developmental changes in the human visual system as reflected by the latency of the pattern reversal VEP. Electroencephalography and Clinical Neurophysiology 56: 1–15

Mushin J, Hogg C R, Dubowitz L M S, Skouteli H, Arden G B 1984 Visual evoked responses to LED photostimulation in newborn infants. Electroencephalography and Clinical Neurophysiology 58: 317–320

Placzek M, Mushin J, Dubowitz L M S 1985 Maturation of the visual evoked response and its correlation with visual acuity in neurologically normal and abnormal preterm infants. Developmental Medicine and Child Neurology 27: 448–454

Porciatti V 1984 Temporal and spatial properties of the pattern-reversal VEPs in infants below 2 months of age. Human Neurobiology 3: 97–102

Purpura D P 1977 Developmental pathobiology of cortical neurons in immature human brain. In: Gluck L L (ed) Intrauterine asphyxia and the developing human brain. Medical Year Book Publishers, Chicago

Sokol S 1976 Visually evoked potentials: theory, techniques and clinical applications. Survey of Ophthalmology 21: 1–44

Umezaki H, Morrell F 1970 Developmental study of photic evoked responses in premature infants. Electroencephalography and Clinical Neurophysiology 28: 55–63

Watanabe K, Iwase K, Hara K 1972 Maturation of visual evoked responses in low-birthweight infants. Developmental Medicine and Child Neurology 14: 425–435

Weiss I P, Barnet A B, Reutter S A 1982 Visual evoked potentials to flash in high-risk premature infants. In: Ross Laboratory Conference on Perinatal Intracranial Haemorrhage. Ross Laboratories, Columbus, Ohio, pp 1204–1228

Whiting S, Jan J E, Wong P, Flodmark O, Farrell K, McCormick A 1985 Permanent cortical visual impairment in children. Developmental Medicine and Child Neurology 27: 730–739

17. Somatosensory evoked potentials

Dr N. Gibson and Dr M. I. Levene

Somatosensory evoked potentials (SEPs) are the least well evaluated evoked response used in the neonatal period. There is however evidence from studies in adults (Brunko & Zegers de Beyl 1987, de Weerd et al 1985) and children (Lutschg et al 1983, Frank et al 1985) that they may be the most sensitive predictor of the quality of outcome following hypoxic or ischaemic cerebral insult and therefore this technique is likely to be used more frequently for non-invasive assessment of neural function in the newborn infant. The close proximity of the sensory and motor axons within the deep periventricular white matter is also likely to make SEPs useful in the assessment of cerebral function in premature infants with periventricular leukomalacia. Unfortunately, as yet, there is little consensus as to the methodology of this technique.

METHODS

The technique relies on the measurement of electrical potentials at several levels from the sensory pathway in response to stimulation of a peripheral sensory nerve. Mechanical stimuli were first used (Hrbek et al 1969) but electrical stimulation is now favoured. The stimulus can be applied to the fingers (Desmedt et al 1976) or directly over a mixed sensory/motor nerve. The median nerve is preferred by most but the posterior tibial nerve has also been used in the infant (Gilmore et al 1987). The stimulus can be applied by a hand-held device to the wrist with the cathode proximal, or by fixed electrodes with the cathode over the median nerve and the anode on the dorsum of the hand. The impulse current is increased until a definite twitch of the thumb is elicited (normally 10–20 mA in a full-term infant). Stimulus times vary between 0.1 and 0.5 ms with a frequency of 3–5 Hz. The evoked potentials can be collected for 50 ms, 100 ms or more, following each stimulus prior to analysis. The signals are then put through a bandpass system to filter spurious signals below 5–10 Hz and above 3000 Hz. A large number of stimuli (250–2000) are computer-averaged to damp down random (higher voltage) EEG waves and are displayed on a screen.

The evoked potentials are recorded by a number of electrodes applied over the spinal cord and scalp. The usual positions are the ipsilateral Erb's point (midportion of clavicle), cervical vertebrae and the contralateral cortex. All refer to a common electrode usually over the frontal midline area at the hairline. These electrodes allow measurement of potentials at various levels of the sensory pathway and determination of absolute and interwave latencies as well as waveforms.

THE RESPONSE

The sensory stimulus elicits a series of measurable potentials from the brachial plexus, spinal cord, subcortical and cortical generators. In Europe they are designated by their polarity — positive (downward) and negative (upward) deflections — and by their average latency. The American system is the opposite of this — positive up and negative down. In adults early negative peaks measured at Erb's point (N9) and over lower cervical vertebrae (N11, N13) are thought to represent brachial plexus and spinal cord potentials. In adults a sharp-peaked negative wave of 20 ms latency is recorded from the contralateral scalp electrode and is referred to as N20. This is thought to be cortically generated. The generators of N14, P15 and other possible 'thalamic' potentials are disputed (Chiappa et al 1979, Allison et al 1980). Confusingly, in infancy the nomenclature is different as the short latency cortical potentials are labelled N1 and N2 referring to the first and second negative waves and P0 and P1 for the first two positive deflections. It is suggested that N1 is equivalent to the adult N20.

Like the auditory brain response (ABR) and visual evoked response (VER), the SEP waveform varies with maturity and becomes better developed with gestational age before reaching adult values at around 8 years (Desmedt et al 1976). The latencies shorten in the first two years as myelination rapidly proceeds and then lengthen as the child grows. To date there are only limited normal data in neonates and infants (Gorke 1986, Willis et al 1984). Full-term babies have well-developed cervical potentials but the cortical response shows a positive peak at 15–16 ms, rising to N1 at 24–26 ms (Willis et al 1984) and a slow drop before the longer latency potentials become obvious. In immature infants the responses are of long latency and are difficult to reproduce. Hrbek (1973) described the appearance of a very long slow cortical wave in infants of less than 30 weeks gestation. With increasing maturity this wave sped up and became more discrete (Fig. 17.1). With advancing age the cortical response attains greater complexity and shorter latency as shown in Fig. 17.2. The median value of N1 latency at 1 month of age is 26.1 ms reducing to 16.6 ms at 10 months (Gorke 1986). Willis et al report slightly faster latencies but this probably reflects differences in methodology. Latencies of the other waves also decreased with advancing postnatal age (Willis et al 1984).

The effects of drugs and neurobehavioural states on the cortical potentials are unclear but there is evidence that short latency potentials are little affected in REM sleep (Desmedt et al 1980). Considerably more work is needed to clarify methodology and to provide reliable and reproducible normal data in pre-term, full-term neonates as well as infants.

is not clear whether the infants were premature or full-term. They found a clear relationship between abnormalities seen in the SEP and depression of the Apgar scores. The characteristic changes included abnormal waveforms with increased latencies or flatness of the response and a decrease or absence of responses ipsilaterally and in the midline. The more severely asphyxiated infants had the most marked abnormalities of the SEP.

Willis et al (1984) reported prolonged N1 peak latency in two babies with extensive germinal matrix haemorrhage–intraventricular haemorrhage, and Gorke (1986) found that in infants, prolongation of N1 predicted neurological disturbance, especially motor handicap. He also reported three infants with cerebral palsy but without abnormalities on their evoked potentials. Laureau et al (1986) used SEPs to monitor the effects of treatment on infants with congenital hypothyroidism.

Spinal cord trauma is associated with difficult delivery and is discussed in Chapter 35. Confirmation of this diagnosis is difficult and the SEP may be particularly useful in determining the level of cord injury. The absence of reproducible potentials above midthoracic level on posterior tibial stimulation in the presence of normal median nerve potentials locates the cord lesion above the sixth thoracic level but below the sixth cervical level (Bell & Dykstra 1985).

CLINICAL APPLICATIONS

Hrbek et al (1977) reported changes in evoked potentials in neonates suffering from perinatal asphyxia. Unfortunately it

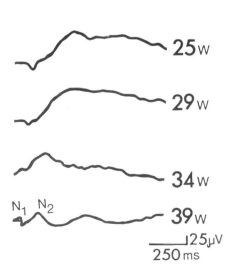

Fig. 17.1 Changing pattern of somatosensory evoked potentials (SEP) in premature infants from 25 to 39 weeks (w) of gestational age. (Redrawn from Hrbek et al 1973.)

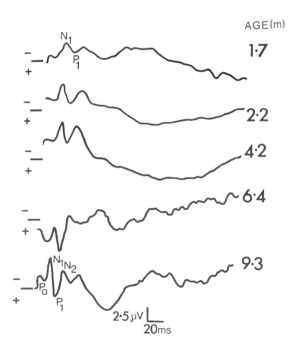

Fig. 17.2 The development of the somatosensory evoked potentials (SEP) over the first 9 months from full-term birth. The five waveforms represent different infants with their ages shown in months. (Redrawn from Gorke 1986.)

REFERENCES

Allison T, Goff W R, Williamson P D, VanGilder J C 1980 On the neural origin of early components of the human somatosensory evoked potential. In: Desmedt J E (ed) Clinical uses of cerebral, brainstem and spinal somatosensory evoked potentials. Progress in Clinical Neurophysiology, No. 7. Karger, Basel, pp 51–68

Bell H J, Dykstra D D 1985 Somatosensory evoked potentials as an adjunct to diagnosis of neonatal spinal cord injury. Journal of Pediatrics 106: 298–301

Brunko E, Zegers de Beyl D 1987 Prognostic value of early cortical somatosensory evoked potentials after resuscitation from cardiac arrest. Electroencephalography and Clinical Neurophysiology 66: 15–24

Chiappa K H, Young R R, Goldie W D 1979 Origins of the components of human short latency somatosensory evoked responses. Neurology 29: 598

Desmedt J E, Brunko E, Debecker J 1976 Maturation of the somatosensory evoked potentials in normal infants and children, with special reference to the early N1 component. Electroencephalography and Clinical Neurophysiology 40: 43–58

Desmedt J E, Brunko E, Debecker J 1980 Maturation and sleep correlates of the somatosensory evoked potential. In: Desmedt J E (ed) Clinical uses of cerebral, brainstem and spinal somatosensory evoked potentials. Progress in Clinical Neurophysiology, No. 7. Karger, Basel, pp 146–161

De Weerd A N, Looijenga A, Veldhuizen R J, Van Huffelen A C 1985 Somatosensory evoked potentials in minor cerebral ischaemia: diagnostic significance and changes in serial records. Electroencephalography and Clinical Neurophysiology 62: 45–55

Frank L M, Furgiuele T L, Etheridge J E 1985 Prediction of chronic vegetative state in children using evoked potentials. Neurology 35: 931–934

Gilmore R L, Brock J, Hermansen M C, Baumann R 1987 Development of lumbar spinal cord and cortical evoked potentials after tibial nerve stimulation in the preterm newborn: effects of gestational age and other factors. Electroencephalography and Clinical Neurology 68: 28–39

Gorke W 1986 Somatosensory evoked cortical potentials indicating impaired motor development in infancy. Developmental Medicine and Child Neurology 28: 633–641

Hrbek A, Hrbkova M, Lenard H-G 1969 Somatosensory, auditory and visual evoked responses in newborn infants during sleep and wakefulness. Electroencephalography and Clinical Neurophysiology 26: 597–603

Hrbek A, Karlberg P, Olssohn T 1973 Development of visual and somatosensory evoked responses in preterm newborn infants. Electroencephalography and Clinical Neurophysiology 34: 225–232

Hrbek A, Karlberg P, Kjellmer I, Olssohn T, Riha M 1977 Clinical applications of evoked electroencephalographic responses in newborn infants. I. Perinatal Asphyxia. Developmental Medicine and Child Neurology 19: 34–44

Laureau E, Vanane M, Hebert R, Letarte J, Glorieux J, Desjardins M, Dussault J M 1986 Somatosensory evoked potentials and auditory brainstem responses in congenital hypothyroidism. I. A longitudinal study before and after treatment in six infants detected in the neonatal period. Electroencephalography and Clinical Neurophysiology 64: 501–510

Lutschg J, Pfenninger J, Ludin H P, Vassella F 1983 Brainstem auditory evoked potentials and early somatosensory evoked potentials in neurointensively treated comatose children. American Journal of Disease in Children 137: 421–426

Willis J, Seales D, Frazier E 1984 Short latency somatosensory evoked potentials in infants. Electroencephalography and Clinical Neurophysiology 59: 366–373

Magnetic resonance spectroscopy

18. Magnetic resonance spectroscopy

Dr P. A. Hamilton,
Dr P. Hope and Prof E. O. R. Reynolds

Cerebral haemorrhage and ischaemia are very common causes of death in infants admitted to neonatal intensive care units and of permanent neurodevelopmental disability in those who survive. Haemorrhage, which is particularly prevalent in very pre-term infants, usually arises in the germinal matrix and often spreads into the ventricles. Germinal matrix haemorrhage–intraventricular haemorrhage (GMH–IVH) has been extensively studied by ultrasound imaging and much is now known about its pathogenesis and evolution. Ischaemic injury is more difficult to study: the early changes do not show up on ultrasound scans and although increased ('ischaemic') echodensities appear a day or two after the insult in some infants, the correlation between these echodensities and autopsy-proven ischaemic lesions is poor (Hope et al in press); only much later, when cystic periventricular leukomalacia (PVL) or other loss of brain tissue has developed, does it become certain that serious ischaemic injury has taken place.

Techniques are therefore required which can be used to explore the early changes of ischaemic injury, so that the aetiology and mechanisms involved can be studied, the outcome determined, and methods of prevention and treatment tested. The need for the development of such techniques is currently being brought more sharply into focus by accumulating evidence that birth asphyxia is the most common cause of perinatally acquired permanent neurodevelopmental disability in newborn infants (Alberman 1982), and also that ischaemic injury is a more important cause than GMH–IVH of disabilities in pre-term infants (Stewart et al 1983, de Vries et al 1985, Sinha et al 1985) — who provide the major work-load of any neonatal intensive care unit.

Magnetic resonance spectroscopy is one technique that shows considerable promise for the investigation of ischaemic injury, as well as for exploring a wide range of other normal and abnormal metabolic processes in the brain and other organs of the body.

MAGNETIC RESONANCE SPECTROSCOPY

Magnetic resonance spectroscopy has been established for many years as a valuable analytical technique in laboratory chemistry, but it is only in recent years that studies of animals and human subjects have become feasible (Gadian 1982). This development depended on the production of the large and powerful superconducting magnets that are necessary for the provision of a sufficiently strong and uniform field. The principle depends on the tendency of certain atomic nuclei with magnetic moments (e.g. ^{31}P, ^{1}H, ^{13}C, ^{23}Na, ^{19}F) to line up along the field. This alignment can be disturbed by applying a suitable radiofrequency pulse at right angles to the field. When the pulse ceases the nuclei return to their previous alignment and in so doing emit small magnetic resonance radiofrequency signals which can be detected. The exact frequencies of the signals define the chemical compounds present in the sample or tissue being investigated and the signal intensity is proportional to concentration. In practice, the part of the body to be examined is normally placed within the horizontal bore of the magnet and a succession of radiofrequency pulses is transmitted into the tissue from a surface coil, which also acts as an aerial to detect signals returning from the tissue. The signals are then processed to optimize signal-to-noise ratio and a spectrum is generated. Because the technique is non-invasive and without known hazard (provided care is taken to avoid the presence of ferrous metal near the magnet) it is particularly suited to the study of infants and children.

Magnetic resonance can also be exploited by using the signals from hydrogen atoms to produce an image in a manner analogous to computed X-ray tomography and this is discussed in detail in Chapter 8.

PHOSPHORUS (^{31}P) MAGNETIC RESONANCE SPECTROSCOPY OF THE BRAIN

The atomic nucleus most frequently studied so far in the living organism is phosphorus (^{31}P), which is of particular interest for the investigation of ischaemic injury since the relative concentrations of the mobile phosphorus compounds that are important in energy metabolism can be measured, notably adenosine triphosphate (ATP), phosphocreatine (PCr) and inorganic orthophosphate (Pi); moreover, intracellular pH (pH$_i$) can be calculated from the difference in frequency between the PCr and Pi resonances. In conditions where oxygen supply or utilization is inadequate, alterations in the concentrations of the metabolites and pH$_i$ are to be expected. In particular, as energy failure develops, the concentration of PCr will fall, in order to maintain ATP levels through the creatine kinase reaction, and the concentration of Pi will rise, causing a fall in the PCr/Pi ratio (Fig. 18.1). Later when energy failure is severe the concentration of ATP will also fall.

Following the demonstration that these changes were easy to detect experimentally in the rabbit (Delpy et al 1982), and the development of a transport system which allowed infants to be studied safely (Chu et al 1986), ^{31}P spectra have been obtained at University College London (UCL) from normal full-term and pre-term infants so as to define changes with maturation of the brain. Studies have also been performed on infants who were small for gestational age and infants with a variety of cerebral abnormalities, especially those known or suspected to be associated with ischaemic injury. Similar studies have been performed in Philadelphia (Younkin et al 1984). Full details of the methods used at UCL have been given elsewhere (Cady et al 1983, Hope et al 1984, Hope & Reynolds 1985). Briefly, an Oxford Research Systems TMR 32-200 spectrometer was used, with the infant's head lying on a surface coil designed to supply the exciting radiofrequency pulses and to detect the magnetic resonance signals returning from the infant's brain. Calculations showed that these signals were acquired largely from the adjacent temporo–parietal cortex.

The spectra were usually produced from the sum of 768 pulses obtained over 30 minutes: more recently 256 pulses over 10 minutes have sufficed. The major findings may be summarized as follows.

Normal pre-term and full-term infants

Figure 18.2 shows spectra from two healthy infants without evidence of cerebral abnormalities, one born at 28 weeks of gestation and the other at full-term. Seven peaks can be seen in each spectrum, which are attributable, from left to right, to phosphomonoesters, Pi, phosphodiesters, PCr, and the γ, α and β peaks of magnesium-complexed nucleotide triphosphates, mainly ATP (Gadian 1982). The broad signal underlying the central peaks is due largely to mobile phospholipids (Cerdan et al 1986). The two spectra appear similar except that the PCr peak is larger, and the Pi peak smaller, in the full-term than in the pre-term infant. Absolute concentrations of metabolites cannot at present be calculated from the spectra but concentration ratios are simple to obtain (from the heights of the steps in the integral curve) and the results from studies of 18 infants are given in Table 18.1. It is evident that PCr/Pi increased with maturation of the brain (see also Fig. 18.3). The increase appeared due both to a rise in PCr and a fall in Pi (since PCr/ATP tended to rise and Pi/ATP to fall). Even at full-term, however, PCr/Pi was much lower than expected in adult brain tissue (Bottomley et al 1984). PCr/Pi is related via the creatine kinase reaction to the free-energy change of hydrolysis of ATP and can be regarded as an index of the phosphorylation potential ([ATP]/[ADP][Pi]) or 'energy state' of tissue (Gadian 1982, Tofts & Wray 1985). It appears therefore that this energy state is lower in the pre-term infant than later on in development. A similar maturational change has been found in the newborn rat by Tofts & Wray (1985) who discuss the possible explanations. No significant changes in the other phosphorus metabolite ratios or in pH$_i$ were found (Table 18.1). The trend towards a fall in phosphomonoester/ATP was, however, as expected, since this ratio falls with age in the newborn rat and guinea pig and is low in adult brain tissue in man and other species (Bottomley et al 1984, Tofts & Wray 1985). The main constituent of the phosphomonoester peak is thought to be phosphoethanolamine, which is a major precursor of membrane phospholipid and myelin and is often present in high concentration in rapidly growing tissue (Gyulai et al 1984, Maris et al 1985).

Small-for-gestational-age (SGA) infants

SGA infants are at increased risk of neurodevelopmental disorders. Preliminary studies have been done on eight infants with birth weights below the third centile (weighing 830–1759 g at 30–38 weeks of gestation) to determine whether abnormalities of ^{31}P spectra were present indicating deranged

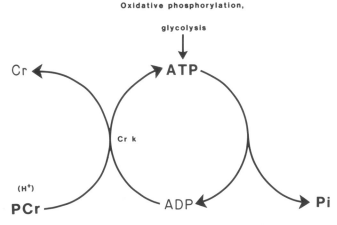

Fig. 18.1 Creatine kinase (Cr k) reaction. Any tendency for the concentration of adenosine triphosphate (ATP) to fall due to inadequate oxidative phosphorylation and glycolysis is buffered by the creatine kinase reaction. The net effect is a fall in the concentration of phosphocreatine (PCr) and a rise in that of inorganic orthophosphate (Pi). ATP, PCr and Pi can be measured by ^{31}P magnetic resonance spectroscopy.

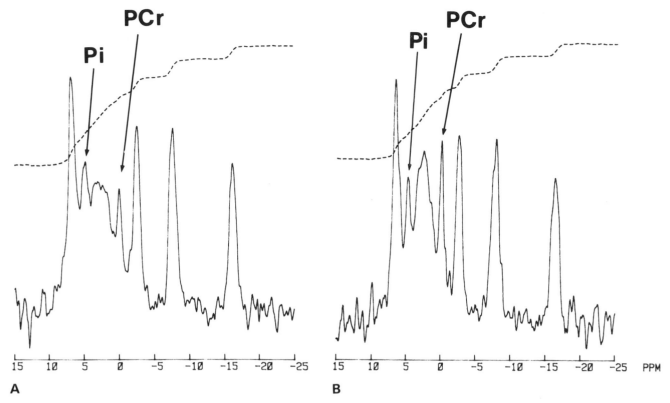

A

B

Fig. 18.2 Phosphorus spectra from two normal infants: (a) born at 28 weeks of gestation and studied 7 days after birth; (b) born at 40 weeks and studied aged 1 day. The x-axis is chemical shift (frequency relative to that of phosphocreatine (PCr), in p.p.m.) and the y-axis is signal intensity: the dashed lines are the integrals of the spectra (concentration is proportional to the height of the steps in the integral curves). The peaks are attributable, from left to right to phosphomonoesters, inorganic orthophosphate (Pi), phosphodiesters, phosphocreatine (PCr), and the γ, α and β phosphorus nuclei of adenosine triphosphate (ATP). The PCr/Pi ratio in the pre-term infant (a) was 0.74 and in the full-term one (b), 1.19. (Data of Hamilton et al 1986a.)

energy metabolism, or changes in the phosphomonoester or phosphodiester regions which might reflect abnormalities in cell synthesis. The infants' perinatal courses were uncomplicated, none had abnormal neurological signs and ultrasound scans of their brains were normal. No evidence was found of any abnormalities in the spectra and pH_i was also normal (Hamilton et al 1986b).

Table 18.1 Changes in phosphorus metabolite concentration ratios and intracellular pH with gestational plus postnatal age in 18 normal infants

	Gestational plus postnatal age (weeks)		
	28	42	r
PCr/Pi	0.77 ± 0.24	1.09 ± 0.24	0.72*
PCr/ATP	0.96 ± 0.39	1.08 ± 0.40	0.22
Pi/ATP	1.22 ± 0.41	1.00 ± 0.41	−0.39
PME/ATP	3.15 ± 1.04	2.67 ± 1.04	−0.34
PDE/ATP	2.20 ± 1.14	2.21 ± 1.15	0.01
ATP/total P	0.095 ± 0.022	0.097 ± 0.022	0.002
pH_i	6.98 ± 0.34	7.11 ± 0.34	0.30

Mean values ± 95% confidence limits from the regressions of metabolite ratios and pH_i on gestational plus postnatal are given. PME = phosphomonoesters; PDE = phosphodiesters; pH_i = intracellular pH.
*$P < 0.001$.
(Data of Hamilton et al 1986.)

Birth asphyxia

Studies of 10 infants who had been severely asphyxiated during delivery (Hope et al 1984) and subsequent experience have shown that the PCr/Pi ratio in brain tissue was often low and sometimes the concentration of ATP was reduced as well, indicating severe energy failure. An example of a ^{31}P spectrum from a birth-asphyxiated infant is shown in Fig. 18.4. Intriguingly, spectra on the first day of life usually proved to be normal: PCr/Pi then progressively fell to minimal values at about 5 days of age and in surviving infants returned to normal by about 2 weeks. Surprisingly, the fall in PCr/Pi was often accompanied by an intracellular alkalosis. The explanation for these changes is by no means clear. Acute cerebral hypoxia or ischaemia in newborn experimental animals causes severe temporary energy failure, and a fall in pH_i due to the production of lactic acid (Hope et al 1987). Recovery takes place over the course of about one hour. We presume that the brains of birth-asphyxiated infants would have shown similar changes if it had been possible to study them during the acute insult and that they were in the phase of recovery from it when the first spectra were obtained. Demands for energy may at this time have been reduced, since the infants were often

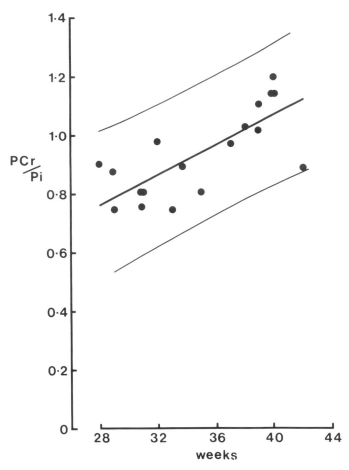

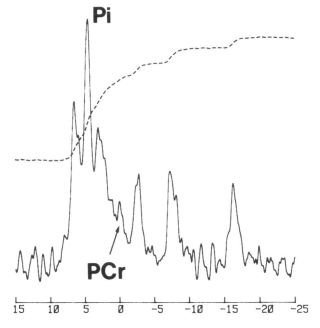

Fig. 18.4 Spectrum from an infant born at 38 weeks of gestation and studied aged 2 days. She had been severely asphyxiated during delivery; the ultrasound scan showed diffuse echodensities. PCr/Pi was very low (0.29) and ATP/total phosphorus was also reduced (0.07). She subsequently died.

Fig. 18.3 Relationship between PCr/Pi ratio and gestational plus postnatal age in 18 normal infants. The regression line and 95% confidence limits are shown. (Data of Hamilton et al 1986a.)

comatose. The subsequent development of 'secondary' energy failure can most readily be accounted for by a progressive increase in the intracellular concentration of adenosine diphosphate (ADP). ADP is normally present in neonatal brain tissue in a concentration of about 25 μmol.l^{-1}, well below the level of detection in ^{31}P spectra. Calculations based on the creatine kinase reaction demonstrate that a two- or three-fold rise in ADP concentration would account for much of the observed fall in PCr/Pi, as shown by Hope et al (1984). The most probable explanations for the rise in ADP concentration are that oxidative phosphorylation had become inadequate due to insufficient oxygen supply to brain tissue or that the mitochondrial respiratory electron transport chain had been damaged. Following asphyxia, oxygen supply can be curtailed by many influences, including capillary endothelial swelling and progressive cerebral oedema (Siesjo 1978). Damage to the electron transport chain could result from mitochondrial disruption due for example to massive calcium entry into cells (Meldrum 1983), or to the toxic action of excitatory neurotransmitters (Schwarcz & Meldrum 1986). The technique of near-infrared spectrophotometry allows measurement in cerebral tissue of the concentrations of oxyhaemoglobin, reduced haemoglobin, and oxidized cytochrome aa_3 — the terminal enzyme of the electron transport chain, which passes the electrons to molecular oxygen (Jobsis 1977, Wyatt et al 1986). Simultaneous observations of ^{31}P spectra and these variables should soon provide information about whether oxygen supply or electron transport is the more deranged in infants with progressive energy failure. Preventive measures and treatment can then be put on a more secure basis.

Periventricular leukomalacia (PVL) and cerebral infarction

PVL is an important cause of brain damage in pre-term infants and is due to hypoxic–ischaemic damage to the periventricular region of the brain. It may be suspected when ultrasound scans show increased echodensities (Nwaesi et al 1984, Levene et al 1985, Trounce et al 1986), although this is neither an invariable nor a reliable finding (Hope et al in press). Fig. 18.5 shows parasagittal scans and ^{31}P spectra from an infant with PVL. The spectrum 3 days after birth was abnormal, with a low PCr/Pi ratio; subsequently periventricular cysts appeared in brain tissue, although the spectrum had by then become normal. Findings in other infants with PVL and cerebral infarction due to arterial obstruction usually demonstrate a similar progression, with the implication that the initiating event often took place close to the time of birth. (See also Chapter 29.)

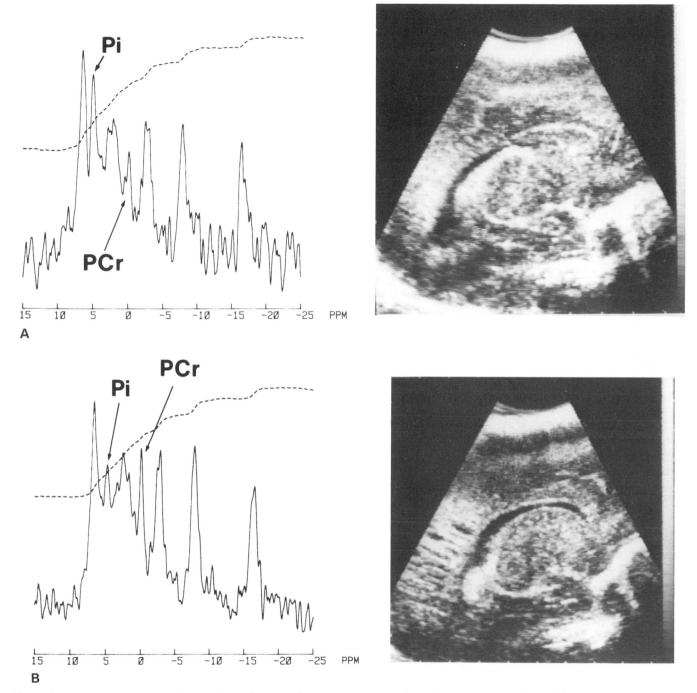

Fig. 18.5 Spectra and parasagittal ultrasound scans from an infant born at 33 weeks of gestation. (**a**) at 3 days of age: PCr/Pi was low, 0.60; the echodensities posterior to the lateral ventricle (left) are consistent with periventricular leukomalacia. (**b**) at 10 days (spectrum) and 20 days (scan). PCr/Pi was normal, 0.85; the scan shows periventricular cysts. (Data of Hamilton et al 1986.)

Congenital abnormalities and inborn errors of metabolism

Studies of infants with a variety of congenital abnormalities have revealed no abnormalities of ^{31}P spectra or pH_i. Two infants with organic acidurias were found to have very gross energy failure, possibly due to interference with the tricarboxylic acid cycle (Hope & Reynolds 1985). In the future, with the introduction of ^1H and ^{13}C spectroscopy,

it is likely that much will be learnt about the pathogenesis and treatment of inborn errors of metabolism.

Prognosis

Two studies have been done to find out whether ^{31}P spectra provide useful prognostic information; firstly, a study of infants with cerebral 'ischaemic' echodensities, and secondly, an investigation of the relationship between the magnetic resonance data and early neurodevelopmental outcome in 65 infants who had reached an age of at least one year.

Infants with 'ischaemic' echodensities

Certain patterns of increased echodensity detected by ultrasound scanning are often attributed to ischaemic injury (Levene et al 1985, Trounce et al 1986). However, an autopsy study has shown that false-positive and false-negative ultrasound diagnoses of ischaemic damage are very common (Hope et al 1988). A magnetic resonance study was therefore undertaken to investigate whether evidence of impaired energy metabolism was detectable in the brains of infants with increased echodensities and, if so, whether infants with a particularly bad prognosis could be identified (Hamilton et al 1986). Only infants whose echodensities appeared consistent with ischaemic injury were studied; infants with very marked echodensities that were attributable largely to blood in brain tissue (and are often due to venous infarction associated with GMH–IVH, Gould et al 1987) were not included; nor were infants whose echodensities persisted for less than 48 hours. Of 27 infants selected for study, 14 had diffuse bilateral echodensities, usually associated with birth asphyxia; 10 had echodensities consistent with PVL; and 3 had echodensities consistent with major arterial infarctions. The infants were

mostly severely ill but 3 appeared clinically normal. In some infants, ^{31}P spectra obtained soon after the echodensities appeared were normal (Fig. 18.6) and others showed a reduced PCr/Pi ratio and sometimes a reduced ATP level as well (Figs 18.4–18.7). Ultrasound scanning was continued in the surviving infants and the development of cerebral atrophy, defined as cysts or other loss of brain tissue, which carried a bad prognosis, was noted. Fig. 18.8 shows that low values for PCr/Pi were strongly associated with death or cerebral atrophy. The difference in adverse outcome between infants whose PCr/Pi ratios were in the normal range and those with ratios below it was highly significant ($P < 0.001$). The results of this study showed that the immediate prognosis for infants with increased echodensities whose PCr/Pi ratios were reduced was much worse than among infants whose ratios lay within the normal range.

Magnetic resonance data and early neurodevelopmental outcome

The progress of a heterogeneous group of 65 infants studied in the first week of life by ^{31}P spectroscopy because of definite or possible cerebral abnormalities has been assessed at one year of age (Reynolds & Hamilton in press). Their neonatal diagnosis included convulsions, asphyxia, polycythaemia, inborn errors of metabolism, meningitis, hydrocephalus, and abnormalities detected by ultrasound. All had repeated neurodevelopmental testing using methods that have been described elsewhere (Stewart

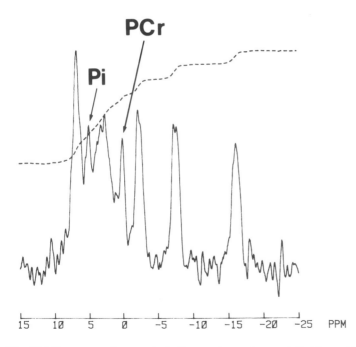

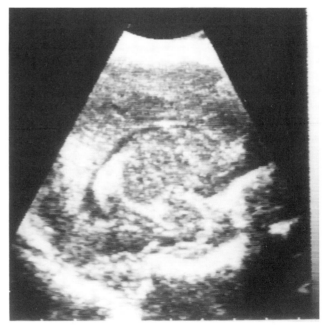

Fig. 18.6 Spectrum and parasagittal ultrasound scan from an infant born at 32 weeks of gestation and studied 8 days after birth. The scan shows echodensities very similar to those in Fig. 18.5 but PCr/Pi was normal (0.84) and no cysts or other evidence of cerebral atrophy developed. (Data of Hamilton et al 1986a.)

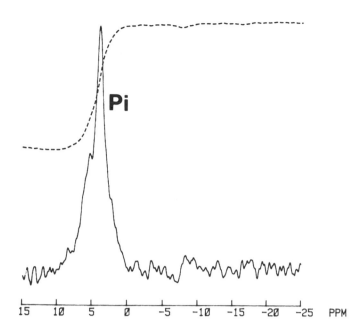

Fig. 18.7 Spectrum from an infant born at 27 weeks of gestation and studied aged 8 days. He had suffered an extremely severe asphyxial episode aged 5 days; PCr and ATP were virtually absent. He subsequently died. (Data of Hamilton et al 1986a.)

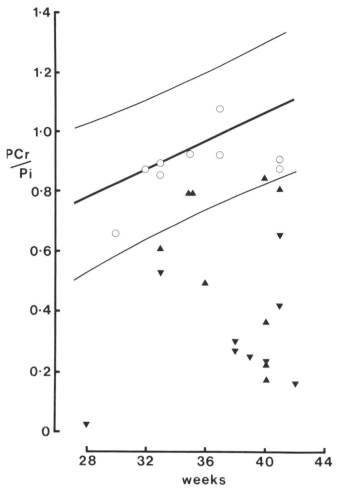

Fig. 18.8 PCr/Pi ratios from 27 infants with increased cerebral echodensities. The regression line and 95% confidence limits from normal infants (Fig. 18.3) are shown for comparison. ○ survived without cerebral atrophy; ▲ survived with cerebral atrophy; ▼ died. (Data of Hamilton et al 1986a.)

et al 1983). Outcome is related in Table 18.2 to the lowest PCr/Pi ratio recorded. It can be seen that infants whose ratios were low were much more likely to die or to suffer cerebral palsy with a low GQ than infants whose ratios were normal ($P < 0.001$).

CONCLUSIONS

Magnetic resonance spectroscopy is a valuable non-invasive technique for exploring cerebral energy metabolism in newborn infants. The major findings so far may be summarized as follows;

1. In normal infants spectral peaks were detectable from adenosine triphosphate (ATP), phosphocreatine (PCr), inorganic orthophosphate (Pi), phosphodiesters and phosphomonoesters. Brain intracellular pH (derived

Table 18.2 PCr/Pi ratio and early neurodevelopmental outcome in 65 infants

	Died	Cerebral palsy		Normal
		GQ[a] <85	GQ >85	
PCr/Pi				
Normal ($n = 42$)	5	6	8	23
Low[b] ($n = 23$)	16	5	1	1

[a]General quotient (Griffiths 1954).
[b]Below 95% confidence limits (Fig. 18.3).

from the frequencies of the PCr and Pi peaks) was about 7.1. Systematic changes took place during gestation in the concentrations of some of the phosphorus metabolites, indicating an increasing phosphorylation potential and a reduction in the concentration of phosphomonoester (probably phosphoethanolamine). Findings in healthy infants who were small-for-gestational-age appeared no different from those in infants who were appropriately grown.

2. Evidence of energy failure (impaired oxidative phosphorylation) was found in the brains of infants with a variety of conditions of suspected or proven hypoxic–ischaemic injury, including birth asphyxia, periventricular leukomalacia and cerebral infarction. Following birth asphyxia, there was often a period of some hours before energy failure developed, suggesting the possibility of effective early treatment.

3. Certain inborn errors of metabolism caused very gross energy failure.

4. Evidence of severe energy failure was closely associated with subsequent death, loss of brain tissue and poor neurodevelopmental progress.

In the future, spectroscopy of other atomic nuclei, especially protons (^{1}H) for measuring lactate and amino acids (such as GABA), and ^{13}C for studying metabolic pathways, seem certain to provide further important information about intracellular metabolism in the brains and other organs of newborn infants and older individuals. The combination of magnetic resonance imaging with spectroscopy, which is possible with the newest machines, will allow spectra to be obtained from selected regions within organs.

ACKNOWLEDGEMENTS

We thank Mr R. Aldridge, Mr E. B. Cady, Dr A. M. de L. Costello, Mr D. T. Delpy, Dr Ann L. Stewart, Prof D. R. Wilkie, F.R.S. and Dr J. S. Wyatt, with whom this work was performed, and the staff of the Neonatal Unit and Department of Medical Physics and Bioengineering. Supported by grants from the MRC, DHSS, the National Fund for Research into Crippling Diseases, the Muscular Dystrophy Group and the Wellcome Trust.

REFERENCES

Alberman E D 1982 The epidemiology of congenital defects: a pragmatic approach. In: Adinolfi M et al (eds) Paediatric research: a genetic approach. SIMP Heinemann, London, pp 1–28

Bottomley P A, Hart H R, Edelstein W A et al 1984 Anatomy and metabolism of the normal human brain studied by magnetic resonance at 1.5 tesla. Radiology 150: 441–446

Cady E B, Costello A M de L, Dawson M J et al 1983 Non-invasive investigation of cerebral energy metabolism in newborn infants by phosphorus nuclear magnetic resonance spectroscopy. Lancet i: 1059–1062

Cerdan S, Subramanian H, Hilberman M et al 1986 ^{31}P NMR detection of mobile dog brain phospholipids. Magnetic Resonance in Medicine 3: 432–439

Chu A, Delpy D T, Thalayasingam S 1986 A transport and life support system for newborn infants during NMR spectroscopy. In: Rolfe P (ed) Neonatal physiological measurements. Butterworth, London, pp 409–415

Delpy D T, Gordon R E, Hope P L et al 1982 Noninvasive investigation of cerebral ischaemia by phosphorus nuclear magnetic resonance. Pediatrics 70: 310–313

de Vries L S, Dubowitz L M S, Dubowitz V et al 1985 Predictive value of cranial ultrasound in the newborn baby: a reappraisal. Lancet ii: 1154–1156

Gadian D G 1982 Nuclear magnetic resonance and its applications to living systems. Clarendon, Oxford

Gould S J, Howard S, Hope P L, Reynolds E O R 1987 Periventricular intraparenchymal cerebral haemorrhage in preterm infants: the role of venous infarction. Journal of Pathology 151: 197–202

Griffiths R 1954 The abilities of babies. University of London Press, London

Gyulai L, Bolinger L, Leigh J S, Barlow C, Chance B 1984 Phosphorylethanolamine — the major constituent of the phosphomonoester peak observed by ^{31}P-NMR in the developing dog brain. FEBS Letters 178: 137–142

Hamilton P A, Hope P L, Cady E B, Delpy D T, Wyatt J S, Reynolds E O R 1986a Impaired energy metabolism in the brains of newborn infants with increased cerebral echodensities. Lancet i: 1242–1246

Hamilton P A, Hope P L, Cady E B, Delpy D T, Wyatt J S, Reynolds E O R 1986b Phosphorus metabolites and intracellular pH in the brains of normal and growth retarded infants. Proceedings of the Society for Magnetic Resonance in Medicine, Fifth annual meeting, Montreal, pp 295–296

Hope P L, Reynolds E O R 1985 Investigation of cerebral energy metabolism in newborn infants by phosphorus nuclear magnetic resonance spectroscopy. Clinics in Perinatology 12: 261–275

Hope P L, Costello A M de L, Cady E B et al 1984 Cerebral energy metabolism studied with NMR spectroscopy in normal and birth asphyxiated infants. Lancet ii: 336–339

Hope P L, Gould S J, Hamilton P A, Costello A M de L, Reynolds E O R 1986 Precision of ultrasound diagnosis of pathologically verified lesions in the brains of very preterm infants. Developmental Medicine and Child Neurology (in press)

Hope P L, Cady E B, Chu A C M, Delpy D T, Gardiner, R M, Reynolds E O R 1987 Brain metabolism and intracellular pH during ischaemia and hypoxia: an in vivo ^{31}P and ^{1}H nuclear magnetic resonance study in the lamb. Journal of Neurochemistry 49: 75–82

Jobsis F F 1977 Noninvasive monitoring of cerebral and myocardial oxygen sufficiency and circulatory parameters. Science 198: 1264–1267

Levene M I, Williams J L, Fawer C-L 1985 Ultrasound of the infant brain. SIMP Blackwell, Oxford

Maris J M, Evans A E, McLaughlin A C et al 1985 ^{31}P nuclear magnetic resonance spectroscopic investigation of human neuroblastoma in situ. New England Journal of Medicine 312: 1500–1505

Meldrum B S 1983 Metabolic factors during prolonged seizures and their relation to nerve cell death. Advances in Neurology 34: 261–275

Nwaesi C G, Pape K E, Martin D J, Becker L E, Fitz C R 1984 Periventricular infarction diagnosed by ultrasound: a postmortem correlation. Journal of Pediatrics 105: 106–110

Reynolds E O R, Hamilton P A 1987 Magnetic resonance spectroscopy of the brain and early neurodevelopmental outcome. In: Kubli F, Patel N, Schmidt W, Linderkamp O (eds) Perinatal events and brain damage in surviving children. Springer-Verlag, Berlin, pp 245–253

Schwarcz R, Meldrum B 1986 Excitatory amino acid antagonists provide a therapeutic approach to neurological disorders. Lancet ii: 140–143

Siesjo B K 1978 Brain energy metabolism. Wiley, Chichester

Sinha S K, Davies J M, Sims D G, Chiswick M L 1985 Relation between periventricular haemorrhage and ischaemic brain lesions diagnosed by ultrasound in very preterm infants. Lancet ii: 1154–1156

Stewart A L, Thorburn R J, Hope P L, Goldsmith M, Lipscomb A P, Reynolds E O R 1983 Ultrasound appearance of the brain in very preterm infants and neurodevelopmental outcome at 18 months of age. Archives of Disease in Childhood 58: 598–604

Tofts P, Wray S 1985 Changes in brain phosphorus metabolites during the post-natal development of the rat. Journal of Physiology 359: 417–429

Trounce J Q, Fagan D, Levene M I 1986 Intraventricular haemorrhage and periventricular leucomalacia: ultrasound and autopsy correlation. Archives of Disease in Childhood 61: 1203–1207

Wyatt J S, Cope M, Delpy D T, Wray S, Reynolds E O R 1986 Quantification of cerebral oxygenation and haemodynamics in sick newborn infants by near infrared spectrophotometry. Lancet ii: 1063–1066

Younkin D P, Delivoria-Papadopoulos M, Leonard J et al 1984 Unique aspects of human newborn cerebral metabolism evaluated with phosphorus nuclear magnetic resonance spectroscopy. Annals of Neurology 16: 581–586

PART 3

Management

Developmental abnormalities

Structural abnormalities of the developing brain may occur as the result of an abnormality in development (malformation) or be due to an external influence which damages the brain at some stage in its development. These may be vascular, infectious or toxic and may produce anatomical and/or functional effects. Major malformations of the developing brain are reviewed in Chapter 19 and the genetic implications of many of these conditions are discussed in Chapter 20. The effects of vascular, infections and toxic insults on structural brain development are reviewed elsewhere but the functional effects of teratogens on the developing brain are discussed in Chapter 21. The diagnosis of developmental abnormalities in the fetus and newborn are considered in Section 2. The most common major developmental abnormality of the brain is a neural tube disorder. In view of the particular nature of this group of conditions it is considered as a separate entity in Section 8.

19. Congenital developmental malformations

Prof G. Lyon and Dr A. Beaugerie

Congenital malformations of the brain are among the most important and common disorders apparent at birth or detected within the first year of life. Most malformations can be appreciated on the basis of a clear understanding of the development of the central nervous system (CNS). In this process, the end of the fifth fetal month can be considered a turning point in the development of the fetal brain (Evrard et al 1984, Lyon et al 1984). Abnormalities in development can be conveniently divided into malformations which arise before 20 weeks of gestational age, and those occurring after this time. Although CNS development is described in detail in Part 1 of this book, some aspects relevant to the understanding of congenital malformations will be reiterated here.

During the first 20 weeks of fetal life, the neural tube closes and the telencephalic vesicles are formed. Nerve cells are generated in the germinal matrix, adjacent to the intracerebral cavities, and migrate to their final position. The majority of authors agree that in most areas of the telencephalic and cerebellar cortex the neuronal guidance is "gliophilic", although this view has been challenged. (See page 12 for a review). In the telencephalon, young neurones migrate along radial glial fibres (Rakic 1972, Gadisseux & Evrard 1985) from the ventricular and subventricular zones to their final sites in the cortical plate. The oldest cells in the cortex occupy layer I (Cajal-Retzius cells) and the innermost layer of the developing cortex (subplate, layer VII) (Marin-Padilla 1983). Neurones generated later occupy successively more superficial positions in the interval between the two primitive layers (Angevine & Sidman 1961, Rakic 1982). Neurones forming layer VI and V of the mature cortex are formed first and those which will constitute layer II are the last to migrate. This inside-out pattern of cortical formation has important implications for the interpretation of telencephalic developmental disorders.

Disorders affecting the brain during this period are either genetically determined or acquired. The morphological changes will affect:

1. The organogenesis of the brain, i.e. the separation of the telencephalon into two hemispheres, the formation of the corpus callosum and other interhemispheric commissures, the optic vesicles, the olfactory tracts.
2. The formation of neurones in the ventricular zone, and/or their migration in the cortical plate, resulting in a reduction of the overall neuronal population (developmental microcephaly) and/or an abnormality in the final position (heterotopias), and in the tangential and radial arrangement of cortical neurones.

The last trimester of pregnancy is a period of intense neuronal maturation and growth. Multiple synaptic contacts are established. Glial cells are formed in great number and multiply actively. Myelination starts in some areas. Secondary and tertiary cortical gyri appear and brain volume increases markedly. Developmental abnormalities result essentially from acquired, destructive processes, of ischaemic haemorrhagic and infectious origin, which may be limited to the cortex (microgyria) or involve a large part of the brain (porencephaly, hydranencephaly).

Fetal intoxications (especially alcohol) and probably also viral infections, endocrine disorders and genetically determined diseases may also act more subtly on cellular growth, synaptogenesis and neuronal function to give rise to moderate microcephalies and mental retardation.

It should be remembered that most inborn errors of metabolism with the notable exception of Zellweger's disease, do not affect the fetal brain to such a degree as to cause a prenatal developmental defect because of the total or partial protection of the fetus by the mother's enzymatic machinery. The typical example is that of phenylketonuria.

DISORDERS OF THE FIRST 20 WEEKS

Brain malformations dating from this period are numerous. Only the most frequent and well-defined entities, which are recognizable during life, are considered here.

A definitive categorization of all developmental abnormalities of the brain, particularly of the cerebral cortex, during this period is not feasible. Numerous morphological variations are apt to arise, depending both on the nature and time of action of the pathogenic agent. One is, however, justified in delineating some major types (see Table 19.1). For each of them, the chronology and in some instances the mechanism of the disorder can be deduced from a careful morphological analysis.

We are, however, still far from understanding clearly their pathophysiology. At the present state of our knowledge, only a few developmental abnormalities dating from this period of fetal life, are undoubtedly due to a single gene defect. A genetically determined hereditary disorder is unquestionable in Zellweger's disease, very probable in some of the developmental microcephalies and Fukuyama's disease, and possible in some lissencephalies and arhinencephalies. Different causes may combine to produce the same developmental change (for instance in the arhinencephalies and type I lissencephaly). On the other hand, a specific metabolic disorder, Zellweger's disease, results in stereotyped, constant, multifocal changes in the brain. To add to the complexity of the aetiological problem the familial occurrence of some developmental disorders may be related to entirely different mechanisms, including a single gene defect, a chromosomal aberration with a balanced translocation in one parent, and possibly a persistent maternal viral infection.

It is now possible, with modern imaging techniques, to detect many developmental abnormalities during life, and new refinements will increase the accuracy of in-vivo

Table 19.1 Classification of the congenital brain malformations occurring in the first 20 weeks of gestation (neural tube defects are considered separately in Section 7)

Abnormalities of telencephalic division
  Arhinencephaly–holoprosencephaly
    Alobar
    Lobar
    Isolated arhinencephaly
  Agenesis of the corpus callosum
  Atrophy of the corpus callosum
  Septo–optic dysplasia
Abnormalities of neurogenesis
  Microcephaly
    Primary
      Microcephalia vera
      Autosomal dominant form
    Secondary
Disorders of neuronal migration
  Lissencephaly
    Type I (Bielschowsky)
    Type II (Walker-Warburg)
    Others
  Periventricular heterotopia
  Hypermigration
Microdysgenesis
Cerebellar disorders
  Disorders of the vermis
    Dandy–Walker malformation
    Joubert' disease
  Cerebellar hypoplasia/aplasia
Developmental megalencephalies

morphological analysis (Ch. 7). A clue may also be given by associated, more or less specific, facial dysmorphias as is the case in arhinencephaly and classical lissencephaly. There is, however, no constant relationship between somatic and cerebral changes and the syndromes described in the literature are subject to many variations. For a given brain malformation, abnormal facial features may or may not be present, are frequently non-specific, and for a given constellation of facial abnormalities, the cerebral defects may vary quite widely.

Despite these uncertainties, much progress has been made recently in the understanding of early brain malformations. Different factors have contributed to this clarification, among which are a better knowledge of the normal development of the cerebral and cerebellar cortex, occasional but very useful studies of developmental anomalies in the human fetus, improvement in brain imaging techniques and finally experiments in animals using teratogenic agents such as X-rays, methylazoxymethanol, 6-hydroxydopamine, and parvoviruses. Unfortunately, no animal mutant is available for the dynamic study of human telencephalic malformations. The cortical abnormality in the reeler mutant mouse is unique (Caviness 1982) but of little practical value for the understanding of human disease.

ABNORMALITIES IN TELENCEPHALIC DIVISION AND COMMISSURAL FORMATION

Arhinencephaly–Holoprosencephaly

This condition is characterized by a profound anomaly in hemispheric cleavage, an absence of olfactory tracts and bulbs, and usually a partial fusion of the basal ganglia. There are various degrees (Yakovlev 1959, Robain & Gorce 1972, Friede 1975).

In its major form, 'alobar holoprosencephaly', the brain forms an undivided monoventricular mass, closed posteriorly by a membrane, which is usually distended by a large cyst. There may be stenosis of the aqueduct of Sylvius. The optic chiasm is atrophic and the eyes are close to the midline, or there may be cyclopia. The abnormal cortical cyto-architecture resembles that of the allocortex.

In 'lobar holoprosencephaly', the anterior part of the brain is undivided and monoventricular but a shallow sagittal fissure exists posteriorly with normal temporo–occipital horns. The cortical cyto-architecture does not show major changes (Fig. 19.1). Finally, arhinencephaly may consist only in the absence of olfactory tract and bulbs.

Clinical features

In its major form, alobar holoprosencephaly, this condition is associated with typical facial anomalies. These include extreme hypotelorism or even cyclopia, a flat nose or a nasal-like tubular appendix (proboscis) protruding above or

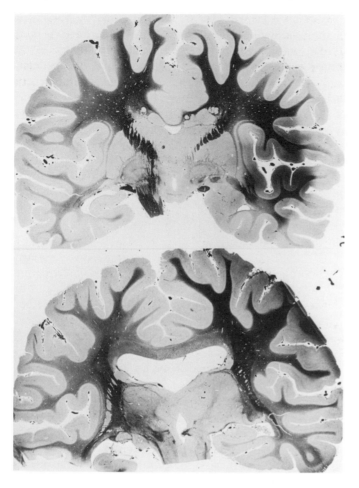

Fig. 19.1 Prosencephaly in a 12-year-old boy with mental retardation, hypotelorism and anosmia. Two coronal sections stained for myelin showing an undivided ventricular cavity in the antero–superior part of the brain. The temporal horns are well differentiated. There is an incomplete interhemispheric fissure anteriorly and partial fusion of the thalami with absence of the olfactory tracts. The cortex is normal.

and the only abnormalities are hypotelorism and anosmia. These are often clinically unsuspected, unless the interorbital distance is measured on a skull X-ray or the sense of smell is tested systematically in mentally retarded children. Otherwise, in the 'formes frustes', the diagnosis of arhinencephaly comes as an unexpected finding on the CT scan in a child with mental retardation.

Aetiology

The incidence of arhinencephaly is about 1/5000 live births and is much higher among spontaneous abortuses. Most cases of holoprosencephaly are sporadic and their cause is unknown. Many patients are born into families of low socio-economic status. There are no known environmental teratogens in man but in animals the condition can be induced by a variety of chemical agents. Holoprosencephaly is not infrequently associated with a trisomy-13 syndrome and more rarely with a deletion of the short arm of chromosome 18 or other chromosomal aberrations.

It may occur among siblings and has been found in monozygotic twins. The affected siblings may have different facial abnormalities. In one of our families, one child had a cleft palate, trigonocephaly, hypotelorism and mental retardation, while the other only had mental retardation and hypotelorism. An autosomal recessive mode of inheritance is probable in some families. An autosomal dominant mode of inheritance has been reported more rarely (Burck 1982). In such instances, the affected parent has a 'form fruste' of the disease which may be easily overlooked when not searched for specifically. Whether severe forms, without chromosomal aberration, represent new mutations of a dominant gene is open to question. It should be noted that mental retardation and other neurological abnormalities are frequently found in the families of sporadic cases.

Isolated agenesis of olfactory tracts (olfactory aplasia)

Absence of olfactory tracts and bulbs, without other brain malformation, is the cause of anosmia in otherwise normal or mentally retarded children. It may represent the mildest form of arhinencephaly. In the X-linked Kallman's syndrome, anosmia is associated with hypogonadism and mental retardation. Another syndrome characterized by anosmia, ichthyosis and hypogonadism is transmitted as an autosomal recessive trait (Esterlyn 1968).

Agenesis of the corpus callosum

Neuropathology and pathophysiology

The formation of the corpus callosum starts during the 16th week of gestation. It has been shown in various animals including primates, that callosal neurones and callosal projections to the contralateral hemisphere undergo a pro-

between the orbits, a cleft lip and cleft palate. Microcephaly is usual but the presence of aqueductal stenosis may lead to hydrocephalus with marked dilatation of the posterior membrane and head enlargement. Transillumination of the posterior half of the skull is remarkable in these cases.

Skeletal, cardiac and other developmental abnormalities may be present. Evidence of hypothalamo–pituitary dysfunction may exist (diabetes insipidus, chronic hypernatremia). The condition is rapidly lethal, although some children survive for several months.

In minor forms of arhinencephaly, children present with mental retardation and lesser facial dysmorphias including hypotelorism (reduction of the interpupillary distance and of the interorbital distance on skull X-rays), trigonocephaly, and cleft palate. Anosmia is always present. In infants it can theoretically be detected by the failure to block α rhythm on an EEG tracing when the child inhales pyridine, a non-irritant product with a strong odour.

In some cases, facial features are quite uncharacteristic

gressive reorganisation, changing from an early widespread distribution within the tangential plane, to a more limited mature distribution. The restriction of axonal projections appears to be due to the selective elimination of early formed callosal collaterals, without accompanying death of neurones. In primates, callosal neurones are confined to the IIIrd cortical layer and to a lesser degree to layer V and VI in certain regions within the plane of the cortex (for references see Stanfield 1984 and Schwartz & Goldman-Rakic 1982).

Agenesis of the corpus callosum is a common condition and is due to failure of a relatively normal complement of callosal fibres to cross the midline in the 'massa commisuralis' but instead course caudally, condensed in a thick longitudinal bundle (Probs't bundle), beneath the cingulum and above the fornix (Fig. 19.10). The septum pellucidum is absent. The so called 'agenesis' of the corpus callosum is in fact a failure of commissuration (Rakic & Yakovlev 1968) (Fig. 19.2). As a result of this defect, the third ventricle ascends dorsally towards the interhemispheric fissure, the frontal horns of the lateral ventricles are displaced laterally, narrowed, often with a concave medial profile, and the occipital portion of the lateral ventricle is enlarged, probably because of the absence of the posterior fibres of the corpus callosum and the narrowing of the anterior part or the lateral ventricles. The pericallosal sulcus and other sulci of the medial aspect of the hemisphere which normally run longitudinally above the corpus callosum are replaced by radially oriented sulci.

The anterior commissure and the hippocampal com-

missure are generally absent, and there may be hypoplasia of the pyramidal tracts, suggesting in some cases a more diffuse developmental defect of projection fibres in the central nervous system. The pathophysiology of this defect is obscure. It can be postulated that exogenous or genetic factors act to force callosal fibres to change their polarity of growth.

Agenesis of the corpus callosum is either an isolated abnormality or part of a more complex developmental encephalopathy. The callosal defect may be partial, involving preferentially the posterior part of the commissure. Exceptionally it is associated with a midline interhemispheric lipoma.

Clinical features

The morphological characteristics of agenesis of the corpus callosum are easily demonstrated on the CT scan and on prenatal or postnatal ultrasound scans. The latter method and magnetic resonance imaging show nicely the abnormal vertical sulci of the medial part of the hemisphere (see Fig. 8.5, p. 126). This finding is important to differentiate in the fetus a callosal defect from a fetal hydrocephalus; a condition in which there is also, at least initially, a dilatation of the posterior part of the lateral ventricles.

An isolated agenesis can exist in perfectly normal individuals. Perceptual abnormalities resulting from the absence of an interhemispheric transport of information observed after postnatal section of the corpus callosum are usually, however, detectable.

In many cases of apparently isolated agenesis of the corpus callosum, mental retardation is present and not unusually there are minor somatic malformations, such as hypertelorism, ocular abnormalities, cleft palate, and malformation of digits. Malformations and mental retardation may also be found in members of the family.

The discovery of the condition in a child with mental retardation strongly suggests the prenatal origin of the mental insufficiency but genetic counselling in these cases is difficult. The great majority of cases are sporadic but when agenesis of the corpus callosum and mental retardation are both present, the latter may recur in the sibship without the commissural defect.

Familial cases have been reported with a possible autosomal recessive or X-linked recessive mode of inheritance (Menkes et al 1964). In certain familial cases, episodes of hypothermia have been observed (Pineda & Gonzalez 1984).

Agenesis of the corpus callosum is also a more or less constant element of a number of complex developmental syndromes and these are discussed in Chapter 20.

Familial atrophy of the corpus callosum

Isolated or familial cases of extreme atrophy of the corpus callosum and cerebral white matter have been reported

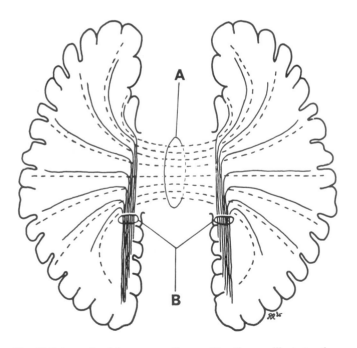

Fig. 19.2 Agenesis of the corpus callosum. The diagram illustrates the failure of commissuration. Instead of crossing the midline (A dashed lines), the fibres of the corpus callosum form abnormal longitudinal bundles (B solid lines). (Reproduced with permission from Rakic & Yakovlev 1968.)

in the literature (Chattha & Richardson 1977). Extreme atrophy is frequently familial whereas agenesis is usually sporadic.

We have studied two siblings with extreme atrophy (not absence) of the commissural fibres of the corpus callosum as well as atrophy of the hemispheric white matter, degeneration of subcortical axons, absence of pyramids, cataracts and myopathy. The radiological appearance was that of agenesis except for the presence of a normal supracallosal sulcus. In this familial disease the diffuse involvement of projection fibres in the brain, could represent an exaggeration of the normal phenomenon of restriction and degeneration of axonal collaterals in the corpus callosum and other cerebral tracts during development (Lyon et al in prep.). Another example of extreme atrophy of the corpus callosum is illustrated in Fig. 19.3.

Septo-optic dysplasia

Septo-optic dysplasia (SOD) was first described by the pathologist de Morsier and is sometimes referred to as the de Morsier syndrome. It is a rare sporadic condition characterized by defects of the anterior prosencephalic structures, particularly the septum pellucidum, bilateral optic nerve hypoplasia and varying degrees of pituitary insufficiency (Landrieu & Evrard 1979). Developmental abnormalities reported under this denomination are, however, so variable that their specificity can be questioned. In a review of

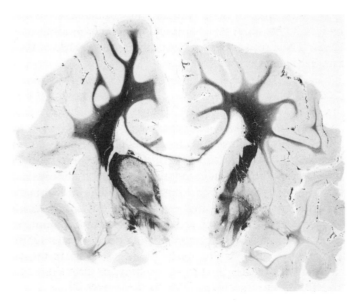

Fig. 19.3 Familial atrophy of the corpus callosum in a 6-month-old infant with severe mental retardation and a brother who has the same disease. Coronal section of the brain (myelin stain) shows marked atrophy of the corpus callosum and cingulum. The supracallosal sulcus is present. Morphology of the frontal horns and third ventricle is as in agenesis of the corpus callosum. (Courtesy of Drs C Allaire and J Journel.)

published cases in whom CT or pneumo-encephalographic data were available, 60% of 178 patients were found to have cerebral abnormalities. These were mainly midline defects of the septum pellucidum, corpus callosum and/or basal ganglia, but hydrocephalus, cerebral atrophy, cerebellar hypoplasia and porencephaly were also described in more than one case (Morishima & Aranoff 1986). Of the patients with bilateral optic nerve hypoplasia who had evaluation of pituitary function (145 cases), 62% had evidence of pituitary insufficiency. This ranged from the isolated deficiency of one hormone to panhypopituitarism. Only 30% of cases had the three features of optic nerve hypoplasia, hypopituitarism and midline cerebral defects.

ABNORMALITIES OF NEUROGENESIS

Microcephaly

Primary developmental microcephalies

Any acquired disorder of the developing brain may result in a stunting of its growth. A microcephaly* may also be the consequence of a primary genetically determined abnormality of brain development. We will consider these primary developmental microcephalies in some detail (Robain & Lyon 1972, Lyon et al 1984).

In these conditions, the reduction in brain volume is the result of a numerical reduction of the final population of telencephalic neurones. This may occur because of an insufficiency in the production of neurones or, less probably, by an exaggeration of the normal phenomenon of spontaneous cell death, which serves normally as a regulatory mechanism to determine the final cell population in the central nervous system. An arrest of cell growth probably also plays a role. Primary developmental microcephalies constitute a heterogeneous group.

Microcephalia vera. One clinical entity stands out, for which we reserve the term microcephalia vera. This condition can be defined as an autosomal recessive inherited disorder (or group of disorders) exclusively characterized by a marked congenital microcephaly with mental retardation, in the absence of any motor or sensory deficit. Fine motor skills are normal and there is no dysmorphic or other extraneurological abnormality. The intellectual deficit is severe but these children are usually pleasant and sociable. Life expectancy is not significantly affected. The brain has a normal appearance on CT scans. The syndrome may be genetically heterogeneous. Its cause is unknown.

There are few good neuropathological studies (Norman 1958). The convolutional pattern is simplified but not disrupted, the ventricular and commissural systems are

*The word microcephaly is used to designate a small brain (micrencephaly) as well as a small skull.

normal. Changes in the cortex are slight. An excessive vertical columnization of the superficial part of the cortex and an apparent reduction of layers II and III are usually reported. In one case there was a premature disappearance of the periventricular matrix zone in a 26-week-old fetus (Evrard et al 1984).

As a practical conclusion any child with a major congenital isolated microcephaly and a normal CT scan can be classified in the provisional group of microcephalia vera and the parents should be informed of the risk of an autosomal recessive inherited disease.

As for other developmental abnormalities, prenatal diagnosis of microcephalia vera is usually not possible before the 20th week of pregnancy (Lyon & Evrard 1987).

Other types of primary developmental microcephalies are associated with facial dysmorphia, and various neuro-sensorial or visceral defects. They may be related to chromosomal abnormalities, or be an element in specific sporadic or hereditary malformation syndromes. A quite different entity consists in a dominant form of microcephaly (head circumference between 3 and 7 standard deviations below the mean with normal intelligence (see Ch. 20).

Microbrains. We have studied seven neonates born at full-term with a normal body weight and length, who died shortly after birth, and whose brains weighed between 16 and 50 g, i.e. 7 to 20 times less than normal. Except for acromicria in one neonate and a congenital nephropathy in another, there was no other significant abnormality and the cause of death could not been determined. Two cases were in one sibship.

There was no evidence of destructive brain lesions. The gyral pattern was somewhat simplified and the cyto-architecture of the cerebral cortex and other grey matter structures was normal. There was a marked overall reduction (up to 30%) in the number of cortical neurones. As the number of neurones in each vertical column was normal, it was thought that the extreme microcephaly was the consequence of a reduction in the number of adjacent verticular columns ('radial microbrains') (Evrard 1986). Microbrains are very rare and have probably more than one cause but it should be known that they may be familial. They provide the demonstration that during brain development the mechanisms that control neurogenesis and migration, may be completely independent.

Secondary microcephalies of prenatal origin

In this situation, microcephaly may be detected in the last weeks of pregnancy or the head circumference is normal at birth and microcephaly develops after several weeks or months. Such secondary microcephalies result from acquired prenatal infections, ischaemia, endocrine disturbances, toxic or traumatic disorders, or are related to chromosomal aberrations or genetic diseases, such as phenylketonuria and lysosomal disorders. In most of the inherited metabolic con-ditions, the mother provides a complete or partial protection against the enzymatic defect, whose adverse consequences on the brain appear only after birth. A prenatal viral infection may also be responsible for secondary microcephaly. This is the case for HIV (AIDS) encephalitis (see Ch. 36), and possibly for the syndrome of basal ganglia calcification, brain atrophy and permanent lymphocytosis (Goutières & Aicardi 1982), which is probably due to a persistent viral infection.

Finally, some of the secondary microcephalies remain of unknown origin. It is possible that, as yet, undeter-mined conditions such as genetic factors, viral infections, intoxications or metabolic abnormalities affecting the brain before birth, may give rise to subtle inhibitions of cellular growth and synaptogenesis, which result in a slow stunting of postnatal brain growth.

DISORDERS OF NEURONAL MIGRATION

A number of fetal encephalopathies are due to, or associated with, a disturbance in the migration of neocortical neurones, occurring before 20 weeks of gestation. A massive failure of neuronal migration always results in abnormalities in the gyral pattern. Such is the case in the group of disorders referred to as the lissencephalies.

Lissencephalies (agyria)

Lissencephaly can be produced by different migrational disorders, among which two well-defined entities can be delineated: the 'classical' lissencephaly of Bielschowsky (Type I) and the Walker–Warburg lissencephaly (Type II). Both have characteristic clinical and radiological features and may possibly be suspected on prenatal ultrasound scans. Their recognition is most important because of their familial nature.

Type I lissencephaly (Bielschowsky)

Neuropathology and pathophysiology. Sulci and gyri are absent or nearly so over the neocortical surface, except for a verticalized Sylvian fissure (Fig. 19.4). In the neocortex, the first neurones to be generated migrate normally but instead of forming the fifth and sixth layers, they are situated superficially under the molecular layer. All subsequently formed neurones do not achieve a normal migration and form a thick diffuse heterotopic band of cells occupying the greatest part of the white matter. This gives a characteristic 'four-layered pattern' to the hemispheric mantle (Figs. 19.5 and 19.6). The allocortex is generally spared.

The basic developmental defect is an abrupt and complete arrest of migration of cortical neurones between 12 and 16 weeks of gestation. The neocortical abnormality is constantly accompanied by hetcrotopias of the inferior olives, which constitute additional proof of the chronology

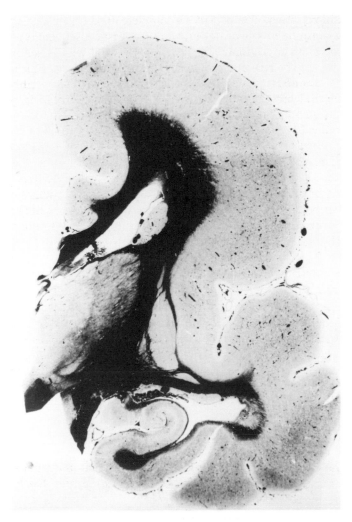

Fig. 19.4 Type I (Bielschowsky) lissencephaly. Coronal section of one hemisphere (myelin stain) showing a smooth brain surface with Sylvian fissure, cingulate sulcus and hippocampus. The 'cortex' appears very thick (unstained).

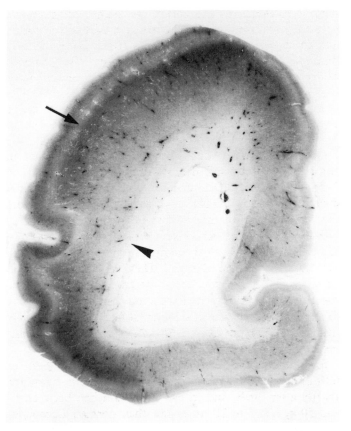

Fig. 19.5 Type I lissencephaly (same case as Fig. 19.4). The superficial 'true cortex' (large pyramidal cells typical of layer V of the normal cortex) is separated by a poorly cellular band representing the upper part of the white matter (arrow) from the underlying thick array of heterotopic neurones. There is a thin rim of periventricular white matter (arrowhead). Cellular stain.

of the disorder, as olivary cells migrate from the rhombic lip between the 8th and 16th week of fetal life. The basic derangement leading to this type of lissencephaly is not known.

Clinical features. Hydramnios is frequent. Mental retardation is profound, infantile spasms or other types of seizure are usual. Head circumference is generally reduced and there may be abnormal facial features including a high forehead, with vertical soft tissue ridging and furrowing when crying, a small anteverted nose, upslanted palpebral fissures, and micrognathia which are characteristic of the Miller–Dieker syndrome (Dobyns et al 1984), which may also be associated with other gyral abnormalities. Other skeletal, cardiac and genital abnormalities may be present. In the rare Norman–Roberts syndrome, other facial changes such as a sloped forehead and a prominent nasal bridge are also said to be associated with lissencephaly (Dobyns et al 1984). Facial features may, however, be entirely normal.

Most children die before the age of 3 years. Several siblings may be affected.

The changes on the CT scan or MRI are diagnostic (Fig. 19.7). A smooth cerebral surface, a large vertical

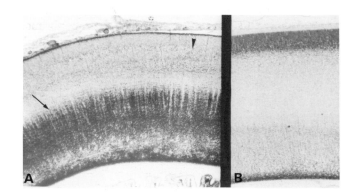

Fig. 19.6 Type I lissencephaly in a 16-week-old fetus. An older sibling had been previously affected. (a) Massive arrest of subcortical neurones (arrow). Only a few cells with the morphology of neurones of layer V and VI have migrated normally. They are located superficially under the molecular layer (arrowhead). (b) Normal 16-week-old fetal brain for comparison (cellular stain). (Dr J. Gadisseux, in preparation).

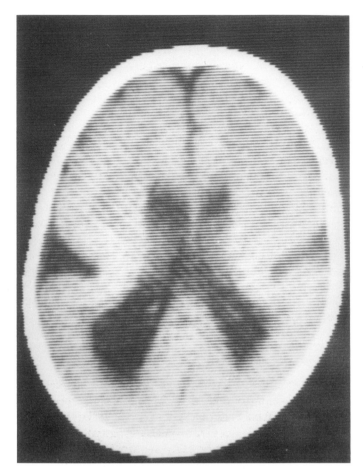

Fig. 19.7 CT scan showing Type I lissencephaly. Note the smooth cerebral surface and the typical appearance of the Sylvian fissure.

Sylvian fissure and moderately dilated lateral ventricles with a thick 'cortex' are very characteristic. In addition the EEG frequently shows typical rapid rhythms. Prenatal ultrasound diagnosis is difficult and cannot be attempted before 30 weeks of gestation (Evrard et al 1984).

Aetiology. Most cases have been sporadic but two siblings have been affected in a number of families. An abnormality of chromosome 17 (17p monosomy) has been reported in sporadic as well as familial cases of the disease (Dobyns et al 1984, Stratton et al 1984). A balanced translocation has occasionally been found in one parent. Recurrence of the disease in siblings may therefore occur in relation to an aberration of chromosome 17. When no such defect is found the possibility of an autosomal recessive mode of inheritance must be considered. No clinical differences seem to exist between the cases with and without abnormalities of chromosome 17.

Type II lissencephaly (Walker–Warburg or HARD(E) syndrome)

Recognition of this disease during life is possible and important because of its frequent familial occurrence. It is not yet clear if Walker's lissencephaly is due to an autosomal recessively inherited trait, or to a persistent viral infection. It is characterized by a complex array of abnormalities in the brain and eyes (Walker 1942, Chan et al 1980, Dobyns et al 1985) and has been alternatively referred to as the HARD(E) syndrome. This is an acronym referring to the major features of the condition: hydrocephalus, agyria, retinal dysplasia, and less consistently encephalocele.

Neuropathology and pathophysiology. We have examined six cases of this condition. A smooth cerebral surface, fetal hydrocephaly and absence of the cerebellar vermis are its main macroscopic characteristics (Fig. 19.8), which are easily seen on the CT scan. The interhemispheric fissure is present but partly coalescent and the corpus callosum is short. The microscopic features are specific. The meninges may be thickened and adherent to the cortex. The cortical ribbon is divided in irregular masses by penetrating vessels and glial septa. Some groups of neurones are clearly heterotopic (Fig. 19.9). There is a diffuse cerebellar microgyria and in the brainstem persistence of the corpus ponto-bulbare (a transient grey structure existing between the 10th and 20th week, formed by neurones which will migrate to the pons and inferior olives) is usual. Various ocular lesions are present, usually thought to stem from 20 to 24 weeks of gestational age.

This complex pathological picture points to a progressive destructive disorder active between 16 and 24 weeks of

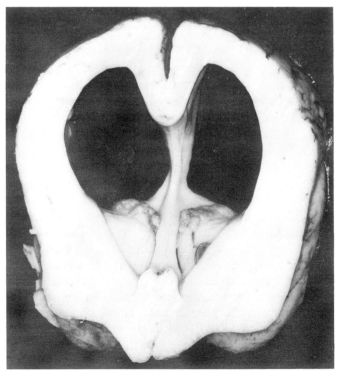

Fig. 19.8 Walker–Warburg (Type II) lissencephaly. There is an entirely smooth cerebral surface with a shallow interhemispheric fissure due to partial coalescence of the medial surface of the brain. Hydrocephaly is obvious and the cerebellar vermis was absent.

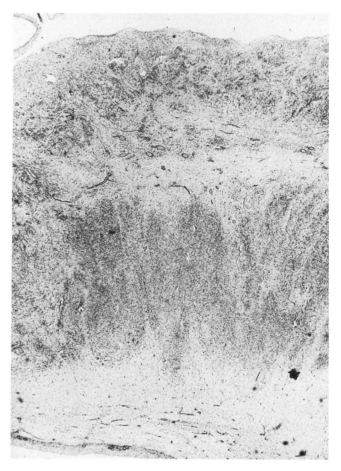

Fig. 19.9 Walker–Warburg lissencephaly (cellular stain). Note the typical appearance of the neocortex; the cortical band is broken into irregularly shaped blocks. The deepest neuronal masses are clearly heterotopic.

gestation. We suggest that an abnormality of the meninges results in a communicating hydrocephalus which is in turn responsible for the vermian agenesis. The involvement of cortical vessels explains the ischaemic scarring of the cortex and the cerebellar microgyria (see below).

Clinical features. The association of fetal hydrocephalus, vermian aplasia, and ocular abnormalities is strongly suggestive of this syndrome. There may be an occipital meningocele or ventriculo–meningocele. Ophthalmological findings are quite variable and include retinal dysplasia, microphthalmia, vitreous abnormalities, retinal detachment, changes in the anterior chamber, cataracts, corneal opacities, glaucoma and coloboma. We do not know of any characteristic dysmorphic features. The condition is usually rapidly lethal and has a strong tendency to be familial. Two or more siblings are frequently affected.

Skeletal muscles must be examined histologically because identical or similar developmental abnormalities of the brain have been described in *Fukuyama's disease*, a frequently familial condition associating a congenital muscle dystrophy, and a developmental encephalopathy, and in the *cerebro-musculo-ocular* syndrome (Towfighi et al 1984, Dobyns et al 1985) which is not always clearly separable from Type II lissencephaly. Muscle changes have been reported in a typical instance of Warburg–Walker's syndrome (Pavone 1986).

Aetiology. The cause of this familial disease is unknown. An autosomal recessive inherited disorder is an obvious possibility and it should be noted that the metabolic disturbance in Zellweger's disease also results in a complex developmental encephalopathy and ocular lesions somewhat similar to those in Walker's lissencephaly. A persistent viral disease infecting successive siblings is another most interesting hypothesis. The brain lesions are consistent with this aetiology and some have suggested that the intrafamilial recurrence rate is not compatible with an autosomal recessive disorder (Williams et al 1984). However, it has been pointed out (Dobyns 1985, Fukuyama & Ohsawa 1984) that in Fukuyama's disease, an autosomal recessive hereditary condition, brain lesions are very similar to those of Walker's lissencephaly.

Zellweger's hepato–cerebro–renal disease

This disorder is described in detail in Chapter 40. It is important to note that this autosomal recessively inherited metabolic disease gives rise to a constant and stereotyped developmental anomaly, essentially characterized by discontinuous subcortical and intracortical neuronal heterotopias, a unique change in the inferior olives, and Purkinje cell heterotopias.

Minor disorders of neuronal migration

Periventricular heterotopias and intrameningeal neuronal heterotopias, are minor, non-specific abnormalities of neuronal migration found in some children with mental retardation. Although they cannot be held responsible for any type of neurological dysfunction, they are probably indicative of a more diffuse developmental disorder which remains undetectable with ordinary neuropathological methods.

Periventricular heterotopias

In this condition a limited number of neurones have not undergone migration and remain in the vicinity of the germinal layer in the periventricular region. They constitute small round masses in which the neurones achieve a good degree of differentiation and maturation and have a tendency to be arranged concentrically. The heterotopic masses may protrude into the ventricular lumen (Fig. 19.10) and be detectable on CT scans or MRI. Even when they are not associated with developmental changes, they are practically always seen in children with mental retardation; a fact that

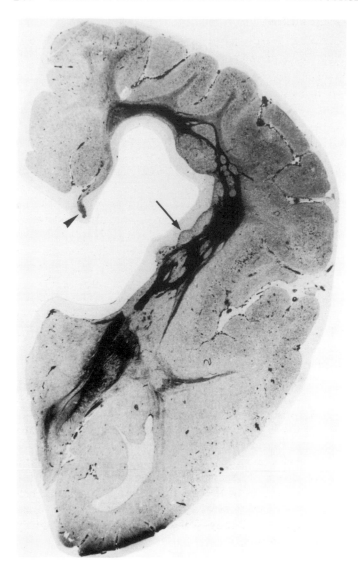

Fig. 19.10 Probable Aicardi's syndrome. Coronal section of one hemisphere (myelin stain) showing agenesis of the corpus callosum with Probst bundle (arrowhead). Periventricular heterotopias are seen protruding into the ventricular lumen (arrow).

Neuronal heterotopias in the meninges and hypermigration

In this type of developmental abnormality, well-differentiated neurones stream vertically across the molecular layer in a limited area and invade the meninges (Robain & Lyon 1972, Caviness et al 1978). This curious phenomenon of 'hypermigration' is probably due to focal destruction of the basal lamina at the surface of the brain. It has interesting neurobiological implications, as it suggests that the integrity of the basal lamina may be a factor governing the final positioning of migratory neurones at some distance from the surface of the brain. This phenomenon has no specificity. It has been found in the brain of mentally retarded or dyslexic children, in severe microcephaly, and frequently in the fetal–alcohol syndrome. It has been reproduced experimentally in the rat using 6-hydroxydopamine (Lidov & Molliver 1982) and found in a strain of mutant mice (Sherman et al 1987).

MICRODYSGENESIS

The finding of minor, limited abnormalities or variations in the usual cortical pattern in some cases of dyslexia (Galaburda & Kemper 1979) and primary (idiopathic) epilepsy (Meencke & Janz 1984) has led some authors to ascribe these disorders to a developmental defect of the brain.

The problem of cortical microdysgenesis is complex. Some of the reported findings probably have no pathological significance and represent minimal variations of the normal cortical pattern. It is quite understandable that, under normal conditions, a few neurones do not reach their specified target (Lyon & Gastaut 1985). On the other hand, some types of microdysgenesis may be an indicator of a minor diffuse developmental defect. It is, however, unwise to create artificial and unwarranted clinico–pathological correlations. The need for a careful and systematic study of a sufficient number of control brains is essential to solve this problem.

Some 'minor' cortical dysgeneses must have a pathological significance. For instance, the only abnormality in the brain of a mentally retarded child that we have recently studied was the inverted polarity of practically all pyramidal cells (10 to 15% of pyramidal cells are inverted in normal brains).

CEREBELLAR HYPOPLASIA OR ATROPHY

Cerebellar hypoplasia or atrophy (a distinction between these two mechanisms is usually impossible) is found in various syndromes.

Total or partial absence of the vermis

This abnormality may occur in association with hydrocephalus. The inferior two-thirds of the vermis are absent in Dandy–Walker syndrome, which is usually a sporadic condition.

probably indicates some other more subtle developmental defect undetectable with standard methods.

Periventricular heterotopias may also be an element in a more complex neuropathological constellation (Fig. 19.10). In *Aicardi's syndrome* they are associated with an agenesis of the corpus callosum and cortical abnormalities. The other elements of this sporadic syndrome restricted to girls are severe mental retardation, infantile spasms with hypsarrhythmia and a lacunar chorioretinopathy. We have described periventricular heterotopias together with incomplete opercularization of the Sylvian fissure in two siblings affected with a hereditary intestinal malformation (Nezelof et al 1976).

In Joubert's disease, an autosomal recessive condition, and in Walker–Warburg lissencephaly (p. 238) this structure is usually undetectable. In the Dandy–Walker syndrome and possibly in the Walker–Warburg type of lissencephaly, the absence of the vermis has been ascribed to a pre-existing fetal hydrocephalus, but this is a debatable hypothesis. In Joubert's disease the mechanism is unknown. In the congenital non-progressive cerebellar ataxias and in Hagberg's disequilibrium syndrome (Hagberg et al 1972), the vermis, and to a lesser extent the cerebellar lobes are hypoplastic.

Dandy–Walker malformation

The original description of this condition recognized the association of hydrocephalus, posterior fossa cyst and hypoplasia of the cerebellar vermis. In a recent review of 40 cases Hirsch et al (1984) conclude that although hydrocephalus commonly occurs in the Dandy–Walker malformation, it is a secondary complication and the underlying defect occurs between 3 and 4 postovulatory weeks. The abnormality affects the structures destined to occupy the posterior fossa. Hirsch et al (1984) found that the ventricles were normal in size in 80% of infants with the Dandy–Walker malformation diagnosed at birth. Cerebrospinal fluid (CSF) flow studies showed that in over 80% of children, fluid flowed from the fourth ventricle into the subarachnoid space although this was usually considerably slower than normal. It has been suggested that the foramen of Magendie is abnormal and CSF flows only through the foramina of Luschka. The development of hydrocephalus occurs when CSF flow becomes further impaired possibly by intracranial haemorrhage (Hirsch et al 1984). Dilatation of the fourth ventricle is usually associated with secondary hypoplasia of the cerebellar hemispheres which are pushed apart, and absence or extreme hypoplasia of the cerebellar vermis. Dandy-Walker syndrome should be distinguished from an arachnoid cyst of the posterior fossa.

The incidence of the Dandy–Walker malformation is 1 in 25–35 000 live births and is very generally sporadic. It may be associated with other cerebral malformations, most commonly agenesis of the corpus callosum. The condition usually presents with increasing head size and hydrocephalus occurs in 90% of cases at various stages. Hirsch and colleagues have drawn attention to the presence of facial angiomas in a proportion of cases. Diagnosis may be made prenatally by ultrasound (p. 113) and the characteristic appearance on antenatal or postnatal scanning is triangular enlargement of the posterior fossa, often without significant ventricular dilatation. The lateral sinus is in an abnormally high position. Treatment is considered in Chapter 46 and prognosis may be reasonably good; 59% of cases in one study had an IQ of 80 or more (Hirsch et al 1984).

Joubert's disease

This disease (Joubert et al 1969, Bolthauser et al 1981, Harmant et al 1983) is an autosomal recessive hereditary disorder characterized by a unique respiratory syndrome and agenesis of the cerebellar vermis. The respiratory abnormality which is present from birth and occurs during waking and sleep, is characterized by frequent bouts of extreme tachypnoea (120–200 breaths per minute) followed by periods of central apnoea exceeding 10 seconds (and possibly up to 60 seconds and more). Abnormal pendular eye movements are usually present. A small occipital meningocele may be found and psychomotor retardation is always evident. Head circumference is normal or moderately increased but there is no progressive hydrocephalus. The CT scan shows an absence of the cerebellar vermis and in some instances a ventriculo–meningocele and moderate ventricular dilatation. Infants with Joubert's disease may die during an apnoeic spell. In those who survive, the respiratory abnormality usually disappears before the end of the first year but mental deficiency is constant and there may be some degree of ataxia. No treatment for the respiratory syndrome is available.

Neuropathological changes include complete absence of the cerebellar vermis with persistence of the floculus, pachygyria of the inferior olive, and heterotopias of Purkinje cells in the neocerebellar white matter. The lateral sinus is in an abnormally high position. The aetiology of the disease and the mechanism of the respiratory syndrome are unknown. Absence of the greatest part of the vermis, anomalies of the inferior olives and Purkinje cell heterotopias, as well as a high position of the lateral sinus, are also found in Dandy–Walker's syndrome, a manifestly different condition.

Cerebellar hypoplasia

Interestingly this is not an exceptional finding in children with apparently isolated mental retardation. The telencephalon in these cases is normal on the CT scans and at autopsy. Such cases may be familial and therefore genetic counselling should be very cautious. The curious association of an asymptomatic cerebellar atrophy and a morphologically normal brain in a mentally retarded child could be due to genetic factors or possibly to a persistent viral infection. Experimentally, parvoviruses are known to induce a cerebellar atrophy by destruction of the actively dividing external granular layer, with only minimal involvement of the brain (Kilham & Margolis 1964).

DEVELOPMENTAL MEGALENCEPHALIES

Progressive megalencephalies in some of the hereditary metabolic diseases are well documented. Non-progressive, usually moderate, megalencephalies occur occasionally in some specific disorders such as von Recklinghausen's disease, and X-linked mental retardation.

Cryptogenetic non-progressive megalencephalies constitute a heterogeneous group. They are frequently associated with mental retardation and may be familial with either an autosomal recessive, dominant or X-linked hereditary transmission. The genetic advice in sporadic cases of mental retardation with megalencephaly should therefore always be cautious. In many of these cases, the ventricles are moderately enlarged and the difference between a fixed hydrocephalus may be difficult to determine. Dominantly inherited isolated megalencephalies (head circumference exceeding 5 to 7 standard deviations) with normal intelligence occur in some families.

We have encountered two sporadic cases of extreme prenatal increase in brain volume. In one child, head circumference was 42 cm at birth and 47 cm at 5 months with a normal body length. Psychomotor retardation was severe. Death occurred at 6 months of age. Brain weight was 1150 g. There was no histological abnormality on examination of the brain, except for the absence of an external granular layer which at 6 months suggests acceleration of brain maturation.

Hemimegalencephalies

There are several diseases with hypertrophy of one cerebral hemisphere. A well-defined condition, which will be referred to here as *dysplastic hemimegalencephaly* (Townsend et al 1975, King et al 1985), is characterized by the presence of numerous giant, occasionally multinucleated nerve cells of neuronal and glial origin, somewhat similar to those seen in tuberous sclerosis. These diffusely invade the cortex, subcortical white matter and basal ganglia of one hemisphere. There is an asymmetrical macrocephaly, mental retardation, unilateral or secondarily generalized intractable seizures, at times a hemiplegia, without other dysmorphic features. Hemispherectomy has been suggested as a cure for the intractable seizures (King et al 1985). This condition may be due to a non-transmissible somatic mutation. Hemimegalencephaly is a feature of the *linear nevus sebaceus syndrome* (Barth et al 1977, Vigevano et al 1984), in which a facial midline linear nevus sebaceus (or organoid nevus) of Jadassohn is associated with partial seizures or infantile spasms, mental retardation, hemimacrocrania and various ocular abnormalities. We are not aware of any pathological study of this disease.

Hypertrophy of one cerebral hemisphere may be a feature of the probably heterogeneous '*idiopathic congenital hemihypertrophy syndrome*' in which there is a unilateral overgrowth of the body. This still obscure condition is not infrequently associated with Wilms tumour or adrenal or hepatic neoplasms. Chromosomal mosaicism

has been reported (Viljoen et al 1984). Vascular nevi and hemangiomas have been described in some cases, which are frequently, but not always convincingly, reported as examples of the Klippel–Trelaunay syndrome. Autopsy in one case has not shown any histological abnormality of the hypertrophic hemisphere (Matsubara et al 1983).

DISORDERS OCCURRING AFTER 20 WEEKS

The study of encephalopathies arising after 20 weeks is of great interest because they represent an important proportion of cerebral palsies and mental retardation. Most of them are the result of ischaemic necrosis, haemorrhage and/or the action of infectious agents. These mechanisms are also discussed in Chapters 30 and 36.

The cause of circulatory disturbance in the fetal brain is usually obscure. Neuropathological data indicate that systemic hypotension may play a role. A systemic circulatory collapse usually gives rise to bilateral but sometimes also to a predominantly unilateral brain infarction. Thrombosis of the sylvian artery has been reported by Larroche and Amit (1966), but evidence of arterial lesions or thrombosis is often lacking. Arterial emboli constitute another possible mechanism to account for unilateral lesions but are rarely found at autopsy perhaps because they usually rapidly lyse. This is described in more detail in Chapter 30.

Cytomegalovirus, the rubella virus, and possibly other viruses are apt to cause or favour ischaemic necrosis of the fetal brain (see Ch. 36). Brain haemorrhage due to feto–maternal platelet immunization is a rare cause of porencephalic brain cysts (Pearson et al 1964) see also p. 341.

Neuropathological evidence indicates that most ischaemic lesions date from 20 to 24 weeks of gestational age. The last days of pregnancy also appear to be a period of predilection for brain infarction. Depending on the intensity, duration and topography of the failure of brain perfusion, different types of lesion occur, ranging from micropolygyria to the extreme destructions of hydranencephaly and multicystic leukomalacia.

MICROGYRIA (MICROPOLYGYRIA)

Macroscopic changes of the surface of the brain are currently used to classify brain malformation. It should be realized, however, that lissencephalies agyrias, pachygyrias and microgyrias, are secondary to alterations in the cortical cyto-architecture, and that different types of cortical abnormality may lead to a similar change over the surface of the brain.

Abnormally small gyri of developmental origin (to be differentiated from ulegyria, which results from localized perinatal ischaemic brain scarring) are seen for instance in Zellweger's disease, Fukuyama's disease, in long-standing hydrocephalus and other conditions, as well as in micro-polygyria. In microgyria also, the appearance of the brain surface is rather variable. The gyri are usually enlarged with numerous minute indentations of their surface (Fig. 19.11).

Consequently, a good classification for the microgyrias (as well as of lissencephalies) must be based on the abnormal pattern of the neocortex.

Ischaemic postmigratory microgyria

This is by far the most frequent type of microgyria. In the usual four layered type the morphological hallmark is a narrow tangential midcortical band devoid of neurones, which is caused by destruction of the lower part of layer III, layer IV and partly or totally layer V (Fig. 19.12).

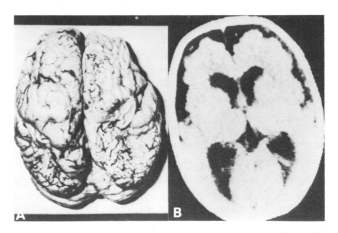

Fig. 19.11 Microgyria. (a) Macroscopic appearance of the brain surface. (b) CT scan of the same case.

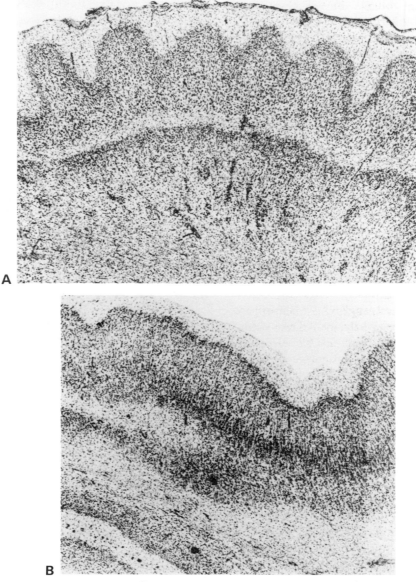

Fig. 19.12 Microgyria. (a) Cortex. Above the characteristic midcortical aneuronal zone, the abnormally convoluted neocortex contains normal layer II (last to migrate) and layer III. (b) Transition with normal cortex. The aneuronal band which is seen here to be continuous with layer IV and V of the normal cortex, results from destruction of these layers.

The well-known susceptibility of the midcortical layers to ischaemia and anoxia (laminar necrosis) and the presence of gliosis and calcification in the aneuronal band are good evidence of the ischaemic nature of the malformation. Above the aneuronal band, the cortical ribbon, usually excessively folded, contains normal layers II and III, which are formed by the last neurones to migrate. It can be concluded that cortical neurones have normally achieved their migration, and microgyria can therefore be considered as a postmigratory ischaemic defect dating from 20 to 24 weeks of gestation (Lyon & Robain 1967, Richman et al 1973, Evrard & Caviness 1974, Marques-Dias et al 1984).

This interpretation is corroborated by a frequently associated cerebellar microgyria. Segments of the cerebellar cortex, approximately situated at the limits of the adjoining vascular territories of two cerebellar arteries are profoundly modified. Cerebellar folia are atrophic, coalescent and arranged in complex patterns. However, the different cellular layers — external granular layer, Purkinje cells, internal granular layer — are present in normal relative position. In a child having died at the age of 18 months, the external granular layer had migrated normally. Such findings also point to the period of 20–24 weeks of gestation for the origin of the malformation.

In the unlayered type of microgyria (Ferrer 1984) the midcortical acellular band is not detectable. The cortical ribbon is narrowed by the disappearance of the inferior cortical layers and displays excessive infolding with fusion of adjacent molecular layers, without any evidence of disturbance of neuronal migration. This pattern may or may not be associated with the 'four-layered' type.

The possibility that ischemic microgyria may at times originate before the end of migration has been suggested by McBride & Kemper (1982). From experiments in rats, Dvorak & Fet (1977) concluded that a microgyric '4-layered' cortex can arise from damage to the brain during neuronal migration. The correlation between the cortical changes these authors have induced in the rat by freezing and human ischaemic polymicrogyria is, however, doubtful.

Microgyria can involve the greater part of both hemispheres, only one hemisphere, or be restricted to small cortical segments. Such is the case for the cortex bordering porencephalic cysts. A tentative explanation of the gyral pattern in postischaemic microgyria has been given by Richman et al 1975 and Ferrer (1984).

Clinical features

Children with diffuse microgyria are mentally retarded and frequently epileptic. In unilateral hemispheric microgyria, partial motor seizures may be a prominent feature. To our knowledge, cases of congenital hemiplegia related to unilateral microgyria have not been documented but such a correlation seems possible. Microgyria is recognizable on the CT scan and MRI, as has for instance been shown in

one of our cases at autopsy (Fig. 19.11). Periventricular calcifications (usually an indication of a congenital CMV infection) are not rare but the interpretation of the radiological appearance of the brain in microgyria lacks uniformity and specificity. Further correlation between pathology and radiology, as well as further advances in radiological techniques are needed to define the radiological appearance of this malformation. This is of great importance as ischaemic postmigratory microgyria is always an acquired accidental lesion.

Other types of microgyria

An excessive infolding of the cortical ribbon with an abnormal appearance of the brain surface, without the typical pattern described above, can be observed in Zellweger's disease, Fukuyama's disease, Miller–Dieker syndrome and other conditions. In most such cases the anomaly of the gyral pattern is produced by a disturbance of neuronal migration.

PORENCEPHALY

The term porencephaly has been indiscriminately applied to any large cystic defect in the cerebral hemispheres of young children. In our opinion congenital intraparenchymal cystic cavities of pre- or peri-natal origin, correspond to two different pathological conditions, both of which generally result from ischaemic or haemorrhagic necrosis or are related to fetal infections which may act in part by means of a vasculitis or a functional circulatory disturbance (Lyon & Van Coster 1987) (see Ch. 30 and 36).

Paraventricular porencephaly

A paraventricular focus of cystic necrosis is usually restricted to the territory of the middle cerebral artery. The cavity is clearly separated from the lateral ventricle which is only moderately dilated. Because of brain atrophy, the segment of the cerebral surface overlying the cyst may be at a distance from the skull, permitting a localized enlargement of the subarachnoid spaces (small secondary arachnoid cyst). This is a non-progressive defect.

Congenital expanding porencephaly

A circumscribed diverticulation of one or both lateral ventricles as a result of focal destructive lesions, to which we propose that the term congenital expanding porencephaly be applied.

This type of porencephaly is a unilateral or bilateral prenatal defect produced by the ischaemic necrosis of the brain usually in the territory of the middle cerebral artery, a brain haemorrhage, the cause of which may be a platelet feto-maternal iso-immunization (Pearson et al 1964) or by periventricular leukomalacia (personal observations). In the central part of the necrotic zone, the cerebral mantle undergoes resorption, and atrophy. In extreme cases, only a thin glial membrane remains (Figs. 19.13 and 19.14). This produces a localized and progressive outpouching of the lateral ventricle. When the cortex bordering the porencephalic cyst shows evidence of less severe ischaemic insult — typical microgyria or other patterns of cortical ischaemic scarring (ulegyria) — it can be assumed that the defect originates between 20 and 24 weeks of gestation, or in the third trimester of pregnancy.

Porencephalies give rise to hemiplegias, diplegias or tetraplegias. Mental retardation occurs but in unilateral porencephaly intelligence may be normal. Congenital porencephalies as defined above, are generally not associated with passive ventricular dilatation. In many cases they constitute active, expanding ventricular diverticulations capable of inducing asymmetrical macrocephaly, a rise in intracranial pressure and progressive neurological signs. On one occasion it was possible to witness the formation of a porencephalic cyst at approximately 20 weeks of gestation and its subsequent prenatal expansion (Isler 1982). Shunting of the cyst results in marked improvement of clinical signs.

The pathophysiology of this condition has recently been reviewed (Tardieu et al 1981). In most cases there is no evidence that the intracranial pressure is increased. The reduced elasticity of the atrophic segment of the ventricular wall probably initiates the ventricular herniation under conditions of normal CSF pressure. The compressed atrophic brain segment is stretched to a point at which it offers the same resistance as normal tissue. The increased surface of the dilated part of the ventricle allows the application of a force on the ventricular wall that is in proportion to the size of the cavity, as has been postulated in normal pressure hydrocephalus (Adams et al 1965). Consequently progressive compression is exerted on the apparently normal brain tissue around the porencephalic defects. Shunting

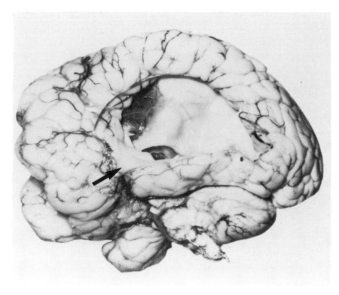

Fig. 19.14 Major form of porencephaly. Lateral view of one hemisphere showing the remnant of the membrane limiting the porus (destroyed at autopsy) marked with arrow.

usually permits the stretched cerebral mantel to regain a near-normal volume.

Unilateral expanding hydrocephalus

We have observed two cases of a condition which differs somewhat from the classical expanding porencephalies. One lateral ventricle is globally dilated, without segmental outpouching, and expands progressively to produce an asymmetrical megalencephaly and signs of raised intracranial pressure, which may become evident only after several years (Fig. 19.15). The aetiology of these 'unilateral expanding

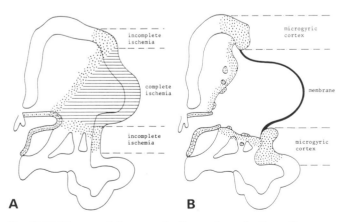

Fig. 19.13 Diagram of the events leading to the major form of porencephaly. (a) Complete resorption of the central zone of ischaemia. (b) Persistence only of a glial membrane with outpouching of the lateral ventricle and microgyric cortex bordering the porus.

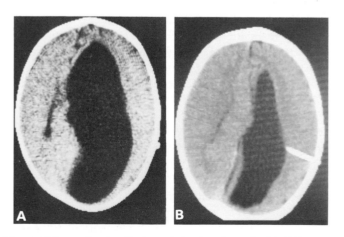

Fig. 19.15 Expanding hemihydrocephaly. An 18-month-old child presenting with signs of raised intracranial pressure but no focal deficit. (a) Before ventriculo–peritoneal shunting there was global dilatation of the right ventricle, contralateral displacement of the interhemispheric fissure and left ventricle and hemimacrocrania. (b) 6 months after shunting there is now marked reduction in ventricular volume and displacement of the midline and contralateral structures. After one year the right ventricle had recovered to near normal size.

hydrocephalies' is obscure. They could be related to diffuse moderate periventricular leukomalacia, and represent a form of the expanding porencephalies. A stenosis of one foramen of Monro can also be postulated but has not been demonstrated in our patients. Ventriculo-peritoneal shunting has given excellent results.

Hydranencephaly and multicystic leukomalacia

These defects represent the most severe expression of the failure of perfusion of the brain before birth (or fetal encephalitis), with subsequent major neurological deficits. In hydranencephaly the brain is severely damaged and reduced to a thin membrane in the irrigation territory of the carotid artery, with relative preservation of limited segments of the posterior part of both hemispheres, which are irrigated by the posterior cerebral artery. Serial fetal ultrasounds in a pregnant woman who experienced a circulatory collapse at 30 weeks of gestation demonstrated the progressive resorption of the anterior two-thirds of both hemispheres (Evrard et al 1984). Neonates with hydranencephaly may be microcephalic or show progressive hydrocephalus in relation to an aqueductal stenosis which is probably due to the presence of blood in the ventricles at the time of the destruction of the parenchyma. During the first days after birth, they may show surprisingly little evidence of neurological dysfunction including apparently normal eye fixation and pursuit. Hydranencephaly and multicystic leukomalacia are described in detail in Section 8.

Occipital encephaloceles

The vast majority of encephaloceles are located in the occipital region. Their estimated frequency is 2–3/10 000 live births. Considered for a long time to be the expression of a defect of the closure of the neural tube, it appears now that many cases are of a different nature. The malformation results from the extracranial evagination of normally formed brain tissue during the 20th gestational week, under the pressure of a prenatal hydrocephalus (Evrard & Caviness 1974). Prenatal ultrasound examination has revealed the formation of an occipital encephalocele at 21–25 weeks in a fetus found to have pre-existing hydrocephalus since the 20th week of gestation (Evrard et al 1984).

The neurological status of infants with occipital encephalocele can be relatively satisfactory. The skull is frequently small with underdevelopment of the frontal area. CT scan and MRI as well as transillumination are necessary to evaluate the defect. Associated malformations, especially ocular lesions, may occur.

Genetic factors probably play a role in the aetiology of occipital encephalocele. Recurrence in sibships of an occipital encephalocele or of a congenital hydrocephalus, myelomeningocele or anencephaly have been reported. Although there is no precise statistical estimation of the recurrence risk, parents should be advised as to this possibility and close ultrasound surveillance and evaluation of the level of alpha-fetoprotein in the amniotic fluid should be systematic in successive pregnancies. Treatment and outcome are discussed in Chapter 26.

Occipital encephalocele also occurs in Meckel–Gruber's syndrome, Joubert's syndrome and Walker's lissencephaly.

Action of viruses and other infectious agents

This vast problem cannot be considered here in any detail. A few points can be made by way of summary: the mode of action of rubella virus, cytomegalovirus (HIV) and *toxoplasma gondii* on the fetal brain is poorly understood; other, as yet unknown viruses (possibly parvoviruses or retroviruses) may be shown to be the cause of prenatal encephalopathies. Careful analysis of human and experimental neuropathological material using immunocytological and in situ hybridization techniques will probably provide valuable information on these points. A major problem in the prevention of the fetal encephalitidies, will be to determine why only a small minority of fetuses from infected mothers are affected.

Possible methods of action of a virus on the fetal brain are indicated in Table 19.2. The effects of viruses on the developing nervous system is discussed fully in Chapter 36.

Table 19.2 Possible methods of action of a virus on the fetal brain

On the mother
  Maternal toxi-infection
  Placentitis (CMV) } Disturbance in fetal brain circulation

On the fetus
  Chromosomal alteration (Johnson 1982)
  Acute cytolysis of nerve cells (direct infection or immune mechanisms)
    On dividing cells in the germinal layer. Mitotic inhibition.
    (? rubella, ? CMV, parvoviruses in animals)
      → microcephaly or cerebellar aplasia
      → ? disturbance of neuronal migration
    On postmitotic nerve cells
      → tissue necrosis, microcephaly
  Persistant viral infection (CMV, rubella)
      → subacute or chronic disease in child
  Cytopathology (functional alteration) without cytolysis (Southern & Oldstone 1986)
  Action on brain circulation
    Vasculitis (by direct infection or immune mechanisms)
      (rubella, CMV)
    Disorder of brain perfusion due to other mechanisms (CMV ?)
      → microgyria, porencephaly

REFERENCES

Adams R D, Fisher C M, Hakim S et al 1965 Symptomatic occult hydrocephalus with 'normal' cerebrospinal fluid pressure: a treatable syndrome. New England Journal of Medicine 273: 117–126

Angevine J B, Sidman R L 1961 Autoradiographic study of cell migration during histogenesis of cerebral cortex of the mouse. Nature 192: 766–768

Barth P G, Valk J, Kalsbeeck G L 1977 Organoid nevus syndrome (linear nevus sebaceus of Jadassohn): clinical and radiological study of a case. Neuropädiatrie 8: 418–428

Bolthauser E, Herdan M, Dumermuth G, Isler W 1981 Joubert syndrome: clinical and polygraphic observations in a further case. Neuropediatrics 12: 181–191

Burck V 1982 Genetic counselling in holoprosencephaly. Helvetia Paediatrica Acta 37: 231–237

Caviness V S 1982 Neocortical histogenesis in normal and reeler mice: a developmental study based upon ^{3}H thymidine autoradiography. Developmental Brain Research 4: 293–301

Caviness V S, Evrard P, Lyon G 1978 Radial neuronal assemblies, ectopia and necrosis of developing cortex. Acta Neuropathologica (Berlin) 41: 67–72

Chan C C, Egbert P R, Herrick M K, Urich H 1980 Oculo cerebral malformations: a reappraisal of Walker's lissencephaly. Archives of Neurology 37: 104–108

Chattha A, Richardson E 1977 Cerebral white-matter hypoplasia. Archives of Neurology 34: 137–141

Dobyns W B 1985 Walker–Warburg syndrome, (Letter to the editor). Neurology 35: 1082

Dobyns W B, Stratton R F, Greenberg F 1984 Syndromes with lissencephaly. American Journal of Medical Genetics 18: 509–526

Dobyns W B, Kirkpatrick J B, Hittner H M, Roberts R M, Kretzer F L 1985 Walker–Warburg and cerebro–oculo–muscular syndromes and a new syndrome with type II lissencephaly. American Journal of Medical Genetics 22: 157–195

Dvorak K, Fet J 1977 Migration of neuroblasts through partial necrosis of the cerebral cortex in newborn rats. Contribution to the problems of morphological development and developmental period of cerebral microgyria. Acta Neuropathologica (Berlin) 38: 203–212

Esterlyn N B 1968 The ichthyosiform dermatoses. Journal of Pediatrics 42: 990–1004

Evrard P 1986 Personal communication

Evrard P, Caviness V S 1974 Extensive developmental defect of the cerebellum associated with posterior fossa ventriculocele. Journal of Neuropathology and Experimental Neurology 33: 385–399

Evrard P, Lyon G, Gadisseux J F 1984 Le développement prénatal du système nerveux et ses perturbations: mécanismes généraux. Progrès en Néonatologie. Karger (Bâle) 4: 71–85

Ferrer I 1984 A Golgi analysis of unlayered polymicrogyria. Acta Neuropathologica 65: 69–76

Friede R L 1975 Developmental Neuropathology, 1st edition. Springer-Verlag, Wien

Fukuyama Y, Ohsawa M 1984 A genetic study of the Fukuyama type congenital muscular dystrophy. Brain and Development 6: 373–390

Gadisseux J F, Evrard P 1985 Glial-neuronal relationship in the developing central nervous system. Developmental Neuroscience 7: 12–32

Galaburda A M, Kemper T L 1979 Cytoarchitectonic abnormalities in developmental dyslexia: a case of study. Annals of Neurology 6: 94–100

Goutières F, Aicardi J 1982 Acute neurological dysfunction associated with destructive lesions of the basal ganglia in children. Annals of Neurology 12: 328–332

Hagberg D, Sanner G, Steen M 1972 The desequilibrium syndrome in cerebral palsy. Acta Paediatrica Scandinavia 226: 7–63

Harmant-van Rijckevorsel G, Aubert-Tulkens G, Moulin D, Lyon G 1983 Le syndrome de Joubert. Etude clinique et anatomo-pathologique. Revue Neurologique 139: 715–724

Hirsch J-F, Pierre-Kahn A, Renier D, Sainte-Rose C, Hoppe-Hirsch E 1984 The Dandy–Walker malformation: a review of 40 cases. Journal of Neurosurgery 61: 515–522

Isler W 1982 Personal communication

Johnson R T 1982 Viral infections of the nervous system. Raven Press, New York, p 206

Joubert M, Eisenring J J, Robb J P, Andermann F 1969 Familial agenesis of the cerebellar vermis. Neurology 19: 813–825

Kilham L, Margolis G 1964 Cerebellar ataxia in hamsters inoculated with rat virus. Science 143: 1047–1048

King M, Stephenson M K, Ziervogel M, Doyle D, Galbraith S 1985 Hemimegalencephaly. A case for hemispherectomy? Neuropediatrics 16: 46–55

Landrieu P, Evrard P 1979 La dysplasie septo-optique: étude clinique et éléments d'un conseil génétique. Journal de Génétique Humaine 27: 329–341

Larroche J C, Amiel C 1966 Thrombose de l'artère sylvienne à la période néonatale. Archives Françaises de Pédiatrie 23: 257–274

Lidov H G, Molliver M E 1982 The structure of the cerebral cortex in the rat following prenatal administration of 6-hydroxydopamine. Developmental Brain Research 3: 81–108

Lyon G, Evrard P 1987 Neuropédiatrie. Masson, Paris, p 65

Lyon G, Gastaut H 1985 Considerations on the significance attributed to unusual cerebral histological findings recently described in eight patients with primary generalized epilepsy. Epilepsia 26: 365–367

Lyon G, Robain O 1967 Encéphalopathies circulatoires prénatales et paranatales. Acta Neuropathologica (Berlin) 9: 79–98

Lyon G, Van Coster R 1987 Porencephaly and arachnoid cysts. In: Johnson R T (ed) Current therapy in neurologic diseases. 2nd edn. Decker B C, Toronto, pp 77–82

Lyon G, Evrard P, Gadisseux J F 1984 Les anomalies du développement du télencéphale humain pendant la période de cytogenèse–histogenèse. In: Minkowski A, Relier J P (eds) Progrès en néonatologie. Karger S, Basel, pp 70–84

Lyon G, Arita F, Misson J P, Ferrière G 1988 A new familial disease with extreme atrophy of corpus callosum and cerebral white matter due to a failure of axonal growth (in preparation)

McBride M C, Kemper K L 1982 Pathogenesis of four layered microgyric cortex in man. Acta Neuropathologica 57: 93–98

Marin-Padilla M 1983 Structural organization of the human cerebral cortex prior to the appearance of the cortical plate. Anatomy and Embryology 168: 21–40

Marques-Dias M J, Harmant-van Rijckevorsel G, Landrieu P, Lyon G 1984 Prenatal cytomegalovirus disease and cerebral microgyria: evidence for perfusion failure, not disturbance of histogenesis, as the major cause of fetal cytomegalovirus encephalopathy. Neuropediatrics 15: 18–24

Matsubara O, Tanaka M, Ida T, Okeda R 1983 Hemimegalencephaly with hemihypertrophy (Klippel-Trenaunay-Weber syndrome). Virchows Archives CA 400: 155–162

Meencke H J, Janz D 1984 Neuropathological findings in primary generalized epilepsy: a study of eight cases. Epilepsia 25: 8–21

Menkes J H, Philipart M, Clarck D B 1964 Hereditary partial agenesis of the corpus callosum. Archives of Neurology 11: 198–208

Morishima A, Aranhoff G S 1986 Syndrome of septo–optic–pituitary dysplasia: the clinical spectrum. Brain and Development 8: 233–239

Nezelof G, Jaubert F, Lyon G 1976 Syndrome familial associant grêle court, malrotation intestinale, hypertrophie du pylore et malformation cérébrale. Annales d'Anatomie Pathologique (Paris) 21: 401–412

Norman R M 1958 Micrencephaly. In: Greenfield J G (ed) Neuropathology. Edward Arnold, London, pp 322–323

Pavone L 1986 Hydrocephalus, lissencephaly, ocular abnormalities and congenital muscular dystrophy: a Warburg syndrome variant? Neuropediatrics 17: 206–211

Pearson H A, Shulman N R, Marder V J 1964 Isoimmune neonatal thrombocytopenic purpura: clinical and therapeutic considerations. Blood 23: 154–177

Pineda M, Gonzalez E 1984 Familial agenesis of the corpus callosum with hypothermia and apneic spells. Neuropediatrics 15: 63–67

Rakic P 1972 Mode of cell migration to the superficial layers of fetal monkey neocortex. Journal of Comparative Neurology 145: 61–84

Rakic P 1982 Early developmental events: cell lineage, acquisition of neuronal positions and areal and laminar developments. In: Rakic P, Goldman-Rakic P S (eds) Development and modifiability of the cerebral cortex. MIT Press, Cambridge, MA, pp 437–451

Rakic P, Yakovlev P 1968 Development of corpus callosum and cavum septi in man. Journal of Comparative Neurology 132: 45–72

Richman D P, Stewart R M, Caviness V S 1973 Microgyria, lissencephaly and neuron migration to cerebral cortex: an architectonic approach. Neurology 23: 413

Richman D P, Stewart R M, Hutchinson J W, Caviness V S 1975 Mechanical model of brain convolutional development. Science 189: 18–21

Robain O, Gorce F 1972 Arhinencéphalie. Etude clinique, anatomique et étiologique de 13 cas. Archives Françaises de Pédiatrie 29: 861–879

Robain O, Lyon G 1972 Les micrencéphalies familiales par malformation cérébrale. Acta Neuropatholgica (Berlin) 20: 96–109

Schwartz M L, Goldman-Rakic P S 1982 Single cortical neurones have axon collaterals to ipsilateral and contralateral cortex in fetal and adult primates. Nature 299: 154–155

Sherman G F, Galaburda A M, Behan P O, Rosen G D 1987 Neuroanatomical anomalies in autoimmune mice. Acta Neuropathologica (Berl) 74: 239–242

Southern P, Oldstone A 1986 Medical consequences of persistent viral infection. New England Journal of Medicine 314: 359–367

Stanfield B B 1972 Postnatal reorganization of cortical projections: the role of collateral elimination. Trends in Neuroscience 7: 37–41

Stratton R F, Dobyns W B, Airhart S D, Ledbetter D M 1984 New chromosomal syndrome: Miller–Dieker syndrome and monosomy 17p13. Human Genetics 67: 193–200

Tardieu M, Evrard P, Lyon G 1981 Progressive expanding congenital porencephalies: a treatable cause of progressive encephalopathy. Pediatrics 68: 198–202

Towfighi J, Sassani J W, Suzuki K, Ladda R L 1984 Cerebro–ocular dysplasia–muscular dystrophy (COD–MD) syndrome. Acta Neuropathologica (Berlin) 65: 110–123

Townsend J J, Nielsen S L, Malamud N 1975 Unilateral megalencephaly: hamartome or neoplasm? Neurology 25: 448–453

Vigevano F, Aicardi J, Lini M, Pasquinelli A 1984 Linear nevus sebaceous syndrome: 11 cases from a multicentric study. Boll. Lega. It. Epil. 45/46: 59–63

Viljoen D, Pear J, Beighton P 1984 Manifestations and natural history of idiopathic hemihypertrophy: a review of eleven cases. Clinical Genetics 26: 81–86

Walker A E 1942 Lissencephaly. Archives of Neurology and Psychiatry 48: 13–29

Williams R S, Swisher C N, Jennings M, Ambler M, Caviness V 1984 Cerebro–ocular dysgenesis (Walker–Warburg syndrome): neuropathologic and etiologic analysis. Neurology 34: 1531–1541

Yakovlev P L 1959 Pathoarchitectonic studies of cerebral malformations. Journal of Neuropathology and Experimental Neurology 18: 22–55

20. Genetics of neurodevelopmental abnormalities

Dr I.D. Young

Major malformations, defined as those which interfere with viability or physical well-being, are observed in approximately 3% of newborn children (Kalter & Warkany 1983). A further 3% have an anomaly which manifests after the neonatal period. Abnormalities of the central nervous system feature prominently among these malformations occurring in 3 to 4% of early spontaneous abortions (Creasy & Alberman 1976) and in approximately 1 in 200 live births (Leck 1974).

These figures may well be underestimates since many neurodevelopmental anomalies will go undetected without careful diagnostic evaluation and expert neuropathology. Postmortem examination of the brain in several large series of mentally retarded patients has identified a cerebral malformation in up to 65% of cases (Palo et al 1966).

Increasingly the parents of a child with an abnormality wish to know not only why it happened but whether it will happen again. For many central nervous system malformations the recurrence risk is low but in some situations a relatively high risk will apply. In the following few pages, data concerning the genetic aspects of most of the more common central nervous system malformations will be presented. It should be remembered, however, that for several malformations, particularly those occurring in isolation, information is scanty and every case should be fully assessed on an individual basis.

Patterns of inheritance

It is traditional to consider these under three headings — chromosomal, single gene and multifactorial. The principles underlying these different mechanisms are well established and discussed in detail in many excellent texts. A particularly enlightening review is provided by Hunter (1983).

Chromosomal abnormalities

The normal human has 46 chromosomes consisting of 22 pairs of autosomes and a single pair of sex chromosomes. At meiosis each pair separates independently into the gamete thus providing for very extensive reassortment of genetic material from generation to generation. Additional rearrangement results from exchange of genetic material between the pairs of homologous chromosomes during the first stage of meiosis.

Regrettably this complex biological process is prone to error so that a gamete may carry an unbalanced chromosome complement, i.e. additional or missing genetic material. The resulting zygote may be so abnormal that miscarriage ensues. Alternatively a viable but abnormal fetus may result.

Almost every infant receiving an unbalanced autosomal complement will be mentally retarded and many will have a central nervous system malformation as outlined in the following pages. How chromosome abnormalities cause malformations is unknown. Loss or addition of genetic material is likely to result in deficiency or excess of structural proteins, receptors or enzymes critical for development at a specific stage in embryogenesis.

The degree of chromosome imbalance may be large or small, with somewhat unpredictable outcome. Thus, loss of a tiny amount of chromosome material ('tiny' in terms of the light microscope but massive when considered at the molecular level) from the short arm of chromosome 5 results in very severe handicap in surviving infants — the Cri Du Chat syndrome. Yet many children with an additional number 21 chromosome are only mildly or moderately retarded.

Recent progress in cytogenetics has permitted the identification of microdeletions, just visible with the light microscope. For example subtle abnormalities of the short arm of chromosome 17 have been detected in several cases of lissencephaly (Dobyns et al 1984). These new developments stress the importance of careful cytogenetic studies in all children with unexplained central nervous system malformations. When an abnormality is found, chromosome studies in the parents will usually be indicated.

Single gene defects

Almost 4000 entities showing single gene inheritance have been identified (McKusick 1986). Recognition of these disorders is vital if parents are to be counselled correctly. Children with multiple congenital abnormalities, frequently associated with mental retardation, present a particularly difficult diagnostic problem, which has been eased to some extent by the development of computerized databases (Winter et al 1984).

How a single mutant gene produces multiple abnormalities is unclear. Possible clues are provided by the concept of the developmental field, defined as a set of embryonic primordia which react identically to an insult, which may be genetic or environmental in origin (Opitz 1985). An example is afforded by the cerebral, ocular and facial abnormalities associated with holoprosencephaly. Thus organs which develop at the same time, or in close proximity, or from a common origin such as neural crest or axial mesoderm, may be susceptible to a single underlying insult but with widespread effects. Clearly much has yet to be learned and it is hoped that the recent advances in molecular genetics will unravel some of the secrets of the complex processes linking genotype with phenotype.

Multifactorial inheritance

There is evidence that many congenital malformations, such as isolated facial clefting and congenital heart disease, result from the interaction of adverse environmental factors upon a genetically predisposed background. Various mathematical models have been proposed to explain the observed incidence of the relevant malformation in first-, second- and third-degree relatives. The most widely quoted model is that of a normally distributed liability (which includes both genetic and environmental factors). A superimposed threshold effect explains the quasicontinuous variation observed at the clinical end, i.e. the patient either has or has not a facial cleft.

Whilst the mathematical principles are complex, their application is relatively straightforward since empirical risk data, which usually closely parallel theoretical predictions, are now available for most malformations believed to show this pattern of inheritance. Figures for use in neural tube defects are discussed elsewhere. Perhaps the most important point to note in relation to multifactorial inheritance is that little or nothing can be done to alter or influence an individual's genes, so that attention should focus on the environmental component. This has been admirably illustrated by the work of Professor Smithells and colleagues (1981) in their study of neural tube defect prophylaxis using periconceptional vitamin supplementation (Ch. 23).

Definitions in dysmorphology

It is worth dwelling briefly on some of the terms and concepts used to describe abnormalities (Spranger et al 1982), for not only does their use impose a discipline on those applying them, but in many instances selection of the correct term will enhance understanding of underlying aetiology and genetic implications for other family members.

A malformation is a morphological defect of an organ resulting from an intrinsically abnormal developmental process. Thus the organ is doomed from conception. In most cases an encephalocele will represent an example of a malformation.

A deformation is an abnormal form or shape or position caused by mechanical forces. Apparent microcephaly may occur as a result of constraint of the developing skull by an abnormally shaped uterus (Smith 1981).

A disruption is a morphological defect of an organ resulting from interference with an originally normal developmental process. Thus severe anoxia or intra-uterine infection may disrupt normal cerebral development causing a secondary malformation such as porencephaly.

A dysplasia is an abnormal organization of cells into tissue. Examples of neurodevelopmental abnormalities which represent dysplasias include schizencephaly and pachygyria.

A sequence is a pattern of multiple anomalies derived from a single prior anomaly, e.g. the sequelae of a myelomeningocele such as lower limb paralysis, talipes and congenital hip dislocation.

A syndrome is a pattern of multiple anomalies, causally related and not representing a sequence or field defect. Strictly this term should be reserved for patterns of abnormalities which cannot be satisfactorily explained embryologically. The term is, however, used very loosely. Numerous syndromes include cerebral malformations as will be illustrated in the following text.

An association is a non-random occurrence in two or more individuals of multiple anomalies not believed to be a field defect, sequence or syndrome. An example is the Schisis association discussed under neural tube defects.

NEURAL TUBE DEFECTS

Neural tube defects (NTDs) comprise a significant proportion of the workload at most genetic clinics. Occurring in isolation they are believed to show multifactorial inheritance. Empirical risks are well established and are widely available in genetics texts (Baraitser 1982, Bundey 1985). In keeping with the principles of multifactorial inheritance, the recurrence risk is directly related to the incidence of the condition in the population, varying from 8.9% for siblings in an area of high incidence such as Northern Ireland (Nevin & Johnstone 1980) to 2.5–3.0% in areas of relatively low incidence such as south–east England (Seller 1981) and Canada (Hunter 1984). Average risk figures which are widely quoted for relatives are given in Table 20.1.

NTDs, in particular encephaloceles, occur in several syndromes, a subject discussed at length by Cohen &

Table 20.1 Risks used in genetic counselling for neural tube defects

Affected relative	Risk (%)
First degree	
One sibling	5
Two siblings	10–12
Parent	4
Second degree	
Aunt, Uncle	
Nephew, Niece	2
Half sibling	
Third degree	
Cousin	
Great uncle or aunt	1

There is a suggestion that these risks may be slightly greater when the affected relative is related through the matrilineal line, and slightly lower when through the patrilineal line.

Lemire (1982). They are also found in several chromosome abnormalities, in particular trisomy 18: of the 23 babies with trisomy 18 born in Leicestershire during the years 1980–5 inclusive, 2 had a lumbosacral meningomyelocele. Single gene disorders in which an NTD may occur are summarized in Table 20.2. It is particularly important that these are recognized since the recurrence risk will be much greater than for an isolated NTD.

Other conditions in which NTDs may occur include the ADAM complex (Keller et al 1978) and the Schisis association (Czeizel 1981). Rupture of the amnion before 45 days of gestation tends to be associated with gross disruption of the developing embryo which may have anencephaly or an anterior or posterior encephalocele (Higginbottom et al 1979). The term 'Schisis association' was proposed in view of the observation that NTDs, oral clefts, omphaloceles and diaphragmatic herniae tend to occur with one another more often than would be expected by chance. The incidence of schisis type abnormalities in siblings in Czeizel's series was 7 out of 190 (3.7%). (See also Section 7.)

HYDROCEPHALUS

Congenital hydrocephalus is a relatively common anomaly with incidence approaching 1 per 1000 births. When not associated with a chromosome abnormality, neural tube defect or single gene defect, the recurrence risk is relatively low, indicating that environmental factors play a major aetiological role. Several family studies have derived an empirical recurrence risk of approximately 1–2% for siblings of an index case with non-syndromal hydrocephalus (Carter et al 1968, Lorber & De 1970, Burton 1979, Adams et al 1982).

There have been many reports of hydrocephalus due to aqueduct stenosis showing X-linked recessive inheritance (Halliday et al 1986). Many of the affected male infants have flexed fingers and flexed adducted thumbs. When more than one male in a family is affected, counselling would be as for sex-linked recessive inheritance. When only one male is affected and aqueduct stenosis has been confirmed, empirical recurrence risks of 4–7% have been obtained (Burton 1979, Howard et al 1981, Halliday et al 1986).

Hydrocephalus has been noted in a large number of syndromes (Smith 1982) so that every individual in whom hydrocephalus is diagnosed merits careful examination. The assistance of a dysmorphology database is particularly valuable in these situations (Winter et al 1984). Important additions to the list in Smith's textbook include the FG syndrome (Opitz & Kaveggia 1974) characterized by macrocephaly, agenesis of the corpus callosum and imperforate anus; the hydrolethalus syndrome (Salonen et al 1981) featuring congenital heart defects and polydactyly; and the Walker–Warburg syndrome, also known as the HARD(E) syndrome (Pagon et al 1983) in which hydrocephalus is associated with agyria, retinal dysplasia and an encephalocele (see p. 238).

HYDRANENCEPHALY

This is characterized by complete or almost complete absence of the cerebral hemispheres in the presence of intact meninges and a relatively normal skull. Thus hydranencephaly represents a good example of a disruption, resulting from destruction of normal brain by infective, teratogenic or vascular agents. The vast majority of cases represent sporadic events within a family.

Table 20.2 Single gene disorders in which neural tube defects (NTD) may occur

Condition	Type of NTD	Inheritance	Associated features
Craniotelencephalic dysplasia (Hughes et al 1983)	Frontal encephalocele	Autosomal recessive	Craniosynostosis, lissencephaly
Cryptophthalmos syndrome (Smith 1982)	Occipital encephalocele	Autosomal recessive	Cryptophthalmos, urogenital abnormalities
Frontofacionasal dysplasia (Gollop et al 1984)	Frontal encephalocele	Autosomal recessive	Facial dysmorphism with clefts and deformed nostrils
Kousseff syndrome (Kousseff 1984)	Sacral meningocele	Autosomal recessive	Congenital heart disease
Meckel's syndrome (Smith 1982)	Occipital encephalocele	Autosomal recessive	Polydactyly, polycystic kidney disease
Roberts syndrome (Smith 1982)	Frontal encephalocele	Autosomal recessive	Cleft lip, phocomelia
Sacral defects (Yates et al 1983)	Anterior sacral meningocele	Autosomal or sex-linked dominant	Partial sacral agenesis
Warburg's syndrome (Pagon et al 1983)	Occipital encephalocele	Autosomal recessive	Hydrocephalus, lissencephaly, retinal dysplasia

However, there are a few reports of familial hydranencephaly. Hamby et al (1950) reported male and female siblings who both had hydranencephaly and talipes; the male also had absent fibulae and the female showed exstrophy of the bladder with absent kidneys. Fowler et al (1972) described five female siblings who had hydranencephaly, hydrocephalus and arthrogryposis. Necropsy studies revealed abnormal vascularization of the central nervous system parenchyma. More recently Siber (1984) reported probable sex-linked recessive inheritance of a syndrome featuring micro-encephaly, microphthalmia with corneal opacities, spastic quadriplegia, hypospadias and cryptorchidism.

The paucity of familial examples and the impressive evidence for an underlying destructive aetiology indicate that most cases of hydranencephaly are not genetic in origin. In the absence of a significant family history it is certainly reasonable to offer a very low recurrence risk.

PORENCEPHALY

The situation with porencephaly is similar to that for hydranencephaly. The term is used to describe any cavity or cerebrospinal fluid (CSF) filled cyst in the brain. The pathogenesis, which spans both intra-uterine and postnatal life, includes developmental arrest of unknown aetiology and destruction by agents such as trauma and infection.

Most cases are believed to be environmental in origin and are sporadic. However, there have been at least two recent reports of familial porencephaly. Berg et al (1983) described two families, one showing autosomal dominant and the other autosomal recessive inheritance. The other report (Airaksinen 1984), describing affected male and female siblings, was consistent with autosomal recessive inheritance.

In view of these reports caution should be exercised in offering genetic counselling. However, as with hydranencephaly, the vast majority of cases appear not to be genetic so that the provision of a very low recurrence risk would be appropriate.

DANDY–WALKER MALFORMATION

This refers to a developmental abnormality in which hydrocephalus is associated with a posterior fossa cyst continuous with the fourth ventricle and hypoplasia or complete absence of the cerebellar vermis. The genetic aspects have recently been reviewed at length by Murray et al (1985).

The condition shows marked aetiological heterogeneity. It has been noted in several chromosome abnormalities including triploidy and trisomy for chromosomes 5p, 8p, 8q, 9, 13 and 18. It is also found in several single

gene disorders as listed in Table 20.3. Murray et al (1985) noted that in approximately 18% of cases the Dandy–Walker malformation is associated with another midline abnormality such as congenital heart disease, cleft lip or neural tube defect, raising the possibility that the Dandy–Walker malformation may be a manifestation of a field defect involving midline structures. In such a situation the recurrence risk normally quoted for the other malformation would seem appropriate.

When the Dandy–Walker malformation occurs in isolation the recurrence risk appears to be low. Pooling the results from two studies (Burton 1979, Murray et al 1985) gives a risk of 1% for siblings (1 affected out of 98). However, there seems to be a slightly increased risk of around 7% that siblings may have other midline defects. Murray et al make the excellent point that the small number of published affected sib pairs with the Dandy–Walker malformation could be examples of a very rare autosomal recessive form but are just as likely to represent the visible end of the spectrum of multifactorial inheritance.

MACROCEPHALY AND MEGALENCEPHALY

Macrocephaly, an enlarged head, is often associated with megalencephaly, an enlarged brain, and is found in a large number of syndromes succinctly summarized by Baraitser (1982) under four headings:

1. The overgrowth disorders such as Sotos syndrome and Weaver's syndrome (Smith 1982).
2. Skeletal dysplasias such as achondroplasia, pyknodysostosis and craniometaphyseal dysplasia.
3. Neurocutaneous syndromes such as neurofibromatosis in which approximately 27% of patients have a head circumference above the 97th centile (Riccardi 1981). Rarer examples include the syndrome of macrocephaly, pseudopapilloedema and multiple haemangiomata re-

Table 20.3 Syndromes featuring the Dandy–Walker malformation

Syndrome	Inheritance	Associated features
Aase–Smith (Patton et al 1985)	Autosomal dominant	Cleft palate, hand abnormalities, joint contractures
Aicardi (Aicardi et al 1965)	Sex-linked dominant	Chorioretinitis, infantile spasms
Coffin–Siris (Smith 1982)	Autosomal recessive (?)	Coarse facies, Hirsutism, small 5th fingers
Joubert (Joubert et al 1969)	Autosomal recessive	Cerebellar vermis agenesis, episodic hyperpnoea
Meckel (Smith 1982)	Autosomal recessive	Encephalocele, polycystic kidneys, polydactyly
Warburg (Pagon et al 1983)	Autosomal recessive	Agyria encephalocele, retinal dysplasia

ported by Riley & Smith (1960) and the Zonana syndrome of macrocephaly, multiple lipomata and haemangiomata (Zonana et al 1976).

4. Neurometabolic storage disorders such as GM gangliosidosis, the mucopolysaccharidoses and the leucodystrophies such as Canavan's disease and Alexander's disease.

Most children with isolated or primary megalencephaly are of normal intelligence with little or no neurological impairment, and the majority of these children are likely to have 'benign familial megalencephaly' which shows autosomal dominant inheritance. Day & Schutt (1979) investigated 18 children with megalencephaly, of whom 3 were mentally retarded. The parents of 13 of the children with normal intelligence were examined; 10 fathers and 1 mother were found to have large heads.

Lorber & Priestley (1981) reported 109 children referred for investigation of a large head, who were found to have primary or non-syndromal megalencephaly. Only 7 were retarded. At least 43 of these children, and the authors admit that this may have been an underestimate, had a relative with head circumference above the 98th percentile.

One family with benign familial macrocephaly has been described in which 3 of 5 individuals, all of whom were of normal intelligence, had dilated ventricles (Asch & Myers 1976). Schreier et al (1974) described a family in which 12 individuals had macrocephaly, of whom 10 were of normal or superior intelligence whilst the remaining 2 had dilated ventricles in association with developmental delay. Gragg (1971) reported 2 megalencephalic brothers whose parents were normal.

The last three reports indicate that megalencephaly and macrocephaly may well be genetically heterogeneous. However, familial reports featuring severe retardation or neurological disability are few. The prognosis in the relatively common autosomal dominant familial megalencephaly fully justifies its prefix of 'benign'.

MICROCEPHALY

This presents a particularly difficult problem in genetic counselling. Defined as a head circumference of more than 2 or 3 standard deviations below the mean for age, sex and body size, it has numerous causes, both environmental and genetic.

Microcephaly occurs in a very large number of chromosome abnormalities, as reviewed in full by Warkany (1981). It also occurs in a formidably long list of syndromes, many showing single gene inheritance, which are fully covered by Smith (1982). Thus, in addition to cytogenetic investigations, every child with microcephaly should be carefully examined, with investigations including careful fundoscopy and neurological assessment, since a large number of conditions include microcephaly with ocular

and/or neurological abnormalities (Bundey 1985). It is also important to remember that microcephaly can be caused by maternal phenylketonuria so that a maternal Guthrie test should also be considered.

In isolation, microcephaly can show autosomal recessive and autosomal dominant inheritance. Autosomal recessive microcephaly, also known as primary or true microcephaly, is characterized by an amiable personality, receding forehead parallel with the slope of the nose, micrognathia and ears which appear large. Usually the mental retardation is not accompanied by other neurological abnormalities (Qazi & Reed 1973). In autosomal dominant microcephaly, the degree of intellectual impairment is less (Haslam & Smith 1979). One family has been described in which affected individuals showed short stature (Burton 1981).

When confronted by an isolated case of non-syndromal microcephaly for which there is no clear chromosomal or environmental explanation, it is customary to offer an empirical recurrence risk of between 10 and 20% (Bartley & Hall 1978, Opitz et al 1978). If the parents are consanguineous this risk should probably be raised to 1 in 4. These empirical risk estimates indicate that approximately half of the isolated cases of non-syndromal or true microcephaly are autosomal recessive.

HOLOPROSENCEPHALY

Holoprosencephaly and its associated facial dysmorphism represent a severe malformation complex or field defect in which the embryonic forebrain shows impaired midline cleavage. Arhinencephaly, in which the olfactory tracts and bulbs are absent represents the mild end of the spectrum. At the other end is alobar holoprosencephaly in which the facies may show premaxillary agenesis (hypotelorism, flat nose and absent philtrum), cebocephaly (hypotelorism with single nostril), ethmocephaly (hypotelorism with a proboscis) or cyclopia (single central eye).

The aetiological heterogeneity of holoprosencephaly has been reviewed in depth by Cohen (1982). It is a common finding in certain chromosome abnormalities such as trisomy 13 and deletion of the long arm of 13 (13q–). It is also seen but less common in trisomy 18, deletion of the short arm of 18 (18p–) and triploidy. Thus chromosome studies are strongly indicated in all children with this abnormality.

Several pleiotropic single gene disorders also feature holoprosencephaly, in particular Meckel's syndrome, which shows autosomal recessive inheritance (see Table 20.2). Arhinencephaly occurs in Kallmann's syndrome of anosmia and hypogonadism (Kallmann et al 1944), in Perrin's syndrome of anosmia, mental retardation, hypogonadism and congenital ichthyosis (Perrin et al 1976) and Varadi's syndrome of polydactyly, facial clefting and retardation (Varadi et al 1980).

Holoprosencephaly may also occur in an otherwise normal infant with normal chromosomes. In most instances it is an isolated event in the family. However, affected siblings born to healthy parents have been reported (DeMyer et al 1963, Hintz et al 1968) thus indicating that some cases may result from autosomal recessive inheritance. A few families showing probable autosomal dominant inheritance have also been described (Dallaire et al 1971, Cantu et al 1978). Roach et al (1975) studied 30 families in each of which there was at least one child with holoprosencephaly. The study was a little unsatisfactory since only half of the affected children had been karyotyped. An empirical risk of 6% for siblings was derived. Thus it would be reasonable to offer a risk of up to 6% for siblings of an isolated case. In families in which there is evidence for dominant inheritance of holoprosencephaly, the penetrance is reduced so that the risk to first-degree relatives is 23 to 35% (Benke & Cohen 1983).

AGENESIS OF THE CORPUS CALLOSUM

Agenesis of the corpus callosum has many causes and is frequently associated with other central nervous system malformations (Jellinger et al 1981). The point has been made (Baraitser 1982) that the large majority of published cases are isolated with only a handful of familial cases having been reported. Thus it is certainly reasonable to offer a low recurrence risk for siblings and offspring, although the author is not aware of any family studies which have been undertaken to clarify the proportion of cases likely to be genetic in origin.

Chromosome abnormalities in which agenesis of the corpus callosum has been documented include trisomy for chromosomes 8, 8p, 11q, 13 and 18. This abnormality also occurs in several single gene disorders as listed in Table 20.4, which also includes published reports of 'private' syndromes featuring agenesis of the corpus callosum. These include examples of autosomal dominant, autosomal recessive and sex-linked recessive inheritance thereby illustrating 1. the importance of taking a careful family history in all cases and 2. the difficulties involved in offering complete reassurance that the problem will not recur.

LISSENCEPHALY

This is the term used to describe a smooth brain lacking gyri and sulci. Pachygyria refers to abnormally thick and broad gyri. Lissencephaly and pachygyria may sometimes occur in different parts of the same brain.

Table 20.4 Syndromes and published reports featuring familial agenesis of the corpus callosum

Reference	Features	Retardation	Inheritance
Aicardi syndrome (Aicardi et al 1965)	Infantile spasms, chorioretinal lacunae	Severe	X-linked dominant
Andermann's syndrome (Andermann et al 1972)	Progressive motor neuropathy	Mild	Autosomal recessive
Acrocallosal syndrome (Schinzel 1982)	Macrocephaly, polydactyly, syndactyly	Severe	Autosomal recessive
FG syndrome (Opitz & Kaveggia 1974)	Macrocephaly, imperforate anus	Severe	X-linked recessive
Naiman & Fraser 1955	Epilepsy, microcephaly	Severe	Autosomal recessive
Ziegler 1958	Myoclonic epilepsy	Severe	Autosomal or sex-linked recessive
Menkes et al 1964	Convulsions, spastic quadreplegia	Severe	Sex-linked recessive
Dogan et al 1967	Strabismus, scoliosis	Severe	Autosomal or sex-linked recessive
Shapira & Cohen 1973	Convulsions, microcephaly	Mild	Autosomal recessive
Cao et al 1977	Infantile spasms, spastic quadriplegia	Severe	Autosomal recessive
Lynn et al 1980	Macrocephaly	Mild	Autosomal dominant
Kaplan 1983	Ptosis, Hirschsprung's disease	Severe	Sex-linked recessive
Wilson et al 1983	Hypotonia	Severe	Autosomal or sex-linked recessive
Pineda et al 1984	Episodic apnoea and hypothermia	Severe	Autosomal recessive
Young et al 1985	Macrocephaly, malrotation	Moderate	Autosomal recessive

Syndromes featuring lissencephaly have been reviewed by Dobyns et al (1984, 1985), and are summarized in Table 20.5. At least two types of lissencephaly exist. In Type I the cerebral cortex is thickened and consists of only four rather than the normal six layers. The brain is microcephalic. In Type II lissencephaly the brain shows disorientated neurones with absent lamination and sparse cell columns. This type of lissencephaly is usually associated with hydrocephalus and other cerebral malformations.

One of the many notable developments of the last few years has been the demonstration, with the help of high-resolution cytogenetic studies, that patients with the Miller–Dieker syndrome (Miller 1963, Dieker et al 1969) are lacking chromosome material in the region of band 17p13 (Dobyns et al 1984). Thus all children with lissencephaly should be subjected to careful cytogenetic study.

Both Dobyns et al (1984) and Warkany (1981) stress that isolated lissencephaly has often recurred so that parents of an affected child, whose chromosomes have been found to be normal, should be alerted to a possible recurrence risk of 25%. Some cases of lissencephaly may well be environmental in origin but until the situation becomes clearer or family studies provide a suitable empirical recurrence risk, it will be very difficult to exclude autosomal recessive inheritance in any particular situation.

Table 20.5 Syndromes with lissencephaly

Syndrome	Inheritance	Associated features
Cerebro-oculo-muscular dystrophy (Krijgsman et al 1980)	Autosomal recessive	Hydrocephalus, encephalocele, muscular dystrophy
Craniotelencephalic dysplasia (Hughes et al 1983)	Autosomal recessive	Craniosynostosis, encephalocele
Miller–Dieker (Dobyns et al 1984)	Chromosomal deletion (17p13)	Convulsions, microcephaly, severe retardation
Neu-Laxova (Mueller et al 1983)	Autosomal recessive	Microcephaly, small digits, early lethality
Norman-Roberts (Dobyns et al 1984)	Autosomal recessive	Microcephaly, convulsions, severe retardation
Warburg (HARD±E) (Pagon et al 1983)	Autosomal recessive	Encephalocele, hydrocephalus, retinal dysplasia

CEREBELLAR ABNORMALITIES

Partial or complete absence of the cerebellar vermis occurs in association with the Dandy–Walker malformation as discussed previously. It also occurs in Joubert's syndrome (Joubert et al 1969) in which episodic hyperpnoea is associated with jerky eye movement, ataxia and mental retardation. Inheritance is autosomal recessive. Leber's amaurosis (King et al 1984) and chorioretinal colobomata (Laverda et al 1984) have been noted in infants with Joubert's syndrome as have polydactyly and lingual abnormalities (Egger et al 1982).

Hypoplasia of the cerebellar hemispheres and vermis has also been described, albeit rarely, in siblings (Norman 1940, Wichman et al 1985). Cerebellar hypoplasia has been recorded in siblings with a lethal multiple congenital anomaly syndrome comprising unilobular lungs, polydactyly, renal hypoplasia and sex reversal (Rutledge et al 1984, Donnai et al 1986). Absence of the cerebellar granular layer has been described in siblings in association with mental retardation and tapetoretinal degeneration by Hunter et al (1982).

The clinical diversity apparent in these reports of genetic disorders featuring cerebellar abnormalities illustrates that caution should be exercised when discussing possible recurrence risks. Bundey (1985) suggests that when no definite entity can be identified, it is appropriate to offer a recurrence risk of 1 in 8 for idiopathic congenital ataxia.

Prenatal diagnosis

Considering the complexity of the human brain it is not too surprising that understanding of its genesis is far from complete. It seems probable that many hundreds of genes are involved in the development of the central nervous system, errors in any one of which may result in serious problems.

It will be evident that every child with a structural CNS abnormality merits careful genetic assessment if correct risk information is to be given to the parents. Empirical risks are not ideal since they have usually been derived from large samples and may not be applicable to an individual case. Without them, however, it can be very difficult to counsel those families in which there is an isolated case of a neurodevelopmental abnormality which is aetiologically heterogeneous.

Progress in ultrasonography (Ch. 7) has demonstrated that many serious cerebral malformations may be diagnosed during the second trimester of pregnancy. Abnormalities detected in this way include the Dandy–Walker malformation (Dempsey & Koch 1981), Joubert's syndrome (Campbell et al 1984a), microcephaly (Nguyen The et al 1985), hydrocephalus, holoprosencephaly, hydranencephaly and porencephaly (Campbell et al 1984b). Given the prevailing uncertainty about the genetic contribution to many of the severe neurodevelopmental abnormalities it would seem an act of both compassion and prudence to offer prenatal diagnosis to the parents of any child with an unexplained cerebral malformation.

REFERENCES

Adams C, Johnston W P, Nevin N C 1982 Family study of congenital hydrocephalus. Developmental Medicine and Child Neurology 24: 493–498

Aicardi J, Lefebvre J, Lerique-Koechlin A 1965 A new syndrome: spasms in flexion, callosal agenesis, ocular abnormalities. Electroencephalography and Clinical Neurophysiology 19: 609–610

Airaksinen E M 1984 Familial porencephaly. Clinical Genetics 26: 236–238

Andermann F, Andermann E, Joubert M, Karpati G, Carpenter S, Melancon D 1972 Familial agenesis of the corpus callosum with anterior horn cell disease: a syndrome of mental retardation, areflexia and paraplegia. Transactions of the American Neurological Association 97: 242–244

Asch A J, Myers G J 1976 Benign familial macrocephaly: report of a family and review of the literature. Pediatrics 57: 535–539

Baraitser M 1982 The genetics of neurological disorders. Oxford University Press, Oxford

Bartley J A, Hall B D 1978 Mental retardation and multiple congenital abnormalities of unknown etiology: frequency of occurrence in similarly affected sibs of the proband. Birth Defects Original Article, Series XIV (6B): 127–137

Benke P J, Cohen M M 1983 Recurrence of holoprosencephaly in families with a positive history. Clinical Genetics 24: 324–328

Berg R A, Aleck K A, Kaplan A M 1983 Familial porencephaly. Archives of Neurology 40: 567–569

Bundey S 1985 Genetics and neurology. Churchill Livingstone, Edinburgh

Burton B K 1979 Recurrence risks for congenital hydrocephalus. Clinical Genetics 16: 47–53

Burton B K 1981 Dominant inheritance of microcephaly with short stature. Clinical Genetics 20: 25–27

Campbell S, Tsannatos C, Pearce J M 1984a The prenatal diagnosis of Joubert's syndrome of familial agenesis of the cerebellar vermis. Prenatal Diagnosis 4: 391–395

Campbell S, Smith P, Pearce J M 1984b The ultrasound diagnosis of neural tube defects and other cranio–spinal abnormalities. In: Prenatal diagnosis (Proceedings of the Eleventh Study Group of the Royal College of Obstetricians and Gynaecologists). Royal College of Obstetricians and Gynaecologists, London, pp 245–259

Cantu J M, Fragosa R, Garcia-Cruz D, Sanchez-Corona J 1978 Dominant inheritance of holoprosencephaly. Birth Defects Original Article, Series XIV (6B): 215–220

Cao A, Cianchetti C, Signorini E, Loi M, Sanna G, De Virgiliis S 1977 Agenesis of the corpus callosum, infantile spasms, spastic quadriplegia, microcephaly and severe mental retardation in three siblings. Clinical Genetics 12: 290–296

Carter C O, David P A, Laurence K M 1968 A family study of major central nervous system malformations in South Wales. Journal of Medical Genetics 5: 81–106

Cohen M M 1982 An update on the holoprosencephalic disorders. Journal of Pediatrics 101: 865–869

Cohen M M, Lemire R J 1982 Syndromes with cephaloceles. Teratology 25: 161–172

Creasy M R, Alberman E D 1976 Congenital malformations of the central nervous system in spontaneous abortions. Journal of Medical Genetics 13: 9–16

Czeizel A 1981 Schisis association. American Journal of Medical Genetics 10: 25–35

Dallaire L, Clarke Fraser F, Wiglesworth F W 1971 Familial holoprosencephaly. Birth Defects Original Article, Series VII (7): 136–142

Day R E, Schutt W H 1979 Normal children with large heads — benign familial megalencephaly. Archives of Disease in Childhood 54: 512–517

de Grouchy J, Turleau C 1984 Clinical atlas of human chromosomes, 2nd edn. John Wiley, New York

Dempsey P J, Koch H J 1981 In utero diagnosis of the Dandy–Walker syndrome: differentiation from extra-axial posterior fossa cyst. Journal of Clinical Ultrasound 9: 403–405

DeMyer W, Zeman W, Palmer C G 1963 Familial alobar holoprosencephaly (arrhinencephaly) with median cleft lip and palate. Neurology 13: 913–918

Dieker H, Edwards R H, ZuRhein G, Chou S M, Hartman H A, Opitz J M 1969 The lissencephaly syndrome. Birth Defects Original Article, Series V (2): 53–64

Dobyns W B, Stratton R F, Greenberg F 1984 Syndromes with lissencephaly. 1. Miller–Dieker and Norman–Roberts syndromes and isolated lissencephaly. American Journal of Medical Genetics 18: 509–526

Dobyns W B, Kirkpatrick J B, Hittner H M, Roberts R M, Kretzer F L 1985 Syndromes with lissencephaly. II. Walker–Warburg and cerebro–oculo–muscular syndromes and a new syndrome with type II lissencephaly. American Journal of Medical Genetics 22: 157–195

Dogan K, Dogan S, Lovrenčić 1967 Agenesis of the corpus callosum in two brothers. Lijecnicki Vjesnik 89: 377–385

Donnai D, Young I D, Owen W G, Clark S A, Miller P F W, Knox W F 1986 The lethal multiple congenital anomaly syndrome of polydactyly, sex reversal, renal hypoplasia, and unilobular lungs. Journal of Medical Genetics 23: 64–71

Egger J, Bellman M H, Ross E M, Baritser M 1982 Joubert–Boltshauser syndrome with polydactyly in siblings. Journal of Neurology, Neurosurgery and Psychiatry 45: 737–739

Fowler M, Dow R, White T A, Green C H 1972 Congenital hydrocephalus–hydrencephaly in five siblings, with autopsy studies: a new disease. Developmental Medicine and Child Neurology 14: 173–188

Gollop T R, Kiota M M, Martins R M M, Lucchesi E A, Alvarenga E 1984 Frontofacionasal dysplasia: evidence for autosomal recessive inheritance. American Journal of Medical Genetics 19: 301–305

Gragg G W 1971 Familial megalencephaly. Birth Defects Original Article, Series VII (1): 228–230

Halliday J, Chow C W, Wallace D, Danks D M 1986 X linked hydrocephalus: a survey of a 20 year period in Victoria, Australia. Journal of Medical Genetics 23: 23–31

Hamby W B, Krauss R F, Beswick W F 1950 Hydranencephaly: clinical diagnosis. Presentation of seven cases. Pediatrics 6: 371–383

Haslam R H A, Smith D W 1979 Autosomal dominant microcephaly. Journal of Pediatrics 95: 701–705

Higginbottom M C, Jones K L, Hall B D, Smith D W 1979 The amniotic band disruption complex: timing of amniotic rupture and variable spectra of consequent defects. Journal of Pediatrics 95: 544–549

Hintz R L, Menking M, Sotos J F 1968 Familial holoprosencephaly with endocrine dysgenesis. Journal of Pediatrics 72: 81–86

Howard F M, Till K, Carter C O 1981 A family study of hydrocephalus resulting from aqueduct stenosis. Journal of Medical Genetics 18: 252–255

Hughes H E, Harwood-Nash D C, Becker L E 1983 Craniotelencephalic dysplasia in sisters: further delineation of a possible syndrome. American Journal of Medical Genetics 14: 557–565

Hunter A G W 1983 The genetics of congenital malformations. Clinical Neurosurgery 30: 139–156

Hunter A G W 1984 Neural tube defects in Eastern Ontario and Western Quebec: demography and family data. American Journal of Medical Genetics 19: 45–63

Hunter A G W, Jurenka S, Thompson D, Evans J A 1982 Absence of the cerebellar granular layer, mental retardation, tapetoretinal degeneration and progressive glomerulopathy: an autosomal recessive occulo–renal–cerebellar syndrome. American Journal of Medical Genetics 11: 383–395

Jellinger K, Gross H, Kaltenbäck E, Grisold W 1981 Holoprosencephaly and agenesis of the corpus callosum: frequency of associated malformations. Acta Neuropathology 55: 1–10

Joubert M, Eisenring J J, Robb J P, Andermann F 1969 Familial agenesis of the cerebellar vermis. A syndrome of episodic hyperpnea, abnormal eye movements, ataxia and retardation. Neurology 19: 813–825

Kallmann F J, Schoenfeld W A, Barrera S E 1944 The genetic aspects of primary eunochoidism. American Journal of Mental Deficiency 48: 203–236

Kalter H, Warkany J 1983 Congenital malformations. New England Journal of Medicine 308: 424–431

Kaplan P 1983 X linked recessive inheritance of agenesis of the corpus callosum. Journal of Medical Genetics 20: 122–124

Keller H, Neuhauser G, Durkin-Stamm M V, Kaveggia E G, Schaaff A, Sitzmann F 1978 ADAM complex (amniotic deformity, adhesions, mutilations): a pattern of craniofacial and limb defects. American Journal of Medical Genetics 2: 81–98

King M D, Dudgeon J, Stephenson J B P 1984 Joubert's syndrome with retinal dysplasia: neonatal tachypnoea as the clue to a genetic brain–eye malformation. Archives of Disease in Childhood 59: 709–718

Kousseff B G 1984 Sacral meningocele with conotruncal heart defects: a possible autosomal recessive trait. Pediatrics 74: 395–398

Krijgsman J B, Barth P G, Stam F C, Slooff J L, Jaspar H H J 1980 Congenital muscular dystrophy and cerebral dysgenesis in a Dutch family. Neuropaediatrie 11: 108–120

Laverda A M, Saia O S, Drigo P, Danieli E, Clementi M, Tenconi R 1984 Chorioretinal coloboma and Joubert syndrome: a nonrandom association. Journal of Pediatrics 105: 282–284

Leck I 1974 Causation of neural tube defects: clues from epidemiology. British Medical Bulletin 30: 158–163

Lorber J, De N C 1970 Family history of congenital hydrocephalus. Developmental Medicine and Child Neurology 12 (suppl 22): 94–100

Lorber J, Priestley B L 1981 Children with large heads: a practical approach to diagnosis in 557 children. with special reference to 109 children with megalencephaly. Developmental Medicine and Child Neurology 23: 494–504

Lynn R B, Buchanan D C, Fenichel G M, Freemon F R 1980 Agenesis of the corpus callosum. Archives of Neurology 37: 444–445

McKusick V A 1986 Mendelian inheritance in man, 7th edn. Johns Hopkins University Press, Baltimore

Menkes J H, Philippart M, Clark D B 1964 Hereditary partial agenesis of corpus callosum. Archives of Neurology 11: 198–208

Miller J Q 1963 Lissencephaly in 2 siblings. Neurology 13: 841–850

Mueller R F, Winter R M, Naylor C P E 1983 Neu–Laxova syndrome: two further case reports and comments on proposed subclassification. American Journal of Medical Genetics 16: 645–649

Murray J C, Johnson J A, Bird T D 1985 Dandy–Walker malformation: etiologic heterogeneity and empiric recurrence risks. Clinical Genetics 28: 272–283

Naiman J, Fraser F C 1955 Agenesis of the corpus callosum: a report of two cases in siblings. Archives of Neurology and Psychiatry 74: 182–185

Nevin N C, Johnstone W P 1980 A family study of spina bifida and anencephalus in Belfast, Northern Ireland (1964–1968). Journal of Medical Genetics 17: 203–211

Nguyen The E, Pescia G, Deonna T, Bakarić O 1985 Early prenatal diagnosis of genetic microcephaly. Prenatal Diagnosis 5: 345–347

Norman R M 1940 Primary degeneration of the granular layer of the cerebellum: an unusual form of familial cerebellar atrophy occurring in early life. Brain 63: 365–379

Opitz J M 1985 The developmental field concept. American Journal of Medical Genetics 21: 1–11

Opitz J M, Kaveggia E G 1974 The FG syndrome. An X-linked recessive syndrome of multiple congenital anomalies and mental retardation. Zeitschrift fur Kinderheilkunde 117: 1–18

Opitz J M, Kaveggia E G, Durkin-Stamm M V, Pendleton E 1978 Diagnostic/genetic studies in severe mental retardation. Birth Defects Original Article, Series XVI (6B): 1–38

Pagon R A, Clarren S K, Milam D F, Hendrickson A E 1983 Autosomal recessive eye and brain anomalies: Warburg syndrome. Journal of Pediatrics 102: 542–546

Palo J, Lydecken K, Kivalo E 1966 Etiological aspects of mental deficiency in autopsied patients. American Journal of Mental Deficiency 71: 401–405

Patton M A, Sharma A, Winter R M 1985. The Aase–Smith syndrome. Clinical Genetics 28: 521–525

Perrin J C, Idemoto J Y, Sotos J F, Maurer W F, Steinberg A G 1976 X-linked syndrome of congenital ichthyosis, hypogonadism, mental retardation and anosmia. Birth Defects Original Article, Series XII (5): 267–274

Pineda M, Gonzalez A, Fabregues I, Fernandez-Alvarez E 1984 Familial agenesis of the corpus callosum with hypothermia and apneic spells. Neuropediatrics 15: 63–67

Qazi Q H, Reed T E 1973 A problem in diagnosis of primary versus secondary microcephaly. Clinical Genetics 4: 46–52

Riccardi V M 1981 Von Recklinghausen neurofibromatosis. New England Journal of Medicine 305: 1617–1627

Riley H D, Smith W R 1960 Macrocephaly, pseudopapilledema and multiple haemangiomata. Pediatrics 26: 293–300

Roach E, DeMyer W, Conneally P M, Palmer C, Merritt A D 1975 Holoprosencephaly: birth data genetic and demographic analyses of 30 families. Birth Defects Original Article, Series XI (2): 295–313

Rutledge J C, Friedman J M, Harrod M J E et al 1984 A new lethal multiple congenital anomaly syndrome. American Journal of Medical Genetics 19: 255–264

Salonen R, Herva R, Norio R 1981 The hydrolethalus syndrome: delineation of a 'new' lethal malformation syndrome based on 28 patients. Clinical Genetics 19: 321–330

Schinzel A 1982 Four patients including two sisters with the acrocallosal syndrome (agenesis of the corpus callosum in combination with preaxial hexadactyly). Human Genetics 62: 382

Schreier H, Rapin I, Davis J 1974 Familial megalencephaly or hydrocephalus? Neurology 24: 232–236

Seller M J 1981 Recurrence risks for neural tube defects in a genetic counselling clinic population. Journal of Medical Genetics 18: 245–248

Shapira Y, Cohen T 1973 Agenesis of the corpus callosum in two sisters. Journal of Medical Genetics 10: 266–269

Siber M 1984 X-linked recessive microcencephaly, microphthalmia with corneal opacities, spastic quadriplegia, hypospadias and cryptorchidism. Clinical Genetics 26: 453–456

Smith D W 1981 Recognizable patterns of human deformation. W B Saunders, Philadelphia

Smith D W 1982 Recognizable patterns of human malformation, 3rd edn. W B Saunders, Philadelphia

Smithells R W, Sheppard S, Schorah C J et al 1981 Apparent prevention of neural tube defects by periconceptional vitamin supplementation. Archives of Disease in Childhood 56: 911–918

Spranger J et al 1982 Errors of morphogenesis: concepts and terms. Journal of Pediatrics 100: 160–165

Varadi V, Szabo L, Papp Z 1980 Syndrome of polydactyly, cleft lip/palate or lingual lump, and psychomotor retardation in endogamic gypsies. Journal of Medical Genetics 17: 119–122

Warkany J, Lemire R J, Cohen M M 1981 Mental retardation and congenital malformations of the central nervous system. Year Book Medical Publishers, Chicago

Wichman A, Frank M, Kelly T E 1985 Autosomal recessive congenital cerebellar hypoplasia. Clinical Genetics 27: 373–382

Wilson W G, Kennaugh J M, Kugler J P, Reynolds J F 1983 Agenesis of the corpus callosum in two brothers. Journal of Medical Genetics 20: 416–418

Winter R M, Baraitser M, Douglas J M 1984 A computerised data base for the diagnosis of rare dysmorphic syndromes. Journal of Medical Genetics 21: 121–123

Yates V D, Wilroy R S, Whitington G L, Simmons J C H 1983 Anterior sacral defects: an autosomal dominantly inherited condition. Journal of Pediatrics 102: 239–242

Young I D, Trounce J Q, Leven M I, Fitzsimmons J S, Moore J R 1985 Agenesis of the corpus callosum and macrocephaly in siblings. Clinical Genetics 28: 225–230

Ziegler V E 1958 Bösartige, familiäre, frühinfantile Krampfkrankheit, teilweise verbunden mit familiärer Balkenaplasie. Helvetica Paediatrica Acta 13: 169–184

Zonana J, Rimoin D L, Davis D C 1976 Macrocephaly with multiple lipomas and haemangiomas. Journal of Pediatrics 89: 600–603

21. Functional teratogenic effects on the developing brain

Prof D. F. Swaab and Dr M. Mirmiran

Probably because of the thalidomide tragedy, our awareness of the dangers of drug ingestion has cautioned us against the indiscriminate use of medicines mainly during the initial stage of pregnancy. However, even medicines that do not cause any gross physical malformations may cause microscopic defects or alter the intricate structure or chemical composition of fetal brain tissue, also during the second part of pregnancy, to such an extent that permanent behavioural deviations later develop. The latter field, which is known as 'functional or behavioural teratology' is the subject of this chapter. In the Netherlands some 80% of pregnant women take medicines, whereas in a prospective study in the UK 35% of pregnant women took drugs (Rubin et al 1986). Most of these drugs are of the type that easily cross the placenta. They readily reach the fetal brain, since the blood–brain barrier at this stage of development is not capable of preventing their passage. The same holds for addictive compounds taken by the mother, e.g heroin, morphine, methadone, alcohol, marihuana and cigarette smoking.

There are several reasons why such effects of medicines were not recognized until recently, the most important one being that chemical compounds do not generally give rise to a syndrome in the child that can easily be recognized by the clinician as being specific to a particular compound taken by the mother during pregnancy. 'Functional teratology' is rather expressed much later in life by cognitive disturbances, mental retardation, reproductive or motor defects, disturbed language development or sleep disturbances. This, and the long time-interval between the use of medicines and the functional disturbances often makes it difficult to establish the relationship with intra-uterine sequelae of chemicals.

CHEMICALS AFFECTING BRAIN DEVELOPMENT

Many different chemicals might affect the developing brain. In fact, all those chemical compounds which are of importance for adult brain function appear to be involved in brain development as well (Swaab 1980). At present this is established for sex hormones, corticosteroids, thyroid hormones, and neurotransmitters. Substances which alter the balance of any of these neuro-active compounds during the vulnerable periods in ontogeny are therefore capable of altering brain development in a permanent way.

Sex hormones

In the rat sex hormones act during the perinatal period by affecting maturation of the brain, both structurally and functionally, inducing in this way a sexual differentiation of the brain. For example, a light microscopically evident sexual dimorphism occurs in the size of a part of the nucleus preopticus medialis (the sexual dimorphic nucleus of the preoptic area, SDN-POA), which is determined in the rat by the levels of testosterone present around the time of birth (Gorski et al 1978, Jacobson et al 1980). The SDN-POA has recently been described by us in the human brain. The volume of this nucleus is 2.5 times as large in men as it is in women and contains 2.2 times as many cells (Swaab & Fliers 1985). Sex hormones coming from the fetus probably constitute in normal development, the biological basis for sex-related brain and behavioural differences in animals as well as in humans. It is therefore a matter of considerable concern that progestagens, oestrogens and/or combinations thereof have frequently been prescribed to pregnant women (Reinish & Karow 1977), in the mistaken belief that they would prevent impending miscarriages. In the USA 1–4.5 million pregnant women used diethylstilboestrol (DES) from 1945 until 1971. It was taken off the market due only to a probable carcinogenic effect on the cervix and vagina in female offspring (Herbst et al 1981). However, not only are these drugs ineffective in sustaining pregnancy but their use entails a real possibility of inducing personality disorders in the offspring. Oestrogen-exposed children have been found between 4 and 21 years of age to be generally less self-confident, less sensitive, and more dependent and group oriented than normal children (Reinisch & Karow 1977). In addition, a high percentage (25%) of infertility and possible interference with sexual function was found following intra-uterine exposure to oestrogens (Beral & Colwell 1981, Stenchever et al 1981). Prenatal administration of oestrogen and progesterone in boys has been reported to influence noticeably certain aspects of postnatal psychosexual development (i.e. 'masculinity', 'aggressiveness', and athletic abilities) (Yalom et al 1973). Recent studies show that DES daughters have an increased incidence of bisexuality and homosexuality (Ehrhardt et al 1985). It is worth mentioning that sexual differentiation of the brain is not only affected by sex hormones. Similar developmental effects affecting sexual differentiation have been described for serotonin, noradrenaline (see later) and dopamine-related drugs (Hull et al 1984), nicotine (Lichtensteiger & Schlumpf 1985), alcohol (McGivern et al 1984), cimetidine (Anand & Van Thiel 1982), morphine (Vathy et al 1983), barbiturates (Reinisch & Sanders 1982), and maternal stress (Dörner 1979). When pregnant rats are exposed to stress, the SDN-POA of the male offspring becomes permanently smaller, i.e. of female size (Anderson et al 1985). Consequently, all types of neuro-active compounds might affect sexual differentiation of the brain. This is another characteristic of the functional teratology of chemical compounds that makes this field hard to study; different compounds, when given during development, may lead to similar aspects of functional sequelae in later life.

Corticosteroids

Corticosteroids are used during pregnancy, for example in cases of allergic reactions, and to promote lung development in the child in cases of imminent parturition. However, in quite a number of patients this treatment did not seem to have the expected effect (Gariete et al 1981). In addition, animal experiments indicate that exposure to corticosteroids can retard brain development and affect behaviour in later life (Balazs et al 1975, Taeusch 1975, Sobel 1978, Dahlof et al 1980, Johnson et al 1981. Marton & Szondy (1982) found a retardation of psychomotor development, which persisted at least up to 2 years of life in prematurely born children who had been exposed to corticosteroids. A good prospective study is badly needed in this area.

Thyroid hormones

Thyroid hormones have been injected directly into the amniotic fluid to enhance fetal lung maturation (Mashiach et al 1978). No follow-up investigation of these children has been carried out to our knowledge, although it is known from animal experiments that such treatment may hamper brain development (Balazs 1979).

Neurotransmitters

Recent research indicates also that *neurotransmitters* which can be subdivided into the following groups: acetylcholine, biogenic amines, amino acids and peptides are essential for normal brain development.

Acetylcholine

Pyridostigmine (an acetylcholinesterase inhibitor), when administered to neonatal rats, induces premature puberty and increased male sexuality in both sexes of the offspring (Hinz et al 1978). Nicotine (an acetylcholine receptor agonist) enhances cell death in the rat fetal brainstem (Kraus et al 1981) while neonatal administration of chlorisodamine (a nicotine-receptor blocker) prevented the normal postnatal increase in volume and cell number of the mouse superior cervical ganglion (Black & Geen 1974). This might be one of the mechanisms by which smoking of the pregnant mother may have a permanent effect on brain development and school performance of the child (Butler & Goldstein 1973, Abel 1980).

Biogenic amines

Apart from the serotonin-reuptake blocker (chlorimipramine) and the alpha-adrenergic agonist (clonidine), see later, there are many examples of medicines which, if used during pregnancy, impair normal brain development by upsetting the balance of the monoamines and/or influencing the sensitivity of the receptors. In animal experiments, reserpine (used as an antihypertensive drug as well as a tranquillizer) decreases the monoamine levels in the brain and has been shown to induce permanent brain and behavioural changes in the offspring. These include reduced formation of neurones, hyperactivity, and increased susceptibility to audiogenic seizures. Amphetamine, which increases the release of catecholamines in the brain, is used as a dieting aid but is also given to children in cases of enuresis nocturna or minimal brain dysfunction. Offspring of pregnant rats treated with such drugs show behavioural changes, most notably an inability in adulthood to adapt to new surroundings. Alpha-methyldopa (a false transmitter precursor for noradrenaline) and propranolol (a beta-adrenergic blocker), when taken by the pregnant mother, result in a reduced head circumference in the human neonate. The use of neuroleptics such as chlorpromazine (a dopamine antagonist) during pregnancy has been reported to lead to extrapyramidal disturbances in the newborn child, while in animal experiments it impaired learning ability (for references on this section see Swaab & Mirmiran 1984). p-Chlorophenylalanine, which blocks serotonin synthesis, affects cell division in regions of the posterior diencephalon known to become innervated by serotonergic fibres (Lauder et al 1983, Lauder & Krebs 1984a,b). Barbiturates, which also stimulate dopamine receptors (Yanai & Feigenbaum 1981), are commonly used as hypnotics, sedatives, anticonvulsants and for preventing neonatal jaundice. They may induce a withdrawal syndrome lasting as long as 3 months (Thornburg & Moore 1976). In animal studies, barbiturates have been shown to impair reproductive function and maze-learning ability of the offspring (Middaugh et al 1975, Clemens et al 1979, Gupta et al 1980). Beta-mimetics, such as ritodrine, that are used frequently to prevent premature delivery, may lead to less good school performance of the children later on in life (Hadders-Algra et al 1986).

Amino acids

Many compounds influencing amino acid transmitters are used during pregnancy and postnatal development. Prenatal or early postnatal treatment of rats with the often used tranquillizer diazepam (which acts upon gamma-aminobutyric acid (GABA)-benzodiazepine receptor complex) produces long-lasting effects on brain enzymes and behavioural disturbances such as hyperactivity, lack of acoustic startle reflexes, and sleep disturbances (Fonseca et al 1976, Jakoubek 1978, Kellog et al 1980, Livezey et al 1985). It also reduces choline uptake in the male rat frontal cortex (Grimm 1984), induces a permanent decrease in noradrenaline level, turnover and release in the hypothalamus (Simmons et al 1984, Kellogg & Retell 1986), and a permanent decline in diazepam binding sites (Livezey 1985). Diphenylhydantoin, administered to the pregnant rat, caused increased levels of GABA in adulthood (Vorhees 1985). Diazepam administration during pregnancy in humans results in low Apgar scores, depressed respiration and impaired suckling (Patrick et al 1972, Cree et al 1973). Long-term follow-ups of such children are lacking. Dairy cow milk formulae might be too low in taurine to secure optimal brain development (Gaull 1985).

Peptides

Little is known about the possible long-term effects on brain development of this recently discovered group of neurotransmitters. They were originally thought to be simply hormones produced by the hypothalamus but later appeared to have important central effects as well (for review, see Swaab 1982, Boer & Swaab 1985).

Oxytocin is routinely used in obstetrics and may cause fetal distress, including a rise in core temperature and possibly retarded motor and speech development. Observations in the rat revealed a permanent decrease in water metabolism following administration of oxytocin to the developing rat (for references see Boer & Swaab 1983). Vasotocin administered to kittens induced delayed eye-opening and brain lipid content while locomotion was diminished and periods of active sleep were enhanced (Goldstein 1984). Vasopressin, which may permanently alter osmoregulation following perinatal administration (Boer & Swaab 1983, Boer et al 1984), and its analogues have been given to mentally retarded children (Waggoner

et al 1978, Anderson et al 1979, Eisenberg et al 1984a,b), and for the treatment of enuresis nocturna (Stegner et al 1986). DGAVP has been given to children following brain trauma (Wit et al 1986). Such children should consequently be followed up for possible long-term sequelae due to the peptide treatment in development. One of the problems of such a long-term follow-up is, however, that not enough experimental studies have been done yet to tell the clinician which functions might be disturbed due to the administration of neuropeptides.

Postnatal treatment with thyrotropin-releasing hormone (TRH) increased rat hypothalamic weight and impaired T-maze learning (Stratton et al 1976). Corticotropin-releasing factor (CRF) accelerated eye-opening, enhanced rearing in an open-field and impaired body temperature regulation. Substance P increased pain perception and induced upregulation of its receptors (Handelmann et al 1984), while neonatal exposure to a high level of ACTH 4-10 u impairs adult learning behaviour (McGivern et al 1986).

Opioids and compounds influencing this system have strong effects on brain development. Methadone exposure of developing rats caused, for example, a delay in reflex development, eye-opening, somatic and brain growth, a regional alteration of catecholamines, hyperactivity, increased emotionality, learning disabilities and dysfunction of thermoregulation and nociception. In children whose mothers had been exposed to opioids, abstinence symptoms were found, a high rate of mortality, sleep disturbances, delays in the sensorimotor development, retardation in somatic growth, smaller head circumference, delays in walking, problems in visual and auditory systems, aberrations in neuro-ontogeny, less alert, poor attention spans, hyperactivity, learning disabilities and social problems (Zagon & McLaughlin 1984).

Naloxone, an opiate antagonist, is administered clinically to normalize fetal heart rate (Goodlin 1981). Animal experiments have implicated naloxone as the cause of a permanent impairment of sensitivity to thermal stimuli (Sandman et al 1979) and of maze-learning ability (Vorhees 1981). Beta-endorphin, used during delivery as an analgesic (Oyama et al 1980), induces similar disturbances in the rat (Sandman et al 1979). This treatment causes a reduced beta-endorphin immunocytochemical staining in various brain regions (Moldow et al 1981).

MECHANISMS OF ACTION OF CHEMICALS ON THE DEVELOPING BRAIN

Drugs taken by the pregnant mother may impair the developing child's brain in different ways:

1. This action may be *indirect*, as in the case of aspirin which, when taken by the pregnant mother, may result in a higher incidence of intracranial bleeding and perinatal mortality (Collins 1981, Rumack et al 1981). Another action of this kind is the alcohol-induced impairment of

umbilical circulation producing hypoxia and acidosis in the fetus (Mukherjee & Hodgen 1982). Prenatal exposure to barbiturates might also influence brain development indirectly by altering liver metabolism of sex hormones (Reinisch & Sanders 1982).

2. Drugs may affect brain development by interacting *directly* with the formation of the neuronal and glial network, e.g. by affecting cell division, cell death, cell migration, or the formation of neurites, synapses and receptors. Most, if not all, medicines appear to affect

Cell division is reported to be slowed down by a number of medicines, both in vivo and in vitro. Barbiturates were found to cause a 30% reduction in the number of cerebellar Purkinje cells and a 15% reduction in hippocampal pyramidal cells. Other compounds which have similar deleterious effects include corticosteroids, chlorpromazine, alcohol, reserpine, thyroid hormone and sex hormones (for references see Swaab & Mirmiran 1984). Indirect evidence for decreased brain cell division is provided by the smaller head circumferences which have been found at birth following treatment with sex hormones (Huisjes H J, personal communication); with alpha-methyldopa or propranolol, and diphenylhydantoin, or by the use of alcohol during human pregnancy (for references see Swaab & Mirmiran 1984).

Cell death is augmented by nicotine (Kraus et al 1981), accelerated by alcohol exposure prior to birth in the rat (Yanai 1981), and delayed by morphine in the chick embryo (Meriney et al 1985).

Cell migration may be disturbed by alcohol (Jones et al 1976), anticonvulsants (Trice & Ambler 1985) and monosodium glutamate (Marani et al 1982).

The formation of neurites and synapses is known to be affected by sex hormones, corticosteroids, morphine, methadone, anticonvulsive agents and by alcohol (for references see Swaab & Mirmiran 1984).

Receptors may also be permanently altered by neuroactive compounds given during development. Haloperidol, which blocks dopamine receptors, induced in this way a permanent decrease in the number of dopamine receptors in the striatum (Rosengarten & Friedhoff 1979). L-Dopa, which increases dopamine synthesis, permanently increased receptor density (Friedhoff et al 1977). Prenatal morphine exposure in the rat increases the adult number and affinity of spinal cord opiate receptors (Kirby 1984), while prenatal exposure to diazepam results in enduring reductions in diazepam binding sites in the rat thalamus (Livezey et al 1985).

3. The third mechanism involves effects of medicines on spontaneous behavioural states, namely wakefulness, quiet sleep and rapid eye movement (REM) sleep. In a study at our institute in which the long-term effect of REM sleep ('active' sleep, AS) deprivation on brain and behaviour development was studied, experimental suppression of AS during early postnatal life by means of clomipramine or clonidine in rats revealed a clear-cut reduction of cortical size, a higher level of open field activity, deficient masculine sexual behaviour, and disturbed sleep patterns in adulthood (Mirmiran et al 1981, 1983a, Swaab & Mirmiran 1984). These results, and those of others using different pharmacological as well as non-pharmacological approaches, argue in favour of AS as a mediating factor for normal brain maturation (Mitler 1971, Juvanes & Nowaczyk 1975, Saucier & Astick 1975), in which, of course, several mechanisms as discussed before may be involved.

The specific reduction of cortical weight, together with decreased protein content, in the absence of any significant change in cell number, was highly reminiscent of the picture seen in rats reared under sensorially impoverished conditions (Rozenzweig & Bennett 1978). Furthermore, concomitant AS deprivation by means of clonidine neutralizes the effect that environmental enrichment normally exerts upon cortical growth (Mirmiran & Uylings 1983). Another intriguing finding is that prolonged AS deprivation by means of clonidine even prior to the period of enrichment rearing interferes with the expected extra brain growth (Mirmiran et al 1983b). Apparently, cortical mechanisms underlying 'plasticity' in later life can be adversely affected by the absence of AS and/or noradrenaline disturbances in early development. Such a phenomenon may implicate abnormal sleep patterns as a potential contributory factor to learning deficiences in humans as well.

The drugs used in the AS-deprivation studies, namely clomipramine (Anafranil) and clonidine (Catapresan) are also used in clinical practice (for treating depression, hypertension, migraine, nocturnal enuresis, sleep apnoea, opiate withdrawal, minimal brain dysfunction, etc.). A recent follow-up study examined the effects of prenatal clonidine treatment of hypertensive mothers on the development of children who are now 6–8 years of age. In the exposed group compared with non-treated hypertensives an excess of sleep disturbances was found (Huisjes et al 1986), indicating that animal experiments in the field of functional teratology might give useful clues on the functions that have to be examined in children by means of long-term follow-up studies.

CLINICAL AWARENESS AND ANIMAL EXPERIMENTS REQUIRED

It is both surprising and a source of concern that practically no follow-up studies appear to have been carried out on the possible long-lasting functional consequences of treatments during human pregnancy. A wide variety of chemical compounds having comparable effects upon monoamine systems and/or AS, as described above, are currently in clinical use (cf. Swaab & Mirmiran 1984) and many consequently cause functional deficits. Effects of chemicals administered during development might even be carried over to following generations (Friedler 1974), possibly by affecting automodulation of genes (Campbell & Zimmerman 1982).

It is important to point out that almost all drugs used during gestation easily cross the placenta, and their level in the fetus (especially in the brain) may even be higher than in the maternal circulation (Mirkin & Singh 1976). In addition, humans are often more sensitive than animals to teratogenicity of drugs (Council on Environmental Quality 1981). One report does demonstrate a prolonged disturbance of sleep in babies born from heroin-addicted mothers (Davis & Glass 1980). Similar sleep disturbances might be responsible for the smaller head circumferences in boys, up to 4 years of age, born to mothers treated with alpha-methyldopa during late gestation (Moar et al 1978, Ounsted et al 1980). A problem is that long-term follow-up without a strong indication of what behaviour or function has to be studied in later life will most probably fail to find disturbances. The sleep disturbances found in children where the mother used clonidine during pregnancy (Huisjes et al 1986) indicate that animal experimental studies might allow a selection of the right functions to study in human follow-up studies. This means that systematic search for functional teratological effects of chemicals should be encouraged.

The direct and indirect effects of a variety of clinically used drugs upon the development of the brain have been discussed here. Taken together, the literature on this subject points to a potential health hazard not only during the first trimester of pregnancy but also throughout the entire period of gestation, and during lactation. The possibility that similar mechanisms are still present in later development cannot be excluded at present. Obstetricians, neonatologists, and paediatricians should, therefore, be aware that the immediate beneficial effects of many drugs may be offset by the induction of permanent behavioural and psychological defects within the children's developing brains. This is a relevant consideration, e.g. in cases involving children suffering from minimal brain dysfunction who are often subjected to extremely high doses of imipramine or amphetamine-like drugs (for review, see Gross & Wilson 1974) even though improvement often occurs eventually even in the absence of any medication whatsoever. The same point can be made, of course, for the treatment of nocturnal enuresis by means of antidepressants. It is an unfortunate commentary at the present time that the mothers themselves are often more aware of the potential dangers inherent in the use of medicines during pregnancy than are the physicians who prescribe them. Since recent work indicates the functional developmental effects of anaesthetics (Chalon et al 1981, Blair et al 1984, Koëter & Rodier 1986, Rodier & Koëter 1986, Rodier et al 1986), it should be a point of concern not only for operations on pregnant mothers but also for pregnant staff in operating and recovery rooms. We suggest that the investigation of the link between experimental and clinical medicine in this area, namely the question of functional teratological sequelae of medications administered during early development, ought to be encouraged (Swaab 1985, Swaab & Mirmiran 1985). For those diseases that have to be treated during pregnancy it is of utmost importance to select, in the future, only those compounds which combine high therapeutic potencies with low functional teratological side effects.

ACKNOWLEDGEMENTS

We are grateful to Mrs W. Chen-Pelt and Mrs O. Pach for their secretarial help.

REFERENCES

Abel E 1980 Smoking during pregnancy: a review of effects on growth and development of offspring. Human Biology 52: 593–625

Anand S, Van Thiel D H 1982 Prenatal and neonatal exposure to cimetidine results in gonadal and sexual dysfunction in adult males. Science 218: 493–494

Anderson D K, Rhees R W, Fleming D E 1985 Effects of prenatal stress on differentiation of the sexually dimorphic nucleus of the preoptic area (SDN-POA) of the rat brain. Brain Research 332: 113–118

Anderson L T, David R, Bennet K, Dancis J 1979 Passive avoidance learning in Lesch–Nyhan disease: effect of 1-desamino-8-arginine vasopressin. Life Sciences 24: 905–910

Balazs R 1979 Cerebellum: certain features of its development and biochemistry. In: Cuenod M, Kreuzberg G W, Bloom F E (eds) Development and chemical specificity of neurons. Progress in Brain Research, No. 51. Elsevier Biomedical Press, Amsterdam, pp 357–372

Balazs R, Patel A J, Hajos F 1975 Factors affecting the biochemical maturation of the brain: effects of hormones during early life. Psychoneuroendocrinology 1: 25–36

Beral V, Colwell L 1981 Randomized trial of high doses of stilboestrol and ethisterone therapy in pregnancy: long-term follow-up of the children. Journal of Epidemiology and Community Health 35: 155–160

Black I B, Geen S C 1974 Inhibition of the biochemical and morphological maturation of adrenergic neurons by nicotinic receptor blockade. Journal of Neurochemistry 22: 301–306

Blair V W, Hollenbeck A R, Smith R F, Scanlon J W 1984 Neonatal preference for visual patterns: modification by prenatal anesthetic exposure? Developmental Medicine & Child Neurology 26: 476–483

Boer G J, Swaab D F 1983 Long-term effects on brain and behavior of early treatments with neuropeptides. In: Zbinden G, Cuomo G, Racagni B, Weiss B (eds) Application of behavioral pharmacology in toxicology. Raven Press, New York, pp 251–263

Boer G J, Swaab D F 1985 Neuropeptide effects on brain development to be expected from behavioral teratology. Peptides 6 (suppl 2): 21–28

Boer G J, Kragten R, Kruisbrink J, Swaab D F 1984 Vasopressin fails to restore postnatally the stunted brain development in the Brattleboro rat, but affects water metabolism permanently. Neurobehavioral Toxicology and Teratology 6: 103–109

Butler N R, Goldstein H 1973 Smoking in pregnancy and subsequent child development. British Medical Journal 4: 573–575

Campbell J H, Zimmerman E G 1982 Automodulation of genes: a proposed mechanism for persisting effects of drugs and hormones in mammals. Neurobehavioral Toxicology and Teratology 4: 435–439

Chalon J, Tang Ch-K, Ramanathan S, Eisner M, Katz R, Turndorf H 1981 Exposure to halothane and enflurane affects learning function of murine progeny. Anesthesia and Analgesia 60: 794–797

Clemens L G, Popham T V, Rupport P H 1979 Neonatal treatment of hamsters with barbiturates alters adult sexual behavior. Developmental Psychobiology 12: 49–59

Collins E 1981 Maternal and fetal effects of acetaminophen and salicylates in pregnancy. Obstetrics and Gynecology 58 (suppl 578): 62S

Council on Environmental Quality 1981 Chemical hazards to human reproduction. Government Printing Office, Washington

Cree J R, Meyer S, Hailey D M 1973 Diazepam in metabolism and effect on the clinical condition and thermogenesis of the new-born. British Medical Journal 4: 251–255

Dahlof L G, Larsson K, Hard E 1980 Sexual differentiation and adult sexual behavior of male offspring of mothers treated with corticosteroids during pregnancy. Neuroscience Letters 5 (suppl): 128

Davis M M, Glass P 1980 Fetal exposure to narcotics: neonatal sleep as a measure of nervous system disturbances. Science 209: 619–621

Dörner G 1979 Psychoneuroendocrine aspects of brain development and reproduction. In: Zichella L, Pancheri P (eds) Psychoneuro-endocrinology in reproduction: an interdisciplinary approach. Elsevier, Amsterdam, pp 43–54

Ehrhardt A A, Meyer-Bahlburg H F L, Rosen L R et al 1985 Sexual orientation after prenatal exposure to exogenous estrogen. Archives of Sexual Behavior 14: 57–75

Eisenberg J, Hamburger-Bar R, Belmaker R H 1984a The effect of vasopressin treatment on learning in Down's syndrome. Journal of Neural Transmission 60: 143–147

Eisenberg J, Chazan-Gologorsky S, Hattab J, Belmaker R H 1984b A controlled trial of vasopressin treatment of childhood learning disorder. Biological Psychiatry 19: 1137–1141

Fonseca N M, Sell A B, Carlini E A 1976 Differential behavioral responses of male and female adult rats treated with five psychotropic drugs in the neonatal state. Psychopharmacology 46: 263–268

Friedhoff A J, Bonnet K A, Rosengarten H 1977 Reversal of two manifestations of dopamine receptor supersensitivity by administration of L-dopa. Research Communications in Chemical Pathology and Pharmacology 16: 411–423

Friedler G 1974 Long-term effects of opiates. In: Dancis J, Hwang J C (eds) Perinatal pharmacology: problems and priorities. Raven Press, New York, pp 207–219

Gariete T J, Freeman R K, Linzey E M, Braly P S, Dorchester W L 1981 Perspective randomised study of corticosteroids on the management of premature rupture of the membranes and the premature gestation. American Journal of Obstetrics and Gynecology 141: 508–515

Gaull G E 1985 Introduction: an overview of early malnutrition and brain development. In: Arima M, Suzuki Y, Yabuuchi H (eds) The developing brain and its disorders. Karger, Tokyo, pp 279–289

Goldstein R 1984 The involvement of arginine vasotocin in the maturation of the kitten brain. Peptides 5: 25–28

Goodlin R C 1981 Naloxone and its possible relationship to fetal endorphin levels and fetal distress. American Journal of Obstetrics and Gynecology 136: 16–19

Gorski R A, Gordon J H, Shryne J E, Southam A M 1978 Evidence for a morphological sex difference within the medial preoptic area of the rat brain. Brain Research 148: 333–346

Grimm V E 1984 A review of diazepam and other benzodiazepines in pregnancy. In: Yanai J (ed) Neurobehavioral teratology. Elsevier, Amsterdam, pp 153–162

Gross M B, Wilson W C 1974 Minimal brain dysfunction. Brunner/Mazel, New York

Gupta C, Sonawane B R, Yaffe S J, Shapiro B H 1980 Phenobarbital exposure in utero: alternations in female reproductive function in rats. Science 208: 508–510

Hadders-Algra M, Touwen B C L, Huisjes H et al 1986 Long-term follow-up of children prenatally exposed to ritodrine. British Journal of Obstetrics 93: 156–161

Handelmann G E, Selsky J H, Helke C J 1984 Substance P administration to neonatal rats increases adult sensitivity to substance P. Physiology and Behavior 33: 297–300

Herbst A L, Hubby M M, Azizi F, Makii M M 1981 Reproductive and gynecologic surgical experience in diethylstilbestrol-exposed daughters. American Journal of Obstetrics and Gynecology 141: 1019–1028

Hinz G, Döcke F, Dörner G 1978 Long-term changes of sexual function in rats treated neonatally with psychotropic drugs. In: Dörner G, Kawakami M (eds) Hormones and brain development, Elsevier, Amsterdam, pp 121–127

Huisjes H J, Hadders-Algra M, Touwen B C L 1986 Is clonidine a behavioural teratogen in the human? Early Human Development 13: 1–6

Hull E M, Nishita J K, Bitran D, Dalterio S 1984 Perinatal dopamine-related drugs demasculinize rats. Science 224: 1011–1013

Jacobson C D, Shryne J E, Shapiro F, Gorski R A 1980 Ontogeny of the sexually dimorphic nucleus of the preoptic area. Journal of Comparative Neurology 193: 541–548

Jakoubek B 1978 The effect of ACTH and/or tranquillizers on the development of brain macromolecular metabolism. In: Dörner G, Kawakami M (eds) Hormones and brain development. Elsevier/North Holland Biomedical Press, Amsterdam, pp 259–264

Johnson J W C, Mitzner W, Beck J C et al 1981 Long-term effects of betamethasone on fetal development. American Journal of Obstetrics and Gynecology 141: 1053–1064

Jones K L, Smith D W, Hanson J W 1976 The fetal alcohol syndrome: clinical delineation. Annals of the New York Academy of Sciences 273: 130–137

Juvanes P, Nowaczyk T 1975 Effects of early postnatal α-methyl-dopa treatment on behavior in the rat. Psychopharmacologia 42: 95–97

Kellogg C K, Retell T M 1986 Release of [³H]norepinephrine: alteration by early developmental exposure to diazepam. Brain Research 366: 137–144

Kellogg C, Tervo D, Ison J, Parisi T, Miller R K 1980 Prenatal exposure to diazepam alters behavioral development in rats. Science 207: 205–207

Kirby M L 1984 Alterations in fetal and adult responsiveness to opiates following various schedules of prenatal morphine exposure. In: Yanai J (ed) Neurobehavioral teratology. Elsevier, Amsterdam, pp 235–248

Koëter H B W M, Roder P M 1986 Behavioral effects in mice exposed to nitrous oxide or halothane: prenatal vs postnatal exposure. Neurobehavioral Toxicology and Teratology 8: 189–194

Kraus H F, Campbell G A, Fowler A C, Farber J P 1981 Maternal nicotine administration and fetal brain stem damage: a rat model with implications for sudden infant death syndrome. American Journal of Obstetrics and Gynecology 140: 743–746

Lauder J M, Wallace J A, Wilkie M B, DiNome A, Krebs H 1983 Roles for serotonin in neurogenesis. Monographs in Neural Sciences (Karger, Basel) 9: 3–10

Lauder J M, Krebs H 1984a Neurotransmitters in development as possible substrates for drugs of use and abuse. In: Yanai J (ed) Neurobehavioral teratology. Elsevier, Amsterdam, pp 289–314

Lauder J M, Krebs H 1984b Humoral influences on brain development. Advances in Cell Neurobiology 5: 3–50

Lichtensteiger W, Schlumpf M 1985 Prenatal nicotine affects fetal testosterone and sexual dimorphism of saccharin preference. Pharma-cology Biochemistry and Behavior 23: 439–444

Livezey G T, Radulovacki M, Isaac L, Marczynski T J 1985 Prenatal exposure to diazepam results in enduring reductions in brain receptors and deep slow wave sleep. Brain Research 334: 361–365

McGivern R F, Clancy A N, Hill M A, Noble E P 1984 Prenatal alcohol exposure alters adult expression of sexually dimorphic behavior in the rat. Science 224: 896–898

McGivern R F, Rose G, Berka C, Clancy A N, Beckwith B E 1986 Neonatal exposure to a high level of ACTH(4-10) impairs adult learning performance. Physiological Psychology

Marani E, Rietveld W J, Boon M E 1982 Monosodium glutamate accelerates migration of hypothalamic perikarya at puberty. Histo-chemistry 75: 145–150

Marton I S, Szondy M 1982 Possible neuroendocrine hazards of prenatal steroid exposure. In: Endröczi et al (eds) Neuropeptides, neurotransmitters and regulation of endocrine processes, pp 535–543

Mashiach S, Barkai G, Sack J et al 1978 Enhancement of fetal lung maturity by intra-amniotic administration of thyroid hormone. American Journal of Obstetrics and Gynecology 130: 289–293

Meriney S D, Gray D B, Pilar G 1985 Morphine-induced delay of normal cell death in the avian ciliary ganglion. Science 228: 1451–1452

Middaugh L D, Santos C A, Zemp J W 1975 Effects of phenobarbital given to pregnant mice on behavior of mature offspring. Developmental Psychobiology 8: 305–313

Mirkin B L, Singh S 1976 Placental transfer of pharmacologically active molecules. In: Mirkin B L (ed) Perinatal pharmacology and therapeutics. Academic Press, New York, pp 1–69

Mirmiran M, Uylings H B M 1983 The environmental enrichment effect upon cortical growth is neutralized by concomitant pharmacological suppression of active sleep in female rats. Brain Research 261: 331–334

Mirmiran M, van de Poll N E, Corner M A, Van Oyen H, Bour H 1981 Suppression of active sleep by chronic treatment with chorimipramine during postnatal development: effects upon adult sleep and behavior in the rat. Brain Research 204: 129–146

Mirmiran M, Scholtens J, Van de Poll N E, Uylings H B M, Van der Gugten J, Boer G J 1983a Effects of experimental suppression of active (REM) sleep during early development upon adult brain and behavior. Developmental Brain Research 7: 277–286

Mirmiran M, Uylings H B M, Corner M A 1983b Pharmacological suppression of REM sleep prior to weaning counteracts the effectiveness of subsequent environmental enrichment on cortical growth in rats. Developmental Brain Research 7: 102–105

Mitler M 1971 Some developmental observations on the effects of prolonged deprivation of low voltage fast wave sleep in the deer mouse. Developmental Psychobiology 4: 293–311

Moar V A, Jefferies M A, Mutch L M M, Ounsted M K, Redman C W G 1978 Neonatal head circumference and the treatment of maternal hypertension. British Journal of Obstetrics and Gynaecology 85: 933–937

Moldow R L, Kastin A J, Hollander C S, Coy D H, Sandman C A 1981 Brain beta-endorphin-like immunoreactivity in adult rats given beta-endorphin neonatally. Brain Research Bulletin 7: 638–686

Mukherjee A B, Hodgen G D 1982 Maternal ethanol exposure induces transient impairment of umbilical circulation and fetal hypoxia in monkeys. Science 218: 700–702

Ounsted M K, Moar V A, Good F J, Redman G W G 1980 Hypertension during pregnancy with and without specific treatment: the development of the children at the age of four years. British Journal of Obstetrics and Gynaecology 87: 19–24

Oyama T, Matsuki A, Taneichi T, Ling N, Guillemin R 1980 Beta-endorphin in obstetric analgesia. American Journal of Gynecology 137: 613–616

Patrick M J, Tilstone W J, Reavey P 1972 Diazepam and breast feeding. Lancet i: 542

Reinisch J M, Karow W G 1977 Prenatal exposure to synthetic progestins and estrogens: effects on human development. Archives of Sexual Behavior 6: 257–288

Reinisch J M, Sanders S A 1982 Early barbiturate exposure: the brain, sexually dimorphic behavior and learning. Neuroscience and Biobehavioral Reviews 6: 311–319

Rodier P M, Koëter H B W M 1986 General activity from weaning to maturity in mice exposed to halothane or nitrous oxide. Neurobehavioral Toxicology and Teratology 8: 195–199

Rodier P M, Aschner M, Lewis L S, Koëter H B W M 1986 Cell proliferation in developing brain after brief exposure to nitrous oxide or halothane. Anesthesiology 64: 680–687

Rosengarten H, Friedhoff A J 1979 Enduring changes in dopamine receptor cells of pups from drug administration to pregnant and nursing rats. Science 203: 1133–1135

Rosenzweig M R, Bennett E L 1978 Experimental influences in brain anatomy and brain chemistry in rodents. In: Gottlieb G (ed) Studies on the development of behavior and the nervous system, 4. Academic Press, New York, pp 289–327

Rubin P C, Craig G F, Gavin K, Sumner D 1986 Prospective survey of use of therapeutic drugs, alcohol, and cigarettes during pregnancy. British Medical Journal 292: 81–83

Rumack C M, Guggenheim M A, Rumack B H, Peterson R G, Johnson M L, Braithwaite W R 1981 Neonatal intracranial hemorrhage and maternal use of aspirin. Obstetrics and Gynecology 58: 52S–56S

Sandman C A, McGivern R F, Berka C, Walker M, Coy D H, Kastin A J 1979 Neonatal administration of beta-endorphin produces 'chronic' insensitivity to thermal stimuli. Life Sciences 25: 1755–1760

Saucier D, Astick L 1975 Effets de l'alpha-methyl-dopa sur le sommeil du chat nouveau-né. Evolution comportementale au cours du 1er mois postnatal. Psychopharmacologia 42: 299–303

Simmons R D, Kellogg C K, Miller R K 1984 Prenatal diazepam exposure in rats: long-lasting, receptor-mediated effects on hypothalamic norepinephrine-containing neurons. Brain Research 293: 73–83

Sobel E H 1978 Effects of neonatal stunting on the development of rats:

early and late effects of neonatal cortisone on physical growth and skeletal maturation. Pediatric Research 12: 945–947

Stegner H, Dittmann R W, Steen S, Commentz J C 1986 DDAVP (desmopressin) treatment in primary enuresis nocturna. Acta Endocrinologica (Suppl) 274: 108

Stenchever M A, Williamson R A, Leonard J et al 1981 Possible relationship between in utero diethylstilbestrol exposure and male fertility. American Journal of Obstetrics and Gynecology 140: 186–193

Stratton L O, Gibson C A, Kolar K G, Kastin A J 1976 Neonatal treatment with TRH affects development, learning and emotionality in the rat. Pharmacology, Biochemistry and Behavior 5 (suppl 1): 65–67

Swaab D F 1980 Neuropeptides and brain development: a working hypothesis. In Di Benedetta C, Balazs R, Gombos G, Procellati P (eds) A multidisciplinary approach to brain development (Proceedings of the International Meeting, Selva di Fasano). Elsevier/North Holland Biomedical Press, Amsterdam, pp 181–196

Swaab D F 1982 Neuropeptides: their distribution and function in the brain. In Buijs R M, Pévet P, Swaab D F (eds) Chemical transmission in the brain. Progress in Brain Research, No. 55. Elsevier, Amsterdam, pp 97–122

Swaab D F 1985 Influence of fetal and neonatal environment on physical, psychological and intellectual development: workshop summary. In Marois M (ed) Prevention of physical and mental congenital defects. B. Epidemiology, early detection and therapy, and environmental factors. Alan Liss, New York, pp 463–467

Swaab D F, Fliers E 1985 A sexually dimorphic nucleus in the human brain. Science 228: 1112–1115

Swaab D F, Mirmiran M 1984 Possible mechanisms underlying the teratogenic effects of medicines on the developing brain. In Yanai J (ed) Neurobehavioral teratology. Elsevier, Amsterdam, pp 55–71

Swaab D F, Mirmiran M M 1985 The influence of chemicals and environment on brain development: 'behavioral teratology'. In Marois M (ed) Prevention of physical and mental congenital defects. B. Epidemiology, early detection and therapy, and environmental factors. Liss, New York, pp 447–451

Taeusch H W 1975 Glucocorticoid prophylaxis for respiratory distress syndrome: a review of potential toxicity. Journal of Pediatrics 87: 617–623

Thornburg J E, Moore K E 1976 Pharmacologically induced modifications of behavioral and chemical development. In Mirkin B L (ed) Perinatal pharmacology and therapeutics. Academic Press, New York, pp 269–354

Trice J E, Ambler M 1985 Multiple cerebral defects in an infant exposed in utero to anticonvulsants. Archives of Pathology and Laboratory Medicine 109: 521–523

Vathy I U, Etgen A M, Rabii J, Barfield R J 1983 Effects of prenatal exposure to morphine sulfate on reproductive function of female rats. Pharmacology, Biochemistry and Behavior 19: 777–780

Vorhees C V 1981 Effects of prenatal naloxone exposure on postnatal behavioral development of rats. Neurobehavioral Toxicology and Teratology 3: 295–301

Vorhees C V 1985 Fetal anticonvulsant syndrome in rats: effects on postnatal behavior and brain amino acid content. Neurobehavioral Toxicology and Teratology 7: 471–482

Waggoner R W, Slonim A E, Armstrong S H 1978 Improved psychological status of children under dDAVP therapy for central diabetes inspidus. American Journal of Psychiatry 135: 361–362

Wit J M, Hijman R, Jolles J et al 1986 Effect of desglycinamide-arginine-vasopressine (DGAVP) on cognitive functions in children with memory disorders. In: Neuropeptides and brain function (May 28–30, Utrecht, The Netherlands). Abstract book

Yalom I D, Green R, Fisk N 1973 Prenatal exposure to female hormones. Effect on psychosexual development in boys. Archives of General Psychiatry 28: 554–561

Yanai J 1981 Comparison of early barbiturate and ethanol effects on the CNS. Substance Alcohol Actions Misuse 2: 79–91

Yanai J, Feigenbaum J J 1981 Lessened sensitivity to apomorphine induced hypothermia following prenatal exposure to phenobarbital. IRCS Medical Science 9: 965

Zagon I S, McLaughlin P J 1984 An overview of the neurobehavioral sequelae of perinatal opioid exposure. In Yanai J (ed) Neurobehavioral teratology. Elsevier, Amsterdam, pp 197–234

Defects of the neural tube

As a group, the neural tube defects, are the most common major congenital malformations diagnosed at birth. Although its incidence has fallen in recent years this is still one of the most difficult problems of diagnosis and management facing obstetricians and paediatricians. For this reason we have devoted an entire section to defects of the neural tube which encompasses all aspects of its diagnosis, management and prevention.

The terminology used to describe this condition has caused confusion. Spina bifida was the term first used by Tulp in 1652 to describe clefting of the vertebral structures. Spinal dysraphism is a general term referring to any abnormality of the spine and is not specific to neural tube disorders. Rachischisis literally means split spine and as such is not a particularly useful term. The terms craniorachischisis and myeloschisis are more meaningful as they are descriptive and refer to the basic abnormality of the brain and spinal cord respectively (Brocklehurst 1976). Craniorachischisis is discussed in the section on anencephaly. Myeloschisis refers to a completely open neural tube, usually involving the thoraco–lumbar spine.

A major facet of the diagnosis of neural tube defects is careful consideration of the risk of recurrence in subsequent pregnancies. Careful genetic counselling is mandatory for each pregnancy in families affected by this condition. The risk of recurrence is discussed in detail in Chapter 20.

22. The spectrum of neural tube defects

Dr M. I. Levene

The neural tube is formed with the fusion of the neural folds which occurs early in embryological development, towards the end of the third week. The cranial end of the neural tube will form the brain and the caudal end will form the spinal cord. The embryological development of the spinal cord and brain are described in detail in Part 1 of this book and are only briefly reiterated here. Once formed the neural tube becomes submerged below the dorsal surface of the embryo by proliferation of the mesodermal tissue which interposes itself between the neural tube and the ectoderm (days 19–21). Final closure of the tube occurs rostrally (the anterior neuropore) at approximately 24 days and caudal closure (posterior neuropore) occurs approximately two days later. Brain development occurs rapidly from the time of closure of the anterior neuropore. The vertebrae develop from ectodermal tissue and the vertebral arches normally enclose the cord from cervical to low sacral level by 11 weeks of embryonic development. Disorders of this process are referred to as neural tube defects (NTD) and show a wide spectrum from anencephaly with myeloschisis to the very common isolated defect of a single vertebral arch with no other abnormality. NTDs with intact skin are referred to as spina bifida occulta and there are a number of clinically important conditions in this group. The main categories of NTD considered in cranio–caudal sequence are:

Anencephaly
Encephalocele
Spina bifida cystica
Spina bifida occulta

ANENCEPHALY

This lethal condition is the most severe form of neural tube defect and is due to failure in the development of structures associated with the anterior neuropore. The defect is believed to occur between 18 and 24 days from conception. Anencephaly usually occurs with some degree of spinal dysraphism although this may not be obvious on clinical inspection. In a proportion of these infants, complete exposure of the neural tube also occurs and this condition is referred to as craniorachischisis totalis. Anencephaly occurs more commonly in females than males and polyhydramnios (presumably due to failure of the fetus to swallow) complicates some affected pregnancies.

The anencephalic infant is usually born with absence of all definable structures above the brainstem. The frontal, parietal and squamous parts of the occipital bone do not develop. The orbits and eyes are well developed but the optic nerves end blindly within the orbits. The neural tissue appears as an amorphous mass with little definable structure (Fig. 22.1). In addition to the absent cerebral hemispheres, the hypothalamus and cerebellum are usually grossly abnormal. The anterior pituitary is always intact (Friede 1975) but the adrenal glands are invariably hypoplastic. Some infants with anencephaly breathe, swallow and cry, indicating that at least some brainstem structures are intact. The spinal cord of anencephalics is thinner than normal and is always histologically abnormal (Friede 1975). The medulla oblongata and spinal cord may also be absent in craniorachischisis.

ENCEPHALOCELE

In this condition there is a variable degree of cerebral herniation through a midline defect of the skull. Its incidence has been variously estimated as 1 per 5000 (Lemire 1983) and 1–3 per 10 000 live births (Friede 1975). The former figure is more representative of Western countries. It is more common in female infants than males and has a higher prevalence amongst the Chinese. Rarely, it is inherited as a recessive condition in the Meckel–Gruber syndrome. This condition includes microphthalmia, cleft lip and palate, polydactyly and large polycystic kidneys. Encephalocele may be part of a variety of other syndromes as discussed in Chapter 20.

Encephalocele is included amongst the NTDs as it is

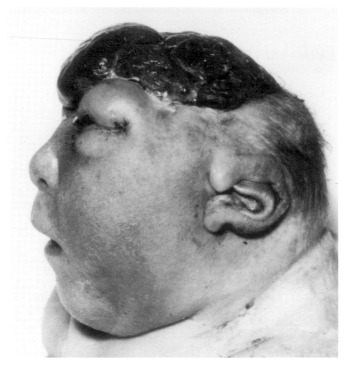

Fig. 22.1 Anencephaly.

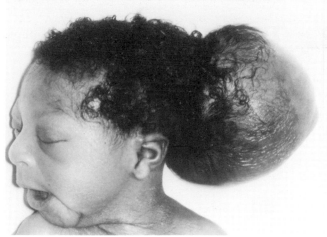

Fig. 22.2 Encephalocele with microcephaly. Excision of the sac which contained brain tissue was performed shortly after birth and the infant at 3 years is of normal intelligence, without cerebral palsy but has severe visual impairment.

probably the result of failure of the anterior neuropore to develop normally. It is, however, difficult to explain the abnormality purely on embryological grounds and its precise pathogenesis is unclear. It has been suggested that encephalocele occurs due to herniation of brain through the skull at about 20 weeks of gestation as the result of hydrocephalus and is not a defect of neural tube development at all. This may certainly be the explanation for some cases and is discussed further in Chapter 19.

Encephaloceles are skin covered and in 75–80% of cases occur in the occipital region (Fig. 22.2), usually involving the squamous portion of the occipital bone, but the basal part may also be involved. Anterior encephaloceles most commonly involve the bridge of the nose (60%) and in a further 30% the nasal cavity (Ziter & Bramwit 1970). Rarely, the cribriform plate or ethmoid bones are involved and exceptionally the base of the skull may be affected with brain tissue protruding into the pharynx. A classification for encephalocele is shown in Table 26.1, page 295. It may be difficult clinically to distinguish an encephalocele from a cranial meningocele. The latter contains no brain and is usually smaller. Rarely they may occur away from the midline over the parietal bone.

The skull defect is usually small but the skull often shows more extensive bony abnormalities. The amount of brain in the sac is very variable but may be massive. The infant with a large lesion may be microcephalic but in a proportion of infants hydrocephalus develops. Cerebral cortex, ventricular structures and cerebellum (in occipital lesions) are often found within the sac. Agenesis of the

corpus callosum may occur together with encephalocele. Treatment is considered in Chapter 26 and recurrence risk on p. 251.

SPINA BIFIDA

The term spina bifida is widely used to refer to disruption of the vertebral arches with or without involvement of the meninges and spinal cord. The original description referred to spina dorsi bifida, in distinction to the very rare spina ventralis bifida in which there is clefting of the body of the cervical or thoracic vertebrae and is often associated with an enterogenous cyst. The term spina bifida can be subdivided into open and closed lesions. Spina bifida aperta refers to the open lesion where the skin over the exposed neural tube is completely deficient. Spina bifida cystica refers only to the lesion covered by a membrane which later epithelializes and technically this term should be used only when epithelialization is complete. In practice, spina bifida cystica is the term most commonly used to refer to the open lesion. Spina bifida occulta (p. 270) describes the skin-covered lesion where the NTD is hidden or only evident by relatively subtle midline abnormalities.

Spina bifida cystica

The first detailed description of the anatomy of spina bifida cystica was by von Recklinghausen in 1886. The spine is abnormal with absence of the vertebral arches, broadening of the vertebrae and lateral displacement of pedicles and a widened spinal canal (Friede 1975). The abnormality can affect most of the spine but 80–90% of lesions involve the lumbar or lumbo–sacral region. Sacral and cervical lesions are also relatively common. Spina bifida confined to the thoracolumbar, total thoracic or total cervico–thoracic regions are virtually never seen (Barson 1970). Multiple lesions are very uncommon and were present in only 1% of cases reported by Fisher et al (1952). Females are more commonly affected than males.

Iniencephaly. This is an uncommon and fatal condition referring to the association of spina bifida cystica involving the cervical spine with severe retroflexion of the infant's head and a bony defect of the foramen magnum (Fig. 22.3). It may be associated with severe meningomyelocele or in less severe cases is confined to a skin-covered spina bifida occulta lesion. This condition in a milder form may be related to the Klippel–Feil syndrome.

Spina bifida cystica can be subdivided into two distinct entities, myelomeningocele and meningocele.

Myelomeningocele

Approximately 80% of infants born with spina bifida cystica have myelomeningocele. This condition is usually extensive and involves a meningeal cyst which often ruptures during delivery. The neural tube is almost always broad-based and the neuro–ectodermal tissue stands proud of the skin, oozing cerebrospinal fluid (CSF) (Fig. 22.4). If untreated the membrane may heal and eventually becomes epithelialized, completely enclosing the myelomeningocele.

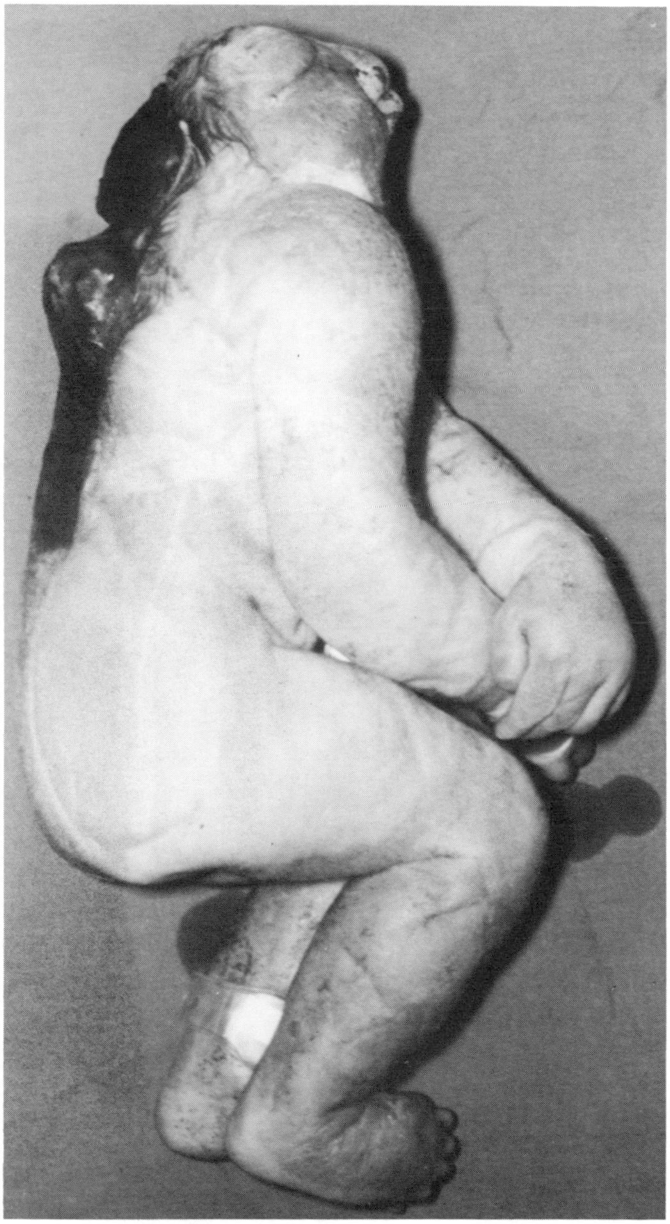

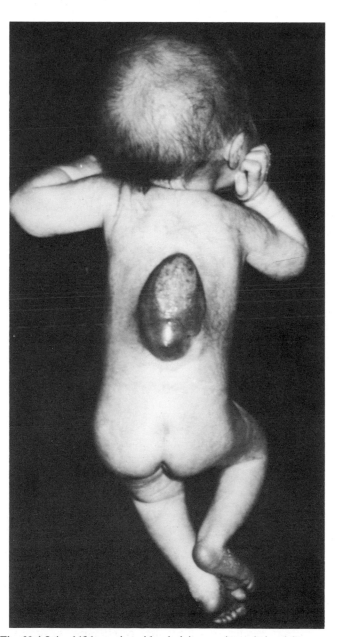

Fig. 22.3 Iniencephaly with rachischisis. Note the marked retroversion of the head.

Fig. 22.4 Spina bifida cystica with a bulging meningocele involving the thoracolumbar region.

The term 'closed' is slightly misleading as the neural tube itself, although eventually covered with skin, remains open with complete and irreparable damage to the involved nervous tissue.

The myelomeningocele is often part of a more complicated abnormality involving other types of dysraphic abnormalities. In an autopsy study of 100 cases of this condition, there was evidence of co-existent hydromyelia (dilatation of the central canal) and/or syringomyelia (extension of the central canal into the cord parenchyma) in 43% of cases (Emery & Lendon 1973). They also found evidence of cord duplication (diplomyelia) in 36% of cases.

Myelomeningocele is usually associated with very severe neurological abnormality and the assessment of motor and sensory levels are described in Chapter 26. In one series only a third of cervical lesions were associated with paralysis (usually of the upper limbs). The lower the myelomeningocele on the spinal axis, the more prevalent was sphincter involvement. Of cases with sacral lesions, 90% had some sphincter paralysis (Laurence 1964).

Meningocele

In this condition the spine is usually intact and it is not associated with neurological deficit. In general, the bony defect in meningocele is less extensive than that of myelomeningocele and rarely involves more than 2–3 vertebrae. Meningocele most commonly involves the lower lumbar or sacral region and is often covered with skin. The sac of the meningocele consists of both arachnoid and dural meninges and contains CSF.

It may be impossible at birth to distinguish clinically a meningocele from the myelomeningocele without obvious neurological signs. Examination of the lesion by real-time ultrasound (p. 146) may demonstrate the spinal cord to be intact and not tethered. Surgical management is discussed in Chapter 26.

Spina bifida occulta

This is a common condition and in one report, 16% of 7- and 8-year-old children had radiological evidence of a bifid 5th lumbar vertebra, falling to an incidence of 2% in adults (Sutow & Pryde 1956). Failure of the vertebral arches to fuse is an insignificant lesion except that it may indicate more extensive but hidden involvement of the spinal cord. The significance of spina bifida occulta is that some lesions are associated with neurological involvement and subsequent development of bladder or motor dysfunction. The most common forms of spina bifida occulta are:

Dermal sinus
Lipomyelomeningocele
Dermoid cyst
Diastematomyelia
Hydromyelia

Often, the only clinical indication of spina bifida occulta in the neonatal period is a relatively subtle cutaneous abnormality anywhere over the spine or midline scalp. Powell et al (1975) reported that 3% of newborn infants had skin abnormalities associated with spina bifida occulta. Till (1968) found a midline hairy patch (Fig. 22.5) and skin dimple or sinus to be the most common cutaneous abnormalities seen in a group of 85 patients with spina bifida occulta. Other midline abnormalities seen were lipomatous swellings, capillary naevi and cutis aplasia. Conversely, in a group of 73 patients (children and adults) with neurological complications of spina bifida occulta, 23% had no evidence of skin lesions (Anderson 1975).

Dermal sinus

A dermal sinus is a deep epithelium-lined tract, sometimes containing hair, that ascends from its external opening over the spine or scalp to terminate at a deeper level, sometimes communicating with the dura. They are most

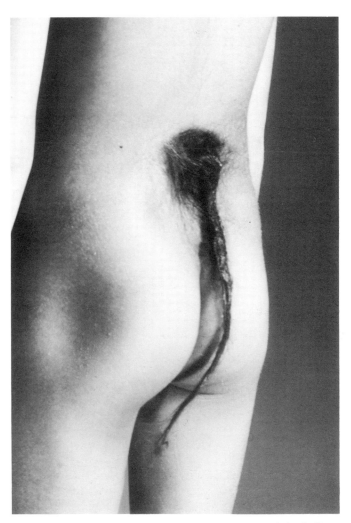

Fig. 22.5 Hairy patch. This child had an excessively long hairy 'tail' with underlying spina bifida occulta.

common in the lumbar or sacral region (63%) and in one report 27% occurred in the occipital area (Powell et al 1975). Cervical sinuses occur rarely. The importance of this condition is meningitis when the sinus communicates with the meninges. Some terminate in an epidermal or dermoid inclusion cyst, and lipomata may also be present at their bases. Vertebral abnormalities are usually present if the sinus extends into the spinal canal. Investigation and management are discussed on p. 299.

Lipomyelomeningocele

Patients with this condition have a fatty swelling over the spine present at birth (Fig. 22.6) and this should always be referred for neurosurgical opinion (p. 298). Despite their presence at birth they are rarely associated with early neurological abnormality but Dubowitz et al (1965) reported the acute onset of gross weakness of one leg at the age of three weeks in an infant with lipomyelomeningocele. The lesion usually overlies the sacral or lumbar region and a deep stalk passes intradurally to the conus medullaris or nerves of the cauda equina. The eventual development of neurological signs is attributed to tethering of the cord (see Ch. 26). Sacrococcygeal teratomas may rarely be confused with a lumbosacral lipoma (Lemire et al 1971).

Diastematomyelia

In this condition the cord is divided into two segments by a bony spur or fibrous tissue protruding from the dorsal surface of the vertebral body into the spinal canal (Friede 1975). It is commonly associated with complicated forms of myelomeningocele. If part of spina bifida occulta, the lesion rarely presents in the neonatal period.

Hydromyelia

This is a dilatation of the central canal of the spinal cord and is usually found in the lumbo–sacral region. It may be an incidental finding at autopsy but is more commonly associated with spina bifida.

ARNOLD–CHIARI MALFORMATION

This condition almost invariably occurs in the presence of spina bifida cystica and is commonly associated with hydro-cephalus. The original description of the Arnold–Chiari malformation is well reviewed by Brocklehurst (1976) and was first described by Cleland in 1883. In the 1890s Chiari described the lesion in a series of reports and recorded four different types. Type I refers to herniation of the cerebellar tonsils seen in raised intracranial pressure and Type II is similar to that described by Cleland and is the only type strongly associated with spina bifida. In 1894, Arnold

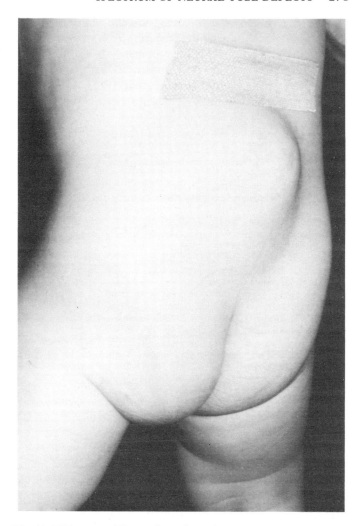

Fig. 22.6 Skin-covered lipomyelomeningocele.

described a case of cerebellar deformation in association with severe spina bifida and subsequently his students coined the term 'Arnold–Chiari' malformation, ignoring the contribution of Cleland.

In the newborn the malformation involves herniation of the cerebellar vermis or occasionally one or other tonsil through the foramen magnum, together with deformity of the brainstem. The fourth ventricle may be displaced into the upper cervical canal. It is virtually only seen in cases of myelomeningocele, and is invariably present in this condition. Generally, the severity of the Arnold–Chiari malformation corresponds to the severity of the lumbo–sacral spina bifida (Friede 1975). Abnormalities of the skull bones are also a constant feature of this condition. There are craniolacuna of the squamous bones of the cranial vault, an enlarged foramen magnum and a shallow posterior fossa best seen on a lateral skull radiograph. This malformation is not seen with spina bifida occulta.

The cause of the Arnold–Chiari malformation is not generally agreed. Neither the traction theory (pulling of the brainstem and cerebellum through the foramen magnum due to a tethered spinal cord) nor the pulsion theory (hydrocephalus impacting the posterior fossa structures into the foramen magnum) can be supported. It is most likely that it is due to a primary developmental disturbance of the structures of the posterior fossa (Friede 1975).

Hydrocephalus commonly complicates spina bifida cyst-ica but it is not necessarily due to the Arnold–Chiari malformation and it may be present without evidence of hydrocephalus (see Ch. 46). Overall, hydrocephalus occurs in 80% of cases of lumbar spina bifida cystica, 70% of thoraco–lumbar, 50% of sacral and 43% of lesions confined to the high thoracic region (Laurence 1960).

REFERENCES

Anderson F M 1975 Occult spinal dysraphism: a series of 73 cases. Pediatrics 55: 826–835

Arnold J 1894 Myelocyste, Transposition von Gewebskeimen und Sympodie. Beiträge zur pathologischen Anatomie und zur allgemeinen. Pathologie 16: 1

Barson A J 1970 Spina bifida: the significance of the level and extent of the defect to the morphogenesis. Developmental Medicine and Child Neurology 12: 129–144

Brocklehurst G 1976 Spina bifida for the clinician. Clinics in Developmental Medicine, No. 57. Spastics International Medical Publications/Heinemann, London

Cleland J 1883 Contribution to the study of spina bifida, encephalocele and anencephalus. Journal of Anatomy and Physiology 17: 257

Dubowitz V, Lorber J, Zachary R B 1965 Lipoma of the cauda equina. Archives of Disease in Childhood 40: 207–213

Emery J L, Lendon R G 1973 The local cord lesion in neurospinal dysraphism (meningomyelocele). Journal of Pathology 110: 83–86

Fisher R G, Uihlein A, Keith H M 1952 Spina bifida and cranium bifidum: study of 530 cases. Proceedings of the Mayo Clinic 27: 33–38

Friede R L 1975 Developmental Neuropathology. Springer-Verlag, Vienna

Laurence K M 1960 The natural history of spina bifida cystica. Proceedings of the Royal Society of Medicine 53: 1055–1056

Laurence K M 1964 The natural history of spina bifida cystica: detailed analysis of 407 cases. Archives of Disease of Childhood 39: 41–57

Lemire R J 1983 Neural tube defects: clinical correlations. Clinical Neurosurgery 30: 65–77

Lemire R J, Graham C B, Beckwith J B 1971 Skin-covered sacrococcygeal masses in infants and children. Journal of Pediatrics 79: 948–954

Powell K R, Cherry J D, Hougen T J, Blinderman E E, Dunn M C 1975 A prospective search for congenital dermal abnormalities of the craniospinal axis. Journal of Pediatrics 87: 744–750

Sutow W W, Pryde A W 1956 Incidence of spina bifida occulta in relationship to age. American Journal of Diseases in Children 91: 211–217

Till K 1968 Spinal dysraphism: a study of congenital malformation of the back. Developmental Medicine and Child Neurology 10: 470–477

von Recklinghausen F 1886 Untersuchungen über die Spina bifida. Virchows Archiv für Pathologische Anatomie und Physiologie und für klinische Medizin 105: 243

Ziter F, Bramwit D 1970 Nasal encephalocele and gliomas. British Journal of Radiology 43: 136–138

23. Epidemiology of neural tube defects

Prof R. W. Smithells

An epidemic is an event that comes upon (epi) the people (demos), but epidemiology has come to describe the patterns of disease in populations, even when the diseases are endemic — as are neural tube defects (NTD).

The fundamental unit of epidemiology is prevalence, which measures how often something happens. Prevalence, once determined, can be studied in the three basic dimensions of time, place and person:

Time — does the prevalence vary from day to day, year to year, season to season?
Place — does the prevalence vary from street to street, from city to city, from country to country?
Person — does the prevalence vary between people of differing age, sex, ethnic origin, blood group, occupation and a thousand other personal variables?

Superimposed upon these three basic dimensions are the interactions within and between them. Thus, within the dimension of time, seasonal variations in NTD prevalence have been recorded, but have subsequently disappeared. Within the dimension of person, social class differences tend to disappear as NTD prevalence falls. Interactions between place and person may be studied when people migrate. Does their NTD prevalence reflect the place they come from or the place they go to?

Techniques for analysing epidemiological data have become increasingly sophisticated as statisticians have become ever more ingenious in their efforts to overcome the unavoidable imperfections of 'controls' in human studies and to make heterogeneous data look more homogeneous than they are. But closer to the heart of the problem are the difficulties of ascertainment — of establishing the facts with sufficient completeness and precision — so that the statisticians are not given sows' ears with which to construct silk purses.

ASCERTAINMENT

It is essential to discuss some of the problems of ascertainment before describing epidemiological phenomena. The first prerequisite is to define the conditions which are to be ascertained. That is to say, what (for epidemiological purposes) is a neural tube defect? The embryology of the neural tube is described in Chapter 1. Failure of closure of the neural tube will result in a bony defect of the skull and/or spinal column with protrusion of meninges and/or neural tissue. Hence NTDs includes anencephaly, iniencephaly, encephalocele, myelocele and cranial or spinal meningocele. The most severe failures of neural tube closure result in varying degrees of cranio–spinal rachischisis.

The recognition of such a lesion is not, of itself, sufficient. It is necessary to know what other defects were (or were not) present. On the one hand, a wide variety of defects, including diaphragmatic hernia and exomphalos (omphalocele), commonly accompany anencephaly and are probably of no special significance. On the other hand, the association of polydactyly, cleft palate and congenital heart disease with encephalocele strongly suggests the diagnosis of Meckel syndrome, a genetic disorder (autosomal recessive).

That much is easy but there are less certain areas. Spinal dysraphism is a term that includes a wider range of developmental anomalies than NTDs, but these additional lesions are relatively rare, often not recognizable at birth, and therefore difficult to ascertain. They are therefore, by convention, not regarded as 'NTDs'. Isolated hydrocephalus is a condition of very varied causation, and even congenital hydrocephalus may not be diagnosed at birth. Although there is now good evidence of an increased frequency of hydrocephalus in the siblings of babies with spina bifida or anencephaly (Lorber 1984) it can result from prenatal infection (toxoplasmosis), drugs (etretinate, isotretinoin) or an X-linked recessive gene, and is therefore not classified as a neural tube defect for epidemiological purposes.

Ascertainment of the defect therefore requires proper examination of the infant or fetus at birth or postmortem. This is particularly difficult to achieve when the pregnancy has been terminated and almost unattainable after spontaneous abortion. Neural tube defects diagnosed by ultrasound scan during pregnancy need to be confirmed by examination of the aborted fetus. This is necessary not only to identify additional defects which may be significant but also because fetal ultrasonography is fallible. A particularly common error is to interpret a swelling in the cervical region as an encephalocele, only to find that it is a cystic hygroma, usually in association with X0 chromosomes and other features of Turner's syndrome. The distinction may not be as easy as it sounds, but no communication will be demonstrable with the skull or spinal canal if the lesion is a cystic hygroma, nor will the cystic spaces be lined by neuro-epithelium. In this example the error of ascertainment will have no profound epidemiological consequences. However, advice about recurrence risks and prenatal tests in future pregnancies will be quite inappropriate if the true nature of the lesion is not recognized.

Ascertainment of other data to be analysed must be carried out with equal care and attention to detail. Are we interested in racial differences? To identify parents as 'Indian' will not do, for India is the home of many ethnic groups. Most seem to have a low prevalence of NTDs, but the Sikhs are the exception, not only in India but elsewhere in the world (Searle 1959, Baird 1983). Are we interested in possible links between NTDs and drugs? (A possible link between spina bifida and the anticonvulsant valproate has been suggested by Robert et al 1984 and Lindhout & Schmidt 1986.) To record drugs given 'in the first trimester' will not do. For the first 2 weeks of 'pregnancy', as conventionally calculated from the mother's last menstrual period, the mother is not pregnant at all, and drugs given after six weeks of 'pregnancy' (four weeks conceptional age) are too late to influence neural tube closure.

Routine recording and notification of birth defects are notoriously incomplete, even for lesions as obvious at birth as NTD (Knox et al 1984). A big change in prevalence of any phenomenon (for example, a measles epidemic) may be reflected even by incomplete notification but small changes in numbers notified are at least as likely to reflect changes in notification practice as real changes in prevalence. The particular problems which result from prenatal diagnosis of NTD and termination of pregnancy are discussed later. Ascertainment tends to be more complete from a relatively small population (say 20–30 000 annual births) which can be closely monitored than from larger populations.

This by no means exhausts the difficulties of ascertaining birth defects but it is necessary to stress the difficulties because much epidemiological research is flawed by the inaccuracy and incompleteness of the basic data. It is only another example of the computer dictum, 'garbage in, garbage out'. Those who do the computing are not always in a position to know whether they have been presented with fact or fiction.

Most of the epidemiological studies of NTDs have concerned themselves with anencephaly and spina bifida because they are the most common forms of NTD, the most immediately recognizable at birth and (in more recent times)

the most readily diagnosed prenatally. Many of the classic studies were carried out in the UK in the 1950s and 1960s, when NTD prevalence was high and prenatal diagnosis had not arrived (Record & McKeown 1949). More recent research has concentrated on the changes in epidemiological patterns since the earlier studies were published.

Temporal variations

Changes in NTD prevalence in time could, in theory, be significant from day to day, from millenium to millenium, or anything in between. The practical constraints on such studies include the size of the population monitored and the length of time over which monitoring has taken place. A large study population will yield relatively large numbers of cases but accuracy of diagnosis and completeness of ascertainment tend to suffer. A small study population yields relatively small numbers of cases. Collaborative ventures such as the International Clearinghouse for Birth Defects are intended to mitigate the problem of numbers. However, the pooling of data could disguise a significant phenomenon affecting only one or two of the contributing registries.

It is obvious that a monitoring system that has only been functional for 10 years is in no position to comment on long-term secular trends. Of the short-term temporal changes in NTD prevalence, the most striking 20–30 years ago were seasonal swings, most marked for anencephaly and showing a greater prevalence of affected births in the winter months than in the summer (McKeown & Record 1951). This suggested a teratogenic factor operative maximally in the spring and has been incorporated into a number of hypotheses involving infective and nutritional factors. However, the seasonal variations noted in Scotland and in Birmingham (England) subsequently disappeared (Leck & Record 1966). Data from Liverpool suggested that the slight seasonal changes in spina bifida births resulted from seasonal changes in mean length of gestation rather than from changes in spina bifida conceptions (Smithells & Chinn 1965).

Longer-term secular trends can only be determined from long-established registries (of which there are few) or from suitable hospital records. Data from North America (MacMahon & Yen 1971, Biggar et al 1976) indicate that in Boston (Massachusetts), Providence (Rhode Island) and Rochester (New York), all on the eastern seaboard of the United States, the prevalence of both anencephaly and spina bifida increased about two-and-a-half-fold between 1910–20 and 1930–34, with a return to the earlier levels by 1960–70 (Fig. 23.1). Data from eastern Canada show a similar decline between 1950 and 1970 but earlier records are not available (Elwood 1976).

An equally striking epidemicity of anencephaly, on a rather shorter time-cycle, was recorded in Birmingham

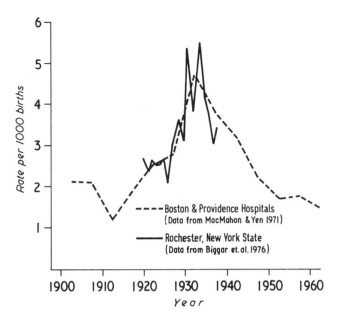

Fig. 23.1 Spina bifida prevalence rates in Eastern USA, 1900–65.

(England) over the period 1936 to 1965 (Fig. 23.2) (MacMahon et al 1951, Leck 1966).

More recently, a decline in NTD prevalence in the United Kingdom has been evident since about 1972. This decline clearly preceded any significant impact from prenatal diagnosis and termination of affected pregnancies. However, as increasing proportions of NTDs have been dealt with in this way it has become increasingly difficult to be sure what is happening to true prevalence. What is clear is that an observed decline, whilst clearly a welcome phenomenon, is not necessarily a permanent one. Reports from Hungary (Cziezel 1983) and South Australia (Simpson & Robertson 1985) have indicated a possible increase in prevalence in recent years.

The interpretation of temporal changes is difficult but even the long-term variations are too rapid to be attributable to genetic factors. Environmental factors must be responsible for these phenomena.

Geographical variations

International and intranational variations in NTD prevalence have always been striking. Celtic peoples in Ireland and South Wales have the unenviable distinction of recording higher NTD rates than anywhere else in the world. Rates in excess of 1% of all births have been recorded in some Welsh mining valleys in the past (Laurence et al 1967). A large international study published in 1966 (Stevenson et al 1966) revealed a more than 10-fold difference in NTD prevalence between the highest and the lowest rates. This study was based on hospital births, not population data, which introduces some selection bias, but there is no reason to doubt the magnitude of the differences.

More surprising is the varying NTD prevalence within one country as small as England. Here prevalence increases as one travels north and west, and two- or three-fold differences in prevalence have been demonstrated in areas less than 300 km apart. Here again, environmental differences seem to offer the most likely explanation.

A correlation between NTD prevalence and geology in Britain was noted long ago (Penrose 1957). The mountains of Scotland, Wales and north-west England are very ancient in comparison with the chalks and gravels of south-east England. These geological differences are reflected in the characteristics of the local water supplies, the 'soft' waters of the mountainous districts having a greater capacity for solutes. The correlation is significant nationally (Stocks 1970) but more local studies in north-west England (Fielding & Smithells 1971) and South Wales (Lowe et al 1971) suggested that a causal relationship was improbable.

Geographical variations inevitably raise the question as to whether the different prevalence rates are attributable to factors which are characteristic of the place or of the people who live there. Migrants to countries with higher or lower NTD prevalences than in their country of origin tend to retain their ancestral prevalence rates initially, though not necessarily in later generations (Naggan & MacMahon 1967, Naggan 1971). The Irish, for example, tend to have rather high rates wherever they live, whereas Negro peoples tend to have low rates. These observations suggest that genetic factors may contribute to the causation of NTD but they could also relate to those aspects of the environment which we take with us — our general life-style and personal habits.

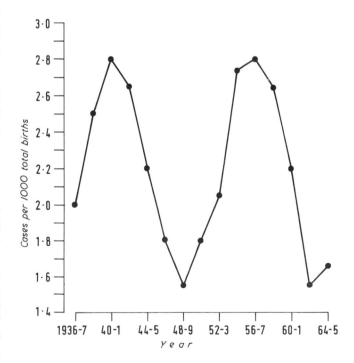

Fig. 23.2 Anencephaly prevalence rates in Birmingham, 1936–65 (data from MacMahon et al 1951, Leck 1966).

It seems unlikely that features of the local environment — water supply, air pollution, background radiation — are of major importance.

Personal variations

The characteristics of humans are countless and each is a unique event. Comparisons on the basis of single attributes are therefore inevitably crude and it is not surprising that comparable studies have sometimes yielded conflicting results. For example, we may consider the relationship of maternal age and parity to NTD prevalence. Some studies have shown a higher prevalence in younger mothers and first-born children; some in older mothers and later birth order; some in both; and some in neither. A reasonable conclusion is that maternal age and parity do not play a significant part in the aetiology of NTDs.

So far as ethnic differences are concerned, reference has already been made to the low prevalence in Negroes and to the high prevalence in the Irish and in Sikhs. Low rates are also characteristic of Jewish people (Leck 1969). In New Zealand, rates are higher in the non-Maori than in the Maori population (Borman et al 1986).

Differences in NTD prevalence between social classes have been evident in many places except, recently, where prevalence has reached very low levels (Strassburg et al 1983, Borman et al 1986). Within the UK, the social class difference has persisted, although the social class gradient has changed to reflect the changing social structure in Britain (see Fig. 23.3). It could be said that in the 1950s, social classes I and II (professional and managerial) were the 'haves', and classes III–V were varying degrees of 'have-nots'. Now, social classes I–IV have, and only class V, the unskilled (and in many cases unemployed) workers are left behind. This social class gradient is common to most birth defects and is by no means unique to NTDs.

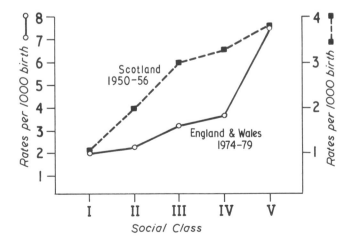

Fig. 23.3 Birth prevalence by social class of anencephaly in Scotland 1950–56 (Record 1961), and of anencephaly and spina bifida in England and Wales 1974–79 (Office of Population Censuses and Surveys 1982).

THE IMPACT OF PRENATAL DIAGNOSIS

The introduction of prenatal diagnostic tests for NTD has made epidemiological studies much more difficult. Ascertainment by traditional methods is now likely to be seriously deficient and the interpretation of standard data almost impossible. In the UK, the voluntary system for reporting birth defects applies only to those in 'viable' infants, i.e. those born after 28 weeks of gestation. Even in this group, notification of NTD is seriously incomplete (Knox et al 1984).

Many obstetricians use ultrasound scans as part of routine antenatal care (see Ch. 25). These will detect all cases of anencephaly and many cases of spina bifida. Many also routinely screen maternal serum for alpha-fetoprotein (AFP), and this will also lead to detection of many NTDs (see Ch. 24). Those that remain undetected until later will be predominantly:

1. in mothers who present late in pregnancy;
2. in mothers who decline antenatal tests;
3. small, skin-covered lesions.

If pregnancy is terminated (the present legal limit in England and Wales is 28 weeks), birth defects are not notifiable. Documentation relating to the termination requires only a statement about the grounds upon which the pregnancy *will be* terminated, and the grounds upon which it *was* terminated, which in these cases will be 'substantial risk of serious defect'. There is no requirement to state that a defect was present, let alone what the defect was.

In the USA, NTDs have become so uncommon that maternal AFP screening may not make economic sense, although obstetric ultrasound is widely used (see Ch. 25). In Ireland, a predominantly Roman Catholic country, prenatal diagnosis and termination of pregnancy are not widely practised. In the UK, however, it is probably fair to say that at least 50% of NTD pregnancies will be terminated; that determined efforts could get this figure up to 90%; and that overall the figure is currently in the region of 60–70%. It follows that in future, epidemiological studies of NTDs *must* incorporate ascertainment of terminated pregnancies. Without that, NTD prevalence could return to its former high levels without anybody noticing.

WHAT USE IS EPIDEMIOLOGY?

Epidemiology is first and foremost a tool of preventive medicine. Originally applied to infectious diseases, then to industrial diseases, the epidemiological approach has now been applied to a wide variety of medical and surgical disorders, accidents (and non-accidents) and birth defects. The hope is that appropriate studies will reveal phenomena that may in turn lead to the identification of aetiological factors and thence to prevention.

Some of the most impressive events in medical history have resulted from observed associations, without benefit of methodology or statistical analysis. A perceived link between cholera and place led to the padlocking of the Broad Street pump. A perceived link between a population subgroup and relative immunity to smallpox led to vaccination.

Prevention of NTDs

The epidemiological features of NTDs have provided the basis for a number of hypotheses. Considered together with data on NTD prevalence in first-, second- and third-degree relatives, they indicate that NTDs are not attributable to any single cause but are of multifactorial origin. Among the factors which have been suggested as possibly contributing to causation are infections (to explain seasonal variations), something related to soft water (to explain geographical variations) and nutritional factors (to explain social class and other variations). Some nutritional hypotheses postulate teratogenic substances in the diet, including canned meats (Knox 1972), tea (Fedrick 1974), and blighted potatoes (Renwick 1972). Others propose a dietary deficiency, particularly of folic acid and/or other vitamins (Smithells et al 1983). Only two of these hypotheses have been put to the test. Total avoidance of potatoes in pregnancy did not lead to a reduced NTD recurrence rate, suggesting that the hypothesis in its original form was invalid (Lorber 1974, Nevin & Merrett 1975).

Intervention studies using vitamin supplements for women at increased risk of NTD (by virtue of previously affected children) have been carried out by two research groups. In South Wales, Laurence et al (1981) gave folic acid 2 mg twice daily or placebo in a randomized study. The number of mothers studied was small and interpretation of the results was further complicated by an apparently high rate of non-compliance, as judged by serum folate levels. Nevertheless, all NTD recurrences were in mothers who were either in the placebo group or were folic acid 'non-compliers'. The same workers had previously reported an apparently beneficial effect of dietary counselling on NTD recurrence (Laurence et al 1980).

In a non-randomized, multicentre study, Smithells et al (1983) used a multivitamin preparation (Pregnavite Forte F, Bencard) including folic acid, to be taken for not less than 4 weeks before conception and continued until well after the normal time of neural tube closure. Supplemented mothers had (and continue to have) a significantly lower rate of NTD recurrence than do unsupplemented mothers with similar histories and resident in the same areas. Further experience with this vitamin supplement continues to support the belief that it substantially reduces NTD recurrence, especially in areas of high prevalence (Seller & Nevin 1984, Seller 1985). The non-randomized nature of the trial raises the possibility that the difference in observed recurrence rate between supplemented and unsupplemented mothers could be attributable to selection bias but a careful search for evidence of such bias failed to reveal any (Wild et al 1986). This topic is also discussed on p. 281.

Further studies of vitamin supplementation and of possible preventive mechanisms currently in progress should resolve some residual problems. Meanwhile, the possibility of primary prevention of a major birth defect should encourage further research in this direction.

CONCLUSION

Epidemiological study of NTDs suggests that:

1. Most are of multifactorial causation.
2. Where prevalence is high (3/1000 births or more), environmental factors are important; seasonal, social class and other variations are demonstrable; primary preventive measures appear effective.
3. Where prevalence is low (1/1000 births or less), environmental factors are less important, and primary prevention will only stem from knowledge we do not yet possess.

ACKNOWLEDGEMENTS

I wish to express my thanks to Miss Anna Durbin for artwork and Miss Christine Hildyard for secretarial help.

REFERENCES

Baird P A 1983 Neural tube defects in the Sikhs. American Journal of Medical Genetics 16: 49–56
Biggar R J, Mortimer E A Jr, Haughie G E 1976 Descriptive epidemiology of neural tube defects, Rochester, New York, 1918–1938. American Journal of Epidemiology 104: 22–27
Borman G B, Smith A H, Howard J K 1986 Risk factors in the prevalence of anencephalus and spina bifida in New Zealand. Teratology 33: 221–230
Cziezel A 1983 Spina bifida and anencephaly. British Medical Journal 287: 429
Elwood J M 1976 Aetiology of anencephaly and spina bifida. British Medical Journal 1: 218
Fedrick J 1974 Anencephalus and maternal tea drinking: evidence for possible association. Proceedings of the Royal Society of Medicine 67: 6–10
Fielding D W, Smithells R W 1971 Anencephalus and water hardness in South-West Lancashire. British Journal of Preventive and Social Medicine 25: 217–219
Knox E G 1972 Anencephalus and dietary intakes. British Journal of Preventive and Social Medicine 26: 219–223
Knox E G, Armstrong E H, Lancashire R 1984 The quality of notification of congenital malformations. Journal of Epidemiology and Community Health 38: 296–305
Laurence K M, Carter C O, David P A 1967 Major central nervous

system malformations in South Wales. I. Incidence, local variation and geographic factors. British Journal of Preventive and Social Medicine 21: 146–160

Laurence K M, James N, Miller M, Campbell H 1980 Increased risk of recurrence of pregnancies complicated by fetal neural tube defects in mothers receiving poor diets, and possible benefit of dietary counselling. British Medical Journal 281: 1592–1594

Laurence K M, James N, Miller M H, Tennant G B, Campbell H 1981 Double-blind randomised controlled trial of folate treatment before conception to prevent recurrence of neural tube defects. British Medical Journal 282: 1509–1511

Leck I 1966 Changes in the incidence of neural tube defects. Lancet ii: 791–792

Leck I 1969 Ethnic differences in the incidence of malformations following migration. British Journal of Preventive and Social Medicine 23: 166–173

Leck I, Record R G 1966 Seasonal incidence of anencephalus. British Journal of Preventive and Social Medicine 20: 67–75

Lindhout D, Schmidt D 1986 In-utero exposure to valproate and neural tube defects. Lancet i: 1392–1393

Lorber J 1974 The potato trial. Link 30: 7

Lorber J 1984 The family history of uncomplicated congenital hydrocephalus: an epidemiological study based on 270 probands. British Medical Journal 289: 281–284

Lowe C R, Roberts C L, Lloyd S 1971 Malformations of the central nervous system and softness of local water supplies. British Medical Journal 2: 357–361

McKeown T, Record R G 1951 Seasonal incidence of congenital malformations of the CNS. Lancet i: 192–196

MacMahon B, Yen S 1971 Unrecognised epidemic of anencephaly and spina bifida. Lancet i: 31–33

MacMahon B, Record R G, McKeown T 1951 Secular changes in the incidence of malformations of the central nervous system. British Journal of Preventive and Social Medicine 5: 254–258

Naggan L 1971 Anencephaly and spina bifida in Israel. Pediatrics 47: 577–586

Naggan L, MacMahon B 1967 Ethnic differences in the prevalence of anencephaly and spina bifida in Boston. New England Journal of Medicine 227: 1119–1123

Nevin N C, Merrett J D 1975 Potato avoidance during pregnancy in women with a previous infant with either anencephaly and/or spina bifida. British Journal of Preventive and Social Medicine 29: 111–115

Office of Population Censuses and Surveys 1982 Congenital malformations and parents' occupations. Monitor MB3 82/1

Penrose L S 1957 Genetics of anencephaly. Journal of Mental Deficiency Research 1: 4–15

Record R G 1961 Anencephalus in Scotland. British Journal of Preventive and Social Medicine 15: 93–105

Record R G, McKeown T 1949 Congenital malformations of the central nervous system. I. A survey of 930 cases. British Journal of Social Medicine 4: 183–219

Renwick J H 1972 Hypothesis — anencephaly and spina bifida are usually preventable by avoidance of a specific but unidentified substance present in certain potato tubers. British Journal of Preventive and Social Medicine 26: 67–88

Robert E, Lofkvist E, Mauguiere F 1984 Valproate and spina bifida. Lancet ii: 1392

Searle A G 1959 The incidence of anencephaly in a polytypic population. Annals of Human Genetics (London) 23: 279–287

Seller M J 1985 Periconceptional vitamin supplementation to prevent recurrence of neural tube defects. Lancet i: 1392–1393

Seller M J, Nevin N C 1984 Periconceptional vitamin supplementation and the prevention of neural tube defects in South-East England and Northern Ireland. Journal of Medical Genetics 21: 325–330

Simpson D, Robertson E 1985 Vitamins and neural tube defects. Medical Journal of Australia 142: 706

Smithells R W, Chinn E R 1965 Spina bifida in Liverpool. Developmental Medicine and Child Neurology 7: 258–268

Smithells R W, Nevin N C, Seller M J et al 1983 Further experience of vitamin supplementation for prevention of neural tube defect recurrences. Lancet i: 1027–1031

Stevenson A C, Johnson H A, Stewart M I P, Golding D R 1966 Congenital malformations: a report of a study of series of consecutive births in 24 centres. Bulletin of the World Health Organisation 34(1): 1–125

Stocks P 1970 Incidence of congenital malformation in the regions of England and Wales. British Journal of Preventive and Social Medicine 24: 67–77

Strassburg M A, Greenland S, Portigal L D, Sever L E 1983 A population-based case-control study of anencephalus and spina bifida in a low-risk area. Developmental Medicine and Child Neurology 25: 632–641

Wild J, Read A P, Sheppard S et al 1986 Recurrent neural tube defects, risk factors and vitamins. Archives of Disease in Childhood 61: 440–444

24. Prenatal diagnosis of neural tube defects

Dr J.E. Haddow

Neural tube defects (NTDs) are a family of congenital malformations including anencephaly, spina bifida and encephalocele, all of which result from a defect in neural tube closure during embryogenesis at between the 17th and 27th day of gestation. Worldwide, NTDs occur with varying frequency, depending upon a number of factors that include, most prominently, geographical location and race (Leck 1974). The birth prevalence is greatest in the UK, especially in the west of Scotland, Wales and Northern Ireland, where between 4 and 8 cases were reported per 1000 live births in the 1970s. In the USA the birth prevalence varies between approximately 0.5 and 2 per 1000 live births, the highest rate being found among the white population on the east coast and the lowest among the black population on the west coast (Greenberg et al 1983). In both the UK and the USA, the birth prevalence has declined over the past 15 years and only a fraction of this decline can be accounted for by prenatal intervention (see Ch. 23). During this same period prenatal diagnostic techniques, both biochemical and biophysical, have been developed and made available to high-risk families, and prenatal biochemical screening directed at the pregnant population-at-large has gradually been introduced. This chapter examines some of the relevant characteristics of NTDs and summarizes the laboratory and screening programmes now applied to diagnosing this group of disorders.

MORBIDITY AND MORTALITY ASSOCIATED WITH NTDs

Anencephaly

The most extreme of the neural tube malformations, anencephaly results from failure of the neural tube to fuse in the cranial region, leading to abnormal forebrain development, failure of the cranial bones to fuse, and degeneration of exposed neural tissue. Pituitary and, by extension, adrenal function is compromised, and the resulting failure in hormonal production is thought to contribute to delayed onset of labour and postterm delivery. Polyhydramnios occurs frequently in association with anencephalic pregnancies, leading to diagnostic studies in cases where the defect has not already been discovered by other screening techniques. The fetus with anencephaly is most often female, the M:F ratio being 1:3, and the condition is not compatible with extra-uterine survival. It has been argued that identifying anencephaly in utero is not of great value because the condition is lethal but at least two immediate considerations oppose this view: 1. the unexpected delivery of an anencephalic infant is devastating to the family and upsetting to delivery room personnel, and 2. Caesarean sections are often performed unnecessarily when anencephaly has not been recognized, due to the delayed onset of labour.

Encephaloceles

These lesions result from failure of neural tube fusion in the cranial region but are less extensive than anencephaly. The least severe are cranial meningoceles, where the defect contains meninges but no neural tissue. Encephaloceles contain both meninges and brain tissue, are usually skin-covered, and are associated with varying degrees of morbidity and mortality. Encephaloceles are most often occipital (75%), with frontal (15%) and parietal (10%) following in that order, and 20% of all conceptuses with encephalocele are stillborn. The prognosis is more favourable if the lesion is frontal and less favourable if there is microcephaly resulting from extensive herniation of brain tissue. In one-third of cases encephaloceles are associated with spina bifida. One population-based study (Field 1974) reports that, among liveborns with encephalocele, 47% survived and, among survivors, severe mental retardation occurred in 35% and mild to moderate mental retardation in 23%.

Spina bifida

When the neural tube fails to fuse in the spinal region, spina bifida results. Occasionally, the defect contains only meninges (meningocele) but most often both meninges and neural elements are present (meningomyelocele). About 80% of spina bifida cases are classified as 'open' (i.e. covered with only a thin membrane), the remainder being covered either by a thick membrane or by skin. Although most frequently located in the lumbar region, these lesions can be found at any point along the spine, and prognosis for both morbidity and mortality depends upon the location of the defect as well as its size, extent of neural involvement, and whether it is 'open' or 'closed'. Hydrocephalus is a frequent companion to meningomyelocele, being reported as an associated anomaly in up to 95% of the cases. Spina bifida occurs twice as often in females as in males.

The most consistent handicapping conditions associated with spina bifida result from damage to the neural elements of the spinal cord at or below the level of the defect and include lower limb paralysis, bowel and bladder dysfunction, and sensory loss. Surgical management of the lesion itself has improved in recent years, thereby reducing the risk of infection, and management of bladder dysfunction has also become more effective in avoiding urinary tract infections. No way has been found, however, to avoid or to reverse peripheral nervous system damage. Recently, it has been claimed that neurological function might be preserved by delivering infants with spina bifida via Caesarean section, but a second group of investigators has presented data that fail to substantiate this observation. Management of hydrocephalus has also improved to the point where brain function is better preserved; the major remaining problems result from shunt blockage and infection that require shunt removal and replacement.

Morbidity and mortality data for spina bifida have been difficult to pinpoint because the cases that finally arrive at specialty centres for management include an adequate representation of neither the very serious (or lethal) nor of the mild. A population-based study on the survival and handicap of infants with spina bifida was carried out in Oxfordshire, England by Althouse & Wald (1980) on 213 affected infants born between 1965 and 1972 (a time when prenatal diagnosis was not yet available). The five-year survival was 36% (39/107) for open lesions, 60% (30/50) for closed lesions, and 18% (10/56) for unclassified lesions. Among those surviving for five years with open or unclassified lesions (49), 84% were severely handicapped, 10% were moderately handicapped and 6% had no handicap. Among those survivors with closed lesions (30), 37% were severely handicapped, 33% were moderately handicapped and 30% had no handicap. Survivors with open lesions spent an average of more than six months in the hospital and had an average of six major surgical procedures during the first five years of life, as opposed to approximately four months hospitalization and three surgical procedures for survivors with closed lesions. Adams et al (1985) carried out a second population-based survey in Atlanta, Georgia, USA on the one-year survival of 154 infants with spina bifida born between 1972 and 1979. Among the 86 infants

with open lesions, 64% were alive after one year; 73% of the 32 with closed lesions and 45% of the 36 with unclassified lesions also survived for that length of time.

WHAT CAUSES NTDs?

Inheritance

A clearly defined explanation as to why neural tube defects occur has not yet been established but information is accumulating that may ultimately provide a better understanding. For the moment, NTDs are thought to result from a combination of genetic and environmental factors, referred to as multifactorial inheritance. This inheritance pattern is characterized by a recurrence risk that is a multiple of the population's occurrence risk and that increases with each succeeding affected pregnancy (Cowchock et al 1980). If a woman's pregnancy has been affected by anencephaly, her risk for having a succeeding NTD-associated pregnancy increases by a factor of 10 over the background for her population. If that woman then has a second pregnancy affected by anencephaly, her risk for having a subsequent NTD-associated pregnancy becomes 20 times that of the background population. In each of these respects, the inheritance pattern is different from that which can be defined by Mendelian laws, where recurrence risk of a given disorder is defined strictly by the presence of the gene in the family and where the risk remains constant for each pregnancy, no matter how many previous pregnancies have been affected by that disorder. Within families, a woman's risk for having an NTD-affected pregnancy is highest when a first-degree relative is affected, and the risk diminishes successively if a second- or third-degree relative is affected. In this last category, the risk is barely above the population background (Toriello & Higgins 1983). The exact genetic risk is shown in Fig. 20.1, page 251.

Associated conditions and other risk factors

Certain of the chromosome disorders are, on occasion, associated with spina bifida (e.g. trisomy 13, trisomy 18, and triploidy), and a few autosomal recessive disorders occasionally demonstrate encephaloceles (e.g. Meckel syndrome, Robert syndrome, cryptophthalmos) (Cohen & Lemire 1982). Various drugs acting as teratogens have also been documented as producing neural tube defects in a proportion of exposed pregnancies including: aminopterin (anencephaly), valproate (spina bifida), and warfarin (encephalocele). Women with poorly controlled insulin-dependent diabetes mellitus are at several times greater risk than the general population of having a pregnancy affected with NTD, and lower blood levels of some vitamins (most notably folate) have been identified in women with NTD pregnancies.

Vitamins and NTDs

As an extension of the observation concerning vitamin levels and NTD pregnancies, two trials of periconceptional vitamin supplementation of high-risk women have been reported, the first a randomized study utilizing folate and the second a non-randomized study utilizing a multivitamin preparation that included folate. In both instances, a reduction in the NTD recurrence rate was reported among vitamin supplemented women but problems existed which prevented either study from providing a definitive conclusion (Wald & Polani 1984). The first study provided appropriate randomization of the women but was too small, while the second contained elements of potential bias that could have influenced the outcome, even though the number of study subjects was adequate. The possibility that vitamins (especially folate) may influence neural tube formation is important to pursue until a firm conclusion can be drawn. Not only might it become possible to define the mechanism of neural tube malformations better from the standpoint of developmental biology (if a vitamin were found to be involved) but also it might become possible to reduce the occurrence of this group of disorders through routine vitamin supplementation of all women in the pregnancy age group. A randomized trial is now underway in the UK, Hungary, and elsewhere aimed at providing a more conclusive answer as to whether vitamins are protective and, if so, whether folate is the active agent. Should a vitamin influence be proven, this would represent the first example wherein a major group of birth defects could be prevented through simple dietary supplementation. (See also Ch. 23.)

MEASURING ALPHA-FETOPROTEIN (AFP) IN AMNIOTIC FLUID TO DETECT OPEN NTDs

In the absence of a defined cause and treatment to prevent the development of NTDs, a search began in the early 1970s for a biochemical test to detect these lesions at a time in fetal development that would allow the option of pregnancy termination. Brock & Sutcliffe (1972), in Edinburgh, developed an electro-immunodiffusion assay ('rocket') with sufficient sensitivity to measure the normally occurring background concentrations of alpha-fetoprotein (AFP) in amniotic fluid and then analysed a group of frozen, stored amniotic fluid samples obtained from pregnancies whose outcomes were subsequently known either to be associated with neural tube defect or to be unaffected. AFP levels in the open NTD pregnancies were distinctly higher than in the controls and this observation initiated a new era of prenatal diagnosis.

Sources of AFP in amniotic fluid

The investigators selected AFP for study because it is the major circulating serum protein in the fetus (occurring in higher concentration than any of the other serum proteins during the early weeks of gestation). Also, it is feto-specific (only trace amounts are found in normal, non-pregnant adult sera), unlike the other major circulating fetal proteins, which are immunologically identical to their adult counterparts (e.g. albumin, transferrin, alpha_1-antitrypsin). Amniotic fluid normally contains measurable amounts of most of the serum proteins common to both fetus and adult (Haddow et al 1978) but the major origin of all except AFP is the maternal circulation. For this reason, protein measurements such as albumin or transferrin cannot act as markers for fetal events, since any fetal contribution would be masked by that from the mother.

The background AFP levels in amniotic fluid that are normally found during the second trimester result from filtration through the fetal kidney and excretion in fetal urine. Amniotic fluid AFP concentrations change steadily throughout the second trimester, becoming progressively lower with the passage of time, and it is necessary to define this background pattern as a first step towards interpreting amniotic fluid AFP measurements in diagnostic samples. Figure 24.1 displays median AFP values in amniotic fluid during the second trimester, along with values that represent an acceptable upper range cut-off for pregnancies not associated with fetal malformations. When an open defect is present on the surface of the fetus, AFP transudates directly into amniotic fluid, nearly

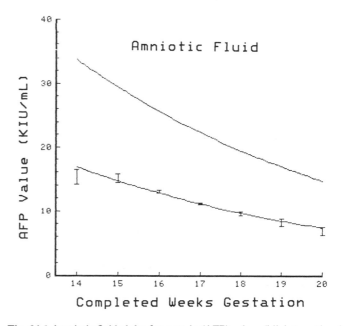

Fig. 24.1 Amniotic fluid alpha-fetoprotein (AFP) values (kilointernational Units/ml) during the second trimester in pregnancies not affected by neural tube defects or other open malformations. Vertical lines with bars at the ends indicate median values and 95% confidence limits for each completed gestational week between 14 and 20. The upper line represents a typical cut-off (two multiples of the median) for defining an abnormal result. Median AFP values in amniotic fluid normally decrease by approximately 13% per gestational week during the second trimester.

always in amounts sufficient to be clearly distinguishable from background. The distributions of AFP concentrations in amniotic fluid are shown in Figure 24.2 for unaffected, open spina bifida, and anencephalic pregnancies. Values for the three distributions are expressed as multiples of the median for the unaffected pregnancies to avoid the need to display separate graphs for each gestational week. There is little overlap between affected and unaffected pregnancies, meaning that AFP measurements in amniotic fluid are a sensitive way to detect these lesions. The specificity of this testing will be addressed later in greater detail. It is worth emphasizing that amniotic fluid AFP levels will be elevated only when the neural tube defect is open, and, thus, approximately 20% of spina bifida cases and many of the encephaloceles will not be detectable by this diagnostic approach. Anencephaly is, for practical purposes, always open. Transudation can also occur from some other types of defects such as open ventral wall defects, and for that (and other) reason(s) amniotic fluid AFP elevations cannot be considered specific as diagnostic markers for open NTDs. Elevated amniotic fluid AFP levels are, as well, a characteristic of a different type of fetal disorder, congenital nephrosis, a serious hereditary condition that usually ends in death before one year of age. In this disorder, AFP is filtered through the kidney in abnormally large amounts, and, in Finland, where congenital nephrosis is relatively common and open NTDs relatively uncommon, amniotic fluid AFP measurements are utilized diagnostically primarily to detect this renal disorder.

Introduction of AFP testing for diagnostic purposes

Following the report by Brock & Sutcliffe that amniotic fluid AFP levels were higher in the presence of open NTDs, confirmatory studies rapidly appeared, and AFP assays began to be set up for diagnostic use in prenatal diagnostic laboratories in Europe, North America, and Australia. Initially, attention focused on women who had already had an NTD-affected pregnancy and who were thereby recognized to be at high risk (between a 1 in 20 and a 1 in 50 chance) for a recurrence of the disorder in subsequent pregnancies. Because of their risk these women were felt to be suitable candidates for amniocentesis, a procedure that itself carries an estimated risk for fetal loss of somewhere between 1 in 200 and 1 in 100. In some centres, high-risk women were identified through a retrospective search of birth and clinic records, so that they could be made aware of the availability of the new diagnostic approach. When health workers contacted the women in one district, it was discovered that most had undergone sterilization procedures as a result of the affected pregnancy and that, with few exceptions, none had been given adequate information about the nature of the disorder or recurrence risks. By contrast, most women with NTD-affected pregnancies that occurred following the availability of amniotic fluid AFP testing were receptive to utilizing the test for future pregnancies, rather than opting for sterilization, and nearly all of the women were anxious to receive as much information as possible about the nature of the disorder.

False-positive AFP values

Unaffected pregnancies may occasionally be associated with amniotic fluid AFP elevations (false-positives), a situation that has been a source of considerable concern to those interpreting amniotic fluid AFP measurements for diagnostic purposes (Haddow 1983). The most common

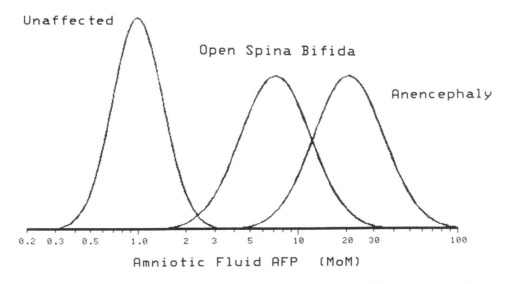

Fig. 24.2 Distributions of amniotic fluid alpha-fetoprotein (AFP) values in unaffected, open spina bifida, and anencephalic pregnancies. All values are expressed as multiples of the median for the unaffected population. The median value for open spina bifida pregnancies is about 7 multiples of the median (MoM), and for anencephalic pregnancies, about 21 MoM. Distributions for all three populations are log Gaussian. There is little overlap.

cause of false-positives is contamination of the amniotic fluid sample with fetal blood as a complication of amniocentesis. Blood-staining of an amniotic fluid specimen does not automatically mean that the amniotic fluid AFP level will be elevated, since the blood comes from the maternal circulation in most instances. When, however, the amniotic fluid AFP level is raised in the presence of blood-staining, it is most important to document whether fetal blood is present (by some test such as the Kleihaur test or counterimmuno-electrophoresis for haemoglobin F) and then interpret the amniotic fluid AFP result cautiously. It may be necessary to repeat the amniocentesis after about 10 days to obtain an amniotic fluid AFP measurement that is no longer influenced by fetal blood contamination from the original procedure. A further complication to identifying fetal blood contamination arises when the amniotic fluid sample is centrifuged and the cells removed before being sent to the AFP laboratory. In those cases, haemoglobin F measurements can be carried out on the supernatant and, if positive, can lead to further documentation of blood contamination by seeking information from personnel directly involved with the amniocentesis. In recent years, acetylcholinesterase measurements and detailed sonographic studies have provided considerable help in sorting out false-positive amniotic fluid AFP results, and their roles will be dealt with in more detail later in this chapter.

Sensitivity and specificity of AFP measurements for open NTDs

A multicentre collaborative study was undertaken in the UK, organized by Wald & Cuckle (1979), to evaluate the sensitivity and specificity of amniotic fluid AFP testing for open NTD, and that study provided extensive information relating to the interpretation of AFP test results, especially the likelihood of a positive amniotic fluid AFP result being true versus false. The study report emphasized the importance of considering a priori risk when estimating the odds of a true versus false-positive AFP test result at or above a given cut-off and put into perspective the pitfalls arising from measuring AFP in amniotic fluid samples obtained from women whose reason for having amniocentesis was having chromosome or other studies unrelated to neural tube defects. For example, a woman whose NTD risk was 20 per 1000 by virtue of a previous affected pregnancy might have a 4 to 1 chance of having an affected pregnancy, given a positive amniotic fluid AFP result, while a woman with the population background risk of 2 per 1000 might have only a 1 in 3 chance, given the same positive amniotic fluid AFP test result. These odds ratios do not take into account other variables, such as fetal blood-staining (or other more recent information such as acetylcholinesterase measurements or sonography). However, they still form the baseline for revised odds calculations that allow additional risk data to be taken

into account; and at each stage of odds revision, the risk of a false-positive remains relatively higher for the woman whose a priori risk is low.

Gel acetylcholinesterase analysis

As prenatal laboratories gained an appreciation for the extent and nature of AFP false-positives in amniotic fluid, considerable attention became directed at finding ways to deal with this problem. A significant advance in identifying false positive amniotic fluid AFP test measurements was made in 1979 (Smith et al), when acetylcholinesterase (AChE) was discovered to be present in amniotic fluid samples from NTD pregnancies but not from unaffected pregnancies. The investigators reasoned that AChE, a neural enzyme, might leak across the exposed fetal neural membranes into amniotic fluid and might, thereby, act as a more specific marker for open NTDs. AChE is one of a family of cholinesterases that are present in various human tissues, all of which react with acetylthiocholine as a substrate in vitro. AChE can be separated from other cholinesterases by gel electrophoresis, and its action on acetylthiocholine can be selectively inhibited by a chemical (BW284C51), two properties which allow it to be assayed readily. In Figure 24.3 a typical slab gel AChE study is shown, demonstrating the normally occurring pseudocholinesterase band near the origin of amniotic fluid sample application and, in the samples from the open NTD pregnancies, the faster moving AChE band. When this second band is discovered, it is important to carry out another gel study to test whether the second band can be inhibited by BW284C51, because,

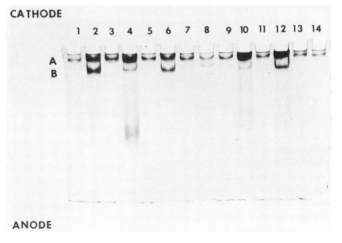

Fig. 24.3 Slab gel electrophoresis amniotic fluid acetylcholinesterase study, including samples from unaffected and open neural tube defect pregnancies. Amniotic fluid samples are applied at the cathodal end of the gel, and each of the numbers arranged horizontally designates a different patient sample. The band in the 'A' position is pseudocholinesterase, and the 'B' band is acetylcholinesterase. Samples 2, 6 and 12 are associated with open spina bifida cases, and samples 4, 8 and 10 are from open ventral wall defect pregnancies. Acetylcholinesterase bands are less pronounced in this latter category of disorders.

on rare occasions, a second pseudocholinesterase band may appear in this location, representing a potentially false-positive result. AChE is not present in maternal blood in measurable amounts but is found in low concentrations in fetal blood. Data on AChE from a number of prenatal laboratories were assembled collaboratively shortly after the original observation (Wald & Cuckle 1981), leading to the conclusion that amniotic fluid AChE testing was comparable in sensitivity to AFP for open NTDs and that approximately 90% of the false-positive AFP test results could be eliminated by demonstrating a negative AChE test result. Most of the remaining false-positive test results could be explained by heavy contamination of the amniotic fluid sample by fetal blood. Acetylcholinesterase measurements are now applied diagnostically as part of the laboratory routine to sort out false-positive amniotic fluid AFP test results and have contributed greatly to solving problem cases. Unlike AFP, however, AChE does not cross into the maternal circulation in sufficient amounts to be measured either quantitatively or qualitatively and so cannot be utilized for screening.

Limitations on the proportion of open NTDs identified by testing high-risk women

Given that the prime target population for amniotic fluid AFP testing included pregnant women known to be at risk for an NTD pregnancy by virtue of a positive history, it became theoretically possible to identify between 2 and 5% of all NTD pregnancies occurring in a given period, assuming that all high-risk women opted to have such testing performed. This meant that between 95 and 98% of all NTD pregnancies would still not be detectable, because they occurred in women with no previously known risk. For this reason the question was raised as to whether it might be possible to detect AFP in maternal blood, thereby allowing the general population of pregnant women to be tested.

MEASURING AFP IN MATERNAL SERUM TO DETECT OPEN NTDs

Sources of AFP in maternal serum and measurement techniques

AFP concentrations in maternal serum are normally considerably lower than in amniotic fluid during the second trimester (about 1/200th), requiring a more sensitive assay system. Radio-immunoassay (RIA) has been the method employed by most laboratories, and this technique is capable of detecting the levels of maternal serum AFP normally found during the 16–20 weeks gestational age period when such testing is usually carried out. AFP crosses into the maternal circulation by diffusion across the amnion (Haddow et al 1979) and also by diffusion or transport directly across the placenta (from the fetal circulation). In fetal blood, AFP concentration averages 1 500 000 µg/l, in amniotic fluid 8000 µg/l, and in maternal blood 40 µg/l at the 16th week of gestation. Both the placenta and the amnion, therefore, represent barriers between the fetal and maternal compartments, and it is surprising that maternal serum AFP levels are influenced by raised amniotic fluid AFP levels sufficiently to allow separation of affected and unaffected pregnancies. Given these physiological conditions one might speculate that raised maternal serum AFP levels would be quite non-specific for detecting open NTDs and also that they might be less sensitive than amniotic fluid measurements in detecting open NTDs; both of these speculations would be correct. Maternal serum AFP levels can be raised by feto–maternal haemorrhage, multiple gestation, or by a distressed or dying fetus, all of which are events that occur regularly during the second trimester. At the same time, NTD detection efficiency is appreciably lower than in amniotic fluid, and one probable reason for this is the restricted diffusion of AFP across the amnion, coupled with a relatively high background transplacental contribution of AFP to the maternal circulation.

The relationship between maternal serum AFP levels and open NTDs

Simultaneous reports by Wald et al and Brock et al in 1974 documented that maternal serum AFP levels were higher in pregnancies affected with anencephaly or spina bifida than in unaffected pregnancies. This finding, because of its potential application to all pregnancies, was immediately translated into a multicentre collaborative study, once again in the UK. The results of that study, published in 1977 (Wald & Cuckle), established the scientific and mathematical basis for maternal serum AFP testing upon which subsequently developed maternal serum AFP screening programmes worldwide have been modelled.

Expressing maternal serum AFP measurements

At the outset the collaborative study data from the 20 participating centres were converted from mass units (nanograms/ml) into multiples of the median (MoM) to overcome difficulties arising from differing laboratory reference ranges and to avoid the need for presenting individual normative data for each gestational week. When the collaborative study was carried out, mass unit standards varied widely between laboratories, so that a maternal blood sample might be analysed as having 30 ng/ml AFP in one laboratory and 45 ng/ml in another, both values being correct within the context of the individual laboratories' reference ranges. Wald & Cuckle obtained maternal serum AFP reference ranges from each of the participating centres for 14–22 weeks of gestation, identified the median value for unaffected singleton pregnancies for each gestational week, and then expressed all of the maternal serum AFP test results as a multiple of that median. In addition to the immediate analytic benefit derived from this treatment of the data, it became apparent that fewer maternal serum AFP measurements were required for establishing reliable median values than for establishing means. Furthermore, even when laboratories differed widely in precision, a given MoM (unlike a given standard deviation) would remain constant for defining the sensitivity of the testing process to detect open NTDs. This approach to unifying and simplifying the data proved so successful that MoM have now become the common currency routinely used for expressing maternal serum AFP measurements.

Optimal maternal serum AFP screening

Maternal serum AFP screening was discovered to have poor sensitivity when the gestational dates were under 15 weeks. The optimal time in gestation for screening was found to be at between 16 and 18 weeks, with screening sensitivity still satisfactory, albeit somewhat lower, at between 19 and 21 weeks gestation. A typical pattern of second trimester maternal serum AFP values for unaffected singleton pregnancies is shown in Figure 24.4, including both median values and cut-off values at 2.0 MoM. Because median maternal serum AFP values for unaffected singleton pregnancies rise at the rate of about 15% per week during the second trimester, accurate gestational dating is of considerable importance to the screening process. If a

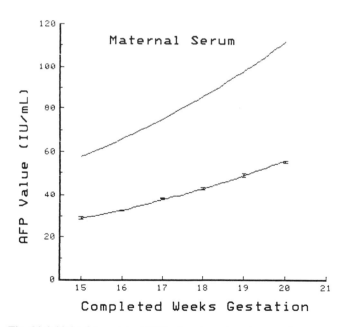

Fig. 24.4 Alpha-fetoprotein (AFP) values in maternal serum from singleton pregnancies without open fetal malformations during the second trimester. Vertical lines with bars at the ends indicate median values and 95% confidence limits for each completed gestational week between 15 and 20, the upper line representing a typical cut-off (two multiples of the median) for defining a positive screening test result. Median maternal serum AFP values normally increase by about 15% per gestational week during the second trimester.

pregnancy is assigned incorrectly advanced dates, then the maternal serum AFP value will appear lower than it really is; the converse is true when a pregnancy is misdated in the other direction.

Sensitivity and specificity of maternal serum AFP screening

Maternal serum AFP measurements were demonstrated to provide between 70 and 80% detection sensitivity for open spina bifida and about 90% detection sensitivity for anencephaly, depending upon the screening cut-off level selected for defining the group of pregnancies labelled as being at high risk. The sensitivity of maternal serum AFP screening was found to be limited by the extent of overlap between values found in affected and unaffected populations (Fig. 24.5), leading to the conclusion that no matter how well the assay was performed or how accurately the pregnancies were dated, a proportion of open NTDs could not be detected. This same lack of specificity in defining a high-risk population meant that maternal serum AFP measurements could not under any conditions be considered diagnostic. A positive maternal serum AFP screening result would simply be a first step, leading to a diagnostic process designed to provide a more definitive answer.

Follow-up testing for pregnancies with elevated maternal serum AFP screening test results

Screening programmes now functional in various locations have established maternal serum AFP screening cut-offs suited to their individual populations; the cut-offs selected are nearly always between 2.0 and 3.0 MoM and define high-risk groups for further study that range between 1 and 5%. Gestational dates for all of the pregnancies found to be above the cut-off are confirmed sonographically, and, if found to differ from dates calculated from the last menstrual period, the revised dates are used to reinterpret the maternal serum AFP value. Often, this step alone places the woman back into the low-risk category (Haddow et al 1983). Often, multiple gestation is discovered during the sonographic study, and these are also removed from the high-risk category, since twin pregnancies give rise to twice the concentration of maternal serum AFP, triplets to three times the maternal serum AFP concentration, and so forth. Maternal serum AFP elevations are found, on occasion, in conjunction with fetal death, and ultrasound identifies this condition, as well. Anencephaly is clearly visible by ultrasound and can be identified as part of the routine type of sonographic study carried out for pregnancy dating. Most open ventral wall defects (gastroschisis and omphalocele) can also be visualized by sonography carried out at this stage of the maternal serum AFP screening process.

Sonographic studies (see Ch. 25) are part of the evaluative

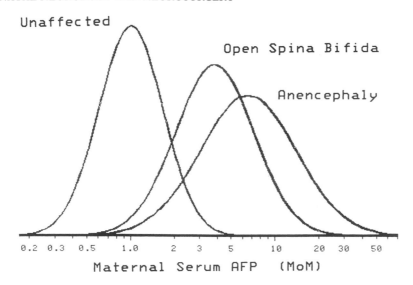

Fig. 24.5 Distributions of maternal serum alpha-fetoprotein (AFP) values in unaffected open spina bifida and anencephalic pregnancies. All values are expressed as multiples of the median (MoM) for the unaffected singleton population. The median value for the open spina bifida population is about 4 MoM, and for anencephalic pregnancies, about 7 MoM. All three populations have log Gaussian distributions. Considerable overlap exists for the three population curves, open spina bifida overlapping more than anencephaly with unaffected pregnancies.

protocol for women with maternal serum AFP elevations in all screening centres, and some of the centres recommend analysing second blood samples for maternal serum AFP, as well. The net effect of these procedures is that between half and two-thirds of the women originally defined as being at risk for open NTDs by the maternal serum AFP measurement are subsequently either removed from that category or diagnosed as having a fetal malformation. The women whose maternal serum AFP elevations are still not explained then become candidates for amniocentesis, totalling between 0.5 and 2% of the original screened population, depending upon the cut-off used to define the high-risk group. For these women, the immediate focus of concern is open spina bifida, a malformation that is reliably detected by only the most extensively trained and experienced sonographic personnel.

Open NTD risk among women whose elevated maternal serum AFP values cannot be explained

As a group, the women recommended for amniocentesis after maternal serum AFP screening actually have a higher open spina bifida risk than women who have had a previous affected pregnancy. Fetal open spina bifida has been identified at the rate of between 1 in 10 and 1 in 30 amniocenteses performed, depending once again on the local prevalence of that malformation and the screening cut-off employed. Amniotic fluid samples are analysed for alpha-fetoprotein (as discussed earlier) and for acetylcholinesterase.

Differing implications for false-positive maternal serum AFP, as opposed to amniotic fluid AFP, test results

Although the term 'false-positive' is commonly used to describe pregnancies that are not affected with open neural tube defects but that have either a positive screening test (elevated maternal serum AFP value) or a positive diagnostic test (elevated amniotic fluid AFP value), the implication of that term is fundamentally different as it applies to the two situations. The purpose of the screening test is to capture as great a proportion of the pregnancies with fetal malformations as possible from the pregnancy population at large, while at the same time including as few unaffected pregnancies as possible. The extent of overlap of maternal serum AFP values between the affected and unaffected populations, and the point at which the cut-off is set to select women for further studies combine to determine the sensitivity and specificity of the screening process, and, to maximize sensitivity, this process purposely includes a proportion of the unaffected pregnancies, because it is possible through subsequent diagnostic testing to discover those that do and those that do not have fetal malformations. For that reason women with elevated maternal serum AFP values might more appropriately be said to have 'screening positive' results, whatever the subsequent testing demonstrates.

The more traditionally understood definition of false-positive occurs when the AFP measurement is elevated in amniotic fluid in the presence of a pregnancy unaffected by a fetal malformation. This condition carries potentially grave consequences because amniotic fluid AFP testing is considered diagnostic, and a falsely elevated test result can lead to the unaffected pregnancy being terminated. Although laboratory error can be the reason for a false-positive, the most frequent explanation is contamination of the amniotic fluid sample with fetal blood. This means that amniotic fluid AFP values also overlap between affected and unaffected populations, albeit to a much lesser extent than maternal serum AFP distributions.

THE ROLE OF ULTRASOUND IN DETECTING OPEN NTDs

Evaluating how ultrasound can contribute to open NTD identification is more complex than evaluating the contribution of alpha-fetoprotein testing because the reliability of sonographic interpretation is more dependent upon each individual operator's skill and experience, unlike the standardized, systematized, and centralized biochemical testing process by which AFP is analysed and interpreted. To complicate such assessment further, ultrasound equipment has undergone a series of refinements in recent years that have substantially improved resolution, making studies carried out even several years ago difficult to interpret in the context of current technology. From the outset, it is important to distinguish between what might reasonably be expected from sonographic studies carried out routinely in physician offices or outpatient radiology units, as opposed to detailed sonographic studies performed on high-risk pregnancies by highly experienced specialists at referral centres.

The ability of ultrasound to visualize NTDs

It is possible to visualize all of the major neural tube malformations sonographically but the ease with which the defect can be identified differs greatly, depending upon the type of lesion present (anencephaly, encephalocele, or spina bifida). Unlike anencephaly, which is easily seen even during a routine scan, spina bifida requires careful positioning and detailed segmental cross-sectional scanning of individual spines and is fully discussed in Chapter 25.

Sensitivity and specificity for detecting NTDs in high-risk pregnancies

Roberts et al (1983), in Wales, carried out a six-year study (1977–83) to evaluate how effectively diagnostic ultrasound could be applied to diagnosing NTDs in women known to be at high risk (on the basis either of a positive family history or a raised maternal serum AFP). During the course of the study, 57 cases of anencephaly were identified and none were missed. Diagnostic success was lower for spina bifida, where 22 out of 38 cases were identified. Distinct improvement, however, was shown in spina bifida identification during the course of the study; only a third of the cases

were found during the first three years, as opposed to 80% during the final three years. This latter diagnostic sensitivity more accurately reflects what might now be expected in referral centres. False-positive spina bifida diagnoses were made in 53 out of the 2361 women studied but only four of the false-positive diagnoses were made in the last three years of the study. This again reflects increasing skill and experience of the operators. Detailed diagnostic sonographic studies are now capable of providing valuable information about the presence or absence of spina bifida, especially in pregnancies known to be at high risk. Both false-positive and false-negative results do occur on occasion, however, and this needs to be borne in mind during the interpretive and decision-making process.

Sensitivity of sonography as a screening test for NTDs

A blinded screening study was reported from Scandinavia in 1983 (Persson et al) comparing routine ultrasound screening with maternal serum AFP screening as a means of detecting open NTDs. Maternal serum AFP was measured by a semiquantitative technique in this study, and a single cut-off of 100 µg/l was selected, regardless of gestational age. Ultrasound was performed routinely on all of the pregnancies in a central facility without knowledge of family history or maternal serum AFP test result. Sonography identified the one case of anencephaly and two of three encephaloceles but missed five cases of open spina bifida, one meningocele, and one encephalocele. Maternal serum AFP identified the case of anencephaly, two of the three encephaloceles, and four of the five cases of open spina bifida. Under these screening conditions, therefore, maternal serum AFP screening was comparable in sensitivity for detecting anencephaly and encephalocele but substantially more sensitive for detecting open spina bifida.

Fetuses with open spina bifida have small biparietal diameter measurements during the second trimester

In the early phase of maternal serum AFP screening for open spina bifida, investigators were concerned that sonographic estimates of gestational age might not be correct in the presence of an open spina bifida fetus because of hydrocephalus associated with the spinal defect. Biparietal diameter measurements, if larger than average for the true gestational age, would incorrectly advance pregnancy dates. If, based on this information, maternal serum AFP measurements were then to be reinterpreted, the net effect would be for the values to appear lower than they really were, thereby decreasing the sensitivity of the screening process. When open spina bifida pregnancy biparietal diameter measurements were analysed, however, it was discovered that they were actually smaller during the second trimester, on average, than those from unaffected pregnancies (Wald et al 1980). This observation meant not only that concerns about correcting menstrual dates by biparietal measurements could be set aside but also that dating pregnancies by BPD measurements before maternal serum AFP screening could actually increase screening sensitivity for detecting open spina bifida. Ultrasound dating of pregnancies now includes measuring additional parameters, such as femur length and abdominal circumference. These other measurements appear not to be altered in spina bifida pregnancies and so do not influence the sensitivity of maternal serum AFP screening for open spina bifida in either direction.

Using routine sonography to improve sensitivity and specificity of maternal serum AFP screening

One discrete application of ultrasound screening to open spina bifida identification, therefore, deserves special consideration. If all pregnancies were to have biparietal diameter measurements performed routinely before maternal serum AFP screening, both the sensitivity and specificity of the maternal serum AFP testing process for open NTDs (and especially open spina bifida) detection would improve measurably, due to: 1. more precise gestational dating; 2. identification of fetal deaths and multiple gestation; and 3. the effect produced on maternal serum AFP interpretation by smaller biparietal measurements in open spina bifida pregnancies (Wald et al 1982). In Figure 24.6, distributions of maternal serum AFP concentrations are modelled for unaffected and open spina bifida populations, first when gestational dates are calculated from the last menstrual

period and then from biparietal diameter measurements. The bell-shaped distribution of unaffected pregnancies pulls in slightly after sonography, while the entire population of open spina bifida pregnancies moves to the right, away from the unaffected pregnancies.

Two recently described anatomical features associated with heads of open spina bifida fetuses

Recently, two anatomical characteristics were observed in ultrasound studies of the heads of open spina bifida fetuses (Nicolaides et al 1986): scalloping of the frontal bones (the lemon sign) and anterior curving of the cerebellar hemispheres with obliteration of the cisterna magna (the banana sign). It is possible that these characteristics may make open spina bifida identification more accessible to screening by routine sonography.

PRENATAL SCREENING AND DIAGNOSTIC SERVICES FOR OPEN NTD DETECTION

A considerable body of specialized knowledge is now available that offers the potential for identifying the majority of open neural tube defects prenatally, and in many areas of the world some or all of this knowledge has been converted into service activities. Health care delivery systems vary widely in their designs, however, from centralized to highly decentralized, and delivery of these new services therefore requires individual planning, tailored to suit the constraints (financial and otherwise) of each system. In areas where maternal serum AFP screening has been introduced, it has been found consistently helpful

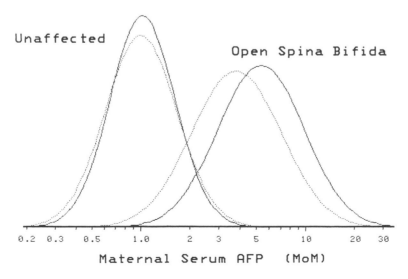

Fig. 24.6 Distributions of maternal serum alpha-fetoprotein (AFP) values in unaffected and open spina bifida pregnancies. Dotted lines represent pregnancies dated by last menstrual period, and unbroken lines depict pregnancies dated by sonographic measurements of biparietal diameters. Sonographic dating produces a tightening of the unaffected population maternal serum AFP distribution and also causes the distribution for open spina bifida pregnancies to be moved to the right.

to have a programme in place to co-ordinate laboratory and patient service activities. Positive maternal serum AFP screening results need to be reported by telephone to health personnel caring for the pregnant woman, along with more detailed information about the meaning of those results. Guidance is often necessary for subsequent testing, and the process needs to be monitored and test results reinterpreted, when appropriate. Amniotic fluid test results require similar management and, if the test results are positive, genetic counselling is necessary, together with a review of available options. Follow-up counselling and information need to be made available, so that the woman can plan how to deal with the question of future pregnancies.

Programme personnel are responsible for monitoring current medical literature and communicating with other programme centres so that new information and patient literature can be made available promptly. Health personnel involved with the primary care of pregnant women need to be able to utilize programme personnel as an ongoing resource for patient-related information. This arrangement not only keeps the screening and diagnostic process orderly but also helps to maintain a sense of confidence and security among health care providers as regards laboratory and ultrasound testing services.

Knowledge continues to accumulate at a rapid rate involving all aspects of prenatal detection of open NTDs and it is unrealistic to expect primary health care providers individually to maintain the special and evolving body of information necessary for this narrow but very important area of pregnancy care. Although the need for programme development began with maternal serum AFP screening, it is now apparent that a variation of this same principle can be applied to ultrasound screening and diagnostic services for open NTDs, as well.

REFERENCES

Adams M M, Greenberg F, Khoury M J, Marks J S, Oakley G P 1985 Survival of infants with spina bifida — Atlanta 1972–1979. American Journal of Diseases of Children 139: 514–517

Althouse R, Wald N J 1980 Survival and handicap of infants with spina bifida. Archives of Disease in Childhood 55: 845–850

Brock D J H, Sutcliffe R G 1972 Alpha-fetoprotein in the antenatal diagnosis of anencephaly and spina bifida. Lancet ii: 197–199

Brock D J H, Bolton A E, Scrimgeour J B 1974 Prenatal diagnosis of spina bifida and anencephaly through maternal plasma-alpha-fetoprotein measurement. Lancet i: 767–769

Campbell S, Pryse-Davies J, Coltart T M, Seller M J, Singer J D 1975 Ultrasound in the diagnosis of spina bifida. Lancet i: 1065–1066

Cohen M M, Lemire R J 1982 Syndromes with cephaloceles. Teratology 25: 161–172

Cowchock S, Ainbender E, Prescott G et al 1980 The recurrence risk for neural tube defects in the United States: a collaborative study. American Journal of Medical Genetics 5: 309–314

Field B 1974 The child with encephalocele. Medical Journal of Australia 1: 700–703

Greenberg F, James L M, Oakley G P 1983 Estimates of birth prevalence rates of spina bifida in the United States from computer generated maps. American Journal of Obstetrics and Gynecology 145: 570–573

Haddow J E 1983 Proteins in amniotic fluid: diagnostic and clinical considerations, with special emphasis on alpha-fetoprotein. In: Proteins in body fluids, amino acids, and tumor markers: diagnostic and clinical aspects. Alan R Liss, New York, pp 173–185

Haddow J E, Cowchock S F, Macri J N, Munson M, Baldwin P, Aldrich N 1978 Second trimester amniotic fluid protein values from normal, neural tube defect, and fetal demise pregnancies after exclusion of maternal blood contamination by testing for pregnancy-associated macroglobulin. Pediatric Research 12: 243–248

Haddow J E, Macri J N, Munson M E 1979 The amnion regulates movement of fetally derived alpha-fetoprotein into maternal blood. Journal of Laboratory and Clinical Medicine 94: 344–347

Haddow J E, Kloza E M, Smith D E, Knight G J 1983 Data from an alpha-fetoprotein screening program in Maine. Obstetrics and Gynecology 62: 556–560

Leck I 1974 Causation of neural tube defects: clues from epidemiology. British Medical Bulletin 30: 158–163

Nicolaides K H, Gabbe S G, Campbell S, Guidetti R 1986 Ultrasound screening for spina bifida: cranial and cerebellar signs. Lancet ii: 72–74

Persson P H, Kullander S, Gennser G, Grennert L, Laurell C B 1983 Screening for fetal malformations using ultrasound and measurements of α-fetoprotein in maternal serum. British Medical Journal 286: 747–749

Roberts C J, Hibbard B M, Roberts E E, Evans K T, Laurence K M, Robertson I B 1983 Diagnostic effectiveness of ultrasound in detection of neural tube defects. Lancet ii: 1068–1069

Smith A D, Wald N J, Cuckle H S, Stirrat G M, Bobrow M, Lagercrantz H 1979 Amniotic fluid acetylcholinesterase as a possible diagnostic test for neural tube defects in early pregnancy. Lancet i: 685–690

Toriello H V, Higgins J V 1983 Occurrence of neural tube defects among first-, second- and third-degree relatives of probands: results of a United States study. American Journal of Medical Genetics 15: 601–606

Wald N J, Cuckle H S 1977 Collaborative study on alpha-fetoprotein in relation to neural tube defects. Lancet i: 1323–1332

Wald N J, Cuckle H S 1979 Second report of the UK collaborative study on alpha-fetoprotein measurement in antenatal diagnosis of anencephaly and open spina bifida in early pregnancy. Lancet ii: 651–662

Wald N J, Cuckle H S 1981 Report of the Collaborative Acetylcholinesterase Study. Amniotic fluid acetylcholinesterase electrophoresis as a secondary test in the diagnosis of anencephaly and open spina bifida in early pregnancy. Lancet ii: 321–324

Wald N J, Polani P E 1984 Neural tube defects and vitamins: the need for a randomized clinical trial. British Journal of Obstetrics and Gynaecology 91: 516–523

Wald N J, Brock D J H, Bonnar J 1974 Prenatal diagnosis of spina bifida and anencephaly by maternal serum alpha-fetoprotein measurement. Lancet i: 765–767

Wald N, Cuckle H, Boreham J, Stirrat G 1980 Small biparietal diameter of fetuses with spina bifida: implications for antenatal screening. British Journal of Obstetrics and Gynaecology 87: 219–221

Wald N, Cuckle H, Boreham J, Turnbull A C 1982 Effect of estimating gestational age by ultrasound cephalometry on the specificity of α-fetoprotein screening for open neural-tube defects. British Journal of Obstetrics and Gynaecology 89: 1050–1053

25. Prenatal ultrasound assessment of neural tube defects

Dr G. Pilu and Prof J. C. Hobbins

Anencephaly was the first congenital anomaly recognized in utero by ultrasound (Campbell et al 1972). The diagnosis is easy, as one relies on the demonstration of the absence of the cranial vault. As the fetal head can be positively identified by modern ultrasound equipment as early as the first trimester, it is likely that anencephaly is recognizable even in this period.

SPINA BIFIDA

We are not aware of cases of spina bifida occulta diagnosed in utero by ultrasound. It seems unlikely that such lesions can be detected even by the most experienced operators. Open defects can be recognized by demonstrating the defect of the neural arches and overlying soft tissues (Fig. 25.1). The accuracy of ultrasound in predicting fetal spinal lesions is a critical issue. It is clear that the predictive value of the technique largely depends upon the quality of the equipment, the experience of the operator, and the amount of time dedicated to any single patient. No data are available with regard to routine scanning (level-one) examinations. However, there is little doubt that the sensitivity of these examinations is quite low. In 10 years of activity at the Prenatal Pathophysiology Unit of the Bologna University, which acts as a second-level centre for an area where almost 30 000 deliveries per year occur, only those cases with overt and severe hydrocephalus were referred from level-one facilities. Level-two examinations on patients at risk for either familial history or elevated alpha-fetoprotein yield a much greater accuracy. The use of sonography for antenatal detection of spina bifida was first suggested by Campbell et al (1975).

In the original report, ultrasound was successful in identifying one affected fetus and ruling out lesions in one normal fetus and failed to recognize a lumbo–sacral defect in a third fetus. Ten years later, the same group reported a sensitivity and specificity of level-two ultrasound very close to 100% (Pearce et al 1985). A similar trend was reported

by Roberts et al (1983), who described the results of a large multicentric study performed in South Wales. The sensitivity of the technique was 30% in the first three years and rose to 80% in the following three years. The false-positive rate decreased from 57% to 9% in the second period of the study. Both the increased experience of the operators and the introduction of high-resolution, real-time ultrasound equipment were probably responsible for this dramatic diagnostic improvement.

We have recently focused our attention on the evaluation of intracranial anatomy in fetuses with spina bifida. Table 25.1 shows our preliminary results. It has been known for a long time that the hydrocephalus, even if it is commonly seen at birth, is a late finding in fetuses with spina bifida.

Only 10 of 14 cases prospectively examined (71%) had overt ventriculomegaly attested to by an abnormal size of the bodies of lateral ventricles (Jeanty et al 1981) at the first examination. However, two of the remaining cases had enlarged atria (Pearce et al 1985) and all had a disproportion between the ventricular lumen at the level of the atria and the corresponding choroid plexus (Chinn et al 1983). Almost all infants with spina bifida have some degree of Arnold–Chiari Type II malformation and autopsy studies indicate a decreased cerebellar weight (Variend & Emery 1973). Recent sonographic studies in newborns have demonstrated that in infants with spina bifida, the cisterna magna is either diminished in size or obliterated (Goodwin & Quisline 1983). These observations directly prompted a study of the fetal posterior fossa. We found that the cisterna

Table 25.1 Ultrasound evaluation of intracranial anatomy in 14 fetuses with spina bifida

Lateral ventricles		
Overt hydrocephalus (abnormal ventricular ratio)	10/14	(71%)
Enlarged atria	12/14	(85%)
Choroid plexus/atrial lumen disproportion	14/14	(100%)
Posterior fossa		
Obliterated cisterna magna	14/14	(100%)
Abnormal or not measurable cerebellar transverse diameter	13/14	(92%)

magna could be consistently recognized by sonography in all cases before 29 weeks (Pilu et al 1986a). We have also developed a nomogram of the normal dimensions of the transverse diameter of the cerebellum (CTD) which was measured in an axial scan angled posteriorly as in Figure 25.2. In a group of 14 spina bifida fetuses prospectively examined, the cisterna magna appeared obliterated in all cases. The cerebellum was always unusually difficult to visualize (Fig. 25.3). The CTD was below the fifth percentile in 76% of cases, and in 15% the measurement could not be obtained due to an extreme alteration of the posterior fossa contents. Only one fetus had a CTD within the normal range. The results of our study indicate that evaluation of intracranial anatomy can positively assist the diagnosis of spina bifida. Qualitative evaluation of the atria of lateral ventricles, and qualitative and quantitative evaluation of the posterior fossa structures can be performed easily and rapidly and may prove to be useful for screening spina bifida in level-one ultrasound examinations.

As anencephaly is an invariably fatal lesion, termination of pregnancy can be offered at any time in pregnancy (Chervenak et al 1984a). When the diagnosis of spina bifida is made before viability, termination of pregnancy can be offered to the parents. When this option is not chosen, and in those cases recognized later on in gestation, an attempt to identify the site and extent of the lesion should be made to assess a tentative prognosis. Options should be discussed with the couples. Several reports indicate that birth injury is frequent in fetuses with spina bifida and represents a major prognostic shortcoming (Stark & Drummond 1970, Ralis & Ralis 1972, Ralis 1975) and caesarean delivery has been recommended (Chervenak et al 1984b).

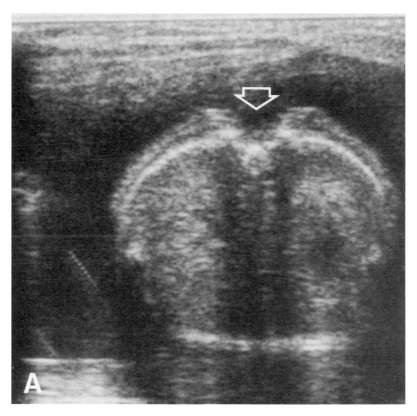

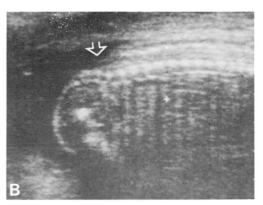

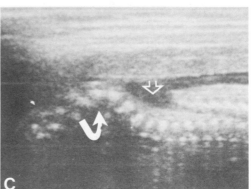

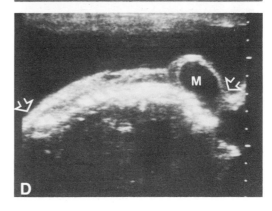

Fig. 25.1 Ultrasound appearances of spina bifida. (**a**) Transverse cross-section of the trunk in a 30-week-old fetus with spina bifida demonstrating the typical U-shaped appearance of the defective vertebrae (arrow). Note the absence of soft tissue above the lesion. (**b–d**) Longitudinal scans of the trunk in fetuses with spinal lesions (open arrows) of different location and severity. In (**b**), a small sacral lesion is demonstrated. In (**c**), a thoraco–lumbar lesion with associated kyphoscoliosis (curved arrow) is shown. In (**d**), a full-length defect of the spine, running from C1 to S5 is seen. Spina bifida is inferred by the absence of the spinal cord mimicking normal soft tissues arise from an associated myelomeningocele that is particularly evident as a cystic mass in the cervical region (M).

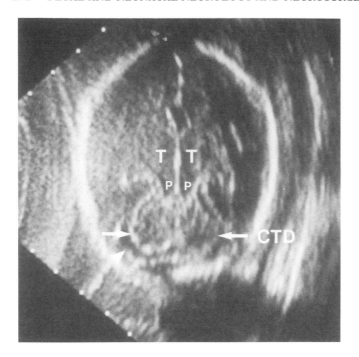

Fig. 25.2 Suboccipito–bregmatic scan in a normal 22-week-old fetus. This view was used for the measurement of the cerebellar transverse diameter (CTD). Note the prominent cisterna magna (arrowhead). T = thalami: P = cerebral peduncles.

ENCEPHALOCELE

The term encephalocele (or cephalocele) indicates a protrusion of intracranial contents through a bony defect of the skull. The incidence is about 1 in 2000 births (Schulman 1979). The aetiology is unknown. The observation that encephaloceles may occur in families with a history of neural tube defects (Warkany 1971) suggests that the anomalies are somewhat related. Encephaloceles may occur either as isolated defects or as a part of genetic and non-genetic syndromes (see Ch. 20). In most cases, the lesion arises from the midline in the occipital area, less frequently from the parietal or frontal bones. Encephaloceles are characterized by the presence of brain tissue inside the lesion. When only meninges protrude, the term cranial meningocele should be used. Encephaloceles often cause impaired cerebrospinal fluid circulation and hydrocephalus. Massive encephaloceles may be associated with microcephaly. The outcome is mainly related to the presence or absence of brain tissue inside the lesion. Encephaloceles carry a neonatal mortality rate of about 40% and an incidence of intellectual impairment and neurological sequelae of 80%. Infants with cranial meningoceles develop a normal intelligence in 60% of cases (Lorber 1971).

Fetal encephaloceles should be suspected when a paracranial mass is seen on sonography. The diagnosis of

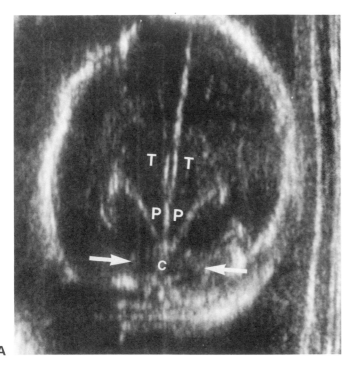

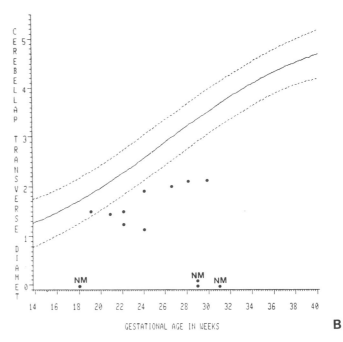

CUBIC REGRESSION OF CEREBELLAR TRANSVERSE DIAMETER

A

B

Fig. 25.3 Cerebellar transverse diameter. (a) Suboccipito–bregmatic scan in a 20-week-old fetus with spina bifida. The cisterna magna is obliterated and the cerebellum is poorly defined. The CTD (arrows) is below the normal limits for gestational age. The low position of the cerebellum results in a typical elongation of the cerebral peduncles (P). The fetus had a spinal defect involving the tract L4–S3. T = thalami. (b) Measurements of the CTD in 13 fetuses with spina bifida plotted against the curve obtained in 215 normal fetuses (NM = not measurable).

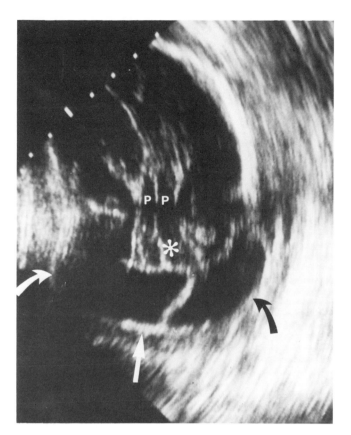

Fig. 25.4 Encephalocele. Low axial scan of the head of a 27-week-old fetus with encephalocele. The cerebellum (*) is entirely displaced outside the cranial cavity and inside the meningeal sac (arrows). P = cerebral peduncles.

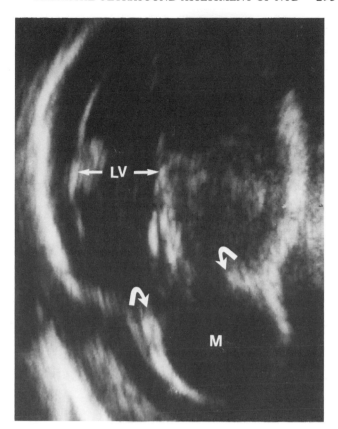

Fig. 25.5 Axial scan of the head of a 35-week-old fetus with a cranial meningocele (M). The dropout of echoes at the level of the occiput (curved arrows) does not represent a bony defect but is due to acoustic shadowing cast by the curvature of the calvarium. After birth, the defect was found to have a diameter of only 2 mm. The lateral ventricles (LV) are enlarged. (Reproduced with permission from Pilu et al 1986b.)

encephaloceles is easy, as the presence of brain tissue inside the sac is striking on ultrasound (Fig. 25.4). Differentiation of a cranial meningocele from soft tissue oedema or a cystic hygroma of the neck may be difficult (Nicolini et al 1983). In a recent series, a proper diagnosis could be made in almost all cases by demonstrating the bony defect of the skull (Pearce et al 1985). Our experience is not in agreement with these results. In most of our cases of pure cranial meningocele, the bony defect was found at birth to have a size of a few millimetres. Such defects easily fall below the lateral resolution power of current ultrasound equipment, and furthermore, they are often obscured by the acoustic shadowing cast by the curvature of the calvarium (Fig. 25.5). Other clues can be searched for to assist in a correct diagnosis. Cranial encephaloceles are often associated with ventriculomegaly. Cystic hygromas arise from the region of

the neck, have multiple internal septations and a thick wall, and are often associated with general soft-tissue oedema and hydrops. Some encephaloceles protrude through the base of the skull inside the pharynx. These lesions are obviously inaccessible to prenatal ultrasound identification unless derangement of intracranial morphology is present. As encephaloceles are often associated with other anomalies, a careful investigation of the entire fetal anatomy is recommended.

Termination of pregnancy can be offered before viability. In continuing pregnancies, a caesarean delivery should be considered to avoid birth trauma. However, as infants with massive encephalocele and microcephaly have a dismal prognosis, conservative management is recommended in these cases (Chervenak et al 1984c).

REFERENCES

Campbell S, Johnstone F D, Holt E M, May P 1972 Anencephaly: early diagnosis and active management. Lancet ii: 1226
Campbell S, Pryse-Davies J, Coltart T M, Seller M, Singer J D 1975 Ultrasound in the diagnosis of spina bifida. Lancet i: 1065

Chervenak F A, Farley M A, Walters L, Hobbins J C, Mahony N H 1984a When is termination of pregnancy during the third trimester morally justifiable? New England Journal of Medicine 310:501

Chervenak F A, Duncan C, Ment L R et al 1984b Perinatal management of myelomeningocele. Obstetrics and Gynecology 64: 86

Chervenak F A, Isaacson G, Mahoney M J et al 1984c Diagnosis and management of fetal cephaloele. Obstetrics and Gynecology 64: 86

Chinn D H, Callen P W, Filley R A 1983 The lateral cerebral ventricle in early second trimester. Radiology 148: 529

Goodwin I, Quisline R G 1983 The neonatal cisterna magna: ultrasonic evaluation. Radiology 149: 691

Jeanty P, Dramaix-Wilmet M, Delbeke D, Rodesch F, Struyven J 1981 Ultrasonic evaluation of fetal ventricular growth. Neuroradiology 21: 127

Lorber J 1971 Results of treatment of myelomeningocele. Developmental Medicine and Child Neurology 13: 279

Nicolini U, Ferrazzi E, Massa E, Minonzio M, Pardi G 1983 Prenatal diagnosis of cranial masses by ultrasound: report of five cases. Journal of Clinical Ultrasound 11: 170

Pearce J M, Little D, Campbell S 1985 The diagnosis of abnormalities of the fetal central nervous system. In: Sanders R C, James A E (eds) The principles and practice of ultrasound in obstetrics and gynecology. Appleton Century-Crofts, Norwalk, pp 243–256

Pilu G, DePalma L, Romero R, Bovicelli L, Hobbins J C 1986a The fetal subarachnoid cisterns: an ultrasound study with report of a case of congenital communicating hydrocephalus. Journal of Ultrasound in Medicine 5: 365

Pilu G, Rizzo N, Orsini L F, Bovicelli L 1986b Antenatal recognition of cerebral anomalies. Ultrasound in Medicine and Biology 12: 319

Ralis Z A 1975 Traumatizing effect of breech delivery on infants with spina bifida. Journal of Pediatrics 87: 613

Ralis Z, Ralis H M 1972 Morphology of peripheral nerves in children with spina bifida. Developmental Medicine and Child Neurology 14 (suppl 27): 109

Roberts C J, Evans K T, Hibbard B M et al 1983 Diagnostic effectiveness of ultrasound in detection of neural tube defects: the South Wales experience of 2509 scans (1977–1982) in high-risk mothers. Lancet ii: 1068

Schulman K 1979 Encephalocele. In: Bergsma D (ed) Birth defect compendium. 2nd edn. Alan R Liss, New York, pp 390–391

Stark G, Drummond M 1970 Spina bifida as an obstetric problem. Developmental Medicine and Child Neurology 12 (suppl 22): 157

Variend S, Emery J L 1973 The weight of cerebellum in children with myelomeningocele. Developmental Medicine and Child Neurology 15 (suppl 29): 77

Warkany J 1971 Congenital malformations: notes and comments. Year Book Medical Publishers, Chicago

26. Surgical management of the infant and outcome

Mr J. Punt

The spectrum of neural tube defects spans some of the most minor to the most devastating congenital malformations encountered at birth. An understanding of the appropriate neurosurgical management, possible implications and probable outcome is crucial to the neonatal physician as the one who must recognize the lesion, initiate neurosurgical referral and make preliminary explanation to the parents. With these prerequisites in mind this chapter reviews current management and prognosis of the open and closed neural tube defects.

ENCEPHALOCELE

Encephaloceles have been classified by Suwanwela & Chaturaporn (1966) according to site (see Table 26.1). The position of the encephalocele can be further subdivided according to site; 70% are occipital and 15% fronto–ethmoidal. In certain Far Eastern countries, notably Thailand, this ratio is reversed and fronto–ethmoidal lesions predominate.

The diagnosis usually declares itself at birth, though

Table 26.1 Classification of encephalocele according to Suwanwela & Chaturaporn 1966

Cranial vault
  Occipital
  Interfrontal
  Parietal
  Anterior or posterior fontanelle
  Temporal

Fronto–ethmoidal (sinupital)
  Naso–frontal
  Naso–ethmoidal
  Naso–orbital

Basal
  Transethmoidal
  Spheno–ethmoidal
  Transphenoidal
  Spheno–orbital

larger lesions may be recognized prenatally by ultrasound. Management commences with general examination to exclude other congenital anomalies especially cardiac (dextrocardia), respiratory (pulmonary hypoplasia and laryngomalacia), genitourinary (renal agenesis) and the occasional concomitant myelomeningocele (Reigel 1982). The site and size of the mass and condition of the overlying skin are noted and the occipito–frontal circumference charted. For occipital encephaloceles the only special investigation required is ultrasound scanning of the intracranial contents to determine ventricular size and configuration and the presence of any concomitant cerebral malformation such as holoprosencephaly, Dandy–Walker malformation and Chiari malformation. The sac is examined by transillumination and by ultrasound to determine its contents, brain tissue being present in 25 to 80% of cases (Mealey et al 1970). For fronto–ethmoidal and basal encephaloceles more detailed examination with computerized tomography of the brain and skull base in axial and coronal planes is indicated to define the skull defect and its contents more precisely. The neurological examination is usually normal at birth.

Large occipital encephaloceles are repaired shortly after birth, the general condition of the baby permitting, as they are distressing for parents and make handling and feeding of the child difficult. Small occipital lesions may be left for a few weeks to enable the child to weather any immediate perinatal crisis and to allow bonding with the parents.

Frontal and basal encephaloceles are repaired after the first few weeks of life when the child has regained birth-weight and is thriving, or may be delayed until such time as any definitive craniofacial corrective procedures are contemplated; a staged procedure is often indicated.

The objective of surgery is to remove the offending mass, to obtain watertight dural closure and good skin cover, and to restore a normal contour to the head. The surgical techniques involved are well described (Reigel 1982, Hendrick 1985). Closure of an occipital encephalocele is carried out in the prone position and the anaesthetist should be prepared for blood loss from venous sinuses, as well as air embolism via the latter, and cardiac disturbances if the brainstem is disturbed. Frontal and basal encephaloceles are closed transcranially by a major bifrontal craniotomy often accompanied by combined or staged procedures with plastic surgical, craniofacial surgical and otorhinolaryngological colleagues. Although attempts should be made to preserve the contents of an occipital encephalocele (Guthkelch 1970) this is often impractical and the contents are frequently non-functional (Urich 1976). Some surgeons have devised elaborate procedures to retain the contents of even large occipital encephaloceles in the fear of losing functioning tissue but those children have a poor prognosis anyway.

The herniated tissue in frontal and basal lesions can be sacrificed by amputation and in the case of the smaller nasal lesions the extracranial portion usually shrivels up thereafter. Immaculate dural closure is vital. Postoperatively the child is held and fed normally. A careful watch is kept for the development of hydrocephalus both clinically and on serial ultrasound examination. Of children with occipital lesions, 60 to 70% require shunt placement but this is rarely needed with frontal or basal lesions.

Unlike myelomeningocele there is no realistic option but to repair the lesions, except for the occasional baby with a lethal extracranial abnormality, as untreated the condition is rarely fatal.

The family are given appropriate counselling regarding outcome and the need for careful neurodevelopmental follow up. They are offered genetic counselling (see Ch. 20).

Follow-up entails monitoring of head growth, visual assessment in the case of occipital lesions and serial developmental evaluations so that any potential handicaps are identified early and appropriate action taken. Large occipital bone defects are repaired by rib-graft cranioplasty at around 5 years of age.

Outcome

In frontal and basal encephaloceles the prognosis for neurodevelopmental progress is usually excellent (Nakamura et al 1974); for occipital lesions it is much more guarded (Matson 1969). For the latter, outcome relates to four factors: the presence or absence of brain tissue in the sac; the development of hydrocephalus; the state of development of the brain as judged by the presence of microcephaly; and the presence of concomitant cerebral malformations such as microgyria, holoprosencephaly, heterotopia, agenesis and optic pathway dysgenesis. Of children with no brain tissue in the sac, 60 to 80% develop normally (Guthkelch 1970, Lorber 1967) as opposed to only 10 to 25% when brain tissue is present in the sac. Only 30% of those with hydrocephalus but no herniated neural tissue have normal intellect (Mealey et al 1970). The 20% of children with microcephaly nearly all show developmental retardation if the head circumference remains below the 10th centile (Guthkelch 1970, Lorber 1967).

MYELOMENINGOCELE

'The most complex, treatable, congenital anomaly consistent with life' (Bunch et al 1972) usually becomes apparent at the moment of birth despite the possibility of prenatal diagnosis by elevated levels of alpha-1-fetoprotein in maternal serum (see Ch. 24) and by prenatal ultrasound examination (Ch. 25).

The first step in management is careful clinical assessment, assuring that the baby is warm and not influenced by any sedative medications given to the mother. General examination will reveal any associated anomalies of the cardiovascular, pulmonary or gastrointestinal systems but these are exceptional. The child is first placed prone and the level of the lesion, any additional lesions, and the appearance of the exposed neural tissue observed. Lesions which are very flat with little sac are more difficult to close. Those in which a considerable cranio–caudal extent of the neuraxis is exposed, with an open 'filleted' appearance of the spinal cord, often with an open central canal are associated with particularly severe neurological abnormalities and are more correctly called myeloschisis. The thoraco–lumbar junction is the most frequent level (45%); followed by lumbar (20%), lumbo–sacral (20%) and sacral (10%), with more rostral lesions being unusual (5%). Multiple lesions at skin level are rare but do occur. A concomitant spinal deformity, either scoliosis, kyphosis or 'telescoping' is noted. Next, with the baby supine, a careful examination of motor function is made; note is taken of any spontaneous movements occurring with crying (see Table 26.2). All stimulation should be confined to the shoulders or head as purely reflex movement may result from stimulation of paralysed lower limbs. Muscle bulk and development of the limbs and trunk are noted. A sensory level is determined using an open nappy-pin moved from caudal to rostral segments (Fig. 26.1). Asymmetry of sensorimotor level and a sensory level more rostral to the motor level are the rule. Each lesion is in its own way as individual as its owner. Sphincter function is assessed by observing anal tone and noting whether urine dribbles continuously from the urethra. Any orthopaedic deformities of hips, knees and feet are noted. Finally the occipito–frontal circumference is measured and charted.

No special neuroradiological procedures are usually required apart from cranial ultrasound examination to determine ventricular size. If, however, there is a gross

Table 26.2 The root innervation responsible for flexion and extension of the joints of the lower limbs

	Flexion	Extension
Hip	L1–2	S1–2
Knee	L5–S1	L3–4
Ankle	L4–5	S1–2
Toes	S2–3	L4–S1

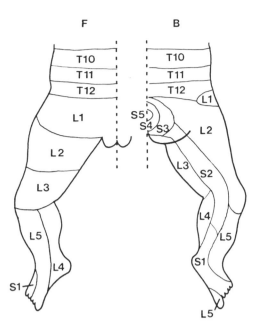

Fig. 26.1 Dermatomes of the lower limbs (F = Front, B = Back).

discrepancy between the level of the open lesion and the neurological level then the presence of a second occult lesion should be suspected and consideration given to full neuroradiological evaluation of the spine, preferably by ultrasound (Ch. 9). Ultrasonography of the genitourinary tract is useful but is usually normal at birth.

Following clinical assessment a prediction of minimum disability can be made on the basis of the sensorimotor level and associated features. Unless there is gross hydrocephalus or a very dysmorphic baby, potentially normal intellect should be assumed. The decision to treat the child actively or conservatively involves a veritable cosmos of medical, ethical, philosophical and social variables which will not be debated here; they are well-covered elsewhere (Ch. 48 and Black 1979).

Active treatment consists of closure of the lesion on the first day of life to prevent serious infection of the central nervous system, to obtain watertight closure of the dura and to provide good skin cover. Before operation the child is nursed prone with a moist saline dressing on the sac. Under general anaesthesia, in the prone position, the sac is opened directly into the intradural compartment and the neural placode mobilized. Dural flaps are then raised and closed over the placode in watertight fashion to create as capacious a sac as possible. The subcutaneous tissues and skin are closed without drainage and a light dressing applied (Humphreys 1985). Using this technique, as opposed to the older one of a circumferential incision around the base of the sac, elaborate skin flaps are rarely needed. Occasionally for the flatter lesions plastic surgical involvement will, however, be required. Postoperatively the baby is fed normally and nursed prone in a way that will minimize soiling of the

wound until it is healed in 7 to 10 days time. Prophylactic antibiotics are not indicated.

In the neonatal period two further associated anomalies may manifest themselves; hydrocephalus and the Chiari malformation.

Although virtually all children with myelomeningocele have ventriculomegaly, only a variable proportion develop progressive hydrocephalus requiring surgical treatment. The more rostral the skin lesion the more likely and the more prominent is the hydrocephalus: overall 80% require treatment but only 50% of those with purely sacral lesions are affected.

Hydrocephalus usually becomes apparent within the first two weeks of life and requires treatment within one month of closure of the sac. Treatment is by insertion of a ventriculo-peritoneal shunt (Ch. 46). Some children with pronounced hydrocephalus at birth should undergo simultaneous shunt placement and myelomeningocele closure; there is some evidence that this is less hazardous than sequential procedures (Epstein et al 1985). Dysraphic children suffer a disproportionately high incidence of shunt infections (Hoffman et al 1982).

The Chiari malformation, universally present, may produce bulbar paresis in the neonatal period even in the presence of a functioning shunt. The first symptoms are progressive slowing down of the child's feeding with nasal regurgitation and change in the pitch of the cry. It is the mother and the nurse who detect these symptoms which, if not promptly recognized by the surgeon, progress to stridor, quadriparesis and respiratory arrest following which useful recovery is unusual (Hoffman et al 1975, Park et al 1983). Neuroradiological investigation is not required but urgent neurosurgical intervention by way of decompressive cervical laminectomy with wide opening of the dura to a level caudal to the displaced cerebellum is indicated. This may entail removal of all the cervical laminae: the dura is either left open or grafted with dural substitute. The posterior fossa bone should not be removed as this is not only unnecessary but rewards the unwary with horrendous bleeding from caudally displaced venous sinuses.

Following surgical closure and shunt placement, full orthopaedic and urological assessments are made. The parents are given instructions on the various aspects of the condition and may benefit from introduction to a parents' association. Genetic counselling is offered in view of the 2 to 4% recurrence risk of neural tube defects in subsequent siblings (Ch. 20). Thereafter the child is managed ideally in a combined clinic.

A number of children for whom conservative treatment is deemed preferable will return after a few months well and thriving but with progressive hydrocephalus. They should receive consideration of shunt placement and full orthopaedic and urological support. Secondary delayed closure of the myelomeningocele may be indicated but this is a most unpleasant surgical procedure.

Outcome

Since the report of the London Committee in 1885 (Marsh et al 1885), prolonged survival without any special active treatment has been well described. From detailed surveys in South Wales, Laurence (1966) has established the most complete natural survival history of untreated cases: namely 30% at 1 year, 20 at 2 years and somewhat fewer thereafter. Deaths in the first few months are mainly from meningitis and ventriculitis; subsequent mortality is due to untreated hydrocephalus and, in older children, renal failure (Lawrence 1964). Only 3.5% survive without physical handicap and with intelligence quotients above 85 (Laurence 1966). Recent personal experience indicates that the survival rate of untreated cases is currently higher than experienced in the past and probably relates to changing views and practices regarding aggressive terminal care for neonates.

For reasons that are not totally clear the prognosis for those children treated actively appears to be more favourable in North America than in Britain. The five-year survival rates of around 50% quoted from the earlier English studies (Sharrard et al 1967, Lorber 1971) have been superceded by figures of over 80% and rising in more recent North American series (Leonard & Freeman 1981, Mclone et al 1981). With regards to quality of survival, the English experience has been grim: in the large unselected Sheffield series (Lorber 1971) only 1% of the total and 4% of the survivors were without handicap; 15% had a moderate handicap and 49% were severely disabled. Only 40% of the handicapped survivors could attend ordinary schools and barely 7% were expected to become self-sufficient. By contrast, many North American authors have found grounds for optimism (O'Brien & McLanahan 1981, Reigel 1982) with most children becoming ambulatory with appropriate orthopaedic and orthotic assistance (Krupka et al 1978).

The prognosis for mobility relates not surprisingly to the segmental level of the lesion, especially the sensory level (Hunt et al 1973). The prognosis for intellect appears to relate to the presence of hydrocephalus: 87% of those without hydrocephalus having intelligence quotients greater than 80 compared with 63% when hydrocephalus is present (Soare & Raimondi 1977). It is more likely that final intellect relates to shunt complications, especially infections, rather than to hydrocephalus per se (McLone et al 1982). Although the majority have a neurogenic bladder the management has been revolutionized by the advent of intermittent catheterization (Lapides et al 1972). Of one group aged 16 to 24 years, 18% were sexually active (Shurtleff & Sousa 1977).

What is absolutely clear is that there is no single approach which will be acceptable to all physicians of all affected children of every family in a wide range of societies and cultures; there are clearly fundamentally different philosophical standpoints between those who select children to die and those who select them to live accepting that comprehensive care will be required for life (Black 1979).

OCCULT SPINAL DYSRAPHISM

This term embraces all those conditions in which there has been disordered closure of the neural tube or its coverings but in which the resultant lesion is skin-covered. The older term of spina bifida occulta is inappropriate as 10 to 20% of the population have a single deficient lamina in the lumbo–sacral spine and the mention of spina bifida is terrifying to parents.

The importance of this group of lesions lies in their propensity to produce neurological, urological and orthopaedic sequelae later in childhood or adolescence (James & Lassman 1972). Most affected children are neurologically normal at birth and it is the finding of a cutaneous blemish that alerts the neonatal physician or nurse to their presence. All newborn children should have the midline of the neuraxis positively examined for the presence of the relevant stigmata which include skin-covered meningoceles, subcutaneous fatty pad, angiomatous and telangiectatic patches, hairy tufts, congenital 'scars', dermoid and dermal sinuses. With regard to the last, many babies have a postanal pit which is of no great import. A pathological sinus is one which is relatively rostral in the natal cleft, eccentrically placed, or is associated with another of the described cutaneous stigmata. They are to be distinguished from the dermoid sinus which is clearly a punctate orifice, variably tethered to the underlying tissues from which clear fluid, hairs and dermoid matter may emerge. The majority of lesions are sited in the lumbo–sacral region. The finding of any of these skins calls for neurosurgical referral. Clinical examination usually confirms the absence of neurological signs but this should not deter formal neuroradiological evaluation.

Plain spine radiographs are of no value in the neonatal period in determining the need for further more extensive examinations as the neural arches are cartilaginous and thus relatively radiolucent, so defective laminae and spinous processes will not be revealed. Formal imaging of the spinal neuraxis is, therefore, performed either by computerized tomography-assisted myelography or, more recently, by ultrasonography or magnetic resonance imaging. These procedures can be postponed until beyond the immediate perinatal period but should be performed within the first few months of life. The purpose of investigation is to define or exclude any intraspinal lesion. The most frequently encountered abnormalities are the lipomyelomeningocele, the thick filum terminale, diastematomyelia and dermoid cysts. Less commonly found are fibrous bands and adhesions, hydromyelia, neurenteric cysts and hamartomatous masses. The entire length of the spine should be examined as multiple lesions are occasionally discovered. The Chiari malformation is not, however, a concomitant finding, in marked contrast to myelomeningocele in which it is universally present.

Any orthopaedic deformities are formally assessed and the genitourinary tract is evaluated by ultrasound, urine culture and plasma creatinine estimation. These aspects are typically normal at birth.

Following global assessment, a decision is made regarding the required neurosurgical action. Traditionally many neurosurgeons, especially those without particular knowledge of, or interest in, paediatric matters have only advised intervention in children with established and progressive neurological abnormalities. It is my view, in common with most paediatric neurosurgeons, that surgery for the lesions of occult spinal dysraphism is indicated to prevent serious neurological, urological and orthopaedic disabilities developing (Till 1969, Hoffman et al 1976). There can be little advantage to the child in allowing preventable abnormalities to develop before operating, especially as they may arise quite unpredictably and acutely or, more frequently, may evolve slowly and subtly. There is now little doubt that prophylactic surgery in infancy is correct for diastematomyelia, thick filum terminale and dermoid cysts and sinuses; the last in particular may lead to serious intraspinal sepsis if ignored. The common surgical goal is untethering of the neural tissue.

The role of prophylactic surgery for lipomyelomeningocele is more hotly debated. Previously, the subcutaneous fatty mass has been variously regarded as of mainly cosmetic significance, or alternatively as not amenable to surgical intervention. It is now quite clear that the majority of children harbouring this lesion, and normal at birth, will acquire serious disabilities by adolescence (Anderson 1975, McLone et al 1983). Thus of 56 children aged under 6 months at presentation to the Hospital for Sick Children, Toronto, 35 were normal compared with 41 aged over 6 months, only 12 of whom were normal (Hoffman et al 1985). Better understanding of the anatomy of this lesion (Chapman 1982, Chapman & Davis 1983) has led to a rational surgical technique consisting of thorough untethering of the lesion, reduction of the fatty mass and generous duraplasty. Technical improvements and adjuncts, such as the operating microscope, the Cavitron Ultrasonic Aspirator, the surgical laser and reliable dural substitutes have all contributed to

a real increase in surgical expertise. There are now good medium-term follow-up studies (Mclone et al 1983, Schut et al 1983, Hoffman et al 1985) showing that children undergoing appropriate prophylactic repair in infancy fare better than those having delayed repair or conservative management. The place of prophylactic surgery in this most difficult lesion is, therefore, becoming established though really long-term evaluations into adolescence are still awaited.

For those children with established deficits, combined follow-up clinics and services as for those with myelomeningocele are appropriate.

Genetic counselling of parents is required as there is a significantly enhanced risk of open neural tube defects in subsequent siblings.

SACRAL AGENESIS

In this rare spinal anomaly varying degrees of absence of the sacrum are associated with neurological abnormalities ranging from total flaccid paraplegia with sphincter paralysis to mild foot deformities (Reigel 1982, Pang 1985). The severely affected neonate has the characteristic flattened buttocks, short gluteal cleft, narrow pelvis and prominent iliac crests with absent sacrum on rectal examination. Motor abnormalities frequently exceed sensory features. In severe cases, associated anomalies elsewhere in the neuraxis, axial skeleton and cardiorespiratory, gastrointestinal and genitourinary systems are found (Sarnat et al 1976, White & Klauver 1976, Andrish et al 1979, Mariani et al 1979). Of affected infants, 16% have diabetic mothers (Passarge & Lenz 1966).

Full general, orthopaedic, neurological and urological assessments are required and the child is best managed in a combined clinic. Although the major therapeutic thrust is directed towards appropriate compensatory procedures to cope with the orthopaedic and urological disabilities, the occasional child will show neurological deterioration and should then be assessed neuroradiologically by ultrasound, magnetic resonance imaging or computerized tomographic myelography to exclude a concomitant tethered spinal cord, diastematomyelia or dural stenosis (Williams & Nixon 1957, Pang & Hoffman 1980).

REFERENCES

Anderson F M 1975 Occult spinal dysraphism: a series of 73 cases. Pediatrics 55: 826–835
Andrish J, Kalanchi A, MacEwen G D 1979 Sacral agenesis: A clinical evaluation of its management, heredity, and associated anomalies. Clinical Orthopaedics and Related Research 139: 52–57
Black P 1979 Selective treatment of infants with myelomeningocele. Neurosurgery 5: 334–338

Bunch W H, Cass A S, Benson A S, Long D N 1972 Modern management of myelomeningocele. Warren H. Green, St Louis
Chapman P H 1982 Congenital intraspinal lipomas: anatomic considerations and surgical treatment. Child's Brain 9: 37–47
Chapman P H, Davis K R 1983 Surgical treatment of spinal lipomas in childhood. In: Raimond A J (ed) Concepts in pediatric neurosurgery, No. 3. S. Karger, Basel, pp 178–190

Epstein N E, Rosenthal A D, Zito J 1985 Shunt placement and myelomeningocele repair: simultaneous vs sequential shunting. Review of 12 cases. Child's Nervous System 1: 145–147

Guthkelch A N 1970 Occipital cranium bifidum. Archives of Disease in Childhood 45: 104–109

Hendrick E B 1985 Encephaloceles. In: Wilkins R H, Rengachary S S (eds) Neurosurgery. McGraw-Hill, New York, pp 2087–2091

Hoffman H J, Hendrick E B, Humphreys R P 1975 Manifestations and management of Arnold–Chiari malformation in patients with myelomeningocele. Child's Brain 1(4): 255–259

Hoffman H J, Hendrick E B, Humphreys R P 1976 The tethered spinal cord: its protean manifestations, diagnosis and surgical correction. Child's Brain 2: 145–155

Hoffman H J, Hendrick E B, Humphreys R P 1982 Management of hydrocephalus. Monographs in Neural Sciences 8: 21–25

Hoffman H J, Taecholarn C, Hendrick E B, Humphreys R P 1985 Journal of Neurosurgery 62: 1–8

Humphreys R P 1985 Spinal dysraphism. In: Wilkins R H, Rengachary S S (eds) Neurosurgery. McGraw-Hill, New York, pp 2041–2052

Hunt G, Lewin W, Gleave J, Gairdner D 1973 Predictive factors in open myelomeningocele with special reference to sensory level. British Medical Journal iv: 197–201

James C C M, Lassman L P 1972 Spinal dysraphism: spina bifida occulta. Butterworth, London

Kupka J, Geddes N, Carroll N C 1978 Comprehensive management in the child with spina bifida. Orthopedic Clinics of North America 9: 97–113

Lapides J, Diokno A C, Silber S J, Lowe B S 1972 Clean, intermittent self-catheterisation in the treatment of urinary tract disease. Journal of Urology 107: 458–461

Laurence K M 1964 The natural history of spina bifida cystica: detailed analysis of 407 cases. Archives of Disease in Childhood 39: 41–57

Laurence K M 1966 The survival of untreated spina bifida cystica. Developmental Medicine and Child Neurology (Suppl)11: 10–19

Laurence K M, Tew B J 1966 Follow-up of 63 survivors from the 425 cases of spina bifida cystica born in South Wales between 1956 and 1962. Developmental Medicine and Child Neurology (Suppl)13: 1–3

Leonard C O, Freeman K M 1981 Spina bifida: a new disease. Pediatrics 68: 136–137

Lorber J 1967 The prognosis of occipital encephalocele. Developmental Medicine and Child Neurology (Suppl)13: 75–86

Lorber J 1971 Results of treatment of myelomeningocele: an analysis of 524 unselected cases with special reference to possible selection for treatment. Developmental Medicine and Child Neurology 13: 279–303

McLone D, Raimond A J, Sommers R 1981 The results of early treatment of 100 consecutive newborns with myelomeningocele. Kinder Chir 34(2): 115–117

McLone D, Czyzewski D, Raimondi A S 1982 The effects of complications on intellectual function in 173 children with myelomeningocele. Surgery of the developing nervous system. Grune and Stratton, New York, pp 49–60

McLone D G, Mutlver S, Naidich T P 1983 Lipomeningoceles of the conus medullaris. In: Raimondi E J (ed) Concepts in pediatric neurosurgery, No. 3. S. Karger, Basel, pp 170–177

Mariani A J, Stern J, Khan A U, Cass A S 1979 Sacral agenesis: an analysis of 11 cases and review of the literature. Journal of Urology 122: 684–686

Marsh H, Gould A P, Clutton H H, Parker R W 1885 Report of a Committee of the Society nominated Nov. 10 1882 to investigate spina bifida and its treatment by the injection of Dr Morton's iedoglycerine solution. Transactions of the Clinical Society of London 18: 339

Matson D D 1969 Neurosurgery of infancy and childhood. 2nd edn. Charles C Thomas, Springfield, Illinois. pp 61–75

Mealey J Jr, Dzenitis A J, Hockey A A 1970 The prognosis of encephaloceles. Journal of Neurosurgery 22: 209–218

Nakamura T, Grant J A, Hubbard R F 1974 Nasoethmoidal meningoencephalocele. Archives of Otolaryngology 100: 62–64

O'Brien M S, McLanahan C S 1981 Review of the neurosurgical management of myelomeningocele at a Regional Pediatric Medical Center. In: Concepts in pediatric neurosurgery, No. 1. S. Karger, Basel, pp 202–215

Pang D 1985 Sacral agenesis. In: Wilkins R H, Rengachary S S (eds) Neurosurgery. McGraw-Hill, New York, pp 2075–2077

Pang D, Hoffman H J 1980 Sacral agenesis with progressive neurological deficit. Neurosurgery 7: 118–126

Park T S, Hoffman H J, Hendrick E B, Humphreys R P 1983 Experience with surgical decompression of the Arnold–Chiari malformation in young infants with myelomeningocele. Neurosurgery 13: 147–152

Passarge E, Lenz H 1966 Syndrome of caudal regression in infants of diabetic mothers: observations of further cases. Pediatrics 37: 672–675

Reigel D H 1982a Spina bifida. In: Pediatric neurosurgery: surgery of the developing nervous system. Grune & Stratton, New York, pp 23–47

Reigel D H 1982b Encephalocele. In: Pediatric neurosurgery: surgery of the developing nervous system. Grune & Stratton, New York, pp 49–60

Reigel D H 1982c Sacral agenesis and diastematomyelia. In: pediatric neurosurgery: surgery of the developing nervous system. Grune & Stratton, New York, pp 79–89

Sarnat H B, Case M E, Graviss R 1976 Sacral agenesis: neurologic and neuropathologic features. Neurology 26: 1124–1129

Schut L, Bruce D A, Sutton L N 1983 The management of the child with a lipomyelomeningocele. Clinical Neurosurgery 30: 446–476

Sharrard W J W, Zachary R B, Lorber J 1967 Survival and paralysis in open myelomeningocele with special reference to the time of repair of the spinal lesion. Developmental Medicine and Child Neurology (Suppl)13: 35–50

Shurtleff D B, Sousa J C 1977 The adolescent with myelodysplasia: development, achievement, sex and deterioration. In: McLaurin R L (ed) Myelomeningocele. Grune & Stratton, New York, pp 809–835

Soare P, Raimondi A J 1977 Intellectual and perceptual motor characteristics of treated myelomeningocele children. American Journal of Diseases of Children 131: 199–204

Suwanwela C, Chaturaporn H 1966 Frontoethmoidal encephalocele. Journal of Neurosurgery. 25: 172–182

Till K 1969 Spinal dysraphism: a study of congenital malformations of the lower back. Journal of Bone and Joint Surgery (British) Volume 51: 415–422

Urich H 1976 Malformations of the nervous system, perinatal damage and related conditions in early life. In: Blackwood W, Corsellid J A W (eds) Greenfields's Neuropathology. 3rd edn. E. Arnold, London, pp 361–469

Weaver D W 1985 Genetics of developmental defects. In: Wilkins R H, Rengachary S S (eds) Neurosurgery. McGraw-Hill, New York, pp 2025–2040

White R I, Klauber G T 1976 Sacral agenesis: analysis of 22 cases. Urology 8: 521–525

Wilkins R H, Rengachary S S (eds) Neurosurgery. McGraw–Hill, New York, pp 2025–2040

Williams D I, Nixon H H 1957 Agenesis of the sacrum. Surgery, Gynecology and Obstetrics 105: 84–88

Haemorrhage and ischaemia

Haemorrhage of the neonatal brain has attracted much attention probably because of its striking appearance and presumed severe implications. That haemorrhage is very common in the neonatal brain is undisputed but the fact that it is often benign is sometimes not appreciated. Intracranial haemorrhage is a generic term used to refer to a heterogeneous group of conditions. We have elected to divide them into those arising from the germinal matrix (Ch. 28) and all the other types which are discussed in Chapter 27 under separate subheadings. Intraparenchymal haemorrhage is an important condition and probably does not have a single aetiology. We have discussed the possible pathogenesis of this condition on p. 317. Cerebral haemorrhage may be confused with bleeding into a primarily ischaemic lesion and cerebral lesions of ischaemic nature are discussed in Chapter 29. It is now well recognized that the fetus is also susceptible to haemorrhagic and ischaemic insults and encephalopathy primarily of circulatory origin affecting the fetal brain is discussed in Chapter 30. Sequelae, mainly ventricular dilatation, are particularly common following either haemorrhagic or ischaemic cerebral insults and these are reviewed in Chapter 31. Management of posthaemorrhagic hydrocephalus is reviewed in Section 15.

27. Intracranial haemorrhage

Dr L.S. de Vries, Dr J-C. Larroche and Dr M.I. Levene

Haemorrhages involving the neonatal brain are among the most frequent and important conditions affecting the newborn. Intracerebral haemorrhage is more common in the neonatal period than at any other time but there is also a wide spectrum of types of haemorrhagic lesions, with differing aetiologies and varying prognostic significance. Table 27.1 lists the types of haemorrhage reported in the newborn brain and their sites of origin and these will be discussed separately. Haemorrhage arising from the germinal matrix at the head of the caudate nucleus and often rupturing into the ventricle is particularly common in immature infants. This is referred to as germinal matrix haemorrhage–intraventricular haemorrhage (GMH–IVH) and is discussed in the next chapter.

The term intraventricular haemorrhage is non-specific and refers to blood in the cerebral ventricles due to any cause. It may commonly arise from germinal matrix and choroid plexus haemorrhage and very rarely be secondary to bleeding into cerebral parenchyma. Exceptionally, bleeding may originate from rupture of an arterio–venous malformation (Schum et al 1979, Heafner et al 1985, McClellan et al 1986).

With the introduction of modern imaging techniques in the late 1970s intracranial haemorrhage could be studied in living infants and information on its pathogenesis and outcome in surviving children assessed. Before that,

information could only be obtained from autopsy material which would bias the findings towards the more severe degrees of haemorrhage. Despite the obvious limitations of postmortem studies, a definite trend can be observed over the last 45 years. In 1938 Craig analysed 126 postmortem examinations in which intracranial haemorrhage was seen. He found subdural haematoma to be common, occurring in almost half of all cases. A similar assessment 40 years later from Hammersmith Hospital autopsies during the years 1978 and 1979 showed a considerable decline in the proportion of subdural haemorrhages, with a corresponding marked increase in the percentage of GMH–IVH (Levene 1985). This is due to a marked reduction in the number of fatal subdural haemorrhages associated with more careful obstetric management of the second stage of labour and the relative increase in cases of GMH–IVH associated with longer survival of very premature infants supported by neonatal intensive care who are most at risk of GMH–IVH.

SUBDURAL HAEMORRHAGE

Fatal subdural haemorrhage is now rare but the incidence of this condition in surviving infants is difficult to ascertain. Various computerized tomography studies have reported subdural haemorrhage to account for 4–11% of infants with intracranial haemorrhage (LeBlanc & O'Gorman 1980, Bergman et al 1985). It may be associated with few clinical signs and remain undiagnosed.

Subdural haemorrhage may be due to a number of different pathological causes.

Dural tear

This was usually associated with rapid delivery of the infant's head or trauma associated with difficult forceps delivery. The dura mater divides the brain into three compartments — the two cerebral hemispheres and the cerebellum. The main folds are the falx cerebri and the tentorium cerebelli. The major venous sinuses are

Table 27.1 Localization and site of origin of various types of intracranial haemorrhage

Type of haemorrhage	Site of origin
Subdural	–
Subarachnoid	Primary
	Secondary to intraventricular haemorrhage
	Subarachnoid haematoma
Intraventricular	Germinal matrix
	Choroid plexus
	Cerebral parenchyma
Intraparenchymal	Periventricular white matter
	Thalamus
	Arterio-venous malformation
Intracerebellar	–

contained within these folds and dural tears are likely to cause extensive bleeding from the adjacent sinus. The fetal head withstands the compressive effects of labour well if the mechanical forces are applied evenly. With passage of the head through the birth canal the head moulds to a long occipito–frontal diameter. If delivery is too rapid then the mechanical forces are less well tolerated and there will be sudden changes in head shape. This causes stretching and possibly tearing of the dura. As long-axis stretching is most common it is the vertical part of the tentorium which is most stressed and liable to rupture (Fig. 27.1). Subdural haemorrhage in the posterior fossa usually arises from rupture of the vein of Galen, straight or lateral sinuses. Tears of the falx cerebri are rare and occasionally subdural haemorrhage is associated with sinus thrombosis (Craig 1938). Welch & Strand (1986) have suggested that some extensive subdural haemorrhages are due to arterial bleeding.

Occipital osteodiastasis

Subdural haemorrhage may be associated with vaginal breech delivery in which there is excessive extension of the infant's neck. This causes separation of the squamous and lateral portions of the occipital bone (osteodiastasis) and direct injury to structures within the posterior cranial fossa (Wigglesworth & Husemeyer 1977). Exceptionally this may occur due to parietal diastasis.

Bridging vein rupture

The most common cause of subdural haemorrhage is rupture of the superior cerebral bridging veins (Page & Wigglesworth 1979). These lesions occur most commonly over the cerebral convexity (Fig. 27.2) and may be seen in association with subarachnoid haemorrhage. Convexity subdural haemorrhages may be more common in infants with coagulation disorders or those undergoing exchange transfusions (Morgan et al 1983). The term convexity haemorrhage is used because the precise origin of the bleeding is unclear and compression of the brain may occur with eventual infarction thus making determination of the origin of the lesion difficult.

Subdural haemorrhage may also occur in infants due to shaking associated with non-accidental injury and following meningitis, particularly if due to *Haemophilus influenzae*. These are, however, rarely seen in the neonatal period.

Clinical findings

These may be non-specific and depend on the severity and localization of the haemorrhage. A large subtentorial bleed may cause lethargy, bulging fontanelle, bradycardia, seizures and skew deviation of the eyes. Massive haemorrhage may be associated with shock, coma and rapid demise. Asphyxia is a common accompaniment of subdural haemorrhage and the clinical features of the two may be similar. Larroche (1977) has pointed out that most full-term infants with subdural haemorrhage have associated diffuse cerebral necrosis or infarction, implying that the brain has sustained widespread insult and damage. Clinical signs may reflect more diffuse involvement.

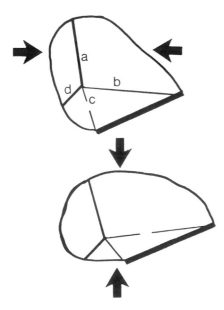

Fig. 27.1 Dural tears associated with compressional stress to the neonatal head. Upper diagram shows the effect of occipito–frontal compression with greatest strain on the vertical part of the tentorium (c). Lower diagram shows the effect of compression between vault and base with greatest strain on the horizontal part of the tentorium (b). Falx cerebri (a), line of junction of tentorium and falx (d). (Redrawn from Holland 1922.)

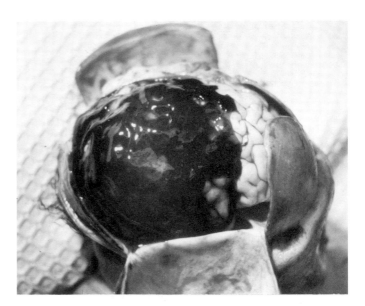

Fig. 27.2 Subdural haematoma over the right cerebral hemisphere. After reflection of the brain, thick blood clot remained over the cerebral convexity. (Reproduced with permission from Larroche 1984.)

Convexity subdural haemorrhage may present with generalized or multifocal seizures. Occasionally, focal neurological signs are seen, in particular a difference in tone between the two sides. Volpe (1977) suggests that the most distinctive sign of compression is a non-reactive or sluggish pupil due to third cranial nerve compression. It is likely that most infants with mild subdural bleeding have no symptoms or signs at all.

Diagnosis

Ultrasound is not very reliable in diagnosing or excluding small subdural lesions. Large convexity haemorrhages, particularly when causing displacement of midline structures, should be detected on ultrasound examination, or the echo-free subdural effusion may be seen (see Ch. 9).

Computerized tomography (CT) is a more sensitive technique for detecting smaller lesions but even with this technique, distinction between small subdural haemorrhage and normal appearance may be impossible (Ludwig et al 1980). Subdural bleeding should be considered in all asphyxiated infants and as its compressive effects are treatable, CT examination is recommended whenever this possibility is considered. Infants with CT evidence of posterior fossa haemorrhage may have either subdural or cerebellar haemorrhage and distinction between the two may be difficult. The two conditions appear to occur with equal frequency in the neonate (Scotti et al 1981) but intracerebellar haemorrhage is more common in premature infants and subdural is more likely in full-term infants (Menezes et al 1983). Figure 27.3 shows an example of subdural haemorrhage due to tentorial tear diagnosed by CT.

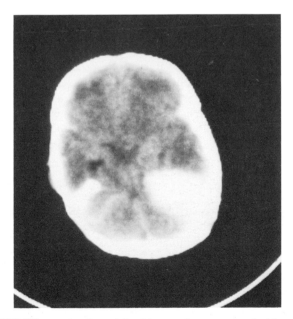

Fig. 27.3 CT scan showing subdural haemorrhage associated with tearing of the left fold of the tentorium cerebelli.

Treatment

Convexity haemorrhages, particularly if causing a midline shift, should be decompressed by subdural tap. It is, however, important to distinguish clinical signs arising from diffuse cerebral involvement as occurs in asphyxia from focal abnormalities arising from haemorrhage. Treatment directed towards a minor collection will not improve the clinical signs or eventual prognosis in the presence of more diffuse cerebral injury. Craniotomy may be necessary if the collection is not accessible to needling through the fontanelle. The management of massive subdural haemorrhage in the posterior cranial fossa is by craniotomy and aspiration of clot. The management of less severe subdural haemorrhage is expectant.

Prognosis

In the most severe cases the prognosis is poor but normal survivors have been reported following surgical evacuation of a large posterior fossa haemorrhage (Menezes et al 1983). Approximately half of infants with subdural haemorrhage diagnosed by CT are neurologically abnormal at follow-up, presumably due to associated cerebral injury.

SUBARACHNOID HAEMORRHAGE

Subarachnoid haemorrhage (SAH) may be primary or secondary to blood tracking through the ventricular system usually from an intraventricular haemorrhage and is described elsewhere (p. 311). Blood exits from the fourth ventricle through the foramina of Luscka and Magendie into the subarachnoid space. Primary haemorrhage is due to either leakage from the fine vessels of the leptomeningeal plexus or to rupture of the larger veins within the subarachnoid space.

Minor focal SAH is commonly seen in autopsy specimens, particularly in premature infants. These small lesions are probably clinically insignificant. It may be impossible to distinguish subpial haemorrhage macroscopically from that confined to the subarachnoid space and this distinction can only be made histologically (Friede 1972). The aetiology of both conditions is probably hypoxic and develops due to oozing from veins. Subarachnoid haemorrhage may occur in full-term babies due to coagulopathy secondary to vitamin K deficiency (Chaou et al 1984). The incidence of primary SAH diagnosed by CT scanning has been reported to be 7% of 118 infants of birth-weight less than 1800 g (Shinnar et al 1982). It is quite unlike SAH seen in adults which is a devastating condition due to rupture of an arterial aneurysm.

Larroche (1977) described 33 cases of a much more extensive form of primary SAH occurring over the cerebral convexity often involving the temporal lobes (Fig. 27.4).

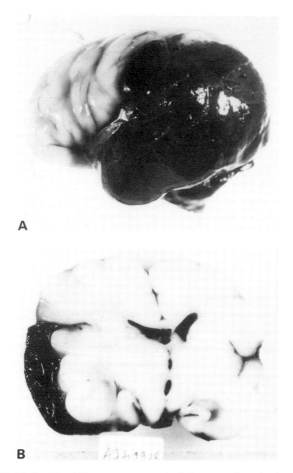

Fig. 27.4 Subarachnoid haematoma over the left temporal, parietal and occipital lobes (**a**). Coronal section (**b**) shows a small GMH–IVH with subarachnoid haematoma compressing and displacing the left hemisphere. (Reproduced with permission from Larroche 1984.)

This lesion has a sharply defined border and may be very extensive, causing severe haemorrhagic necrosis to underlying cortical and subcortical structures due to a compressive effect. The convexity lesion was mainly seen in infants with bleeding disorders and particularly those having an exchange transfusion. The underlying cause of this condition is unclear but arterial occlusion cannot be excluded.

Clinical findings

The majority of infants with SAH are asymptomatic. Massive convexity SAH may cause symptoms similar to large subdural haemorrhage with coma and shock. Large convexity lesions may also produce focal signs. The classical symptom associated with this type of haemorrhage is convulsion. Convulsions are usually generalized and often multifocal. The infants usually behave and feed remarkably normally between seizures. Nystagmus and apnoeic episodes have also been reported to be associated with SAH. Asphyxia often accompanies significant SAH

and the symptoms may be related to this more generalized abnormality.

Diagnosis

Traditionally the diagnosis has been made by lumbar puncture. A non-traumatic tap with free flow of blood-stained cerebrospinal fluid (CSF) which does not clear in successive tubes strongly suggests the diagnosis of SAH but this will not distinguish primary from secondary haemorrhage. Ultrasound has little role in the diagnosis or exclusion of SAH and CT is much more sensitive to the diagnosis (see Ch. 8).

Prognosis

The prognosis is generally thought to be good even in infants presenting with seizures (Rose & Lombroso 1970) but Fenichel et al (1984) reported that only 5 out of 10 infants with the CT diagnosis of SAH were subsequently normal. The follow-up period in these infants was short and further information is awaited. Posthaemorrhagic hydrocephalus may occur following primary SAH but this is not common.

CHOROID PLEXUS HAEMORRHAGE

Bleeding from the choroid plexus is a common cause of intraventricular haemorrhage (IVH). Larroche (1977) has reported minor bleeding into the choroid plexus to be associated with or cause IVH in 25% of cases. In another postmortem study Friede (1975) found choroid plexus haemorrhage in only 7% of neonatal brains. The most frequent site of bleeding is into the posterior tufts at the level of the glomus. Autopsy studies emphasize that choroid plexus haemorrhage occurs most commonly in full-term infants (Donat et al 1978, Lacey & Terplan 1982) and may arise following birth asphyxia. More recent studies using real-time ultrasound report that 59% of all intracranial haemorrhages seen in very-low-birth-weight infants were due to bleeding from the choroid plexus (Reeder et al 1982).

Diagnosis

There are no recognized clinical features of choroid plexus haemorrhage and the diagnosis can be made by ultrasound (Fig. 27.5) or CT examination.

INTRACEREBELLAR HAEMORRHAGE

Primary haemorrhage into the cerebellum is well recognized (Fig. 27.6). Diffuse microscopic haemorrhages are seen in

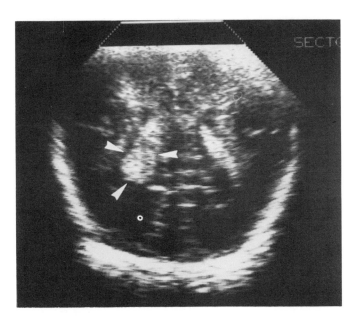

Fig. 27.5 Choroid plexus haematoma (arrows) adherent to the left choroid plexus, diagnosed on ultrasound scan. (Reproduced with permission from Levene et al 1984.)

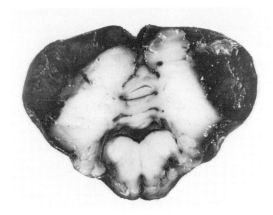

Fig. 27.6 Bilateral cerebellar haematoma in an infant born at 28 weeks of gestation.

premature infants and not uncommonly in association with periventricular haemorrhage or rarely with meningo–encephalitis (Larroche 1977). They usually arise either within the cerebellar cortex or less commonly in the subependymal layer of the roof of the fourth ventricle (Pape & Wigglesworth 1979). It has been suggested that bleeding into the cerebellar folia is related to poor vascularization of the cerebellar cortex (Pape & Wigglesworth 1979). Large primary cerebellar haematomas are much less common and have been diagnosed in life in both premature (Grunnet & Shields 1975, Martin et al 1976, Peterson et al 1984) and full-term infants (Rom et al 1978, Ravenel 1979, Fishman et al 1981). Bleeding disorders or severe rhesus iso-immunization have been reported to be common aetiological factors.

Secondary haemorrhages have been described due to occipital osteodiastasis associated with breech delivery (Wigglesworth & Husemeyer 1977) or a face-mask applied by a tight-fitting band around the back of the infant's head (Pape et al 1976). The tight band caused distortion of the occipital bone and probably mechanical trauma to the cerebellum with venous infarction.

Diagnosis

Clinical features include apnoea and bradycardia, seizures, opisthotonus and nystagmus. These features are similar to those described for infants with subdural haemorrhage arising in the posterior cranial fossa and these two conditions may be extremely difficult to distinguish even by imaging techniques (Scotti et al 1981). Diagnosis may be made by CT examination or ultrasound (Fig. 27.7).

Management

Suboccipital craniotomy has been performed successfully in a few full-term infants (Rom et al 1978, Ravenel 1979) but conservative management has also been advocated with apparent good outcome (Fishman et al 1981).

THALAMIC HAEMORRHAGE

This may be primary or due to extension of haemorrhage arising from the germinal matrix. The latter condition is rarely seen and is most likely to occur in the most immature infants. Primary haemorrhage into the thalamus has been described and there may be secondary rupture

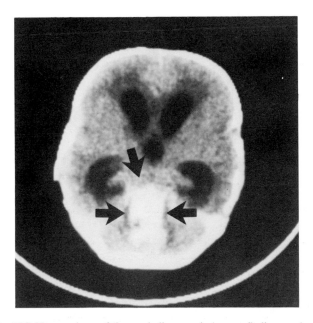

Fig. 27.7 Haemorrhage of the cerebellar vermis (arrowed) diagnosed on CT scan in a full-term infant. Posthaemorrhagic ventricular dilatation is also present. (Courtesy of Dr K. Simpson.)

into the lateral ventricle (Trounce et al 1985). The cause of this type of lesion is unknown but does not appear to be due to an arterio–venous malformation, trauma or coagulopathy. Haemorrhagic infarction of the thalamus (Fig. 27.8) may be indistinguishable macroscopically from primary haemorrhage.

Very rarely, haemorrhage into the basal ganglia may occur due to micro-angiomas. Alonso et al (1984) have reported two such cases occurring in neonates.

Diagnosis

A specific clinical syndrome associated with primary thalamic haemorrhage has been described. The condition presents in previously well babies at about 7 to 14 days with acute onset of seizures. Most had dramatic eye signs including sunsetting and eye deviation downwards and outwards to the side of the thalamic lesion. The abnormal eye posture is due to the close proximity of the haemorrhage to the fronto–mesencephalic pathway of the optic tract. Facial palsy is also seen in a proportion of infants.

Diagnosis may be confirmed by CT (Fig. 27.9) or ultrasound examination. Cerebral angiography is necessary to exclude micro-angiomas but this is rarely indicated. Confusion has arisen between this condition and infants with the appearance of bilateral 'bright' thalamic lesions as illustrated on p. 143 (Kotagel et al 1983, Donn et al 1984, Kreusser et al 1984, Voit et al 1985, Shen et al 1986). All these cases occurred in full-term infants sustaining severe asphyxia who were profoundly neurologically abnormal from birth. Autopsy showed these to be due to haemorrhagic necrosis (Kreusser et al 1984). These case reports appear to be fundamentally different to the 'benign' intrathalamic haemorrhage reported by Trounce et al (1985).

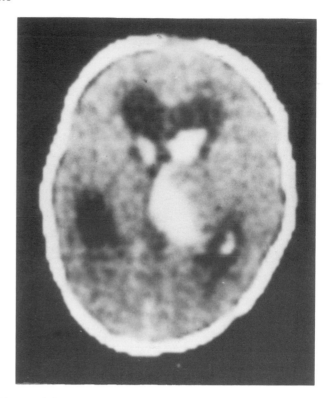

Fig. 27.9 Primary thalamic haemorrhage in a previously healthy infant. Secondary intraventricular clot with ventricular dilatation is also present on the CT scan.

Prognosis

The infants with unilateral thalamic haemorrhage showed abnormal neurological signs for some time but the majority of infants have no neurodevelopmental abnormality at 18 months. In contrast, all asphyxiated infants with a bilateral bright thalamic appearance are dead or severely handicapped.

PARENCHYMAL HAEMORRHAGE

The distinction between a primary haemorrhagic process extending from an intraventricular bleed and bleeding into previously ischaemic periventricular tissue is difficult and is discussed in detail in the next section. In addition, confusion between primary parenchymal haemorrhage and cerebral artery infarction may easily occur. Distinction between these two conditions is possible and cerebral artery infarction is discussed later in Chapter 29.

Most of the reported cases of primary intraparenchymal haemorrhage have been associated with fetal or neonatal coagulopathy (Bleyer & Skinner 1976, Zalneraitis et al 1979, Chaou et al 1984, Motohara et al 1984, Whitelaw et al 1984, Morales & Stroup 1985, Sadowitz & Balcom 1985, Sia et al 1985). The most common cause for the bleeding disorder is vitamin K deficiency. This occurs

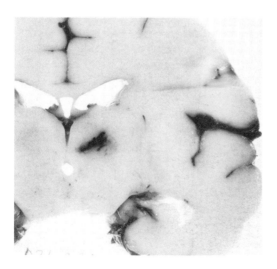

Fig. 27.8 Haemorrhagic infarction within the right thalamus in a premature infant with congenital listeriosis. Subarachnoid haemorrhage is also visible in the Sylvian fissure.

in solely breast-fed infants who are not given vitamin K at birth. It is now clear that a single prophylactic vitamin K injection will protect the full-term infant from significant haemorrhage due to vitamin K deficiency. Other causes include iso-immune thrombocytopoenia and specific clotting factor deficiency. Alpha-1-antitrypsin deficiency may present with intracranial haemorrhage associated with coagulation disorders (Jenkins et al 1982, Hope et al 1982, Payne & Hasegawa 1984) and bleeding associated with this condition is readily treated with intramuscular vitamin K. Bowerman et al (1985) have reported intraparenchymal haemorrhage following heparinization for extracorporeal membrane oxygenation therapy. Intracranial haemorrhage appears to be particularly common in premature infants treated with this technique (Cilley et al 1986). Very rarely, parenchymal haemorrhage in infants may occur due to an intracerebral tumour (Palma et al 1979) or an arterio-venous malformation of which the vein of Galen aneurysm is the best known. McClellan et al (1986) have recently reported a case of localized haematoma (Fig. 27.10a) in the fronto-parietal area due to aneurysmal rupture of the middle cerebral artery (Fig. 27.10b).

Diagnosis

Clinical features usually suggest a bleeding disorder as multiple petechial haemorrhages are present on the infant's skin. The infant may only show minor neurological disturbances including lethargy and irritability. Seizures are common. Diagnosis is confirmed by ultrasound (Fig. 27.11) or CT examination.

Management

Haemorrhage due to vitamin K deficiency is a preventable condition if synthetic vitamin K is given routinely to all infants at birth. Vitamin K should be given to infants with intracerebral haemorrhages and other clotting disorders should be treated as appropriate. Platelet transfusion may be necessary in infants with severe thrombocytopoenia. Specific neurological treatment is only necessary if progressive ventriculomegaly occurs.

Prognosis

From the case reports published up to the present time it appears that approximately one-third of infants die, one-third are handicapped and one-third are subsequently neurologically normal.

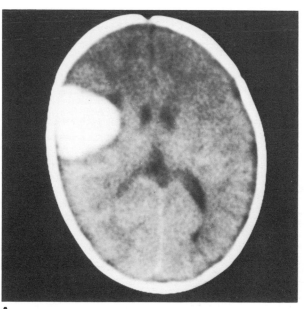
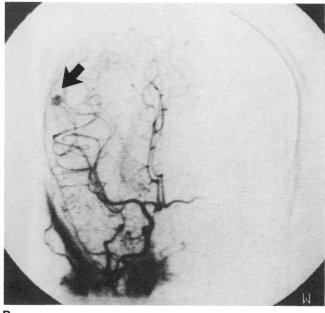

A B

Fig. 27.10 Parenchymal haematoma in the right fronto–parietal lobe seen on CT scan (a). Angiography (b) shows an arterial aneurysm (arrow) in an ascending branch of the right middle cerebral artery. (Reproduced with permission from McLellan et al 1986.)

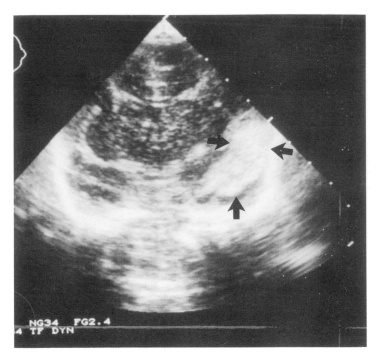

Fig. 27.11 Primary parenchymal haemorrhage diagnosed by ultrasound and involving the right temporal lobe (arrowed). (Courtesy of Dr Keith Dodd.)

REFERENCES

Alonso A, Taboada D, Alvarez J A, Vidal-Sampedro J, Vieito X 1984 Spontaneous hematomas caused by microangiomatosis of the basal ganglia. Child's Brain 11: 202–211

Bergman I et al 1985 Intracerebral hemorrhage in the full-term neonatal infant. Pediatrics 75: 488–496

Bleyer W A, Skinner A L 1976 Fatal neonatal hemorrhage after maternal anticonvulsant therapy. Journal of the American Medical Association 235: 626–627

Bowerman R A, Zwischenberger J B, Andrews A F, Bartlett R H 1985 Cranial sonography of the infant treated with extracorporeal membrane oxygenation. American Journal of Roentgenology 145: 161–166

Chaou W-T, Chou M-L, Eitzman D V 1984 Intracranial hemorrhage and vitamin K deficiency in early infancy. Journal of Pediatrics 105: 880–884

Cilley R E, Zwischenberger J B, Andrews A F, Bowerman R A, Roloff D W, Bartlett R H 1986 Intracranial hemorrhage during extracorporeal membrane oxygenation in neonates. Pediatrics 78: 699–704

Craig W S 1938 Intracranial haemorrhage in the new-born. Archives of Disease in Childhood 13: 89–124

Donat J F, Okazaki H, Kleinberg F, Reagan T J 1978 Intraventricular hemorrhages in full-term and premature infants. Mayo Clinic Proceedings 53: 437–441

Donn S M, Bowerman R A, DiPietro M A, Gebarski S S 1984 Sonographic appearance of neonatal thalamic–striatal haemorrhage. Journal of Ultrasound in Medicine 3: 231–233

Fenichel G M, Webster D L, Wong W K T 1984 Intracranial hemorrhage in the term newborn. Archives of Neurology 41: 30–34

Fishman M A, Percy A K, Cheek W R, Speer M E 1981 Successful conservative management of cerebellar hematomas in term neonates. Journal of Pediatrics 98: 466–468

Friede R L 1972 Subpial hemorrhage in infants. Journal of Neuropathology and Experimental Neurology 31: 548–556

Friede R L 1975 Developmental neuropathology. Springer-Verlag, Vienna

Grunnet M L, Shields W O 1975 Cerebellar hemorrhage in the premature infant. Journal of Pediatrics 88: 605–608

Heafner M D et al 1985 Intraventricular hemorrhage in a term neonate secondary to a third ventricular AVM. Journal of Neurosurgery 63: 640–643

Holland E 1922 Cranial stress in the foetus during labour and on the effects of excessive stress on the intracranial contents. Journal of Obstetrics and Gynecology of the British Empire 29: 549–569

Hope P L, Hall M A, Millward-Sadler G H, Normand I C S 1982 Alpha-1-antitrypsin deficiency presenting as a bleeding diathesis in the newborn. Archives of Disease in Childhood 57: 68–79

Jenkins H R et al 1982. Alpha-1-antitrypsin deficiency, bleeding diathesis, and intracranial haemorrhage. Archives of Disease in Childhood 57: 722–723

Kotagel S, Toce S, Kotagel P, Archer C 1983 Symmetrical bithalamic and striatal hemorrhage following perinatal hypoxia in a term infant. Journal of Computer Assisted Tomography 7: 353–355

Kreusser K L, Schmidt R E, Shackelford G D, Volpe J J 1984 Value of ultrasound for identification of acute hemorrhagic necrosis of thalamus and basal ganglia in an asphyxiated term infant. Annals of Neurology 16: 361–363

Lacey D J, Terplan K 1982 Intraventricular hemorrhage in full-term neonates. Developmental Medicine and Child Neurology 24: 332–337

Larroche J-C 1977 Developmental pathology of the neonate. Excerpta Medica, Amsterdam

Larroche J-C 1984 Perinatal brain damage. In: Adams J H, Corsellis J, Duchen L W (eds) Greenfield's Neuropathology. Edward Arnold, London, pp 451–489

LeBlanc R, O'Gorman A M 1980 Neonatal intracranial hemorrhage: a clinical and serial computerized tomographic study. Journal of Neurosurgery 53: 642–651

Levene M I 1985 Diagnosis and management of intraventricular haemorrhage in the neonate. World Pediatrics and Child Care 1: 7–12

Levene M I, Williams J L, Fawer C-L 1985 Ultrasound of the infant brain. Clinics in Developmental Medicine 92

Ludwig B, Brand M, Brockerhoff P 1980 Postpartum CT examination of the heads of full term infants. Neuroradiology 20: 145–154

McLellan N J, Prasad R, Punt J 1986 Spontaneous subhyaloid and retinal haemorrhages in an infant. Archives of Disease in Childhood 61: 1130–1132

Martin R, Roesmann U, Fanaroff A 1976 Massive intracerebellar hemorrhage in low birth weight infants. Journal of Pediatrics 89: 290–292

Menezes A H, Smith D E, Bell W E 1983 Posterior fossa hemorrhage in the term neonate. Neurosurgery 13: 452–456

Morales W J, Stroup M 1985 Intracranial hemorrhage in utero due to isoimmune neonatal thrombocytopenia. Obstetrics and Gynecology 65: 205–215

Morgan M E I, Hensey O J, Cooke R W I 1983 Convexity cerebral haemorrhage in the neonate: in vivo ultrasound diagnosis. Archives of Disease in Childhood 58: 814–818

Motohara K et al 1984 Severe vitamin K deficiency in breast-fed infants. Journal of Pediatrics 105: 943–945

Palma P A et al 1979 Intraventricular hemorrhage in the neonate born at term. American Journal of Diseases in Children 133: 941–944

Pape K E, Wigglesworth J S 1979 Haemorrhage, ischaemia and the perinatal brain. Clinics in Developmental Medicine 69/70, Spastics International Medical Publications, London

Pape K E, Armstrong D L, Fitzhardinge P M 1976 Central nervous system pathology associated with mask ventilation in the very low birth weight infant: a new etiology for intracerebellar hemorrhages. Pediatrics 58: 473–483

Payne N R, Hasegawa D K 1984 Vitamin K deficiency in newborns. Pediatrics 73: 712–716

Peterson C M, Smith W L, Franklen E A 1984 Neonatal intracerebellar hemorrhage: detection by real-time ultrasound. Radiology 150: 391–392

Ravenel S D 1979 Posterior fossa hemorrhage in the term newborn: report of two cases. Pediatrics 64: 39–42

Reeder J D, Kaude J V, Setzer E S 1982 Choroid plexus hemorrhage in premature neonates: recognition by sonography. American Journal of Neuroradiology 3: 619–622

Rom S, Serfontein G L, Humphreys R P 1978 Intracerebellar hematoma in the neonate. Journal of Pediatrics 93: 486–488

Rose A L, Lombroso C T 1970 Neonatal seizure states: a study of clinical, pathological, and electroencephalographic features in 137 full-term babies with a long-term follow-up. Pediatrics 45: 404–425

Sadowitz P D, Balcom R 1985 Intrauterine intracranial hemorrhage in an infant with isoimmune thrombocytopenia. Clinical Pediatrics 24: 655–657

Schum T R, Meyer G A, Grausz J P 1979 Neonatal intraventricular hemorrhage due to an unruptured arteriovenous malformation: a case report. Pediatrics 64: 242–244

Scotti G, Flodmark O, Harwood-Nash D C, Humphries R P 1981 Posterior fossa hemorrhages in the newborn. Journal of Computer Assisted Tomography 5: 68–72

Shen E Y, Huang C C, Chyou S C, Hung H Y, Hsu C H, Huang F Y 1986 Sonographic finding of the bright thalamus. Archives of Disease in Childhood 61: 1096–1099

Shinnar S, Molteni R A, Gammon K, D'Souza B J, Altman J, Freeman J 1982 Intraventricular hemorrhage in the premature infant: a changing outlook. New England Journal of Medicine 306: 1464–1468

Sia C G, Amigo N C, Harper R G, Farahani G, Kochen J 1985 Failure of cesarian section to prevent intracranial hemorrhage in siblings with isoimmune neonatal thrombocytopenia. American Journal of Obstetrics and Gynecology 153: 79–81

Trounce J Q, Dodd K L, Fawer C-L, Fielder A R, Punt J, Levene M I 1985 Primary thalamic haemorrhage in the newborn: a new clinical entity. Lancet i: 190–192

Voit T, Lemburg P, Stork W 1985 NMR studies in thalamic–striatal necrosis. Lancet ii: 445

Volpe J J 1977 Neonatal intracranial hemorrhage: pathophysiology, neuropathology, and clinical features. Clinics in Perinatology 4: 77–102

Welch K, Strand R 1986 Traumatic parturitional intracranial hemorrhage. Developmental Medicine and Child Neurology 28: 156–164

Whitelaw A G, Haines M E, Bolsover W, Harris E 1984 Factor V deficiency and antenatal intraventricular haemorrhage. Archives of Disease in Childhood 59: 997–999

Wigglesworth J S, Husemeyer R P 1977 Intracranial birth trauma in vaginal breech delivery: the continued importance of injury to the occipital bone. British Journal of Obstetrics and Gynaecology 84: 684–691

Zalneraitis E L, Young R S K, Krishnamoorthy K S 1979 Intracranial hemorrhage in utero as a complication of isoimmune thrombocytopenia. Journal of Pediatrics 95: 611–614

28. Germinal matrix haemorrhage and intraventricular haemorrhage

Dr L.S. de Vries, Dr J-C. Larroche and Dr M.I. Levene

The terminology used to describe haemorrhage in and around the lateral ventricles is confusing and lacks a clear consensus view. Intraventricular haemorrhage is an imprecise term used to describe bleeding within the ventricular cavities but arising from any site. It may be impossible to distinguish on ultrasound examination the presence of liquid-phase blood in the lateral ventricle. Consequently, the distinction between unruptured germinal matrix haemorrhage (GMH) and intraventricular haemorrhage (IVH) can often not be confidently made by this imaging technique. The generic term periventricular haemorrhage is also widely used to refer to haemorrhage originating in the germinal matrix, often with involvement of the lateral ventricles and on occasions extending into the periventricular white matter. It is now clear that haemorrhage occurring de novo in the periventricular white matter, without germinal matrix bleeding also occurs not infrequently and this condition might be referred to more accurately as periventricular haemorrhage. For these semantic reasons we have chosen to use the term 'germinal matrix haemorrhage–intraventricular haemorrhage' (GMH–IVH) to refer to a common form of intracranial haemorrhage usually seen in premature infants. Throughout this section the term GMH–IVH is used in a general sense to describe the condition that other authors have described by a variety of other terms but which we believe to refer to the same condition. There is now growing evidence that a proportion (probably a majority) of haemorrhagic lesions in the cerebral parenchyma have quite a different pathophysiological basis from GMH–IVH and are ischaemic in origin. This is discussed in detail on page 317.

PATHOLOGY

Ruckensteiner & Zollner in 1929 were the first to recognize that in premature infants, blood in the ventricles commonly occurred as the result of haemorrhage in the subependymal germinal matrix. Despite an abundant literature on the subject, the mechanism by which this lesion develops is still incompletely understood. The subependymal germinal matrix is a transient structure and is initially the site of vigorous neuroblast and glioblast mitotic activity. When cell division is complete and after the majority of the neurones have completed their migration, the relative size of the periventricular germinal matrix progressively decreases but a conspicuous mass of cells persist over the head and body of the caudate nucleus until 33 to 34 weeks of gestation. In addition, residual matrix tissue persists in the roof of the temporal horn and in the external wall of the occipital horn. Anteriorly the germinal matrix is supplied by Heubner's artery, a branch of the lateral striate arteries and the anterior choroidal artery. In premature infants, Takashima & Tanaka (1978) have demonstrated by micro-angiography, the relative underdevelopment of the vascular bed supplying this region and in beagle puppies, arterial flow through the germinal matrix has been shown to be low (Pasternak et al 1982). In contrast, the venous drainage of the developing cerebral hemispheres via the deep system of Galen is more highly developed. The compactly arranged cells which comprise the germinal matrix at the end of the second trimester are mainly small immature neurones or glial cells with scanty cytoplasm.

From 8 to 18 weeks after conception and during the rapid mitotic activity of the subependymal germinal matrix, the density of capillaries within this structure increases. After this time the number of vascular lumina per unit of surface area decreases whilst a spectacular proliferation of capillaries occurs in the cortical plate (Larroche in preparation). Even on electron microscopy the capillaries are indistinguishable from small veins. By 20 weeks the 'capillary unit' (that is the endothelial cell, pericyte, basal lamina and glial-end foot) is morphologically mature (Povlishock et al 1977, Larroche in preparation). This unit does, however, differ from the mature capillary structure in some respects. The capillary wall is often thicker and the cytoplasm shows a greater number of organelles including vacuoles, microvilli and rod-shaped bodies. This last substructure may be related to thromboplastic and clotting activity. Under normal circumstances the cerebral capillaries are very resistant to rupture (Goldstein 1979) but in infants who have been asphyxiated, electron microscopy has revealed swollen glial-end feet, cloudy basal lamina and dislocation of endothelial cells with extravasation of blood (Larroche in preparation).

In cases of germinal matrix haemorrhage, small thrombi and fibrin deposits and/or rupture of small vessels have been described on light microscopy (Larroche 1964, 1977). The capillaries enter directly into the major vein branches usually at right angles to the large vessels and rupture at the capillary–vein junction has been reported by Hambleton & Wigglesworth (1976). In addition, in most cases of GMH–IVH described at autopsy, the main tributaries of the internal cerebral veins (thalamo–striate, terminal, frontal, septal and choroidal veins) are severely dilated. Towbin (1968) and Rorke (1982) have described ischaemic infarcts which predate or accompany the haemorrhage. In these pale areas, we have found proliferation of glial cells which are positive for a specific protein for glial cells (GFAP).

Ninety per cent of haemorrhages occur into the germinal matrix at the head of the caudate nucleus adjacent to the foramen of Monro as illustrated in Figure 28.1 (Leech & Kohnen 1974). Bleeding sites may be multiple and in some cases develop in the roof of the temporal horn and posteriorly in the germinal matrix of the external wall of the lateral ventricle. Bleeding may also extend into the caudate nucleus and other adjacent structures. Germinal matrix haemorrhage is bilateral in half of affected brains but left-sided lesions may be slightly more common (Donn & Bowerman 1985). Blood may also extend into the ventricle from primary bleeding of the tela choroidea and from the choroid plexus.

Blood in the ventricular system may remain in the liquid phase but when it is present in large amounts clots develop. In severe cases a cast of clot involving the lateral, third and fourth ventricular system forms and if the infant survives, ventricular dilatation is almost inevitable (see p. 347).

Alternatively, multiple small clots may develop which are suspended in the liquid phase of the intraventricular blood and these may also cause obstruction to cerebrospinal fluid (CSF) drainage. Blood commonly collects in the subarachnoid spaces of the posterior fossa and may extend into the basal cistern.

INCIDENCE

Although prenatal haemorrhage is well documented (see Ch. 30) it occurs rarely and GMH–IVH is essentially a postnatal event. Its incidence after birth reflects the population from which the data are drawn and reports on its frequency vary from 31% (DeCrespigny et al 1982) to 90% (Bejar et al 1980) in premature infants. Neither of these figures represents the true frequency of this condition. The incidence of GMH–IVH is directly related to the maturity of the infant and for infants weighing below 1500 g (approximating to 30 weeks of gestation) it is about 50%. The incidence of haemorrhage appears to increase with reducing gestational age below 30 weeks (see Fig. 28.2). With advancing gestational age, GMH–IVH becomes progressively less common.

The true incidence in infants of 35 weeks of gestation and above is difficult to derive as most infants born at this maturity are healthy and are not referred to neonatal units

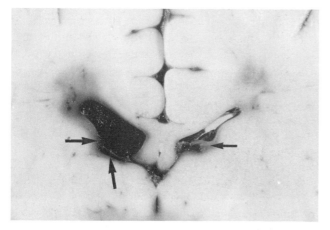

Fig. 28.1 Bilateral germinal matrix haemorrhage (arrowed) with rupture into the left lateral ventricle which is filled with clot.

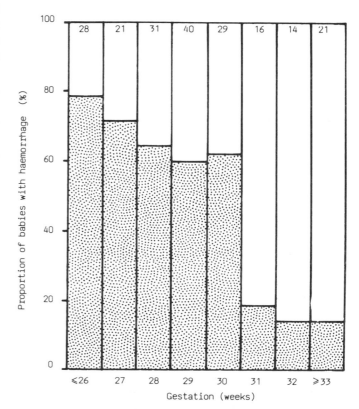

Fig. 28.2 Incidence of GMH–IVH in extremely premature infants by gestational age. The number at the top of each column refers to the number of infants in each group.

for intensive care or intracranial scanning. Those that are referred are clearly highly selected and the incidence of GMH–IVH in this group will not be representative of the whole population. Although GMH–IVH is uncommon in mature infants it is well documented (Cartwright et al 1979, Palma et al 1979, Mitchell & O'Tuama 1980, Scher et al 1982, Fenichel et al 1984). By 35 to 36 weeks, involution of the subependymal germinal matrix is almost complete and bleeding in this area is uncommon. The overall incidence diagnosed by ultrasound is 5% of an unselected group of full-term infants (Hayden et al 1985). It was bilateral in approximately one-half of cases and the infants sustaining GMH–IVH were no iller than other infants of similar gestation without haemorrhage.

These mature infants described in isolated case-reports are likely to be symptomatic for the attending clinicians to perform scans and it is not surprising that in these infants the majority of lesions are extensive and some involve the cerebral parenchyma. Asphyxia may precede the haemorrhage in mature infants but this is not invariable and often there are no obvious risk factors. Intraventricular haemorrhage in full-term infants has been reported to be due to choroid plexus or tela choroidea haemorrhage, vascular malformations or extension of parenchymal haemorrhagic infarcts and these are all discussed in Chapter 29. In general, extensive IVH occurring in full-term infants is very unusual.

TIMING

As discussed above, GMH–IVH is generally a condition that occurs after birth. The age at onset of haemorrhage has until relatively recently been inferred from autopsy material and was likely to reflect a bias towards the most severe cases. Indirect methods designed to time the onset of GMH–IVH have depended on analysis of the proportion of radio-actively labelled red cells (Tsiantos et al 1974) or the proportion of mature erythrocytes in the intracerebral clot found at autopsy (Emerson et al 1977). These studies suggested that most bleeds occurred within the first 48 hours after birth.

Real-time ultrasound allows frequent scanning of high-risk infants and a number of groups have now reported the accurate timing of the onset of GMH–IVH. These studies confirm that most haemorrhages occur in the first week of life (Bejar et al 1980, DeCrespigny et al 1982, Levene et al 1982, Thorburn et al 1982, Dolfin et al 1983, Szymonowicz & Yu 1984, McDonald et al 1984a, Ment et al 1984a) and the majority within the first three days of life. Some infants appear to have very early or prenatal onset of their GMH–IVH but in the majority of reports the lesions were fairly equally distributed between the first, second and third days of life. Late onset GMH–IVH is not uncommon and 15% of very-low-birth-weight infants develop haemorrhage

after two weeks of life (Trounce et al 1986). Hecht et al (1983) reported 17 infants with late onset of haemorrhage after one week of age and all but two were confined to the region of the germinal matrix. If late GMH–IVH occurs it is usually benign with little likelihood of adverse outcome.

Repeated ultrasound scans have shown that in 10 to 20% of infants, progression in the initial size of the GMH–IVH occurs over 24 to 48 hours, illustrated in Fig. 28.3 (Shankaran et al 1982, Levene & De Vries 1984). The mechanism by which this happens is speculative and is discussed more fully on p. 317.

AETIOLOGY

Much has been written about the risk factors predisposing to periventricular haemorrhage but there is little that is undisputed. It is agreed that PVH is a condition of prematurity related to rupture of small vessels within the germinal matrix. It is also widely accepted that the presence of respiratory distress syndrome and complications of it are important related factors. It is not particularly fruitful to analyse every study but of more interest to discuss those major factors reported from careful research which throw light on the aetiology of GMH–IVH. Confusion has arisen concerning the predisposing cause of GMH–IVH because of the poor design and methodology of many studies. Early reports analysed risk factors only in children who died with GMH–IVH. Others have not timed the onset of bleeding and consequently the cause and effect of haemorrhage may become confused. The most useful studies are those which have accurately timed the onset of GMH–IVH and analysed risk factors only up until the time of haemorrhage.

Obstetric factors

The role of obstetric factors in causing GMH–IVH is at most minor. It is certainly true that the better the obstetric care and management of labour so the better the condition the infant will be in at birth. There are, however, surprisingly few studies that suggest prenatal events are a major risk factor in the development of GMH–IVH.

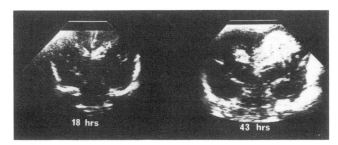

Fig. 28.3 Extension of intraventricular haemorrhage. The timing of the scans are shown in hours from birth. There has been progressive involvement of the right parenchymal region. (Reproduced with permission from Levene & De Vries 1984.)

Antepartum haemorrhage

There have been no positive reports that there is a direct association between either placental abruption or placenta praevia and GMH–IVH.

Mode of delivery

The question as to whether mode of delivery influences survival and morbidity is yet to be answered. As there are no controlled studies of vaginal delivery and caesarean section, information as it stands may be misleading. Most reports do not find elective caesarean section when the woman is not in labour to protect the infant from developing GMH–IVH (Levene et al 1982, Bada et al 1984, Strauss et al 1985). Another study found caesarean section to lower the incidence of GMH–IVH compared with vaginal delivery but neither reduced the severity of haemorrhage, nor reduced the mortality rate (DeCrespigny & Robinson 1983). A protective effect of caesarean section has been claimed by others (Thorburn et al 1982, Tejani et al 1984) but in the former study the majority of infants delivered by section was significantly greater, thus reducing the likelihood of GMH–IVH occurring.

Breech versus vertex delivery

Only two of seven studies support the contention that infants born by the breech have a significantly higher incidence of haemorrhage (Thorburn et al 1982, Horbar et al 1983) and the latter study did not substantiate on multivariate analysis the independent effect of presentation. Five well-conducted studies have found no significant difference in the incidence of GMH–IVH between infants born vaginally and those presenting either by the breech or vertex (Lavene et al 1982, DeCrespigny & Robinson 1983, Bada et al 1984, Tejani et al 1984, Strauss et al 1985).

Intrapartum monitoring

In a study of monitoring in labour, the product of which subsequently developed severe GMH–IVH with parenchymal involvement, there were significantly increased numbers of ominous fetal heart rate patterns, although the numbers reported were small (Strauss et al 1985). Other studies have shown no predictive benefit from cardiotocography in labour (Levene et al 1982, Beverley et al 1984a, Tejani et al 1984).

Condition at birth

No report has found that cord blood gases predict the risk of GMH–IVH (Beverley & Chance 1984, Beverley et al 1984a, Tejani et al 1984) and Apgar scores have infrequently been correlated with the development of haemorrhage (Beverley

et al 1984a, Strauss et al 1985). The majority of reports find no such association (Levene et al 1982, Thorburn et al 1982, DeCrespigny & Robinson 1983, Beverley & Chance 1984, Hawgood et al 1984). Szymonowicz et al (1984) have found that severe facial bruising, a feature of birth trauma, was a strong predictor of infants likely to develop more severe forms of haemorrhage.

Place of birth

It has been suggested that infants born outside a perinatal centre and transported in have a higher incidence of GMH–IVH (Clark et al 1981, Levene et al 1982, Hawgood et al 1984). The transported infants are highly selected as those who are in good condition at birth may not be referred, thus biasing the group towards those with more severe illness and who are more likely to have intracerebral haemorrhage. Clark et al (1981) studied a group of very-low-birth-weight infants in a geographically well-defined area. All infants born outside the perinatal centre were referred in and there was no selection on the basis of severity of illness. Only 29% of the inborn infants had GMH–IVH compared to 79% of those outborn.

Respiratory distress syndrome

This is the most consistently recognized risk factor predisposing to GMH–IVH in premature infants. The association between massive intracranial haemorrhage (many of which were GMH–IVH in origin) and the presence of respiratory distress syndrome (RDS) was first made by Harrison et al (1968). They attributed the haemorrhage to severe hypoxia consequent on the lung disease. Subsequently the association has been confirmed by other groups (Cooke 1981, Levene et al 1982, Thorburn et al 1982, Perlman et al 1983, Szymonowicz et al 1984) but there is probably not a causal relationship between RDS and haemorrhage. Infants with severe RDS require mechanical ventilation and are subject to complications associated with this form of treatment. It has been suggested that hypercapnia, pneumothorax and the fluctuating pattern of systemic blood pressure cause GMH–IVH and these are discussed below. Cooke et al (1981) have suggested that acute blockage of the endotracheal tube is the most important factor in the genesis of GMH–IVH.

Hypercapnia and acidosis

Hypercapnia is a potent vasodilator of newborn intra-cerebral arterioles (Archer et al 1986) and this is an important factor in the development of germinal matrix haemorrhage. A number of studies have reported hypercapnia to be an important independent factor in the evolution of GMH–IVH (Dykes et al 1980, Cooke 1981, Levene et al 1982, Szymonowicz et al 1984). Levene et al (1982) found that 81% of low-birth-weight infants who had both hypercapnia ($P_{a,CO_2}>6$ kPa) and severe acidosis (pH<7.1) developed GMH–IVH and more than half of these infants had moderate or severe degrees of haemorrhage.

Metabolic acidosis has also been reported to be an important independent variable in the development of GMH–IVH (Cooke 1981, Levene et al 1982, Hawgood et al 1984) although others have not confirmed this (Thorburn et al 1982).

Infusion of sodium bicarbonate to treat metabolic acidosis has been claimed to be an important cause of GMH–IVH (Simmons et al 1974, Anderson et al 1976, Wigglesworth et al 1976). The rapid or large infusion of hypertonic base induces osmotic gradients between blood and brain causing cerebral shrinkage and subsequent haemorrhage. It has been calculated that an infusion of 10 ml of molar concentration sodium bicarbonate over less than four hours will produce such a gradient (Finberg 1977). Subsequent prospective studies also suggested that rapid infusion of hyperosmolar sodium bicarbonate was associated with a significantly increased incidence of GMH–IVH (Papile et al 1978, Hawgood et al 1984). Dykes et al (1980) found that administration of sodium bicarbonate after the first day of life was also a significant risk factor in the development of GMH–IVH. A controlled study of bicarbonate infusion in high-risk premature infants could not confirm it as a cause of GMH–IVH (Corbet et al 1977). These studies did not account for the timing of the haemorrhage and confusion between cause and effect is possible. There are no reports looking at risk factors up to the time of haemorrhage which suggest that sodium bicarbonate has a direct role in the causation of GMH–IVH but dosage of this agent is now considerably less than previously reported. Unless large volumes of sodium bicarbonate or other hyperosmolar solutions are used these substances are unlikely to produce GMH–IVH by a direct effect.

Pneumothorax

Pneumothorax has frequently been reported to cause or be an important factor in the development of GMH–IVH (Dykes et al 1980, Lipscomb et al 1981, Peabody 1981, Hill et al 1982, Thorburn et al 1982, Szymonowicz et al 1984) although a number of other equally careful studies have failed to substantiate this association (Cooke et al 1981, Levene et al 1982).

In a prospective study GMH–IVH was usually found to have developed within six hours of the clinical diagnosis of pneumothorax (Hill et al 1982). In each infant in whom blood pressure was measured there was an increase in diastolic pressure and a fall in pH at the time of pneumothorax. Hill et al (1982) suggest that GMH–IVH occurs as the direct result of the increase in blood pressure consequent on the development of pneumothorax.

Blood pressure

It is generally thought that ill premature infants cannot regulate their cerebral blood flow constant in the presence of changes in systemic blood pressure and consequently rapid changes cause either ischaemia or haemorrhage in the vulnerable germinal matrix (Lou et al 1979, Pape & Wigglesworth 1979). A number of studies have attempted to relate loss of autoregulation to the development of haemorrhage (Milligan 1980, Ment et al 1981, Ahmann et al 1983) but all have major methodological problems and do not prove the hypothesis.

Acute changes in blood pressure due to rapid infusions of blood or plasma and leading to GMH–IVH have been reported (Dykes et al 1980, Milligan 1980, McDonald et al 1984a, Hawgood et al 1984). Goddard-Finegold et al (1982) have developed an animal model for GMH–IVH and produce the lesion by rapid volume expansion in puppies who had been previously rendered hypotensive. This did not occur following infusion in untreated normotensive animals. Perlman et al (1983) have shown that GMH–IVH occurred mainly in infants who were ventilated and who showed an unstable pattern of blood pressure characterized by rapid beat-to-beat fluctuations. This was only seen in infants after 12 hours of age. They suggested that the fluctuating blood pressure pattern led to similar changes in cerebral blood flow which caused rupture of the germinal matrix vessels. This pattern is usually seen in infants who actively breathe against the positive-pressure inspiration of mechanical ventilation and they have subsequently shown a fall in the incidence of GMH–IVH if spontaneous breathing is abolished by neuromuscular relaxation (Perlman et al 1985). The abolition of acute rises in blood pressure occurring in infants with RDS has also been shown to occur after phenobarbitone injection (Wimberley et al 1982).

The role of increased intracerebral venous pressure has also been suggested to be an important cause of GMH–IVH (Reynolds et al 1979). Little is known of the relationship between RDS and venous pressure but anatomical evidence exists for severe venous stasis in the right atrium, jugular veins and deep venous system of Galen in neonatal respiratory disease. Increased intracranial venous pressure observed during the course of mechanical ventilation has been reported by Vert et al (1975) and others have also reported increased pressure in the right atrium (Perlman & Volpe 1986). Toubas et al (1978) have described an increase in central venous pressure in hypothermic experimental animals.

Extravascular pressure

The brain loses extracellular fluid over the first few days of life and it has been suggested that shrinkage predisposes to vessel rupture due to a lower tissue hydrostatic pressure and an acute increase between intra- and extra-vascular pressure gradients (DeCourten & Rabinowicz 1981). Others have shown that prevention of postnatal water loss from the brain by prolactin injection prevents intracerebral haemorrhage (Coulter et al 1985).

Coagulation defects

It has been postulated by a variety of researchers that after capillary rupture has occurred, bleeding is more likely to continue in the presence of coagulation disturbances (Chessels & Wigglesworth 1972, Foley & McNicol 1977, Thorburn et al 1982, Setzer et al 1982, Beverley et al 1984b, McDonald et al 1984b). Few studies have examined clotting before the onset of haemorrhage and results are conflicting. Beverley et al (1984b) found no significant differences at birth in a variety of coagulation studies in infants who later developed GMH–IVH but at 48 hours of age there were significant differences in activated partial thromboplastin time and the activity of clotting factors II, III and X between the non-haemorrhage and GMH–IVH groups. They could not, however, show a relationship between the timing of GMH–IVH and the severity of coagulopathy. Conversely, McDonald et al (1984b) found a significant association between coagulopathy in the first few hours of life and subsequent GMH–IVH or extension of intracranial haemorrhage.

Indomethacin, a potent prostaglandin synthetase inhibitor, is widely used in premature infants to close a patent ductus arteriosus. It has been suggested that the drug may also inhibit platelet aggregation and exacerbate germinal matrix haemorrhage. Corazza et al (1984) found that indomethacin significantly prolonged the bleeding time within two hours of its administration but they and others (Maher et al 1985) could find no convincing link between indomethacin administration and the initiation or maximal size of haemorrhage.

Patent ductus arteriosus (PDA)

It has been reported that infants with PDA are at increased risk of developing GMH–IVH due to haemodynamic disturbances associated with the ductal shunt (Perlman et al 1981, Martin et al 1982). Additionally, once the ductus has been surgically ligated there is a sudden increase in systemic blood pressure (Marshall et al 1982) which may cause germinal matrix haemorrhage. Other studies have shown no correlation between GMH–IVH and PDA (Ment et al 1984a) or acute onset or extension of an existing GMH–IVH lesion after surgical ligation of the ductus (Strange et al 1985). It is unlikely that PDA or its treatment is a major factor in the development of GMH–IVH.

Other factors

A recent report claims that flush solutions containing benzyl alcohol as a preservative cause GMH–IVH (Hiller et al 1986). A study over two consecutive periods showed a 66% incidence of GMH–IVH before cessation of benzyl alcohol, falling to 43% after the preservative was withdrawn. In addition, the extent of the lesions was less in the second period. Clearly iatrogenic causes of GMH–IVH must always be suspected as new treatments are commonly introduced into neonatal medicine in an uncontrolled manner.

A unifying hypothesis

GMH–IVH may occur when the structural integrity of the vessel wall is compromised and then ruptures following subsequent changes in intravascular pressure or blood flow. An additional hypothetical factor may be alterations in extravascular pressure. Various factors may be associated with acute changes in intravascular pressure including mechanical ventilation, pneumothorax and rapid transfusion of hypotensive infants. The changes in blood pressure and consequently in blood flow through the germinal matrix are most likely to occur in the presence of hypercapnia and hypoxia as these factors maximally dilate the cerebral arterioles. Prostaglandins play an important role in the vascular tone of the germinal matrix vessels and factors may act at this level to predispose the infant to changes in local blood flow predisposing to rupture of compromised vessels. Once rupture has occurred, coagulopathy will exacerbate bleeding which may then become more extensive and rupture into the lateral ventricles. This mechanism is summarized in Figure 28.4.

HAEMORRHAGIC PARENCHYMAL INVOLVEMENT

It is often impossible at autopsy to determine the underlying pathogenesis of haemorrhagic involvement of the cerebral parenchyma, and this is all the more difficult by means of imaging techniques. Furthermore, it is likely that there are a number of mechanisms by which parenchymal involvement may occur. Understanding these mechanisms is necessary in order to prevent this complication from occurring.

Direct extension

The origin of the germinal matrix haemorrhage which is usually thought to arise from capillaries, may cause extensive bleeding with clot formation in the ventricle but it would be surprising if this causes direct breach of the ependyma with white matter involvement at the time of the GMH in previously normal tissue. Alternatively, it is possible that some GMH lesions are due to arteriole bleeding with greater hydrostatic force but at present there is no evidence that either mechanism is the cause of parenchymal involvement in infants without previous white matter injury.

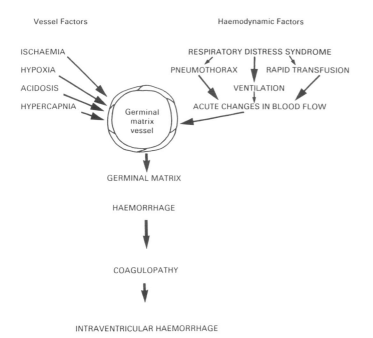

Fig. 28.4 Model for the development of GMH and IVH which is dependent on both vessel and haemodynamic factors.

Secondary bleeding

This probably occurs in infants in whom the periventricular white matter has been previously compromised by concomitant injury, most likely to be ischaemic infarction as occurs in PVL (see p. 328). Evidence for this has been provided by positron emission tomography (Volpe et al 1983). Armstrong & Norman (1974) have shown that one-quarter of infants with periventricular infarction had bleeding into the infarcted area. If this occurred in the presence of intraventricular haemorrhage then direct haemorrhagic extension might be mistakenly diagnosed.

Venous infarction

The deep periventricular white matter is served by a fan-shaped leash of short and long medullary veins which flow vertically into subependymal veins (Takashima & Tanaka 1978, Takashima et al 1986) and this is illustrated in Figure 28.5. Venous infarction has been reported to be due to thrombosis of the sagittal sinus but may also occur following intraventricular clot formation (Pape & Wigglesworth 1979). Clot distending the ventricle may cause obstruction of these veins with increasing congestion and reduction in venous return. This may eventually lead to venous infarction due to stasis. Takashima et al (1986) have speculated, on the basis of autopsy material, that haemorrhagic infarction in the periventricular white matter may be due to venous thrombosis in some cases. We have previously reported ultrasound evidence for extension of GMH–IVH in 15% of infants with this form of haemorrhage

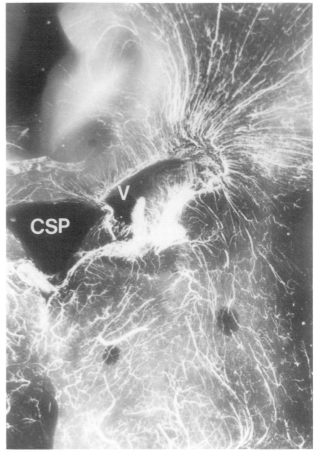

Fig. 28.5 Microvenography showing the fan-shaped leash of veins in the deep periventricular white matter of a 28-weeks-gestation neonate. V = ventricle, CSP = cavum septi pellucidi. (Reproduced with permission from Takashima et al 1986.)

over a period of up to 48 hours (Levene & De Vries 1984). The initial lesion is one of distension of the ventricle with clot and subsequently extension of echodensity into the periventricular white matter occurs (Fig. 28.3). There is some evidence for this mechanism from pathological specimens (Pape & Wigglesworth 1979) and an example is shown in Figure 28.6. This lesion, if it occurs, is likely to have a slower evolution and will be seen in conjunction with (usually) distension of a lateral ventricle with a haematoma.

Vaso-active agents

It has been suggested that blood within the lateral ventricle liberates vaso-active compounds which induce local arterial spasm within the periventricular arteries to produce ischaemia with subsequent infarction. The time scale for the evolution of this lesion will be similar to that of venous infarction (White et al 1975, Edvinsson et al 1986). To date there is no good evidence for this mechanism in the newborn and it remains speculative.

We believe that the majority of cases of parenchymal

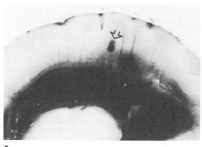
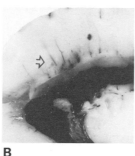

Fig. 28.6 Close-up of the two hemispheres from a 30-weeks-gestation infant showing distension of both lateral ventricles with clot. There is congestion of the veins draining the deep periventricular white matter. Note also the white spots of PVL (arrowed) and the secondary bleeding into the necrotic tissue.

extension are due to underlying ischaemic injury in the periventricular white matter as suggested by Rushton et al (1985). In some cases, particularly where intraventricular clot distends the lateral ventricle, secondary venous infarction of the periventricular white matter occurs and if the infant survives, a large porencephalic cavity may develop (see p. 346).

DIAGNOSIS

Clinical

This is discussed in detail in Chapter 00, and will be summarized briefly here. Before the introduction of scanning techniques, GMH–IVH was thought to be a devastating condition with obvious clinical signs. Volpe (1977) described two clinical manifestations; a rapidly evolving catastrophic deterioration and less commonly a slower saltatory course. Lazzara et al (1978) reported the main physical signs associated with GMH–IVH diagnosed by CT to include a tense fontanelle and either increase or decrease in spontaneous activity. In another study decerebrate posturing was seen in one half of infants who were shown to have GMH–IVH on CT scans but clonic seizures were seen equally frequently in the group of infants without haemorrhage (Krishnamoorthy et al 1977).

With the introduction of routine scanning techniques it was recognized that the majority of infants with GMH–IVH showed no obvious symptoms. Burstein et al (1979) reported that the frequency of 'silent' haemorrhage was as high as 68% in a group of very-low-birth-weight infants.

More recently, comprehensive neurological assessment methods have been introduced (Dubowitz et al 1981) and a variety of clinical signs have been found to correlate with the presence of GMH–IVH, including impaired visual tracking, abnormal popliteal angle, later development of roving eye movements, decrease in tone, and poor motility (p. 55). Others have also found infants with GMH–IVH to have increased tone in the lower limbs (particularly popliteal angle) and hypotonia of the neck (particularly flexor

muscles) and upper limb girdle muscles. In addition, those with GMH–IVH had brisker tendon reflexes and clonus of the ankle (Stewart et al 1983a).

Imaging

Computerized tomography was first used to diagnose GMH–IVH in 1976 (Pevsner et al 1976) but is not appropriate for routine clinical use. Several years later ultrasound was shown to be a sensitive method of diagnosing GMH–IVH and has now become widely used as a convenient and safe method for detecting this condition. The role of these two techniques in diagnosing haemorrhage is fully discussed in Chapters 8 and 9.

Electro-encephalography

Cukier (1972) first described a specific EEG abnormality associated with GMH–IVH. This was referred to as a positive rolandic sharp wave and the association has been confirmed subsequently by other workers (Blume & Dreyfus-Brisac 1982). Unfortunately, this abnormality appears not to be sensitive for uncomplicated GMH–IVH (Watanabe et al 1983, Clancy et al 1984) nor specific (Lombroso 1982). Positive rolandic sharp waves have also been reported in periventricular leukomalacia (Lombroso 1982, Marret et al 1986) and this particular EEG pattern is common when GMH–IVH is associated with severe leukomalacia. Therefore, the EEG may not be a useful method for diagnosing GMH–IVH alone but may be of value in prognosis because of frequently associated parenchymal lesions. The role of this technique is fully discussed in Chapter 13.

PREVENTION OF GMH–IVH

Since 1981 a profusion of papers have been published claiming that a variety of drugs prevent the development of GMH–IVH in infants or animal models (Table 28.1). Different studies on a number of agents such as phenobarbitone and vitamin E produced conflicting results and the whole area is at present confused and confusing. The question is not can GMH–IVH be prevented but do these methods prevent neurological handicap, and to date little data exists to answer this question.

Table 28.1 Agents used in controlled studies in the prevention of GMH–IVH in premature infants

Ethamsylate
Fresh frozen plasma
Indomethacin
Pancuronium
Prolactin
Phenobarbitone
Tranexamic acid
Vitamin E

General methods

It has been noted that hypercapnia vasodilates cerebral arterioles and together with failure of autoregulation there may be a predisposition to germinal matrix haemorrhage. Lou et al (1982) have retrospectively analysed the P_{a,CO_2} following elective intubation and resuscitation in a group of very premature infants. They suggested that hyperventilation might re-establish autoregulation in these babies and consequently prevent GMH–IVH. No infant developed haemorrhage whose early P_{a,CO_2} was less than 25 mmHg, and haemorrhage tended to occur in the infants with the highest P_{a,CO_2} levels measured in the first hour. All the infants with early GMH–IVH were born vaginally. The authors claim that the severity of the infant's lung disease was not the reason for the differences in P_{a,CO_2} and the reduced incidence of GMH–IVH. These results must be treated with caution in view of the retrospective and uncontrolled nature of this study.

A group in Melbourne (Szymonowicz et al 1986) have attempted to modify early neonatal management in order to reduce the incidence of GMH–IVH in infants with birth weight below 1250 g. They achieved significant improvement in measurements of pH, body temperature and blood pressure measured on admission to the neonatal unit, and subsequently found significantly lower arterial carbon dioxide tensions and higher blood pressure measurements. Infants treated by these methods had a 36% incidence of GMH–IVH compared with a 60% incidence in infants of the same birth-weight treated by less aggressive means in a previous period. This was a highly significant reduction in the incidence of haemorrhage ($P<0.001$). They claim that changes in neonatal management may account for apparent reduction in the incidence of GMH–IVH in drug studies, particularly if these are not performed blind.

Phenobarbitone

This was the first agent claimed to prevent GMH–IVH. Donn et al (1981) gave two loading doses of 10 mg/kg intravenously 12 hours apart and adjusted the maintenance dose to achieve a serum level of 20–30 μg/ml by the third day of life. GMH–IVH occurred in only four of the 30 (13%) infants in the phenobarbitone group compared with 14 of 30 (47%) of the control infants ($P=0.01$). They reported their results again after studying a total of 105 babies and continued to show an impressive reduction in the incidence of GMH–IVH in the treated group (Donn et al 1982). This study was not performed blind and the neonatal staff knew which infants received the drug.

They suggested a number of mechanisms by which phenobarbitone may have protected the brain, including a reduction in cerebral metabolic rate, reduction in catecholamine release, inactivation of oxygen free radicals, reduction in vasogenic and cytotoxic oedema, an anticonvulsant effect, reduction in raised intracranial pressure and enzyme induction. They did not specify which one or number of these mechanisms produced the apparent protective effect. In addition to these mechanisms Wimberley et al (1982) have shown that anticonvulsant doses of phenobarbitone reduce blood pressure fluctuations in premature infants but this effect is very transient.

Two further non-blind studies have claimed that phenobarbitone may reduce the incidence of GMH–IVH (Ruth 1985, Anwar et al 1986). In the former study, although the number of infants with GMH–IVH in the phenobarbitone-treated group (8/25) was reduced compared with the controls (14/27), this did not reach statistical significance. The administration of phenobarbitone to mothers in premature labour has been reported (Morales & Koerten 1986, Shankaran et al 1986) and these studies showed a statistically significant reduction in the overall incidence of GMH–IVH in the treated group. Shankaran et al (1986) found no infants in the phenobarbitone group sustained moderate or severe haemorrhage compared with 6 of 13 in the control group ($P<0.01$). Surprisingly, in this study the cord serum level of phenobarbitone was 8.85 μg/ml, on average three times lower than that of the original study by Donn et al. Morales & Koerten (1986) achieved higher levels of phenobarbitone in the infants (ranging from 15 to 17 μg/ml).

In contrast to these studies, four other reports have failed to reproduce the protective effect of phenobarbitone (Morgan et al 1982, Whitelaw et al 1983, Bedard et al 1984, Kuban et al 1986). These reports were prospective and three were randomized blind control studies. The dosages used were similar to those of Donn's original study. Unfortunately, Donn et al (1981) did not report early serum levels before three days of age and it is not possible to know whether the original study achieved higher levels in the first 48 hours of life, when the majority of haemorrhages would be expected to occur. Whitelaw et al (1983) also reported that in spontaneously breathing infants the loading dose of phenobarbitone was associated with a high incidence of respiratory failure within hours of using the drug; a previously unrecognized side-effect.

The study performed by Kuban et al (1986) from Boston must be considered to be the definitive work thus far. They designed the study to have a 90% power of showing a 50% reduction in the occurrence of GMH–IVH. They enrolled 280 infants in the study and showed that the phenobarbitone-treated infants had a significantly *higher* incidence of haemorrhage ($P=0.003$). There were also more severe haemorrhages in the phenobarbitone-treated group. The balance of evidence does not support the use of phenobarbitone to prevent GMH–IVH in premature infants.

Ethamsylate

As GMH–IVH occurs due to capillary bleeding from

the germinal matrix, Morgan et al (1981) suggested that ethamsylate, a drug known to reduce capillary bleeding, may prevent this form of haemorrhage. They enrolled 70 very-low-birth-weight infants in a double blind controlled study using 0.1 mg/kg of drug or placebo. There was a significantly reduced incidence of GMH–IVH in ethamsylate-treated infants but the frequency of larger bleeds was no different between the two groups. They subsequently enrolled more infants (not in a randomized manner) and claimed that there was a reduction in neurological abnormalities at follow-up, as well as a reduction in the number of ventriculo–peritoneal shunts needed to treat posthaemorrhagic hydrocephalus (Cooke & Morgan 1984). It has been suggested that as well as the platelet effect, ethamsylate reduces the synthesis of prostaglandins (Ment et al 1984b) which may protect the germinal matrix from rapid fluctuations in cerebral blood flow. The results of a multicentre trial assessing the effect of ethamsylate in the prevention of GMH–IVH has recently been reported (Benson et al 1986). In a carefully conducted double blind study they showed that ethamsylate does appear to have a protective effect in both reducing the incidence of IVH and in limiting the size of the eventual lesion.

Tranexamic acid

Another drug which reduces fibrinolytic activity of the germinal matrix is tranexamic acid and this has also been assessed for its ability to prevent GMH–IVH. In a double blind controlled study of 100 very-low-birth-weight infants, no reduction in either the incidence or severity of haemorrhage was found (Hensey et al 1984).

Vitamin E

Chiswick et al (1983) from Manchester have claimed that early treatment with vitamin E protects against intraventricular haemorrhage in premature infants. They attempted to distinguish, by ultrasound scanning, ruptured from unruptured germinal matrix haemorrhage and on this basis showed an apparent protective effect of vitamin E on the frequency of GMH–IVH. However, when the combined incidences of both germinal matrix haemorrhages *and* intraventricular haemorrhages were compared there was no difference in the incidence of GMH–IVH between the two groups. It is not possible using ultrasound to make the distinction Chiswick claims (Levene et al 1985) but they have subsequently reported the results of a larger prospective study (Sinha et al 1987). Unfortunately, this study was not carried out in a blind manner but they found that both inborn and outborn babies pretreated with vitamin E had a lower incidence of IVH and parenchymal haemorrhage.

Speer et al (1984) have also assessed the efficacy of vitamin E in preventing PVH and claimed it was effective in reducing the incidence of this condition but a third study of infants weighing less than one kilogram at birth showed the opposite effect (Phelps 1984). In this study, 14 of 43 infants pretreated with vitamin E developed severe haemorrhage compared with only 4 of 42 given placebo.

It is suggested that vitamin E stabilizes endothelial membranes, thus limiting the extent of haemorrhage (Chiswick et al 1983, Speer et al 1984) but, alternatively, it has been suggested that it prevents mitochondrial damage by its activity in scavenging oxygen free radicals (Ment 1985, Sinha et al submitted). In addition, it has been shown that superoxide dismutase (a powerful oxygen free radical scavenger) reduces the incidence of PVH in an animal model (Ment et al 1985a).

Recently, evidence has accumulated in the United States suggesting that a particular form of parenteral vitamin E (E-Ferol) causes thrombocytopenia, renal dysfunction and cholestatic liver failure (Bove et al 1985). It is not clear whether this is a direct effect of the vitamin preparation or occurs as a result of the vehicle in which the drug is administered. In view of the potential hazards of this agent and doubt as to its efficacy in preventing GMH–IVH we cannot recommend it for routine use in premature infants.

Pancuronium

Pancuronium, a non-depolarizing neuromuscular blocker, has also been shown to prevent GMH–IVH in premature infants with marked beat-to-beat fluctuations in blood pressure (Perlman et al 1985). This pattern occurs in infants who actively expire against a positive-pressure inspiratory breath of the mechanical ventilator. Perlman et al recognized a group of infants with the fluctuating blood pressure pattern and paralysed a randomly selected proportion of them. GMH–IVH developed in all 10 spontaneously breathing infants but only 5 of 14 given pancuronium developed haemorrhage, and in 4 of these 5 GMH–IVH developed after the paralysis had worn off. On closer examination of their data only 20 of the 166 (12%) infants they studied actually developed GMH–IVH, an incidence well below that reported previously by Volpe in a population of very-low-birth-weight infants (Tarby & Volpe 1982). This must raise the question of how representative of high-risk infants was their cohort.

Two previous studies of pancuronium failed to show any significant reduction in the incidence of GMH–IVH (Pollitzer et al 1981, Greenhough et al 1984). Further information must be obtained on the safety and efficacy of neuromuscular blockade in the prevention of GMH–IVH before it becomes routinely accepted.

Indomethacin

Indomethacin is a potent prostaglandin synthetase inhibitor and inactivates prostaglandin and other prostaglandin-like compounds. In an animal study Ment et al (1983) found that indomethacin significantly reduced the incidence of GMH–IVH induced by a hypotension/hypertension technique. The pretreated puppies had significantly less fluctuation in blood pressure and indomethacin appeared to damp down lability of blood pressure. This same group has subsequently shown that indomethacin significantly reduced the incidence of GMH–IVH in premature infants (Ment et al 1985b). The treated infants received 0.1 mg of indomethacin 12 hourly for five doses and the first dose was given within approximately six hours of birth. The authors speculate that indomethacin inhibits the vasodilatory prostaglandins and limits acute changes in blood pressure and this is the mechanism by which the incidence of haemorrhage is reduced.

Fresh frozen plasma

Beverley et al (1985) have reported a reduction in the incidence of GMH–IVH from 41% to 14% by means of early infusion of 10 ml/kg of fresh frozen plasma (FFP) on admission to the neonatal unit and then again at 48 hours from birth. This was highly statistically significant ($P=0.022$). The mechanism by which FFP prevents haemorrhage is unclear. They did not find that it reduced the frequency of clotting abnormalities in these infants but did not report blood pressure data. It is possible that the reduction in incidence of severe GMH–IVH was related to prevention of cerebral ischaemia due to the effects of the FFP stabilizing the cerebral circulation. Further studies comparing FFP with a similar colloid solution without clotting factors may resolve this question.

PROGNOSIS

Outcome following GMH–IVH can be considered in terms of mortality and handicap in surviving infants. Unfortunately there have been surprisingly few good follow-up studies of infants who have sustained GMH–IVH and it is difficult to draw clear conclusions from these studies.

Mortality

Death in extremely premature infants may be due to a variety of causes including lung disease, sepsis, necrotizing enterocolitis and brain haemorrhage. At autopsy cerebral haemorrhage may be found but this may not be the primary cause of death and deciding what single insult killed the infant may be impossible. In general, it appears that the more severe the degree of haemorrhage, the higher is the mortality (Thorburn et al 1981, Shankaran et al 1982, Smith et al 1983). Haemorrhage confined to the region of the germinal matrix does not increase the risk of death but intraparenchymal involvement has a high mortality. Approximately one-half (Martin et al 1984, Ahmann et al 1983) to three-quarters (Thorburn et al 1981, Trounce et al 1986) of infants with intraparenchymal lesions die.

Neurodevelopmental outcome

Early studies reporting outcome are biased towards those cases with the most obvious clinical presentation as it was only those who had CT scans performed (Kosmetatos et al 1980, Krishnamoorthy et al 1979). Studies in which all very premature infants had regular ultrasound scans provide more accurate follow-up data. There appears to be little increased risk of handicap in infants with grade I haemorrhage confined to the region of the germinal matrix, compared with similar infants without GMH–IVH (Shankaran et al 1982, Papile et al 1983, Stewart et al 1983b). Some authors have also suggested that moderate haemorrhage (clot in the lateral ventricles with no parenchymal extension) does not significantly increase the risk of adverse outcome compared with mild GMH–IVH (Papile et al 1983, Stewart et al 1983, Dubowitz et al 1984). However, others have suggested a definite trend between the size of GMH–IVH and incidence of severe disability (Catto-Smith et al 1985). They report that two-thirds of infants with this form of haemorrhage had major disability; an incidence higher than most other follow-up studies.

The underlying aetiology of parenchymal haemorrhage is discussed in the next section but follow-up studies agree that there is a high incidence of adverse neurodevelopmental outcome whatever the cause. Major handicap ranges from 85% to 100% of infants with parenchymal involvement (Shankaran et al 1982, Stewart et al 1983, Papile et al 1983, Dubowitz et al 1984, Catto-Smith et al 1985, TeKolste et al 1985). McMenamin et al (1984) have suggested that outcome following this form of haemorrhage is much worse in infants weighing less than 1000 g at birth compared with larger babies. Furthermore, they found that survivors of large parenchymal lesions all had more significant handicap than those surviving less extensive parenchymal involvement. It is important to note that despite extensive haemorrhage and early signs of cerebral palsy the eventual disability may be mild and the child should be able to attend a normal school (Fawer et al 1983).

Clinical assessment at full-term in prematurely born infants is also useful in predicting outcome and has been shown to be a better predictor of poor outcome than neonatal ultrasound abnormalities (Dubowitz et al 1984). Of the 62 infants considered normal at 40 weeks, 91% were assessed as normal at one year.

EEG has been reported to predict outcome (Clancy et al 1984). In one study all infants with at least one severely abnormal EEG suffered adverse outcome (death or significant disability).

REFERENCES

Ahmann P A, Dykes F D, Lazzara A, Holt P J, Giddens D P, Carrigan T A 1983 Relationship between pressure passivity and subependymal/intraventricular hemorrhage as assessed by pulsed Doppler ultrasound. Pediatrics 72: 665–669

Anderson J M et al 1976 Hyaline membrane disease, alkaline buffer treatment, and cerebral intraventricular haemorrhage. Lancet i: 117–119

Anwar M, Kadam S, Hiatt I M, Hegyi T 1986 Phenobarbitone prophylaxis of intraventricular hemorrhage. Archives of Disease in Childhood 61: 196–197

Archer L N J, Evans D H, Paton J Y, Levene M I 1986 Controlled hypercapnia and neonatal cerebral artery Doppler ultrasound wave-forms. Pediatric Research 20: 218–221

Armstrong D, Norman M G 1974 Periventricular leucomalacia in neonates: complications and sequelae. Archives of Disease in Childhood 49: 367–375

Bada H S, Korones S B, Anderson G D, Magill H L, Wong S P 1984 Obstetric factors and relative risk of neonatal germinal layer/intraventricular hemorrhage. American Journal of Obstetrics and Gynecology 148: 798–804

Bedard M P, Shankaran S, Slovis T L, Pantoja A, Dayal B, Poland R L 1984 Effect of prophylactic phenobarbital on intraventricular hemorrhage in high-risk infants. Pediatrics 73: 435–439

Bejar R, Curbelo V, Coen R W, Leopold G, James H, Gluck L 1980 Diagnosis and follow-up of intraventricular and intracerebral hemorrhages by ultrasound studies of infant's brain through the fontanelles and sutures. Pediatrics 66: 661–673

Benson J W T et al 1986 Multicentre trial of ethamsylate for prevention of periventricular haemorrhage in very low birthweight infants. Lancet ii: 1297–1300

Beverley D W, Chance G 1984 Cord blood gases, birth asphyxia and intraventricular haemorrhage. Archives of Disease in Childhood 59: 884–897

Beverley D W, Chance G W, Inwood M J, Schaus M, O'Keefe B 1984a Intraventricular haemorrhage: timing of occurrence and relationship to perinatal events. British Journal of Obstetrics and Gynaecology 91: 1007–1013

Beverley D W, Chance G W, Inwood M J, Schaus M, O'Keefe B 1984b Intraventricular haemorrhage and haemostasis defects. Archives of Disease in Childhood 59: 444–448

Beverley D W, Pitts-Tucker T J, Congdon P J, Arthur R J, Tate G 1985 Prevention of intraventricular haemorrhage by fresh frozen plasma. Archives of Disease in Childhood 60: 710–713

Blume W T, Dreyfus-Brisac C 1982 Positive rolandic sharp waves in neonatal EEG: types and significance. Electroencephalography and Clinical Neurophysiology 53: 227–282

Bove K et al 1985 Vasculopathic hepatotoxicity associated with E-Ferol syndrome in low-birth-weight infants. Journal of the American Medical Association 254: 2422–2430

Burstein J, Papile L A, Burstein R 1979 Intraventricular hemorrhage in premature newborns: a prospective study with CT. American Journal of Roentgenology 132: 631–635

Cartwright G W, Culbertson K, Schreiner R L, Garg B P 1979 Changes in clinical presentation of term infants with intracranial hemorrhage. Developmental Medicine and Child Neurology 21: 730–737

Catto-Smith A G, Yu V Y H, Bajuk B, Orgill A A, Astbury J 1985 Effect of neonatal periventricular haemorrhage on neurodevelopmental outcome. Archives of Disease in Childhood 60: 8–11

Chessells J M, Wigglesworth J S 1972 Coagulation studies in preterm infants with respiratory distress and intracranial haemorrhage. Archives of Disease in Childhood 47: 564–570

Chiswick M L et al 1983 Protective effect of vitamin E (dl-alpha-tocopherol) against intraventricular haemorrhage in premature babies. British Medical Journal 287: 81–84

Clancy R R, Tharp B R, Enzman D 1984 EEG in premature infants with intraventricular hemorrhage. Neurology 34: 583–590

Clark C E, Clyman R I, Roth R S, Sniderman S H, Lane B, Ballard R A 1981 Risk factor analysis of intraventricular hemorrhage in low birth weight infants. Journal of Pediatrics 99: 625–628

Cooke R W 1981 Factors associated with periventricular haemorrhage in very low birth weight infants. Archives of Disease in Childhood 56: 425–431

Cooke R W I, Morgan M E I 1984 Prophylactic ethamsylate for periventricular haemorrhage. Archives of Disease in Childhood 59: 82–84

Cooke R W I, Morgan I M, Coad N A G 1981 Pneumothorax, mechanical ventilation, and periventricular haemorrhage. Lancet i: 555

Corazza M S, Davis R F, Merritt A, Bejar R, Cvetnic W 1984 Prolonged bleeding time in preterm infants receiving indomethacin for patent ductus arteriosus. Journal of Pediatrics 105: 292–296

Corbet A J, Adams J M, Kenny J D, Kennedy J, Rudolph A J 1977 Controlled trial of bicarbonate therapy in high-risk premature newborn infants. Journal of Pediatrics 91: 771–776

Coulter D M, La Pine T R, Gooch M 1985 Treatment to prevent postnatal loss of brain water reduces the risk of intracranial hemorrhage in the beagle puppy. Pediatric Research 19: 1322–1326

Cukier F, Andre M, Monod N, Dreyfus-Brisac C 1972 Apport de l'EEG au diagnostic des hemorrhagies intra-ventriculaires du premature. Revue Electroencephalographie et Neurophysiologique Clinique 2: 318–322

DeCourten G M, Rabinowicz T 1981 Intraventricular hemorrhage in premature infants: reappraisal and a new hypothesis. Developmental Medicine and Child Neurology 23: 389–403

DeCrespigny L Ch, Robinson H P 1983 Can obstetricians prevent neonatal intraventricular haemorrhage? Australian and New Zealand Journal of Obstetrics and Gynaecology 23: 146–149

DeCrespigny L, Mackay R, Muston L J, Roy R N D, Robinson P H 1982 Timing of neonatal cerebroventricular haemorrhage with ultrasound. Archives of Disease in Childhood 57: 231–233

Dolfin T, Skidmore M B, Fong K W, Hoskins E M, Shannon A T 1983 Incidence, severity and timing of subependymal and intraventricular hemorrhages in preterm infants born in a perinatal unit as detected by serial real-time ultrasound. Pediatrics 71: 541–546

Donn S M, Bowerman R A 1985 Unilateral germinal matrix hemorrhage in the newborn. Journal of Ultrasound in Medicine 4: 251–253

Donn S M, Roloff D W, Goldstein G W 1981 Prevention of intraventricular haemorrhage in preterm infants by phenobarbitone: a controlled trial. Lancet ii: 215–217

Donn S M, Roloff D W, Goldstein G W 1982 Phenobarbitone and neonatal intraventricular haemorrhage. Lancet i: 1240–1241

Dubowitz L M S, Levene M I, Morante A, Palmer P, Dubowitz V 1981 Neurologic signs in neonatal intraventricular hemorrhage: a correlation with real-time ultrasound. Journal of Pediatrics 99: 127–133

Dubowitz L M S, Dubowitz V, Palmer P G, Miller G, Fawer C-L, Levene M I 1984 Correlation of neurologic assessment in the preterm newborn infant with outcome at one year. Journal of Pediatrics 105: 452–456

Dykes F D, Lazzara A, Ahmann P, Blumenstein B, Schwartz J, Brann A W 1980 Intraventricular hemorrhage: a prospective evaluation of etiopathogenesis. Pediatrics 66: 42–49

Edvinsson L, Lou H C, Tvede K 1986 On the pathogenesis of regional cerebral ischaemia in intracranial haemorrhage: a causal influence of potassium? Pediatric Research 20: 478–480

Emerson P et al 1977 Timing of intraventricular haemorrhage. Archives of Disease in Childhood 52: 183–187

Fawer C-L, Levene M I, Dubowitz L M S 1983 Intraventricular haemorrhage in a preterm neonate: discordance between clinical course and ultrasound scan. Neuropediatrics 14: 242–244

Fenichel G M, Webster D L, Wong W K T 1984 Intracranial hemorrhage in the term infant. Archives of Neurology 41: 30–34

Finberg L 1977 The relationship of intravenous infusions and intracranial hemorrhage — a commentary. Journal of Pediatrics 91: 777–778

Foley M E, McNicol G P 1977 An in-vitro study of acidosis, platelet function, and perinatal cerebral intraventricular haemorrhage. Lancet i: 1230–1232

Goddard-Finegold J, Armstrong D, Zeller R S 1982 Intraventricular hemorrhage following volume expansion after hypovolaemic hypotension in the newborn beagle. Journal of Pediatrics 100: 796–799

Goldstein G W 1979 Relation of potassium transport to oxidative metabolism in isolated brain capillaries. Journal of Physiology 286: 185–195

Greenhough A, Wood S, Morley C J, Davis J A 1984 Pancuronium prevents pneumothoraces in ventilated premature babies who actively expire against positive pressure inflation. Lancet i: 1–3

Hambleton G, Wigglesworth J S 1976 Origin of intraventricular haemorrhage in the preterm infant. Archives of Disease in Childhood 51: 651–659

Harrison V C, Heese H, Klein M 1968 Intracranial haemorrhage associated with hyaline membrane disease. Archives of Disease in Childhood 43: 116–120

Hawgood S, Spong J, Yu V Y H 1984 Intraventricular hemorrhage: incidence and outcome in a population of very low birth weight infants. American Journal of Diseases of Children 138: 136–139

Hayden C K, Shattuck K E, Richardson C J, Ahrendt D K, House R, Swischuk L E 1985 Subependymal germinal matrix hemorrhage in full-term neonates. Pediatrics 75: 714–718

Hecht S T, Filly R A, Callen P W, Wilson-Davis S L 1983 Intracranial hemorrhage: late onset in the preterm neonate. Radiology 149: 697–699

Hensey O J, Morgan M E I, Cooke R W I 1984 Tranexamic acid in the prevention of periventricular haemorrhage. Archives of Disease in Childhood 59: 719–721

Hill A, Perlman J M, Volpe J J 1982 Relationship of pneumothorax to occurrence of intraventricular hemorrhage in the premature newborn. Pediatrics 69: 144–149

Hiller J L et al 1986 Benzyl alcohol toxicity: impact on mortality and intraventricular hemorrhage among very low birthweight infants. Pediatrics 77: 500–506

Horbar J D, Pasnick M, McAuliffe T L, Lucey J F 1983 Obstetric events and risk of periventricular hemorrhage in premature infants. American Journal of Diseases of Children 137: 678–681

Kosmetatos N, Dinter C, Williams M L, Lourie H, Berne A S 1980 Intracranial hemorrhage in the premature: its predictive features and outcome. American Journal of Diseases of Children 134: 855–859

Krishnamoorthy K S et al 1977 Evaluation of neonatal intracranial hemorrhage by computerized tomography. Pediatrics 59: 165–172

Krishnamoorthy K S, Shannon D C, DeLong G R, Todres I D, Davis K R 1979 Neurologic sequelae in the survivors of neonatal intraventricular hemorrhage. Pediatrics 64: 233–237

Kuban C K et al 1986 Neonatal intracranial hemorrhage and phenobarbital. Pediatrics 77: 443–450

Larroche J-C 1964 Les hemorrhagies cerebrales intraventriculaires chez le premature: anatomie et physiopathologie. Biology Neonatorum 7: 26–35

Larroche J-C 1977 Developmental pathology of the neonate. Excerpta Medica, Amsterdam

Larroche J-C Structure of the capillaries of the subependymal matrix in the developing human fetus. (In preparation)

Lazzara A, Ahmann P A, Dykes T D, Brann A, Schwartz J F 1978 Clinical predictability of intraventricular hemorrhage in preterm infants. Annals of Neurology 4: 187

Leech R W, Kohnen P 1974 Subependymal and intraventricular hemorrhage in the newborn. American Journal of Pathology 77: 465–475

Levene M I, De Vries S H 1984 Extension of neonatal intraventricular haemorrhage. Archives of Disease in Childhood 59: 631–636

Levene M I, Fawer C-L, Lamont R F 1982 Risk factors in the development of intraventricular haemorrhage in the preterm neonate. Archives of Disease in Childhood 57: 410–417

Levene M I, Williams J L, Fawer C-L 1985 Ultrasound of the infant brain. Clinics in Developmental Medicine, No. 92, Blackwell Scientific Medical Publications, Oxford

Lipscomb A P et al 1981 Pneumothorax and cerebral haemorrhage in preterm infants. Lancet i: 414–416

Lombroso C T 1982 Neonatal electroencephalography. In: Niedermeyer E, daSilva F L (eds) Electroencephalography. Urban & Schwarzenberg, Baltimore

Lou H C, Lassen N A, Friis-Hansen B 1979 Is arterial hypertension crucial for the development of cerebral haemorrhage in premature infants? Lancet i: 1215–1217

Lou H C, Phibbs R H, Wilson S L, Gregory G A 1982 Hyperventilation at birth may prevent early periventricular haemorrhage. Lancet i: 1407

McDonald M M et al 1984a Timing and antecedents of intracranial hemorrhage in the newborn. Pediatrics 74: 32–36

McDonald M M et al 1984b Role of coagulopathy in newborn intracranial hemorrhage. Pediatrics 74: 26–31

McMenamin J B, Shackelford G D, Volpe J J 1984 Outcome of neonatal intraventricular hemorrhage with periventricular echodense lesions. Annals of Neurology 15: 285–290

Maher P, Lane B, Ballard R, Piecuch R, Clyman R I 1985 Does indomethacin cause extension of intracranial hemorrhages: a preliminary study. Pediatrics 75: 497–500

Marret S, Parain D, Samson-Dollfus D, Jeannot E, Tessart C 1986 Positive rolandic sharp waves and periventricular leukomalacia in the newborn. Neuropediatrics 17: 199–202

Marshall T A, Marshall F, Reddy P P 1982 Physiologic changes associated with ligation of the ductus arteriosus in preterm infants. Journal of Pediatrics 101: 749–753

Martin C G, Snider A R, Katz S M, Peabody J L, Brady J P 1982 Abnormal cerebral blood flow patterns in preterm infants with a large patent ductus arteriosus. Journal of Pediatrics 101: 587–593

Martin D J, Pape K E, Daneman A 1984 The site of neonatal periventricular hemorrhage: an important prognostic sign of mortality and morbidity. Annals of Radiology 27: 243–246

Ment L R 1985 Prevention of neonatal intraventricular hemorrhage. New England Journal of Medicine 312: 1385–1387

Ment L R, Ehrenkranz R A, Lange R C, Rothstein P T, Duncan C C 1981 Alterations in cerebral blood flow in preterm infants with intraventricular hemorrhage. Pediatrics 68: 763–769

Ment L R, Stewart W B, Scott D T, Duncan C C 1983 Beagle puppy model of intraventricular hemorrhage: randomized indomethacin prevention trial. Neurology 33: 179–184

Ment L R et al 1984a Intraventricular hemorrhage in the preterm neonate: timing and cerebral blood flow changes. Journal of Pediatrics 104: 419–425

Ment L R, Stewart W B, Duncan C C 1984b Beagle puppy model of intraventricular hemorrhage: ethamsylate studies. Prostaglandins 27: 245–256

Ment L R, Stewart W B, Duncan C C 1985a Beagle puppy model of intraventricular hemorrhage: effect of superoxide dismutase on cerebral blood flow and prostaglandins. Journal of Neurosurgery 62: 563–569

Ment L R et al 1985b Randomized indomethacin trial for prevention of intraventricular hemorrhage in very low birthweight infants. Journal of Pediatrics 107: 937–943

Milligan D W A 1980 Failure of autoregulation and intraventricular haemorrhage in preterm infants. Lancet i: 896–898

Mitchell W, O'Tuama L 1980 Cerebral intraventricular hemorrhages in infants: a widening age spectrum. Pediatrics 65: 35–39

Morales W J, Koerten J 1986 Prevention of intraventricular hemorrhage in very low birth weight infants by maternally administered phenobarbitol. Obstetrics and Gynaecology 68: 295–299

Morgan M E I, Benson J W T, Cooke R W I 1981 Ethamsylate reduces the incidence of periventricular haemorrhage in very low birth weight babies. Lancet ii: 830–831

Morgan M E I, Massey R F, Cooke R W I 1982 Does phenobarbitone prevent periventricular haemorrhage in very low birth weight babies? A controlled trial. Pediatrics 70: 186–189

Palma P A, Miner M E, Morriss F H, Adcock E W, Denson S E 1979 Intraventricular hemorrhage in the neonate born at term. American Journal of Diseases of Children 133: 941–944

Pape K E, Wigglesworth J S 1979 Haemorrhage, ischaemia and the perinatal brain. Clinics in Developmental Medicine, No. 69/70, Heinemann Medical Books, London

Papile L-A, Burstein J, Burstein R, Koffler H, Koops B 1978 Relationship of intravenous sodium bicarbonate infusions and cerebral intraventricular hemorrhage. Journal of Pediatrics 93: 834–836

Papile L-A, Munsick-Bruno G, Schaefer A 1983 Relationship of cerebral intraventricular hemorrhage and early childhood neurologic handicap. Journal of Pediatrics 103: 273–277

Pasternak J F et al 1982 Regional blood flow in the newborn beagle pup: the germinal matrix is a 'low-flow' structure. Pediatric Research 16: 499–503

Peabody J L 1981 Mechanical ventilation of the newborn . . . good news . . . bad news. Critical Care Medicine 9: 710–713

Perlman J M, Volpe J J 1986 Are venous circulatory abnormalities important in pathogenesis of intraventricular hemorrhage in preterm infants? Annals of Neurology 20: 434–435

Perlman J M, Hill A, Volpe J J 1981 The effect of patent ductus arteriosus on flow velocity in the anterior cerebral arteries: ductal steal in the premature newborn infant. Journal of Pediatrics 99: 767–771

Perlman J M, McMenamin J B, Volpe J J 1983 Fluctuating cerebral blood flow velocity in respiratory distress syndrome: relation to the development of intraventricular hemorrhage. New England Journal of Medicine 309: 204–209

Perlman J M, Goodman S, Kreusser K L, Volpe J J 1985 Reduction in intraventricular hemorrhage by elimination of fluctuating cerebral blood flow velocity in preterm infants with respiratory distress syndrome. New England Journal of Medicine 312: 1353–1357

Pevsner P H, Garcia-Bunuel R, Leeds N, Finkelstein M 1976 Subependymal and intraventricular hemorrhage in neonates: early diagnosis by computed tomography. Radiology 119: 111–114

Phelps D L 1984 Vitamin E and CNS hemorrhage. Pediatrics 74: 1113–1114

Pollitzer M J, Reynolds E O R, Shaw D G, Thomas R M 1981 Pancuronium during mechanical ventilation speeds recovery of the lungs of infants with hyaline membrane disease. Lancet i: 346–348

Povlishock J T, Martinez A J, Moossy J 1977 The fine structure of blood vessels of the telencephalic germinal matrix in the human fetus. American Journal of Anatomy 149: 439–452

Reynolds M L, Evans C, Reynolds E O R, Saunders N R, Durbin G M, Wigglesworth J S 1979 Intracranial haemorrhage in the preterm sheep fetus. Early Human Development 3/2: 163–186

Rorke L B 1982 Pathology of perinatal brain injury. Raven Press, New York

Ruckensteiner E, Zollner F 1929 Uber die Blutungen im Gebiete der Vena terminalis bei Neugeborenen. Frankfurt Z fur Pathologie 37: 568–578

Rushton D I, Preston P R, Durbin G M 1985 Structure and evolution of echodense lesions in the neonatal brain: a combined ultrasound and necropsy study. Archives of Disease in Childhood 60: 798–808

Ruth V 1985 Brain protection by phenobarbitone in very low birthweight (VLBW) prematures — a controlled trial. Klinikum Pediatric 197: 170–171

Scher M S, Wright F S, Lockman L A, Thompson T R 1982 Intraventricular hemorrhage in the full-term neonate. Archives of Neurology 39: 769–772

Setzer E S, Webb I B, Wassenaar J W, Reeder J D, Mehta P S, Eitzman D 1982 Platelet dysfunction and coagulopathy in intraventricular hemorrhage in the premature infant. Journal of Pediatrics 100: 599–605

Shankaran S, Slovis T L, Bedard M P, Poland R L 1982 Sonographic classification of intracranial hemorrhage: a prognostic indicator of mortality, morbidity and short-term neurologic outcome. Journal of Pediatrics 100: 469–475

Shankaran S et al 1986 Antenatal phenobarbital for the prevention of neonatal intracerebral hemorrhage. American Journal of Obstetrics and Gynecology 154: 53–57

Simmons M A, Adcock E W, Bard H, Battaglia F C 1974 Hypernatraemia and intracranial hemorrhage in neonates. New England Journal of Medicine 291: 6–10

Sinha S, Davies J, Toner N, Bogle S, Chiswick M 1987 Vitamin E supplementation reduces the incidence of periventricular haemorrhages in very preterm babies. Lancet i: 466–471

Smith W L, McGuinness G, Cavanaugh D, Courtney S 1983 Ultrasound screening of premature infants: longitudinal follow-up of intracranial hemorrhage. Radiology 147: 445–448

Speer M E, Blifeld C, Rudolph A J, Chadda P, Holbein B M, Hittner H M 1984 Intraventricular hemorrhage and vitamin E in very low birth weight infant: evidence for efficacy of early intramuscular vitamin E administration. Pediatrics 74: 1107–1112

Stewart A L, Thorburn R J, Lipscomb A P, Amiel-Tison C 1983a Neonatal neurologic examinations of very preterm infants: comparison of results with ultrasound diagnosis of periventricular hemorrhage. American Journal of Perinatology 1: 6–11

Stewart A L, Thorburn R J, Hope P L, Goldsmith M, Lipscomb A P, Reynolds E O R 1983b Ultrasound appearance of the brain in very preterm infants and neurodevelopmental outcome at 18 months of age. Archives of Disease in Childhood 58: 598–604

Strange M J et al 1985 Surgical closure of patent ductus arteriosus does not increase the risk of intraventricular hemorrhage in the preterm infant. Journal of Pediatrics 107: 602–604

Strauss A, Kirz D, Modanlou H D, Freeman R K 1985 Perinatal events and the very low-birth weight infant. American Journal of Obstetrics and Gynecology 151: 1022–1027

Szymonowicz W, Yu V Y H 1984 Timing and evolution of periventricular haemorrhage in infants weighing 1250 g or less at birth. Archives of Disease in Childhood 59: 7–12

Szymonowicz W, Yu V Y H, Wilson F E 1984 Antecedents of periventricular haemorrhage in infants weighing 1250 g or less at birth. Archives of Disease in Childhood 59: 13–17

Szymonowicz W, Yu V Y H, Walker A, Wilson F 1986 Reduction in periventricular haemorrhages in preterm infants. Archives of Disease in Childhood 61: 661–665

Takashima S, Tanaka K 1978 Microangiography and vascular permeability of the subependymal matrix in the premature infant. Canadian Journal of Neurological Science 5: 45–50

Takashima S, Mito T, Ando Y 1986 Pathogenesis of periventricular white matter hemorrhages in preterm infants. Brain and Development 8: 25–30

Tarby T J, Volpe J J 1982 Intraventricular hemorrhage in the premature infant. Pediatric Clinics of North America 29: 1077–1089

Tejani N, Rebold B, Tuck S, Ditroia D, Sutro W, Verma U 1984 Obstetric factors in the causation of early periventricular–intraventricular hemorrhage. Obstetrics and Gynecology 64: 510–515

TeKolste K A, Bennett F C, Mack L A 1985 Follow-up of infants receiving cranial ultrasound for intracranial hemorrhage. American Journal of Diseases of Children 139: 299–303

Thorburn R J, Lipscomb A P, Stewart A L, Reynolds E O R, Hope P L, Pape K E 1981 Prediction of death and major handicap in very preterm infants by brain ultrasound. Lancet i: 1119–1121

Thorburn R J, Lipscomb A P, Stewart A L, Reynolds E O R, Hope P L 1982 Timing and antecedents of periventricular hemorrhage and of cerebral atrophy in very preterm infants. Early Human Development 7: 221–238

Toubas P L, Hof R P, Heymann M, Rudolph A 1978 Effects of hypothermia and rewarming on the neonatal circulation. Archives Francaises Pediatrie (Suppl) 35: 84–92

Towbin A 1968 Cerebral intraventricular haemorrhage and subependymal matrix infarction in the fetus and premature newborn. American Journal of Pathology 52: 121–134

Trounce J Q, Rutter N, Levene M I 1986 A prospective study of the incidence of periventricular leukomalacia and intraventricular haemorrhage in the preterm neonate. Archives of Disease in Childhood 61: 1196–1202

Tsiantos A et al 1974 Intracranial hemorrhage in the prematurely born infant: timing of clots and evaluation of clinical signs and symptoms. Journal of Pediatrics 85: 854–859

Vert P, Nomin P, Sibout M 1975 Intracranial venous pressure in the newborn: variations in physiological state and in neurologic and respiratory distress. In: Stern L (ed) Intensive care in the newborn. Masson, New York

Volpe J J 1977 Neonatal intracranial hemorrhage: pathophysiology, neuropathology and clinical features. Clinical Perinatology 4: 77–102

Volpe J J, Herscovitch P, Perlman J M, Raichle M E 1983 Positron emission tomography in the newborn: extensive impairement of regional blood flow with intraventricular hemorrhage and hemorrhagic involvement. Pediatrics 72: 589–601

Watanabe K, Hakemada S, Kuroyanagi M, Yamazaki T, Takeuchi T 1983 Electroencephalographic study of intraventricular hemorrhage in the preterm newborn. Neuropediatrics 14: 225–230

White R P, Hagen A A, Morgan H, Dawson W N, Robertson J T 1975 Experimental study on the genesis of cerebral vasospasm. Stroke 6: 52–57

Whitelaw A, Placzek M, Dubowitz L, Lary S, Levene M I 1983 Phenobarbitone for prevention of periventricular haemorrhage in very low birth weight infants. Lancet ii: 1168–1170

Wigglesworth J S, Keith I H, Girling D J, Slade S A 1976 Hyaline membrane disease, alkali and intraventricular haemorrhage. Archives of Disease in Childhood 51: 755–759

Wimberley P D, Lou H C, Pederson H, Hejl M, Lassen N A, Friis-Hansen B 1982 Hypertensive peaks in the pathogenesis of intraventricular hemorrhage in the newborn: abolition by phenobarbitone sedation. Acta Paediatrica Scandinavica 71: 537–542

29. Cerebral ischaemic lesions

*Dr L.S. de Vries, Dr J-C. Larroche and
Dr M.I. Levene*

Brain ischaemia occurs as the result of a variety of perinatal insults. During intrapartum asphyxia cerebral hypoperfusion occurs in the presence of hypoxia and produces a typical pathological and clinical appearance which is discussed in Chapters 32 and 33. In this section we will refer to the more specific condition of cerebral ischaemia associated with vascular compromise. This may develop in the watershed area between the vascular territory of two arterial beds as occurs in leukomalacia or following infarction of the whole or a branch of a major cerebral artery.

LEUKOMALACIA

Leukomalacia literally means 'softening of the white matter' and has been recognized as a pathological entity for longer than periventricular haemorrhage but has until recently been relatively neglected as an important cause of neurodevelopmental sequelae. The aetiology of leukomalacia is basically ischaemic and can occur in different forms. In the last few years it has become possible to diagnose ischaemic lesions with the use of real-time ultrasound. The modern sector scanners give a wide view of the periventricular white matter and higher frequency transducers give excellent resolution of pathological processes within this area. Consequently, recent studies using this equipment have rapidly advanced our understanding of this condition.

Historical review

Ischaemic lesions in general and periventricular leukomalacia (PVL) in particular have commonly been diagnosed at autopsy, before the era of the newer imaging techniques. PVL has been known to pathologists for more than a century and was first described by Virchow in 1867, who noted yellowish white areas in the periventricular white matter, which he associated with infection and he named the condition 'congenital interstitial encephalitis'.

Parrot (1873) reviewed the condition around the same time in a series of reports and pointed out that the problem was more common in premature infants and he therefore assumed that the immature white matter might be especially vulnerable in this age group. A major advance in understanding this condition occurred in 1962 when Banker & Larroche described the pathological changes in 51 infants. They introduced the name periventricular leukomalacia to describe their observation of the periventricular 'white spots' seen macroscopically (Fig. 29.1) and the softening (malacia) of the white matter (leucos). Perinatal anoxia was noted in the clinical history of all their cases and they were the first to point out that the condition was vascular in origin. Van den Bergh (1969) and De Reuck et al (1972) further stressed the vascular origin of these lesions and attributed the cause to hypoperfusion of the boundary zones between ventriculofugal and ventriculopetal arteries. This hypothesis was supported by Armstrong & Norman in 1974 who showed that haemorrhages could occur as a secondary

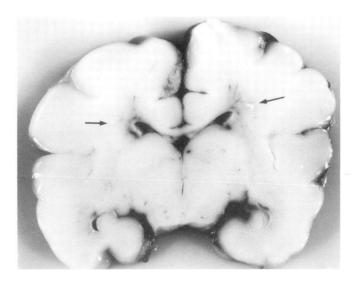

Fig. 29.1 Bilateral 'white spots' (arrowed) of periventricular leukomalacia. Histologically glial proliferation and calcification were present. Small bilateral germinal matrix haemorrhage (GMH) is also present.

process into these ischaemic lesions (Fig. 29.2). Leech & Atvord (1974) reported that the lesions could extend beyond the periventricular region into the subcortical white matter. Takashima & Tanaka (1978) performed postmortem cerebral angiography and showed that the boundary zones between the ventriculofugal and ventriculopetal arteries were affected in the infants with PVL. Takashima et al (1978) performed similar studies in more mature infants and showed a relatively avascular triangle in the white matter at the depth of the sulcus. These areas corresponded well with the site of the subcortical lesions seen in more mature infants. They therefore suggested that the distribution of these cystic lesions was related to the maturity of the vascular supply.

Pathology

Macroscopical examination shows a typical distribution of the periventricular lesions involving the external angle of the lateral ventricles (centrum semiovale), the corona radiata, the optic radiation and the temporal auditory radiation (Fig. 29.3).

Histological findings depend on the duration between the insult and the time of death. The earliest changes consist of coagulation necrosis, characterized by loss of architecture and this can be found within 5–8 hours following an insult. A few days later, nuclear debris, astrocytes and macrophages are noted to fill the periphery of the necrotic area. These macrophages can remain for months or years. The centre of the necrotic area may liquefy, resulting in small cavities, usually not communicating with the lateral ventricles (Fig. 29.4). Calcified capillaries can sometimes be noted in the periphery of these areas. Cavitation is not always observed and gliosis and persisting macrophages may be noted instead. Thinning of the white matter with enlargement of the lateral ventricles is present in both cases.

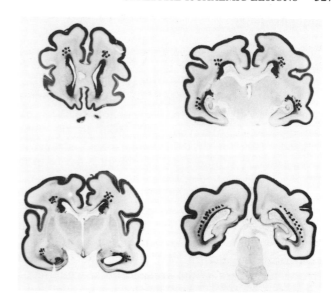

Fig. 29.3 Distribution of periventricular leukomalacia (PVL) lesions. The sites of prediliction of white matter lesions are superimposed on brain sections stained with cresyl violet. (From Larroche 1984. Reproduced with permission of Edward Arnold.)

The incidence of PVL in these pathology studies varies between 7 and 34% (Armstrong & Norman 1974, Pape & Wigglesworth 1979) but this increases to over 80% if only those infants are taken who required ventilation and survived beyond the first 7 days of life (Shuman & Selednik 1980).

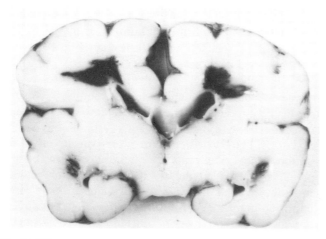

Fig. 29.2 Haemorrhagic necrosis into bilateral periventricular leukomalacic lesions.

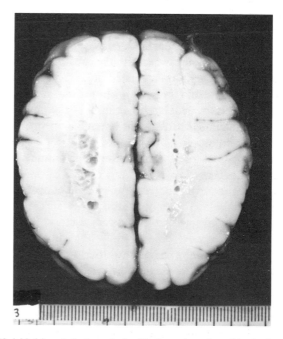

Fig. 29.4 Multicystic leukomalacia. Horizontal section of brain from an infant of 29 weeks of gestation who survived for 5 weeks. (From Larroche 1984. Reproduced with permission of Edward Arnold.)

Pathophysiology

The generally accepted concept that PVL is caused by hypoperfusion, has so far only been supported by a few animal studies. Abramovicz (1964) obliterated the basilar artery and ligated one or both common carotid arteries in mature cats. Subsequently, he was able to show patchy infarcts close to the ventricular wall in the centrum semiovale. Gilles et al (1976) administered intraperitoneal *E. coli* endotoxin to neonatal kittens for 6 days and found telencephalic leuko-encephalopathy at postmortem. The severity of the lesions appeared to be related to the dose of the endotoxin. Other groups used dogs as an animal model. Young et al (1982) produced systemic hypotension either by withdrawal of blood, or by injecting *E. coli* into the peritoneum and showed a significant reduction in cerebral blood flow in the periventricular white matter in these dogs, while the blood flow to the cortical and deep grey matter was preserved. Ment et al (1985a) supported these findings. They further noted a regional increase in glucose utilization in the periventricular white matter and therefore assumed uncoupling between local cerebral blood flow and glucose metabolism in the periventricular white matter. This uncoupling was also noted by Cavazutti & Duffy (1982) who looked at hyperaemia following hypoxia. They found that the compensatory hyperaemia was less pronounced in the periventricular white matter while an extremely high rate of glycolysis was found in this area, compared with other regions of the brain. Prostaglandin E2, a potent vasodilator, was also carefully studied by Ment et al (1985b) following hypotension and the concentration of prostaglandin E2 was shown to increase to a lesser extent in the periventricular white matter than in the cortex and grey matter.

These animal studies suggest that hypoperfusion alone could be an oversimplification in explaining the pathophysiology of PVL. Other related factors, such as compensatory hyperaemia following hypoxia, as well as a secondary rise in prostaglandin levels and regional increase in glucose metabolism following hypotension may all play an important role.

Few relevant studies, which could help to clarify the pathophysiology of PVL, have been carried out in humans. An important contribution came from Lou et al (1979) who performed radio-active xenon studies in sick premature infants in order to measure the cerebral blood flow. Using this method they were able to show the apparent lack of cerebral autoregulation in compromised neonates. In these infants there was a marked reduction in cerebral blood flow coincident with hypotension.

Changes in cerebral blood flow velocity, detected by continuous wave Doppler, have been observed in infants with severe respiratory distress syndrome, following a pneumothorax and following the use of indomethacin and in several other conditions (Perlman & Volpe 1985, Perlman

et al 1985, Cowan et al 1986). These studies are discussed in more detail in Chapter 11. Cowan et al (1986) and Evans et al (1987), using pulsed Doppler, recently studied changes in cerebral blood flow velocity following the administration of indomethacin and noted a marked reduction in cerebral blood flow velocity. The Doppler studies reported so far have looked at infants who had problems related to haemorrhagic lesions and not at infants who developed PVL. It is possible that pulsed Doppler studies which are now in progress will give us valuable information about changes in cerebral blood flow velocity before the onset of PVL. Positron emission tomography also holds promise in the assessment of PVL but data are so far only available in relatively normal infants, studied from the first week of life to 6 months of age, showing a change in distribution of active brain metabolism (Chugani & Phelps 1986) and in infants with large intraparenchymal haemorrhages (Volpe et al 1983).

Diagnosis and evolution of PVL

With the use of newer imaging techniques it is now well recognized that many infants with PVL do survive. Valuable information about the timing, the evolution of the ultrasound changes and the possible risk factors has recently been reported (Chow et al 1985, Dolfin et al 1984).

Correlation with autopsy findings has been found to be very good (Nwaesei et al 1984, Fawer et al 1985a, Trounce et al 1986a). False-negatives were only noted in a few cases who had not been scanned on a regular basis before death occurred (Nwaesei et al 1984).

The evolution of the ultrasound changes has been described in detail in Chapter 9. Areas of increased echogenicity are usually seen within 24 to 48 hours following an acute clinical episode. This increase in echogenicity was initially thought to be due to haemorrhages occurring in the ischaemic areas, following restoration of the circulation. Several authors have now shown that non-haemorrhagic infarction is also able to give this echogenic appearance (Martin et al 1983, Delaporte et al 1985, Trounce et al 1986a). This can be confirmed at autopsy or by the use of a CT scan within a week following the lesions (Fig. 29.5).

It is assumed that severe congestion may cause this increase in echogenicity. The densities can resolve over a period of one week and the ultrasound scan may subsequently appear normal, until the dense areas reappear 2–4 weeks later with breakdown into cystic lesions several days later. The densities can also persist until the cavitation occurs. The cysts appear in clusters in the area of previous echogenicity. They vary in diameter between a few millimetres to over a centimetre and are only rarely noted to communicate with the ventricles (Fig. 29.6a). The cysts remain for several weeks but tend to become smaller and are usually not visible once the infant is 2–3 months old (Fig. 29.6b). When the cysts become less apparent,

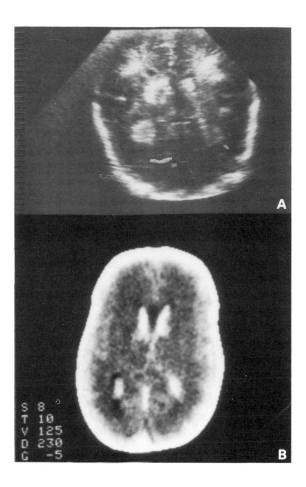

dilatation of the lateral ventricles can be noted (Bozynski et al 1985). The outline of the cysts may disappear completely as was observed in a child with PVL who died at 8 months of age. Histological examination showed gliosis, delayed myelination and mild ventricular dilatation (Trounce et al 1986a).

While it is relatively uncommon for a child to develop extensive cystic lesions, many infants develop increased echogenicity in the external angle of the lateral ventricle without or with less apparent echogenicity around the occipital horns (McMenamin et al 1984, Di Pietro et al 1986, Guzzetta et al 1986). A small number of these cases develop very small localized cysts in the centrum semiovale (Fig. 29.7). These cysts are usually unilateral and few in number and can only be visualized with a 7.5 MHz transducer. Trounce et al (1986b) defined these periventricular densities as prolonged 'flares' if they remained for at least 14 days (see Chapter 9). They subsequently resolve but mild ventricular dilatation can be observed in some of these infants when they are scanned again between 6 and 9 months of age and this can be asymmetrical in those where the flare was asymmetrical to start with. Subsequent widening of the interhemispheric fissure has also been recorded in a few infants with flares in the neonatal period, possibly indicating some degree of atrophy. In a few infants who died, gliosis has been observed at autopsy and it is therefore likely that these flares represent a milder degree of PVL (McMcnamin et al 1984, Trounce et al 1986a). There is still discussion about the relevance of the flares which are seen in so many infants (15–20%).

Other techniques have recently become available to aid early prediction as to the significance of these areas of increased echogenicity. Continuous 24-hour, 4-channel

Fig. 29.5 Non-haemorrhagic periventricular leukomalacia (PVL). Coronal ultrasound scan (**a**) showing intraventricular haemorrhage (IVH) and areas of increased echodensity in the periventricular white matter. CT scan (**b**) of the same infant in the acute phase showing no evidence of blood in the deep periventricular white matter.

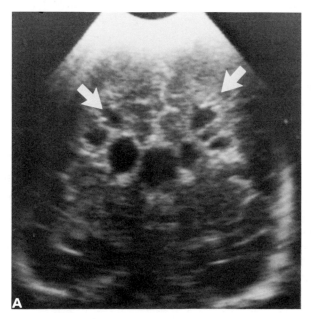
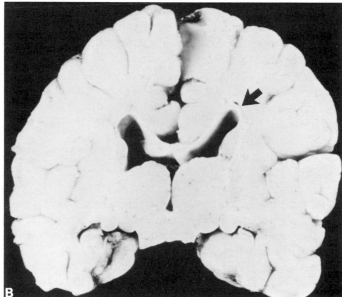

Fig. 29.6 Evolution of cystic periventricular leukomalacia (PVL) lesions. Coronal ultrasound scan (**a**) showing multiple echofree cavities (arrows) in the white matter. The infant died 3 months later and at autopsy the brain showed collapse of the cavities (**b**) which were only just visible (arrow).

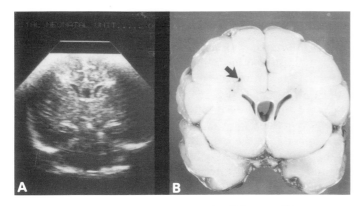

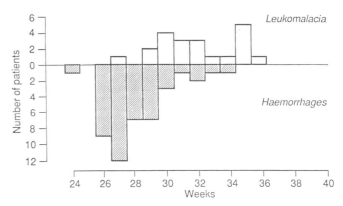

Fig. 29.7 Cystic periventricular leukomalacia (PVL). (a) Midcoronal ultrasound scan showing echodense areas in the periventricular white matter with small cysts on the left side. (b) Postmortem correlate showing a small cyst on the left (arrowed) with discoloration and softening of the periventricular white matter on the right.

Fig. 29.8 Age in postmenstrual weeks at the onset of haemorrhagic and ischaemic lesions.

EEG recordings show marked abnormalities (seizures, low amplitude) in those infants who have densities which subsequently evolve into extensive cystic lesions. The EEG findings of those with transient periventricular densities and subsequently normal development are, however, normal (see Ch. 13). Magnetic resonance spectroscopy (see Ch. 18) is also of value in predicting the importance of these early echodensities. Hamilton et al (1986) showed that all infants with flares who had a PCr/Pi ratio below the normal range either died or developed extensive cystic lesions, while most of those with normal ratios did not develop extensive cystic lesions.

Timing

The onset of PVL usually occurs in the perinatal period but any severe deterioration in the condition of the infant, such as necrotizing enterocolitis or septicaemia, occurring up until 40 weeks postmenstrual age, can still lead to this condition (Rushton et al 1985, De Vries et al 1986) (Fig. 29.8). This is in contrast to GMH–IVH which is known to occur rarely beyond the first week of life (Partridge et al 1983, Fawer et al 1984). PVL may also be due to insults occurring in utero (Barth 1984, Larroche 1986) and this is discussed in more detail in Chapter 30.

Incidence

The first reports of PVL described the ultrasound findings in a small number of cases only. However, recently, several population studies have been performed, reporting an incidence of between 2.3 and 17.8% (Levene et al 1983, Sinha et al 1985, Weindling et al 1985a, Trounce et al 1986b) (Table 29.1). The incidence will vary with the type of patient admitted to the intensive care unit (Larroche et al 1986), the type of transducer used (5 or 7.5 MHz), the number of ultrasound examinations performed, and the

definition used to describe PVL. Those authors who find a low incidence have restricted the term PVL to infants who developed extensive cystic lesions, while those giving a higher incidence have also included localized cystic lesions restricted to the centrum semiovale (Fawer et al 1985b). Trounce et al (1986b) reported a 9.5% incidence of cystic PVL. If prolonged flares were included in the PVL category, the incidence increased to 26%. The incidence of flares was found to be 12.5%. A study performed at the Hammersmith Hospital in 1984 and 1985 showed a similar incidence of PVL (23.9%). The ultrasound appearance of flare was seen in 15.8% and cystic PVL in 7.9%. Extensive cystic lesions, both in the trigone and in the centrum semiovale were noted in only 2.7% of all the infants. We feel that this distinction is of significance, in relation to later outcome (see later). An incidence of periventricular infarction of 48% was reported by Nwaesei et al (1984) who studied those infants who died beyond 21 days of life.

SUBCORTICAL LEUKOMALACIA

Cystic lesions have also been observed to develop further away from the lateral ventricles in the subcortical white matter as shown in Figure 29.9 (Pfister-Goedeke & Boltshauser 1982, De Vries & Dubowitz 1985, Trounce & Levene 1985).

Table 29.1 Incidence of ultrasound diagnosed periventricular leukomalacia (PVL) from seven studies

Author	Incidence (%)	Group selection
Levene et al 1983	7.5	<1500 g
Bozynski et al 1985a	5	<1201 g
Weindling et al 1985	8	<1500 g or 34 wks
Fawer et al 1985a	16.8	<34 wks
Sinha et al 1985	17.8	<33 wks
Trounce et al 1986a	26*	<1501 g
Calvert et al 1986	2.3	<1501 g

* This figure refers to both cystic PVL (12.5%) and prolonged flare (13.5%) added together.

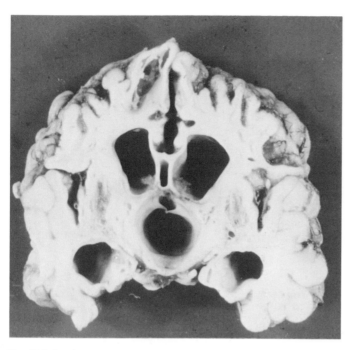

Fig. 29.9 Cystic subcortical leukomalacia. There is an irregular cavity in the subcortical region on the left side.

These cystic lesions have also been described as multicystic encephalopathy or included in studies describing infants with PVL (Pfister-Goedeke & Boltshauser 1982). The term subcortical leukomalacia was again introduced by Banker & Larroche (1962) who described this condition in 2 full-term infants who formed part of the cohort of 51 infants diagnosed as having leukomalacia at autopsy. The appearance of these cystic lesions was first shown during life using pneumo-encephalography, by Taboada et al (1980), who found rounded dilated lateral and third ventricles in 9 microcephalic infants. In an attempt to explain the apparent conservation of the thickness of the cerebral parenchyma they performed pneumo-encephalographic studies, needling the anterior fontanelle. Using this method they were able to show separate subcortical cysts. CT scans of these infants merely showed areas of decreased attenuation and dilatation of the ventricles.

Pathophysiology

The progression of arterial development in the immature brain is in a continual state of remodelling during fetal life and through the first few months after birth. In the early part of the third trimester PVL occurs in the watershed region of the periventricular white matter and further development provides secure anastomoses within this region. During this time the brain is relatively smooth with shallow sulci and a rich leptomeningeal vascular supply to the cortical and subcortical regions. Elegant studies by Takashima et al (1978) have shown how further cerebral development exposes the subcortical region to ischaemic

injury. In conjunction with the disappearance of the primitive vascular supply to the subcortex, the sulci deepen and the vascular supplies to cortical and subcortical areas extend deeper towards the lateral ventricles. This leaves a new triangular watershed area of white matter at the depth of the sulci exposed to the effects of ischaemia (Fig. 29.10). With further development of the arterial bed, new vessels will grow in to supply this region, thereby reducing its vulnerability. Regional differences in energy metabolism during brain maturation have also been suggested as a causative mechanism for leukomalacia (Farkas-Bargeton & Diebler 1978) and the regional differences in cerebral metabolism at different gestational ages can now be studied further with the use of positron emission tomography (Chugani & Phelps 1986).

Ultrasonography can show the evolution of subcortical leukomalacia non-invasively, as was first described by Pfister-Goedeke & Boltshauser (1982). The evolution of the ultrasound changes is described fully in Chapter 9. The cysts occur within 2–3 weeks following the insult and tend to be larger in diameter than in the infants with PVL (Fig. 29.11). The cysts are noted to persist far beyond 40 weeks postmenstrual age and can be recognized by ultrasonography as long as the fontanelle permits this form of examination to be performed.

Other techniques such as visual evoked responses (VERs) and continuous EEG recordings have made us aware of the severity of subcortical lesions compared with periventricular lesions (De Vries et al in press). VERs performed at 40 weeks of postmenstrual age were absent in infants with subcortical lesions while they were present in those with periventricular lesions (see Ch. 16). EEG recordings were severely abnormal in the acute stages and abnormalities were still present at 40 weeks in infants with

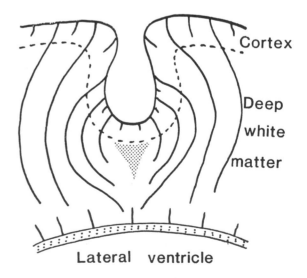

Fig. 29.10 A coronal section through cortex, white matter and lateral ventricle. There is a watershed area of subcortical white matter (stippled) exposed to ischaemic injury. (Redrawn from Takashima et al 1978.)

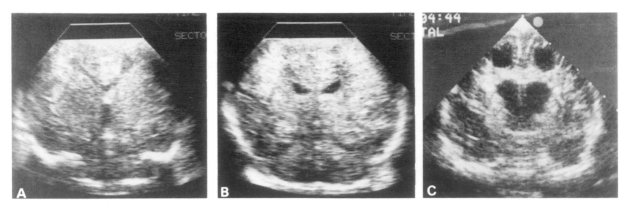

Fig. 29.11 Evolution of subcortical leukomalacia on ultrasound scans: (**a**) coronal scan showing a 'fuzzy' brain with slit-like ventricles; (**b**) same infant 5 days later showing increased echodensity around the lateral ventricles; (**c**) scan at 7 months of age showing multiple subcortical cysts and ventricular dilatation.

subcortical leukomalacia (SCL), while abnormalities seen in the infants with PVL were only present in the acute phase with complete recovery at 40 weeks of postmenstrual age in most infants (see Ch. 13).

Risk factors

So far, little work has been carried out to identify the risk factors for leukomalacia. The number of infants reported in most original studies was too small to draw any valid conclusions. Weindling et al (1985a) stressed that 4 of their 8 infants with PVL had a history of antepartum haemorrhage (APH). APH was also common among infants studied by Calvert et al (1986) who found APH or placental abruption in 6 of 15 cases. Sinha et al (1985) were the first to study a cohort of infants to identify factors related to ischaemic lesions. They found birth asphyxia, antepartum haemorrhage, recurrent apnoea and septicaemia, all strongly associated with the presence of PVL, and pointed out that all these factors are associated with hypotension. Trounce et al (1987) also looked at a large cohort of premature infants. They were unable to identify hypotension as an independent risk factor, despite continuous recording of the arterial blood pressure in many of the high-risk infants. Hypercarbia, pneumothorax, surgery and hyperbilirubinaemia were identified as independent risk factors. They were further able to show that immaturity was closely related to GMH–IVH but there was no such relationship with PVL. Risk factors for PVL appear to be much more multifactorial than has been reported for GMH-IVH. A wide variety of different risk factors can be found in infants with extensive cystic lesions. A total of 22 infants with extensive cystic lesions were studied at the Hammersmith Hospital between 1982 and 1986. A history of pre-eclamptic toxaemia (PET) was present in 4 of the 12 infants with PVL. In the 8 infants with cysts extending into the subcortical white matter, 4 had a history of antepartum haemorrhage (APH), 4 of severe birth asphyxia (2 associated with APH); 3 developed necrotizing

enterocolitis (NEC), 1 in association with a Gram-negative septicaemia. These risk factors are summarized in Fig. 29.12. The insults suffered seemed to be more obvious among those infants with subcortical cysts than in those with only periventricular lesions. No obvious cause could be related to the development of PVL in 2 infants and 3 other infants had moderate respiratory distress syndrome (RDS) requiring ventilation but without any further recognized complications.

In contrast to previous authors, we noted a significant difference in gestational age between infants with PVL and those with SCL. In the cohort studied at the Hammersmith Hospital, periventricular lesions were only seen in premature infants (28–31 weeks of gestation), while subcortical cysts occurred either in more mature infants or in pre-term infants who suffered an insult several weeks after birth (33–38 weeks of postmenstrual age). This difference would fit in with the cerebral angiography studies performed by Takashima et al (1978) discussed earlier. Our findings therefore suggest that a premature infant (28–31 weeks) would be especially at risk of developing PVL, while those infants above 32 weeks of gestation are more

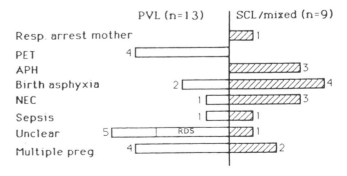

Fig. 29.12 Comparison of risk factors of infants with periventricular leukomalacia (PVL) and with subcortical leukomalacia (SCL). PET = pre-eclamptic toxaemia, APH = antepartum haemorrhage and NEC = necrotizing enterocolitis.

prone to developing cysts extending into the subcortical white matter.

Another potentially important risk factor for the infant is being one of a multiple pregnancy. Of 22 infants with extensive cystic lesions seen at Hammersmith Hospital, 7 were of multiple pregnancies. Of the 7 infants, 2 were one of triplets. Infants who are part of multiple pregnancies are already compromised in utero and therefore may be more susceptible to subsequent insult in the neonatal period (see Ch. 30).

Outcome

Several follow-up studies have been reported relating neurodevelopmental outcome to the presence of intracranial haemorrhages as diagnosed by CT or ultrasonography (Thorburn et al 1981, Catto-Smith et al 1985). Most of these studies were performed with linear array equipment utilizing a 5 or a 3.5 MHz transducer. These studies suggested that the size of the haemorrhages and the presence of ventricular dilatation were of prognostic significance (Palmer et al 1982, Stewart et al 1983). Catto-Smith et al (1985) and McMenamin et al (1984) noted that the presence of large intraparenchymal lesions carried a poor prognosis. These studies, however, were performed before the ultrasound diagnosis of PVL was commonly made. It is therefore likely that cases of PVL were missed or that densities seen in the acute phase were interpreted as parenchymal haemorrhages. Stewart et al (1983) stressed the predictive value of cerebral atrophy, diagnosed when irregular ventricular dilatation was noted in association with normal or delayed head growth. They assumed this to be due to ischaemia and cerebral infarction. De Vries et al (1985) compared the neurodevelopmental outcome of infants with a large intraventricular and/or intraparenchymal haemorrhage with infants who developed extensive cystic leukomalacia. They noted that 43% of the infants with large haemorrhages were normal, compared with none of those with extensive cystic lesions. Infants who developed a porencephalic cyst following a parenchymal haemorrhage developed hemiplegia but all had a normal intellect. Of 23 infants with large haemorrhages only 3 were severely handicapped with quadriplegia and severe mental retardation. These 3 infants also showed associated ischaemic lesions on their ultrasound scans. The presence of ischaemic lesions was thus of more predictive value than the size of the haemorrhage.

Neurodevelopmental outcomes of 82 infants with extensive cystic lesions who have so far been reported in the literature show a much more uniform picture (Bowerman et al 1984, Bozynski et al 1985, Weindling et al 1985b, Calvert et al 1986, Fawer et al 1987). Most infants have developed cerebral palsy, with or without associated seizures, visual and auditory impairment and a variable degree of mental retardation. Graziani et al (1986) reported 3 infants with

diffuse cystic lesions who were normal at follow-up. Fawer et al (1985b) have reported 6 infants who either developed transient dystonia (3) or were completely normal following the ultrasound diagnosis of cystic leukomalacia. The cysts, however, were small in size and restricted to the external angle of the lateral ventricle. It seems therefore important to make a distinction between extensive cystic lesions which usually occur throughout both hemispheres and infants who develop a few small cysts, usually unilateral and restricted to the external angle of the lateral ventricle (Fawer et al 1987).

No distinction has been made so far between infants with periventricular lesions and those with subcortical lesions. Trounce & Levene (1985) and De Vries & Dubowitz (1985) noted a marked difference between the outcome in infants with periventricular lesions and those with subcortical lesions. A total of 22 infants have been diagnosed as having extensive cystic lesions at the Hammersmith Hospital between 1982 and 1986 (De Vries et al in press). Of these, 16 have survived and are now 9 months of chronological age or more (Fig. 29.13). Neurological examination at 40 weeks of postmenstrual age showed severe abnormalities, such as marked irritability, increased tone and abnormal finger and toe posture (see Ch. 3). It was, at this stage, not possible to make a distinction between infants with periventricular cysts and those with subcortical cysts. Eight infants with PVL are now between 9 months and 3 years of age and 6 of these have developed spastic diplegia with mild to moderate mental retardation. All these developed a marked squint but maintained their vision. The 2 remaining infants developed hypsarrythmia at 6 months of age and were subsequently noted to develop quadriplegia. This more severe course may be related to the development of the hypsarrythmia. The 8 infants who had subcortical lesions (SCL) or both subcortical and periventricular cysts (mixed) had an even worse outcome. They developed quadriplegia and severe mental retardation. Six were cortically blind and one has very poor vision at 13 months of age. Three infants have associated seizure activity. The DQ was below 50 in all these

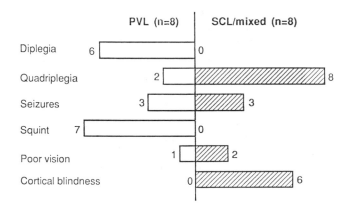

Fig. 29.13 Neurodevelopmental outcome of periventricular and subcortical leukomalacias (PVL and SCL) in relation to the distribution of the cystic lesions.

infants. This marked difference in later outcome fitted in well with magnetic resonance imaging findings, performed later in the first year of life. Infants with PVL showed delayed myelination, especially around the irregularly dilated occipital horns. Subsequent scans did, however, show progression of myelination (Fig. 29.14). The children with subcortical lesions, however, showed persistence of the cystic lesions and little or no myelination. There was also evidence of marked cortical atrophy indicating that the initial lesions were much more extensive than could be visualized by ultrasonography in the neonatal period. At follow-up very little if any progression of myelination was noted (Fig. 29.15).

The outcome of the infants with flares has so far only been reported by McMenamin et al (1984). They were able to study 32 infants with small intraparenchymal echodensities (IPE), which were bilateral in 50% of the cases. Of the infants, 22 survived and complete resolution was noted in 19, while small cysts were noted in the other 3: 14 infants had a normal outcome, 6 showed mild deficits, 2 moderate and none was severely handicapped. A total of 59 infants with periventricular densities were studied at the Hammersmith Hospital over a 2-year period. Transient dystonia was noted in 49% of the infants, and 4 infants developed spastic diplegia. The incidence of dystonia was significantly higher than in the controls, born during the same period, but without any ultrasound abnormalities

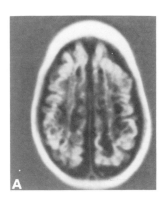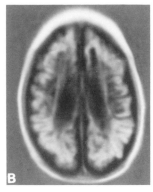

Fig. 29.15 Magnetic resonance imaging scans of an infant with subcortical leukomalacia (same child as illustrated in Fig. 29.11). (a) Inversion recovery at midventricular level (6 months corrected age) showing multiple subcortical cysts. No myelination is seen. (b) Same child at 12 months at a higher level. The cysts remain visible with still no evidence of myelination.

(8.6%). Preliminary follow-up data from Leicester shows that the risk of cerebral palsy is higher in infants with prolonged flare but not as high as those with cavitating PVL.

These studies would imply that flares or non-cavitating parenchymal densities are less predictive but they should not be disregarded as they probably represent mild periventricular leukomalacia.

CEREBRAL ARTERY INFARCTION

Infarction of a major artery or a branch arising from it is now recognized in an increasing number of newborn infants. Bleeding into an infarcted area occurs relatively often and we believe that many infants previously thought to have had 'primary parenchymal haemorrhage' have in fact sustained neonatal 'stroke' with secondary haemorrhage. Knowledge of this condition and use of appropriate imaging techniques should allow their differentiation.

Cerebral infarction in the neonate has been defined as a severe disorganization or even complete disruption of both grey and white matter caused by embolic, thrombotic or ischaemic events (Barmada et al 1979). Friede (1975) has reviewed the earlier pathology literature on this condition and described 5 cases of his own. These were all wedge-shaped haemorrhagic lesions involving cortical, subcortical and deep periventricular white matter. Friede (1975) could only positively identify these lesions as infarctive histologically.

Larroche (1977) described the pathological appearance of cerebral artery infarction in 6 cases. In those infants dying in the acute stage of the condition, the hemisphere was swollen and deeply congested. There was involvement of both white matter and cortex, with secondary haemorrhagic infarction in some cases (Fig. 29.16). In those infants who survived for longer, contraction of the affected area was seen with softening and multiple cystic degeneration giving

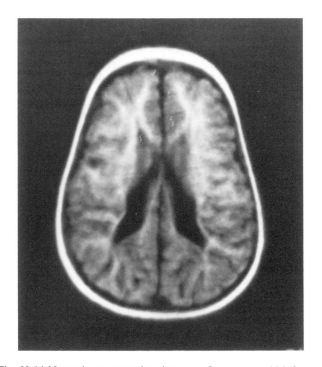

Fig. 29.14 Magnetic resonance imaging scan of a one-year-old infant who, during the neonatal period had developed cystic periventricular leukomalacia (PVL) in the occipital region. The inversion recovery scan at midventricular level shows delay in myelination, particularly around the irregularly dilated occipital horns.

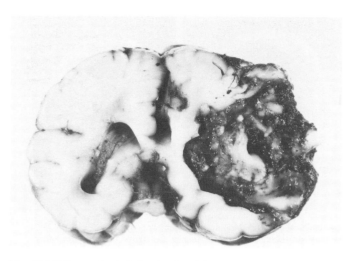

Fig. 29.16 Haemorrhagic infarction involving cortex and white matter in the distribution of the middle cerebral artery. The infant had received an exchange transfusion and the infarction may have been due to an embolus during this procedure.

a honeycomb appearance on sectioning. The extent of the atrophic process was thought to reflect the level of arterial infarction. In some cases, infarction occurred very early in fetal life and these brains showed extensive porencephalic cyst formation. This is discussed in more detail in Chapter 30. Barmada et al (1979) reported cerebral infarction in over 5% of infants examined at autopsy. This incidence is unusual in our experience and may reflect a particularly high-risk population.

Aetiology

Stroke in the newborn does not appear to be the same condition as is seen in older children and adults. In children the most common cause of stroke is haemorrhage (either arterio–venous malformation, aneurysm or tumour) and arterial occlusion less frequently (Eeg-Olofsson & Ringheim 1983). Haemorrhagic stroke is virtually unrecorded in the newborn, although venous infarction due to sinus thrombosis is well recognized but less frequently seen at autopsy than cerebral artery occlusion.

The causes of neonatal stroke fall into three groups: embolization, thrombosis and ischaemia (Mannino & Trauner 1983). Embolic causes are the most commonly reported (Barmada et al 1979) and twin-to-twin transfusion as well as congenital heart disease is well recognized. Emboli from a patent ductus arteriosus or the placenta (Cocker et al 1965) have also been reported. Temporal artery catheterization has been related to ipsilateral cerebral infarction (Bull et al 1980) and disseminated intravascular coagulation and sepsis have also been associated with the development of thrombotic arterial infarction. Clancy et al (1985) report that asphyxia and polycythaemia were additional important predisposing factors and described one infant who had sustained severe and prolonged hypertension before the stroke. Maternal cocaine abuse has been considered to cause stroke in one affected infant (Chasnoff et al 1986).

Although neonatal stroke is most commonly seen in full-term infants it has been reported at autopsy in premature neonates (Barmada et al 1979). The diagnosis of arterial infarction made by imaging techniques in premature infants must be made with caution as other conditions such as periventricular leukomalacia can give the appearances reported to be the result of cerebral infarction by Ment et al (1984).

The introduction of modern imaging techniques has confirmed the pathologist's impression that neonatal stroke occurs commonly. A total of 69 cases have been reported where the diagnosis was made in life (Billard et al 1982, Hill et al 1983, Mannino & Trauner 1983, Voorhies et al 1984, Mantovani & Gerber 1984, Ment et al 1984, Nanni et al 1984, Clancy et al 1985, Levy et al 1985, Chasnoff et al 1986, Trauner & Mannino 1986, Levene 1987). Lesions involving the left hemisphere are three to four times more common than those of the right hemisphere. Middle cerebral artery infarction occurs twice as commonly as involvement of any other artery. The anterior cerebral artery is rarely recognized to be affected but this may reflect the silent nature of symptoms related to involvement of this vessel. We estimate the incidence of 'neonatal stroke' to be one in 5000 full-term infants (Levene 1987).

Diagnosis

Acute onset of seizures is the most common presenting feature. Billard et al (1982) reported onset of fits between 8 and 60 hours after birth in all 8 of their cases and fits occurred in 10 of 11 reported by Clancy et al (1985). Among infants presenting with seizures, cerebral infarction is recognized to be an important cause (Levene & Trounce 1986, Levy et al 1985). The convulsions are usually of the focal clonic variety but multifocal tonic or subtle seizures may all be seen. Many of the infants show no major clinical neurological abnormality between seizures. Infants with middle cerebral artery infarction often show marked asymmetry between the two sides which may persist to appear as a hemiparesis in the older child. Infants with posterior cerebral artery infarction may develop abnormal eye signs which later can be shown to be due to homonymous hemianopia.

Ultrasound diagnosis is possible but this modality is unreliable. If haemorrhagic infarction is present the focal increased echodensity is obvious but Hill et al (1983) have reported increased echoes from non-haemorrhagic infarcted areas. Sometimes extensive stroke may show relatively subtle changes on ultrasound. For this reason CT is of more value but a normal scan within 48 hours of birth does not exclude this condition. At least two scans over one week are necessary before the condition can be excluded. The classical appearance is a wedge-shaped area of low attenuation with irregular margins. If bleeding occurs into the infarcted region, areas of high attenuation may be seen on CT scan examination (Fig. 29.17a). Rescanning some months later shows full-thickness loss of cerebral tissue in the same distribution (Fig. 29.17b). A mass effect may be seen due to severe oedema surrounding the infarcted area. Later scans may reveal multifocal cavity formation. It has been reported that complete occlusion of the common or internal carotid arteries may be associated with no focal abnormalities on the CT (Voorhies et al 1984). The infants described in this study had all suffered very severe perinatal asphyxia and are not typical of most infants with cerebral artery infarction.

Radionuclide brain scanning is also of value in diagnosing cerebral artery infarction and is particularly useful if there is marked oedema around the infarcted lesion. Gamma-emitting technetium is retained only in areas of damaged blood–brain barrier and thus will delineate the area of vascular damage (Fig. 29.18). O'Brien et al (1979) performed technetium scans on 85 asphyxiated full-term infants and found uptake in the region of the middle cerebral artery in 20% of cases. It has been reported that technetium brain scans may be negative in the first week following cerebral infarction (Harwood-Nash & Fitz 1976).

Electro-encephalography has also been used in the diagnosis of neonatal stroke (Billard et al 1982, Mantovani & Gerber 1984, Clancy et al 1985, Levy et al 1985). This investigation revealed focal abnormalities in almost all patients. These included persistent localized voltage reduction, focal slowing, sharp waves and focal seizure activity.

Cerebral arteriography is a highly invasive procedure in infancy and is unnecessary in most cases. Less invasive

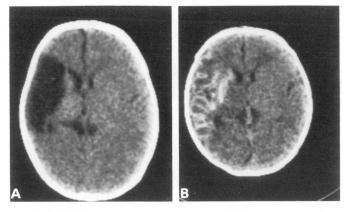

Fig. 29.17 Middle cerebral artery infarction. (a) CT scan at one week showing some increased attenuation in the region of the right middle cerebral artery, probably due to secondary haemorrhage. (b) Same patient 9 months later showing large porencephalic cavity in the region of the previous infarct.

digital intravenous angiography has been used in the diagnosis of neonatal occlusive vascular disease (Voorhies et al 1984). Contrast medium is injected via an umbilical venous catheter which has been advanced to lie near the right atrium. This technique, although relatively safe, is probably not necessary as surgical treatment to remove an embolus is not feasible.

Prognosis

The outlook in most cases is relatively good. Intellectual development is usually normal but spastic hemiplegia is the most important sequel, particularly following infarction of the middle cerebral artery. Homonymous hemianopia

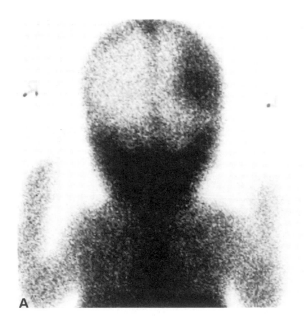
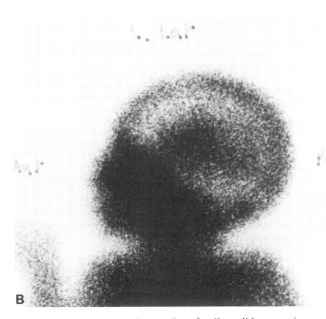

Fig. 29.18 Radionuclide technetium scan of an infant with middle cerebral artery infarction. There is retention of radionuclide tracer (arrowed) in the region supplied by the left middle cerebral artery on coronal (a) and sagittal (b) planes.

may follow posterior cerebral artery infarction. Published follow-up data from case reports suggest that over half of all infants surviving neonatal stroke are entirely normal at 12–18 months of age. Trauner & Mannino (1986) found that 8 out of 10 infants with neonatal cerebral infarction were normal at 2–5 years. The 2 children in whom neurological deficits were found were only mildly affected.

The overall prevalence of cerebral palsy is approximately one in 2000 children. On the basis of the estimated incidence of perinatal cerebral vascular infarction it might be expected that this condition is the cause of the neurological deficit in 20% of children with cerebral palsy (Levene 1987).

REFERENCES

Abramovicz A 1964 The pathogenesis of perinatal brain damage and their conditions of occurrence in primates. Advances in Neurology 27: 85–95

Armstrong D, Norman M G 1974 Periventricular leukomalacia in neonates: complications and sequelae. Archives of Disease in Childhood 49: 367–375

Banker B Q, Larroche J-C 1962 Periventricular leukomalacia of infancy: a form of neonatal anoxic encephalopathy. Archives of Neurology 7: 386–410

Barmada M A, Moossy J, Shuman R M 1979 Cerebral infarcts with arterial occlusion in neonates. Annals of Neurology 6: 495–502

Barth P G 1984 Prenatal clastic encephalopathies. Clinical Neurology and Neurosurgery 86: 65–75

Billard C, Dulac O, Diebler R 1982 Ramollissement cerebral ischemique du nouveau-ne: une etiologie possible des etats de mal convulsifs neonatals. Archives Francaises de Pediatrie 39: 677–683

Bowerman R A, Donn S M, DiPietro M A, D'Amato C J, Hicks S P 1984 Periventricular leukomalacia in the preterm infant: sonographic and clinical features. Radiology 151: 383–388

Bozynski M E, Nelson M N, Matalon T A S, Genaze D R, Rosati-Skertich C, Naughton P M, Meier W A 1985 Cavitary periventricular leukomalacia: incidence and short term outcome in infants weighing <1200 grams at birth. Developmental Medicine and Child Neurology 27: 572–577

Bull M J, Schreiner R L, Garg B P, Hutton N M, Lemons J A, Gresham E L 1980 Neurologic complications following temporal artery catheterization. Journal of Pediatrics 96: 1071–1073

Calvert S A, Hoskins E M, Fong K W, Forsyth S C 1986 Periventricular leukomalacia: ultrasonic diagnosis and neurological outcome. Acta Paediatrica Scandinavica 75: 489–496

Catto-Smith A G, Yu V Y H, Bajuk B, Orgill A A, Astbury J 1985 Effect of neonatal periventricular haemorrhage on neurodevelopmental outcome. Archives of Disease in Childhood 60: 8–11

Cavazutti M, Duffy T E 1982 Regulation of cerebral blood flow in normal and hypoxic newborn dogs. Annals of Neurology 11: 247–257

Chasnoff I J, Bussey M E, Savich R, Stack C M 1986 Perinatal cerebral infarction and maternal cocaine use. Journal of Pediatrics 108: 456–459

Chow P P, Morgan J G, Taylor K J W 1985 Neonatal periventricular leukomalacia: a real-time sonographic diagnosis with CT correlation. American Journal of Radiology 145: 155–160

Chugani H T, Phelps M E 1986 Maturational changes in cerebral function in infants determined by 18FDG positron emission tomography. Science 231: 840–843

Clancy R, Malin S, Laraque D, Baumgart S, Younkin D 1985 Focal motor seizures heralding stroke in fullterm neonates. American Journal of Diseases in Childhood 139: 601–606

Cocker J, George S W, Yates P O 1965 Perinatal occlusion of the middle cerebral artery. Developmental Medicine and Child Neurology 7: 235–243

Cowan F 1986 Indomathacin, patent ductus arteriosus, and cerebral blood flow. Journal of Pediatrics 109: 341–344

Delaporte B, Labrune M, Imbert M C, Dahan M 1985 Early echographic findings in non-haemorrhagic periventricular leukomalacia in the premature infant. Pediatric Radiology 15: 82–84

De Reuck J, Cattha A S, Richardson E P 1972 Pathogenesis and evolution of leukomalacia in infancy. Archives of Neurology 27: 229–236

De Vries L S, Dubowitz L M S 1985 Cystic leukomalacia in preterm infants: site of lesion in relation to prognosis. Lancet ii: 1075–1076

De Vries L S, Dubowitz L M S, Dubowitz V, Kaiser A, Lary S, Silverman M, Whitelaw A, Wigglesworth J W S 1985 Predictive value of cranial ultrasound: a reappraisal. Lancet ii: 137–140

De Vries L S, Regev R, Dubowitz L M S 1986 Late onset cystic leukomalacia. Archives of Disease in Childhood 61: 298–299

De Vries L S, Connell J C, Pennock J M, Oozeer R C, Dubowitz L M S, Dubowitz V Neurological, electrophysiological and MRI abnormalities in infants with extensive cystic leukomalacia. Neuropediatrics (in press)

DiPietro M A, Brody B A, Teele R L 1986 Peritrigonal echogenic 'blush' on cranial sonography: pathologic correlates. American Journal of Radiology 146: 1067–1072

Dolfin T, Skidmore M B, Fong K W, Hoskins E M, Shennan A T, Hill A 1984 Diagnosis and evolution of periventricular leukomalacia a study with real-time ultrasound. Early Human Development 9: 105–109

Eeg-Olofsson O, Ringheim Y 1983 Stroke in children: clinical characteristics and prognosis. Acta Paediatrica Scandinavica 72: 391–395

Evans D M, Levene M I, Archer L N J 1987 The effect of indomethain on cerebral blood-flow velocity in premature infants. Developmental Medicine and Child Neurology 29: 776–782

Farkas-Bargeton E, Diebler M F 1978 A topographical study of enzyme maturation in human cerebral neocortex: a histochemical and biochemical study. Architectonics of the cerebral cortex. Raven Press, New York

Fawer C-L, Calame A, Anderegg A 1984 Real-time ultrasonography in the neonate: a systematic study of high risk infant population. Helvetica Acta Paediatrica 39: 34–45

Fawer C-L, Calame A, Perentes E, Anderegg A 1985a Periventricular leukomalacia: a correlation study between real-time ultrasound and autopsy findings. Neuroradiology 27: 292–300

Fawer C-L, Calame A, Furrer M-T 1985b Neurodevelopmental outcome at 12 months of age, related to cerebral ultrasound appearances of high risk preterm infants. Early Human Development 11: 123–132

Fawer C-L, Diebold P, Calame A 1987 Periventricular leukomalacia and neurodevelopmental outcome in preterm infants. Archives of Disease in Childhood 62: 30–36

Friede R 1975 Developmental neuropathology. Springer, Vienna

Gilles F H, Leviton A, Kerr C S 1976 Endotoxin leukoencephalopathy in the telencephalon of the newborn kitten. Journal of the Neurological Sciences 27: 183–191

Graziani L J, Pasto M, Stanley C et al 1986 Neonatal neurosonographic correlates of cerebral palsy in preterm infants. Paediatrics 78: 88–95

Guzzetta F, Shackelford G D, Volpe S, Perlman J M, Volpe J J 1986 Periventricular intraparenchymal echodensities in the premature newborn: critical determinant of neurologic outcome. Pediatrics 78: 995–1006

Hamilton P A, Hope P L, Cady F B, Delpy D T, Wyatt J S, Reynolds E O R 1986 Impaired energy metabolism in brains of newborn infants with increased cerebral echodensities. Lancet i: 1242–1246

Harwood-Nash D C, Fitz C R 1976 Neuroradiology in infants and children. CV Mosby Publications, St Louis

Hill A, Martin D J, Danemann A, Fitz C R 1983 Focal ischaemic cerebral injury in the newborn: diagnosis by ultrasound and correlation with computed tomographic scans. Pediatrics 71: 790–793

Larroche J-C 1977 Developmental pathology of the neonate. Excerpta Medica, Amsterdam

Larroche J-C 1986 Fetal encephalopathies of circulatory origin. Biology of the Neonate 50: 61–74

Larroche J-C, Bethmann O, Beadoin M, Couhard M 1986 Brain damage in the premature infant: early lesions and new aspects of sequelae. Italian Journal of Neurological Sciences (Suppl) 5: 43–52

Leech R W, Atvord E C 1974 Morphologic variation in periventricular leukomalacia. American Journal of Pathology 74: 591–600

Levene M I 1987 Neonatal neurology. Churchill Livingstone, Edinburgh

Levene M I, Trounce J Q 1986 Cause of neonatal convulsions: towards more precise diagnosis. Archives of Disease in Childhood 61: 78–79

Levene M I, Wigglesworth J S, Dubowitz V 1983 Hemorrhagic periventricular leukomalacia: a real-time ultrasound study. Pediatrics 71: 794–797

Levy S R, Abrams I F, Marshall P C, Rosquette E E 1985 Seizures and cerebral infarction in the full-term newborn. Annals of Neurology 17: 366–370

Lou H C, Lassen N A, Friis-Hansen B 1979 Impaired autoregulation of cerebral blood flow in the distressed newborn infant. Journal of Pediatrics 94: 118–121

McMenamin J B, Shackelford G D, Volpe J J 1984 Outcome of neonatal IVH with periventricular echodense lesions. Annals of Neurology 15: 285–290

Mannino F L, Trauner D A 1983 Stroke in neonates. Journal of Pediatrics 102: 605–610

Mantovani J F, Gerber G J 1984 'Idiopathic' neonatal cerebral infarction. American Journal of Diseases of Children 138: 359–362

Martin D J, Hill A, Fitz C R, Daneman A, Havill D A, Becker L E 1983 Hypoxic/ischaemic cerebral injury in the neonatal brain: a report of sonographic features with computed tomographic correlation. Pediatric Radiology 13: 307–312

Ment L R, Duncan C C, Ehrenkrantz R A 1984 Perinatal cerebral infarction. Annals of Neurology 16: 559–568

Ment L R, Stewart W B, Duncan C C, Pitt B R, Rescigno A, Cole J 1985a Beagle puppy model of perinatal cerebral infarction: acute changes in cerebral blood flow and metabolism during hemorrhagic hypotension. Journal of Neurosurgery 63: 441–447

Ment L R, Stewart W B, Duncan C C, Cole J, Pitt B R 1985b Beagle puppy model of perinatal cerebral infarction: acute changes in cerebral prostaglandins during hemorrhagic hypotension. Journal of Neurosurgery 63: 899–904

Nanni G S, Kaude J V, Reeder J D 1984 Ischemic brain infarct in a neonate: ultrasound diagnosis and follow-up. Journal of Clinical Ultrasound 12: 229–231

Nwaesei C G, Pape K E, Martin D J, Becker L E, Fitz C R 1984 Periventricular infarction diagnosed by ultrasound: a postmortem correlation. Journal of Pediatrics 105: 106–110

O'Brien M J, Ash J M, Gilday D L 1979 Radionucleide brain scanning in perinatal hypoxia. Developmental Medicine and Child Neurology 21: 161–168

Palmer P, Dubowitz L M S, Levene M I, Dubowitz V 1982 Developmental and neurological progress of preterm infants with intraventricular haemorrhage and ventricular dilatation. Archives of Disease in Childhood 57: 748–753

Pape K E, Wigglesworth J S 1979 Haemorrhage, ischaemia and the perinatal brain. Clinics in Developmental Medicine, No. 69/70. Spastics International Medicine Publications, Heinemann, London

Parrot J 1873 Etude sur la ramollisement de l'encephale chez la nouveau-ne. Arch Physiol Norm Pathol 5: 59–73, 176–195, 283–330

Partridge J C, Babcock D S, Steichen J J, Bokyung K H 1983 Optimal timing for diagnostic ultrasound in low birth weight infants for detection of intracranial haemorrhage and ventricular dilatation. Journal of Pediatrics 102: 281–287

Perlman J M, Volpe J J 1985 Episodes of apnea and bradycardia in the preterm newborn: impact on cerebral circulation. Pediatrics 76: 333–338

Perlman J M, Goodman S, Kreussen K L, Volpe J J 1985 Reduction of intraventricular hemorrhage by elimination of fluctuating cerebral blood flow velocity in preterm infants with respiratory distress syndrome. New England Journal of Medicine 312: 1353–1357

Pfister-Goedeke L, Boltshauser E 1982 Postnatale Entwicklung einer multilokularen zystischen Encephalopathie beim Neugeborenen. Helvetica Paediatrica Acta 37: 59–65

Rushton D I, Preston P R, Durbin G M 1985 Structure and evolution of echodense lesions in the neonatal brain. Archives of Disease in Childhood 60: 798–808

Shuman R M, Selednik L J 1980 Periventricular leukomalacia: a one year autopsy study. Archives of Neurology 37: 231–235

Sinha S K, Davies J M, Sims D G, Chiswick M L 1985 Relation between periventricular haemorrhage and ischaemic brain lesions diagnosed by ultrasound in very preterm infants. Lancet ii: 1154–1155

Stewart A L, Thorburn R J, Hope P L, Goldsmith M, Lipscomb A P, Reynolds E O R 1983 Ultrasound appearance of the brain in very preterm infants and neurodevelopmental outcome at 18 months of age. Archives of Disease in Childhood 58: 598–604

Taboada D, Alonso A, Olague R, Mulas F, Andres V 1980 Radiological diagnosis of periventricular and subcortical leukomalacia. Neuroradiology 20: 33–41

Takashima J, Tanaka K 1978 Development of cerebral architecture and its relationship to periventricular leukomalacia. Archives of Neurology 35: 11–16

Takashima J, Armstrong D, Becker L E 1978 Subcortical leukomalacia: relationship to development of the cerebral sulcus and its vascular supply. Archives of Neurology 35: 470–472

Thorburn R J, Lipscomb A P, Stewart A L, Reynolds E O R, Hope P L, Pape K E 1981 Prediction of death and major handicap in very preterm infants by brain ultrasound. Lancet i: 1119–1121

Trauner D A, Mannino F L 1986 Neurodevelopmental outcome after neonatal cerebrovascular incident. Journal of Pediatrics 108: 459–461

Trounce J Q, Levene M I 1985 Diagnosis and outcome of subcortical cystic leukomalacia. Archives of Disease in Childhood 60: 1041–1044

Trounce J Q, Rutter N, Levene M I 1986a Periventricular leucomalacia and intraventricular haemorrhage in the preterm neonate. Archives of Disease in Childhood 61: 1196–1202

Trounce J Q, Fagan D, Levene M I 1986b Intraventricular haemorrhage and periventricular leukomalacia: ultrasound and autopsy correlation. Archives of Disease in Childhood 62: 1203–1207

Trounce J Q, Shaw O E, Levene M I, Rutter N 1988 Clinical risk factors and periventricular leucomalacia. Archives of Disease in Childhood 63: 17–22

Van den Bergh R 1969 The periventricular intracerebral blood supply. In: Meyer J, Lechner H, Eichhorn O (eds) Research of the cerebral circulation. Ch Thomas, Springfield, pp 52–65

Virchow R 1867 Zur pathologishen Anatomie des Gehirns. I. congenitale Encephalitis und Myelitis. Virchows Archives 38: 129–142

Volpe J J, Herscovitch P, Perlman J M, Raichle M E 1983 PET in the newborn: extensive impairment of regional cerebral blood flow with intraventricular hemorrhage and hemorrhagic intracerebral involvement. Pediatrics 72: 589–601

Voorhies T M, Lipper E G, Lee B C P, Vanucci R C, Auld P A M 1984 Occlusive vascular disease in asphyxiated newborn infants. Journal of Pediatrics 105: 92–96

Weindling A M, Wilkinson A R, Cook J, Calvert S A, Fok T-F, Rochefort M J 1985a Perinatal events which precede periventricular haemorrhage and leukomalacia in the newborn. British Journal of Obstetrics and Gynaecology 92: 1218–1223

Weindling A M, Rochefort M J, Calvert S A, Fok T-F, Wilkinson A 1985b Development of cerebral palsy after sonographic detection of periventricular cysts in the newborn. Development Medicine and Child Neurology 27: 800–806

Young R S K, Hernandez M J, Yagel S K 1982 Selective reduction of blood flow to white matter during hypotension in newborn dogs: a possible mechanism of periventricular leukomalacia. Annals of Neurology 12: 445–448

30. Fetal encephalopathy of circulatory origin

Dr L.S. de Vries, Dr J-C. Larroche and
Dr M.I. Levene

The conditions described in the previous four chapters are not confined to the newborn and pathologists have described similar disorders in fetal brains for many years. More recently imaging techniques, particularly ultrasound, have made it possible to detect these lesions and in some cases to time their onset in relation to the development of complications in pregnancy. In addition the demonstration of ischaemic or haemorrhagic lesions immediately after birth has led many investigators to suggest, not unreasonably, that the origins of these conditions were in prenatal life and, depending on the scan appearances, possibly well before the onset of labour. Unfortunately, most descriptions are individual case reports or series from high-risk populations and little is known of the true prevalence of these conditions.

It is now clear that a wide variety of pathological conditions arise from circulatory impairment and may occur at any time during fetal development. The classification of these lesions may be based on their appearances or upon aetiological mechanisms. Larroche (1986) in a recent review has classified fetal encephalopathies of circulatory origin according to their circumstances or settings in which the lesions developed. This classification is summarized in Table 30.1 and falls into four main groups referring to the origin of the circulatory compromise: maternal, fetal, placental and an idiopathic group. It is of note that the

Table 30.1 A classification schema for the mechanisms causing circulatory disorders of the fetal brain

Maternal Conditions
  1. Systemic disorders
  2. Trauma
  3. Gas poisoning
  4. Coagulopathy

Fetal Conditions
  1. Multiple pregnancy
  2. Cerebral artery occlusion
  3. Coagulopathy

Complications of Placenta and Cord

Idiopathic

same insult at different times may lead to different types of lesion and morphologically identical lesions may be due to a variety of causes.

MATERNAL CONDITIONS

Systemic disorders

In the older pathology literature, multicystic encephalomalacia has been reported in children born to mothers who had suffered anaemia (Norman 1952), severe anoxia (Scharpe & Hale 1953), severe hypertensive pre-eclamptic toxaemia (Courville 1959) and renal disease complicated by seizures in the second trimester (Rizzuto & Martin 1967).

More recently ultrasound imaging has been used to show a close temporal relationship between maternal circulatory disturbances and the development of cerebral pathology in the fetus. Erasmus et al (1982) performed ultrasound examinations of a fetus one week after the mother had suffered an anaphylactoid reaction following a bee sting and showed an increase in fetal biparietal diameter. The child was born 5 weeks after this episode and died 4 weeks later. At autopsy, the brain was atrophic with numerous cavitations and old haemorrhages were present in both germinal matrices.

Severe respiratory failure requiring ventilatory support in a mother known to be 20 weeks pregnant has been shown to cause extensive multicystic lesions and hydrocephalus (Goodlin et al 1984). The fetus had a normal ultrasound scan one week before the mother's illness and 12 weeks later repeat scans showed extensive abnormalities, similar to those found at autopsy and described above. It is likely that the utero–placental and fetal circulations were impaired during the episode of maternal cardiovascular collapse. Fetal intraventricular haemorrhage has been diagnosed in utero by ultrasound following a series of maternal seizures in a 28-year-old epileptic woman (Minkoff et al 1985). It is recommended that careful ultrasound examination of the fetal brain be performed following any episode during pregnancy where maternal circulatory compromise may have occurred. This is particularly important if the mother has been mechanically ventilated before the elective delivery of her baby.

Maternal trauma

Direct trauma to the mother can lead to injury of the fetus. Both cephalohaematoma and subdural haemorrhage have been described following blunt trauma to the maternal abdomen (Grylack 1982, Amiel-Tison & Grenier 1985). A case of multicystic encephalomalacia following repeated kicking to the maternal abdomen in the first trimester in an attempt to induce abortion has been reported by Barth (1984) and a description of the 'battered fetus' with intraventricular haemorrhage has been reported by Morey et al (1981). Gunn & Becroft (1984) have subsequently reported 20 stillborn infants with unexplained intracranial haemorrhage (80% of which were subdural) but found no evidence for either direct or indirect trauma. Interestingly, all the infants were born to immigrant mothers from the Pacific Islands and these lesions were not seen in stillborn infants from other racial groups. There appears to be an, as yet, unrecognized factor associated with the development of subdural haemorrhages in this population.

Severe maternal traumas such as occur in automobile or aeroplane accidents have also been reported to cause fetal cerebral injury but it is often difficult to know whether the injury has been due to direct fetal trauma or subsequent maternal shock. Lesions reported in the fetus to be due to extensive maternal trauma include bilateral middle cerebral artery infarction (Coignet et al 1979), multicystic encephalomalacia (Ferrer & Navaro 1978) and hydranencephaly (Fowler et al 1971). Larroche (1986) has reported three cases of fetal cerebral injury following car accidents involving the mother but without obvious physical injury to her. In one case a healthy mother had three normal ultrasound scans before a car accident at 34 weeks of gestation. She was not physically injured but deeply stressed. At 37 weeks a subsequent scan showed dilated ventricles in an otherwise normal fetus. The infant, who was born shortly after the incident, died 7 minutes after birth and one hemisphere showed multicystic malacia and probable posthaemorrhagic hydrocephalus (Fig. 30.1). Another case of a low-velocity deceleration head-on car crash involving a 37-week pregnant woman demonstrated the vulnerability of the fetus (Chetcuti & Levene 1987). The mother was wearing a lap-sash seat belt and was admitted to hospital apparently uninjured but complaining of abdominal pain. The infant was delivered by caesarian section following the discovery of fetal bradycardia and he subsequently developed renal failure and postasphyxial encephalopathy with seizures. Extensive placental abruption was noted. In this case and others the effect of deceleration probably caused placental abruption with severe circulatory disturbance to the fetus resulting in cerebral ischaemic injury. A retrospective analysis from Melbourne (Pepperell et al

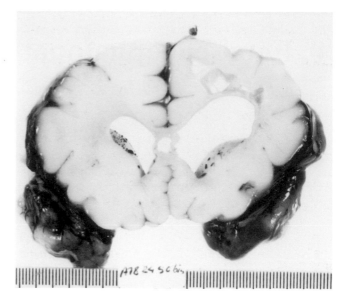

Fig. 30.1 Multicystic leukomalacia (right side) and posthaemorrhagic hydrocephalus (with a degree of cerebral atrophy) in the brain of a fetus whose mother sustained an automobile accident but who suffered no direct trauma. (Reproduced with permission from Larroche 1986.)

1977) examined the circumstances behind 27 fetal deaths from road traffic accidents involving women in the third trimester of pregnancy. Of the 14 who wore seat belts, 12 developed placental abruption. Of the 13 not wearing seat belts, only 2 had placental abruption although the maternal injuries were more severe in this group.

Myers (1975) has demonstrated that psychological stress to a pregnant monkey may cause anoxic–ischaemic brain injury to her fetus, and it is likely that similar lesions may occur in human newborn infants. Catecholamine release in response to the maternal stress may compromise placental perfusion and consequently damage the brain.

Gas poisoning

Maternal carbon monoxide poisoning has been reported to cause extensive cerebral injury in the fetus involving either grey or white matter (Beaudoing et al 1969). Ginsberg et al (1974) exposed juvenile monkeys to carbon monoxide inhalation and found the animals developed a bilateral symmetrical destructive leuko-encephalopathy but with relative sparing of the globus pallidus and hippocampus. The extent of the injury appeared to depend on the severity of metabolic acidosis and the degree of systemic hypotension during the carbon monoxide exposure. The physiological and biochemical factors underlying the difference in susceptibility between mother and fetus have been described in detail by Longo (1977) who noted in an animal model a slower washout of carbon monoxide from the fetus compared with the mother.

Butane gas poisoning in the mother at 30 weeks of gestation has been reported to cause multicystic encephalomalacia (Fig. 30.2) with severe damage to the brainstem and cerebellum of the fetus (Gosseye et al 1982). It is unlikely that the gas itself has a toxic effect but rather causes severe maternal and fetal hypoxia with consequent hypotension leading to extensive cerebral injury.

Maternal coagulopathy

A bleeding tendency in the mother may cause a clotting abnormality in her fetus. Maternal anticoagulants and idiopathic thrombocytopoenic purpura are the two most common forms of this disorder. Robinson et al (1980) reported a case of subdural haemorrhage in the fetus of a woman who had been anticoagulated with warfarin. A case has also been reported of parenchymal haemorrhage occurring in both occipital hemispheres in a fetus of a woman with idiopathic thrombocytopoenic purpura (Levene 1987).

FETAL CONDITIONS

Multiple pregnancy

Twins, particularly if monozygotic, appear to have a considerably higher risk of cerebral injury than the singleton fetus (Stevenson & McGowan 1942, Smith & Rodeck 1975, Melnick 1977, Schinzel et al 1979). Cerebral lesions reported in twins include multicystic encephalomalacia (Yoshioka et al 1979, Choulot et al 1982, Szymonowicz et al 1986), microcephaly (Durkin et al 1976, Schinzel et al 1979), porencephaly (Schinzel et al 1979, Jung et al 1984), hydranencephaly (Schinzel et al 1979, Jung et al 1984), cerebellar necrosis (Melnick 1977), periventricular

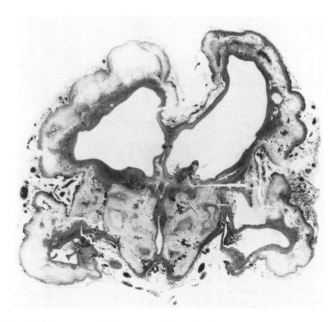

Fig. 30.2 Severe and diffuse encephalomalacia in the brain of a fetus whose mother had sustained butane gas intoxication. (Reproduced with permission from Larroche 1986.)

leukomalacia (Szymonowicz & Yu 1985) cerebral venous (Manterola et al 1966) and arterial infarction (Szymonowicz et al 1986). Szymonowicz et al (1986) have reviewed the literature and found 53 cases of a surviving monozygotic twin whose pair had died in utero and 72% had an abnormality of the central nervous system. Recently, cases have been reported where the diagnosis of cerebral injury was made in utero by ultrasound examination (Hughes & Miskin 1986, Szymonowicz et al 1986).

The incidence of single fetal demise in a twin pregnancy varies between 0.5% (Bernischke 1961) and 6.8% (Litschgi & Stucki 1980, Dudley & D'Alton 1986). The incidence of neurological sequelae in the surviving twin was reported to be 20% where the co-twin had died in utero (D'Alton et al 1984) but a more recent review of 14 published reports indicated that 46.2% of the liveborn twins suffered major morbidity or death (Enborn 1985). This figure is probably an overestimate as the reports were gathered retrospectively.

A variety of well-described mechanisms exist for this high risk of cerebral involvement. In monochorionic placentae, anastomoses frequently exist (Bernischke 1961, Galea et al 1982) and necrotic or thromboplastic material may pass from one to twin to the other. In some cases there is clear evidence from arteriographic studies of embolization from the dead twin to the live fetus through the shared circulation (Yoshioka et al 1979). The development of disseminated intravascular coagulation due to death of one fetus with release of thromboplastins leading to bleeding in the surviving twin has been described (Moore et al 1969). Other possible aetiologies include an episode of severe maternal hypotension leading to death of one fetus and ischaemic brain damage in the survivor.

The most severe form of cerebral injury is hydranencephaly. Norman (1980) reported a case in which the brain of one twin showed cortical disorganization with polymicrogyria. This case illustrates the importance of the time factor in determining the morphology of the lesions. Early impairment disturbs morphogenesis whilst later compromise is more likely to lead to clastic lesions. We have seen a case of an infant born with extensive embolic cutis aplasia and agenesis of the corpus callosum together with a fetus papyraceous co-twin. Ultrasound scanning had dated fetal death at 12 to 16 weeks and the skin lesions in the surviving twin were probably of this duration with extensive scarring in places. It is likely that the congenital cerebral anomaly developed as the result of early embolization at the time of development of the corpus callosum in the early part of the second trimester.

Abnormal neurological signs may be obvious at birth but the infant can behave remarkably normally despite major cerebral malformations. In one case, delivery occurred at 33 weeks of gestation, 4 weeks after the death of the co-twin. Extensive lesions seen on ultrasound were present at birth in the survivor (Fig. 30.3). Szymonowicz et al (1986) recommend prompt delivery of the survivor following in-utero

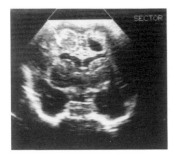
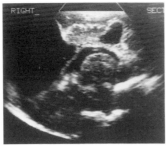

Fig. 30.3 Encephalomalacia and cerebral atrophy in a surviving monozygotic twin whose co-twin died at 29 weeks of gestation. Midcoronal ultrasound scan (left) showing cerebral atrophy and a cystic lesion above the right ventricle. Parasagittal view (right) of the same infant; a huge cavity is noted behind the occipital horn of the lateral ventricle.

demise of the co-twin to prevent the development of these extensive lesions. It is possible, however, that damage may have occurred before appropriate obstetric action can be taken (D'Alton et al 1984). A history of death in utero of one fetus of a multiple pregnancy should alert the physician to the risk to surviving fetuses and regular ultrasound scans should be performed during pregnancy and after delivery to detect these lesions.

Arterial occlusion

Infarction of a cerebral artery has been discussed in detail in Chapter 29 but the first pathological descriptions of cerebral infarction were made in fetal brains (Larroche & Amiel 1966, Larroche 1977) and most cases of infarction recognized in the newborn probably have their origins in fetal life. Infarction has been reported to be due to emboli from placental or fetal veins and they reach the brain through the large left-to-right shunt present during fetal life (Clark & Linnell 1954, Cocker et al 1965). In other cases, thrombus or blood clot was not identified within the feeding cerebral artery and the cause of the infarction was not obvious.

The pathological changes seen at autopsy are dependent on the duration from infarction to death. Recent softening of no more than a few days in duration was described by Clark & Linell (1954) in an infant who died 90 minutes after birth. Serial sections through the dissected middle cerebral artery identified an 'embolus' which was thought to have arisen from the placenta. Larroche has reported a number of infants with infarction of a major cerebral artery occurring before birth (Larroche & Amiel 1966, Larroche 1977, 1984). In one case (illustrated in Fig. 30.4) the affected hemisphere was smaller than the other and was the site of palpable softening, which contained multiple cavities in the region of the affected middle cerebral artery. The underlying tissue contained glial cells, macrophages and encrusted neurones. The thalamus and basal ganglia of the damaged hemisphere were partially cavitated. The cerebral peduncles, pons and medulla oblongata were asymmetrical with marked atrophy

of the pyramidal tract suggesting that the vascular accident had occurred long before birth. Dissection of the affected middle cerebral artery showed successive areas of total and partial occlusion of the lumen by an old and well-organized parietal thrombus at the origin of the vessel. Like the lesions seen in infants, the condition in the fetus is usually unilateral and most commonly involves the middle cerebral artery.

Early vascular compromise due to infarction is probably a relatively common cause of major cerebral malformations. These include areas of polymicrogyria and cerebral clefts (Norman 1980), porencephaly and microgyria (Stewart et al 1978). Bilateral occlusion of the carotid arteries is the most serious form of cerebral infarction and this leads to hydranencephaly (Yakovlev & Wadsworth 1946). The midbrain and hindbrain are usually preserved due to vertebral artery perfusion.

Fetal coagulopathy

An abnormality of coagulation affecting the fetus and not the mother is a common cause of fetal intracranial haemorrhage and iso-immune thrombocytopoenia is probably the most common haematological problem (Zalneraitis et al 1979, Naidu et al 1983, Paichak et al 1984, Magny et al 1984, Sadowitz & Balcom 1985). Furthermore, it has been shown that elective caesarian section does not protect the

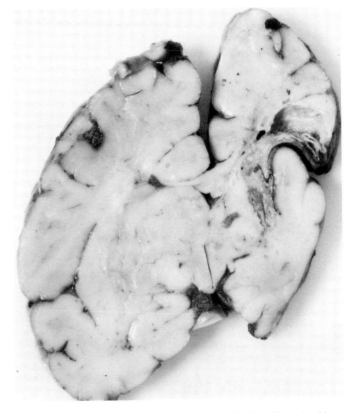

Fig. 30.4 Intra-uterine middle cerebral artery occlusion. There is old infarction with multicystic softening and atrophy of the right hemisphere. (Reproduced with permission from Larroche 1986.)

fetus from developing the haemorrhage (Morales & Stroup 1985, Sia et al 1985). Intracranial haemorrhage occurring before delivery has been recognized on ultrasound scans (McGahan et al 1984, Minkoff et al 1985, Mintz et al 1985) and by CT scan of the maternal pelvis (McGahan et al 1984). Intracerebral haemorrhage has also been described in a case of hydrops fetalis due to haemolytic disease (Bose 1978) and in a case of non-immune hydrops fetalis without blood-group incompatability (illustrated in Fig. 30.5, Larroche 1977). Inherited clotting factor deficiencies leading to intraparenchymal haemorrhages have also been reported (Whitelaw et al 1984).

We recently studied an infant with iso-immune thrombocytopoenia in whom there was evidence of recurrent intraparenchymal bleeding in utero, associated with periventricular leukomalacia. Ultrasonography performed following an elective caesarian section at 35 weeks of gestation showed two intraparenchymal haematomas, one more recent than the other, and periventricular cysts. It is likely that the leukomalacia occurred due to hypotension following the blood loss in utero. Intravascular platelet transfusion before an elective caesarian section has been advised under these circumstances (Daffos et al 1984). Fetal thrombocytopoenia in viral infections such as rubella may also be associated with intracerebral bleeding and white matter softening (Boreau & Larroche 1966).

Prenatal GMH–IVH

Germinal matrix haemorrhage and/or intraventricular haemorrhage (GMH–IVH) is a distinct entity which has

been reported to occur in approximately 5% of stillborn infants coming to autopsy (Hemsath 1934, Harcke et al 1972, Leech & Kohnen 1974). It is thought to be due to disturbances in cerebral circulation and the fetal aspects are therefore discussed in this section. More recently, a number of case reports have appeared describing the diagnosis of IVH by CT or ultrasound scans before delivery (see Fig. 30.6 McGahan et al 1984, Minkoff et al 1985, Mintz et al 1985). These isolated cases have been related to maternal seizures or intra-uterine growth retardation, as well as coagulation disorders which have been discussed above.

Some authors have reported the ultrasound diagnosis of GMH–IVH within hours of birth (Bejar et al 1980, Beverley et al 1984, McDonald et al 1984) and suggest that, in these infants, haemorrhage occurred before birth. In another study, almost one-quarter of lesions were present on a scan performed within an hour after delivery (de Crespigny et al 1982). This is not the experience of the majority of other investigators and is discussed in more detail in Chapter 28.

CONDITIONS OF PLACENTA AND CORD

Abnormalities of placenta and cord may also interfere with the fetal circulation and lead to brain damage. Placental abruption, true knots in the umbilical cord or a tight cord around the neck are potential hazards to fetal cerebral circulation, especially during labour and/or delivery. In the past, chronic placental insufficiency and fetal distress with intra-uterine growth retardation commonly led to death in utero or during labour but the brains of these fetuses did not show specific lesions. Myers (1969) reported a case of multicystic encephalomalacia in a monkey with longstanding incomplete placental abruption. It is, of course, not necessary to see macroscopic lesions for serious cerebral damage to have occurred. It is now well accepted

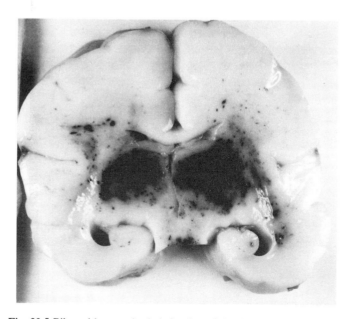

Fig. 30.5 Bilateral haemorrhagic infarction of the thalami from an infant with non-immune hydrops fetalis. There are also minute and scattered petechial haemorrhages in the periventricular white matter. (Reproduced with permission from Larroche 1986.)

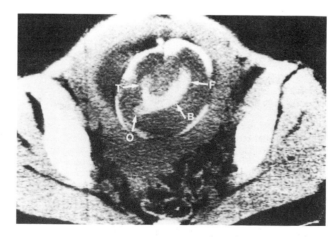

Fig. 30.6 CT scan of the maternal pelvis showing blood distending the lateral ventricle (arrowed) of the fetal brain. T = Temporal horn, O = Occipital horn, B = Body of lateral ventricle, F = Frontal horn. (Reproduced with permission from McGahan et al 1984.)

that severe intra-uterine growth retardation, particularly if the infant is also born prematurely, is associated with a lower intelligence due to restriction of brain growth. This is discussed in more detail in Chapter 5.

IDIOPATHIC CAUSES

We have attempted to relate a variety of neuropathological lesions to circulatory disturbances affecting the fetus. There are, however, a considerable number of examples of similar lesions in which no obvious compromise to the placental or fetal circulation has occurred and the causes of these conditions remain uncertain. With the greater use of more sophisticated methods for studying the fetal circulation, such as Doppler ultrasound (see Ch. 12), further understanding of the cause and effect of these lesions will be achieved.

CONCLUSIONS

Increased awareness of the vulnerability of the fetal brain to circulatory disorders has confirmed that many of the lesions commonly seen in the infant's brain may also occur prenatally. Their appearance depends on the timing of the intra-uterine insult and on the time elapsed between the insult and examination of the brain. It is important to recognize that ultrasound examination of the fetal brain immediately after the insult may reveal no abnormality and repeated examinations may be necessary to reveal cerebral pathology. An awareness of the possibility of these lesions developing following maternal hypoxic–ischaemic or traumatic injury will increase the frequency with which these lesions are diagnosed.

REFERENCES

Amiel-Tison C, Grenier A 1985 Hematome sousdural in utero, consequence d'une chute maternelle. In: La surveillance neurologique au cours de la premiere annee de la vie. Masson, Paris, pp 71–72

Barth P G 1984 Prenatal clastic encephalopathies. Clinical Neurology and Neurosurgery 86: 65–75

Beaudoing A, Gachon J, Butin L P, Bost M 1969 Les consequences foetales de l'intoxication oxycarbonnee de la mere. Pediatrie 24: 539–553

Bejar R, Curbelo V, Coen R W, Leopold G, James H, Gluck L 1980 Diagnosis and follow-up of intraventricular and intracerebral hemorrhages by ultrasound studies of infant's brain through the fontanelles and sutures. Pediatrics 66: 661–673

Bernischke K 1961 Twin placenta in perinatal mortality. New York Medical Journal 61: 1499–1508

Beverley D W, Chance G W, Inwood M J, Schaus M, O'Keefe B 1984 Intraventricular haemorrhage and haemostasis defects. Archives of Disease in Childhood 59: 444–448

Boreau T, Larroche J-C 1966 Note sur la pathologie foeto–neonatale liee a la rubeole. Bulletin of the Federated Societies of Gynaecology and Obstetrics 18: 239–241

Bose C 1978 Hydrops fetalis and in utero intracranial haemorrhage. Journal of Pediatrics 93: 1023–1024

Chetcuti P, Levene M I 1987 Seat belts: a potential hazard to the fetus. Journal of Perinatal Medicine 15: 207–209

Choulot J J, Leclerc M A, Saint-Martin J 1982 Malformation cerebrale et jumeau survivant. Archives Francaises de Pediatrie 39: 105–107

Clark R M, Linell E A 1954 Prenatal occlusion of the internal carotid artery. Journal of Neurology, Neurosurgery and Psychiatry 17: 295–297

Cocker J, George S W, Yates P O 1965 Perinatal occlusion of the middle cerebral artery. Developmental Medicine and Child Neurology 7: 235–243

Coignet J, Palix C, Tommasi C, Raybaud C 1979 Apport de la sonographie dans la souffrance de nouveau-ne. Pediatrie 34: 787–797

Courville C B 1959 Antenatal and paranatal circulatory disorders as a cause of cerebral damage in early life. Journal of Neuropathology and Experimental Neurology 18: 115–139

Daffos F et al 1984 Antenatal treatment of allo-immune thrombocytopenia. Lancet ii: 632

D'Alton M E, Newton E R, Cetrulo C L 1984 Intrauterine fetal demise in multiple gestation. Acta Genetica and Medical Gemellology 33: 43–49

de Crespigny L, Mackay R, Muston L J, Roy R N D, Robinson P H 1982 Timing of neonatal cerebroventricular haemorrhage with ultrasound. Archives of Disease in Childhood 57: 231–233

Dudley D K L, D'Alton M E 1986 Single fetal death in twin gestation. Seminars in Perinatology 10: 65–72

Durkin M V, Kaveggia E G, Pendleton E, Neuhauser G, Opitz J M 1976 Analysis of etiologic factors in cerebral palsy with severe mental retardation. European Journal of Pediatrics 123: 67–81

Enborn J A 1985 Twin pregnancy with intrauterine death of one twin. American Journal of Obstetrics and Gynecology 152: 424–429

Erasmus C, Blackwood W, Wislon J 1982 Infantile multicystic encephalomalacia after maternal bee sting anaphylaxis during pregnancy. Archives of Disease in Childhood 57: 785–787

Ferrer I, Navarro C 1978 Multicystic encephalomalacia of infancy. Journal of the Neurological Sciences 38: 179–189

Fowler M, Brown C, Cabrera K F 1971 Hydranencephaly in a baby after an aircraft accident to the mother: case report and autopsy. Pathology 3: 21–30

Galea P, Scott J M, Goel K M 1982 Feto–fetal transfusion syndrome. Archives of Disease in Childhood 57: 781–794

Ginsberg M D, Myers R E, McDonagh B F 1974 Experimental carbon monoxide encephalopathy in the primate. Archives of Neurology 30: 209–216

Goodlin R C, Heidrick W P, Papenfuss H L, Kubitz R L 1984 Fetal malformations associated with maternal hypoxia. American Journal of Obstetrics and Gynecology 149: 228–229

Gosseye S, Golaire M C, Larroche J-C 1982 Cerebral, renal and splenic lesions due to fetal anoxia and their relationship to malformations. Developmental Medicine and Child Neurology 24: 510–518

Grylack L 1982 Prenatal sonographic diagnosis of cephalhaematoma due to pre-labour trauma. Pediatric Radiology 12: 145–147

Gunn T R, Becroft D M 1984 Unexplained intracranial haemorrhage in utero: the battered fetus? Australian and New Zealand Journal of Obstetrics and Gynaecology 24: 17–22

Harcke H T, Naeye R L, Sturch A, Blanc W A 1972 Perinatal cerebral intraventricular hemorrhage. Journal of Pediatrics 80: 37–42

Hemsath F A 1934 Ventricular cerebral hemorrhage in the newborn infant. American Journal of Obstetrics and Gynecology 28: 343–353

Hughes H E, Miskin M 1986 Congenital microcephaly due to vascular disruption: in utero documentation. Pediatrics 78: 85–87

Jung J H, Graham J M, Schultz N, Smith D W 1984 Congenital hydranencephaly/porencephaly due to vascular disruption in monozygotic twins. Pediatrics 73: 467–469

Larroche J-C 1977 Developmental pathology of the neonate. Excerpta Medica, Amsterdam

Larroche J-C 1984 Perinatal brain damage. In: Adams J H, Corsellis J A N, Duchen L W (eds) Greenfield's Neuropathology. 4th edn. Edward Arnold, London

Larroche J-C 1986 Fetal encephalopathies of circulatory origin. Biology of the Neonate 50: 61–74

Larroche J-C, Amiel C 1966 Thrombose de l'artere sylvienne a la periode neonatale: etude anatomique et discussion pathologique des hemiplegies dites congenitales. Archives Francaises de Pediatrie 23: 257–274

Leech R W, Kohnen P 1974 Subependymal and intraventricular hemorrhage in the newborn. Annals of Pathology 77: 465–475

Levene M I 1987 Neonatal neurology. Churchill Livingstone, Edinburgh

Litschgi M, Stucki D 1980 Course of twin pregnancies after fetal death in utero. Zeitschrift zur Geburtschilfe und Perinatologie 184: 227–230

Longo L D 1977 The biological effects of carbon monoxide on the pregnant woman, fetus and newborn. American Journal of Obstetrics and Gynecology 129: 69–103

McDonald M M et al 1984 Timing and antecedents of intracranial hemorrhage in the newborn. Pediatrics 74: 32–36

McGahan J P, Haesslein H C, Meyers M, Ford K B 1984 Sonographic recognition of in utero intraventricular hemorrhage. American Journal of Radiology 142: 171–174

Magny J F et al 1984 Hemorrhagie cerebrale antenatale et incompatibilitie plaquettaire foeto–maternelle. Archives Francaises de Pediatrie 41: 711–712

Manterola A, Towbin A, Yakovlev P I 1966 Cerebral infarction in the human fetus near term. Journal of Neuropathology and Experimental Neurology 25: 479–488

Melnick M 1977 Brain damage in survivor after death of monozygotic co-twin. Lancet ii: 1287

Minkoff H, Schaffer R M, Delke I, Grunebaum A N 1985 Diagnosis of intracranial hemorrhage in utero after a maternal seizure. Obstetrics and Gynaecology 65: 22S–24S

Mintz M C, Arger P H, Coleman B G 1985 In utero sonographic diagnosis of intracerebral hemorrhage. Journal of Ultrasound in Medicine 4: 375–376

Moore C M, McAdams A J, Sutherland J 1969 Intrauterine disseminated intravascular coagulation: a syndrome of multiple pregnancy with dead twin fetus. Journal of Pediatrics 74: 523–528

Morales W J, Stroup M 1985 Intracranial hemorrhage in utero due to isoimmune neonatal thrombocytopenia. Obstetrics and Gynecology 65: 20S–21S

Morey M A, Begleiter M L, Harris D J 1981 Profile of a battered fetus. Lancet ii: 1294–1295

Myers R E 1969 Cystic brain alteration after incomplete placental abruption in monkey. Archives of Neurology 21: 133–141

Myers R E 1975 Maternal psychological stress and fetal asphyxia: a study in the monkey. American Journal of Obstetrics and Gynecology 122: 47–59

Naidu S, Messmore H, Caserta V, Fine M 1983 CNS lesions in neonatal isoimmune thrombocytopenia. Archives of Neurology 40: 552–554

Norman R M 1952 Mental deficiencies (Proceedings 1st International Congress of Neuropathology, Rome, Vol. 2). Rosenberg Sellier, Turin, pp 276–282

Norman M G 1980 Bilateral encephaloclastic lesions in a 26 week gestation fetus: effect on neuronal migration. Journal of Canadian Scientific Neurology 7: 191–194

Paichak A F, Aster R H, Opitz J M 1984 Effect of maternal–fetal platelet incompatability on fetal development. Pediatrics 74: 570–573

Pepperell R J, Rubinstein E, MacIsaac I A 1977 Motor car accidents during pregnancy. Medical Journal of Australia 1: 203–205

Rizzuto N, Martin L 1967 Le probleme de l'encephalopathie foetale kystique survenant au cours du deuxieme tiers de la grossesse. Biology Neonatorum 11: 115–127

Robinson M J, Cameron M D, Smith M F, Ayers A B 1980 Fetal subdural haemorrhage presenting as hydrocephalus. British Medical Journal 281: 35

Sadowitz P D, Balcom R 1985 Intrauterine intracranial hemorrhage in an infant with isoimmune thrombocytopenia. Clinical Pediatrics 24: 655–657

Scharpe O, Hale E G 1953 Renal impairment, hypertension and encephalomalacia in infant surviving severe intrauterine anoxia. Procedings of the Royal Society of Medicine 46: 1063–1065

Schinzel A, Smith D W, Miller J R 1979 Monozygotic twinning and structural defects. Journal of Pediatrics 95: 921–930

Sia C G, Amigo N C, Harper R G, Farahani G, Kochen J 1985 Failure of caesarian section to prevent intracranial hemorrhage in siblings with isoimmune thrombocytopenia. American Journal of Obstetrics and Gynecology 135: 79–81

Smith J F, Rodeck C 1975 Multiple cystic and focal encephalomalacia in infancy and childhood with brainstem damage. Journal of Neurological Sciences 25: 377–388

Stevenson L D, McGowan L E 1942 Encephalomalacia with cavitary formation in infants. Archives of Pathology 34: 286–300

Stewart R M, Williams R S, Kukl P, Schoenen J 1978 Ventral porencephaly: a cerebral defect associated with multiple congenital anomalies. Acta Neuropathology 42: 231–235

Szymonowicz W, Yu V Y H 1985 Outcome of intrauterine periventricular haemorrhage and leukomalacia. Australian Paediatric Journal 21: 261–264

Szymonowicz W, Preston H, Yu V Y H 1986 The surviving monozygotic twin. Archives of Disease in Childhood 61: 454–458

Whitelaw A, Haines M E, Bolsover W, Harris E 1984 Factor V deficiency and antenatal intraventricular haemorrhage. Archives of Disease in Childhood 59: 997–999

Yakovlev P I, Wadsworth R C 1946 Schizencephalies: a study of congenital clefts in cerebral mantles: clefts with fused lips. Journal of Neuropathology and Experimental Neurology 5: 116–130

Yoshioka H, Kadomoto Y, Mino M, Morikawa Y, Kasebuchi Y, Kasunoki T 1979 Multicystic encephalomalacia in liveborn twin with a stillborn macerated co-twin. Pediatrics 95: 798–800

Zalneraitis E L, Young R S K, Krishnamoorthy K S 1979 Intracranial hemorrhage in utero as a complication of iso-immune thrombocytopenia. Journal of Pediatrics 95: 611–614

31. Intracranial sequelae

Dr L.S. de Vries, Dr J-C. Larroche and Dr M.I. Levene

METABOLIC PROBLEMS

A number of hormonal disturbances or metabolic problems are described in association with various types of intracranial haemorrhage. Inappropriate antidiuretic hormone secretion has been reported in a few premature infants with CT scan diagnosis of intracranial haemorrhage (Moylan et al 1978). Central diabetes insipidus has also been reported in a premature infant with GMH–IVH (Adams et al 1976). This was a transient condition and required short-term treatment with a vasopressin-like agent.

Hyperpyrexia following GMH–IVH is well recognized (Gomes & Weerasuriya 1975) and this is seen particularly in full-term infants and may occur following a variety of different forms of intracranial haemorrhage. Elevated body temperature may persist for weeks and may initially cause confusion with meningitis, particularly if there is a high cerebrospinal fluid (CSF) white cell count with low glucose.

SUBEPENDYMAL PSEUDOCYST

Cyst formation is a relatively common finding in the subependymal region at the head of the caudate nucleus in the newborn (Fig. 31.1). Cavitation within the germinal matrix is referred to as a pseudocyst because it is not lined by epithelium (Larroche 1972a). These commonly develop after small haemorrhage in the region of the germinal matrix and are easily recognized on ultrasound. They may develop following a variety of insults including prenatal infection with rubella or cytomegalovirus (Sha & Alvord 1974). They may also occur as 'normal' events if the rapidly developing germinal matrix outgrows its blood supply. When the pseudocyst occurs following GMH–IVH it has no prognostic significance and if it represents the only cerebral insult the prognosis is excellent.

PORENCEPHALY

Porencephalic cavitation is commonly seen in infants and

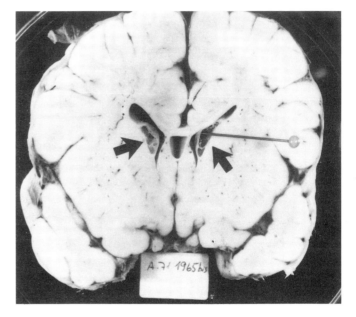

Fig. 31.1 Bilateral subependymal pseudocysts (arrowed) in the germinal matrix.

may be due to a variety of insults, the most common of which is haemorrhage into the periventricular white matter. Encephaloclastic porencephaly refers to a fluid-filled defect lying within the cerebral parenchyma and communicating with the lateral ventricles (Fig. 31.2). In premature infants up to two-thirds of GMH–IVH lesions which involve the cerebral parenchyma will evolve to porencephaly (Pasternak et al 1980) and these can readily be recognized by ultrasound.

The prognosis for infants with posthaemorrhagic porencephaly is that of the underlying pathology, usually haemorrhage or infarction. Massive porencephaly following extensive haemorrhage into the periventricular white matter may cause only minor neurodevelopmental sequelae (Fawer et al 1983). Rarely, the porencephalic cavity progressively expands and this may cause deterioration in cerebral function (Tardieu et al 1981). Although the measured CSF pressure is not elevated, ventriculo–peritoneal shunting can

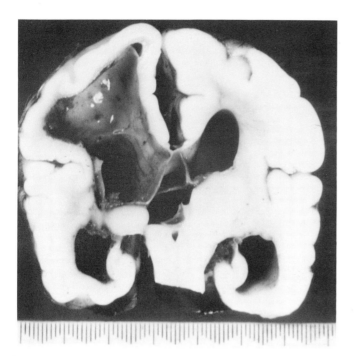

Fig. 31.2 Posthaemorrhagic porencephaly in communication with the left lateral ventricle. Note the haemosiderin staining in the wall of the cavity.

result in remarkable improvement of focal motor deficits and intellectual development. Porencephalic lesions in general are discussed more fully in Chapter 19.

POSTHAEMORRHAGIC VENTRICULAR DILATATION

This is one of the most common and important complications of intracranial haemorrhage. Hydrocephalus occurring after intracranial bleeding was first described by West in 1848, and not reported again for a further 74 years, when Fraser & Dott (1922) described seven cases. In recent years it has been recognized to be a frequent finding in infants following GMH–IVH but it may follow any form of intracranial haemorrhage. Unfortunately, it may be extremely difficult to decide whether dilated ventricles are due to obstruction or cerebral atrophy and there is considerable confusion as to the timing of treatment and the most appropriate management of ventriculomegaly.

Incidence

Congenital hydrocephalus has rarely been recognized to be due to prenatal intracranial haemorrhage secondary to coagulopathy (Zalneraitis et al 1979, Whitelaw et al 1984) or germinal matrix haemorrhage (Hill & Rozdilsky 1979, Larroche 1986) and this is discussed in more detail in Chapter 30.

Before the introduction of routine ultrasound scans, haemorrhage was thought to be the cause of hydrocephalus in only 3% of children (Lorber & Bhatt 1974) and as late as 1977 it was stated that if infants survived GMH–IVH, 80% would develop hydrocephalus (Volpe 1977). With the introduction of real-time ultrasound, ventricular size could be rapidly and accurately diagnosed (Fig. 31.3). To recognize ventricular dilatation ultrasound measurements must be made consistently from the same point on each occasion and a centile chart giving the normal range for ventricular size is shown on p. 144. Surprisingly, few studies have documented the incidence of posthaemorrhagic ventricular dilatation (PHVD) in high-risk infants. Levene & Starte (1981) studied 202 consecutive admissions of all birth-weights to a neonatal intensive care unit and found 25% developed ventriculomegaly, defined as the ventricular index exceeding the 97th centile, following intracranial haemorrhage. Only 3 of their 15 infants with PHVD required a ventricular shunt. Others have reported a 33% incidence of PHVD based on similar diagnostic criteria in infants below 35 weeks of gestation (Szymonowicz et al 1985). The incidence of ventriculomegaly in premature infants with moderate or severe GMH–IVH is reported to vary between 10% (Ment et al 1984) and 54% (Allan et al 1982). The incidence of PHVD depends in part on the clinician's definition but appears to increase with severity of the intracranial haemorrhage and is three times more common in infants with parenchymal involvement than in those with bleeding confined to the region of the germinal matrix (Levene 1987). If premature infants with only minor degrees of germinal matrix or intraventricular haemorrhage are considered, then the incidence of PHVD in this group is 14% (Fishman et al 1984). Posthaemorrhagic ventricular dilatation appears to be very uncommon following primary subarachnoid haemorrhage in the neonatal period (LeBlanc & O'Gorman 1980).

Pathology

In a necropsy study of nine infants with posthaemorrhagic hydrocephalus, Larroche (1972b) found obliterative arachnoiditis at the exit of the fourth ventricle to be the cause of the ventricular dilatation in most of her cases. Only one infant had obstruction at the aqueduct of Sylvius. Most surviving infants with PHVD have a communicating form of obstruction. Hill et al (1984), in an ultrasound study, suggested that small, mobile particulate matter caused blockage to absorptive pathways at the site of the arachnoid granulations. In Leicester we found only 18% of infants with PHVD had a non-communicating form of ventricular dilatation (Levene 1987), presumably due to obliterative arachnoiditis at the base of the skull and Chaplin et al (1980) reported a similar incidence of 17%. In the majority of infants with PHVD it is assumed that the obstruction to CSF occurs over the surface of the brain at the arachnoid granulations but this has not been shown morphologically as the granulations are not visible in premature infants.

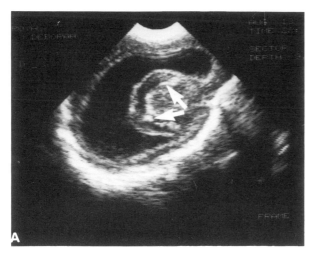
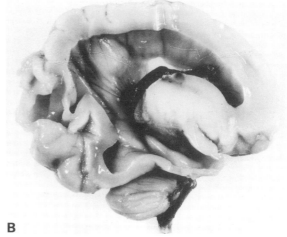

Fig. 31.3 Posthaemorrhagic ventricular dilatation. Parasagittal ultrasound scan (a) showing blood clot in the floor of the lateral ventricle (arrowed). Postmortem specimen in the same infant (b) confirming the dilatation. Blood clot is present on the floor of the ventricle as well as small germinal matrix haemorrhage (GMH). (Courtesy of the ICU, Hopital Port-Royal, Paris.)

Clinical features

In the older literature the clinical signs of hydrocephalus have been well documented but in recent years, with the introduction of reliable imaging techniques, the diagnosis of ventriculomegaly has been made before symptoms develop and treatment is often undertaken in asymptomatic infants.

The most obvious clinical sign is enlarging head size but ventriculomegaly may precede this by days or weeks (Korobkin et al 1975, Volpe et al 1977). In another study the mean age at clinical diagnosis of hydrocephalus was 30 days (Chaplin et al 1980). The rapidly enlarging head is associated with bulging fontanelles, split sutures and congested scalp veins. Neurological signs include impaired vertical gaze, apnoea with bradycardia, sixth cranial nerve palsy, vomiting, seizures and the 'sunset' sign (see p. 522). Increased tone or spasticity is seen in untreated cases during late infancy and particularly involves the lower limbs. In older children, ataxia, tremor and clumsiness are seen.

Diagnosis

A diagnostic problem is the distinction between communicating and non-communicating PHVD as this is difficult with ultrasound and CT examinations. Functional assessment with radionuclide scanning may be helpful. This consists of instilling radiolabelled isotope into the CSF at lumbar puncture or through a ventricular catheter. Repeated gamma camera images show flow of the radioactive tracer through the ventricular and subarachnoid circulation. In children, radio-active tracer injected into the lateral ventricles became apparent over the cerebral convexities by 24 hours (Sty et al 1979). Tracer may also be instilled into the lumbar CSF and various patterns of filling have been seen (Donn et al 1983). In cerebral atrophy there was rapid filling of the ventricles with radio-active material but ventricular emptying was delayed despite signs of activity over the cerebral convexity soon after injection. In communicating hydrocephalus there was prompt ventricular filling but markedly delayed emptying and little activity over the convexity of the brain.

An alternative and simple method for distinguishing communicating from non-communicating PHVD is to perform lumbar puncture. If more than 5 ml of CSF drips from the needle, we assume there to be communication. If, after two attempts by experienced staff, less than this volume of CSF is obtained, the site of obstruction is likely to be at the base of the skull and is non-communicating. In practice this method is safe and coning has not been reported to occur in the neonate. A reduction in size of the lateral ventricle is often seen on ultrasound following removal of a volume of CSF in communicating PHVD.

Posthaemorrhagic ventricular dilatation may be due to obstruction or atrophy and distinction between these two pathological conditions is a major problem. Radionuclide scanning may help (Donn et al 1983) but this technique is not readily available in many centres. The description in children of normal pressure hydrocephalus has further confused the issue and CSF pressure monitoring for up to 48 hours may be the only way of distinguishing the two.

Flodmark et al (1981) diagnosed ventriculomegaly on CT scans as often in infants who had not sustained intracranial haemorrhage as in those who had, and suggested that most cases of persistent ventricular dilatation are due to cerebral atrophy (hydrocephalus ex vacuo). They recommended that any infant with ventriculomegaly but without evidence of rapid head growth or clinical signs of raised intracranial pressure should be considered to be suffering from cerebral atrophy until neurological findings suggest that the ventriculomegaly is progressive. We and others (Graziani et al 1985) are unconvinced that ventriculomegaly following haemorrhage is necessarily dependent on obstruction to CSF pathways. There is evidence that leukomalacia is the cause of dilatation in a relatively high proportion of these infants. Unfortunately, measurement of head growth may not be particularly helpful in distinguishing one pattern from another.

The CT or ultrasound appearance of the lateral ventricles may be of some value. This is discussed in detail in Chapters 8 and 9. We accept asymmetrical ventricular dilatation to be a helpful feature in recognizing cerebral atrophy. More subtle features may also help in distinguishing the two conditions. It has been reported that in cerebral atrophy the lateral ventricles maintain their original shape and simply appear larger. The temporal horn does not tend to become enlarged. Obstructed ventricles appear 'ballooned' with loss of the normal lateral angles (Heinz et al 1980).

Normal pressure hydrocephalus (NPH)

The term NPH has been applied to elderly adult patients with dilated ventricles and signs of dementia, ataxia, disturbances of ocular movements and incontinence who were found to have CSF pressures below 20 cmH$_2$O. In some cases, permanent improvement occurred following ventricular shunting. Normal pressure hydrocephalus has also been reported in the newborn (Hill & Volpe 1981) but this is not the same condition as is seen in adults and the term probably should not be applied to young children. The infant has a compliant cranium and ventriculomegaly can occur due to obstruction without a rise in pressure. Ventricular dilatation and normal CSF pressure are also seen in cerebral atrophy and Hill & Volpe (1981) have failed to distinguish the two adequately.

Prognosis

Assessment of the risk of handicap due to ventricular dilatation as opposed to handicap associated with it is almost impossible. The problem is complicated by multiple factors likely to cause brain damage, including unrelated cerebral pathology, severity of the initial haemorrhage and the adverse effects of treatment. On review of follow-up data from infants with PHVD a number of generalizations can be made. In a review of seven studies reporting the outcome of infants shunted for hydrocephalus following haemorrhage, only 9 of 50 (18%) were neurodevelopmentally normal (Krishnamoorthy et al 1979, Chaplin et al 1980, Palmer et al 1982, Cooke 1983, Liechty et al 1983, Allan et al 1984, Kreusser et al 1985). The reasons for the poor outcome are of course multifactorial and include reluctance to shunt infants except in the most severe cases as well as ventriculitis associated with shunt surgery.

It has been suggested that PHVD in itself is a risk factor in the development of handicap (Palmer

et al 1982, Stewart et al 1983) but it is impossible to separate the size of the underlying haemorrhage from the degree of ventricular dilatation and subsequent outcome. In addition co-existent cerebral atrophy, particularly when due to periventricular leukomalacia, may cause compensatory dilatation and this, rather than obstructive pressure-driven hydrocephalus, determines the poor outcome. Recent studies have suggested that the poor outcome seen in many infants with ventricular dilatation following GMH–IVH is most likely to be due to associated infarction and atrophy (Allan et al 1984, Graziani et al 1985). We have found that 57% of all infants with PVL or parenchymal haemorrhage develop ventricular dilatation by 14 days of age (Trounce et al 1986).

The effect of increased CSF pressure per se rather than the associated parenchymal injury can be assessed by examining the outcome of infants born with congenital hydrocephalus due to anatomical obstruction such as Arnold–Chiari malformation or aqueductal stenosis and without apparent periventricular injury. Generally, the prognosis in this group is surprisingly good. Data from four follow-up studies of infants surviving a variety of forms of congenital hydrocephalus (not posthaemorrhagic) show that 52 of 92 (57%) are considered to be neurodevelopmentally normal by the authors (Lorber 1968, Mealey et al 1973, Hagberg & Naglo 1977, McCullough & Balzer-Martin 1982). In general, the thinner the cerebral mantle the poorer the prognosis but Lorber (1968) reports some infants with extremely thinned mantles who are functioning normally or even above average for intelligence. Ventriculitis occurring in shunted infants is an adverse risk factor (McLone et al 1982). The comparison between PHVD and congenital hydrocephalus is used to emphasize a point but it is clear that the most severely affected infants with spina bifida and hydrocephalus would have died early and the follow-up group represents a relatively lower risk cohort.

Krishnamoorthy et al (1984) report follow-up data on 12 children who developed posthaemorrhagic hydrocephalus following intraventricular haemorrhage but without parenchymal involvement. The outcome in this group was relatively good as only 3 (25%) had substantial neurodevelopmental sequelae and 5 of the 9 normal children received ventricular shunts.

These studies support the concept that if there is no injury to the periventricular white matter, hydrocephalus is relatively well tolerated by the majority of infants and the poor prognosis seen in those surviving haemorrhage is more likely to be related to the extent of the initial lesion and/or the presence of cerebral atrophy.

Our explanation for the observation that dilatation occurs frequently in the presence of IVH is that partial obstruction to CSF pathways occurs as the result of haemorrhage with some transient elevation of CSF pressure. In many ill infants the haemorrhage occurs in association with ischaemic injury to the periventricular white matter. Elevated CSF pressure causes transependymal extravasation of CSF which further compromises the already damaged structures in the periventricular region and this accelerates cerebral atrophy leading to further passive ventricular dilatation. Treatment of the ventriculomegaly will thus have no influence on the subsequent outcome, as handicap was due to PVL and atrophy rather than the relatively minor GMH–IVH with modest ventricular obstruction.

Treatment

There is no consensus on the best method for treating ventriculomegaly following haemorrhage. A variety of methods exist and are discussed below. Unfortunately there have been no controlled studies of methods for treating this problem and the benefits of these treatment regimes are largely anecdotal.

Compressive head wrapping

This method was suggested in the 1970s to prevent hydrocephalus (Epstein et al 1973, Epstein et al 1974, Porter 1975) but it is associated with a marked elevation in intracranial pressure (Epstein et al 1974). Follow-up reports on infants treated by this method have not appeared and compressive head wrapping cannot be recommended.

Isosorbide

This drug is a derivative of mannitol and works by osmotic action. In 14 hydrocephalic children a single dose of isosorbide reduced the CSF pressure on average by 50%, although the effect was short-lived (Hayden et al 1968). Lorber has used this drug extensively in the treatment of many types of infantile hydrocephalus and reports good results (Lorber 1975, Lorber et al 1983). The starting dose is 2 g/kg 6 hourly, reducing to 1–1.5 g/kg 6 hourly after 3 weeks if the results are favourable (Table 31.1). Hypernatraemia develops in about 20% of treated infants (Lorber 1975). Unfortunately, isosorbide appears to be least effective when used for treating posthaemorrhagic hydrocephalus.

Acetazolamide

This drug is a carbonic anhydrase inhibitor and its action in controlling hydrocephalus is not well understood. It probably reduces secretion of CSF by the choroid plexus.

There have been a number of reports on its efficacy in the management of posthaemorrhagic hydrocephalus (Bergman et al 1978, Shinnar et al 1985). The recommended starting dose is 25 mg/kg/day increasing by 25 mg/kg/day up to a maximum dose of 100 mg/kg/day (Table 31.1). It is given orally every 8 hours. Acetazolemide induces metabolic acidosis and careful assessment of acid–base and electrolyte balance is essential. It is necessary to give replacement base in the form of citrate solution. Frusemide (1 mg/kg) is usually given in conjunction with acetazolamide. Shinnar et al (1985) claim that insertion of a shunt was avoided in almost half of their cases but as the study was uncontrolled and spontaneous remission of hydrocephalus is well recognized, the efficacy of this drug must remain questionable. Despite the lack of control data in this study, it is the most convincing paper on the medical management of hydrocephalus yet published.

Glycerol

This is used more commonly in the United States than elsewhere because isosorbide has not been available there (Volpe 1977). Starting dose is 1 g/kg orally every 6 hours, increasing to 2 g/kg after one week (Table 31.1). Electrolytes must be monitored to avoid dehydration. There is little data on the effectiveness of this drug in the management of PHVD.

Lumbar puncture

In infants with communicating hydrocephalus, CSF can be removed and the ventricles decompressed by lumbar puncture tap. A styletted needle must be used and is inserted using aseptic techniques at the L4–5 vertebral interspace. Use of a non-styletted needle may cause an epidermoid spinal tumour (Shaywitz 1972, Halcrow et al 1985). Regular lumbar punctures have been recommended by a number of authors to treat PHVD and claims have been made that it prevents the need for shunting (Goldstein et al 1976, Papile et al 1980). In a study of 12 low-birth-weight infants who survived severe IVH and subsequently developed progressive ventricular dilatation, only 4 required shunting after serial lumbar punctures (Papile et al 1980). They claimed that this treatment prevented hydrocephalus but unfortunately the treatment was uncontrolled and it is interesting to compare their results with a similar group of 15 infants with PHVD who received no treatment (Levene

Table 31.1 Drugs used in the management of posthaemorrhagic ventricular dilatation

Drug	Starting dose	Maintenance dose	Side effects
Isosorbide	2 mg/kg 6 hourly	1–1.5 mg/kg 6 hourly	Hypernatraemia
Acetazolamide	25 mg/kg 24 hourly	100 mg/kg 24 hourly	Metabolic acidosis
Frusemide	1 mg/kg 24 hourly	1 mg/kg 12 hourly	Potassium depletion
Glycerol	1 g/kg 6 hourly	2 g/kg 6 hourly	Dehydration

& Starte 1981). The numbers of infants requiring shunts in the two groups were similar and it is likely that both studies describe the natural history of PHVD and the outcome in Papile's study was not influenced by lumbar puncture treatment. Another report on the effect of regular lumbar punctures claimed that it may temporarily ameliorate progressive ventricular dilatation (Kreusser et al 1985). This study was uncontrolled and the results are difficult to evaluate but half of the 16 infants described required shunts.

The rationale for repeated lumbar puncture taps is to remove blood from the CSF which might otherwise cause obstruction and hydrocephalus. Two studies have attempted to test this hypothesis by performing regular taps in one group of infants with GMH–IVH and compared the number requiring shunts to an untreated control group (Mantovani et al 1980, Anwar et al 1985). There was no difference in the number of infants developing hydrocephalus in either group. This confirms that lumbar puncture cannot remove enough blood from the CSF to prevent ventricular obstruction. There is no evidence that repeated ventricular taps are any more beneficial.

Lumbar punctures should, however, not be completely dismissed as they serve two useful purposes. Firstly, they will establish whether the obstruction is communicating or not (see p. 348). Secondly, subarachnoid opening pressure can be measured at lumbar puncture. When the infant is lying on his side in a semiflexed position, the pressure in the lumbar subarachnoid space should equilibrate with intraventricular pressure, providing the infant is not crying. Measurement of CSF pressure may help to delineate those infants more at risk of periventricular oedema and in whom active treatment is likely to be of most benefit.

Ventricular drainage

This is discussed in detail in Chapter 46. If the methods already described fail to control progressive ventricular dilatation, then a surgical procedure to drain the ventricles will be necessary. A ventriculo–peritoneal shunt is the definitive and long-standing treatment for hydrocephalus but is associated with considerable potential complications, including shunt blockage and infection. Children who remain shunt dependent will require revision with increasing growth. It is to avoid these complications that alternative surgical methods have been described.

The placement of a ventricular catheter to allow prolonged external ventricular drainage has been used successfully in premature infants (Harbaugh et al 1981, Kreusser et al 1984). The majority of infants treated in this manner required subsequent ventriculo-peritoneal shunts but the babies' condition improved sufficiently in a number to allow subsequent surgery to be successfully completed. Disadvantages of this technique are the risk of ascending infection and electrolyte disturbances.

An alternative approach has been to place a subcutaneous reservoir attached to the ventricular catheter (Marlin 1980, McComb et al 1983). This low-profile device is inserted over the skull and the skin is closed over it. Fluid can be removed by needling the reservoir. The advantage of this technique is a lower risk of infection and the reservoir can later be converted to a valve system if necessary.

Practical management of PHVD

There are no generally accepted guidelines as to the management of this condition. The regime suggested here is one that has been used in Leicester for a number of years (Levene 1987). The basic premises include distinction between atrophy and obstruction, avoidance of long-standing intracranial hypertension and ensuring that the infant does not have an unnecessary shunt inserted.

A clear definition of when PHVD occurs is fundamental to the diagnosis (Levene 1981). We use the criterion of Kaiser & Whitelaw (1985) which is dilatation to the point that the ventricular index exceeds the 97th centile by 4 mm or more for the infant's postconceptual age (Fig. 31.4). When this occurs an initial lumbar puncture is performed to establish whether there is communication with the lumbar subarachnoid space. At the same time the CSF pressure is measured. If the obstruction is communicating and the pressure below 15 cmH_2O then no further tap is performed unless the ventricle continues to dilate. If this happens then repeated lumbar puncture taps can be performed but no action taken unless the pressure exceeds 15 cmH_2O. If the pressure is high then we start acetazolamide and if this is unsuccessful repeat lumbar puncture taps are instituted

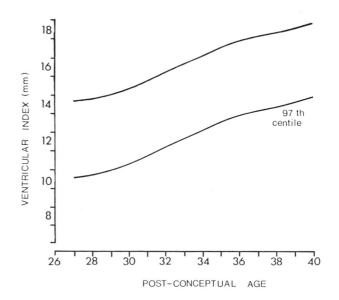

Fig. 31.4 Treatment criteria for posthaemorrhagic ventricular dilatation according to Kaiser & Whitelaw 1985 (upper line). This is 4 mm above the 97th centile for the ventricular index of Levene 1981.

to drain 10 ml of CSF on each occasion and to monitor CSF pressure. If the pressure remains above 15 cmH$_2$0 then a neurosurgical opinion is sought as to the need for a ventriculo–peritoneal shunt once the infant is more than 30 days old. In non-communicating PHVD a ventricular tap to measure pressure will be necessary but otherwise the treatment is similar to that of non-communicating dilatation. The decision to shunt such an infant might be taken relatively earlier to avoid multiple ventricular taps. This method is summarized in Fig. 31.5.

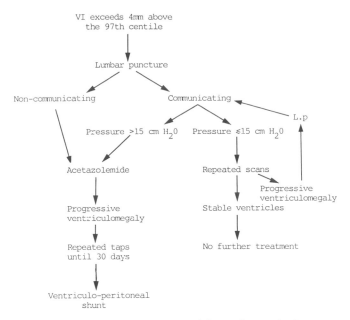

Fig. 31.5 Suggested management protocol for posthaemorrhagic ventricular dilatation. VI = ventricular index, L.p = lumbar puncture.

REFERENCES

Adams J M, Kenny J D, Rudolph A J 1976 Central diabetes insipidus following intraventricular haemorrhage. Journal of Pediatrics 88: 292–294

Allan W C, Holt P J, Sawyer L R, Tito A M, Meade S K 1982 Ventricular dilation after neonatal periventricular-intraventricular hemorrhage. American Journal of Diseases of Childhood 136: 589–593

Allan W C, Dransfield D A, Tito A M 1984 Ventricular dilation following periventricular-intraventricular hemorrhage: outcome at one year. Pediatrics 73: 158–162

Anwar M, Kadam S, Hiatt I M, Hegyi T 1985 Serial lumbar punctures in prevention of post-hemorrhagic hydrocephalus in preterm infants. Journal of Pediatrics 107: 446–450

Bergman E 1978 Medical management of hydrocephalus with aceta-zolemide and frusemide. Annals of Neurology 4: 189–194

Chaplin E R, Goldstein G W, Myerberg D Z, Hunt J V, Tooley W H 1980 Posthemorrhagic hydrocephalus in the preterm infants. Pediatrics 65: 901–909

Cooke R W I 1983 Early prognosis of low birth weight infants treated for progressive posthaemorrhagic hydrocephalus. Archives of Disease in Childhood 58: 410–414

Donn S M, Roloff D W, Keyes J W 1983 Lumbar cisternography in evaluation of hydrocephalus in the preterm infant. Pediatrics 72: 670–676

Epstein F J, Hochwald G M, Ransohoff J 1973 Neonatal hydrocephalus treated by compressive head wrapping. Lancet i: 634–636

Epstein F, Wald A, Hochwald G M 1974 Intracranial pressure during compressive head wrapping in treatment of neonatal hydrocephalus. Pediatrics 54: 786–790

Fawer C-L, Levene M I, Dubowitz L M S 1983 Intraventricular haemorrhage in a preterm neonate: discordance between clinical course and ultrasound scan. Neuropediatrics 14: 242–244

Fishman M A, Dutton R V, Okumura S 1984 Progressive ventriculomegaly following minor intracranial hemorrhage in premature infants. Developmental Medicine and Child Neurology 26: 725–731

Flodmark O, Scotti G, Harwood-Nash D C 1981 Clinical significance of ventriculomegaly in children who suffered perinatal asphyxia with or without intracranial hemorrhage: an 18 month follow up study. Journal of Computer Assisted Tomography 5: 663–673

Fraser J, Dott N 1922 Hydrocephalus. British Journal of Surgery 10: 165–191

Goldstein G W, Chaplin E R, Maitland J, Norman D 1976 Transient hydrocephalus in premature infants: treatment by lumbar punctures. Lancet i: 512–514

Gomes W J, Weerasuriya N 1975 Hyperpyrexia in neonates: a sign of intraventricular haemorrhage. Indian Pediatrics 12: 505–507

Graziani L J, et al 1985 Cranial ultrasound and clinical studies in preterm infants. Journal of Pediatrics 106: 269–276

Hagberg B, Naglo A-S 1977 The conservative management of infantile hydrocephalus. Acta Paediatrica Scandinavica 61: 165–177

Halcrow S J, Crawford P J, Craft A W 1985 Epidermoid spinal cord tumour after lumbar puncture. Archives of Disease in Childhood 60: 978–979

Harbaugh R E, Saunders R L, Edwards W H 1981 External ventricular drainage for control of posthemorrhagic hydrocephalus in premature infants. Journal of Neurosurgery 55: 766–770

Hayden P W, Foltz E L, Shurtleff D B 1968 Effect of an oral osmotic agent on ventricular fluid pressure of hydrocephalic children. Pediatrics 41: 955–967

Heinz E R, Ward A, Drayer B P, Dubois P J 1980 Distinction between obstructive and atrophic dilatation of ventricles in children. Journal of Computer Assisted Tomography 4: 320–325

Hill A, Rozdilsky B 1984 Congenital hydrocephalus secondary to intra-uterine germinal matrix/intraventricular haemorrhage. Developmental Medicine and Child Neurology 26: 524–527

Hill A, Volpe J J 1981 Normal pressure hydrocephalus in the newborn. Pediatrics 68: 623–629

Hill A, Shackelford G D, Volpe J J 1984 A potential mechanism of pathogenesis for early posthemorrhagic hydrocephalus in the premature newborn. Pediatrics 73: 19–21

Kaiser A M, Whitelaw A G 1985 Cerebrospinal fluid pressure during post haemorrhagic ventricular dilatation in newborn infants. Archives of Disease in Childhood 60: 920–924

Korobkin R 1975 The relationship between head circumference and the development of communicating hydrocephalus following intraventricular hemorrhage. Pediatrics 59: 74–77

Kreusser K L et al 1984 Rapidly progressive posthemorrhagic hydrocephalus. Treatment with external ventricular drainage. American Journal of Diseases in Children 138: 633–637

Kreusser K L, Tarby T J, Kovnar E, Taylor D A, Hill A, Volpe J J 1985 Serial lumbar punctures for at least temporary amelioration of neonatal posthemorrhagic hydrocephalus. Pediatrics 75: 719–724

Krishnamoorthy K S, Shannon D C, DeLong G R, Todres I D, Davis

K R 1979 Neurologic sequelae in the survivors of neonatal intraventricular hemorrhage. Pediatrics 64: 233–237

Krishnamoorthy K S, Kuehnle K J, Todres I D, DeLong G R 1984 Neurodevelopmental outcome of survivors with posthemorrhagic hydrocephalus following Grade II neonatal intraventricular hemorrhage. Annals of Neurology 15: 201–204

Larroche J-C 1972a Sub-ependymal pseudocysts in the newborn. Biology of the Neonate 21: 170–183

Larroche J-C 1972b Post-haemorrhagic hydrocephalus in infancy anatomical study. Biology of the Neonate 20: 287–299

Larroche J-C 1986 Fetal encephalopathies of circulatory origin. Biology of the Neonate 50: 61–74

LeBlanc R, O'Gorman A M 1980 Neonatal intracranial hemorrhage. A clinical and serial computerized tomographic study. Journal of Neurosurg 53: 642–651

Levene M I 1981 Measurement of the growth of the lateral ventricles in preterm infants with real-time ultrasound. Archives of Disease in Childhood 56: 900–904

Levene M I 1987 Current reviews in neonatal neurology. Churchill Livingstone, Edinburgh

Levene M I, Starte D R 1981 A longitudinal study of post-haemorrhagic ventricular dilatation in the newborn. Archives of Disease in Childhood 56: 905–910

Liechty E A, Gilmor R L, Bryson C Q, Bull M J 1983 Outcome of high-risk neonates with ventriculomegaly. Developmental Medicine and Child Neurology 25: 162–168

Lorber J 1968 The results of early treatment of extreme hydrocephalus. Developmental Medicine and Child Neurology 16: 21–29

Lorber J 1975 Isosorbide in treatment of infantile hydrocephalus. Archives of Disease in Childhood 50: 431–434

Lorber J, Bhat US 1974 Posthaemorrhagic hydrocephalus. Diagnosis, differential diagnosis, treatment and long-term results. Archives of Disease in Childhood 49: 751–762

Lorber J, Salfield S, Lonton T 1983 Isosorbide in the management of infantile hydrocephalus. Developmental Medicine and Child Neurology 25: 502–511

McComb J G, Ramos A D, Platzker A C, Henderson D J, Segall H D 1983 Management of hydrocephalus secondary to intraventricular haemorrhage in the preterm infant with a subcutaneous ventricular catheter reservoir. Neurosurgery 13: 295–300

McCullough D C, Balzer-Martin A 1982 Current prognosis in overt neonatal hydrocephalus. Journal of Neurosurgery 57: 378–383

McLone D G, Czyzewski D, Raimond A J, Sommers R C 1982 Central nervous system infections as a limiting factor in the intelligence of children with meningomyelocele. Pediatrics 70: 338–342

Mantovani J F et al 1980 Failure of daily lumbar punctures to prevent the development of hydrocephalus following intraventricular hemorrhage. Journal of Pediatrics 97: 278–281

Marlin A E 1980 Protection of the cortical mantle in premature infants with posthaemorrhagic hydrocephalus. Neurosurgery 7: 464–468

Mealey J, Gilmour R L, Bubb M L 1973 The prognosis of overt hydrocephalus at birth. Journal of Neurosurgery 39: 348–355

Ment L R, Duncan C C, Scott D T, Ehrenkranz R A 1984 Posthemorrhagic hydrocephalus. Low incidence in very low birth weight neonates with intraventricular hemorrhage. Journal of Neurosurgery 60: 343–347

Moylan F M, Herrin J T, Krishnamoorthy K, Todres I D, Shannon D C 1978 Inappropriate antidiuretic hormone secretion in premature infants with cerebral palsy. American Journal of Diseases in Children 132: 399–402

Palmer P, Dubowitz L M S, Levene M I, Dubowitz V 1982 Developmental and neurological progress of preterm infants with intraventricular haemorrhage and ventricular dilatation. Archives of Disease in Childhood 57: 748–753

Papile L, Burstein J, Burstein R, Koffler H, Koops B L, Johnson J D 1980 Post-hemorrhagic hydrocephalus in low birth weight infants: Treatment by serial lumbar punctures. Journal of Pediatrics 97: 273–277

Pasternak J F, Mantovani J F, Volpe J J 1980 Porencephaly from periventricular intracerebral hemorrhage in a premature infant. American Journal of Disease in Children 134: 673–675

Porter F N 1975 Hydrocephalus treated by compressive head wrapping. Archives of Disease in Childhood 50: 816–818

Shaw C-M, Alvord E C 1974 Subependymal germinolysis. Archives of Neurology 31: 374–381

Shaywitz B A 1972 Epidermoid spinal cord tumours and previous lumbar punctures. Journal of Pediatrics 80: 638–640

Shinnar S, Gammon K, Bergman E W, Epstein M, Freeman J M 1985 Management of hydrocephalus in infancy: Use of acetazolamide and frusemide to avoid cerebrospinal fluid shunts. Journal of Pediatrics 107: 31–37

Stewart A L, Thorburn R J, Hope P L, Goldsmith M, Lipscomb A P, Reynolds E O R 1983 Ultrasound appearance of the brain in very preterm infants and neurodevelopmental outcome at 18 months of age. Archives of Disease in Childhood 58: 598–604

Sty J R, Babbitt D P, D'Souza B 1979 Pediatric radionuclide ventriculography. Clinics in Nuclear Medicine 10: 417–421

Szymonowicz W, Yu V Y H, Lewis E A 1985 Post-haemorrhagic hydrocephalus in the preterm infant. Australian Paediatric Journal 21: 175–179

Tardieu M, Evrard P, Lyon G 1981 Progressive expanding congenital porencephalies: a treatable cause of progressive encephalopathy. Pediatrics 68: 198–202

Trounce J Q, Rutter N, Levene M I 1986 Periventricular leukomalacia and intraventricular haemorrhage in the preterm neonate. Archives of Disease in Childhood 61: 1196–1202

Volpe J J 1977 Neonatal intracranial hemorrhage: pathophysiology, neuropathology and clinical features. Clinics in Perinatology 4: 77–81

Volpe J J, Pasternak J F, Allan W C 1977 Ventricular dilation preceding rapid head growth following neonatal intracranial hemorrhage. American Journal of Diseases in Children 131: 1212–1215

West C 1848 Lectures on the diseases of infancy and childhood. Longmans, London

Whitelaw A G, Haines M E, Bolsover W, Harris E 1984 Factor V deficiency and antenatal intraventricular haemorrhage. Archives of Disease in Childhood 59: 997–999

Zalneraitis E L, Young R S K, Krishnamoorthy K S 1979 Intracranial hemorrhage thrombocytopenia. Journal of Pediatrics 95: 611–614

Asphyxia and trauma

The most important cerebral complication of full-term delivery is asphyxia. With modern obstetrical methods, trauma has become considerably less common but is still an important cause of neurological injury (see Ch. 35). In this section we have chosen to consider the problem of asphyxia and its management only in the context of the full-term infant. This is because the premature infant shows different effects and pathological sequelae to this condition and these are reviewed elsewhere (see Section 8).

32. Prenatal and intrapartum asphyxia

Prof I. Kjellmer

DEFINITION

The term asphyxia is used with different meanings by different authors. In this survey asphyxia will denote the combination of oxygen lack and acidosis. Oxygen lack without an accompanying acidosis will be termed hypoxia or hypoxaemia.

The word asphyxia itself — meaning 'without pulse' — describes the ultimate form of severe oxygen lack. In the fetus and neonate, however, cardiac events are generally secondary to the problems of gas transport. Therefore, cardiac standstill and organ ischaemia will be the effect of asphyxia rather than the cause during the perinatal period.

INCIDENCE OF ASPHYXIA

Because of widely varying definitions and because of differences in the practical management of pregnancy, labour and delivery, incidence rates for perinatal asphyxia vary. The Collaborative Perinatal Study contains information on more than 49 000 newborn infants (Nelson & Ellenberg 1981). Incidence rates for moderately low Apgar scores at 1 minute (4–6) were 19.7% for babies below 2501 g birth-weight and 13.1% for babies with birth-weight above 2500 g. Babies with very low Apgar scores (0–3) at 1 minute were 15.5% and 4.5% respectively. Babies with moderately low Apgar scores at 1 minute generally do not need active resuscitation while neonates with Apgar scores of 3 or less often will need some cardiopulmonary resuscitation. In a country-wide recent survey of neonatal asphyxia in Sweden, Palme & Ericsson (1986) reported an incidence rate of 2.0% of neonates with very low Apgar scores at 1 minute (3 or less) from a population of 95 000 births.

PHYSIOLOGICAL ADJUSTMENTS TO ASPHYXIA

Haemodynamic

The general train of events elicited by intra-uterine asphyxia on the fetal circulation has been well described in animal preparations. There are reasons to believe that the same principles are also valid for humans. A brief and schematic summary from some recent work gives the following picture (Cohn et al 1974, Edelstone et al 1977, Peeters et al 1979, Fisher et al 1980, Rosén et al 1986a). During asphyxia fetal heart rate falls, mean arterial blood pressure rises, myocardial contractility increases and cardiac output (measured as combined ventricular output) is maintained without much change up to a point when circulatory collapse ensues. Dramatic changes in the distribution of cardiac output take place with an enhanced blood flow reaching the myocardium, the central nervous system and the adrenals at the expense of reduced perfusion in other tissues such as the liver, kidney, intestine, muscle and skin. The perfusion of the fetal placenta is largely preserved and the efficiency of the placental circulation is enhanced by adjustments of the perfusion/perfusion ratio of fetal/maternal blood flow in individual cotyledons (Power et al 1967).

The redistribution of blood flow during periods of asphyxia also implies a redistribution of the well-oxygenated blood from the umbilical vein. Owing to preferential streamlining of that blood in the inferior vena cava the myocardium and the brain receive an increased proportion of the most oxygenated blood available to the fetus (Reuss & Rudolph 1980).

Hormonal

The profound alterations of blood flow and metabolism during asphyxia are the result of complex changes in regulatory mechanisms both from the autonomic nervous system and from the endocrine apparatus. During the stress of normal vaginal birth, the neonate reacts with an impressive release of catecholamines (Lagercrantz & Bistoletti 1977). This surge of catecholamines is further enhanced to values many times higher than ever recorded in adults when the neonate has been the victim of perinatal asphyxia (Nylund et al 1979). Using fetal sheep Jones & Ritchie (1983) collected evidence that many of the fetal circulatory and hormonal responses to hypoxia could be caused by the rise in plasma catecholamines, and Dagbjartsson et al (1985) demonstrated that fetal sheep depended on intact beta-adrenoceptor mechanisms to be able to cope with asphyxia of a moderate degree.

A host of other hormones and vaso-active substances have been reported to be released during birth and particularly during asphyxia. Among these substances are vasopressin, adenine and adenosine, prostaglandin and prostacycline metabolites. Each of these substances may be attributed some very interesting and potent effects on circulation, respiration, metabolism and behaviour. However, definite evaluation of the importance of these substances for fetal adaptation to asphyxia must await further knowledge.

Metabolic

The hallmark of the metabolic response to asphyxia is anaerobic glycolysis. Classic studies demonstrate a linear relationship between the tolerance to asphyxia expressed as time to last gasp and the size of the glycogen depots in liver and myocardium (Dawes et al 1959, Shelley 1961). The time period between cardiac arrest and disruption of ion homeostasis in the rat brain was directly proportional to the blood glucose concentration and thereby to the substrate stores available for immediate anaerobic glycolysis (Hansen 1978). The process of anaerobic glycolysis depends on beta-adrenoceptive mechanisms. However, anaerobic glycolysis implies an enormous waste of energy supplies in comparison to aerobic combustion. The rate of anaerobic glycolysis would have to increase 15 times to maintain the pre-asphyctic rate of ATP regeneration. Obviously, anaerobic glycolysis is a short-term salvage mechanism that soon leads to the accumulation of lactate in tissues and blood. Gradually increasing concentrations of lactic acid together with increasing acidosis have long been recognized as characteristic findings during asphyxia, both when experimentally induced (Dawes et al 1959) and in the clinical situation (Daniel & James 1965).

The inability of anaerobic glycolysis to maintain ATP regeneration during anaerobic conditions results in a decomposition of the energy-rich intracellular phosphates. Saugstad (1975) demonstrated that this process was quantitatively reflected in augmented plasma levels of hypoxanthine. The plasma level of hypoxanthine in the fetus was closely related to the degree of intra-uterine asphyxia (Thiringer et al 1980). The source of hypoxanthine in the lamb fetus proved to be multiple with a dominant release from the liver and skeletal muscle early during asphyxia, at a more severe stage of asphyxia followed by release from myocardium, and only at the most severe stage of asphyxia also a release from the central nervous system (Thiringer et al 1982, 1984).

Cerebral

During asphyxia two major stages can be discerned with regard to the situation of the brain. The first stage occurs initially, before oxygen lack has become complete and is characterized by general mechanisms (mainly circulatory) that tend to keep up oxygen supply to the brain and maintain aerobic metabolism. The second stage is reached when the haemodynamic adjustments fail to compensate for the desaturation and acidification of the blood.

The first stage is characterized by cerebral vasodilatation (Cohn et al 1974) and a pronounced redistribution of blood flow within the central nervous system providing the highest blood flows to brainstem, midbrain and cerebellum (Blomstrand et al 1978, Shapiro et al 1980). During the stage when oxygen delivery to the brain is curtailed in spite of blood flow alterations, an adaptive reduction in cerebral oxygen consumption takes place that is particularly pronounced when acidosis prevails (Kjellmer et al 1974).

When asphyxia is so severe that the brain resorts to breaking down the high-energy phosphate compounds of the cells, severe impairment of the electrical function of the neurones take place. The spontaneous EEG activity has already ceased but at this stage also the cortical evoked EEG potentials vanish (Thiringer et al 1982).

When oxygenation is adequate the fetal brain normally consumes not only glucose but also lactate and hypoxanthine (Mann 1970, Thiringer et al 1982). During asphyxia, however, there occurs a net release from the brain of these two products of anaerobic metabolism.

The disruption of neurophysiological activity during asphyxia is related to different events. The synaptic transmission is impaired because of reduced synthesis and release of excitatory transmitter substances such as noradrenaline and dopamine (Hedner 1978, Silverstein & Johnston 1984). Complete anoxia leads to a reduction of the $Na^+/K^+/ATPase$ activity and the inability of the neuronal cell membrane to maintain electrical stability. Leakage of K^+ ions into the extracellular space of the brain and of Ca^+ ions into the cytosol of the neurones takes place as the ultimate result of the cellular energy crisis (Hansen 1978, 1985, Hansen & Nordström 1979). These events occur at a late stage during asphyxia, immediately before death. For a schematic representation of some major events taking place in the brain during a progressively increasing asphyxia, see Fig. 32.1.

MECHANISMS OF CEREBRAL INJURY DURING ASPHYXIA

'Anoxia not only stops the machine, it wrecks the machinery.' This classical expression by J. S. Haldane (1922) has for many decades influenced our ideas on the mechanisms of brain damage during asphyxia and

CEREBRAL FUNCTIONS IN ASPHYXIA

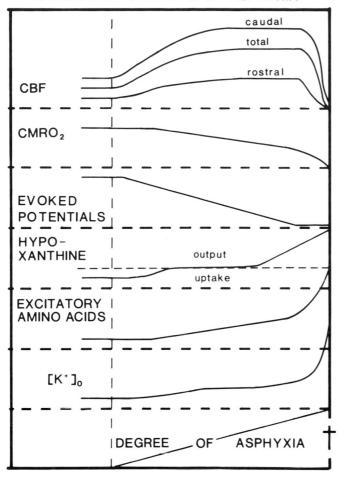

Fig. 32.1 The reactions of cerebral blood flow (CBF), cerebral oxygen uptake ($CMRO_2$), evoked EEG potentials, cerebral uptake and release of hypoxanthine and extracellular concentration in the brain of excitatory amino acids and potassium ions during conditions of gradually increasing perinatal asphyxia leading to death. Data for this scheme were collected from Kjellmer et al 1974 and 1986, Hrbek et al 1974, Thiringer et al 1982 and Hansen 1977.

has led to the non-disputed notion that oxygen lack in itself damages the cells. However, several experimental observations favour the interpretation that oxygen lack in itself cannot be the major reason for cell destruction. Thus, neurones from retina and from the central nervous system can tolerate periods of 20–60 minutes of total anoxia without irreversible injury (Ames & Gurian 1963, Hossman & Kleihues 1973).

Does irreversible damage occur from complete exhaustion of substrates for energy supplies? Less than five minutes of complete ischaemic anoxia is sufficient for the total exhaustion of intracellular ATP (Ljunggren et al 1974). In spite of this the brain is capable of complete recovery of its adenylate charge even after 30 minutes of ischaemic anoxia (Hossman 1983).

Thus asphyctic brain damage appears to not be directly caused by lack of oxygen or complete lack of substrates for

the generation of energy. Instead, other mechanisms for brain damage must be operating.

In the following, three different kinds of potentially brain damaging mechanism shall be discussed, namely development of acidosis, accumulation of cytotoxic amino acids and generation of oxygen-derived free radicals together with calcium ion intoxication.

Acidosis

In clinical asphyxia, acidosis is an inescapable companion of oxygen lack. The same events that impede oxygen transport to the fetus also complicate the delivery of carbon dioxide from the fetus. This results in a carbonic acidosis. The increased rate of anaerobic glycolysis leads to a gradual accumulation of lactic acid and to the development of a non-carbonic acidosis. When the degree of acidosis was experimentally manipulated in the fetal sheep during hypoxia the cerebral activity measured as somatosensory evoked potentials deteriorated significantly more in the acidotic than the non-acidotic state (Hrbek et al 1974). With the same experimental set-up the rate of cerebral oxygen uptake was reduced significantly more when hypoxia was combined with acidosis than hypoxia alone (Kjellmer et al 1974). On the other hand, fetal acidosis induced by infusing lactic acid to achieve arterial pH levels around 6.88 did not lead to severe deterioration of cerebral function in the absence of concomitant hypoxia (Mann et al 1971).

The production of lactic acid within the brain tissue in connection with oxygen lack results in detrimental effects on the brain. Newborn Rhesus monkeys were subjected to complete ischaemia by means of circulatory arrest. Hyperglycaemic animals had higher rates of brain tissue production of lactic acid and also more pronounced deterioration of cerebral function than normo- and hypoglycaemic animals (Myers & Yamaguchi 1976). Adult rats fasted before a period of 30 minutes of incomplete brain ischaemia demonstrated lower cortical concentrations of lactate and significantly better recovery rates of spontaneous EEG and of somatosensory evoked potentials than rats given an i.v. infusion of glucose before ischaemia (Rehncrona et al 1981).

However, in fetal asphyxia both before and during labour the brain is not rendered ischaemic, as in the above-mentioned studies. Rather, the typical reaction is an overall augmentation of cerebral blood flow. To study the influence of glucose availability on brain function during conditions of unrestricted cerebral blood flow, blood glucose concentrations were varied over a fourfold range (from 50 to 200% of normal fetal concentrations) and fetal sheep were subjected to graded asphyxia. Hyperglycaemia was associated with rapid development of lactic acidosis and reduction of cerebral oxygen consumption together with deterioration of the neurophysiological characteristics of the brain (Blomstrand et al 1984). Far from being beneficial during asphyxia, fetal hyperglycaemia thus appears to reduce the tolerance towards asphyxia of the fetal brain.

In summary, acidosis in the well-oxygenated fetus does not cause severe impairment of cerebral blood flow until extremely low levels of pH are reached that are associated with cardiac failure. During asphyxia, acidosis is associated with reduction of cerebral oxygen uptake, impairment of neurophysiological activity and inability to restore energy-rich phosphates and electrical function during postasphyctic stages. The degree of accumulation of lactic acid in brain tissue is negatively related to chances for recovery of cerebral functions.

Accumulation of cytotoxic amino acids

Indirect evidence has accumulated that excitatory amino acids exert toxic effects during experimental brain ischaemia. Selective loss of neurones was demonstrated in regions where glutamate is involved in neurotransmission (Jörgensen & Diemer 1982). When postsynaptic receptors for excitatory amino acids were blocked by a specific blocker, neurone death during anoxia was prevented in tissue cultures (Rothman 1984). When a selective inhibitor of N-methyl-D-aspartate receptors was locally administered to the hippocampus of the rat, the occurrence of ischaemic neuronal damage was effectively inhibited (Simon et al 1984). To these observations direct evidence of high concentrations of excitotoxic amino acids has recently been added (Hagberg et al 1985). Using a microdialysis system these authors investigated the shift of amino acids from intra- to extracellular compartments in the hippocampus of adult rabbits during periods of brain ischaemia. Fig. 32.2 demonstrates the dramatic increase of the concentrations of the excitatory amino acids glutamate and aspartate during ischaemia. These compounds reach concentrations that are neurotoxic (Choi 1985, Olney 1983). It is thus conceivable that brain damage caused by ischaemia is related to the release of excitatory amino acids. It should be noted, though, that two amino acids that inhibit synaptic transmission are also released. Both gamma-aminobutyric acid (GABA) and taurin in high concentrations would tend to counterbalance the hyperstimulation of postsynaptic neurones induced by the excitatory amino acids.

The results described were obtained from experiments on adult animals during complete ischaemia. In perinatal asphyxia, however, cerebral blood flow usually increases until the phase of cardiac standstill. The microdialysis technique was therefore applied to the exteriorized fetal sheep under conditions of induced graded fetal asphyxia (Kjellmer et al 1986, Hagberg et al 1987a). Two microprobes inserted stereotactically permitted sampling of dialysis fluid from the cerebral cortex and from the caudate nucleus. As long as the cerebral blood flow was augmented, asphyxia resulted in only moderate elevation of the excitatory amino acids. When asphyxia was so severe that both cardiac output and

cerebral blood flow fell, a 3–5-fold increase in extracellular concentrations of the excitatory amino acids glutamate and aspartate took place. The rise of amino acid concentrations was higher in the striatum than in the cortex. GABA and especially taurin levels also increased to very high values.

Thus, the fetus during asphyxia responded qualitatively similarly to the ischaemic adult brain but the leakage of excitatory amino acids was less in the asphyctic fetal brain while the release of taurin was very pronounced. The concentrations of excitatory amino acids in the interstitial fluid of the striatum reached potentially neurotoxic levels during circulatory arrest. This finding is particularly relevant in the light of the recent evidence for a transient, perinatal glutamatergic innervation of the globus pallidus in the rat (Greenamyre et al in press).

Generation of oxygen-derived free radicals (OFR) and calcium ion intoxication

During the normal oxidative process a small proportion of the oxygen utilized is converted into free radicals: the

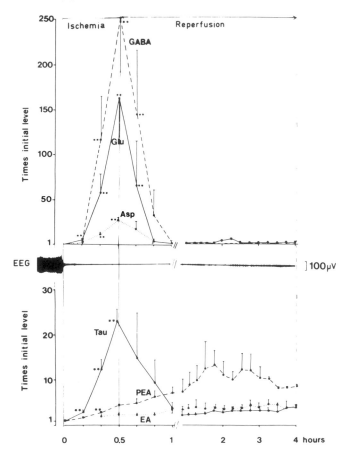

Fig. 32.2 Extracellular amino acids during 30-minute ischaemia. Top: Levels of γ-aminobutyric acid (GABA), dashed line; glutamate (Glu), unbroken line; aspartate (Asp), dotted line. Bottom: levels of taurine (Tau), unbroken line; phosphoethanolamine (PEA), dashed line; and ethanolamine (EA), dotted line. Values are means ± SEM times initial levels, $n = 4$–7. Levels of significance were tested vs initial values, *$P<0.01$. Representative EEG recording from one experiment is displayed. (Reproduced with permission from Hagberg et al 1985.)

superoxide ion and the related species hydrogen peroxide and hydroxyl radical. These potentially destructive agents are extremely reactive and attack membrane structures (cell membranes and mitochondria) and also inflict direct injuries to the cellular DNA (Del Maestro et al 1980). During normal oxidative metabolism several inactivating systems effectively prevent the action of the free radicals. The superoxide dismutase prevents the accumulation of the superoxide radical in concentrations high enough to produce tissue damage and to activate the Haber–Weiss reaction that results in the formation of the most highly reactive radical, the hydroxyl radical (Haber & Weiss 1934, Kontos 1985).

During re-oxygenation after asphyxia or during reperfusion after ischaemia a number of complex, interacting reactions take place that are depicted in simplified form in Fig. 32.3.

During asphyxia, several interacting processes occur that set the stage for the generation of large amounts of free radicals during the re-oxygenation phase. The energy-rich phosphated nucleotides are rapidly consumed (Ljunggren et al 1974) and hypoxanthine is accumulated both in the circulating blood and in tissues, including the brain (Thiringer et al 1980, 1983, 1984). When oxygen is added to a system rich in xanthine and hypoxanthine, free radicals are formed in large quantities provided xanthine oxidase is available (Thomas et al 1978). This enzyme is generally not directly available but can be transformed from xanthine dehydrogenase. The transformation is induced by hypoxia and by a drastic increase in intracellular calcium ion concentration (see later), which in turn is caused by the lack of oxygen (Parks et al 1982, McCord 1985).

The xanthine oxidase system produces superoxide radicals and, both directly and via dismutation, hydrogen peroxide. In the presence of free iron to catalyse the Haber–Weiss reaction these two compounds react to form the hydroxyl radical. Endogenous cerebrospinal fluid contains enough free iron for this process (Halliwell & Gutteridge 1984). In the brain the superoxide radical and hydrogen peroxide both induce transitional relaxation of arteriolar smooth muscle while the hydroxyl radical appears to be responsible for permanent vascular injury (Kontos 1985).

During ischaemia and asphyxia the elevation of tissue hypoxanthine levels is paralleled by a build-up of arachidonic acid as the result of a gradual breakdown of membrane phospholipids. This is induced by an activation of tissue phospholipase via the elevation of intracellular free calcium ion levels (Siesjö 1981). The accumulation of arachidonic acid in neuronal tissue can be partially prevented with calcium entry blockers (Nemoto et al 1983).

During the re-oxygenation phase the accumulated arachidonic acid serves as substrate for two different oxidative enzymatic pathways. The lipo-oxygenase pathway metabo-

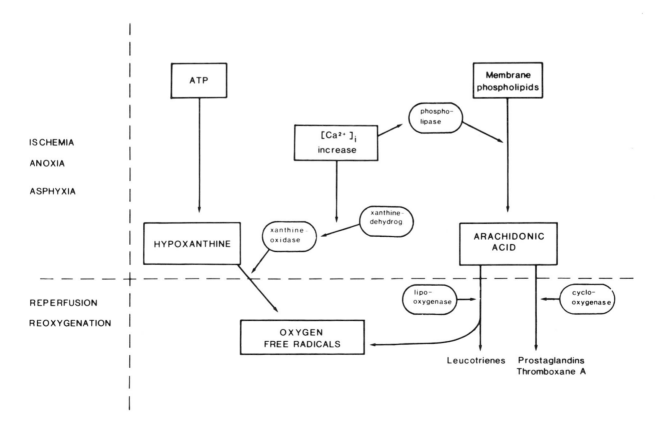

Fig. 32.3 The events resulting in accumulation of hypoxanthine and arachidonic acid in brain tissue during asphyxia and the generation of free oxygen radicals during re-oxygenation.

lizes arachidonic acid to the leukotriene system which effectively contributes to the generation of free oxygen radicals (Chan & Fishman 1978). The free oxygen radicals tend to perpetuate a chain reaction since they accelerate the formation of arachidonic acid via phospholipid degradation and lipid peroxidation.

The cyclo-oxygenase pathway contributes to the formation of a host of prostaglandins. The net vascular effect of prostaglandin formation in the brain will be vasoconstriction, since the postasphyctic brain has only a low capacity to synthesize the vasodilator prostacycline (Raichle 1983) while the production rate of the potent vasoconstrictor thromboxane A_2 is high (Gaudet & Levine 1979). Pretreatment with an inhibitor of cyclo-oxygenase activity (indomethacin) has proved effective in preventing postischaemic brain hypoperfusion (Hallenbeck & Furlow 1979).

There is thus an abundance of indirect, theoretical evidence to suggest a role for oxygen free radicals in postischaemic brain damage. Direct evidence, however, is meagre. Siesjö (1981) reported that the ratio of glutathione to the dimer of glutathione produced by glutathione peroxidase did not change in the postischaemic brain. This was interpreted as evidence against the existence of large amounts of free radicals. On the other hand, our own study using the microdialysis probe on the brain of the fetal sheep has demonstrated a 2–3-fold increase of the extracellular concentration of xanthine during severe asphyxia (Kjellmer et al 1986). This finding suggests an activation of the xanthine oxidase system already during the asphyctic stage and thus also evidence for the formation of free oxygen radicals in the brain. Moreover, studies on the adult rat demonstrated a transient sevenfold increase of the xanthine concentration in brain extracellular fluid upon recirculation after ischaemia (Hagberg et al 1987b), and in the same species an increased tissue concentration of uric acid was found after ischaemia (Kanemitsu et al 1986).

During anoxia–ischaemia both the activation of phospholipase and the conversion of xanthine dehydrogenase to xanthine oxidase depend on the intracellular accumulation of free calcium ions (Fig. 32.3). The overloading of the neurones with calcium ions takes place as a result of the rapid break down of the normal Ca^{2+} gradient across the cell membrane. This occurs within a few minutes of complete ischaemic anoxia resulting in a 200-fold increase of intracellular concentration of free Ca^{2+} (Vykocil et al 1972, Siesjö 1981, White et al 1984).

Inhibition of the neuronal overloading with calcium ions has proved effective in ameliorating postanoxic neuronal injury. Thus, pretreatment with calcium antagonists has improved postischaemic cerebral function in cats (Hoffmeister et al 1979) and dogs (Bircher & Safar 1983, Steen et al 1983, White et al 1983).

The majority of studies on postanoxic brain injury are performed on adult animals after complete cerebral ischaemia. In most instances the experimental animals are pretreated with the drugs tested. During perinatal asphyxia brain circulation is maintained and even augmented for a long period. Very limited practical possibilities exist for pretreatment in the clinical situation. Therefore, Thiringer et al (1987) studied the combined effect of free oxygen radical scavengers and lidoflazine, a calcium channel blocker, given during the resuscitation phase to newborn lambs after severe perinatal asphyxia. The radical scavengers used were mannitol, L-methionin and $MgSO_4$ in a solution of 3% dextran aimed at inactivating both the superoxide and the hydroxyl radicals. Fig. 32.4 summarizes the results. The control animals had a short period of hyperaemia in the brain after resuscitation but within 30 minutes this was converted into cerebral hypoperfusion. Concomitantly, the oxygen uptake of the brain was attenuated. The electrical activity measured both as spontaneous EEG activity and evoked EEG potentials vanished during the period of asphyxia. Return of neurophysiological activity was seen as recovery of evoked potentials. Only 1/12 control animals demonstrated 'cerebral survival' for 2 hours. In contrast, the animals treated with scavengers and lidoflazine during resuscitation retained a high cerebral perfusion rate and

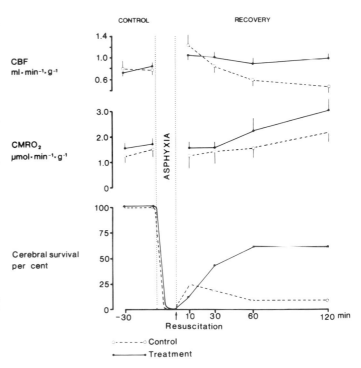

Fig. 32.4 Fetal sheep were acutely asphyxiated by tying the umbilical cord. After 15 minutes, resuscitation was instituted. During resuscitation the treatment group was given a combination of free oxygen radical scavengers and a calcium channel blocker while the control group was given placebo. At 60 and 120 minutes after start of resuscitation the treatment group showed significantly higher cerebral blood flows, cerebral oxygen consumption and higher cerebral survival measured as recovery of evoked EEG potentials. (Modified from Thiringer et al in press.)

an increased metabolic rate of oxygen for 2 hours postresuscitation. These animals also demonstrated a significantly higher success rate in terms of recovery of evoked potentials (8/14). Thus, the combined short-term effect of scavengers and lidoflazine was beneficial for the prevention of postresuscitation cerebral injury.

At present, little information exists on long-term effects of treatment either with radical scavengers or calcium blockers to combat postasphyxial brain damage in the perinatal period in animals, let alone in humans. Pretreatment of 7-day-old rats with flunarizin, a calcium channel blocker, provided significant protection against morphological brain damage 2 weeks after the combined insult of unilateral carotid ligation and exposure to 2 hours of hypoxia (Silverstein et al 1986).

WHY IS THE IMMATURE BRAIN MORE RESISTANT TO HYPOXIA THAN THE MATURE BRAIN?

Robert Boyle (1670) was probably first to produce evidence that the immature animal has a greater tolerance to suffocation than the mature animal. He enclosed newborn rat pups with an adult rat in a jar with a burning candle. He observed that the young animals survived longer than the adult animal after the candle had expired. Numerous studies have later confirmed this original observation. One way to illustrate the phenomenon is shown in Fig. 32.5. Hansen (1977) compared the extracellular concentrations of potassium in the brains of young and adult rats during anoxia. The phase of slowly rising $[K^+]_0$ during anoxia lasted 2 minutes in the adult rat but 25 minutes in the 4-day-old rat. The large difference is partly due to the young rat's ability to preserve cerebral circulation during anoxia and thereby ensure supply of substrate for energy metabolism during anoxia. When circulatory effects were excluded by rendering the brains totally ischaemic the phase

of slowly increasing $[K^+]_0$ was reduced to 10 minutes in the 4-day-old rat — still five times longer than for the adult animal. The higher cerebral tolerance to anoxia and asphyxia in the young animal compared with the adult is thus expressed as a better ion homeostasis during these conditions. The background is probably multiple: the immature brain, with smaller neurones, less branched and with fewer synapses has smaller demands for energy-consuming ion pumping than the adult brain (Hansen 1985). The rate of energy metabolism in the immature rat brain is much lower than in that of the adult (Duffy et al 1975). In the fetal sheep the cerebral metabolic rate of oxygen is further reduced during conditions of oxygen lack and asphyxia (Kjellmer et al 1974). The glycolytic capacity of the immature rat brain allows the regeneration of ATP at about half the normal rate (Hansen & Nordström 1979), compared with only 25% in the adult brain (Nordström & Siesjö 1978).

Thus, for reasons of structure, differentiation and basal energy demands the perinatal brain can withstand a longer period of oxygen lack or asphyxia than can the mature brain. Does this also mean that the risk of postresuscitation brain injury is less the more immature the brain?

From clinical experience, this would appear to be true. While adult patients and children resuscitated after drowning accidents and cardiac standstill have a sinister prognosis (Torphy et al 1984) newborn babies resuscitated after severe perinatal asphyxia and after prolonged periods of oxygen lack show a 50–75% rate of survival with intact cerebral functions (Scott 1976, Nelson & Ellenberg 1981, Celander et al 1985).

The lower risk for severe brain damage in survivors after asphyxia when neonates are compared with adults may be linked to factors such as those related to leakage of excitotoxic amino acids into the extracellular space of the brain. There may even be a phase of active repair of the brain tissue facilitated by neurotrophic factors (Ebendal et al 1980, Thoenen & Edgar 1985). Nieto-Sampedro

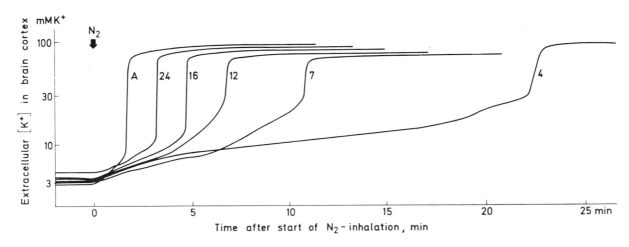

Fig. 32.5 Extracellular potassium concentration in brain cortex of rats at different ages following exposure to nitrogen. The numbers indicate the age (days) of the animal. A = adult. (Reproduced with permission from Hansen 1977.)

and associates (1982, 1985) demonstrated that fluid from 6-day-old brain wound cavities enhanced the survival in tissue cultures of neurones from young rats.

However, it appears likely that there is another major reason why survivors after severe asphyxia have greater chances to preserve brain function when the asphyctic insult strikes a neonate than when an adult is hit. During both childhood and adult life the brain is by far the most exclusively oxygen-dependent organ in the body. In the perinatal period, however, due to lower metabolic demands, the brain is only barely more dependent on oxygen than the myocardium, the liver or the kidneys. Thus, in the perinatal period, the brain is but one of several vital organs that are severely affected by asphyxia. Therefore, survival after asphyxia is much more an all-or-none phenomenon during the perinatal period than during adult life.

DETECTION OF FETAL ASPHYXIA

The connection between thick, meconium-stained amniotic fluid and poor start of breathing in the neonate was observed long ago. Likewise the association between fetal bradycardia and neonatal asphyxia was established long before the advent of modern fetal surveillance. However, it is only during the last few decades that systematic knowledge and experience have been gathered to enable the detection in the clinical situation of most asphyxiated fetuses. And still, it must be realized that most clinical decisions regarding the asphyxiated fetus rest on pure empirical grounds. Our understanding of the underlying mechanisms is very incomplete.

Cardiotocography

The pioneering work of Hon (1959) and Caldeyro-Barcia (1956) introduced the simultaneous recording of the uterine activity and the fetal heart rate. The patterns of changes that may occur during uterine contractions were described and are now in everyday clinical use. To the description of fetal heart rate decelerations, accelerations and changes of basal heart rates was added the concept of heart rate variability, and the ominous significance of a decreased variability with loss of beat-to-beat variation was established (Beard et al 1971).

Much work has been devoted to clarify what mechanisms contribute to the different cardiotocographic (CTG) patterns. Although, there appears to be a consensus of opinion that the early decelerations are caused by vagal hyperactivity, induced by an increased intracranial pressure during contractions, the mechanisms behind late decelerations are incompletely understood.

They are considered indicative of fetal distress and are associated with an increased incidence of fetal acidaemia (Bissonette 1975) and of fetal and neonatal release of cat-echolamines (Lagercrantz & Bistoletti 1977). Nevertheless, neonates delivered by emergency caesarean section because of late deceleration show more often than not lack of evidence for any degree of fetal asphyxia (Bissonette 1975).

Changes of heart rate variability add to the discriminative power of the CTG. In animal experiments it was clarified that variability changed in a predictable way during a sequence of gradually increasing lack of oxygen (Dalton et al 1977, Stånge et al 1977). At the earliest stages of oxygen lack, fetal heart rate variability rose in response to stimulation of alpha-adrenergic receptors (Lilja 1983), while variability decreased to a 'silent pattern' when lack of oxygen was aggravated. In spite of these simple relationships neonates born after exhibiting a silent pattern have a normal arterial pH and normal Apgar score at birth in no less than 60% (Beard et al 1971, Bissonette 1975).

At present, a normal CTG pattern may be taken to indicate fetal well-being and lack of intrapartum asphyxia, while the occurrence of 'abnormalities' in the CTG patterns may not necessarily signify that the fetus is in danger.

That recordings of fetal heart rate only convey an incomplete picture of fetal distress should not come as a surprise. The reason why fetal heart rate has been extensively studied and is now regularly monitored during risk labour is not primarily that it reflects fetal well-being but, instead, that it is the fetal signal most easily accessible.

Consequently, other fetal signals have been sought to reflect fetal distress more truly, either singly or in combination with the CTG. Among several methods, brief mention shall be made to five: fetal scalp pH, fetal breathing movements, fetal electroencephalogram, fetal ECG pattern and blood velocities in large fetal vessels.

Fetal scalp pH assessment

The introduction of fetal scalp pH measurements in clinical practice meant an increased precision of the diagnosis of fetal distress (Saling & Schneider 1967). Serial sampling of micro-amounts of blood from the fetal head enables the obstetrician to separate cases with CTG changes without acidaemia from those with acidaemia. This technique has gained wide acceptance and, together with the CTG, forms the corner-stone of modern fetal surveillance during labour. The limitations of the technique are obvious. It can only be applied after the membranes are ruptured and it is a somewhat laborious, invasive technique.

Fetal breathing

When fetal breathing movements were rediscovered by Dawes et al (1972) they at first appeared very promising for the prediction of fetal asphyxia. A clear relationship was established between lack of breathing movements and fetal asphyxia (Boddy & Dawes 1975). Since fetal breathing movements were obtained by ultrasonography, expectations were that breathing movements should be used for long-term antenatal surveillance of fetuses at risk for asphyxia. These expectations have been fulfilled only partially. The periodicity of the fetal breathing movements, due to shifts between different stages of sleep in utero (Patrick et al 1978, Bowes et al 1981) makes very long periods of observation necessary. The fetal breathing movements normally cease some hours before the start of spontaneous labour. Therefore, lack of fetal breathing movements may signify both the start of normal labour, a peacefully sleeping fetus and impending fetal demise. Because of restricted usefulness, fetal breathing movements have now been introduced as only one out of five different criteria that taken together give a 'biophysical profile' that has proved useful in antenatal surveillance (Manning et al 1980).

Fetal breathing movements express one basic rhythmic function of the central nervous system. There are more direct ways of assessing CNS function. Much effort has been put into obtaining electro-encephalograms from the human fetus during delivery. The achievements are thoroughly reviewed in Chapter 14. Fetal EEG remains an interesting investigative tool but lacks applicability in everyday medicine.

Fetal ECG

The fetal ECG pattern as a means to reveal intra-uterine asphyxia has attracted recent attention by our group (Rosén et al 1985, 1986b). The ordinary CTG equipment uses a built-in filter to exclude low-frequency variations and thereby eliminates the possibility to display true changes of the ST–T segment of the electrocardiogram. By applying ordinary ECG recorders Rosén and coworkers first demonstrated that T wave changes regularly occur during fetal asphyxia in anaesthetized guinea pigs and sheep (Rosén & Kjellmer 1975, Rosén et al 1976) and then that oxygen lack in the awake, chronically instrumented fetal sheep was associated with elevation of the T wave (Greene et al 1982).

This, in turn, was closely related to the release of fetal catecholamines (Rosén et al 1984). An automatized ST-analyser (Lindecrantz 1983) is currently being tested in a large clinical cohort. Some time remains before the place for fetal ECG analysis in practical clinical work can be defined. It is obvious, however, that the place is restricted to fetal surveillance during labour since a scalp lead is a prerequisite for a technically acceptable recording.

Doppler assessment

For the long-term antenatal supervision of the fetal state the ultrasonic Doppler principle has recently come into use. After description of the technique of combining a linear array ultrasonograph with a pulsed Doppler system at a fixed angle (Eik-Nes et al 1980) normal values for blood velocities in the descending aorta and the umbilical vein of human fetuses during the third trimester of normal pregnancy have been produced (Lingman & Maršál 1986). Relations between decreased mean blood velocites in the fetal aorta and several indices of poor perinatal outcome have been established (Hackett et al 1987, Jouppila & Kirkinen 1984). Direct evidence of a linear relationship between reduction of mean blood velocities in fetal aorta and of degree of fetal hypoxia (measured from direct sampling from the umbilical vein) was recently produced (Soothill et al 1986).

The waveform from the velocity curves has also proved useful, as an indirect measure of fetal well-being. In a series of papers Maršál and coworkers demonstrated that the peak velocities during diastole convey much information about fetal distress and probably about placental perfusion. In cases of intra-uterine growth retardation (and presumably chronic fetal hypoxia), end-diastolic blood velocities both in the descending aorta and in the umbilical arteries decrease to zero and even reach negative values (reversed flow) at the end of diastole (Lingman et al 1986, Laurin et al in press). This also means that a simplification of the method, by taking into account only the curve form in terms of 'pulsatility index', disregarding the angle of insonation and thereby the absolute blood velocities is applicable to the umbilical artery. This simplified measure has given promising results in the long-term surveillance of the fetus at risk for chronic hypoxia. (See also p. 169).

DIAGNOSIS OF POSTNATAL ASPHYXIA

When presenting her neonatal scoring system Virginia Apgar described it as a systematic way to evaluate 'neonatal alertness' (Apgar 1953). Nevertheless the Apgar score has become an international standard of postnatal asphyxia (Nelson & Ellenberg 1981). However, when biochemical parameters of oxygen lack have come into use, the Apgar score has been criticized for not being what it never claimed to be. Thus, poor agreement was found between low Apgar scores and low pH values in the umbilical artery at birth (Sykes et al 1982). The lack of concordance between the two methods of assessing the newborn baby was partly resolved when it was demonstrated that neonates with low pH values had higher Apgar scores at 1 and 5 minutes when the catecholamine values were high, while low Apgar scores were associated with the combination of low pH and poor release of catecholamines (Lagercrantz 1982).

Other biochemical parameters of asphyxia are cord blood lactate (Daniel & James 1965) and hypoxanthine (Thiringer 1983). Both substances accumulate in blood during asphyxia and the degree of elevation of both substances can to some extent be regarded as an indicator of the oxygen debt of the neonate.

For research purposes, some measure of the total asphyetic insult is valuable but the practical evaluation in the delivery room of the degree of asphyxia has to rest on the measurement of cord blood pH and, in particular, on the baby's clinical behaviour, time to first gasp, to first cry and to regular breathing, and on the response to resuscitation.

RESUSCITATION OF THE ASPHYXIATED NEONATE IN THE DELIVERY ROOM

Some basic principles should be considered in every delivery whether the baby is asphyxiated or not*:

1. Before the first breath the baby should be held in a drainage position (head low, face down).
2. Suctioning of the oro-pharynx should be a brief procedure to avoid reflex bradycardia and apnoea. Suctioning is only indicated when the infant has thick mucus or meconium-stained fluid in the mouth.
3. Heat loss should be minimized by drying the neonate with a warmed towel — the sensory stimulation often effectively contributes to initiation of respiration.

When a newborn baby does not start regular breathing during the first minute of extra-uterine life the attending midwife or physician must be able to decide whether resuscitation should be initiated.

The key sign to observe, besides respiration, is the heart rate. The decision on resuscitative measures may be made very simple: if the baby does not breathe but has a high heart rate (above 100/min) the apnoea is *primary* and breathing will start spontaneously or after sensory stimulation. If, on the other hand, the baby does not breathe and the heart rate is low (below 100/min) the apnoea is *terminal* and the neonate demands active resuscitation to start breathing. Rarely, the baby's heart rate gives rise to doubt about into which category the situation should be classified — either the heart rate is well above or well below 100/min.

The most effective method for resuscitation of a baby in terminal apnoea is to apply intermittent positive ventilation via bag and tracheal tube. This should be the procedure when the asphyxia has been anticipated (e.g. when a very immature baby is born) and a trained physician attends the delivery. However, a large proportion of neonates with postnatal asphyxia still present themselves unexpectedly. In many situations the physician or the midwife responsible for initial resuscitation has a limited training in the intubation of newborn infants.

Therefore, ventilation by bag and mask is the recommended initial procedure for resuscitation in all situations, except when medical personnel with great experience in intubation are present.

The choice of equipment for bag and mask ventilation can be guided by three recent investigations demonstrating: that round face-masks provide better seal between mask and face than Rendall Baker-type masks and particularly that the type of mask with a flaccid inner portion enables effective sealing (Palme et al 1985); that bags of sufficient volume enabling the inflation pressure to be sustained for a second are most efficient for ventilation (Field et al 1986); and that self-inflating bags with a pop-off device should be equipped with a reservoir in circumstances when ventilation with a high oxygen fraction is desirable (Finer et al 1986).

We use the Laerdal neonatal or paediatric resuscitator with a round, flaccid face-mask as the equipment recommended (Celander et al 1985). The frequency of compression should be about 60/min with some prolonged initial compressions lasting one second each for initial aeration of the lungs. If the neonate does not respond with tachycardia after 2 minutes of bagging the baby should be endotracheally intubated and ventilation continued. When, on the other hand, the neonate responds with tachycardia within 2 minutes, ventilation by bag and mask is continued until spontaneous respiration takes over.

When the baby is born without heartbeats, external cardiac compression is started immediately, concomitantly with ventilation. Cardiac compression is also started in babies with a persistent severe bradycardia despite adequate ventilation. We perform external cardiac massage at a frequency of about 120/min simultaneously with ventilation without attempts to match the two procedures into alternating periods. If these procedures fail to produce clinical improvement within 5–10 minutes, buffer is given intravenously (4 ml/kg NaHCO$_3$, 0.6 M solution) in the umbilical vein slowly, over a 5 minute period. If the baby is still unresponsive epinephrine (0.05 mg/kg) is given, either intratracheally (Lindemann 1984) or via direct cardiac puncture. The scheme of resuscitation is summarized in Table 32.1.

Table 32.1 Scheme for resuscitation

Stage	Condition of infant		Procedures
Primary apnoea	Apnoea	Heart rate above 100/min	O$_2$-flush against baby's face Sensory cutaneous stimulation
Terminal apnoea	Apnoea or gasping	Heart rate below 100/min	Ventilation by bag and mask
	Persistent bradycardia and inefficient ventilation in spite of 'bagging' for 2 min		Endotracheal intubation and ventilation
	Persistent severe bradycardia despite adequate ventilation		External cardiac massage
	Should these steps not result in clearcut improvement		I.v. buffer therapy, intratracheal or intracardiac epinephrine
Note	When the baby is born without heartbeats		Cardiac massage and ventilation immediately at birth

*The routines described represent those applied in Sweden since 1972 in a national training programme for neonatal resuscitation (Celander et al 1985).

How long should resuscitation continue? If the baby does not exhibit any vital signs within 20 minutes in spite of adequately performed resuscitation the procedure is discontinued.

If the baby does not respond with spontaneous breathing movements during a 45 minute period the attempts to resuscitate are abandoned even if occasional heartbeats or a regular bradycardia have been recorded. Prolongation of artificial ventilation in such cases does not result in survival.

ACKNOWLEDGEMENTS

Original work from my own group mentioned in this survey was supported by the Swedish Medical Research Council (Grants 2591, 5654), the 'Expressen' Prenatal Research Foundation, Föreningen Margaretahemmet and Frimurare Barnhusdirektionen, Göteborg.

REFERENCES

Ames A III, Gurian B S 1963 Effect of glucose deprivation on function of isolated mammalian retina. Journal of Neurophysiology 26: 617–634

Apgar V 1953 A proposal for a new method of evaluation of the newborn infant. Anesthesia and Analgesia 32: 260–270

Beard R W, Filshie G M, Knight C A, Roberto G M 1971 The significance of the changes in the continuous fetal heart rate in the first stage of labour. Journal of Obstetrics and Gynaecology of the British Commonwealth 78: 865–881

Bircher N G, Safar P 1983 Cerebral preservation during cardiopulmonary resuscitation (CPR) in dogs. Anesthesiology 59: A93

Bissonette J M 1975 Relationship between continuous fetal heart rate patterns and Apgar score in the newborn. British Journal of Obstetrics and Gynaecology 82: 24

Blomstrand S, Karlsson K, Kjellmer I 1978 Measurement of cerebral blood flow in the fetal lamb with a note on the flow-distribution. Acta Physiologica Scandinavica 103: 1–8

Blomstrand S, Hrbek A, Karlsson K, Kjellmer I, Lindecrantz K, Olsson T 1984 Does glucose administration affect the cerebral response to fetal asphyxia? Acta Obstetrica Gynaecologica Scandinavica 63: 345–353

Boddy K, Dawes G S 1975 Fetal breathing. British Medical Bulletin 31: 3–7

Bowes G, Adamson T M, Ritchie B C, Wilkinson M H, Maloney J E 1981 Development of patterns of respiratory activity in unanesthetized fetal sheep in utero. Journal of Applied Physiology 50: 693–700

Boyle R 1670 New pneumatical experiments about respiration. Philosophical Transactions of the Royal Society, London 5: 2011–2031

Celander O, Kjellmer I, Svenningsen N, Tunell R 1985 A Swedish national programme for resuscitation of newborn babies. In: SAREC report R 2: 1985 — Breathing and warmth at birth. Swedish Agency for Research Cooperation with Developing Countries p 94–103

Caldeyro-Barcia R 1956 The physiology of prematurity. Josiah Macey Jr Foundation, New York

Chan P H, Fishman R A 1978 Transient formation of superoxide radicals in poly-unsaturated fatty acid induces brain swelling. Journal of Neurochemistry 35: 1004–1007

Choi D W 1985 Glutamate neurotoxicity in cortical cell culture is calcium dependent. Neuroscience Letters 58: 293–297

Cohn H E, Sacks E J, Heymann M A et al 1974 Cardiovascular responses to hypoxemia and acidemia in fetal lambs. American Journal of Obstetrics and Gynecology 120: 817–824

Dagbjartsson A, Karlsson K, Kjellmer I, Rosén K G 1985 Maternal treatment with a cardioselective beta-blocking agent — consequences for the ovine fetus during intermittent asphyxia. Journal of Developmental Physiology 7: 387–396

Dalton K J, Dawes G S, Patrick J E 1977 Diurnal, respiratory, and other rhythms of fetal heart rate in lambs. American Journal of Obstetrics and Gynecology 127: 414

Daniel S S and James L S 1965 Lactic acid in the neonatal period in man. Annals of the New York Academy of Sciences 119: 1142

Dawes G S, Mott J C, Shelley H J 1959 The importance of cardiac glycogen for the maintenance of life in foetal lambs and new-born animals during anoxia. Journal of Physiology 146: 516–538

Dawes G S, Fox H E, Leduc B M, Liggins G C, Richards R T 1972 Respiratory movements and rapid eye movement sleep in the foetal lamb. Journal of Physiology 220: 119–143

Del Maestro R F, Thaw H H, Björk J et al 1980 Free radicals as mediators of tissue injury. Acta Physiologica Scandinavica (Suppl) 492: 43–58

Duffy T E, Kohle S J, Vannucci R C 1975 Carbohydrate and energy metabolism in perinatal rat brain: relation to survival in anoxia. Journal of Neurochemistry 24: 271–276

Ebendal T, Olson L, Seiger A, Hedlund K O 1980 Nerve growth factors in the rat iris. Nature (London) 286: 25–28

Edelstone D I, Rudolph A M, Heymann M A et al 1977 Liver and ductus venosus blood flow in fetal lambs in utero. Circulation Research 42: 426

Eik-Nes S H, Brubakk A O, Ulstein M 1980 Measurement of human fetal blood flow. British Medical Journal i: 283–284

Field D, Milner A D, Hopkin I E 1986 Efficiency of manual resuscitators at birth. Archives of Disease in Childhood 61: 300–302

Finer N N, Barrington K J, Al-Fadley F, Peters K L 1986 Limitations of self-inflating resuscitators. Pediatrics 77: 417–420

Fisher D J, Heymann M A, Rudolph A M 1980 Myocardial oxygen and carbohydrate consumption in fetal lambs in utero and in adult sheep. American Journal of Physiology 238: H399–405

Gaudet R J, Levine L 1979 Transient cerebral ischemia and brain prostaglandins. Biochemical and Biophysical Research Communications 86: 893–901

Greenamyre J T, Penney J B, Young A B et al 1987 Evidence for transient perinatal glutamatergic innervation of globus pallidus. Journal of Neuroscience 7: 1022–1030

Greene K R, Dawes G S, Lilja H, Rosén K G 1982 Changes in the ST waveform of the fetal lamb electrocardiogram with hypoxia. American Journal of Obstetrics and Gynecology 144: 950–958

Haber F, Weiss J 1934 The catalytic decomposition of hydrogen peroxide by iron salts. Proceedings of the Royal Society, London A147: 332–351

Hackett G A, Campbell S, Gamsu H, Cohen-Overbeek T, Pearce J M F 1987 Doppler studies in the growth retarded fetus and prediction of neonatal necrotizing enterocolitis, haemorrhage, and neonatal morbidity. British Medical Journal i: 13–16

Hagberg H, Lehman A, Sandberg M, Nyström B, Jacobson I, Hamberger A 1985 Ischaemia-induced shift of inhibitory and excitatory amino acids from intra- to extracellular compartments. Journal of Cerebral Blood Flow and Metabolism 5: 413–419

Hagberg H, Anderrson P, Kjellmer I, Thiringer K, Thordstein M 1987a Extracellular overflow of glutamate, aspartate, GABA and taurine during hypoxia ischemia. Neuroscience Letters 7–8: 311–317

Hagberg H, Andersson P, Lacarewicz J, Jacobson I, Butcher S, Sandberg M 1987b Extracellular adenosine, inosine, hypoxanthine and xanthine in relation to tissue nucleotides and purines in rat striatum during transient ischaemia. Journal of Neurochemistry 49: 227–231

Haldane J S 1922 Respiration. Yale University Press, New Haven

Hallenbeck J M, Furlow T W 1979 Prostaglandin 12 and indomethacin prevent impairment of post-ischemic brain reperfusion in the dog. Stroke 10: 629–637

Halliwell B, Gutteridge J M C 1984 Oxygen toxicity, oxygen radicals, transition metals and disease. Biochemical Journal 219: 1–14

Hansen A J 1977 Extracellular potassium concentration in juvenile and adult rat brain cortex during anoxia. Acta Physiologica Scandinavica 99: 412–420

Hansen A J 1978 The extracellular potassium concentration in brain cortex following ischemia in hypo- and hyperglycemic rats. Acta Physiologica Scandinavica 102: 324–329

Hansen A J 1985 Effect of anoxia on ion distribution in the brain. Physiological Review 65: 101–148

Hansen A J, Nordström C-H 1979 Brain extracellular potassium and energy metabolism during ischemia in juvenile rats after exposure to hypoxia for 24 h. Journal of Neurochemistry 32: 915–920

Hedner T 1978 Central monoamine metabolism and neonatal oxygen deprivation. Acta Physiologica Scandinavica (Suppl) 460: 1–33

Hoffmeister F, Kazda S, Krause H P 1979 Influence of nimodipine on the post-ischemic changes of brain function. Acta Neurologica Scandinavica 60 (Suppl 72): 358–359

Hon E H 1959 The fetal heart rate patterns preceding death in utero. American Journal of Obstetrics and Gynecology 78: 47–56

Hossman K A 1983 Neuronal survival and revival during and after cerebral ischemia. American Journal of Emergency Medicine 1: 191–197

Hossman K A, Kleihues P 1973 Reversibility of ischemic brain damage. Archives of Neurology 29: 375–384

Hrbek A, Karlsson K, Kjellmer I, Olsson T, Riha M 1974 Cerebral reactions during intrauterine asphyxia in the sheep. II. Evoked electroencephalogram responses. Pediatric Research 8: 58–63

Jones C T, Ritchie J W K 1983 The effects of adrenergic blockade on fetal response to hypoxia. Journal of Developmental Physiology 5: 211–222

Jouppila P, Kirkinen P 1984 Increased resistance in the descending aorta of the human fetus in hypoxia. British Journal of Obstetrics and Gynaecology 91: 107–110

Jörgensen M B, Diemer N-H 1982 Selective neuron loss after cerebral ischemia in the rat: possible role of transmitter glutamate. Acta Neurologica Scandinavica 66: 536–546

Kanemitsu H, Tamura A, Sanok, Iwamoto T, Yoshiura M, Iriyama K 1986 Changes of uric acid level in rat brain after focal ischemia. Journal of Neurochemistry 46: 851–853

Kjellmer I, Karlsson K, Olsson T, Rosén K G 1974 Cerebral reactions during intrauterine asphyxia in the sheep. I. Circulation and oxygen consumption in the fetal brain. Pediatric Research 8: 50–57

Kjellmer I, Andersson P, Hagberg H, Ostwald C, Thiringer K 1986 Extracellular accumulation of amino acids and purine catabolites in the brain of asphyxiated fetal sheep. Joint Meeting of Neonatal Societies of UK and Sweden (Abstract). Early Human Development 14: 137

Kontos H A 1985 Oxygen radicals in cerebral vascular injury. Circulation Research 57: 508–516

Lagercrantz H 1982 Asphyxia and the Apgar score. Lancet i: 966

Lagercrantz H, Bistoletti P 1977 Catecholamine release in the newborn infant at birth. Pediatric Research ll: 889–893

Laurin J, Lingman G, Maršál K, Persson P-H Fetal blood flow in pregnancies complicated by intra-uterine growth retardation. Obstetrics and Gynecology (in press)

Lilja H 1983 Fetal cardiac response to hypoxia. Thesis, Gothenburg University

Lindecrantz K 1983 Processing of the fetal ECG: an implementation of a dedicated real time microprocessor system. Technical Report, No 135. Chalmers University of Technology, Göteborg

Lindemann R 1984 Resuscitation of the newborn. Acta Paediatrica Scandinavica 73: 210–212

Lingman G, Maršál K 1986 Fetal central blood circulation in the third trimester of normal pregnancy — a longitudinal study. I. Aortic and umbilical blood flow. Early Human Development 13: 137–150

Lingman G, Laurin J, Maršál K 1986 Circulatory changes in fetuses with imminent asphyxia. Biology of the Neonate 49: 66–73

Ljunggren B, Schultz H, Siesjö B K 1974 Changes in energy state and acid–base parameters of the rat brain during complete compression ischemia. Brain Research 73: 277–289

McCord J M 1985 Oxygen-derived free radicals in postischemic injury. New England Journal of Medicine 312: 159–163

Mann L I 1970 Effects of hypoxia on fetal cephalic blood flow, cephalic metabolism and the electroencephalogram. Experimental Neurology 29: 336–348

Mann L I, Solomon G, Carmichael A, Duchin S 1971 The effect of metabolic acidosis on fetal brain function and metabolism. American Journal Obstetrics and Gynecology 111: 353–359

Manning F A, Platt L D, Sipos L 1980 Antepartum fetal evaluation: development of a fetal biophysical profile. American Journal of Obstetrics and Gynecology 136: 787–795

Myers R A, Yamaguchi M 1976 Effects of serum glucose concentrations on brain response to circulatory arrest. Journal of Neuropathology and Experimental Neurology 35: 301

Nelson K B, Ellenberg J H 1981 Apgar scores as predictors of chronic neurologic disability. Pediatrics 68: 36–44

Nemoto E M, Sjiu G K, Nemmer J P et al 1983 Free fatty acid accumulation in the pathogenesis of cerebral ischemic–anoxic injury. American Journal of Emergency Medicine 1: 175–179

Nieto-Sampedro M, Lewis E R, Cotman C W et al 1982 Brain injury causes a time-dependent increase in neuronotrophic activity at the lesion site. Science 217: 860–861

Nieto-Sampedro M, Needles D L, Cotman C W 1985 A simple, objective method to measure the activity of factors that promote neuronal survival. Journal of Neuroscientific Methods 15: 37–48

Nordström C-H, Siesjö B K 1978 Influence of phenobarbital on changes in the metabolites of the energy reserve of the cerebral cortex following complete ischemia. Acta Physiologica Scandinavica 104: 271–280

Nylund L, Lagercrantz H, Lunell N O 1979 Catecholamines in fetal blood during birth in man. Journal of Developmental Physiology 1: 427–435

Olney J W 1983 In: Fuxe, Roberts, Schwarcz (eds) Excitotoxins. Wennergren, International Symposium Series 39: 82–96

Palme C, Ericsson A 1986 What happened to asphyxic Swedish neonates in 1985? Joint Meeting of Neonatal Societies of UK and Sweden (Abstract) Early Human Development 14: 145

Palme C, Nyström B, Tunell R 1985 The evaluation of the efficacy of face masks in the resuscitation of newborn infants. Lancet i: 207–210

Parks D A, Bulkley G B, Granger N, Hamilton S R, McCord J M 1982 Ischaemia injury to the cat small intestine: role of superoxide radicals. Gastroenterology 82: 9–15

Patrick J, Natale R, Richardson B 1978 Patterns of human fetal breathing activity at 34–35 weeks of gestational age. American Journal of Obstetrics and Gynecology 132: 507–513

Peeters L L H, Sheldon R E, Jones M D Jr, Makowski E L, Meschia G 1979 Blood flow to fetal organs as a function of arterial oxygen content. American Journal of Obstetrics and Gynecology 135: 637–646

Power G G, Longo L D, Wagner Jr H N, Kuhl D E, Forster R E 1967 Uneven distribution of maternal and fetal placental blood flow, as demonstrated using macroaggregates and its response to hypoxia. Journal of Clinical Investigation 46: 2053–2063

Raichle M E 1983 The pathophysiology of brain ischaemia. Annals of Neurology 13: 2–10

Rehncrona S, Rosén I, Siesjö B K 1981 Brain lactic acidosis and ischemic cell damage. I. Biochemistry and neurophysiology. Journal of Cerebral Blood Flow and Metabolism 1: 297–311

Reuss M L, Rudolph A M 1980 Distribution and recirculation of umbilical and systemic venous blood flow in fetal lambs during hypoxia. Journal of Developmental Physiology 2: 71–84

Rosén K G, Kjellmer I 1975 Changes in the fetal heart rate and ECG during hypoxia. Acta Physiologica Scandinavica 93: 59

Rosén K G, Hökegård K-H, Kjellmer I 1976 A study of the relationship between the electrocardiogram and hemodynamics in the fetal lamb during asphyxia. Acta Physiologica Scandinavica 98: 275–284

Rosén K G, Dagbjartsson A, Henriksson B-Å Lagercrantz H, Kjellmer I 1984 The relationship between circulating catecholamines and ST waveform in the fetal lamb electrocardiogram during hypoxia. American Journal of Obstetrics and Gynaecology 149: 190–195

Rosén K H, Lilja H, Hökegård K-H, Kjellmer J 1985 The relationship between cerebral cardiovascular and metabolic functions during labour in the lamb fetus. In: Jones C T (ed) Symposium on the physiological development of the fetus and newborn. Academic Press, London

Rosén K G, Hrbek A, Karlsson K, Kjellmer I 1986a Fetal cerebral, cardiovascular and metabolic reactions to intermittent occlusion of ovine maternal placental blood flow. Acta Physiologica Scandinavica 126: 209–216

Rosén K G, Greene K R, Hökegård K-H, Karlsson K, Lilja H, Lindecrantz K, Kjellmer J 1986b ST waveform analysis of the fetal ECG — a potent method for fetal surveillance? A presentation of experimental and clinical data. In: Cardiovascular and respiratory physiology of the fetus and neonate. Colloque INSERM 133: 67–82

Rothman S 1984 Synaptic release of excitatory amino acid neurotransmitter mediates anoxic neuronal death. Journal of Neuroscience 4: 1884–1891

Saling E, Schneider D 1967 Biochemical supervision of the fetus during labour. Journal of Obstetrics and Gynaecology of the British Commonwealth 74: 799–811

Saugstad O D 1975 Hypoxanthine as a measurement of hypoxia. Pediatric Research 9: 158–161

Scott H 1976 Outcome of very severe birth asphyxia. Archives of Disease in Childhood 51: 712–716

Shapiro H M, Greenberg J H, van Horn Naughton K, Reivich M 1980

Heterogeneity of local cerebral blood flow — PaCO$_2$ sensitivity in neonatal days. Journal of Applied Physiology 49: 113–118

Shelley H J 1961 Glycogen reserves and their changes at birth. British Medical Bulletin 17: 137–143

Siesjö B K 1981 Cell damage in the brain: a speculative synthesis. Journal of Cerebral Blood Flow and Metabolism 1: 155–185

Silverstein F S, Johnston M V 1984 Effects of hypoxia–ischemia on monoamine metabolism in the immature brain. Annals of Neurology 15: 343–347

Silverstein F S, Buchanan K, Hudson C, Johnston M V 1986 Flunarizine limits hypoxia–ischemia induced morphologic injury in immature rat brain. Stroke 17: 477–482

Simon R P, Swan J H, Griffiths T, Meldrum B S 1984 Blockade of N- methyl-D-aspartate receptors may protect against ischemic damage in the brain. Science 226: 850–852

Soothill B W, Nicolaides K H, Bilardo C M, Campbell S 1986 Relation of fetal hypoxia in growth retardation to mean blood velocity in the fetal aorta. Lancet ii: 1118–1120

Stånge L, Rosén K G, Hökegård K-H, Karlsson K, Rochlitzer F, Kjellmer I, Joelsson I 1977 Quantification of fetal heart rate variability in relation to oxygenation in the sheep fetus. Acta Obstetrica et Gynecologica Scandinavica 56: 205–209

Steen P A, Newbury L A, Milde J H et al 1983 Nimodipine improves cerebral blood flow and neurologic recovery after complete cerebral ischemia in the dog. Journal of Cerebral Blood Flow and Metabolism 3: 38–42

Sykes G S, Molloy P M, Johnson P, Gu W, Ashworth F, Stirrat G M, Turnbull A C 1982 Do Apgar scores indicate asphyxia? Lancet i: 494–496

Thiringer K 1983 Cord plasma hypoxanthine as a measure of foetal asphyxia. Acta Paediatrica Scandinavica 72: 231–237

Thiringer K, Saugstad O D, Kjellmer I 1980 Plasma hypoxanthine in exteriorized, acutely asphyxiated fetal lambs. Pediatric Research 14: 905–910

Thiringer K, Blomstrand S, Hrbek A, Karlsson K, Kjellmer I 1982 Cerebral arterio–venous difference for hypoxanthine and lactate during graded asphyxia in the fetal lamb. Brain Research 239: 107–117

Thiringer K, Karlsson K, Rosén K G, Kjellmer I 1984 Contribution of heart muscle, liver, skeletal muscle and placenta to the asphyxial hypoxanthine elevation in the acutely exteriorised fetal lamb. Biology of the Neonate 45: 169–182

Thiringer K, Hrbek A, Karlsson K, Rosén K G, Kjellmer I 1987 Postasphyxial cerebral survival in newborn sheep after treatment with oxygen free radical scavangers and a calcium antagonist. Pediatric Research 22: 62–66

Thoenen H, Edgar D 1985 Neurotrophic factors. Science 229: 238–242

Thomas M J, Mehl K S, Pryor W A 1978 The role of the superoxide anion in the xanthine oxidase induced autooxidation of linoleic acid. Biochemical and Biophysical Research Communications 83: 927–932

Torphy D E, Minter M G, Thompson B M 1984 Cardiorespiratory arrest and resuscitation in children. American Journal of Diseases of Children 138: 1099–1102

Vykocil F, Kritz N, Bures J 1972 Potassium selective microelectrodes used for measuring the extracellular brain K+ during spreading depression and anoxic depolarization in rats. Brain Research 39: 255–259

White B C, Winegar C D, Wilson R F et al 1983 Calcium blockers in cerebral resuscitation. Journal of Trauma 23: 788–793

White B C, Wiegenstein J G, Winegar C D 1984 Brain ischemic anoxia: mechanism of injury. Journal of the American Medical Association 251: 1586–1590

33. The asphyxiated newborn infant

Dr M.I. Levene

In the developed world, birth asphyxia is arguably the most common cause of perinatally acquired severe brain injury in full-term infants. It is a tragedy for a normally developed fetus to sustain cerebral injury during the last hours of prenatal life and then to survive for many more years with major handicap. The clinical term 'asphyxia' is widely used but there is little consensus as to what is meant by it. Hypoxic–ischaemic insult better describes the pathophysiology of intrapartum asphyxia and stresses the two major components of the condition. The cerebral effects of asphyxia are quite different in the mature brain when compared with the brain of a severely premature infant. The neuropathological insults seen in premature infants are predominantly haemorrhagic or ischaemic and intrapartum events only rarely precipitate these conditions — they are discussed in detail in Section 8. Apnoea is a common feature apparent in premature infants at birth. This may cause the Apgar score to be depressed and require the infant to be intubated. Clinicians may then refer to such infants as asphyxiated but with little evidence that the baby has suffered the hypoxic–ischaemic pathophysiological insult inherent in this definition. Because of the fundamental differences in the definition and neuropathological sequelae of asphyxia between pre-term and full-term infants this chapter only mentions perinatal asphyxia with reference to the mature infant.

In the previous chapter asphyxia was defined on a pathophysiological basis referring to a biochemical effect of the process. Clinicians are less able to measure routinely the acid–base status in their infants and therefore must rely on a clinical definition. Donald (1959) defined 'asphyxia neonatorum' as failure to establish spontaneous ventilation at birth but there may be many causes for this, including depression of ventilation due to drugs, trauma and, rarely, neuromuscular disorders affecting the onset of spontaneous breathing.

Virginia Apgar first described the scoring system which now bears her name (Apgar 1953) and proposed that it should be assessed one minute after birth. Later, Drage et al (1964) recommended reassessment 5 minutes after

birth. This system is effective for describing the infant's condition shortly after birth but relates poorly to preceding events and is only a weak predictor of those infants who are later identified as having neurodevelopmental deficits caused by perinatal asphyxia (see p. 389). Like the onset of spontaneous respiration, the Apgar score may be influenced by non- asphyxial factors. Nevertheless, depression of the Apgar score is widely used in diagnosing perinatal asphyxia, and a score of 3 or less at 5 minutes is often taken as indicating severe asphyxial insult (Nelson & Ellenberg 1981, Ergander et al 1983).

Disturbances in the behaviour of the infant following birth give a sensitive indicator of significant asphyxia. It is likely that intrapartum asphyxia severe enough to cause neurodevelopmental handicap will be associated with clinical neurological dysfunction and if no abnormalities occur the infant appears to be at little risk. Unfortunately, postasphyxial encephalopathy must be a retrospective diagnosis and does not appear to correlate well with the Apgar scores (Levene et al 1986). In practice a number of different methods are used to describe 'birth asphyxia' in the newborn infant and care must be taken in comparing incidence and outcome figures.

INCIDENCE

The incidence of birth asphyxia in full-term infants has been variously reported from the United States, Sweden and Britain to be between 2.9 and 9.0 cases per 1000 deliveries (Brown et al 1974, MacDonald et al 1980, Finer et al 1981, Nelson & Ellenberg 1981, Ergander et al 1983, Levene et al 1985a). The incidence in premature babies is very much higher. In two studies, asphyxia was defined as an Apgar score of 3 or less at 5 minutes (Nelson & Ellenberg 1981, Ergander et al 1983), and another included all infants who required intermittent positive-pressure ventilation for more than one minute (MacDonald et al 1980). Two other studies reported the incidence of postasphyxial encephalopathy (PAE). Brown et al (1974) found that 5.9 per 1000 full-term deliveries showed clinical signs due to intrapartum asphyxia, and in Leicester we reported an incidence of 6.0 per 1000 inborn infants (Levene et al 1985a). Moderate and severe postasphyxial encephalopathy occurred in 1.1 and 1.0 per 1000 infants respectively. One-quarter of the infants with PAE born in Leicester showed intra-uterine growth retardation which is comparable to the 29% reported by Finer et al (1981).

There appears to have been a reduction in the incidence of asphyxia in full-term infants over recent years. In the United States, infant mortality (all birth-weights) due to intra-uterine hypoxia and birth asphyxia has fallen from 253 per 1000 births in 1970 to 39 per 1000 by 1981 (Wegman 1984). The incidence of infants with convulsions associated with severe asphyxia, born in Montreal in Canada, and weighing more than 2500 g at birth fell from 1.8 per 1000 in 1960 to 0.7 per 1000 in 1978–80 (Cyr et al 1984). Figures from Paris (Amiel-Tison et al 1980) have shown a dramatic fall in the incidence of mild and moderate encephalopathy in full-term infants over a 4-year period. In 1974, the incidence of this condition was 18.9 per 1000 and for the years 1976–78 it had fallen to 3.9 per 1000. There was, however, no change in the proportion of infants who were stillborn due to intrapartum asphyxia or who had the most severe form of encephalopathy.

PATHOLOGY

Consistent pathological features associated with birth asphyxia have been recognized since the nineteenth century. Ulegyria or gyral scarring was first described by Bressler in 1899 and status marmoratus or état marbre involving the basal ganglia was reported by Anton in 1893. Despite these observations, no single distinct or uniform pathological appearance is recognized following severe hypoxic–ischaemic injury. The brain may be either globally affected with extensive swelling and necrosis or pathological lesions may be more focal and discrete. These heterogeneous and clinically unpredictable appearances are related to the variety of pathophysiological insults to which the fetus is exposed. The majority of pathological lesions seen in the brain following asphyxia have been explained either as ischaemic injury based on a vascular aetiology or due to the vulnerability of certain regions of the brain to metabolic injury.

Vascular injury

Parasagittal injury. Volpe (1977) has drawn attention to the parasagittal injury seen in full-term asphyxiated infants. Cortical necrosis occurring at the junction between the territories of the anterior, middle and posterior cerebral arteries has been produced experimentally in animals (Brierley et al 1969) and recognized at autopsy in the brains of children (Adams et al 1966). These authors have

related this boundary-zone injury to hypotension affecting the region between major arterial distribution. Similar lesions (Fig. 33.1) have been produced in fetal monkeys by inducing maternal hypotension for 1–5 hours (Brann & Myers 1975).

This lesion has been diagnosed during life by means of technetium brain scans (Volpe & Pasternak 1977) or positron emission tomography (Volpe et al 1985). Seventeen infants with evidence of significant postasphyxial encephalopathy were studied within the first 5 days. There was a consistent, symmetrical decrease in cerebral blood flow of up to 50% to the parasagittal regions more marked posteriorly than anteriorly (see Frontispiece II).

Postischaemic vasospasm. Following a period of asphyxia and with restoration of the systemic circulation, reactive hyperaemia initially occurs and cerebral blood flow (CBF) increases to above pre-ischaemic levels (Hossman & Kleihues 1973). In some cases the period of initial hyperaemia rapidly fails and cerebral hypoperfusion develops with CBF falling to 40% of the pre-asphyxial level (Fig. 33.2). This has been referred to as the 'no reflow phenomenon' (Ames et al 1968) and is probably due to vasoconstriction as the result of arteriolar injury and spasm. A second arteriolar abnormality has been described as the 'luxury perfusion' of Lassen (1966). The arterioles become widely dilated, atonic and probably insensitive to changes in carbon dioxide tension. Either of these abnormalities may produce secondary cerebral ischaemia following resuscitation, by vasospastic hypoperfusion or 'steal' of blood away from compromised areas of brain.

Metabolic injury

In certain animal species a cortical pattern of cerebral injury was produced by fetal hypoxia (Windle 1966,

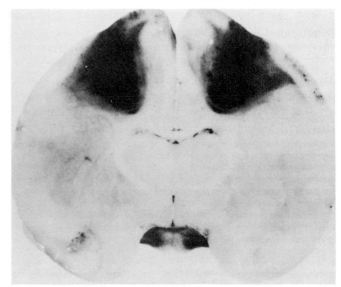

Fig. 33.1 Parasagittal injury. Coronal section through a fetal monkey brain showing an asphyxial injury similar to the parasagittal watershed lesion. (Reproduced with permission from Brann & Myers 1975.)

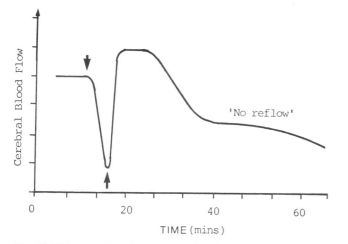

Fig. 33.2 The 'no reflow phenomenon'. Cerebral blood flow (CBF) before, during (marked by arrows) and after acute asphyxia. Following an initial period of hyperperfusion immediately after restoration of the circulation, the CBF falls to below 50% of the initial level.

Myers 1972). Episodes of partial asphyxia produced lesions predominantly in cortical and subcortical structures. Acute and total asphyxia produced a totally different type of injury involving thalamus, brainstem and spinal cord structures (Myers 1972). Cerebral oedema did not occur following acute asphyxia. When episodes of total asphyxia are superimposed upon episodes of partial asphyxia mixed lesions may develop. Myers (1977) has suggested that damage occurs due to anaerobic metabolism in areas of highest metabolic activity with the production of a critical concentration of lactate in excess of 20 μmol/g. This leads to the irreversible cerebral damage seen in the animal experiments. This hypothesis of metabolic injury appears to conflict with the ischaemic injury propounded by Brierley and Volpe. Imbalance between local cerebral metabolic rate and regional blood flow will cause cerebral injury whether absolute blood flow is decreased or not and this explanation will satisfy both observations.

Neuropathology resulting from perinatal asphyxia may affect white or grey matter or both. Involvement of the white matter occurs commonly in immature infants (periventricular leukomalacia) and often in conjunction with periventricular haemorrhage. This condition, together with subcortical leukomalacia, is discussed in detail in Chapter 29 and this section will deal mainly with neuronal necrosis which is commonly seen in full-term infants following asphyxia.

The appearance of the asphyxiated brain depends on the age at which it is examined. Within hours of the insult the brain may appear grossly normal. In the first 48 hours histological examination may be unremarkable but later acidophilic staining of the cytoplasm with pyknosis or nuclear fragmentation is seen (Pape & Wigglesworth 1979). Electron microscopy reveals diffuse change involving both vascular endothelium and neurones. Haemorrhage may be present on removing the brain from the skull.

Subdural bleeding due to tentorial tears may be seen and subarachnoid haemorrhage is particularly common.

Cerebral oedema

Within 24 to 48 hours, gross swelling with marked flattening and widening of the gyri and obliteration of the sulci may occur. The brain at this time is soft and very friable. In some cases cerebral herniation may have occurred with grooving of the uncus and partial cerebellar displacement through the foramen magnum but this is infrequent. On cutting the brain the ventricles are slit-like and little CSF drains out. Protrusion of the infundibulum into the interpeduncular cistern may occur (Larroche 1984).

Brain swelling and intracranial hypertension do not occur in all severely asphyxiated full-term infants (Pryse-Davies & Beard 1973, Levene et al in press) and the factors involved in its development are not clear. Klatzo (1967) has classified brain oedema into two types: cytotoxic and vasogenic. In vasogenic oedema there is an increase in leakiness of the blood–brain barrier allowing entry of serum proteins into the cerebral parenchyma. The resulting increase in intracerebral osmotic pressure leads to accumulation of fluid within the extracellular compartment of the brain. Cytotoxic oedema is due to failure of cellular membrane pumps and there is swelling of the cells. Cytotoxic oedema probably occurs earlier and in response to the initial hypoxic–ischaemic insult and may affect the grey matter in preference to the white (Klatzo 1985). Later, and in response to a less clearly defined insult, the blood–brain barrier opens to proteins. The swollen brain seen at autopsy probably results predominantly from vasogenic oedema and this does not reach maximum effect until 48 hours after birth (Anderson & Belton 1974). In a fetal lamb model vasogenic oedema did not appear to be a significant feature following hypoxic–ischaemic insult at least in the first 24 hours (Tweed et al 1981).

Injury to grey matter

It is rare for isolated lesions to occur in only one area of the brain and multiple or focal sites of involvement are usual but for the sake of clarity neuropathological features will be described under separate subheadings.

Cortex. In the acute stages following asphyxia the cerebral cortex may appear normal but within a week or two it may become fluctuant to touch and occasionally cystic. On cut section the cortex may show a grey-brown discoloration (Larroche 1984). Ulegyria, a macroscopic appearance of gyral sclerosis with widening of the sulci, is seen in some infants who have survived the asphyxial event by months or years (Fig. 33.3). Microscopically, cortical involvement may be focal or diffuse and may preferentially involve certain cortical layers, notably III and V with II being well preserved (Larroche 1984). This may be due to

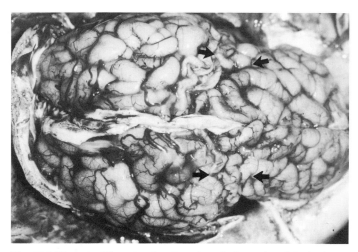

Fig. 33.3 Ulegyria. There is sclerosis and cortical atrophy of the brain in the region between the anterior and middle cerebral arteries (arrows).

relative differences in metabolic rate (Farkas-Bargeton & Diebler 1978). The hippocampus is particularly vulnerable to hypoxic insult and partial or total destruction of pyramid cells within this area is almost invariable following significant cerebral asphyxic injury (Larroche 1977). Other particularly vulnerable areas include the pre- and postcentral gyri and the visual cortex around the calcarine fissure.

Subcortical structures. The region immediately below the cortical ribbon is particularly vulnerable to the effects of perinatal asphyxia due to the temporary vascular watershed exposed in full-term infants. Cortical and subcortical structures at the depths of sulci are particularly likely to develop infarction (Fig. 33.4) and may evolve to subcortical leukomalacia or multiple cystic encephalomalacia.

Basal ganglia. Status marmoratus is the classical neuropathological lesion affecting the basal ganglia and is seen only in infants who survive the asphyxia by many months. This is a visible marble-like appearance of the thalamus and basal ganglia and is due to abnormal myelination. Rorke (1982) states that this is a rare condition, and is uncommonly seen even in infants who survive for many years after severe asphyxial insults. She found lesions confined to the basal ganglia in only 3% of perinatal autopsies but these lesions were relatively commonly seen together with more extensive cerebral injury. The majority of infants with selective damage to the thalamus had frank infarction with or without haemorrhage. Cystic infarction is also seen and in some cases has been related to maternal drug addiction (Rorke 1982). Lesions apparent in the thalamus usually indicate more extensive involvement throughout the central nervous system.

Haemorrhage or haemorrhagic infarction involving the basal ganglia is seen frequently following birth asphyxia in full-term infants (Fig. 33.5). Recently CT scanning has detected bilateral striatal haemorrhage (Kotagel et al 1983), and haemorrhagic infarction (Morimoto et al 1985) during life. In addition, imaging techniques have shown diffuse

echodensity on ultrasound (Kreusser et al 1984, Shen et al 1986) and high attenuation on CT (Shewman et al 1981). Autopsy correlation suggests this may be due to capillary proliferation and microcalcification.

Brainstem. Injuries to the brainstem are usually associated with concomitant lesions to the basal ganglia, as mentioned above. The most vulnerable structure is the inferior colliculus probably due to its high metabolic rate but the reticular formation, lateral geniculate bodies and pontine nuclei may also be involved. Leech & Alvord (1977) found evidence of brainstem lesions in 15 of 16 (93%) brains they examined. Lesions from the diencephalon, through the midbrain, pons, medulla and cord have been described in some infants (Schneider et al 1975). Lesions are rarely evident on macroscopic examination.

Cerebellum. The cerebellum is more resistant to the effects of asphyxia than the cerebrum and pathological involvement following perinatal asphyxia has been reported infrequently. The dentate nuclei, Purkinje cells and internal granular layers appear to be most vulnerable. Interestingly, the external granular layer is usually normal (Larroche 1977). Bilateral lesions may occur in the watershed region between the two superior and inferior cerebellar arteries (Friede 1975). Occipital diastasis may cause local trauma to the cerebellum and is described in Chapter 27. One-third of infants found at postmortem to have obvious brain swelling showed cerebellar herniation (Pryse-Davies & Beard 1973).

Spinal cord. Lesions within the cord are rarely obvious on macroscopic examination but evidence of asphyxial injury is present microscopically. The gracile and cuneate nuclei, nuclei of the medulla oblongata and the anterior horn cells are particularly vulnerable. Trauma to the spinal cord may be associated with intrapartum asphyxia (Chapter 35).

CLINICAL FEATURES

Mature infants exposed to a period of asphyxia usually show a definite and predictable sequence of clinical features. In addition the severity and duration of symptoms depends on the duration of the hypoxic–ischaemic event. The reason for the regular progression is not clear but certainly reflects pathophysiological changes in terms of cerebral blood flow, cerebral metabolism and increase in brain swelling. Some of the clinical features such as differential tone between upper and lower limbs can be explained on the basis of parasagittal vascular injury. Chapter 3 details the clinical assessment and the features seen in infants with birth asphyxia. In this section, discussion is confined to the progression and clinical grading of hypoxic–ischaemic encephalopathy.

Sarnat & Sarnat (1976) were the first to devise a method to describe the progression of symptoms in asphyxiated full-term infants and combined it together with EEG activity. The clinical stages are shown in Table 33.1. Subsequently a number of methods based on the Sarnat's

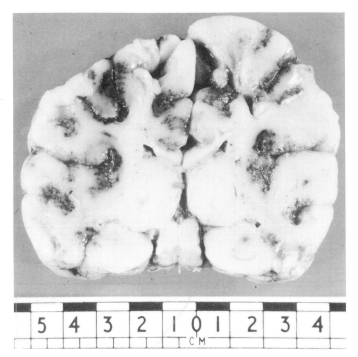

Fig. 33.4 Deep cortical and subcortical haemorrhagic necrosis. The depths of the sulci are most severely involved.

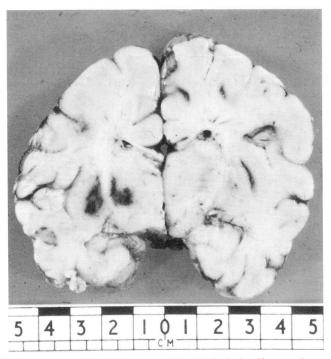

Fig. 33.5 Haemorrhagic infarction of the left basal ganglion. Both the lentiform nucleus and lateral thalamus are involved, with the white matter or the internal capsule being spared.

scheme have been described which can be used to refer to the maximum level of neurological abnormality in mature infants (Amiel-Tison 1979, Finer et al 1981, Fenichel 1983, Levene et al 1985a, Amiel-Tison & Ellison 1986). All these methods utilize a three-point grading system referring to mild, moderate and severe abnormality.

Mild encephalopathy

These infants show no alteration in conscious level but appear to be 'hyperalert'. They spend more time in an awake and restless state, often with staring eyes. They show excessive response to stimulation and are jittery with

Table 33.1 A clinical grading system for post-asphyxial encephalopathy (Sarnat & Sarnat 1976)

	Mild (1)	Moderate (2)	Severe (3)
Level of consciousness	Hyperalert	Lethargic	Stuporose
Neuromuscular control			
Muscle tone	Normal	Mild hypotonia	Flaccid
Posture	Mild distal flexion	Strong distal flexion	Intermittent decerebration
Stretch reflexes	Overactive	Overactive	Decreased or absent
Segmental myoclonus	Present	Present	Absent
Complex reflexes			
Suck	Weak	Weak or absent	Absent
Moro	Strong: low threshold	Weak: incomplete; high threshold	Absent
Oculovestibular	Normal	Overactive	Weak or absent
Tonic neck	Slight	Strong	Absent
Autonomic function	Generalized sympathetic	Generalized parasympathetic	Both systems depressed
Pupils	Mydriasis	Miosis	Variable; often unequal; poor light reflex
Heart rate	Tachycardia	Bradycardia	Variable
Bronchial and salivary secretions	Sparse	Profuse	Variable
Gastrointestinal motility	Normal or decreased	Increased; diarrhoea	Variable
Seizures	None	Common; focal or multifocal	Uncommon (excluding decerebration)

spontaneous or exaggerated Moro reflexes. The infant's passive limb tone is normal but there is usually some mild increase on assessment of active tone. When held in a sitting position, some head lag is noticeable but the tone in the neck extensors is relatively increased compared with the flexors. Limb reflexes are normal or slightly increased but sustained ankle clonus may be elicitable. Clinically apparent seizures do not occur. The sucking reflex is often weak and the infants need encouragement to complete feeds. Sarnat & Sarnat (1976) found the duration of mild encephalopathy to range between 1.5 to 18 hours but we allow up to 48 hours for complete recovery to occur (Levene et al 1985a). Amiel-Tison & Ellison (1986) allow up to 7 days for complete recovery in mild encephalopathy.

Moderate encephalopathy

The main features of this condition are seizures and lethargy with reduction in spontaneous movements. These infants are slower to react to stimuli and their responses may be incomplete. A somewhat higher threshold is usually necessary before reaction is seen. The infants lie in a more hypotonic posture with abducted arms and legs. A consistent feature is differential tone between upper and lower limbs. The arms show much less spontaneous movement and are relatively hypotonic compared with the legs (Volpe & Pasternak 1977). Tendon jerks are exaggerated and the Moro reflex incomplete. Autonomic function is largely parasympathetic with relative bradycardia and constricted pupils. The sucking reflex is poor and feeding incomplete. Tube feeding is usually necessary. Convulsions

occur usually in the second 24-hour period but may be seen earlier. They may be subtle or fragmentary and relatively easy to control pharmacologically. Sarnat & Sarnat (1976) found these infants showed abnormal behaviour for a mean of 4.7 days. Complete recovery (if it occurs) may take several weeks but some improvement is usually seen by the end of the first week.

Severe encephalopathy

These infants are comatose with severe hypotonia and usually require respiratory support from birth. They are profoundly hypotonic with no spontaneous movements. Seizures are frequent and may be prolonged. The most severely asphyxiated infants of this group may have no seizure activity associated with an iso-electric EEG. Tendon jerks and primitive reflexes are usually absent. The infants have no suck reflex but may show abnormal sucking-like seizure movements. Pupils are fixed and dilated or react only sluggishly to light. Infants who die due to asphyxia all have severe encephalopathy. With recovery the infants may show a progression from hypotonia to extensor hypertonicity (Brown et al 1974). Some infants can recover fully but this may take up to 6 weeks.

Both moderate and severe encephalopathy follow a progression of clinical signs. In the first few hours the infant may breathe spontaneously and show increasing tone and movement activity. Seizures initially appear to be subtle and then become more overt and last for a longer time with progression of the encephalopathy. The infant later becomes more hypotonic and enters a period of stabilization although seizures may continue to be a problem. Subsequently, signs of clinical recovery occur in some infants. Others show changes in their pattern of neurological abnormality predictive of severe neurodevelopmental sequelae.

INVESTIGATIONS

The diagnosis of birth asphyxia is usually made on clinical criteria. Evidence for intrapartum compromise such as fetal bradycardia, passage of meconium, cardiotocographic abnormalities, low Apgar scores or delay in establishing respiration will alert the clinician to the condition and the subsequent evolution of clinical signs and symptoms is usually sufficient to make a firm diagnosis of hypoxic–ischaemic encephalopathy. Some infants present late to the clinician and information on intrapartum events may be absent or incomplete. Investigations may be necessary to elucidate the cause of the neurological abnormalities or to monitor a potentially asphyxiated infant who requires neuromuscular paralysis to facilitate mechanical ventilation. A further important role for investigative techniques is to give prognostic information in the acute stages of hypoxic–ischaemic encephalopathy. This is further discussed in the section on outcome.

Imaging

Only ultrasound and computerized tomography (CT) have been widely used to study the neonatal brain following birth asphyxia. Details of these techniques together with examples of pathology are discussed in Chapters 8 and 9. Two main ultrasound abnormalities have been associated with birth asphyxia in full-term infants. These are a generalized increase in echodensity throughout the brain (Babcock & Ball 1983, Martin et al 1983, Skeffington & Pearse 1983, Williams 1983) and echodensity confined to the region of the basal ganglia (Levene et al 1985b, Shen et al 1986). This latter condition (see p. 143) has been reported only rarely and has been assumed to be due to oedema, but Shen et al (1986) report that the increase in echoes persists for over 6 months in some cases; far too long to be due to oedema. Multicystic leukomalacia involving the periventricular region and subcortical leukomalacia have also been diagnosed by ultrasound following severe birth asphyxia (Babcock & Ball 1983, Martin et al 1983, Levene et al 1985b, Trounce & Levene 1985).

Two major CT abnormalities have been reported in asphyxiated infants; haemorrhage and extensive areas of low X-ray attenuation. Asphyxiated infants show a high incidence of intracranial haemorrhage diagnosed by CT ranging from 19 to 73% of at-risk infants (Flodmark et al 1980, Magilner & Wertheimer 1980, Fitzhardinge et al 1981, Gerard et al 1981, Finer et al 1983, Adsett et al 1985, Lipp-Zwahlen et al 1985). Analysis of cumulative data gives an overall risk of haemorrhage of approximately 30%

in infants showing clinical evidence of significant asphyxia. More than half of the lesions are due to subarachnoid haemorrhage.

Areas of low attenuation also occur commonly and are related to the severity of the asphyxial insult (for examples see p. 130). Moderate or severe involvement affecting white matter or cortex occurs in approximately 40% of asphyxiated full-term infants examined by CT scan (Flodmark et al 1980, Magilner & Wertheimer 1980, Schrumpf et al 1980, Fitzharginge et al 1981, Gerard et al 1981, Finer et al 1983, Adsett et al 1985, Lipp-Zwahlen et al 1985). This represents a high-risk group of infants who were selected for scanning in view of the severity of their neurological involvement. Local lesions apparently confined to the thalamus have also been reported on CT scans (Shewman et al 1981, Morimoto et al 1985) and magnetic resonance imaging (Voit et al 1985). These appearances may be due to infarction, oedema or haemorrhage (Kotagel et al 1983). Shewman et al (1981) have shown that the high-attenuation thalamic lesions show considerable enhancement on infusion of radio-opaque dye suggesting that they are due to postischaemic hypervascularity.

Infarction of a major cerebral artery occurs relatively commonly following asphyxia (Voorhies et al 1983) and should be apparent on ultrasound scans (Levene et al 1985b). If infarction is suspected on ultrasound examination, then CT is necessary to confirm the diagnosis (see p. 336). Radionuclide scanning may also be helpful in this diagnosis as well as giving prognostic information (O'Brien et al 1979).

In practice all infants with moderate or severe post-asphyxial encephalopathy should have a routine ultrasound scan performed within 48 hours of birth. Clinically significant and treatable lesions should be suspected by this technique, particularly if midline shift is present. A convexity subdural or subarachnoid haemorrhage will require CT scanning to delineate its precise position and its response to treatment if this is undertaken (Fig. 33.6). In general, CT is of much more value in the assessment of birth asphyxia than ultrasound and a late CT scan (approximately 2 weeks from birth) may be very valuable in the accurate prediction of outcome (see p. 390).

Measurement of intracranial pressure (ICP)

Cerebral oedema may occur as the result of hypoxic–ischaemic insult and the measurement of ICP is necessary to logically manage intracranial hypertension. ICP can be measured either directly or indirectly across the anterior fontanelle. The latter has the obvious advantage of being non-invasive but may also be less accurate.

Indirect methods

A variety of methods have been designed to assess ICP non-invasively. The earliest ones were based on

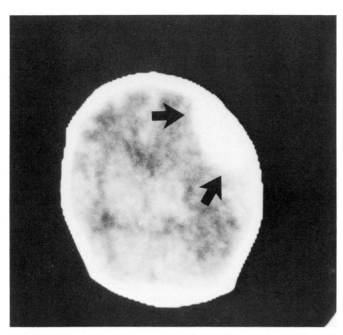

Fig. 33.6 CT scan showing convexity left-sided haemorrhage (arrowed) present in a severely asphyxiated infant. Note the midline shift and extensive areas of low attenuation.

ophthalmic tonometers and required to be hand-held (Davidoff & Chamlin 1959, Edwards 1974, Robinson et al 1977, Lopez-Ibor et al 1982, Menke et al 1982) or fixed to the fontanelle (Wealthall & Smallwood 1974, Salmon et al 1977). These devices were usually of the aplanation variety, whereby a guard-ring with a plunger in its centre was placed against the fontanelle and the spring-loaded plunger made contact with the scalp. The force applied on the plunger by the spring in order for it to remain in the same place as the guard-ring equated with the pressure across the fontanelle membrane (Wealthall & Smallwood 1974).

The best-evaluated method for non-invasively measuring ICP is the Ladd monitor. This device consists of a membrane attached to a plastic blister in which a mirror is adherent to the membrane base. The membrane is stuck over the fontanelle and fibre optic tubes transmit light to the mirror and detect reflections. Increased pressure across the membrane will force the mirror upwards, thus causing a reduction in reflected light. This is detected by a servo mechanism and air is pumped into the blister to force the mirror down again in order for maximum light to be reflected back. The principle is that the pressure within the blister to ensure maximum light reflection approximates to the ICP across the fontanelle (Vidyasagar et al 1978).

The blister is usually applied to the head by self-adhesive foam (Hill & Volpe 1981), velcro tape (Vidyasagar et al 1978) or dental adhesive (Raju & Vidyasagar 1982) after first shaving the fontanelle. A number of validation studies have shown good correlation between transfontanelle ICP and direct subarachnoid or lumbar puncture pressure usually in abnormal children (Hill & Volpe 1981, Donn

& Philip 1978, Wealthall & Smallwood 1974, Salmon et al 1977). Doubt has, however, been expressed as to the reliability of transfontanelle ICP monitoring. A number of studies have shown that the application pressure of the device influences the perceived pressure (Horbar et al 1980, Walsh & Logan 1983), thus making accurate measurement of ICP unreliable. Most published studies do not state the application pressure used. In a study using monkeys, Myerberg et al (1980) found the Ladd device to correlate well with induced changes in ICP but the response time was slow. Kaiser & Whitelaw (1987) have performed careful validation studies on both the Ladd and Wright ICP monitor (Whitelaw & Wright 1982) and have found accurate recording of ICP to be unreliable.

Direct methods

Doubt as to the accuracy of indirect methods has prompted a number of attempts at invasive measurement of ICP in infants. Goitein & Amit (1982) described placement through the fontanelle of a 22-gauge Quick-Cath into the subdural space, and found no complications. Levene & Evans (1983) used a fine subarachnoid catheter inserted percutaneously to monitor ICP and have used this successfully in over 30 infants without complications associated with the technique. More recently McWilliam & Stephenson (1984) published a method for monitoring ICP directly from the anterior horn of the lateral ventricle. To date this has not been described in the neonate.

The advantage of these direct methods lies in their ability to accurately and reliably measure ICP and all appear to be remarkably safe in clinical practice but they should be reserved for use in infants with severe encephalopathy. Published data suggest that only 50% of such infants actually develop raised intracranial pressure and monitoring may not significantly alter outcome in the majority of infants (Levene et al 1987).

Normal ICP

Most normal data are derived from the Ladd device and normal data are shown in Table 33.2. The normal figure of approximately 7 mmHg is in my view a little high and Minns (1984) gives a lower figure of approximately 2 mmHg for normal newborn ICP. Kaiser & Whitelaw (1987) have reported normal lumbar CSF pressure to range from 0 to 5.5 mmHg measured at lumbar puncture. Normally ICP is reported to rise in the first few days of life and Donn & Philip (1978) reported an increase to a mean pressure of 18.5 mmHg at 24 hours from birth in a group of apparently normal premature babies. This must be treated with suspicion and further suggests that the Ladd device overestimates ICP.

Table 33.2 'Normal' data for intracranial pressure in premature and full-term infants

Authors	Measuring device	Gestational age	Intracranial pressure (mmHg)
Robinson et al 1977	Hewlett-Packard APT-16 (hand-held)	Full-term	8.2 ± 2.4
Salmon et al 1977	Hewlett-Packard APT-16 (hand-held)	Full-term	7.4 ± 1.5
Philip et al 1981	Ladd	Prematures	7.9
Philip et al 1981	Ladd	Full-term	9.7 ± 2.2
Raju & Vidyasagar 1982	Ladd	≤ 34 weeks	7.4 ± 1.5
Raju & Vidyasagar 1982	Ladd	> 34 weeks	7.8 ± 1.4
Menke et al 1982	Aplanation tonometer (hand-held)	Full-term	7.0 ± 1.9
Strassburg et al 1984	Aplanation	Full-term	3.1 ± 2.1

Cerebral perfusion pressure

This concept has been used in adults and children to describe the resistance to cerebral perfusion due to elevations in ICP. Cerebral perfusion pressure (CPP) is calculated by subtracting ICP from mean arterial blood pressure (MAP):

$$CPP = MAP - ICP$$

In essence, the driving force of blood through the cerebral arterioles will be reduced by increments in ICP if the MAP remains unchanged.

A critically low CPP has been associated with poor outcome in adults (Rowan et al 1972) and infants (Raju et al 1983). The normal range for CPP in infants has been prone to the same methodological problems inherent in the measurement of ICP. The only normal data are from Raju et al (1982) who measured ICP by the Ladd device and blood pressure by a sphygmomanometer. As discussed above, their normal ICP data may be artefactually high. They suggest that the mean CPP for infants during the first week of life is roughly equal to the gestational age in weeks.

Electrodiagnostic tests

These methods include electro-encephalography (Ch. 13), visual and auditory evoked responses (Ch. 16 and 15) and somatosensory evoked potentials (Ch. 17). These methods are discussed in detail elsewhere. Continuous EEG monitoring is a feasible method for assessing abnormal electrical activity (Coen et al 1982, Eyre et al 1983) and ensuring adequate suppression with anticonvulsant drugs. These methods are also of value in prognosis following hypoxic–ischaemic encephalopathy.

Biochemical methods

A variety of biochemical tests have been used to assess postasphyxial cerebral injury or energy state of the brain. Some studies have looked at biochemical variables in the CSF as a reflection of central nervous system function but more usually blood levels are assayed which measure total body change rather than directly reflecting brain abnormality. It is thought by some that as the blood–brain barrier in neonates is less functionally competent, aerobically derived enzymes may more readily cross into the systemic circulation, thus enabling cerebral function to be monitored more reliably than in older patients. Energy states within the brain can now be assessed non-invasively by magnetic resonance spectroscopy and this is discussed in detail in Chapter 18.

Lactate dehydrogenase

Lactate dehydrogenase (LDH) and hydroxybutyrate dehydrogenase (HBDH) have been used as indicators of neurological damage in asphyxiated newborn infants. Iso-enzyme studies have suggested that the LDH originated from neuronal tissue. Hall et al (1980) found that although infants dying of asphyxia had high levels, prediction of handicap on the basis of elevated LDH was poor. A later study showed that subsequent abnormal neurological features did not correlate with elevated LDH or HBDH levels but those infants handicapped as the result of asphyxia had significantly higher CSF levels in the first few days of life (Dalens et al 1981).

Hypoxanthine

During hypoxia, energy is supplied from ATP which is degraded to AMP and thence to hypoxanthine (Hx). This is discussed in detail on p. 361. Magnetic resonance spectroscopy measures ATP reduction states in vivo in asphyxiated infants and is fully discussed on p. 221. Saugstad (1975) suggested that hypoxanthine is a sensitive and specific measure of energy states following perinatal asphyxia. Various studies have shown there to be a wide overlap between Hx in normal control and asphyxiated fetuses (O'Connor et al 1981). In a study of cord blood Hx measurements, Thiringer (1983) found poor correlation between Hx and low Apgar scores but abnormal clinical findings correlated better. Two infants who showed few abnormal neurological signs in the newborn period but who had high Hx levels both subsequently developed spastic diplegia. Unfortunately, Hx is not a specific measure of cerebral energy breakdown but reflects whole body changes. The liver and brain appear to contribute most to total Hx following severe fetal hypoxia.

Creatine kinase

The enzyme creatine kinase (CK) is derived from brain, heart and skeletal muscle in response to tissue injury. Attempts have been made to separate the three iso-enzymes chemically in order to study changes in the brain-derived enzyme (CK-BB) following asphyxia. Worley et al (1985) have shown CK-BB to be derived from both neurones and astrocytes. A variety of methods, including electrophoretic separation (Cuestas 1980, Walsh et al 1982) and radio-immunoassay (Thompson et al 1980, Worley et al 1985) have been used to measure CK-BB. These methods, particularly electrophoresis, have been criticized because they do not accurately separate the various component CK-BB from cardiac enzyme CK-MB (Hoo & Goedde 1982). Apparent measurements of CK-BB can be badly contaminated by CK-MB, thus rendering results unreliable.

A study from Toronto reported that low levels of CK-BB predicted normality reasonably well and significantly elevated levels found during the first 12 hours of life predicted later neurological abnormality in 92% of cases (Walsh et al 1982). Amato et al (1986) could not, however, find any correlation between levels of CK-BB iso-enzyme in cord blood and depressed Apgar scores at 5 minutes of low umbilical cord pH. The role of CK-BB iso-enzyme in quantifying cerebral injury is not clear. Certainly earlier techniques have failed to separate accurately the various iso-enzymes.

Biochemical tests in general may support the impression of cerebral injury but are of limited value in terms of prognosis. CK-BB in particular must be further evaluated before it is used as a routine test in the assessment of perinatal asphyxia.

COMPLICATIONS

During the acute hypoxic–ischaemic insult, changes occur in the distribution of blood flow in order to preserve circulation to the most vital organs, as described in Chapter 32. In summary, blood flow to brain, heart and adrenals increases in inverse proportion to arterial oxygen content and at the expense of kidneys, liver and gastrointestinal tract. This accounts for the increased vulnerability of some organs to acute asphyxial events and anticipation of complications is important in the appropriate management of such infants.

Kidney

Asphyxia in fetal or newborn animals causes a marked reduction in renal blood flow (Rudolph 1969) with a significant increase in the vascular resistance of the kidney (Alward et al 1978), and renal failure is a relatively common complication of severe hypoxic–ischaemic insult (Dauber et al 1976). Renal failure may also occur due to myoglobinuria following tissue breakdown in asphyxiated infants (Kojima et al 1985).

Gastrointestinal tract

Necrotizing enterocolitis (NEC) is the major complication affecting the bowel in asphyxiated infants. Fitzhardinge (1977) reported one-third of infants with NEC to have suffered asphyxia before its onset. Although NEC is much more common in premature infants, it is also described following asphyxia in full-term infants (Goldberg et al 1983). Abnormal liver function tests are also described in asphyxiated infants (Goldberg et al 1983, Zenardo et al 1985).

Cardiovascular system

Cardiac output

Compromise of myocardial contractility may reduce cardiac output due to decreased stroke volume with subsequent systemic hypotension. In extreme cases, cardiogenic shock and heart failure may occur (Burnard & James 1961, Cabal et al 1980). Acute cardiac dilatation associated with asphyxia may cause functional tricuspid atresia, further impairing cardiac function (Bucciarelli et al 1977). In a group of infants with low Apgar scores and acidosis (pH<7.10) their blood pressure, cardiac output and stroke volume were found to be lower than a similar but non-acidotic group. Dopamine is valuable in increasing blood pressure in asphyxiated infants (Di Sessa et al 1981) by its inotropic effect which improves cardiac output and stroke volume (Walther et al 1985).

Myocardial infarction

Ischaemic necrosis of the papillary muscle following severe birth asphyxia has been found in a high proportion of autopsy specimens (Donnelly et al 1980, De Sa & Donnelly 1984). Evidence for myocardial ischaemia is often present on ECG assessment (Daga et al 1983, Primhak et al 1985).

Lung

Meconium aspiration is a common accompaniment of hypoxic–ischaemic encephalopathy. Hypoxia induces fetal gasping during labour as well as passage of meconium and meconium aspiration occurs before the infant is born. Pulmonary hypertension is a common complication of meconium aspiration and the ensuing systemic hypoxaemia may further compromise cerebral function. Arnold et al (1985) have suggested that some asphyxiated infants develop pulmonary hypertension due to pulmonary embolism.

Metabolism

A variety of metabolic problems may arise in asphyxiated infants including hyponatraemia, hypoglycaemia, hypocalcaemia, metabolic acidosis and hyperammonaemia. Hyponatraemia may occur due to fluid retention as a result of renal compromise or due to inappropriate antidiuretic hormone secretion (IADHS). Perinatal asphyxia causes high levels of circulating ADH (Daniel et al 1978, Speer et al 1984) and fluid retention occurs as a result of this. IADHS is recognized by the combination of dilute plasma and concentrated urine.

Transient hyperammonaemia in association with severe perinatal asphyxia has been described by Goldberg et al (1979). Some of the clinical features seen in these infants and thought to be due to asphyxia, including hyperthermia, hypertension and lack of beat-to-beat variability, may have been caused by the hyperammonaemia. The reason for the transient elevation in serum ammonia is not known.

Haematological complications

Disseminated intravascular coagulation (DIC) occurs commonly following intrapartum asphyxia (Anderson et al 1974, Chessels & Wigglesworth 1970, Chadd et al 1971). Bleeding due to DIC may cause severe secondary complications including intracranial haemorrhage. Anderson et al (1974) could find no evidence that DIC was associated with significant intracerebral thrombus deposition.

REFERENCES

Adams J H, Brierley J B, Connor R C R 1966 The effects of systemic hypotension upon the human brain: clinical and neuropathological observations in 11 cases. Brain 89: 235–268

Adsett D B, Fitz C R, Hill A 1985 Hypoxic–ischaemic cerebral injury in the term newborn: correlation of CT findings with neurological outcome. Developmental Medicine and Child Neurology 27: 155–60

Alward C T, Hook J B, Helmrath T A 1978 Effects of asphyxia on renal function in the newborn piglet. Pediatric Research 12: 225–228

Amato M, Gambon R C, von Muralt G 1986 Accuracy of apgar score and arterial cord-blood pH in diagnosis of perinatal brain-damage assessed by CK–BB isoenzyme measurement. Journal of Perinatal Medicine 14: 335–338

Ames A, Wright R L, Kowada M 1968 Cerebral insult II. The no reflow phenomenon. American Journal of Pathology 52: 437–453

Amiel-Tison C 1979 Birth injury as a cause of brain dysfunction in full-term newborns. In: Korobkin R, Guilleminault L(eds) Advances in perinatal neurology, Vol 1. Spectrum, New York

Amiel-Tison C, Ellison P 1986 Birth asphyxia in the fullterm newborn: early assessment and outcome. Developmental Medicine and Child Neurology 28: 671–682

Anderson J M, Belton N R 1974 Water and electrolyte abnormalities in the human brain after severe intrapartum asphyxia. Journal of Neurology, Neurosurgery and Psychiatry 37: 514–520

Anderson J M, Brown J K, Cockburn F 1974 On the role of disseminated intravascular coagulation in the pathology of birth asphyxia. Developmental Medicine and Child Neurology 16: 581–591

Anton G 1893 Uber die Betheiligung der basalen Gehringaglien bei Bewegungsstorungen und insbesondere bei der Chorea; mit Demonstrationen von Gehirnschaitten. Wiener Klinische Wochenschrift 6: 859–861

Apgar V 1953 A proposal for a new method of evaluation of the newborn infant. Current Researches in Anaesthesia and Analgesia 32: 260–267

Arnold J, O'Brodovich H, Whyte R, Coates G 1985 Pulmonary thromboemboli after neonatal asphyxia. Journal of Pediatrics 106: 806–809

Babcock D S, Ball W 1983 Postasphyxial encephalopathy in full-term infants: ultrasound diagnosis. Radiology 148: 417–423

Brann A W, Myers R E 1975 Central nervous system findings in the new born monkey following severe in utero partial asphyxia. Neurology 25: 327

Bresler J 1899 Klinische und pathologisch-anatomische Beitrage zur Mikrogyrie. Archiv fur Psychiatrie 31: 566–573

Brierley J B, Brown A W, Excell B J, Meldrum B S 1969 Brain damage in the rhesus monkey resulting from profound arterial hypotension. I. Its nature, distribution and general physiological correlates. Brain Research 13: 68–100

Brown J K, Purvis R J, Forfar J O, Cockburn F 1974 Neurological aspects of perinatal asphyxia. Developmental Medicine and Child Neurology 16: 567–580

Bucciarelli R L, Nelson R M, Egan E A, Eitzman D V, Gessner I H 1977 Transient tricuspid insufficiency of the newborn: a form of myocardial dysfunction in stressed newborns. Pediatrics 59: 330–334

Burnard E D, James L A 1961 Failure of the heart after undue asphyxia at birth. Pediatrics 28: 545–547

Cabal L A, Devaskar U, Siassi B, Hodgman J E, Emmanouilides G 1980 Cardiogenic shock associated with perinatal asphyxia in preterm infants. Journal of Pediatrics 4: 705–710

Chadd M A, Elwood P C, Gray O P, Muxworthy S M 1971 Coagulation defects in hypoxic full-term newborn infants. British Medical Journal 4: 516–518

Chessells J M, Wigglesworth J S 1970 Secondary haemorrhagic disease of the newborn. Archives of Disease in Childhood 45: 539–543

Coen R W, McCutchen C B, Wermer D, Gluck F E 1982 Continuous monitoring of the electroencephalogram following perinatal asphyxia. Journal of Pediatrics 100: 628–630

Cuestas R A 1980 Creatine kinase isoenzymes in high-risk infants. Pediatric Research 14: 935–938

Cyr R M, Usher R H, McLean F H 1984 Changing patterns of birth asphyxia and trauma over 20 years. American Journal of Obstetrics and Gynecology 148: 490–498

Daga S R, Prabhu P G, Chandrashekhar L, Lokhande M P 1983 Myocardial ischaemia following birth asphyxia. Indian Pediatrics 20: 567–571

Dalens B, Viallard J-L, Raynauld E-J, Dastuge B 1981 CSF levels of lactate and hydroxybutyrate dehydrogenase as indicators of neurological sequelae after neonatal brain damage. Developmental Medicine and Child Neurology 23: 228–233

Daniel S S, Husain M K, Milliez J, Stark R I, Yeh M-N, James L S 1978 Renal response of the fetal lamb to complete occlusion of the umbilical cord. American Journal of Obstetrics and Gynecology 131: 514–519

Dauber I M, Krauss A N, Symchych P S, Auld P A 1976 Renal failure following perinatal asphyxia. Journal of Pediatrics 88: 851–855

Davidoff L M, Chamlin M 1959 The 'Fontanometer'. Adaptation of the Schiotz tonometer for the determination of intracranial pressure in the neonatal and early periods of infancy. Pediatrics 24: 1065–1068

De Sa D J, Donnelly W H 1984 Myocardial necrosis in the newborn. Perspectives in Pediatric Pathology 8: 295–311

Di Sessa T G, Leitner M, Ti C C, Gluck L, Coen R, Friedman W F 1981 The cardiovascular effects of dopamine in the severely asphyxiated neonate. Journal of Pediatrics 99: 772–776

Donald I 1959 Birth: adaptation from intrauterine to extrauterine life.

In: Holland E, Bourne A (eds) British obstetric practice. Heinemann, London

Donn S M, Philip A G S 1978 Early increase in intracranial pressure in preterm infants. Pediatrics 61: 904—907

Donnelly W H, Bucciarelli R L, Nelson R M 1980 Ischaemic papillary muscle necrosis in stressed newborn infants. Journal of Pediatrics 96: 295–300

Drage J S, Kennedy C, Schwarz B K 1964 The Apgar score as an index of neonatal mortality: a report from the collaborative study of cerebral palsy. Obstetrics and Gynecology 24: 222–230

Edwards J 1974 An intracranial pressure tonometer for use on neonates: preliminary report. Developmental Medicine and Child Neurology (Suppl:) 32: 38–39

Ergander U, Eriksson M, Zetterstrom R 1983 Severe neonatal asphyxia: incidence and prediction of outcome in the Stockholm area. Acta Paediatrica Scandinavica 72: 321–325

Eyre J H, Oozeer R C, Wilkinson A R 1983 Diagnosis of neonatal seizure by continuous recording and rapid analysis of the electroencephalogram. Archives of Disease in Childhood 58: 785–790

Farkas-Bargeton E, Diebler M F 1978 A topographical study of enzyme maturation in human cerebral neocortex: a histological and biochemical study. In: Brazier M A B, Petsche H (eds) Architectonics and the cerebral cortex. Raven Press, New York

Fenichel G M 1983 Hypoxic–ischaemic encephalopathy in the newborn. Archives of Neurology 40: 261–266

Finer N N, Robertson C M, Richards R T, Pinnell L E, Peters K L 1981 Hypoxic–ischaemic encephalopathy in term neonates: perinatal factors and outcome. Journal of Pediatrics 98: 112–117

Finer N N, Robertson C M, Peters K L, Coward J H 1983 Factors affecting outcome in hypoxic–ischaemic encephalopathy in term infants. American Journal of Diseases of Children 137: 21–25

Fitzhardinge P M 1977 Complications of asphyxia and their therapy. In: Gluck L (ed) Intrauterine asphyxia and the developing fetal brain. Year Book Medical Publishers, Chicago

Fitzhardinge P M, Flodmark O, Fitz C R, Ashby S 1981 The prognostic value of computed tomography as an adjunct to assessment of the term infant with postasphyxial encephalopathy. Journal of Pediatrics 99: 777–781

Flodmark O, Becker L E, Harwood-Nash D C, Fitzhardinge P M, Fitz C R, Chuang S H 1980 Correlation between computed tomography and autopsy in premature and full-term neonates that have suffered perinatal asphyxia. Radiology 137: 93–103

Friede R L 1975 Developmental neuropathology. Springer-Verlag, Berlin

Gerard P, Verheggen P, Bachy A, Langhendries J-P 1981 Interet de la tomodensitometrie cerebrale chez les enfants nes asphyxies. Archives Francaises de Pediatrie 38: 591–596

Goitein K J, Amit Y 1982 Percutaneous placement of subdural catheter for measurement of intracranial pressure in small children. Critical Care Medicine 10: 46–48

Goldberg R N, Cabal L A, Sinatra F R, Plajstek C E, Hodgman J E 1979 Hyperammonemia associated with perinatal asphyxia. Pediatrics 64: 336–341

Goldberg R N, Thomas D W, Sinatra F R 1983 Necrotizing enterocolitis in the asphyxiated full-term infant. American Journal of Perinatology 1: 40–42

Hall R T, Kulkarni P B, Sheehan M B, Rhodes P G 1980 Cerebrospinal fluid lactate dehydrogenase in infants with perinatal asphyxia. Developmental Medicine and Child Neurology 22: 300–307

Hill A, Volpe J J 1981 Measurement of intracranial pressure using the Ladd intracranial pressure monitor. Journal of Pediatrics 98: 974–976

Hoo J J, Goedde H W 1982 Determination of brain type creatine kinase for diagnosis of perinatal asphyxia — choice of method. Pediatric Research 16: 806

Horbar J D, Yeager S, Philip A G S, Lucey J F 1980 Effect of application force on noninvasive measurements of intracranial pressure. Pediatrics 66: 455–457

Hossman K A, Kleihues P 1973 Reversibility of ischaemic brain damage. Archives of Neurology 29: 375–385

Kaiser A M, Whitelaw A G L 1987 Noninvasive monitoring of intracranial pressure — fact or fancy? Developmental Medicine and Child Neurology 29: 320–326

Klatzo I 1967 Neuropathological aspects of brain damage. Journal of Neuropathology and Experimental Neurology 26: 1–5

Klatzo I 1985 Brain oedema following brain ischaemia and the influence of therapy. British Journal of Anaesthesia 57: 18–22

Kojima T, Kobayashi T, Matsuzaki S, Iwase S, Yobayashi Y 1985 Effects of perinatal asphyxia and myoglobinuria on development of acute neonatal renal failure. Archives of Diseases in Childhood 60: 908–912

Kotagel S, Toce S S, Kotagel P, Archer C R 1983 Symmetric bithalamic and striatal hemorrhage following perinatal hypoxia in a term infant. Journal of Computer Assisted Tomography 7: 353–355

Kreusser K L, Schmidt R E, Shackelford G D, Volpe J J 1984 Value of ultrasound for identification of acute hemorrhagic necrosis of thalamus and basal ganglia in an asphyxiated term infant. Annals of Neurology 16: 361–363

Larroche J-C 1977 Developmental pathology of the neonate. Excerpta Medica, Amsterdam

Larroche J-C 1984 Perinatal brain damage. In: Adams J H, Corsellis J A N, Duchen L W (eds) Greenfield's neuropathology. Edward Arnold, London

Lassen N A 1966 The luxury perfusion syndrome and its possible relation to acute metabolic acidosis localised within the brain. Lancet ii: 1113–1115

Leech R W, Alvord E C 1977 Anoxic–ischemic encephalopathy in the human neonatal period: the significance of brain stem involvement. Archives of Neurology 34: 109–113

Levene M I, Evans D H 1983 Continuous measurement of subarachnoid pressure in the severely asphyxiated newborn. Archives of Disease in Childhood 58: 1013–1015

Levene M I, Kornberg J, Williams T H C 1985a The incidence and severity of post-asphyxial encephalopathy in full-term infants. Early Human Development 11: 21–28

Levene M I, Williams J L, Fawer C-L 1985b Ultrasound of the infant brain. Spastics International Medical Publications, No. 92, Oxford

Levene M I, Sands C, Grindulis H, Moore J R 1986 Comparison of two methods of predicting outcome in perinatal asphyxia. Lancet i: 67–91

Levene M I, Evans D H, Forde A, Archer L N J 1987 The value of intracranial pressure monitoring in asphyxiated newborn infants. Developmental Medicine and Child Neurology 29: 311–319

Lipp-Zwahlen A E, Deonna T, Micheli J L, Calame A 1985 Prognostic value of neonatal CT scans in asphyxiated term babies: low density score compared with neonatal neurological signs. Neuropediatrics 16: 209–217

Lopez-Ibor B, Garcia-Sola R, Hernandez C, Moro M, Casado E 1982 ICP monitoring during the first week of life in the preterm infant. Monographs in Pediatrics 15: 134–138

MacDonald H M, Mulligan J C, Allan A C, Taylor P M 1980 Neonatal asphyxia. I. Relationship of obstetric and neonatal complications to neonatal mortality in 38 405 consecutive deliveries. Journal of Pediatrics 96: 898–902

McWilliam R C, Stephenson J B P 1984 Rapid bedside technique for intracranial pressure monitoring. Lancet ii: 73–75

Magilner A D, Wertheimer I S 1980 Preliminary results of a computed tomography study of neonatal brain hypoxia–ischaemia. Journal of Computer Assisted Tomography 4: 457–463

Martin D J, Hill A, Fitz C R, Daneman A, Havill D A, Becker L E 1983 Hypoxic/ischaemic cerebral injury in the neonatal brain. Pediatric Radiology 13: 307–312

Menke J A et al 1982 The fontanelle tonometer: a noninvasive method for measurement of intracranial pressure. Journal of Pediatrics 100: 960–963

Minns R A 1984 Intracranial pressure monitoring. Archives of Disease in Childhood 59: 486–488

Morimoto K, Sumita Y, Kitajima H, Mogami H 1985 Bilateral, asymmetrical hemorrhagic infarction of the basal ganglia and thalamus following neonatal asphyxia. No To Shinkei 37: 133–137

Myerberg D Z, York C, Chaplin E R, Gregory G A 1980 Comparison of noninvasive and direct measurements of intracranial pressure. Pediatrics 65: 473–476

Myers R E 1972 Two patterns of perinatal brain damage and their conditions of occurrence. American Journal of Obstetrics and Gynecology 112: 246–276

Myers R E 1977 Experimental models of perinatal brain damage: relevance to human pathology. In: Gluck L (ed) Intrauterine asphyxia and the developing fetal brain. Year Book Medical Publishers, Chicago

Nelson K B, Ellenberg J H 1981 Apgar scores as predictors of chronic neurological disability. Pediatrics 68: 36–44

O'Brien M J, Ash J M, Gilday D L 1979 Radionuclide brain scanning in perinatal hypoxia/ischaemia. Developmental Medicine and Child Neurology 21: 161–173

O'Connor M C, Harkness R A, Simmonds R J, Hytten F E 1981 The measurement of hypoxanthine, xanthine, inosine and uridine in umbilical cord blood and fetal scalp blood samples as a measure of fetal hypoxia. British Journal of Obstetrics and Gynaecology 88: 381–390

Pape K E, Wigglesworth J S 1979 Haemorrhage, ischaemia and the perinatal brain. Spastics International Medical Publications, London

Philip A G S, Long J G, Donn S M 1981 Intracranial pressure. Sequential measurements in full-term and pre-term infants. American Journal of Diseases of Children 135: 521–524

Primhak R A et al 1985 Myocardial ischaemia in asphyxia neonatorum. Acta Paediatrica Scandinavica 74: 595–600

Pryse-Davies J, Beard R W 1973 A necropsy study of brain swelling in the newborn with special reference to cerebellar herniation. Journal of Pathology 109: 51–73

Raju T N, Vidyasagar D 1982 Intracranial and cerebral perfusion pressure: methodology and clinical considerations. Medical Instrumentation 16: 154–156

Raju T N, Doshi U V, Vidyasagar D 1982 Cerebral perfusion pressure studies in healthy preterm and term newborn infants. Journal of Pediatrics 100: 139–142

Raju T N, Doshi U, Vidyasagar D 1983 Low cerebral perfusion pressure: an indicator of poor prognosis in asphyxiated term infants. Brain Development 5: 478–482

Robinson R O, Rolfe P, Sutton P 1977 Non-invasive method for measuring intracranial pressure in normal newborn infants. Developmental Medicine and Child Neurology 19: 305–308

Rorke L B 1982 Pathology of perinatal brain injury. Raven Press, New York

Rowan J O, Johnston H, Harper A M, Jannett W B 1972 Perfusion in intracranial hypertension. In: Borck M, Dietz H (eds) Intracranial pressure. Springer-Verlag, New York

Rudolph A M 1969 The course and distribution of the fetal circulation. In: Wolstenholme G, O'Connor M J A (eds) Foetal autonomy. Churchill, London

Salmon J H, Hajjar W, Bada H S 1977 The fontogram: a noninvasive intracranial pressure monitor. Pediatrics 60: 721–725

Sarnat H B, Sarnat M S 1976 Neonatal encephalopathy following fetal distress. Archives of Neurology 33: 696–705

Saugstad O D 1975 Hypoxanthine as a measurement of hypoxia. Pediatric Research 9: 158–161

Schneider H, Ballowitz L, Schachinger H, Hanefield F, Droszus J-U 1975 Anoxic encephalopathy with predominant involvement of basal ganglia, brain stem and spinal cord in the perinatal period. Acta Neuropathologica 32: 287–298

Schrumpf J D, Sehring S, Killpack S, Brady J P, Hirata T, Mednick J P 1980 Correlation of early neurologic outcome and CT findings in neonatal brain hypoxia and injury. Journal of Computer Assisted Tomography 4: 445–450

Shen E Y, Huang C C, Chyou S C, Hung H Y, Hsu C H, Huang F Y 1986 Sonographic finding of the bright thalamus. Archives of Disease in Childhood 61: 1096–1099

Shewman D A, Fine M, Masdeu J C, Palacios E 1981 Postischemic hypervascularity of infancy: a stage in the evolution of ischemic brain damage with characteristic CT scan. Annals of Neurology 9: 358–365

Skeffington F S, Pearse R G 1983 The 'bright brain'. Archives of Disease in Childhood 58: 509–511

Speer M E, Gormon W A, Kaplan S L, Rudolph A J 1984 Elevation of plasma concentrations of arginine vasopression following perinatal asphyxia. Acta Paediatrica Scandinavica 73: 610–614

Strassburg H M, Klemon F J , Wais U, Goppinger A 1984 Nichtinvasive

hirndruckmessung uber der vorden Fontanelle bei gesunden Sauglingen in den ersten Lebenstagen. Monatsschrift Kinderheilkunde 132: 904–908

Thiringer K 1983 Cord plasma hypoxanthine as a measure of foetal asphyxia: comparison with clinical assessment and laboratory measures. Acta Paediatrica Scandinavica 72: 231–237

Thompson R J, Graham J G, McQueen I N F, Kynoch P A M, Brown K W 1980 Radioimmunoassay of brain type creatine kinase-BB isoenzyme in human tissues and in serum of patients with neurological disorders. Journal of Neurological Science 47: 241–254

Trounce J Q, Levene M I 1985 The diagnosis and outcome of subcortical cystic leukomalacia. Archives of Disease in Childhood 60: 1041–1044

Tweed W A, Pash M, Doig G 1981 Cerebrovascular mechanisms in perinatal asphyxia: the role of vasogenic brain edema. Pediatric Research 15: 44–46

Vidyasagar D, Raju T N, Chiang J 1978 Clinical significance of monitoring anterior fontanel pressure in sick neonates and infants. Pediatrics 62: 996–999

Voit T, Lemburg P, Stork W 1985 NMR studies in thalamic–striatal necrosis. Lancet ii: 445

Volpe J J 1977 Observing the infant in the early hours after asphyxia. In: Gluck L (ed) Intrauterine asphyxia and the developing fetal brain, Year Book Medical Publishers, Chicago

Volpe J J 1987 Neurology of the newborn, 2nd edn. W B Saunders, Philadelphia

Volpe J J, Pasternak J F 1977 Parasagittal cerebral injury in neonatal hypoxic–ischemic encephalopathy: clinical and neuroradiologic features. Journal of Pediatrics 91: 472–476

Volpe J J, Herscovitch P, Perlman J M, Kreusser K L, Raichle M E 1985 Positron emission tomography in the asphyxiated term newborn: parasagittal impairment of cerebral blood flow. Annals of Neurology 17: 287–296

Voorhies T M, Ehrlich M E, Frayer W, Lee B, Vannucci R C 1983 Occlusive vascular disease in perinatal cerebral hypoxia–ischaemia. American Journal of Perinatology 1: 1–5

Walsh P, Logan W J 1983 Continuous and intermittent measurement of intracranial pressure by Ladd monitor. Journal of Pediatrics 102: 439–442

Walsh P, Jedeikin R, Ellis G, Primhak R, Makela S K 1982 Assessment of neurologic outcome in asphyxiated term infants by use of serial CK-BB isoenzyme measurement. Journal of Pediatrics 101: 988–992

Walther F J, Siassi B, Ramadan N A, Wu P 1985 Cardiac output in newborn infants with transient myocardial dysfunction. Journal of Pediatrics 107: 781–785

Wealthall S R, Smallwood R 1974 Methods of measuring intracranial pressure via the fontanelle without puncture. Journal of Neurology, Neurosurgery and Psychiatry 37: 88–96

Wegman M E 1984 Annual summary of vital statistics — 1983. Pediatrics 74: 981–990

Whitelaw A G L, Wright B M 1982 A pneumatic applanimeter for intracranial pressure measurements. Journal of Physiology 336: 3P-4P

Williams J L 1983 Intracranial vascular pulsations in pediatric neurosonology. Journal of Ultrasound in Medicine 2: 485

Windle W F 1966 An experimental approach to prevention or reduction of the brain damage of birth asphyxia. Developmental Medicine and Child Neurology 8: 129–140

Worley G et al 1985 Creatine kinase brain isoenzyme: relationship of cerebrospinal fluid concentration to the neurologic condition of newborns and cellular localization in the human brain. Pediatrics 76: 15–21

Zanardo V, Bondio M, Pesini G, Temporin G F 1985 Serum glutamic–oxaloacetic transaminase and glutamic–pyruvic transaminase activity in premature and full-term asphyxiated newborns. Biology of the Neonate 47: 61–69

34. Management and outcome of birth asphyxia

Dr M.I. Levene

The acute management of birth asphyxia is directed towards resuscitation (see p. 366) and stabilization of the infant's condition. Asphyxia may compromise the functions of a variety of immature systems (p. 379) and anticipation of such complications with appropriate management is essential. The management of the asphyxiated infant must be considered in relation to general systemic complications as well as directing therapy towards the brain. Brain-orientated management is misplaced if systemic hypotension is unrecognized or inadequately treated. Severely asphyxiated infants must be treated in the same manner as the very-low-birth-weight infant, with adequate monitoring and the provision of cerebrally orientated intensive care should this be necessary.

MANAGEMENT: GENERAL METHODS

Respiratory support

Respiratory support may be necessary for comatose infants with severe encephalopathy and those with coincident lung disease, of which meconium aspiration is the most common. Infants with frequent and prolonged convulsions may also need to be supported by mechanical ventilation and this may become necessary as a result of their anticonvulsant management. Careful assessment of arterial blood gas estimates is necessary to provide appropriate support. Spontaneously breathing infants should be electively intubated and ventilated if they develop hypercapnia due to depression of respiratory drive or lung disease ($P_{a,CO_2} < 6$ kPa, >45 mmHg). The fear of inducing respiratory arrest by adequate dosage of anticonvulsants is irrational. The effects of prolonged or frequent seizures make the need to adequately treat this complication essential (see Ch. 41). If fear of the infant requiring mechanical ventilation is a factor in avoiding adequate anticonvulsant therapy, then the infant should be referred to a centre where it can be safely and rapidly undertaken. Hypoxia should also be avoided and although there are no clear guidelines the P_{a,O_2} should be maintained in the range of 10–12 kPa (75–90 mmHg) in mature infants.

Environmental temperature

To prevent cold stress and unnecessary utilization of oxygen to maintain body temperature, the infant should be nursed in the thermoneutral range for his/her birth-weight and postnatal age. Therapeutic hypothermia is discussed on p. 385.

Fluids

Fluid restriction is widely recommended in the management of asphyxiated infants to prevent brain swelling but the evidence that fluid intake contributes to cerebral oedema is lacking. The baby should be given only the volume of fluid necessary to keep just adequately hydrated. This requires at least daily measurement of serum osmolality and urinary concentration (specific gravity), aiming to maintain the serum osmolality in the region of 290 mOsm/l and the urinary specific gravity at 1010. If the infant develops hyponatraemia it is usually due to inappropriate ADH secretion and this is confirmed by demonstrating dilute plasma and concentrated urine. The fluid intake should be restricted until the serum osmolality and serum sodium levels return to normal. Oliguria is managed by maintenance of careful fluid balance. Daily measurement of plasma creatinine is a sensitive method of assessing renal function. Assessment of the state of hydration in oliguric patients is facilitated by measurement of central venous pressure. Acute renal failure is best managed conservatively.

Blood pressure

Hypotension occurs frequently in severely asphyxiated infants and continuous monitoring of arterial blood pressure is essential (Diprose et al 1986). Plasma is often ineffective in restoring normotension and dopamine (5–15 μg.kg⁻¹.min⁻¹) or dobutamine (2.5–5.0 μg.kg⁻¹.min⁻¹) is usually necessary.

Haemostasis

Disturbances in blood clotting are most commonly due to disseminated intravascular coagulation. Management is supportive and there is no place for systemic heparinization. The infant should receive additional vitamin K and may require fresh frozen plasma for replacement of clotting factors or platelet transfusion. Regular haematological checks of clotting function should be performed in all infants with severe birth asphyxia.

Infection

A high index of suspicion for infection must be maintained in all ill infants. Routine use of antibiotics cannot be recommended and should be used only for clinical indications or strongly suspected infection. Early neonatal meningitis may present clinically in a manner similar to birth asphyxia and if there is any doubt a lumbar puncture must be performed.

Prevention of acidosis

Asphyxiated infants are commonly acidotic as a result of hypercapnia and excessive lactate accumulation. Management of the acidosis should be directed towards relieving factors precipitating asphyxia and providing adequate ventilation. Most infants who are efficiently resuscitated at birth correct their acidosis spontaneously and the routine use of alkali therapy cannot be recommended. Arterial pH should be regularly monitored to recognize acidosis early, and treatment depends on whether it is predominantly of respiratory or metabolic origin. In the latter case, slow infusion of 8.4% sodium bicarbonate may be beneficial but first ensure that perfusion and ventilation are adequate.

BRAIN-ORIENTATED MANAGEMENT

Traditionally, the management of asphyxiated infants has been directed towards achieving a stable condition, adequate treatment of seizures and preventing or controlling cerebral oedema. Increased awareness of subtle fits or asymptomatic electroconvulsive seizure activity in infants given neuromuscular relaxing agents has made continuous EEG monitoring more widely used (see p. 184). Adequate control of seizures is essential and this is discussed in Chapter 41.

When analysing the effect of drugs in hypoxic–ischaemic injury the pathogenesis of the injury must be considered in relation to the pharmacological action of the drug. Following perinatal asphyxia, both the primary and the secondary cerebral insults may vary in severity and although interdependent they may not necessarily be sequential. Ideally, in order to predict the likelihood of acute intracerebral sequelae, it is necessary to know for how long the fetus or infant has suffered significant cerebral underperfusion and if there was a period of complete anoxia (cardiac arrest). Once resuscitation has been achieved, further variables include whether or not cerebral hypoperfusion (the 'no-reflow phenomenon') has developed and if intracranial hypertension intervened to further impede cerebral perfusion. The measurement of cerebral blood flow is fundamental to understanding these events but this is not possible in the routine management of the asphyxiated newborn infant (see Ch. 10). Ignorance of the duration of intrapartum asphyxia is common in the clinical setting and this makes assessment and management of birth asphyxia largely empirical.

Glucose

Whether or not to give asphyxiated infants glucose is a highly controversial question. The deleterious effects of glucose on cerebral asphyxia have been reviewed by Myers et al (1983) and they make a strong case for avoiding the infusion of glucose in any potentially asphyxiated fetus or newborn. Although the evidence is scanty, they further suggest that infused glucose may also cause brain damage *following* asphyxia. Damage is caused by the conversion of glucose to lactate under anaerobic conditions.

Glucose and oxygen are the main substrates of brain metabolism and hypoglycaemia may be devastating. Although the place for glucose infusion is unclear, hypoglycaemia must be avoided. Asphyxiated infants should have regular blood glucose stick-test estimations and if the blood glucose of mature infants falls below 2 mmol/l, an infusion of 10% dextrose should be given to correct this. Once the blood glucose has remained above 2 mmol/l for 4 hours, the infusion should be cut back to a 5% solution. Rapid bolus injections of concentrated glucose must be avoided.

Barbiturates

This group of drugs have multiple action on the central nervous system and are still the mainstay of brain-orientated management of the asphyxiated newborn infant. The cerebral effects of barbiturates include:

1. Reduction in cerebral metabolic rate; thiopentone reduces this by up to 50% (Michenfelder 1974).
2. Depression of cerebral function, including suppression of the EEG to the point at which it becomes iso-electric.
3. Reduction in cerebral blood flow due to an increase in cerebral vascular resistance (Pierce et al 1962, Hanson et al 1975).
4. Anticonvulsant effects.
5. Reduction of cerebral oedema (Simeone et al 1979) in part related to reduction in cerebral blood flow.

6. Oxygen free radical consumption (Flamm et al 1978).
7. Biochemical modification of the cell, including stabilization of lysosomal membranes, reduction in intracellular calcium concentrations and modified neurotransmitter release (Steen & Michenfelder 1980).

These effects are dose related and may be specific to one type of barbiturate only.

The benefit of barbiturates in the management of hypoxic–ischaemic injury has been demonstrated in human and animal studies but only when the drug was given *before* the asphyxial event (Campbell et al 1968, Cockburn et al 1969, Goodlin & Lloyd 1970). There has been only one prospective randomized clinical study assessing the cerebral protective effects of a barbiturate (thiopentone) in humans following global asphyxia (cardiac arrest). This study in adults showed no difference between the treated and untreated groups with regard to outcome (Abrahamson et al 1983). Eyre & Wilkinson (1986) have reported the use of thiopentone in six severely asphyxiated neonates. The dosage was sufficient to produce an iso-electric EEG. In two infants the infusion was stopped because of hypotension and in all six the outcome was death or severe handicap.

In a paper entitled 'Brain-orientated intensive care', Svenningson et al (1982) recommended routine use of phenobarbitone within an hour of delivery in all severely asphyxiated infants. Using this as well as other methods, they claim to have reduced the mortality and incidence of neurodevelopmental handicap. It seems unlikely that the effect of phenobarbitone in the dosage used (10 mg/kg) would have any significant protective effect on the brain. It is more likely that these authors, by paying more careful attention to all aspects of the care of asphyxiated infants, have thereby improved the outlook.

The dosage of phenobarbitone should be carefully monitored in asphyxiated infants as toxicity may easily occur. Gal et al (1984) have shown that asphyxiated neonates require about half the maintenance dose compared with non-asphyxiated infants to achieve a similar plasma concentration.

Hypothermia

Hypothermia is known to reduce cerebral metabolic rate below that achieved by dosage of barbiturates which produce an iso-electric EEG (Gisvold & Steen 1985). Hypothermia, in the region of 18–25°C, is used in open-heart surgery and no measurable long-term cerebral sequelae are associated with cardiac arrest for a period of up to 30 minutes. It is well known that asphyxiated newborn animals continue to gasp for a longer time if they are cold, and Miller (1961) has suggested that hypothermia may protect asphyxiated newborns. Reports in the Russian literature also recommend it as a method for treating birth asphyxia (Persianinov et al 1978). Miller (1961) reported

the treatment of 11 newborn infants in whom hypothermia was induced by placing the apnoeic infant in a bath of cold water for up to 17 minutes. The core temperature in some infants fell to 23°C. The neurological outcome was stated to be near-normal in most of these children. This treatment was apparently adopted before efficient methods of resuscitation became available and it attests to the robustness of many newborn infants. Although hypothermia protects the normal brain during cardiac arrest there is no evidence that it will limit cerebral injury after birth asphyxia. This form of treatment is not recommended.

Other drugs

Considerable interest has recently been directed towards the early pharmacological management of hypoxic–ischaemic injury and almost all this work is on adult patients or mature animals. Virtually no controlled studies have been performed in the human newborn and data from immature animals are reviewed in detail in Chapter 28. In the late 1980s there are few positive data indicating the most appropriate methods for treating neonatal asphyxia but this section might point the way to management in the next decade.

Calcium channel blockers

Lidoflazine and nimodipine appear to be the most promising of these agents in improving outcome following complete cerebral ischaemia as occurs after cardiac arrest, but to date no human studies have been reported (Gisvold & Steen 1985). There is no evidence that these drugs protect the neurone but may prevent failure of reperfusion following resuscitation (see p. 362).

Oxygen free radical scavengers

Oxygen free radicals are highly unstable atoms or molecules which may cause membrane damage which further exacerbates cerebral dysfunction. The role of oxygen-derived free radicals in cerebral injury is fully discussed on p. 360.

Prostaglandins

These substances are involved in the basic control of cerebral blood flow. Two opposing systems are in balance and are summarized in Figure 34.1. During asphyxia arachidonic acid accumulates and, following reperfusion, oxidation occurs with the production of vaso-active prostaglandins. Indomethacin, a prostaglandin synthetase inhibitor, reduces the synthesis of both thromboxane and prostacyclin and causes a fall in cerebral blood flow (Cowan 1986, Evans et al 1987), suggesting that prostaglandin is preferentially inhibited with a net effect on cerebral arteriolar vasoconstriction. Hallenbeck & Furlow (1979)

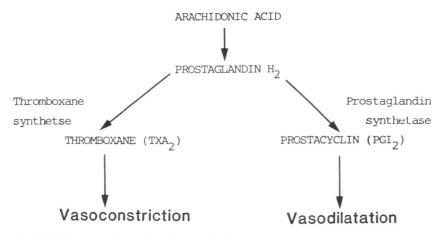

Fig. 34.1 The opposing action of prostaglandins in controlling the cerebral circulation.

have shown that giving both indomethacin and prostacyclin infusion after experimental ischaemic cerebral injury in dogs prevents subsequent impairment of cerebral blood flow (the 'no-reflow phenomenon'). Neither indomethacin nor prostaglandin when given alone has a similar beneficial effect.

Neurotransmitter inhibition

The role of excitatory amino acid accumulation in cerebral injury has been discussed in detail on p. 360. Agents which act as inhibitors of neurotransmitters, have been shown to reduce the cerebral metabolic rate by inhibiting glucose utilization in the rat brain (Wolfson et al 1977) and to prevent neuronal death in tissue culture during anoxia (Rothman 1984). There is evidence that the inhibitors may reduce cerebral blood flow to a greater extent than they reduce metabolic rate thus failing to improve the ratio between metabolism and substrate delivery (Gisvold & Steen 1985).

Naloxone

It has been suggested that hypoxia is associated with the release of endogenous opiates (endorphins) and these contribute to respiratory depression (Wardlow et al 1981) occurring after birth in asphyxiated infants. A number of studies have suggested that the specific opiate antagonist naloxone, given after asphyxia, improves blood flow to the brainstem in lambs (Lou et al 1985) or improves the short-term outcome of rabbits if given before asphyxia (Chernick & Craig 1982). Others, however, have found that naloxone exacerbates cerebral injury in the neonatal rat (Young et al 1984) and the newborn rabbit (Goodlin 1981). Naloxone should be used with caution in asphyxiated human infants.

Cerebral oedema

There is some dispute as to the role of cerebral oedema in contributing to acute cerebral injury following asphyxia. Brann & Myers (1975) have shown evidence of cerebral oedema both macroscopically and microscopically within 2 hours of severe asphyxia in a fetal monkey. In our experience the median time for intracranial hypertension (ICP > 15 mmHg) to develop in the human neonate following severe asphyxia is 26 hours (unpublished data). These data are not of course incompatible but the implication that early cerebral oedema has a role in the primary pathogenesis of brain injury following intrapartum hypoxic–ischaemic injury is unsubstantiated. Cerebral oedema severe enough to cause secondary cerebral hypoperfusion is a complication of asphyxia and adequate treatment of intracranial hypertension will not per se prevent brain injury. Levene et al (1987) have analysed the results of monitoring and treating raised intracranial pressure in full-term asphyxiated infants. In less than 10% of the babies studied could intervention to control intracranial hypertension have had any significant beneficial effect on outcome.

Corticosteroids

The role of steroids in the management of asphyxia is controversial, with little data available for either newborn humans or animals. Studies on 5-day-old rats, whose brains at that age are at a comparable state of development to the full-term human brain, showed that treatment with dexamethasone before asphyxiation resulted in less severe cerebral effects than in untreated animals (Adlard & De Souza 1976). Use of steroids following neonatal asphyxia was ineffective in treating or preventing cerebral oedema (De Souza & Dobbing 1973).

It has been suggested that dexamethasone has its main benefit in treating vasogenic oedema and is less effective in cytotoxic oedema (Yamaguchi et al 1976) but in clinical practice both types of brain swelling probably occur together. Corticosteroids have their major role in the treatment of focal cerebral oedema associated with tumour or abscess, neither of which bears a close resemblance to the generalized brain swelling that occurs following perinatal asphyxia. In addition, there is a body of evidence on the adverse effects of steroids on the developing brain even when used over a short period (Weichsel 1977). Fitzhardinge et al (1974) found measurable differences in neurological function of children who had received hydrocortisone only in the first 24 hours of life, compared with untreated controls. Levene & Evans (1985) found no improvement in cerebral perfusion pressure within 6 hours of giving dexamethasone. There is no good evidence for the beneficial effect of using steroids after an hypoxic–ischaemic insult in the newborn and their use is not recommended. There is however some, as yet, unconfirmed evidence that steroids inhibit the release of arachidonic acid from cell membranes.

Hyperventilation

There is a predictable relationship between $P_{a,CO2}$ and cerebral blood flow. Increasing carbon dioxide tension induces cerebral arteriolar vasodilatation with increase in cerebral blood flow and vice versa (see Fig. 34.2). In adults, for every 0.13 kP_a (1 mmHg) change in P_{CO2}, there is approximately a 3% change in cerebral blood flow over the physiological range for $P_{a,CO2}$ (Bruce 1984). This proportional change diminishes for levels of $P_{a,CO2}$, below 2.7 kPa (20 mmHg). Following perinatal asphyxia the arteriolar response may be less sensitive to changes in $Pa_{,CO2}$ and in some there may be a paradoxical increase in cerebral blood flow with controlled hyperventilation (Sankaran 1984). It is considered unlikely that more extreme degrees of hypocapnia produce cerebral ischaemia in the healthy brain (Bruce 1984).

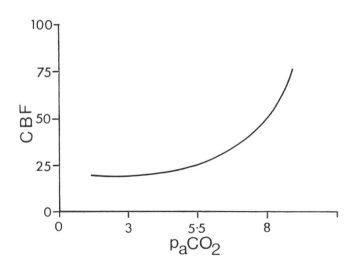

Fig. 34.2 The relationship between arterial carbon dioxide tension (P_{a,CO_2}) and cerebral blood flow (CBF). (Redrawn from Bruce 1984.)

In practice we attempt to maintain the $P_{a,CO2}$ in asphyxiated infants who are mechanically ventilated between 3.5 and 4.0 kPa (26–30 mmHg). A high positive end expiratory pressure (PEEP) level is likely to produce a higher $P_{a,CO2}$ (Stewart et al 1981) and PEEP should be kept as low as possible in asphyxiated infants who are mechanically ventilated.

Osmotic agents

A variety of agents, including mannitol, glycerol and urea, have been used to shrink the swollen neonatal brain. These agents act by inducing a higher osmotic pressure outside the brain than within, thereby causing intracerebral shrinkage. A theoretical hazard is entry of the osmotic agent into the brain through the damaged blood–brain barrier, causing a rebound effect of brain swelling. Mannitol is the only osmotic agent where published data exist on its use in the newborn (Marchal et al 1974). A study of intracranial pressure monitoring reported a fall in ICP and an improvement in cerebral perfusion pressure on each occasion when mannitol was used (Levene & Evans 1985). This appears to be the only agent which is of value in treating brain swelling in the asphyxiated newborn.

Barbiturates

As mentioned above, the barbiturates increase cerebral vascular resistance, thereby reducing cerebral blood flow and it is this action that contributes to lowering intracranial pressure in the swollen brain. It is unlikely that this will improve cerebral perfusion pressure.

OUTCOME

Prediction of outcome in asphyxiated infants is of obvious importance for the parents as they will ask 'will my baby be handicapped?' An accurate and honest answer is available from the results of good follow-up studies. Another important aspect of predicting outcome is the question of when it is appropriate to abandon resuscitative efforts or withdraw intensive care in infants likely to be severely handicapped. The answers to these questions are beginning to emerge but critical review of the assessment methods is necessary and this is discussed in detail in Chapter 5. A major problem in the evaluation of follow-up studies is the failure to distinguish whether the data refer to full-term babies only or a mixture of mature and immature infants. In addition, the problem of defining what is asphyxia influences outcome statistics. For the purpose of this review, only reports from full-term infants will be considered and outcome from different assessment techniques will be discussed separately. The value of any test can be evaluated from its sensitivity and specificity. Sensitivity refers to the percentage of handicapped infants predicted by an abnormal test, and specificity to the percentage of normal infants predicted by a normal test. To evaluate any assessment of outcome both figures should be considered. Wherever it has been possible to calculate these figures they are given in the text.

There is evidence that the prognosis following intrapartum asphyxia has improved over recent years (Finer et al 1983). A Swedish study reported that 50% of infants surviving asphyxia between 1973 and 1976 had significant neurodevelopmental sequelae, in contrast to a 17% incidence of handicap in those born between 1976 and 1979 (Svenningson et al 1982). These authors related the improved outcome to the introduction of brain-orientated intensive care.

Mortality

The mortality rate of liveborn asphyxiated infants depends on the severity of the insult and the intensity of treatment. If asphyxia is defined by depression of the Apgar score, then mortality increases inversely to gestational age and birth-weight. MacDonald et al (1980) report an overall mortality of 46% in severely asphyxiated infants of all gestational ages, and the presence of intra-uterine growth retardation, respiratory distress syndrome and hypothermia were all associated with a significantly higher risk of death. In another study, over half of the infants died, if born with an Apgar score of 0 at birth, or delay in establishing respiration until 20 minutes after birth (Scott 1976). In the well-known study of Nelson & Ellenberg (1981) over 40 000 infants had accurate assessment of Apgar score. Those of birth-weight below 2500 g with severe depression of the Apgar score at 15 and 20 minutes had approximately a 90% chance of dying but this was considerably less in infants weighing more than 2500 g (see Table 34.1). Steiner & Nelligan (1975) have shown that infants who have not established regular breathing 30 minutes after return of the heartbeat, subsequently have a very poor outcome. They suggest that resuscitation under these circumstances should not be continued for longer than this time.

Table 34.1 Risk of death or cerebral palsy (CP) in infants with Apgar scores of 0–3 at varying times from birth (data from Nelson & Ellenberg 1981)

Age (min)	Death in first year <2500 g (%)	CP <2500 g (%)	Death in first year ≥2500 g (%)	CP ≥2500 g (%)
1	26	2	3	0.7
5	55	7	8	0.7
10	67	7	18	5
15	84	0	48	9
20	96	0	59	57

Handicap

Babies may be born apparently dead but if resuscitated rapidly may subsequently be neurologically normal (Steiner & Nelligan 1975, Scott 1976). Handicap probably depends on the duration of asphyxia and the development of cerebrovascular complications. There is probably a continuum of mild to severe handicap culminating in death in those most severely damaged. It is somewhat illogical therefore to consider outcome separately in terms of death and handicap and in the following section adverse outcome usually refers to either of these conditions.

Cardiotocography

Although cardiotocography (CTG) is commonly undertaken during the course of labour, there are few data on the long-term prediction of outcome. Painter et al (1978) followed up 38 full-term infants with 'ominous' fetal heart rate patterns. These infants showed moderate to severely variable patterns with or without late decelerations. Of the 38 infants, 5 were neurologically abnormal at one year of age; 4 in the group had patterns showing severe variability. Surprisingly few of these infants had depressed Apgar scores. A subsequent report stated that none of these children was abnormal in later childhood (Paneth & Stark 1983). Ingemarrson et al (1981) showed that fewer infants were born with depressed Apgar scores over three time periods following the introduction of CTG monitoring but in the high-risk full-term pregnancies there was no statistically significant reduction in neurological sequelae at 2 years although there was a trend towards improvement. This study was undertaken over a period of time when many changes were introduced in both obstetric and neonatal management and no firm conclusions on the prognostic value of abnormal CTGs can be made.

Acidosis

Cord blood lactate measurement, fetal blood sampling and arterial pH assessment at birth or shortly afterwards have been reported to provide diagnostic criteria for intrapartum asphyxia. Sykes et al (1982) have suggested that umbilical artery pH estimates are a reliable method for diagnosing asphyxia when acidosis exists. Low et al (1978) defined fetal acidosis as an umbilical artery buffer base below 34 mmol/l and these infants had on average a lower 1 and 5 minute Apgar score than a control, non-acidotic group. The authors could find no differences in neurological outcome between the acidotic and control group at 12 months of age. Another study, measuring umbilical artery pH in a group of infants of varying gestational ages, defined acidosis as a pH below 7.15. In this study there was also good correlation between fetal acidosis and depressed Apgar scores but only 2% of the acidotic infants were eventually found to have cerebral palsy and both these children had had depressed Apgar scores and major neurological abnormalities in the first week of life. Acidosis appears to be sensitive for predicting outcome but very poorly specific.

Apgar scores

Depression of the Apgar score has traditionally been widely used as a method for determining asphyxia and predicting outcome. The risk of handicap following depression of the Apgar score is best estimated from the data of Nelson & Ellenberg (1981) and is shown in Table 34.1. In full-term infants the risk only becomes significant if the Apgar score remains 0–3 at 20 minutes. Depression of the Apgar score to this degree at 15 minutes is associated with less than 10% risk of subsequent cerebral palsy in surviving infants. In another study, 93% of infants with severely depressed Apgar scores (0 at 1 minute and/or 0–3 at 5 minutes) were normal at follow-up (Thomson et al 1977). Levene et al (1986) identified a group of infants at risk of handicap following intrapartum asphyxia and assessed the sensitivity of various degrees of Apgar score depression (see Table 34.2). They found an Apgar score of 5 or less at 10 minutes to be the most sensitive predictor of outcome and also highly specific. Apgar scores do not reflect how long the infant suffered from intrapartum asphyxia and this is therefore, in most cases, a blunt instrument for predicting outcome.

Onset of spontaneous respiration

The time to establish spontaneous respiration is used by many as an index of the severity of asphyxia. Unfortunately, factors other than hypoxic–ischaemic insult may cause depression of respiration, such as the administration of maternal drugs and neuromuscular disease of the newborn. Steiner & Neligan (1975) reported that ill infants with no spontaneous respiration 30 minutes after birth or recovery from cardiac arrest, and who subsequently survived, developed quadriplegia. This has been confirmed by Koppe & Kleiverda (1984). In a Swedish study, 75% of infants who had not breathed spontaneously by 20 minutes after birth died or were severely handicapped (Ergander et

al 1983). Scott (1976), however, had previously reported a remarkably low risk of handicap in a group of infants who had shown no spontaneous respiration by 20 minutes from birth. In another study almost 70% of mature infants who had required IPPV for more than one minute were normal (Mulligan et al 1980). Fysh et al (1982) reported an infant who did not establish regular respiration for 25 minutes and who had an arterial pH of 6.6 at one hour. This infant was entirely normal at 3 years of age and it is interesting to note that she had neither convulsions nor other neurological abnormality in the newborn period, supporting the contention that the severity of clinical neurological abnormality is the more important predictor of adverse outcome.

Post-asphyxial encephalopathy

Moderate or severe encephalopathy following intrapartum asphyxia has been shown to be a more sensitive predictor of death or severe neurodevelopmental sequelae than depression of the Apgar scores (Levene et al 1986). Different studies have reported an outcome related to the severity of post-asphyxial encephalopathy (PAE) (Sarnat & Sarnat 1976, Finer et al 1981, Finer et al 1983, Low et al 1985, Robertson & Finer 1985, Amiel-Tison & Ellison 1986, Levene et al 1986) and these methods are discussed on p. 373. Although some vary slightly in their definition of the grades of encephalopathy there is remarkable consensus agreement when predicting adverse outcome. Results from five of these studies are shown in Table 34.3. No infant with mild PAE developed significant neurodevelopmental handicap. The one handicapped infant in the study of

Table 34.2 Sensitivity and specificity of six different grades of Apgar depression (Levene et al 1986)

Depression of Apgar score	n	Sensitivity (%)	Specificity (%)
≤3 at 1 min: >5 by 5 min	42	13	38
≤5 at 5 min: >5 by 10 min	35	17	67
≤3 at 5 min: >5 by 10 min	10	13	90
≤5 at 10 min: >5 by 20 min	15	43	95
≤3 at 10 min: >5 by 20 min	5	17	99
≤5 at 20 mins or more	3	13	100

Table 34.3 Proportion of handicapped children depending on their degree of postasphyxial encephalopathy (PAE). Only full-term infants are included

Authors	n	Mild (1)	Moderate (2)	Severe (3)	Duration of follow-up (years)
		Proportion severely abnormal or dead (%)			
Sarnat & Sarnat 1976	21	–	25	100	1
Finer et al 1981	89	0	15	92	3.5
Robertson & Finer 1985	200	0	27	100	3.5
Low et al 1985	42	–[a]	27	50	1
Levene et al 1986	122	1[b]	25	75	2.5 (median)

[a]Mild and moderate PAE considered together.
[b]Handicap due to congenital myopathy.

Levene et al (1986) had congenital myopathy. The incidence of severe handicap or death in the moderate encephalopathy group varied between 15 and 27%. Robertson & Finer (1985) found all infants with severe encephalopathy to have poor outcome but this was not the case in the majority of studies. Surprisingly, up to 25% of infants comatose due to asphyxia survived without significant handicap.

The duration of time that infants show clinical neurological abnormalities following asphyxia correlates well with the risk of handicap. Sarnat & Sarnat (1976) reported that a good outcome was seen in infants with moderate encephalopathy (lethargy, hypotonia and seizures) if abnormal clinical signs had disappeared within 5 days of life. In another study, only infants with neurological signs persisting for more than 6 weeks developed cerebral palsy (Scott 1976).

Lipper et al (1986) have devised a postasphyxial score (PAS) assigned within the first 24 hours based on 17 items; 6 of which are related to tone. The optimal (maximum) score was 39 and no infants with a score of 6 or less survived without severe handicap. The PAS correctly predicted abnormal outcome (sensitivity) at one year in 95% of infants and showed a specificity of 83%. Levene et al (1986) found moderate or severe encephalopathy to predict adverse outcome (handicap or death) in 96% with a specificity of 78%.

The type of abnormal neurological signs may also predict poor outcome. Brown et al (1974) recognize two clinical categories which are particularly associated with death or handicap. In the group with persistent hypotonia, only 16% were normal and in those in whom hypotonia evolved to extensor hypertonia, only 23% were normal. Among infants with a predominant extensor type of abnormality, 56% were normal on follow-up. Apathy in the newborn period had also been reported to occur more frequently in infants with abnormal outcome but no children were found to be severely handicapped in this group (De Souza & Richards 1978). Convulsions may to some extent predict outcome. Approximately half of the asphyxiated infants with neonatal seizures have some functional handicap (see Ch. 41).

It is clear that abnormal neurological behaviour occurring after birth in infants who have suffered intrapartum asphyxia is an excellent predictor of subsequent outcome.

Computerized tomography

This technique (CT) has proven to be a very good predictor of neurodevelopmental outcome. In full-term infants who showed extensive areas of hypodensity (see p. 130 for examples) on their scans, 13 of 17 had major neurodevelopmental sequelae and 11 of 15 with intracranial haemorrhage had a similarly poor outcome (Fitzhardinge et al 1981). Adsett et al (1985) performed CT scans on 43 full-term asphyxiated infants and described the appearances as either normal, areas of patchy or diffusely decreased density or global decrease in density. All 6 infants in the latter group died or were severely handicapped and 20 of 23 with diffuse decrease in density had a similar outcome. The infants were all scanned within the first 2 weeks of life and the sensitivity and specificity of abnormal scans (diffuse or global decrease in density) in the prediction of major handicap or subsequent death were 90% and 80% respectively. Lipper et al (1986) quantified the area of CT hypodensity by planimetry. All infants with a low density score (<0.72) had abnormal neurobehavioural outcomes with microcephaly at one year of age, and predicted outcome with a sensitivity of 91% and specificity of 60%.

Surprisingly in view of these reports, Finer et al (1983) found no correlation between abnormal CT scans and outcome but in this study the scans were performed within 7 days from birth and Lipp-Zwahlen et al (1985) have shown that early scans within the first week had no predictive value. Scans performed after this time correlated well with adverse outcome if they showed areas of low attenuation (hypodensity).

In summary, CT appears to be a particularly good predictor of subsequent outcome in asphyxiated full-term infants but only if the scan is done after the first week of life. This limits the value of this technique in the acute management of the severely asphyxiated infant in whom withdrawal of care is considered.

Electro-encephalography

These techniques are discussed fully in Chapter 13. The EEG abnormalities seen in mature asphyxiated infants and associated with a poor prognosis include iso-electric recordings and periodic patterns (Sarnat & Sarnat 1976, Holmes et al 1982) and persistent low voltage states (Holmes et al 1982). Holmes et al (1983) have shown that some infants with a burst suppression pattern can be stimulated to produce continuous activity and in these infants the prognosis is better. A normal EEG in asphyxiated infants is usually associated with an excellent prognosis (Rose & Lombroso 1970, Sarnat & Sarnat 1976, Watanabe et al 1980). Evoked response electro-encephalograms such as visual, auditory and somatosensory evoked potentials also provide some prognostic information in asphyxia (Hrbek et al 1977, Hecox & Cone 1981).

Intracranial pressure

Continuous measurement of ICP by a subarachnoid catheter gives some prognostic information (Levene et al 1987). No infant with a sustained rise in ICP of 15 mmHg or more lasting for an hour or more survived without major handicap. Infants with sustained elevations in ICP above

10 mmHg generally had a worse prognosis than those without a rise to this level but a cut-off of 10 mmHg was not as sensitive for handicap as a sustained elevation to 15 mmHg.

Interestingly, low cerebral perfusion pressure (CPP) did not predict outcome as well as intracranial hypertension (Levene et al 1987). This is probably because hypotension can cause low CPP without significant cerebral oedema. The hypotension reflects cardiovascular injury with good prognosis rather than cerebral compromise.

Doppler assessment

The measurement of PI (Pourcelot's resistance index; see p. 163) predicts outcome in asphyxiated full-term infants with an 86% accuracy (Archer et al 1986). A low PI (<0.55) predicted adverse outcome with sensitivity and specificity of 100% and 81% respectively. The advantage of this method is that the PI became abnormal within 62 hours of birth and at a median time of 28 hours. This is considerably earlier than any other prognostic method.

Practical guidelines

Resuscitative measures should be abandoned if an infant has no cardiac output for 10 minutes or fails to breathe spontaneously 30 minutes after establishing cardiac output. If there is any doubt, treatment should be continued and the infant brought to the neonatal intensive care unit. Progression of encephalopathy gives useful prognostic information. Infants who recover within 48 hours have an excellent prognosis and the parents should be very strongly reassured. Approximately half of infants with clinically overt seizures will have adverse outcome, this being much more likely in the presence of severe encephalopathy with coma. Early and regular assessment with Doppler may give particularly useful prognostic information in the first 48 hours of life and comatose infants with low PI have a very poor prognosis. If the infant survives into the second week of life, CT scans provide further very good prognostic information. With improvement in our techniques for accurately predicting outcome, important ethical issues must be faced concerning the withdrawal of care and this is discussed further in Chapter 48.

REFERENCES

Abramson N S et al 1983 Thiopental loading in cardiopulmonary resuscitation (CPR) survivors: a randomized collaborative clinical study. Anaesthesiology 51: A101
Adlard B P F, De Souza S W 1976 Influence of asphyxia and of dexamethasone on ATP concentrations in the immature rat brain. Biology of the Neonate 24: 82–88
Adsett D B, Fitz C R, Hill A 1985 Hypoxic–ischaemic cerebral injury in the term newborn: correlation of CT findings with neurological outcome. Developmental Medicine and Child Neurology 27: 155–160
Amiel-Tison C, Ellison P 1986 Birth asphyxia in the fullterm newborn: early assessment and outcome. Developmental Medicine and Child Neurology 28: 671–682
Archer L N J, Levene M I, Evans D H 1986 Cerebral artery doppler ultrasonogrpahy for prediction of outcome after perinatal asphyxia. Lancet ii: 1116–1118
Brann A W, Myers R E 1975 Central nervous system findings in the newborn monkey following severe in utero partial asphyxia. Neurology 25: 327
Brown J K, Purvis R J, Forfar J O, Cockburn F 1974 Neurological aspects of perinatal asphyxia. Developmental Medicine and Child Neurology 16: 567–580
Bruce D A 1984 Effects of hyperventilation on cerebral blood flow and metabolism. Clinical Perinatology 11: 673–680
Campbell A G M, Milligin J E, Talner N S 1968 The effect of pretreatment with pentobarbital, meperidine or hyperbaric oxygen on the response to anoxia and resuscitation in newborn rabbits. Journal of Pediatrics 72: 518–527
Chernick V, Craig R J 1982 Naloxone reverses neonatal depression caused by fetal asphyxia. Science 216: 1252–1253
Cockburn F, Daniel S S, Dawes G S, James L S, Myers R E, Niemann W 1969 The effect of pentobarbital anesthesia on resuscitation and brain damage in fetal rhesus monkeys asphyxiated on delivery. Journal of Pediatrics 75: 281–291
Cowan F 1986 Acute effects of indomethacin on cerebral blood flow velocities. Journal of Pediatrics 109: 341–344
De Souza S W, Dobbing J 1973 Cerebral oedema in developing brain. III. Brain water and electrolytes in immature asphyxiated rats treated with dexamethasone. Biology of the Neonate 22: 388–397
De Souza S W, Richards B 1978 Neurological sequelae in newborn babies after perinatal asphyxia. Archives of Disease in Childhood 53: 564–569
Diprose G K, Evans D H, Archer L N J, Levene M I 1986 Dinamap fails to detect hypotension in very low birthweight infants. Archives of Disease in Childhood 61: 771–773
Ergander U, Eriksson M, Zetterstrom R 1983 Severe neonatal asphyxia: incidence and prediction of outcome in the Stockholm area. Acta Paediatrica Scandinavica 72: 321–325
Evans D H, Levene M I, Archer L N J 1987 The effect of indomethacin on cerebral blood flow velocity in premature infants. Developmental Medicine and Child Neurology 29: 776–782
Eyre J A, Wilkinson A R 1986 Thiopentone-induced coma after severe birth asphyxia. Archives of Disease in Childhood 61: 1084–1089
Finer N N, Robertson C M, Richards R T, Pinnell L E, Peters K L 1981 Hypoxic–ischaemic encephalopathy in term neonates: perinatal factors and outcome. Journal of Pediatrics 98: 112–117
Finer N N, Robertson C M, Peters K L, Coward J H 1983 Factors affecting outcome in hypoxic–ischaemic encephalopathy in term infants. American Journal of Diseases of Children 137: 21–25
Fitzhardinge P M, Eisen E, Lejtonyi C, Metrakos K, Ramsay M 1974 Sequelae of early steroid administration to the newborn infant. Pediatrics 53: 877–883
Fitzhardinge P M, Flodmark O, Fitz C R, Ashby S 1981 The prognostic value of computed tomography as an adjunct to assessment of the term infant with postasphyxial encephalopathy. Journal of Pediatrics 99: 777–781
Flamm E S, Demopoulos H B, Seligman M L, Poser R G, Ransohoff J 1978 Free radicals in cerebral ischaemia. Stroke 9: 445–447
Fysh W J, Turner G M, Dunn P M 1982 Neurological normality after extreme birth asphyxia: case report. British Journal of Obstetrics and Gynaecology 89: 24–26
Gal P, Toback J, Erkan N V, Boer H R 1984 The influence of asphyxia on phenobarbital dosing requirements in neonates. Developmental Pharmacology and Therapeutics 7: 145–152
Gisvold S E, Steen P A 1985 Drug therapy in brain ischaemia. British Journal of Anaesthesia 57: 96–109
Goodlin R C 1981 Naloxone administration and newborn rabbit response to asphyxia. American Journal of Obstetrics and Gynecology 140: 340–341

Goodlin R C, Lloyd D 1970 Use of drugs to protect against fetal asphyxia. American Journal of Obstetrics and Gynecology 107: 227–231

Hallenbeck J M, Furlow T W 1979 Prostaglandin I2 and indomethacin prevent impairment of post-ischemic brain reperfusion in the dog. Stroke 10: 629–637

Hanson J, Anderson R, Sundt T 1975 Influence of cerebral vasoconstricting and vasodilating agents on blood flow in regions of cerebral ischemia. Stroke 6: 642–648

Hecox K E, Cone B 1981 Prognostic importance of brainstem auditory evoked responses after asphyxia. Neurology 31: 1429–1433

Holmes G, Rowe J, Hafford J, Schmidt R, Testa M, Zimmerman A 1982 Prognostic value of the electroencephalogram in neonatal asphyxia. Electroencephalography and Clinical Neurophysiology 53: 60–72

Holmes G L, Rowe J, Hafford J 1983 Significance of reactive burst suppression following asphyxia in full term infants. Clinical Electroencephalography 14: 138–141

Hrbek A, Karlberg P, Kjellmer I, Olsson T, Riha M 1977 Clinical application of evoked electroencephalographic responses in newborn infants. I Perinatal asphyxia. Developmental Medicine and Child Neurology 19: 34–44

Ingemarsson E, Ingemarsson I, Svenningsen N W 1981 Impact of routine fetal monitoring during labor on fetal outcome with long-term follow-up. American Journal of Obstetrics and Gynecology 141: 29–38

Koppe J G, Kleiverda G 1984 Severe asphyxia and outcome of survivors. Resuscitation 12: 193–206

Levene M I, Evans D H 1985 Medical management of raised intracranial pressure after severe birth asphyxia. Archives of Disease in Childhood 60: 12–16

Levene M I, Sands C, Grindulis H, Moore J R 1986 Comparison of two methods of predicting outcome in perinatal asphyxia. Lancet i: 67–91

Levene M I, Evans D H, Forde A, Archer L N J 1987 The value of intracranial pressure monitoring in asphyxiated newborn infants. Developmental Medicine and Child Neurology 29: 311–319

Lipper E G, Voorhies T M, Ross G, Vannucci R C, Auld P 1986 Early predictors of one-year outcome for infants asphyxiated at birth. Developmental Medicine and Child Neurology 28: 303–309

Lipp-Zwahlen A E, Deonna T, Chrzanowski R, Micheli J L, Calame A 1985 Temporal evolution of hypoxic–ischaemic brain lesions in asphyxiated full-term newborns assessed by computerized tomography. Neuroradiology 27: 138–144

Lou H C, Tweed W A, Davies J M 1985 Preferential blood flow increase to the brain stem in moderate neonatal hypoxia: reversal by naloxone. European Journal of Pediatrics 144: 225–227

Low J A, Galbraith R S, Muir D, Killen H, Karchmar J, Campbell D 1978 Intrapartum fetal asphyxia: a preliminary report in regard to long-term morbidity. American Journal of Obstetrics and Gynecology 130: 525–533

Low J A, Galbraith R S, Muir D W, Killen H L, Pater E A, Karchmar E J 1985 The relationship between perinatal hypoxia and newborn encephalopathy. American Journal of Obstetrics and Gynecology 152: 256–260

MacDonald H M, Mulligan J C, Allan A C, Taylor P M 1980 Neonatal asphyxia. I. Relationship of obstetric and neonatal complications to neonatal mortality in 38 405 consecutive deliveries. Journal of Pediatrics 96: 898–902

Marchal C, Costagliola P, Leveau Ph, Dulucq Ph, Steekler R, Bouquier F 1974 Traitement de la souffrance cerebrale neonatale d'origine anoxique par le mannitol. La Revue de Pediatrie 9: 581–589

Michenfelder J D 1974 The interdependancy of cerebral function and metabolic effects following massive doses of thiopental in the dog. Anesthesiology 41: 231–236

Miller J A 1961 Hypothermia in the treatment of asphyxia. New York State Journal of Medicine 61: 2954–2965

Mulligan J C, Painter M J, O'Donoghue P A, MacDonald H M, Allen A C, Taylor P M 1980 Neonatal asphyxia. II. Neonatal mortality and long-term sequelae. Journal of Pediatrics 96: 903–907

Myers R E, Wagner K R, Courten-Myers G M 1983 Brain metabolic and pathologic consequences of asphyxia. In: Milunsky A et al (eds) Advances in perinatal medicine, Vol 3. Plenum Medical Book Co, New York

Nelson K B, Ellenberg J H 1981 Apgar scores as predictors of chronic neurological disability. Pediatrics 68: 36–44

Painter M J, Depp R, O'Donogue P D 1978 Fetal heart rate patterns and development in the first year of life. American Journal of Obstetrics and Gynecology 132: 271–277

Paneth N, Stark R I 1983 Cerebral palsy and mental retardation in relation to indicators of perinatal asphyxia. American Journal of Obstetrics and Gynecology 147: 960–966

Persianinov L S, Rasstrigina N N, Dizny S N 1978 Controlled craniocerebral hypothermia in the complex treatment of posthypoxic states in newborns. Akusherstvo I Ginekologiia 9: 40–45

Pierce E C et al 1962 Cerebral circulation and metabolism during thiopental anesthesia and hyperventilation in man. Journal of Clinical Investigation 41: 1664–1671

Robertson C, Finer N 1985 Term infants with hypoxic–ischaemic encephalopathy: outcome at 3.5 years. Developmental Medicine and Child Neurology 27: 473–484

Rose A L, Lombroso C T 1970 A study of clinical, pathological and electroencephalographic features in 137 full-term babies with a long term follow up. Pediatrics 111: 133–141

Rothman S 1984 Synaptic release of excitatory amino acid neurotransmitter mediates anoxic neuronal death. Journal of Neuroscience 4:1884–1891

Sankaran K 1984 Hypoxic–ischemic encephalopathy: cerebrovascular carbon dioxide reactivity in neonates. American Journal of Perinatology 1: 114–117

Sarnat H B, Sarnat M S 1976 Neonatal encephalopathy following fetal distress. Archives of Neurology 33: 696–705

Scott H 1976 Outcome of very severe birth asphyxia. Archives of Disease in Childhood 51: 712–716

Simeone F A, Frazer G, Lawner P 1979 Ischemic brain oedema: comparative effects of barbiturates and hypothermia. Stroke 10: 8–12

Steen P A, Michenfelder J D 1980 Mechanisms of barbiturate protection. Anesthesiology 53: 183–190

Steiner H, Neligan G 1975 Perinatal cardiac arrest: quality of the survivors. Archives of Disease in Childhood 50: 696–702

Stewart A R, Finer N N, Peters K L 1981 Effects of alterations of inspiratory and expiratory pressures and inspiratory/expiratory ratios on a mean airway pressure, blood gases and intracranial pressure. Pediatrics 67: 474–481

Svenningsen N W, Blennow G, Lindroth M, Gaddlin P O, Ahlstrom H 1982 Brain-orientated intensive care treatment in severe neonatal asphyxia: effects of phenobarbitone protection. Archives of Disease in Childhood 57: 176–183

Sykes G S et al 1982 Do Apgar scores indicate asphyxia? Lancet i: 494–496

Thomson A J, Searle M, Russell G 1977 Quality of survival after severe birth asphyxia. Archives of Disease in Childhood 52: 620–626

Wardlow S L, Stark R I, Daniel S, Frantz A G 1981 Effects of hypoxia on B-endorphin and B-lipoprotein release in fetal, newborn and maternal sheep. Endocrinology 108: 1710–1715

Watanabe K, Miyazaki S, Hara K, Hakamada S 1980 Behavioural state cycles, background EEGs and prognosis of newborns with perinatal hypoxia. Electroencephalography and Clinical Neurophysiology 49: 618–625

Weichsel M E 1977 The therapeutic use of glucocorticoid hormones in the perinatal period: potential neurological hazards. Annals of Neurology 2: 364–366

Wolfson L I, Sakurada O, Sokoloff L 1977 Effects of gammabutyrolactone on local cerebral glucose utilization in the rat. Journal of Neurochemistry 29: 777–781

Yamaguchi M, Shirakata S, Yamasaki S, Matsumoto S 1976 Ischaemic brain edema and compression brain edema. Stroke 7: 77–83

Young R S K, Hessert T R, Pritchard G A, Yagel S K 1984 Naloxone exacerbates hypoxic–ischaemic brain injury in the neonatal rat. American Journal of Obstetrics and Gynecology 150: 52–56

35. Traumatic injuries to the nervous system

Dr D.I. Tudehope and Dr A. Vacca

Injuries may be sustained to the central nervous system in utero or during labour or delivery. This chapter is concerned with injuries sustained from mechanical factors during labour or delivery and excludes those injuries primarily caused by ischaemia. Frequently there is concurrence of hypoxic–ischaemic injury with birth trauma or occurring as a sequel to perinatal central nervous system trauma. Depending on the definition, the incidence of birth injury has been variably reported to be between 2 and 7/1000 live births. In a study of autopsies Valdes-Dapena & Arey (1970) found birth injury in 2% of infants and in 11% of those weighing over 2500 g. As a cause of neonatal mortality, birth injury ranks eighth in overall importance but in infants weighing over 2500 g it ranks fourth. The decreased incidence of birth trauma over recent years has been attributed to changing trends in obstetric management such as avoiding difficult vaginal delivery by caesarean section. Despite its falling incidence, birth injury is still a cause for concern to the obstetrician and neonatal paediatrician. Parents sometimes attribute birth injury to obstetric mismanagement and this may result in litigation. Unfortunately such events encourage the practice of defensive obstetrics and a high caesarean section rate may be a consequence of this. Illingworth (1985) believes it may be inappropriate to ascribe a child's so-called 'brain damage' solely to labour or delivery without considering other causative factors. 'Brain damage' can occur without difficult labour or perinatal hypoxia and despite caesarean section. It is simplistic to relate brain damage to single factors such as breech delivery or hypoxia at birth without considering the many interacting prenatal, perinatal and postnatal factors.

It is difficult to obtain reliable data on the incidence of neural injuries from hospital records but two American surveys deserve a mention. Incidence of major birth injury from data collected in 41 American States between 1973 and 1974 was 0.22/1000 livebirths (Department of Health, Education and Welfare, 1978) and Naeye (1977) analysing data from the US Collaborative Perinatal Project 1959–1966

reported that only 0.5% of total deaths could be directly attributed to birth injury.

RISK FACTORS FOR BIRTH INJURY

The effect of changing patterns of obstetric practice on birth-associated mechanical injuries is difficult to evaluate. However, a number of risk factors for birth injury have been identified (Table 35.1).

Table 35.1 Risk factors for birth injury

Fetal condition
  Prematurity
  Small for gestational age
  Multiple pregnancy
  Fetal distress

Malpresentation
  Breech presentation
  Brow, face, compound presentation

Malposition
  Occipito–posterior arrest
  Deep transverse arrest

Cephalo–pelvic disproportion
  Macrosomia, e.g. IDM, hydrops fetalis
  Macrocephaly
  Contracted pelvis
  Shoulder dystocia
  Severe moulding
  Unengaged head

Prolonged labour
  Delay — cervix fully dilated
  Delay — cervix not fully dilated

Precipitate labour

Maternal factors
  Nulliparity
  Short stature
  Obesity

Inexperienced accoucher

Instrumental delivery

Birth injury occurring with forceps or vacuum extraction is often ascribed to the method of delivery even though the association may be coincidental, not causal. Because risk of injury during birth is much greater when the fetus is already compromised, especially if instrumental assistance is required, all obstetric risk factors should be thoroughly evaluated before embarking on forceps or vacuum extraction.

O'Driscoll et al (1981) studied all cases of subdural haemorrhage found at autopsy in a large series of firstborn infants excluding breech presentation and noted that all of them were associated with forceps delivery. They concluded that serious injury to the forecoming head of a firstborn infant was a direct effect of forceps and that although no instrumental delivery was devoid of risk, the infant was more susceptible when rotation as well as traction was employed. Using computerized X-ray tomography (CT) to diagnose intracranial haemorrhage and examining asymptomatic as well as symptomatic babies, Brockerhoff et al (1981) were unable to establish a relationship between intracranial bleeding and method of delivery but they noted a significant correlation between abnormal neurological signs in the neonate and CT findings of intracranial haemorrhage.

Chiswick & James (1979) analysed the neonatal outcome in 86 Kielland's forcep deliveries and compared the findings with 86 babies born by spontaneous vertex vaginal delivery. They found that all measures of outcome were worse in the Kielland's group but when outcome of the surviving infant's was corrected for fetal asphyxia the only difference of significance was noted in the babies with abnormal neurological behaviour. All babies were normal by 7 days of age.

Following Chiswick & James' report a number of studies were published in support of the use of Kielland's forceps on the basis that neonatal outcome was no worse with these forceps than with other methods of dealing with malpositions of the occiput (Paintin & Vincent 1980, Healy et al 1982).

Most studies on the effect of vacuum extraction on the neonate do not reveal any long-term neonatal sequelae (Bjerre & Dahlin 1974, Carmody et al 1986) but Moolgaoker (1979) reported serious long-term neurological complications in a group of babies where vacuum extraction was attempted before the cervix was fully dilated.

Breech delivery

Perinatal morbidity and mortality are higher in babies presenting by the breech compared with cephalic presentations. Hypoxia due to cord compression or prolapse, asphyxia due to delay in delivery especially of the head, and mechanical trauma associated with manipulations during delivery have been identified as the main causes for the increased morbidity and mortality. Injury to the nervous system may occur when difficulty is encountered with the delivery of the head and excessive traction and rotation forces are required to complete the delivery.

For these reasons there is a tendency to deliver the breech baby by caesarean section but such a trend must be balanced by the increased maternal morbidity in the short- and long-term and by the small but definite increase in maternal mortality associated with caesarean section compared with vaginal delivery. Because premature infants are more prone to trauma and hypoxia, many obstetricians advocate caesarean section as the method of choice for delivery of the pre-term breech. As a consequence, more classical caesarean sections are being performed because the lower segment of the uterus may not be adequately formed to allow delivery of the pre-term infant. For the mature breech, most obstetricians practise selective vaginal delivery, a policy based on the premise that adequate antenatal and intrapartum evaluation will distinguish those patients suitable for vaginal delivery from those best delivered by caesarean section. A major objective of antenatal care is the diagnosis of all breech presentations of at least 34 weeks of gestation. Should the breech presentation persist, size of the fetus in relation to the maternal pelvis can be estimated by clinical and radiological means and the biparietal diameter can be measured by ultrasonography. Fetal anomalies may be detected by fetal X-ray and ultrasound scanning. The decision about the method of delivery should be made by the patient's obstetrician after discussing with her the findings and the anticipated outcome. The decision should be clearly stated in the patient's records so that all obstetric attendants are in no doubt of the procedure to follow. The mother should be advised to enter hospital early, as soon as the membranes rupture or at the onset of contractions.

Most obstetricians prefer spontaneous onset of labour but early artificial rupture of the membranes is not necessarily contra-indicated, provided the breech is well applied to the lower uterine segment (Jaffa et al 1981). Vaginal examination should be performed as soon as the membranes rupture to exclude prolapse of the umbilical cord and to apply an electrode for continuous fetal heart monitoring. Progress in labour is assessed by regular vaginal examinations to assess the dilatation of the cervix. Use of oxytocin to augment labour is controversial and some obstetricians regard delay in labour as an indication of feto–pelvic disproportion, preferring to deliver the baby by caesarean section. Lumbar epidural analgesia has many advantages in the management of breech delivery once labour is established.

Breech delivery is usually conducted with the mother in the lithotomy position with a wedge under one buttock. The delivery should be conducted by an obstetrician experienced in breech delivery. If epidural analgesia has not been used, facilities for general anaesthesia should be available with an anaesthctist standing by.

A paediatrician skilled in resuscitation of the newborn should be present. The aim should be for assisted spontaneous breech delivery, employing a wide episiotomy especially in primigravid patients and using forceps to the aftercoming head (Milner 1975).

SKULL FRACTURE

Because the fetal skull is poorly ossified and readily malleable, considerable distortion may occur without injury to the skull itself. Skull fractures may occur in utero, during labour or during forceps delivery.

Linear fractures are usually frontal or parietal and heal spontaneously without specific treatment. The incidence of linear skull fractures underlying cephalhaematomata has varied from 5 to 25% in reported series (Axton et al 1966).

Depressed skull fractures are generally caused by compression of the fetal head against the maternal pelvis or by forceps delivery (Fig. 35.1). Many skull depressions represent buckling of the inner table of the skull without a break in the continuity of the bone. When a depressed skull

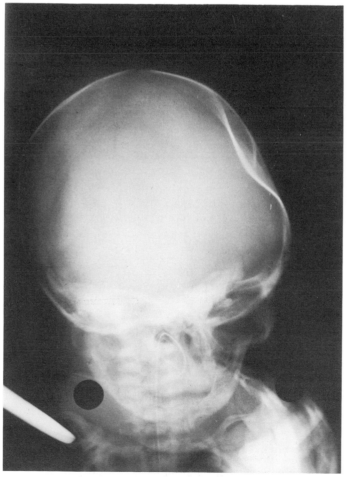

Fig. 35.1 Skull radiograph demonstrating depressed fracture with periosteal elevation of the left parietal bone.

fracture is seen, a cranial ultrasound or CT scan should be performed to diagnose any underlying cerebral contusion or subdural haematoma. Uncomplicated fractures may slowly elevate spontaneously but rarely a breast pump or vacuum extractor may be used to correct the depression. Surgical elevation is recommended if there are bone fragments in the cerebrum, neurological deficit, signs of raised intracranial pressure or failure of spontaneous elevation. Parents are often distressed by the dented appearance of their infant's head, and the cosmetic appearance alone usually warrants surgical attention. Most cases of depressed fractured skull should therefore be elevated.

Because the fracture soon becomes 'sticky', elevation should be performed in the first week of life, as soon as the child is fit for general anaesthesia and when the immediate effects of any birth asphyxia have settled. With early operation it is nearly always possible to elevate the fracture through the anterior fontanelle. This is accessed through a short incision, and using a blunt instrument passed extradurally, the depressed area is 'popped' at its base back into alignment with the surrounding calvarium. If operation is delayed more than about 10 days then a formal craniotomy may be required. Neurosurgical referral at birth is therefore indicated. It is important that the family appreciate that any subsequent neurological or developmental deficits are nearly always the sequel of the concomitant cerebral injury, either traumatic or hypoxic, rather than the result of the fracture per se. Exceptionally the depression may be of such severe degree to be associated with laceration of the dura. In this case, early surgical exploration and repair are crucial to avoid a leptomeningeal cyst and growing skull fracture. For all these reasons, the decision to elevate the skull fracture should be made by the neurosurgeon in consultation with the neonatal paediatrician.

TRAUMATIC INTRACRANIAL HAEMORRHAGE

Intracranial haemorrhage is a well-recognized complication occurring in the perinatal period and may be associated with birth injury. The major varieties of intracranial haemorrhage associated with trauma include extradural, subdural (acute, subacute and chronic), subarachnoid, intraventricular, intracerebral and intracerebellar haemorrhage. These conditions are discussed in detail in Section 8 and will be described briefly here where relevant to birth trauma. Haemorrhage due to trauma may be associated with evidence of other injury such as cephalhaematoma, subgaleal haemorrhage, subconjunctival haemorrhage, retinal haemorrhage, fractured skull or palsies of the brachial plexus or facial nerve.

Extradural haemorrhage

Haemorrhage between the periosteum and the inner surface of skull bone is referred to as extradural haemorrhage and is the intracranial analogue of a cephalhaematoma. This type of bleeding is rare in the newborn since difficult vaginal delivery has been replaced by caesarean section. Takagi et al (1978) in a study of autopsies of 134 babies with intracranial haemorrhage reported that in only 2 of them was the haemorrhage extradural.

The haemorrhage most commonly results from a tear of the middle meningeal artery or major venous sinuses following skull fracture of the temporal bone, most usually associated with forceps delivery. A falling haemoglobin, signs of raised intracranial pressure and asymmetrical or focal neurological signs develop rapidly. Such a clinical course should alert the clinician to the possibility of extradural haemorrhage and the diagnosis can be confirmed by CT scan. Treatment involves formal craniotomy, evacuation of the haematoma, and stopping the source of the bleeding. It is vital that the neurosurgeon and the anaesthetist fully appreciate that the volume of blood that has been lost into the extradural space is enough to deplete the baby's blood volume and that blood transfusion must precede induction of anaesthesia and craniotomy. Failure to recognize this factor and that the hypertensive cardiovascular response to raised intracranial pressure is in effect supporting the baby's blood pressure will lead to serious, possibly fatal, haemodynamic consequences and cardiac dysrrhythmias on elevation of the bone flap. Very occasionally, the presentation may be delayed for days or even weeks, in which case the child may have a dangerous combination of severe anaemia and chronically elevated intracranial pressure.

Subdural haematoma

Subdural haematomas are now uncommon in full-term infants as a result of the avoidance of difficult vaginal births with caesarean section. On the other hand the relative proportion of pre-term infants with subdural haemorrhage has increased over recent years.

The three basic origins of subdural haemorrhages are:

1. Tentorial laceration with rupture of straight sinus resulting in infratentorial haematoma.
2. Falx cerebri laceration and rupture of inferior sagittal sinus giving rise to a haematoma of the longitudinal cerebral fissure.
3. Rupture of superficial cerebral veins with subdural haematoma over the temporal lobe which is usually unilateral and accompanied by subarachnoid blood.

Predisposing factors are believed to be related to excess moulding of the fetal head and include:

Rigid birth canal — nullipara, small pelvis
Labour — precipitous, prolonged
Cephalo–pelvic disproportion
Delivery — instrumental delivery associated with malposition
Presentation — breech, footling, face, brow.

Occipital diastasis was described in five infants who presented by the breech and who died with evidence of significant intracranial birth trauma. There is separation of the squamous and lateral portion of the occipital bones with resultant laceration of the dura, occipital sinus and/or cerebellum. (Wigglesworth & Husemeyer 1977).

Clinical features include:

1. Subdural haematomas over the temporal cerebral convexities may be asymptomatic or present with seizures on days 2 and 3 with or without focal neurological signs. A chronic subdural effusion may develop over several months with or without associated hydrocephalus.
2. Infants with subdural haematomas due to tentorial laceration or laceration of the falx cerebri usually have compression of brainstem and midbrain. Abnormal neurological signs include coma, asymmetrical pupil size, bradycardia, seizures and opisthotonus.
3. Posterior cranial fossa subdural haematoma although uncommon is associated with signs resembling those of intracerebellar haemorrhage.

A full-term infant usually delivered by forceps or breech extraction is initially well but develops lethargy and irritability within the first few days of life. This is accompanied by respiratory difficulties, a tense fontanelle, anaemia, bloody cerebrospinal fluid (CSF) and an increasing head size. Sometimes there are associated ophthalmic signs of nystagmus, skew eye deviation and sixth or seventh nerve palsy.

The diagnosis is made by ultrasound or CT scanning which will define the location and extent of subdural haematoma (Fig. 35.2), and distinguish a posterior cranial fossa haematoma from an intracerebellar haemorrhage.

Prognosis depends on the site of the haemorrhage; convexity subdural haematomata may be successfully drained by subdural taps with good prognosis in 50–80% of survivors (Schipke et al 1954). Diagnostic subdural taps can only be justified if an ultrasound or CT scan is unavailable or if there is rapid clinical deterioration. Infants who survive tentorial or falx cerebri lacerations usually have hydrocephalus and severe functional handicap (Fenichel et al 1984).

Subarachnoid haemorrhage

This is the most common type of intracranial haemorrhage seen in neonates and is described in detail in Chapter 27. It is not usually associated with birth trauma but more commonly with hypoxia and metabolic compromise.

Intracerebellar haemorrhage

Intracerebellar haemorrhage is described in detail on p. 306. It is seen in both full-term and premature infants and may be due to traumatic laceration of the cerebellum.

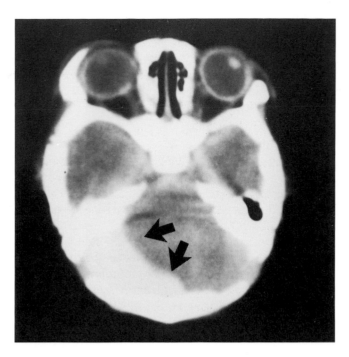

Fig. 35.2 CT scan through the posterior fossa showing right subdural haematoma (arrowed) extending along the tentorium cerebelli.

In infants with birth weight below 1500 g, intracerebellar haemorrhage has been attributed to mechanical deformation of the infant's occiput by a tight-fitting Velcro band used to attach a face-mask for positive-pressure breathing (Pape et al 1976).

In full-term infants the clinical findings of posterior cranial fossa haematoma include difficult labour and delivery, sudden onset of apnoea during the first 24 hours of life, tense bulging fontanelle, falling haematocrit, bloody CSF and cerebral obtundation. The diagnosis is confirmed by CT scan (Rom et al 1978, Fishman et al 1981). In a review of the literature on intracerebellar haematoma, Fishman et al (1981) described 21 cases and reported that 17 of 20 infants treated by surgical evacuation of the haematoma had survived. Thirteen of these infants had a favourable long-term outcome. They also described 4 patients in whom a conservative approach was undertaken and they advocate this as an alternative method of treatment of subdural haematoma. Even managed conservatively, hydrocephalus may still result and necessitate treatment by insertion of a ventriculo–peritoneal shunt.

Intracerebral haemorrhage

This is due to a wide variety of causes as discussed in Section 8. When intracerebral haemorrhage is related to birth trauma there is usually evidence of extracranial injury such as cephalhaematoma, depressed fracture of the skull or subgaleal haematoma. Focal temporal lobe haematomas, almost invariably associated with forceps delivery, may produce signs of progressive intracranial hypertension with focal or generalized seizures and anaemia. Evacuation at formal craniotomy is indicated. Epilepsy, hemiparesis and intellectual handicap are frequent sequelae.

Cerebral contusion refers to a focal region of necrosis and haemorrhage involving the cerebral cortex and subcortical white matter. This lesion is rare because of the low incidence of focal blunt trauma and because the resilience of the neonatal cranium and cerebral mantle has a protective influence on the underlying structures.

Intracranial haemorrhage in utero

Maternal trauma is a well-documented cause of subdural and intraventricular haemorrhage in the fetus occurring before the onset of labour (Crosby 1974). In most reported cases the maternal trauma was severe and caused by automobile accidents, falls or assaults. The fetal intracranial haemorrhage was accompanied by other maternal and fetal injuries. Severe fetal head injuries without maternal uterine rupture have been reported and in a few cases these have followed relatively minor maternal trauma (Poulson & Grabert 1973). Nevertheless fetal subdural haemorrhage without skull fracture or other severe fetal or maternal injury is a very uncommon outcome of non-penetrating blunt maternal trauma as the fetus in utero is well protected by maternal structures and amniotic fluid.

The term 'battered fetus' was first coined by Pugh (1978) who described direct assault on the mother by boot or fist. The fetal intracranial vessels are susceptible to shearing and decelerative forces and fetal intracranial haemorrhage may result from domestic violence, such as shaking, pushing or throwing rather than direct assault. (see also Ch. 30.)

SPINAL CORD INJURY

Although intrapartum injuries to the fetal spinal cord were described in the nineteenth century, the mechanisms of such injuries were not understood until the classic papers of Crothers (1923) and Ford (1925), and Crothers & Putnam (1927). This type of injury was relatively common several decades ago but has become progressively less frequent with improved obstetric practice. Trauma to the cervical cord is a known hazard of breech delivery (80% of cases) but can also occur during cephalic delivery. It particularly occurs in the 'flying fetus' or 'star-gazing fetus' or 'fetus opisthotonus'. The injury may be due to longitudinal stretching of cervical spinal cord in a breech delivery, hyperextension of the head in a breech delivery or transverse presentation or cord traction via the brachial plexus in shoulder dystocia. The presumed mechanism in cephalic deliveries is due to torsional forces in rotation of the head. The apparent rarity of this lesion may reflect the fact that few infants with major spinal cord damage survive the neonatal period and in those who survive with mild injury the lesion may be confused by the attendant spastic quadriplegia.

Towbin (1969) concluded that spinal cord injury was a causal factor in 10% of neonatal deaths. Some infants with spinal cord injury undoubtedly are stillborn. Spinal cord injuries are surprisingly rarely associated with injuries to the vertebral column and its joints. Reid (1983) demonstrated some degree of trauma to the cervical spine in 12% of autopsies but of a lesser degree than was described 20 years previously.

Clinical features

Spinal cord injuries in the neonate may present in different ways (Volpe 1981). The most common involves high cervical cord and brainstem and severe neonatal respiratory failure may manifest from birth or in the first few days of life, necessitating respiratory support. The newborn may exhibit weakness, hypotonia and poverty of movement and later on develop spasticity which is mistakenly labelled as cerebral palsy. The more common, lower cervical cord injuries are characterized by motor, sensory and sphincter involvement. Motor involvement consists of weakness, hypotonia and areflexia in lower limbs and sometimes upper limbs. Intercostal muscles and perhaps diaphragmatic involvement will result in respiratory embarrassment and a 'bell-shaped' chest deformity. The sensory level will usually be at upper trunk or lower neck. Anal sphincter will be atonic and patulous and bladder distension will need to be relieved by suprapubic compression. A Horner's syndrome may develop (Fig. 35.3).

Pathology

The common levels of involvement are mid- or lower cervical and upper thoracic spines. Lesions seen include spinal cord transection in haematomyelia and spinal epidural haemorrhage. These acute lesions are followed by chronic changes with adhesions between dura, meninges and cord and cystic cavities in the cord (Fig. 35.4). At times, damage to the vertebral arteries is demonstrated with haemorrhage into the various coats of the arteries causing narrowing of the lumen and thrombosis, with resultant spinal cord infarction.

Differential diagnosis

This includes myelodysplasia, infantile muscular atrophy, myelitis, neoplasia and infantile botulism. The vertebral elements of the spine can stretch up to 5 cm without body disruption compared with only 6–8 mm for the spinal cord (Towbin 1964). Consequently, if a dislocation or fracture of cervical spine is demonstrated on X-ray it is likely that there is a severe transection of the cervical spinal cord.

Investigations

Myelograms and CT scans of the cervical spinal cord should delineate pathology such as haematomyelia or extradural haematomata (Fig. 35.5). Somatosensory evoked potentials are helpful in determining the level of the spinal injury (see p. 214).

Management

Prevention of such lesions involves appropriate management of breech presentations and dysfunctional labour, avoidance of fetal depression and caesarean section for hyperextension of fetal head with breech presentation.

Once remedial surgical lesions have been excluded, treatment will predominantly be supportive and may involve neurosurgical consultation and spinal immobilization. There are currently no data to support laminectomy and decompression. Because of occasional spontaneous recovery, conservative management with supportive therapy

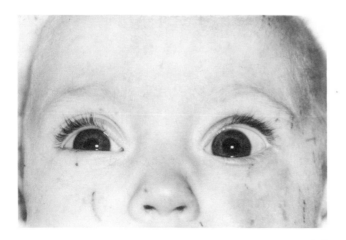

Fig. 35.3 Horner's syndrome. Note the ptosis and pupillary constriction on the right side.

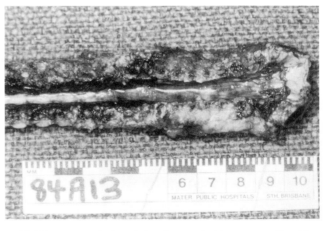

Fig. 35.4 Dissected spinal cord showing cervical haematomyelia with fibrosis.

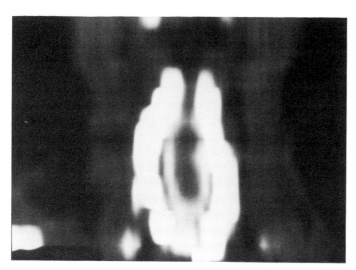

Fig. 35.5 Reconstructed CT scan in longitudinal plane showing haematomyelia in the region of the cervical cord.

(ventilation, prevention of infection and contractures and bladder expression) is recommended. However, this form of therapy can result in difficult ethical and moral decisions.

Prognosis

Survival is dependent on the level of the lesion, with a cervical lesion being almost incompatible with life. The quality of survival for those with lesions of C8–T1 and below depends on the child's multiple medical complications. Of 14 children followed up from 2 to 12 years, 8 died (Koch & Eng 1979).

PERIPHERAL NERVE INJURIES

Nerve injuries in the newborn infant may be due to stretching, compression, twisting, hyperextension or separation of the nervous tissue. The nerve injuries may be classified pathologically as:

Neuropraxis — swelling of nerve
Axonotmesis — complete peripheral
   degeneration with total recovery
Neurotmesis — complete division of
   all structures.

Electromyography and nerve conduction studies can distinguish a neuropraxis from a neurotmesis.

The following nerve injuries occur in the newborn:

FACIAL NERVE PALSY

Theoretically, facial nerve palsy may be due to either an upper or lower motor neurone lesion. In practice, the clinical distinction between these two is extremely difficult.

The lower motor neurone lesion is the most common injury and is usually due to oblique application of forcep blades or prolonged pressure on the maternal sacral promontory in spontaneous deliveries. Rarely, it may result as a postural deformity along with mandibular hypoplasia from the persistent position of the fetal foot against the superior ramus of the mandible. Palsy due to upper motor neurone injury is extremely rare.

Clinical features

The lesion is recognized clinically by inability to close the eye and lack of lower-lip depression on crying on the affected side (Fig. 35.6). These signs must be distinguished from 'asymmetrical crying facies' due to absence of the depressor anguli oris muscle. In this condition, eye closure is normal but there is failure of the mouth to move downward and outward on the affected side when the infant cries (Fig. 35.7). Asymmetry usually remains into adult life but becomes less obvious with time. It is commonly seen in other members of the family.

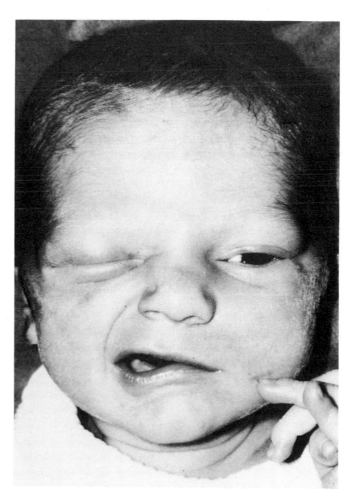

Fig. 35.6 Facial nerve palsy on the left side. When the infant cries he is unable to close the left eye or open the mouth normally on the affected side.

Incidence

The incidence of facial nerve palsy has been variably reported as 1.3/1000 Rubin (1964), 2.5/1000 McHugh et al (1969) and 7.5/1000 livebirths Levine et al (1984). Minor degrees of facial paresis present on the second day of life have been described in 6.4% of all births with the incidence being the same in forceps as manual deliveries (Hepner 1951). The uniformly good prognosis for these infants suggested haemorrhage or oedema into the nerve sheath by intra-uterine pressure on the facial nerve by the sacral promontory. Approximately 75% of cases involve the left face reflecting the relative frequencies of intra-uterine positions.

Management

If the eye cannot be closed, patching and 1% methylcellulose (artificial tears) eye drops should be used to prevent corneal damage. There are no controlled data to indicate the value of massage, electrical stimulation or surgical intervention.

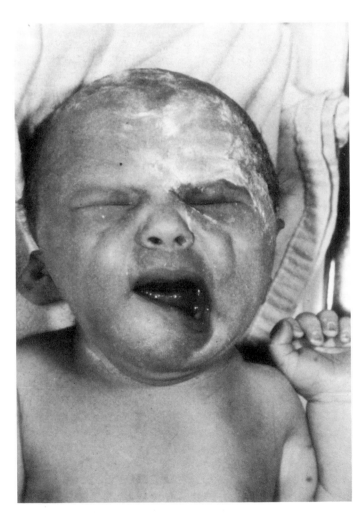

Fig. 35.7 Asymmetrical crying facies on the right side. Compare this with facial palsy.

The prognosis is good, with the majority recovering completely within 1–3 weeks and only rarely do cases have a detectable deficit after 3 months. In the rare cases of severe degeneration of the nerve, regeneration occurs at the rate of approximately 2.5 cm a month. In a recent study neither clinical examination nor electrical or radiological investigations were able to predict pre-operatively, the congenital or traumatic aetiology in 9 cases of neonatal facial paralysis (Narcy et al 1982). In cases of non-regressive facial paralysis in a neonate and when doubt persists after radiological and electrical examinations, the intraparotid portion of facial nerve may be explored in the stylomastoid region. Its absence suggests agenesis of the nerve.

BRACHIAL PLEXUS PALSIES

Injuries to the brachial plexus may be due to excessive lateral flexion, rotation or traction upon the neck. Such trauma may be seen with normal delivery, with impacted shoulders or during delivery of the aftercoming head of a breech. Right-sided palsies are more common than left and bilateral lesions occur in only 10% of cases. Frequently the clavicle is fractured. The injuries are divided into three types:

1. Erb–Duchenne palsy (80% of brachial plexus palsies). This palsy involves the upper brachial plexus (C5, C6) and results in denervation of the deltoid, supraspinatus, biceps and brachioradialis resulting in the classical 'waiters tip' position (Fig. 35.8).
2. Klumpke's paralysis (2.5% of brachial plexus palsies). This palsy involves the lower brachial plexus (C8, T1) and results in denervation of the intrinsic muscles of the hand, flexors of the wrist and fingers and sympathetics, with a 'claw hand' posture. The infant holds his arm loosely at the side of his thorax. The Moro reflex is absent on the affected side.
3. Erb–Duchenne–Klumpke paralysis (7.5% of brachial plexus palsies). This total brachial plexus palsy (C5–T1) involves all nerve fibres and there is complete paralysis of the arm with flaccidity and sensory, trophic and circulatory changes. Paralysis of the diaphragm may be expected in those injuries involving C4 nerve root. When paralysis is bilateral, spinal injury should be suspected. Horner's syndrome occurs in about one-third of patients (Fig. 35.3).

Improvements in obstetric care have reduced the incidence of brachial plexus injury from 1.56 to 0.38/1000 livebirths during the twentieth century but there has not been a significant change in the last decade (Greenvald et al 1984), except for a marked decrease in the severity of palsies. Although the vast majority of cases can be distinguished straight after birth, in one study of 36 babies, 5 were not diagnosed until some weeks after birth (Rossi et al 1982).

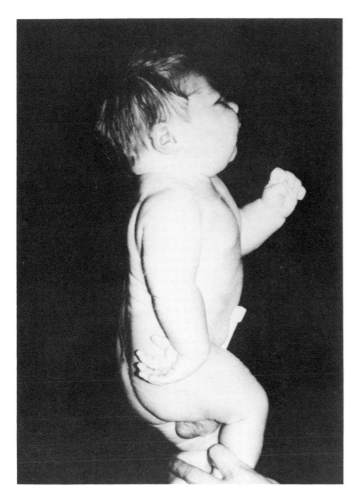

Fig. 35.8 Erb's palsy. The infant's right arm is adducted and internally rotated with the elbow extended and pronated. The wrist and fingers are flexed.

Management and prognosis

The most important measure of treatment is to prevent further stretching on the plexus and subsequent contractures by the use of elbow and shoulder splints. Later on, physiotherapy and mobilization of the joints are practised. There was no correlation between treatment and eventual outcome with physiotherapy in 32 patients and electrotherapy in 5. Nine of 12 infants with complete brachial plexus palsy had persisting nerve palsy at 3 years of age compared with 15% who had lower brachial plexus palsies (Rossi et al 1982). Varying long-term results have been reported. In the Collaborative Perinatal Study, 88% were normal by 4 months of age, 92% by 12 months and 93% by 4 years (Gordon et al 1973). Czurda & Meznik (1977) reported that all patients who made a complete or almost complete recovery did so within 6 weeks of birth. A New Zealand study reported only 80% making a complete recovery by 12 months of age but none of the infants with residual defects having severe sensory or motor deficit of the hand (Hardy 1981).

Clearly, for the majority of infants the current conservative management yields good results. Efforts must now be directed towards improving the 7–15% of patients who do badly. A recommended treatment includes monthly evaluation to document functional return, supervision of the child's exercise programme, and parental support. Babies who do not improve rapidly within 2 to 3 months should have electromyogram and nerve conduction studies (Brown 1984).

Denervation at birth has been demonstrated to impair normal development of muscle contractile properties of the flexor carpi ulnaris muscle. Presently the role of microsurgical reconstruction of these injuries is undergoing evaluation. Treatments attempted include tendon transfers to rotation cuff (Hoffer 1978) and reconstruction of part of the torn brachial plexus with free nerve grafts. Full nerve graft treatment performed in 3 patients at 3 months of age gave excellent functional results when infants were assessed at 28 months of age (Solomon et al 1981).

RADIAL NERVE INJURY

Very occasionally radial nerve paralysis may result from fracture of the humerus, as with difficulty in delivering the arm during breech delivery. It has also been described in association with traumatic fat necrosis over the lateral aspect of the upper arm, presumably secondary to uterine compression. The lesion presents with wrist drop with preservation of grasp reflex and intrinsic hand muscles. All reported cases have recovered within a few weeks or months of life (Feldman 1957).

MEDIAN NERVE PALSY

Diminished grasp has been attributed to median nerve palsy following radial artery puncture in the newborn infant (Pape et al 1978).

SCIATIC NERVE INJURY

All reported cases of sciatic nerve injury have been postnatal and iatrogenic in nature. Infants exhibit limitation of hip abduction and all movements at distal joints. Misplacement of the needle tip during intramuscular injection into the buttock region carries with it the risk of injuring the sciatic nerve and may prove permanent (Gilles & Matson 1970). Injections of hypertonic solutions and drugs into the umbilical artery have caused an ischaemic sciatic neuropathy, presumably attributed to spasm or occlusion of the inferior gluteal artery (San Augustin et al 1962).

LUMBOSACRAL PLEXUS INJURY

Injuries to the lumbar (L2–L4) and sacral (L4–S3) nerve roots may occur with excessive traction in a frank breech delivery. This is extremely rare and occurred in only 3 of Eng's series of 128 neonatal peripheral palsies (Eng 1975). The lesion is distinguished from sciatic nerve palsy and spinal dysraphism by the total paralysis of the lower extremity.

DIAPHRAGMATIC PARALYSIS

Phrenic nerve palsy

This is due to an injury to cervical nerve roots (C3, C4 and C5) supplying the phrenic nerve. In 80–90% of cases it is associated with a complete brachial plexus palsy. Approximately 5% of cases of brachial plexus palsy are associated with diaphragmatic paralysis. Haemorrhage and oedema associated with tearing of the nerve sheath to the predominant nerve root C4 is the usual pathology with complete avulsion confined to the most severe cases. As the newborn infant breathes predominantly with the diaphragm, rather than intercostal muscles, there is often severe respiratory distress, especially when the lesion is bilateral. The more usual unilateral palsy is most common on the right and is confirmed by fluoroscopic demonstration of paradoxical diaphragmatic movement.

The clinical picture is one of early onset respiratory distress suggestive of hypoventilation, often followed by stabilization or clinical improvement. Schifrin (1952) reported 4 infants where diagnosis was not made until 6 weeks of age. Mortality has been reported to be 10–20%, with 50% showing complete recovery in 2–3 months but clinical recovery occurs in the majority even though considerable weakness can still be demonstrated by X-ray (Greene et al 1975). The clinical diagnosis is confirmed by chest X-ray which shows an elevated hemidiaphragm and fluoroscopy screening shows an immobile diaphragm. Management may be divided into non-surgical modalities such as 'rocker bed', electrical pacing, continuous positive airway pressure and intermittent positive-pressure ventilation and surgical plication (Volpe 1981). These are expectant modalities of treatment and are designed to temporize until natural improvement in the neural injury occurs. Green et al (1975) recommended that the infant with diaphragmatic paralysis who requires intermittent positive-pressure ventilation should receive a trial of no longer than 2 weeks and if support is still required plication of the affected diaphragm is recommended.

VOCAL CORD PARALYSIS

This is a rare injury associated with birth.

Unilateral vocal cord paralysis is more frequent and due to stretching of one of the recurrent laryngeal nerves. Left-sided palsies predominate because the recurrent laryngeal nerve arises lower in the neck, has a longer course and loops around the aorta. It usually presents with hoarseness and inspiratory stridor with crying, and is confirmed by laryngoscopy. Treatment is both symptomatic and expectant. With severe lesions gavage feeding and tracheostomy may be necessary.

Bilateral vocal cord paralysis is associated with extremely traumatic deliveries, severe perinatal asphyxia and resultant cerebral palsy. Initially intubation is required and after a period of time tracheostomy may be necessary. Only 29% of congenital vocal cord palsies recover spontaneously (Emery & Fearon 1984).

SYRINGOMYELIA

The cause of the majority of cases of communicating syringomyelia is unknown. Williams (1977) after analysing the results of a questionnaire to the mothers of syringomyelia patients found there was a high incidence of difficult labour usually in nulliparae and forceps deliveries in the births of affected infants. This suggested that birth trauma is a cause of tonsillar descent through the foramen magnum and with the subsequent development of arachnoiditis. Once the tonsils become entrapped in the foramen magnum, the difference between cranial and spinal pressure may, over the course of several years cause further tonsillar descent, thus leading to a communicating syringomyelia. (See also p. 270.)

EYE INJURIES

Retinal haemorrhages represent the most common ophthalmological birth injury. Although incidence figures for retinal haemorrhage vary from 3 to 50% it has been estimated that 3% of newborn infants have retinal haemorrhages at 12 hours of age but that the majority have resolved by 48 hours (Besio et al 1979). These haemorrhages are flame-shaped and radiate from the disc. An ophthalmic review of 234 newborn infants revealed that the retinal haemorrhage in 71 (30.3%) was related to mode of delivery; occurring in 38% of spontaneous vaginal, 25% of forceps deliveries and 3% of caesarean section births.

Retinal haemorrhages are reported to occur more frequently in babies delivered by vacuum extraction than in those delivered by forceps (Egge et al 1981). The cause and significance of retinal haemorrhages in the newborn are unknown although Pajor et al (1964) suggested that amblyopia is a potential association with these haemorrhages due to granular macular changes.

Other reported eye injuries include eversion of the upper lids secondary to face presentation (Rainin 1976), anterior chamber haemorrhage and rupture of Descemet's membrane from misapplication of forceps blades (Pohjanpelto et al 1979) which can give rise to a condition that mimics congenital glaucoma (Kwitko 1969). Angell et al (1981) described eye injuries in 7 patients who had forceps-assisted

delivery with damage to the cornea involving rupture of Descemet's membrane and found that astigmatism was invariably present on the side involved.

REFERENCES

Angell L K, Robb R M, Beison F G 1981 Visual prognosis in patients with ruptures in Descemet's Membrane due to forceps injuries. Archives of Ophthalmology 99: 2137–2139

Axton J H M 1966 Depressions of the skull in the newborn. Nursing Mirror 4: 123

Besio R, Gaballeco G, Meerhoff E 1979 Neonatal retinal hemorrhages and influence of perinatal factors. American Journal of Ophthalmology 87: 74

Bjerre I, Dahlin K 1974 The long term development of children delivered by vacuum extraction. Developmental Medicine and Child Neurology 16: 378

Brockerhoff P, Brand M, Ludwig B 1981 Untrsuchungen zur Ha haufigkeit perinataler Hirnblutungen und deren Abhangigkeit vom Geburtsverlauf mit Hilfe der cranialen Computertomographie. Geburtsch und Frauen heilk 4: 597

Brown K L 1984 Review of obstetrical palsies. Non-operative treatment. Clinical Plastic Surgery 11(1): 181–187

Carmody F, Grant A, Mutch L, Vacca A, Chalmers I 1986 Follow up of babies delivered in a randomised controlled comparison of vacuum extraction and forceps delivery. Acta Obstetrica et Gynaecologica Scandinavica 65: 763–766

Chiswick M L, James D K 1979 Kielland's forceps: association with neonatal morbidity and mortality. British Medical Journal 1: 7–12

Crosby W M 1974 Trauma during pregnancy: maternal and fetal injury. Obstetric and Gynaecological Survey 29: 683–699

Crothers B 1923 Injuries of the spinal cord in breech extraction as an important cause of fetal death and paraplegia in childhood. American Journal of Medical Science 165: 94

Crothers B, Putnam M C 1927 Obstetrical injuries of the spinal cord. Medicine (Baltimore) 6: 41

Czurda R, Meznik F 1977 Therapy and diagnosis of obstetrical lesions of the brachial plexus. Paediatric Pathology 12(2): 137–145

Department of Health, Education and Welfare 1978 Congenital anomalies and birth injuries among live births, United States, 1973–1974. Series 21, No. 31, Hyattsville, Md

Egge K, Lyng G, Maltau J M 1981 Effect of instrumental delivery on the frequency and severity of retinal haemorrhages in the newborn. Acta Obstetrica et Gynaecologica Scandinavica 60: 153–155

Emery P J, Fearon B 1984 Vocal cord palsy in paediatric practice: a review of 71 cases. International Journal of Paediatric Otorhinolaryngology 8(2): 147–154

Eng G D 1975 Neuromuscular diseases. In: Avery G B (ed) Neonatology. Philadelphia, Lippincott, pp 821–837

Feldman G U 1957 Radial nerve palsies in the newborn. Archives of Disease in Childhood 32: 469

Fenichel G M, Webster D L, Wong W K T 1984 Intracranial haemorrhage in the term newborn. Archives of Neurology 41: 30–34

Fishman M A, Percy A K, Cheek W R, Speer M E 1981 Successful conservative management of cerebellar hematomas in terms infants. Journal of Pediatrics 98: 466–468

Ford F R 1925 Breech delivery in its possible relation to injury of the spinal cord, with special reference to infantile paraplegia. Archives of Neurological Psychiatry 14: 742

Gilles F H, Matson D D 1970 Sciatic nerve injury following misplaced gluteal injection. Journal of Pediatrics 76: 247

Gordon M, Rich H, Deutschberger J, Green M 1973 The immediate and long term outcome of obstetric birth trauma. I. Brachial plexus paralysis. American Journal of Obstetrics and Gynecology 117: 51

Greene W, L'Heureux P, Hunt G E 1975 Paralysis of the diaphragm. American Journal of Diseases of Children 129: 1402

Greenvald A G, Schate P C, Shiveley J L 1984 Brachial paralysis birth palsy: a 10 year report on the incidence and prognosis. Journal of Pediatric Orthopedics 4(6): 689–692

Hardy A E 1981 Birth injuries of the brachial plexus: incidence and prognosis. Journal of Bone and Joint Surgery 63B(1): 98–101

Healy D L, Quinn M A, Pepperell R J 1982 Rotational delivery of the fetus: Krielland's forceps and two other methods compared. British Journal of Obstetrics and Gynaecology 89(7): 501–506

Hepner W R 1951 Some observations on facial palsies in the newborn infant: etiology and incidence. Pediatrics 8: 494

Hoffer M M, Wickenden R, Roper B 1978 Brachial plexus birth palsies: results of tendon transfer to the rotator cuff. Journal of Bone and Joint Surgery 60(5): 691–695

Illingworth R S 1985 A paediatrician asks — why is it called birth injury? British Journal of Obstetrics and Gynaecology 92(2): 122–130

Jaffa A J, Peyser M R, Ballas S, Tooff R 1981 Management of term breech presentation in Primigravidae. British Journal of Obstetrics and Gynaecology 88: 721–724

Koch B M, Eng G M 1979 Neonatal spinal cord injury. Archives of Physical and Medical Rehabilitation 60(8): 378–381

Kwitko M L 1968 Anterior segment anomalies. Canadian Journal of Ophthalmology 3: 116

Levine M G, Holroyde J, Woods J R, Siddiqui T A, Scott M, Miodovnik M 1984 Birth trauma: incidence and predisposing factors. Obstetrics and Gynaecology 63: 792–795

McHugh H E, Sowden K A, Levitt M N 1969 Facial paralysis and muscle agenesis in the newborn. Archives of Otolaryngology 89: 157

Milner R D 1975 Neonatal mortality of breech deliveries with and without forceps to the aftercoming head. British Journal of Obstetrics and Gynaecology 82: 783

Moolgaoker A, Ahamed S, Payne P 1979 Comparison of different methods of instrumental delivery based on electronic measurements of compression and traction. Obstetrics and Gynaecology 54: 299

Naeye R L 1977 Causes of perinatal mortality in the US Collaborative Perinatal Project. Journal of the American Medical Association 238: 228

Narcy P, Tran-Ba-Huy E, Morgoloff B, Bobin S, Manac'h Y 1982 Therapeutic indications in facial paralysis of the newborn infant: apropos of 9 cases. Annales d'Oto-laryngologie et de Chiriurgie Cervico-faciale 99(9): 377–382

O'Driscoll K, Meagher D, MacDonald D, Geoghegan F 1981 Traumatic intracranial haemorrhage in first-born infants and delivery with obstetric forceps. British Journal of Obstetrics and Gynaecology 88(6): 577–581

Paintin D B, Vincent F 1980 Forceps delivery — obstetric outcome. In: Beard, Paintin (eds) Outcomes of obstetric intervention in Britain. The Royal College of Obstetricians and Gynaecologists, London

Pajor R, Szabo Z, Poskas E 1964 Control examination at 3 years of age in 227 infants with retinal hemorrhages at birth. Orvosi Hetilap 105: 78

Pape K, Armstrong D, Fitzhardinge P M 1976 Central nervous system pathology associated with mask ventilation in the very low birth weight infant: a new etiology for intracerebellar hemorrhages. Pediatrics 58: 473

Pape K E, Armstrong D L, Fitzhardinge P M 1978 Peripheral median nerve damage secondary to brachial arterial blood gas sampling. Journal of Pediatrics 83: 852

Pohjanpelto P, Niemi K, Sarmela T 1979 Anterior chamber haemorrhage in the newborn after spontaneous delivery. Acta Ophthalmology 57: 443

Poulson A M, Grabert H A 1973 Fetal death secondary to nonpenetrating trauma to the gravid uterus. American Journal of Obstetrics and Gynecology 116: 580–582

Pugh R J 1978 The battered fetus. British Medical Journal 1: 858

Rainin E A 1976 Eversion of upper lids secondary to birth trauma. Archives of Ophthalmology 94: 330

Reid H 1983 Birth injury to the cervical spine and spinal cord. Acta Neurochirurgica (Suppl) 32: 87–90

Rom S, Serfontein G L, Humphreys R P 1978 Intracerebellar haemotoma in the neonate. Journal of Pediatrics 93: 486

Rossi L N, Vassella F, Mumenthaler M 1982 Obstetrical lesions of the brachial plexus. Natural history in 34 cases. European Neurology 21(1): 1–7

Rubin A 1964 Birth injuries: incidence, mechanisms and end results. Obstetrics and Gynecology 23: 218

San Augustin M, Nitowsky H M, Borden J N 1962 Neonatal sciatic palsy after umbilical vessel injection. Journal of Pediatrics 60: 408

Schifrin N 1952 Unilateral paralysis of the diaphragm in the newborn infant due to phrenic nerve injury, with and without associated brachial palsy. Pediatrics 9: 69

Schipke R, Riege D, Scoville W 1954 Acute subdural hemorrhage at birth. Pacdiatrics 14: 468

Solomon K A, Telaranta T, Ryloppy S 1981 Early reconstruction of birth injuries of the brachial plexus. Journal of Pediatric Orthopedics 1(4): 367–370

Takagi T, Nagai R, Wakabayashi S, Mizawa I, Hajashi K 1978 Extradural haemorrhage in the newborn as a result of birth trauma. Childs Brain 4(5): 306–318

Towbin A 1964 Spinal cord and brain stem injury at birth. Archives of Pathology 77: 620

Towbin A 1969 Latent spinal cord and brain stem injury in newborn infants. Developmental Medicine and Child Neurology 11: 54

Valdes-Dapena M A, Arey J B 1970 The causes of neonatal mortality: an analysis of 501 autopsies on newborn infants. Journal of Pediatrics 77: 366

Volpe J J 1981 Neurology of the newborn. W B Saunders, Philadelphia, Ch. 20, p.590

Wigglesworth J S, Husemeyer R P 1977 Intracranial birth trauma in vaginal breech delivery: the continued importance of injury to the occipital bone. British Journal of Obstetrics and Gynaecology 84(9): 684–691

Williams B 1977 Difficult labour as a cause of communicating syringomyelia. Lancet ii: 51–53

Infection

36. Viral and protozoal infections

Prof C. S. Peckham and Dr S. Hall

Sustained or progressive neurological damage in infants and older children may result from fetal or neonatal infection with viruses or protozoa (Table 36.1). Infection may be acquired before birth, during the process of delivery or in the postnatal period. Intra-uterine infection follows invasion of the maternal bloodstream by microorganisms with resultant placental infection and/or transplacental transmission to the fetus. Sometimes the placenta may be infected without fetal spread. Infections may also reach the fetus from the genital tract by the cervical amniotic route, or they may be acquired following exposure to infected cervical secretions or to maternal blood or faeces during delivery. Infection acquired in the neonatal period may have been transmitted via breast milk, transfused blood, by hands or instruments or via the respiratory route from infected contacts such as the mother, other babies, medical attendants or other family members.

Some viruses and protozoa that cross the placenta may cause fetal damage in the form of congenital abnormalities and/or tissue invasion and destruction, both of which may involve the central nervous system (CNS). Tissue destruction may also continue after birth because of the persistence of viable organisms (Haywood 1986). Such chronic infection occurs with rubella, cytomegalovirus (CMV), herpes simplex virus (HSV), varicella–zoster (V–Z) virus, human immunodeficiency virus (HIV), lymphocytic choriomeningitis virus (LCV), *Toxoplasma gondii* and the trypanosomes.

Most infants congenitally infected by these agents have no clinical illness at birth but may later develop neurological signs and symptoms in infancy, childhood, or adult life because of the persistence and activity of the microorganism (Peckham 1972). It is often not possible to identify the cause of these late manifestations because microbiological investigations at this stage cannot distinguish congenital from postnatally acquired infection. The difficulty is compounded by the non-specific nature of the symptoms. For example, it is not possible to diagnose a congenital infection in a 3-year-old child presenting with global retardation who is excreting CMV in the urine or who has a positive toxoplasma dye test.

Some viruses, such as measles, mumps and the enteroviruses, may cause intra-uterine infection but do not persist. Transplacental transmission of human serum parvovirus (B19) is also well documented (Knott & Welply 1984, Bond et al 1986) but it is not known whether infection persists as it does with animal parvoviruses. Apart from congenital poliomyelitis, neurological damage associated with infection with these viruses appears to be due to prematurity (Cherry 1983, Young & Gershon 1983).

Demonstrating the possible role of viruses and protozoa as a cause of fetal damage and/or neurological sequelae can be difficult and is open to misinterpretation. Maternal infection may be missed because it is subclinical or non-specific and mild (CMV infection and toxoplasmosis are typical examples). There is little precise information

Table 36.1 Viruses and protozoa known to infect the human fetus or newborn infant and cause damage to the nervous system

Viruses	Protozoa
Rubella	*Toxoplasma gondii*
Cytomegalovirus	*Trypanosoma cruzi*
Varicella–zoster	*gambiense*
Herpes virus hominis	*rhodesiense*
Human immunodeficiency virus	
Lymphocytic chorioretinitis virus	
Non-polio enteroviruses	
Polio virus	

available on the frequency of infection in pregnancy but in a prospective study of 30 000 pregnancies, carried out in the United States, 5.2% were complicated by at least one clinically recognizable illness, the majority of which were non-specific and 'viral' (Sever & White 1968). In such cases it is unlikely, if the infant is normal at birth or has non-specific symptoms, that investigations for evidence of infection will be done. If symptoms suggestive of congenital infection then present in the older infant or child it may no longer be possible to reach a conclusive diagnosis.

Any study of the gestational effects of a microorganism known to cause mild or subclinical maternal infection must be prospective. This necessitates the serological follow-up of women through pregnancy to identify those who become infected, to measure specific IgM antibodies in cord blood, and to investigate appropriate fetal or neonatal samples for evidence of congenital infection. Where the sensitivity of the laboratory investigation of the neonate is in doubt (as for toxoplasma IgM) or unknown (as for human parvovirus), infants must be followed clinically and serologically for at least the first year. The significance of non-specific outcomes such as abortion, prematurity, neurological or sense organ sequelae can only be made by comparison with a control group of pregnancies matched for confounding variables such as age, parity, social class and ethnic background. Large numbers of women have to be studied because even the most common congenital infection, CMV, occurs in only 1% of pregnancies and in only a proportion of these will transplacental infection take place.

Associating a particular infection with fetal damage may be difficult if the infection is uncommon in pregnancy, even if the maternal infection is symptomatic. Examples include mumps, chickenpox and measles. The likelihood of an association is increased if the organism can be recovered from the fetus or infant, or if there is serological evidence of infection in the neonate. However, unless a series of cases with similar defects or with a characteristic syndrome is reported, as with congenital varicella, evidence of transplacental transmission does not necessarily confirm that the agent was responsible for the defects.

Mumps is an example of an infection whose gestational effects are still a matter of debate. A study of placental infection following mumps vaccine in pregnancy demonstrated that fetal infection could occur (Yamauchi et al 1974) and experimentally acquired hydrocephalus due to aqueduct stenosis may develop in suckling hamsters infected with mumps virus at birth; similar defects have been reported in infants following early childhood mumps (Johnson 1968). The virus readily invades the meninges and brain and insufficient attention has been given to the possibility of fetal mumps infection damaging the central nervous system.

This chapter reviews viral and protozoal infections which, if acquired during pregnancy or the neonatal period, are known to infect the CNS and to result in neurological sequelae. Organisms whose neuropathic effect is speculative or non-specific will not be considered.

VIRUSES
RUBELLA

Rubella infection acquired during early fetal life may result in fetal damage and the birth of an infant with multiple defects including neurological abnormalities. Fetal infection results from a primary rubella infection in pregnancy and reinfection is assumed not to constitute a risk (Dudgeon 1975). The current immunization programme in the UK is based on this important assumption. Maternal infection in pregnancy is not inevitably followed by fetal infection or damage and prospective studies, where evaluation begins from the time of maternal infection, have been carried out in many countries to estimate the risk of damage. A summary of these prospective studies suggests that the risk of damage is about 21% following infection in the first 8 weeks, declining to about 6% at 12 to 16 weeks of gestation (Dudgeon 1976). However, more recent studies based on serological confirmation of rubella in pregnancy have put the risk higher and Miller et al (1982) found that 9 out of 10 infants were infected following maternal infection before the 11th week, and all were damaged. Infection beyond 16 weeks of gestation is only occasionally associated with defects, although cases of deafness have been reported up to 22 weeks of gestation. Well-designed prospective studies of children born after later infection have shown that although rubella infection after this period can result in fetal infection, there is no increased risk of defects (Miller et al 1982, Grilner et al 1983). Infection in early pregnancy is likely to result in multiple defects whereas infection in the third and fourth month usually results in a single defect, sensorineural deafness.

In addition to cataracts, congenital heart disease, deafness and non-specific manifestations presenting in the newborn such as failure to thrive, hepatomegaly, splenomegaly, jaundice, and thrombocytopenic purpura, the CNS is a common site for the infection and neurological defects may be present. These include microcephaly, mental retardation, cerebral palsy, defects of hearing and speech, features of autism, retinal changes and visual disturbances due to cataract and microphthalmos. Seizures and hydrocephalus are rare. With the exception of deafness, CNS involvement rarely occurs in the absence of manifestations involving other systems. Chess (1971) has drawn attention to the high incidence of autistic features in children with congenital rubella deafness and a small number with normal hearing have also been observed with classic autism.

Sensorineural hearing loss is the most frequent rubella defect. It may be moderate or severe, bilateral or unilateral and is often associated with pigmentary retinopathy. Epidemiological studies carried out in the prevaccination era suggested that rubella accounted for 18% of childhood sensorineural deafness (Martin & Moore 1979, Peckham et al 1979).

It is difficult to establish the full impact of congenital rubella on a population; there is not always a history of maternal infection, and in addition congenital rubella is a potentially progressive disorder. Defects may not manifest or even develop until weeks, months or years after birth. The most important example of this is sensorineural deafness (Peckham 1972) but other more unusual forms of this late onset disease include pneumonitis, diabetes mellitus, hypothyroidism, growth hormone deficiency and encephalitis (Marshall 1973).

Meningoencephalitis may occasionally present in infancy or early childhood and rubella virus has been isolated from the cerebrospinal fluid (CSF) which may contain raised protein levels and show pleocytosis (Desmond et al 1967). Infection at this site may be a factor causing further damage to the nervous system. The chronic nature of congenital rubella is demonstrated by the small number of individuals with congenital rubella in whom severe progressive neurological disease resembling subacute sclerosing panencephalitis (SSPE) of measles has been reported in the second decade of life (Johnson 1975, Townsend et al 1975). The clinical features of this disorder are characterized by progressive cerebellar ataxia, spasticity, mental retardation and seizures. In one case, rubella virus was isolated from the brain and high levels of antibody were present in the CSF (Weil et al 1975). The panencephalitis and severe degeneration of the white matter is similar to the lesions seen in SSPE but in rubella encephalitis vascular deposits are also observed (Singer et al 1967).

Diagnosis

In the newborn period a diagnosis of congenital rubella depends on isolation of the virus from urine or nasopharynx or by the demonstration of IgM-specific antibodies. Serological tests for rubella specific IgG are of little value at this age because no distinction can be made between maternal and fetal antibody. The test should therefore be repeated at 6 to 8 months when maternal antibody will have declined. Prenatal diagnosis has been attempted by direct puncture of the umbilical cord with determination of rubella-specific IgM on fetal blood prior to 18 weeks of gestation (Daffos et al 1984), with the recommendation for termination of pregnancy in some cases based on these results.

Prevention

With the development of live attenuated rubella vaccines, rubella in pregnancy has become a preventable condition. There are two possible strategies for vaccination. The first involves the immunization of all infants of both sexes to eliminate the risk of exposure of pregnant women to rubella by interrupting the transmission of infection among children. The second involves selective immunization of adolescent girls to eliminate the risk of rubella occurring in pregnancy. This strategy does not aim to interrupt the transmission of infection within the population, indeed, it builds on the acquisition of natural immunity during childhood and allows for the boosting of vaccine-induced antibody by circulating virus. Universal immunization has a more immediate effect on the prevention of congenital rubella whereas selective immunization requires years to elapse before the impact is felt.

In the UK, rubella vaccine was introduced in 1970 and a policy of selective immunization was adopted in which school-girls between 11 and 14 years of age were offered vaccine (DHSS 1970). This was extended to include susceptible women of child-bearing age, particularly those working with children. In addition, women found to be susceptible to rubella in the antenatal period were offered vaccine postpartum. The recommendation was also made that men whose work brought them into contact with pregnant women, such as medical personnel and medical students, be offered vaccination if they were not immune.

The impact of the UK immunization policy is now becoming apparent but continued surveillance is essential. There has been a marked decline in the number of pregnant women susceptible to rubella infection, from about 18% before the immunization programme to about 5% in 1986, with even lower rates for parous women. The number of terminations for rubella or rubella contact has declined by about 60% and there has been a marked fall in the number of children born with congenital rubella (Smithells et al 1985).

In the US a policy of universal immunization of children was adopted. In 1985 a provisional total of 604 cases of rubella was reported which represented a 20% decline from 1969, the year rubella vaccine was licensed. This decline has been paralleled by a decline in reported cases of congenital rubella syndrome (CDC 1986).

CYTOMEGALOVIRUS INFECTION

Cytomegalovirus (CMV) is one of the herpes group of viruses which includes herpes simplex virus, varicella–zoster virus and Epstein–Barr virus. A unique characteristic of the herpes virus group is their ability to establish latent infection. This is established after a primary infection and periodic episodes of reactivation can occur.

Cytomegalovirus is the most common known congenital infection. The incidence of congenital CMV infection varies in different parts of the world from 0.2 to 2.2% of livebirths and there is no evidence of seasonal variation (Stagno et al 1983). As maternal infections are nearly always asymptomatic and over 90% of congenitally infected infants have no clinically recognizable signs of infection at birth, the vast majority of congenital infections pass unrecognized. Initial studies, largely based on children admitted to hospital, suggested that the prevalance of defects associated with congenital infection was high (Weller et al 1964, McCracken et al 1969). However, more recent prospective studies, following children systematically screened for CMV at birth and found to have infection, have demonstrated that the incidence of adverse sequelae is not as high as originally estimated (Ahlfors et al 1979, Saigal et al 1982, Peckham et al 1983).

It is estimated that 33 000 infants are born with congenital CMV in the United States each year (Stagno & Whitley 1985) and 1800 in England and Wales (Preece et al 1984). Fewer than 10% of congenitally infected infants are symptomatic at birth (Hanshaw & Dudgeon 1978) but the majority of this symptomatic group will have later complications including hearing loss, mental retardation or seizures. Of the remainder who are asymptomatic at birth, a small proportion will also develop long-term neurological sequelae.

Symptomatic congenital infection

The clinical manifestations of congenital infection at birth include pneumonitis, prolonged neonatal jaundice, hepatomegaly, splenomegaly, petechiae, low birth-weight, microcephaly and thrombocytopenia, and periventricular intracranial calcifications may also be present. On follow-up symptomatic neonates are almost invariably found to have permanent brain damage which may include signs of cerebral palsy, epilepsy, mental retardation, chorioretinitis, optic atrophy, delayed psychomotor development, expressive language delay and learning disability. Sensorineural deafness is the most frequent defect.

Microcephaly has been described in a high proportion of severely affected infants with congenital CMV and who also had associated psychomotor retardation. If intracranial calcifications are present the brain is invariably impaired. These periventricular calcifications which are in the subependymal regions are characteristic of severe congenital CMV encephalitis. Cerebral calcifications are rare, however, and occur in fewer than 1% of all CMV-infected infants (Hanshaw et al 1985). Hydrocephalus has been described following obstruction of the fourth ventricle but this is rare and microcephaly is more usual.

Neurological problems are not always obvious in neonates who subsequently develop neurological handicap. Neurological involvement may be progressive and Bray et al (1981) described two children who had normal or minor changes only on computerized tomography but whose condition progressed to severe extensive disease over a 3-month period. Congenital CMV has also been associated with visual defects including optic atrophy, chorioretinitis and strabismus. CMV chorioretinitis cannot be distinguished from that produced by toxoplasmosis on the basis of location or appearance and both can induce central retinal lesions. Unlike toxoplasmosis, however, chorioretinitis has not been reported in isolation in an otherwise asymptomatic child.

Congenital CMV is an important cause of sensorineural deafness. This is probably due to a viral labrynthitis affecting the vestibular and semicircular canals and the epithelial cells of the inner ear, resulting in hydrops of the inner ear (Myers & Stool 1968). CMV has been cultured from the inner ear (Davis et al 1981), and Stagno et al (1977) demonstrated the presence of viral antigen in spiral ganglion neurones and the organ of Corti. The relationship with specific ear damage remains obscure and the mechanism whereby virus is transmitted to the inner ear is not known. Progressive deterioration of hearing may occur, possibly due to viral replication. Williamson et al (1982) reported three children with mild hearing loss diagnosed before 2 years which had progressed to severe bilateral deafness by 3 years. Dahle et al (1979) reported similar findings.

McCracken et al (1969) described the long-term follow-up of 18 children with symptomatic congenital CMV: 16 presented with hepatosplenomegaly and 9 with evidence of CNS involvement. Pass et al (1980) reported the long-term follow-up of 33 infants with symptomatic CMV, 19 of whom presented with evidence of CNS disease. Most deaths occurred in the first year of life and all were in infants with severe CNS disease such as cerebral palsy and microcephaly. The outcome for symptomatic infants was poor, with a mortality rate of about 25% in both series. In the study reported by Pass et al (1980) 10 children died and all but 2 of the remaining 23 showed evidence of CNS disease or auditory damage and were significantly handicapped. Of the 23 survivors, 14 suffered from spasticity, fits and mental retardation, 16 had microcephaly, 7 were deaf but had a normal IQ, and 5 had chorioretinitis or optic atrophy. McCracken et al (1969) reported only 4 to be normal at 9 years, 4 had bilateral sensorineural deafness and 7 severe psychomotor delay with spasticity and/or fits. Williamson et al (1982) followed 17 newborns with symptomatic infection: 9 had severe CNS disease, 6 had hearing loss with normal IQ and only 2 were normal at 4 years. Chorioretinitis was present in 41%. In addition, 3 children had specific language disorders and 4 had learning difficulties despite normal intelligence.

The risk of subsequent damage in symptomatic newborns is unknown, as most studies have based their findings on infants with congenital infection who were referrals into special care baby units. This may have led to selection of the most severely affected infants and to an overestimate of the risk of subsequent handicap. In a prospective study by Saigal et al (1982) in Canada, however, only 1 in 4 children with symptomatic CMV later developed neurological sequelae. In a similarly designed study in London (Preece et al 1984) where 5% of congenitally infected infants were symptomatic, all 5 children developed late sequelae. These later studies were based on children screened at birth and the children were not as severely abnormal in the newborn period as those reported by Pass et al, most of whose patients were referrals into a special unit.

In a study carried out by MacDonald & Tobin (1978), 37 infants were indentified in a prospective survey and 47 referred on clinical grounds. Among those children with symptomatic congenital infection the rate of handicap was high and only 5 (21%) of the 24 with signs of damage to the CNS at birth remained normal. Of the 25 with jaundice, hepatosplenomegaly and/or purpura but no CNS signs, 12 remained normal.

Asymptomatic congenital infection

An important feature of congenital CMV is the observation that a small proportion of clinically normal neonates with congenital infection may later manifest problems, the most common being sensorineural deafness. The risk of a significant bilateral sensorineural hearing loss of greater than 50 dB in this group is about 6% and studies report rates ranging from 0 to 7.8% (Kumar et al 1984). In the majority of cases this loss does not progress after the first year. In a significant number of children with unexplained sensorineural hearing loss the cause may be CMV but it is unlikely that a diagnosis of congenital CMV will be made if the infant was asymptomatic. In a study of children attending a referral centre for speech and hearing, 1644 children under 4 years were screened for CMV viruria and virus was isolated from 9.5% (Peckham 1986). Children with sensorineural hearing loss but no family history of deafness were almost twice as likely to shed CMV in the urine (13%) than children who have normal hearing or a family history of hearing loss. This highlights the importance of CMV infection in the aetiology of hearing loss in children (see Ch. 43).

Other neurological features such as microcephaly, spasticity and fits have been described in children who were asymptomatic at birth.

Psychomotor development

Congenital CMV may cause severe neurological sequelae but it is not clear whether it has a specific effect on intelligence in the absence of neurological problems. Studies of the long-term effect of congenital CMV on mental ability produce conflicting results. Kumar et al (1984) reported the development of 17 asymptomatic congenitally infected infants at a mean age of 7.6 years (range 4.5–10.5 years) using the Weschler Intelligence Scales for Children (WISC-R). The mean IQ of children with congenital infection was not significantly different from that of uninfected or postnatally infected children (Saigal et al 1982) using the Stanford Binet test and a Wide Range of Achievement test

at 3 and 5 years found no significant difference in the IQs of 47 children with congenital CMV and their controls. However, Reynolds et al (1974) using a Stanford Binet IQ assessment when the children were 21–77 months suggested that an adverse effect was likely because 8 out of 18 children with asymptomatic congenital CMV had IQs of 90 or below, compared with 4 out of 18 controls, although the difference was not statistically significant. Their conclusion that asymptomatic congenital CMV caused a tendency to low IQ was based on the distribution of IQ scores in the two groups and not on comparisons of means. The only study to demonstrate an effect of CMV on intellectual development was that reported by Hanshaw et al (1976). The development of 44 congenitally infected children who were asymptomatic at birth was assessed at 3.3–7 years using the Wechsler Preschool Primary Scale of Intelligence. The congenitally infected children had significantly lower mean IQs than their matched controls and a group of random controls. In a recent study, 41 children with congenital CMV infection and their controls were assessed at 2 years of age using the Griffiths Developmental Scale (Pearl et al 1986). The scores achieved by children with asymptomatic congenital CMV were similar to control children. Similar findings were reported by Conboy et al (1986). Thus it appears that about 90% of children with congenital CMV will be neurologically and developmentally normal.

Recurrent maternal infection

Unlike congenital rubella or toxoplasma infection intrauterine transmission of CMV infection can occur following reactivated infection, even in the presence of substantial humeral immunity. Congenital infections resulting from a recurrence of CMV during pregnancy are less likely to result in fetal damage than primary infections (Stagno et al 1982) although defects compatible with congenital CMV infection have been reported in women who were seropositive before conception (Ahlfors et al 1981, Rutter et al 1985).

Diagnosis of congenital CMV

The diagnosis of congenital infection is confirmed by isolation of virus in cell culture from urine or from throat swabs collected in the first 3 weeks of life. Infants who acquire CMV during delivery do not excrete CMV until after 3 weeks of age so that the presence of virus before this time is diagnostic of congenital infection.

The presence of CMV-specific IgM in cord blood or blood samples collected before acquired infection could have occurred is also diagnostic of congenital infection. As CMV is commonly acquired in early infancy it is not possible to distinguish congenital from acquired infection in a child who presents with neurological problems and in whom CMV is cultured from the urine after 3 weeks of age.

Postnatally acquired infection

The rapid acquisition of CMV infection in infants of seropositive mothers within the first 3 months of life, and its relative absence among infants of seronegative mothers, suggests that the mother is the major source of infection. Infection may be acquired during delivery through contact with infected cervical secretions (Reynolds et al 1980) or after birth primarily from breast milk (Stagno et al 1980). A further important source of postnatally acquired infection is transfusion or seropositive blood products (Ballard et al 1979, Yeager et al 1981, Adler et al 1983).

Reynolds et al (1980) reported the early acquisition of CMV infection in 40% of infants born to women known to be shedding the virus in late pregnancy. Infected breast milk is an even more efficient source of early acquired infection. CMV can be isolated from breast milk in about 30% of seropositive women although lower rates of isolation from colostrum are reported (Hayes et al 1972, Stagno et al 1980). In a recent UK study, 33% of infants of seropositive mothers were infected by one year and most of these infections had already occurred by 3 months (Peckham et al 1987). The acquisition of CMV among infants of seropositive mothers who breast-fed was higher than among bottle-fed infants. DNA typing of virus isolates from the mother's milk and infant's urine confirmed that the virus was of maternal origin.

Although neonatally acquired CMV infection has been temporarily associated with pneumonitis (Stagno et al 1981), it is seldom symptomatic. However, CMV infections transmitted by blood transfusion to very-low-birth-weight infants born to seronegative mothers or those with unknown serology, have resulted in acute illness with lymphocytosis, hepatosplenomegaly, respiratory distress and even death (Ballard et al 1979, Yeager et al 1981).

Treatment

To prevent the acquisition of CMV in premature neonates, it is recommended that blood products given to very-low-birth-weight infants should be restricted to CMV-negative donors. It is not known whether expressed human milk from seropositive donors is also a nosocomial source of severe infection in premature neonates who are at risk of infection. It has been recommended that fresh milk from donors fed to premature infants should be appropriately processed to reduce infectivity but this may also decrease the potential benefit of the milk.

There is, as yet, no effective treatment for congenital infection, although high-titre CMV-specific immunoglobulin has been used.

VARICELLA–ZOSTER VIRUS INFECTION

Varicella–zoster (V–Z) is a DNA virus and a member of the herpes group. Varicella is the manifestation of a primary infection and zoster is a reactivated infection. Varicella, or chickenpox, is highly contagious and in developed temperate regions it is almost universally acquired in childhood and infection in pregnancy is infrequent. In semitropical and tropical countries, however, varicella occurs at an older age and a higher proportion of women of child-bearing age are susceptible (Weller 1983).

In a prospective study of clinically recognized infection that occurred in pregnancy between 1958 and 1964, the Collaborative Perinatal Study identified 20 infections attributed to chickenpox among 30 000 pregnancies, 14 of which were substantiated; a minimal rate of infection of 0.5 per 1000 pregnancies (Sever & White 1968). This is likely to be an underestimate since mild and subclinical cases would have been excluded. Herpes zoster may also occur during pregnancy but as it is a disease of older people it is uncommon in women of child-bearing age.

Congenital varicella syndrome

Varicella–zoster virus can infect the placenta and produce areas of necrosis (Garcia 1963) and fetal infection can occur (Young & Gershon 1983). However, this is a rare event and no accurate estimate can be made of the risk of congenital abnormalities associated with chickenpox in early pregnancy. The risk of damage must be extremely low since in prospective studies carried out in the US (Siegel 1973) and England (Manson et al 1960, Bradford Hill et al 1978) there was no statistical association between maternal varicella and abnormal offspring. There is, therefore, no convincing indication for termination of pregnancy.

The congenital varicella syndrome was first described by Laforet & Lynch (1947). They reported an infant with paralysis and muscular atrophy of the right leg, rudimentary digits, cortical atrophy with hypoplasia of the cerebellum, growth retardation and scarred skin lesions on the left leg. The mother had varicella at the eighth week of pregnancy. For more than 20 years no further cases were reported but since 1967 there have been several similar case reports from a number of different countries (Enders 1985). The constellation of abnormalities described in these case reports of infants born to mothers who had varicella in early pregnancy is sufficiently distinctive to suggest that the V–Z virus is teratogenic. The pathognomonic stigmata of the varicella syndrome include cicatricial scars which are often dermatomal in distribution and related to hypoplasia of one or more limbs, and malformed digits. CNS damage may be manifested by convulsions and mental retardation and chorioretinitis and cataracts are typically present.

Several features of the reported cases are consistent with the hypothesis that congenital defects result from viral damage to developing neural tissue in early gestation and the reduction deformity appears to occur secondarily to the degeneration of the nerve supply to that particular area.

Direct proof that V–Z infection of the fetus causes congenital anomalies is still lacking. The link was established because of the similarity of defects reported from different parts of the world and in no case of congenital V–Z syndrome has isolation of the virus from blood, tissue or fluids been reported. The latent persistence of the V–Z virus in infants infected in utero is further supported by reports of children with the congenital V–Z syndrome who develop zoster in early life (Dworsky et al 1980). The development of zoster in the infant or young child suggests intra-uterine infection and a search for residua of congenital damage, particularly chorioretinitis, should be made.

Perinatal chickenpox

Transmission of virus to the fetus later in pregnancy, particularly shortly before or during birth may result in severe systemic illness but without the development of congenital stigmata. Infection may be transmitted transplacentally or acquired postnatally by droplet infection. Infection is considered to be congenital if it occurs within 10 days of birth. Postnatally acquired chickenpox, which begins between 10 and 28 days after birth, is generally mild whereas congenital chickenpox is associated with significant mortality. Congenital chickenpox occurs in about 24% of infants exposed to intra-uterine infection in the 21 days before delivery (Young & Gershon 1983).

When infection occurs in late pregnancy, severe and often fatal disseminated varicella infection may develop in the neonate (Meyers 1974). Infants at greatest risk are those whose mothers develop chickenpox in the last 4 days of gestation or up to 2 days after delivery. The variation in the severity of the disease in neonates is probably influenced by the transfer of maternal antibody across the placenta (Brunell 1967). When maternal infection occurs just before or at delivery, the neonate is infected before circulating antibody is produced by the mother. Mortality among neonates infected under these circumstances is estimated to

be about 31% (Gershon 1975). When birth occurs after the production of circulating maternal antibody, 5 to 21 days before delivery, the neonate appears to be protected against severe disease but may have mild chickenpox at birth or in the first few days of life. Table 36.2 shows the time of maternal illness in relation to outcome in 50 pregnancies complicated by varicella near full-term.

Management

Passive immunization with antivaricella–zoster immunoglobulin (ZIg) is recommended as soon as possible after birth to infants whose mothers had onset of varicella within 5 days of delivery. ZIg, even if given in repeated high doses, does not necessarily prevent varicella in the newborn although it may modify the course of the illness. In a follow-up study of 104 neonates given ZIg prophylaxis (Miller et al 1986), 37 of the 67 born 0 to 15 days after the onset of maternal chickenpox lacked V–Z antibody before receiving ZIg; maternal antibody was absent in all 26 infants born less than 3 days after the onset of maternal rash, and in 11 of the 23 born 3 to 5 days after onset. All 18 infants born 6 or more days after maternal chickenpox were seropositive at birth. Clinical and/or serological evidence of V–Z infection was found in 46 of the 74 (62%) infants who were seronegative before receiving ZIg. In most cases the chickenpox was mild and there were no deaths. Infections occurring in infants with maternal antibody were of similar severity. However, since neonatal deaths from chickenpox were rare before ZIg was introduced in the UK, the risk to infants lacking maternal antibody may have been overestimated.

The antiviral drugs adenine arabinoside (Ara-A) and acylovir have been used in the treatment of severe neonatal varicella but their efficacy is unproven and the long-term effects of the drugs are unknown. To avoid the transmission of infection to other neonates, mothers or hospital personnel, the mother and her infant with varicella or at high risk of contracting the infection should be isolated together and sent home as soon as possible. If maternal infection occurs at or within the first few days of birth it is advisable to isolate the infant from the mother.

Herpes zoster

Herpes zoster is rare in pregnancy but occurs in the presence of maternal antibodies and is not usually associated with a viraemia. There is no evidence to suggest that zoster causes malformations. Isolated case reports of abnormalities associated with herpes zoster in early pregnancy have been described but in these cases mothers had also been exposed to rubella during pregnancy (Brazin et al 1979).

Table 36.2 Maternal varicella near full-term and its effect on the fetus

Onset of maternal infection	Onset of neonatal infection	Outcome			
		Died	Survived	Total	Fatality rate
>5–21 days before delivery	0–4 days (maternal antibody present)	0	27	27	nil
4 days before to 2 days after delivery	5–10 days (maternal antibody absent)	7	16	23	31%

Adapted from Hanshaw et al 1985.

HERPES SIMPLEX VIRUS

In recent years publicity has been given to the increasing prevalence of genital herpes. Whether this represents a true increase or is merely the result of greater awareness of the infection, possibly due to the publicity given to antiviral drugs of low toxicity, is open to debate. In 1984, 19 869 new cases of genital herpes were reported by clinics for sexually transmitted disease in the UK. This represented a marked increase from 14 842 in 1982 and 9576 in 1979 (PHLS 1986). This number is likely to be an underestimate since infection is often asymptomatic and only those cases seen for treatment in clinics for sexually transmitted diseases are notified.

Herpes simplex virus (HSV) is a double-stranded DNA virus which can be classified into types 1 and 2. Traditionally HSV-1 produced lesions above the belt (face, lips, eyes) and HSV-2 below the belt. However, this is not absolute and either type can cause lesions at any site. There appears to have been a change in the pattern of infection and the distinction of HSV-1 causing labial herpes and HSV-2 genital has become less clear (Lancet 1981).

Transplacental infection

Transplacental infection appears to be rare although there have been isolated case reports of primary maternal infection in the first 20 weeks of pregnancy resulting in congenital abnormality (South et al 1969, Florman et al 1973, Komorous et al 1977). These infants suffered from microcephaly, microphthalmia and intracranial calcifications and had cutaneous lesions at birth. Reports of adverse effects following HSV infection in early pregnancy are few and the evidence that HSV is teratogenic remains inconclusive. Early primary infection is not an indication for termination of pregnancy. An increased rate of abortion has been reported in women with genital herpes (Nahmias et al 1971) but this needs further clarification.

Intranatal infection

Neonatal herpes infection is usually acquired when the infant is in contact with infected genital secretions during delivery, or by ascending infection, particularly after prolonged rupture of the membranes. Fetal scalp monitoring has also been associated with neonatal infection (Parvey & Ch'ien 1980). Herpetic vesicles appear at the monitoring site and disseminated infection can result. Clinical evidence of infection usually presents at between 5 and 17 days of life.

Infected neonates have a high frequency of visceral and central nervous system infection and the overall mortality and morbidity is high. Table 36.3 shows the outcome of untreated HSV infection in newborns from data derived from the United States. Infection which appears to be disseminated and presents as hepatitis, pneumonitis, encephalitis or intravascular coagulopathy has a poor prognosis and is associated with a high mortality. Similarly, the outcome is poor when infection is confined to the central nervous system and many of the infants who survive have severe neurological and/or ocular sequelae. If infection is limited to the eye, skin or oral cavity the outcome is better and death is unusual. Although infection is more frequent in premature infants (Nahmias et al 1983) there appears to be no difference in the type, or severity of the disease, nor in its outcome in premature or full-term infants. About 75% of virus isolates typed from infected newborns are HSV-2, the remainder being HSV-1, but there is no apparent difference in the severity of the disease (Visintine et al 1981).

The risk of perinatal HSV infection is unknown and in its clinically recognizable form it is a rare disease. Nahmias et al (1970) estimated that among lower

Table 36.3   Prognosis of untreated neonatal HSV infection*

Clinical groups	No. cases	Deaths (%)	Survivors With sequelae (%)	Without sequelae (%)
Disseminated disease				
without CNS involvement	38	87	3	10
with CNS involvement	78	71	15	14
Localized disease				
CNS	61	37	51	12
Eye	13	–	31	69
Skin	39	10	26	64
Oral cavity	4	–	–	100
Total	233	49	25	20

*Neonates diagnosed at postmortem excluded.
From Nahmias et al 1983.

socio-economic populations in the United States clinically recognized neonatal HSV infection occurred in about 1 in 7500 deliveries, resulting in about 70 cases per year. In Seattle the incidence of neonatal herpes has increased from 2 cases per 100 000 livebirths during 1966–69 to 13.8 per 100 000 during 1978–82 (Sullivan-Bolyai et al 1983). The risk of neonatal infection is reported to be higher following clinically apparent primary genital infection than recurrent infection, possibly due to the higher titres of virus present in the genital tract. Although the protective value of maternal herpes antibodies is limited, it may play some part in decreasing the risk of neonatal infection (Probert et al 1987). Infants born to mothers with onset just before full-term may lack maternal antibodies at birth and suffer from more severe disease.

The management of labour, and the route of delivery remains very controversial in pregnancies complicated by herpes infection and at the present time no unequivocal guidelines can be given.

Neonatal herpes appears to be rare in the UK. In a national enquiry by Dinwiddie and his colleagues (personal communication 1987) 18 cases had been observed by neonatologists over a 5-year period. In the 10 years 1976–85, 136 reports of virus isolates from neonates were received by the Public Health Laboratory Service Communicable Disease Surveillance Centre (unpublished data). There was little annual variation and about 14 cases were reported per year. There has been no clinical follow-up of these cases nor confirmation that they were cases of neonatal HSV infection. Since June 1986 paediatricians in the UK have been asked to notify all cases of neonatal HSV infection to the British Paediatric Surveillance Unit (PHLS 1987). This should provide a more accurate estimate of the number of infants with diagnosed neonatal HSV infection.

The incidence of neonatal herpes may be underestimated because up to 50% of infected neonates lack cutaneous involvement and the diagnosis may therefore be missed (Whitley et al 1980, Yeager et al 1980, Arvin et al 1982). This is particularly so for disseminated infection where the sudden onset of hepatosplenomegaly, thrombocytopenia and liver failure may be assumed to be due to bacterial sepsis. HSV infection should be suspected in newborn infants who have focal seizures or who develop signs suggestive of bacterial sepsis. Early clinical features may include apnoea, hepatomegaly and persistent acidosis. An important feature of neonatal HSV infection, which can be of value in diagnosis, is the relatively high frequency of isolation of the virus from CSF (Barnes et al 1982). This contrasts markedly with encephalitis in older children or adults (Whitley et al 1980).

Data from a prospective study by the National Institute of Allergy and Infectious Disease (IAID) Collaborative Antiviral Study and from cases reported in the literature on more than 400 infants with neonatal herpes, showed that only 10% of mothers had experienced clinically apparent HSV (Whitley et al 1980). A past history of genital HSV was obtained from 13% of mothers who were asymptomatic at delivery and 20% of their sexual partners; in 70% there was no history or evidence of genital HSV.

Post-natal infection

Other important routes of neonatal infection include maternal non-genital infection or infection from other adults or infants in the nursery (Francis et al 1975, Light 1979, Hammerberg et al 1983). Spread between or from individuals other than the mother has been well documented and the source of infection confirmed by DNA 'fingerprinting' (Linneman et al 1978). Hospital staff may pose a risk, and the observation that one-third of the obstetric staff in a unit in Melbourne suffered from one or more labial lesions during a one-year period raises the question of protection of newborns from this source (Hatherley et al 1980a). Hatherley et al (1980b) further investigated the incidence of oral HSV shedding during this period and virus was isolated from the saliva of 10% of 384 asymptomatic obstetric staff. Virus isolation was attempted repeatedly and 27% or more individuals with HSV-1 antibodies excreted HSV at sometime during the study period. Despite these findings, neonatal HSV infection was exceedingly rare.

Management

Antiviral drugs are now used in the treatment of neonatal infection. The IAID collaborative study concluded that although the type of neonatal disease was the major determinant of outcome, regardless of therapy, adenine arabinoside showed a beneficial effect, similar to that found in the treatment of HSV encephalitis in older individuals. A high index of suspicion of HSV infection is required so that a diagnosis can be made early in the course of the disease and treatment can be given as soon as possible. Antiviral chemotherapy has reduced the mortality from neonatal herpes to 25% but the morbidity, especially in infants with central nervous system involvement remains high (Corey & Spear 1986). Acyclovir which is well tolerated in newborns is now used in the treatment of neonatal infection. Trials comparing acyclovir with adenine arabinoside are in progress but acyclovir does not appear to confer any advantage.

The American Academy of Pediatrics (Committee on Fetus and Newborn 1980) recommended that staff with active labial or other HSV infections, should have limited contact with neonates and that those with herpetic whitlow should wear gloves when handling the infant. Some experts have even recommended that staff with active HSV infections should be removed from the nursery until the lesions have dried but such a policy would deprive a hard-pressed nursery of experienced nursing staff and have serious consequences (Kilbrick 1980). A survey of 161 neonatal referral centres in the United States revealed that 83% excluded personnel with overt oral HSV lesions from direct patient care and 27% excluded infected personnel from all hospital work (Kleinman et al 1982). Despite the high incidence of oral herpes lesions and excretion of HSV among asymptomatic hospital staff, the incidence of recognized neonatal HSV infection caused by type 1 HSV is extremely low.

Schreiner et al (1979) reported that although many institutions in the United States did not isolate mothers with oral herpes from their newborn infants the transmission of infection from infected mothers to their infants was 'occasional'. More information was needed to formulate a policy for isolation in these circumstances. There appears to be no reason why such women should not breast-feed their infants. One report suggested that transmission of the virus may have taken place through breast milk; this was not established with certainty (Dunkle et al 1979).

HUMAN IMMUNODEFICIENCY VIRUS

Human immunodeficiency virus (HIV), the cause of the acquired immune deficiency syndrome (AIDS), is a retrovirus and a member of the lentivirus subfamily. It is an RNA virus containing the enzyme reverse transcriptase which enables it to make DNA copies of itself which can then insert into the host cell's genome, causing lifelong infection.

Data from Zaire (Mann et al 1986a) and from the Centers for Disease Control AIDS surveillance programme, to which 394 cases of paediatric AIDS had been reported by December 1986 (CDC 1987) suggest that most paediatric infections in these countries are acquired vertically. While some of these children had received a blood transfusion before the onset of symptoms, most were born to mothers in high-risk groups for AIDS, such as intravenous drug abusers, prostitutes, women from countries where the prevalence of HIV is high or women whose sexual partners were in a high-risk group.

There is good evidence that transplacental infection can occur (Jovaisas et al 1985, Lapoint et al 1985, Di Maria et al 1986, Lifson & Rogers 1986, Sprecher et al 1986). Other possible sources of infection include contact with infected maternal secretions during delivery (Chiodo et al 1986) and breast milk (Ziegler et al 1985). HIV has been isolated from cervical secretions (Vogt et al 1986, Wofsy et al 1986) and there is one report of isolation of HIV from the non-cellular fraction of breast milk (Thirty et al 1985). These routes of infection, however, have not been substantiated. In Africa, postnatal acquisition of HIV infection in infancy has been associated with injections and blood transfusions but this appears to be less common than maternal transmission (Mann et al 1986a, 1986b). As there have been no published

prospective studies of children born to mothers with HIV infection, the rate of perinatal transmission is unknown.

A new dysmorphic syndrome has recently been described in children with symptomatic HIV infections (Marion et al 1986). This is probably related to viraemia in early fetal life but its prevalence among HIV-infected infants is not known.

Neurological features of HIV infection

While the initial reports of the clinical problems of children with HIV infection described severe infections resulting from a compromised immune system (Rubinstein et al 1983, Rogers 1985, Jones & Watson 1986, Rubenstein 1986), the neurological effects of HIV are now being increasingly recognized. There is evidence that the virus can cross the blood–brain barrier and replicate within the CNS. Invasion of the CNS may occur early in the infection and can be asymptomatic or associated with a meningitic syndrome or an acute self-limiting encephalopathy (Carne et al 1985, Carne & Adler 1986).

In one study there were six children with neurological problems who were presumed to have been infected perinatally and all of whom also had clinical AIDS (Belman et al 1985). The age at which neurological signs presented ranged from 6 to 36 months and the most frequent manifestations were acquired microcephaly, encephalopathy and pyramidal tract signs. Three had severe deterioration with dementia and died and three had delayed language and motor milestones, and cognitive impairment. Computed tomographic examination showed varying degrees of cortical atrophy with ventricular dilatation and calcification.

Another related study followed 7 children with AIDS aged from 6 months to 6 years and 9 children with AIDS-related complex (ARC) (Ultmann et al 1985). The acquisition of milestones, particularly motor, was delayed following the onset of AIDS or ARC. Several of the children with AIDS but none of those with ARC lost milestones as their illness developed and cognitive dysfunction became more marked. Although some children had clinical and radiological evidence of CNS involvement, developmental abnormalities in these children are likely to be multifactorial as many of them suffered from environmental deprivation and the adverse effects of prolonged hospital stays.

In another series, three of four children presented with a neurological disorder before any signs of immunodeficiency were apparent (Habibi et al 1986). All four showed regression of milestones after 12–18 months. One child had focal fits and developmental delay, another progressive spastic quadriplegia, and a third global retardation.

Epstein et al (1986) described 36 children, 10 of whom had received HIV-contaminated blood products. Sixteen of 21 with AIDS, 3 of 12 with ARC and 1 of 3 asymptomatic HIV-infected children developed a progressive encephalopathy. Poor outcome was associated with absence of serum neutralizing antibodies. The incubation period preceding onset of neurological symptoms in the perinatal cases was presumed to range from 2 months to 5 years. There was evidence that the encephalopathy resulted from primary, persistent HIV infection of the brain.

Diagnosis and management

A definitive diagnosis of HIV infection cannot be made serologically in the first 15 months of life because the presence of antibody may reflect maternal IgG. The typical immunological aberrations such as reverse T4 to T8 ratios seen in older children and adults are not often present at this age. A specific IgM assay is being developed but is not yet widely available and a definitive diagnosis of HIV in the neonate can only be made by cocultivation of the virus with a permissive cell line or by utilization of specific DNA probes to detect viral genome in lymphocytes. The sensitivity of this approach is not yet known (Parks & Scott 1985, Marion et al 1986).

There is currently no specific effective treatment for HIV infection. It is clear that any antiviral agent will have to cross the blood–brain barrier and that lifelong therapy may be necessary. Management depends on prevention, early diagnosis and treatment of opportunistic infections with special attention to nutritional needs. Major emotional, social and educational problems require practical guidelines including those relating to immunization (CDC 1985, 1986, DHSS 1986). Mothers should be advised against embarking on further pregnancies as there is a substantial risk of delivery of a second infected infant. Mothers known to be seropositive should be warned of a possible risk of transmission by breast milk, although the evidence for this mode of transmission has not been substantiated (Ziegler et al 1985). A general policy for advising against breast-feeding without adequate information could have serious consequences in countries where breast-feeding plays an important role in infant survival.

LYMPHOCYTIC CHORIOMENINGITIS VIRUS

Lymphocytic choriomeningitis virus (LCV) is acquired principally from rodents. Mice and hamsters have been the most frequently implicated sources of infection and apparently healthy animals may shed the virus in faeces and urine for months (Smadel & Wall 1942).

There have been reports of LCV infection in pregnancy associated either with abortion or hydrocephalus, and with chorioretinitis in surviving infants (Sheinbergas et al 1984, Sheinbergas 1976). Perinatal acquisition from a mother infected at full-term with resultant severe neonatal meningitis has also been described (Komrower et al 1955).

Although numbers of cases reported have been small, a diagnosis of congenital LCV should be considered in infants with hydrocephalus and/chorioretinitis, especially if there is a history of a severe influenza-like illness in pregnancy and/or of rodent contact. The diagnosis can be made by viral isolation or serology (Yeager 1983a).

ENTEROVIRUSES

The enteroviruses include polioviruses 1–3; echoviruses 1–34; coxsackie A 1–24; coxsackie B 1–6 and the recently identified enteroviruses 68–71.

Non-polio enteroviruses

Although transplacental transmission of echo and coxsackie viruses occurs, there is no published evidence of an association with central nervous system malformations. The importance of these enteroviral infections lies in their effects on the neonate. Enteroviral illness presenting in the first 5 days of life will almost certainly have been acquired from the mother, transplacentally or intranatally. Infections occurring later are likely to have been acquired from other babies or health care personnel, and outbreaks in hospital nurseries have been well documented.

Table 36.4 Laboratory reports of neonatal viral meningitis 1975–83

Organism	Type	No. cases	(% total)
Coxsackie A	7	1 } 8	
	9	7	
B	1	3	
	2	15	
	3	8 } 48	
	4	17	
	5	4	
	6	1	
Total Coxsackie		56	(36.4)
Echovirus	3	2	
	6	6	
	7	3	
	9	3	
	11	36	
	14	1	
	17	6	
	19	7	
	20	1	
	30	6	
Total Echovirus		69	(44.8)
Herpes simplex		15	(9.7)
Respiratory syncytial virus		1	
Influenza A		1	
Mycoplasma		3	
Rotavirus		2	
Adenovirus		1	
Cytomegalovirus		4	
Total		154	

Enteroviruses are the most common cause of neonatal viral meningitis (NNVM) in England and Wales (Table 36.4) (PHLS 1985). The incidence of NNVM is unknown but the annual number of cases in England and Wales reported by laboratories between 1975 and 1983 ranged from 4 to 40; NNVM accounted for 0.3 to 2.6% of viral meningitis reported at all ages with the higher proportion occurring in more recent years. North American data have also shown an unexplained downward trend in the age of children with enteroviral meningitis from the mid-1970s onwards (Lepow 1978, Sumaya & Corman 1982).

Figure 36.1 demonstrates the annual trends and prevalent serotypes in echovirus and coxsackie virus NNVM in England and Wales between 1975 and 1983. It was notable that these usually coincided with national epidemics of the same types. These epidemiological data have practical clinical significance because knowledge of a prevailing community enterovirus epidemic and of the current circulating type provides a valuable diagnostic aid (Wilfert et al 1983).

Clinical features and diagnosis

Enterovirus infections may be subclinical, mild and non-specific or may present with respiratory illness, gastroenteritis and myocarditis. All enterovirus types can invade the meninges and CNS although coxsackie B types are more likely to be the cause of encephalitis.

The clinical diagnosis of NNVM is difficult because the symptoms are non-specific and may resemble those of bacterial sepsis (Wilfert et al 1983). Fever, anorexia, lethargy, jaundice, vomiting and occasionally tremors, increased tone and seizures may occur. Cerebrospinal fluid (CSF) examination is not always helpful because the changes can overlap those of bacterial meningitis; for example

polymorphonuclear leukocytosis and and hypoglycorrhachia may be present. Diagnostic suspicion would be heightened if there was:

1. a recent pre- or post-partum maternal history of a mild non-specific febrile illness or one of the more characteristic enteroviral syndromes such as aseptic meningitis or hand, foot and mouth disease;
2. a history of such an illness in neonatal nursery staff, or family members;
3. a concurrent enteroviral epidemic in the nursery or community;
4. the season of onset in a temperate climate was in late summer or autumn (although these infections can occur all year round).

Laboratory diagnosis depends principally on virus isolation. The large number of possible serotypes and the need to examine acute and convalescent sera contemporaneously, mean that serological antibody studies are impractical. However, examination of paired sera may be useful in an outbreak where one particular prevalent enterovirus is suspected. Isolation of virus from CSF provides conclusive diagnostic evidence of NNVM but the organism may be present for only a short time (Spector & Straube 1983). It is important, therefore, to take specimens from multiple sites. Virus can be isolated from nose, throat, urine and buffy coat, but excretion persists for the longest time in stools.

Management and prevention

Management of NNVM and encephalitis is mainly non-specific and directed towards correction, where appropriate, of fever, fluid and electrolyte balance, convulsions and cerebral oedema (Cherry 1983). Human normal immuno-globulin (HNIG) has been used both for therapy and prevention in outbreaks of echovirus 11 infection in neonatal nurseries (Nagington et al 1983). The effectiveness of this has been questioned and may depend on the titre of the appropriate neutralizing antibody in the HNIG and on its early administration (Kinney et al 1986).

As non-polio enteroviral vaccines are not available, prevention of NNVM is directed towards control of spread of infection (Cherry 1983, Kinney et al 1986). Any hospitalized infant with known or suspected enterovirus infection should be isolated and strict enteric precautions taken. Staff and parents should not enter the nursery if they develop a feverish illness. In nosocomial outbreaks, cohorting of infants and personnel should be undertaken.

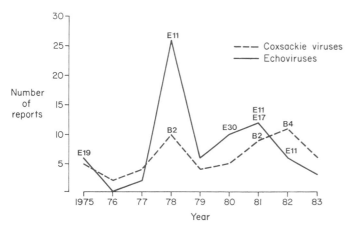

Fig. 36.1 Laboratory reports of neonates with viral meningitis for the years 1975–83. Where the type is indicated there have been four or more reports of that type in a one-year period. (Prepared by Communicable Disease Surveillance Center.)

Neurological sequelae

Enteroviral meningitis acquired early in infancy may result in long-term neurodevelopmental sequelae. It is difficult to compare results of different follow-up studies because some are uncontrolled (Nakao 1970), some are restricted to infection acquired in the neonatal period (Farmer et al 1975) while others include infection acquired at any time during the first year of life (Sells et al 1975, Wilfert et al 1981, Chamberlain et al 1983). Different viral types, degrees of severity of the initial illnesses, lengths of follow-up and methods of assessment of neurological and developmental outcome also make comparison difficult.

In a 6-year follow-up study of neonatally acquired coxsackie B meningoencephalitis, two of three infants with neurological symptoms during their acute illness had severe neurodevelopmental sequelae whereas the physical development, intelligence and visual perception of the 12 without such symptoms was similar to the controls (Farmer et al 1975). In another study, 45 of 48 survivors of infant viral meningitis (40 enteroviral) followed for more than 5 years were in normal schools but their mean performance IQ was 6 points lower than that of the matched controls (Chamberlain et al 1983). Although this difference was statistically significant its practical significance is questionable. The other three survivors had severe sequelae but only one had had an enteroviral infection. In a third controlled study of infants infected in the first 3 months of life and followed for 4 years there were no differences in IQ but their receptive language functioning was significantly lower than the controls (Wilfert et al 1981). This substantiated an earlier study in which delayed language and speech development was the only consistent problem observed (Sells et al 1975).

Although the evidence for long-term sequelae is conflicting it seems reasonable to conclude that children with a history of NNVM/encephalitis merit careful surveillance in their preschool years.

Poliovirus infection

Paralytic poliomyelitis is still a major public health problem in much of the developed world. In countries with high uptake rates of polio vaccine, however, epidemic paralytic poliomyelitis is no longer seen although sporadic cases of both wild and vaccine-associated disease (VAD) continue to be reported (Bell et al 1986, Begg et al 1987). The incidence of neonatal poliomyelitis in the prevaccine era and currently in those parts of the world where the infection is still endemic is not known. It is thought to be uncommon because of protection provided by maternal polioviral antibodies. Of 182 cases of paralytic disease admitted to hospital during an epidemic in Delhi in 1971, the youngest was 2 months but the 7 to 12 month group accounted for one-third of all the cases (Sehgal & Oberoi 1977). Nevertheless, paralytic poliomyelitis presenting in the first month of life and acquired perinatally is well documented (Bates 1955, Sathy et al 1984).

Clinical features, diagnosis and management

There is no evidence to suggest that transplacentally transmitted poliovirus causes malformations (Cherry 1983). Furthermore, while live virus vaccine is contra-indicated in pregnancy there is no evidence that polio vaccine causes fetal malformations or neonatal disease (Cherry 1983), although a recent report described irreparable damage to the anterior horn cells of a 20-week-old fetus whose mother was immune to poliomyelitis before conceiving, but who was inadvertently given oral polio vaccine (OPV) at 18 weeks of gestation (Burton et al 1984).

Poliomyelitis presenting in the first 5 days of life is likely to have been acquired transplacentally or intranatally. It has been estimated that the risk of an infant developing the infection when born to a woman with clinical disease at delivery is 40% (Wyatt 1979). Although asymptomatic neonatal infection probably occurs, most case reports describe severe disease resulting in death or residual paralysis. Fever, listlessness, dysphagia and flaccid paralysis should suggest the diagnosis which can be confirmed by viral isolation. Non-polio enteroviruses should be excluded as coxsackie B and enterovirus 71 can also cause paralytic disease (Cherry 1983, Chonmaitree et al 1981).

Management and prevention are as described for the non-polio enteroviruses with the addition of positive-pressure ventilation if respiratory paralysis occurs. Survivors will require a full course of immunization against poliomyelitis because the serotype with which they have been infected does not prevent subsequent infection with the other two.

Neonatal poliomyelitis immunization has been introduced in countries where the incidence of paralytic disease in infants is high (John 1984, 1985). Vaccine-associated disease in a neonate was first described in 1986 in a report of a child who developed apnoea at 18 days and subsequent permanent monoparesis (Bergeisen et al 1986). Serology and culture confirmed infection with a vaccine strain of poliovirus. The probable source was a one-year-old infant who had been given OPV 34 days previously and who had had diarrhoea. This case report illustrates the need for continued diagnostic vigilance for paralytic poliomyelitis even in developed countries.

PROTOZOAL INFECTIONS

Toxoplasma gondii and the *Trypanosoma cruzi, gambiense* and *rhodesiense* are two species of protozoa known to infect the fetus and neonate and to cause neurological sequelae directly related to invasion of the nervous system. Infections are characterized by transplacental rather than neonatal acquisition and by persistence of infection with continued tissue destruction. Toxoplasmosis is a common, world-wide infection whereas trypanosomiasis, although common, is restricted to parts of Central and South America and Africa.

TOXOPLASMOSIS

Although the highest population rates of *T. gondii* infection recorded in seroprevalence surveys occur in Central America, toxoplasmosis is also common in industrialized nations. In the USA and UK just over half of the population have acquired antibody by middle age (Feldman 1982, Fleck 1969). In France, and to a lesser extent Austria, infection is acquired more rapidly in childhood and adolescence and only 20% of women embarking on pregnancy are susceptible. Indeed, in Paris 96% of pregnant women aged over 35 years were seropositive in one study (Remington & Desmonts 1983).

Although *T. gondii* was first described in 1908 it was not until 1969, with the discovery of the oocyst, that plausible hypotheses could be generated about its mode of transmission (Hutchinson et al 1969). Even now the precise mode of acquisition is not well understood although the infection is thought to be associated with the consumption of raw or undercooked meat or with contact with the faeces of cats who have recently acquired toxoplasma (Hall 1986).

Transplacental infection with toxoplasma probably occurs during the phase of maternal parasitaemia and the organism is unlikely to be acquired intranatally or in the neonatal period. Experimental work has demonstrated the tachyzoite stage of the parasite in milk of infected animals and the offspring can be infected from this source (Pettersen 1984). There is only one report of postnatally acquired infection in a 7-month-old infant where circumstantial evidence implicated goat's milk (Reimen et al 1975).

Although a severely affected infant who had been exposed to maternal toxoplasma infection around the time of conception was recently described (Haentjens et al 1986), the risk of fetal infection is thought (but not proven) to be negligible following reactivated toxoplasmosis among women with evidence of previous infection. France and Austria have national antenatal serological screening programmes for the prevention of congenital toxoplasmosis (CT), the organization of which is based on this precept. However, an open mind should be kept about the role of reactivated infection, especially in women on immunosuppressive therapy, since a diagnosis of CT may not otherwise be considered if the mother is known to be seropositive before pregnancy.

Prospective serological studies show that the incidence of CT varies in different populations, ranging from 1 per 1000 livebirths in Norway to 6 to 7 per 1000 in Vienna (Remington & Desmonts 1983). It is, however, difficult to compare and interpret results from these surveys because of the different ways in which subjects were recruited, followed up and examined. The current incidence of CT in the UK is unknown and only two prospective studies have been undertaken. In London in the 1960s a seroconversion rate of 3 per 1000 pregnancies was reported although none of the 7 affected pregnancies resulted in congenital infection (Ruoss & Bourne 1972). In Scotland in the mid-1970s an incidence of about 0.5 per 1000 livebirths was reported and 3 children were born with CT (Williams et al 1981). In an epidemiological study of symptomatic cases under the age of 4 years reported by reference laboratories for England and Wales for the period 1975 to 1980, only 34 satisfied the diagnostic criteria of CT (Hall 1983).

Women who acquire toxoplasma in pregnancy do not necessarily transmit the infection to the fetus. The only studies relating risk of transmission to stage of pregnancy are from Paris (Remington & Desmonts 1983). The overall transmission rate from mother to infant was 33% but this increased from 14% in the first trimester to 29% in the second and 59% in the third. The risk of severe damage to the fetus was, however, inversely related to the gestational age at acquisition.

Clinical features of congenital toxoplasmosis

Approximately 80–90% of cases of CT are asymptomatic. The 'classic triad' of hydrocephalus, chorioretinitis and intracranial calcification presenting at birth is extremely rare and only 4 such cases were reported in England and Wales between 1975 and 1980 (Hall 1983). In addition to the individual components of the classic triad, a wide variety of non-specific clinical manifestations may occur, including prematurity, dysmaturity, convulsions, hypotonia, jaundice, hepatosplenomegaly, thrombocytopenia and CSF lymphocytosis with elevated protein.

Although hydrocephalus is seen more frequently than microcephaly, the latter can occur in CT. The hydrocephalus, which is of the obstructive type and usually progressive, may be the only clinical manifestation of CT. Chorioretinitis associated with CT may be present at birth in infants who are symptomatic and in those who are otherwise clinically normal (Remington & Desmonts 1983). It may also appear later in life in individuals whose fundi were normal in the neonatal period (Hogan et al 1957, Wilson et al 1980a, Koppe et al 1986).

Follow-up studies of CT are often difficult to interpret. This is due to: the inclusion of cases diagnosed retrospectively so that postnatally acquired infection cannot be excluded, inadequately matched controls, small numbers, the inclusion of treated cases, bias towards symptomatic cases, and inadequate length of follow-up. In the largest follow-up series of untreated infants with symptomatic CT (Eichenwald 1960), 85% were mentally retarded by 5 years of age, 75% had neurological handicap and 50% had impaired vision. Although most infants with CT are asymptomatic, it appears from long-term follow-up studies that a high proportion of this group, like the symptomatic group, will eventually develop sequelae. The most common sequela is chorioretinitis causing serious visual impairment. In a Dutch series, examination at 20 years of age revealed that 9 of 11 individuals in whom CT had been diagnosed at birth (6 were asymptomatic) had developed scars in one or both eyes; 4 had seriously impaired vision and 3 uni-ocular blindness (Koppe et al 1986). In one, the first attack of chorioretinitis was at 18 years. In a North American study, 11 of 13 children with asymptomatic CT at birth developed chorioretinitis at ages ranging from 1 month to 9.3 years (Wilson et al 1980). Three children had unilateral blindness and the remainder had temporarily decreased vision during the episodes, which were often recurrent. These two follow-up studies differed in that there were no significant neurological abnormalities among the Dutch children but in the American series 5 of 13 developed neurological sequelae, although only one was seriously impaired.

The role of asymptomatic CT as a cause of mental retardation is not clear. Only one controlled study, where the cases were prospectively identified, has been published (Saxon et al 1973). This comprised 8 children, 3 of whom had been treated. An average IQ reduction (Slosson Intelligence Test for Children and Adults) of 17 points was recorded among the 5 untreated cases compared with their controls. CT is not usually considered to be a significant cause of sensorineural deafness (Remington & Desmonts 1983) although well-documented cases associated with severe clinical disease have been reported (Eichenwald 1960).

Diagnosis

The diagnosis of congenital toxoplasmosis is often problematic because of the late presentation of sequelae. If a diagnosis of CT is first considered outside infancy it is not possible to distinguish congenital from acquired disease serologically. Other difficulties include the non-specificity of clinical features which are shared by other congenital and neonatal infections and non-infectious conditions. The chorioretinitis of CT is said to be indistinguishable from that of congenital CMV (Hanshaw 1983) and difficult to differentiate from that associated with herpes or congenital syphilis. It is quite unlike the 'salt and pepper' retinopathy of congenital rubella. Although congenital CMV is more common than CT, chorioretinitis is thought to be an extremely rare finding in infants with congenital CMV. This observation, coupled with the extreme rarity of congenital syphilis and neonatal herpes in developed countries should suggest a diagnosis of CT in neonates with chorioretinitis. In CT the intracranial calcifications, like those of HSV infection but unlike those of congenital CMV, are scattered throughout the brain. Intracerebral calcification is not characteristic of congenital rubella or congenital syphilis.

The laboratory diagnosis of CT includes isolation of *T. gondii* from blood or body fluids, histological demonstration of tissue cysts in the placenta or infant, and measurement of specific antibodies. Isolation of the parasite from a

neonate, or histological identification of tissue cysts provide conclusive proof of congenital infection. Parasitaemia can be demonstrated in cord blood or in peripheral blood taken in the first 4 weeks of life in nearly 50% of infants with CT, including asymptomatic cases. Results may, however, not be available for up to 6 weeks.

Serological diagnosis of CT depends on the identification of specific IgM antibody in cord or neonatal blood. Because of the relative insensitivity of toxoplasma IgM assays, the sequential measurement of IgG for at least the first year of life is necessary to demonstrate changes in titre that would differentiate passively acquired maternal antibody and fetal infection. In practice this follow-up serology is rarely done and in an analysis of 'TORCH' requests on infants under 6 months repeat serology was requested in only 9% of cases with positive titres (Leland et al 1983).

The immunofluorescent antibody (IFA) toxoplasma IgM test is only positive in about 25% of sera taken in the first 4 weeks of life from infants with CT, while the IgM ELISA and IgM immunosorbent agglutination assay (ISAGA) both have similar sensitivities of around 80% (Desmonts et al 1981, Naot et al 1981). False-positive results due to cross-reaction with rheumatoid factor and/or antinuclear antibodies may occur with the IgM IFA test but not with IgM ELISA or IgM ISAGA. Regardless of the IgM assay method used, therefore, it is essential that the infant's IgG levels are monitored. This is best done by the Sabin–Feldman dye test which is the definitive reference test for toxoplasma IgG and which alone has sufficient accuracy for the precise quantitative results necessary for the diagnosis of CT. This test is expensive, however, requires special expertise and is often restricted to a few specialized laboratories. ELISA technology for IgG measurement is increasingly available and has a high sensitivity and specificity (Balfour & Harford 1985). Infected infants whose mothers acquired their infection near to delivery may have very low or even absent IgG in cord blood (Remington & Desmonts 1983). Since these late congenital infections are usually clinically 'silent' they are also likely to remain undiagnosed until the first episode of chorioretinitis occurs in later life.

The prenatal management of CT depends on identifying acute infection in pregnancy and then, at least in France, on establishing fetal infection by amniocentesis and fetal blood sampling (Desmonts et al 1985). The antenatal diagnosis of toxoplasmosis raises issues about serological screening programmes which require detailed consideration before they are adopted on a national scale as in France and Austria (Hall 1986, Henderson et al 1984).

Treatment in pregnancy with spiramycin has been most extensively evaluated in France and the data, although needing cautious interpretation because of limitations of study design, suggest that fewer infected babies are born to treated than to non-treated women (Desmonts 1982). Therapy, however, may pose a diagnostic problem in the neonate who should be treated as if CT had been first diagnosed postnatally, especially if there is suspicion of infection from the clinical features and/or from examination of placenta or cord blood.

There are only limited data on the value of treatment for CT diagnosed in the first year of life (Wilson et al 1980b, Remington & Desmonts 1983). Studies have suffered from small numbers, lack of case-control and random allocation of treatment and lack of long-term follow-up. Data suggest that treatment may decrease the frequency and severity of adverse sequelae and it is therefore advocated for all definite cases of CT whether symptomatic or not, as well as in certain circumstances for suspected cases. The wisdom of treating infants with toxic drugs where there is diagnostic doubt and where there is only limited evidence of efficiency has to be questioned. However, in view of the serious and seemingly almost inevitable sequelae of CT it is likely that most clinicians would be reluctant to withhold therapy until further evidence on efficacy has accumulated.

Drugs, dosages and different regimens appropriate for various situations have been described in detail by Remington & Desmonts (1983). In summary, alternate courses of 21 days of pyrimethamine + sulphadiazine with folinic acid and 30–45 days of spiramycin are recommended throughout the first year of life. Twice-weekly peripheral blood cell and platelet counts are necessary during the pyrimethamine courses. Supplementation with corticosteroids is also suggested where there are signs of inflammation such as chorioretinitis, high CSF protein, generalized infection, and jaundice. Treatment is not continued routinely after the first 12 months although it may be reinstated during exacerbations of eye and CNS disease (McCabe & Remington 1983), when pyrimethamine and sulphadiazine plus folinic acid are recommended, for at least one month with repeat courses if necessary. Systemic steroids are indicated if vision is endangered by lesions involving the macula or optic nerve head.

It is important to follow treated infants serologically for several years because treatment has been reported to result in negative IgG antibody levels by the end of the first year and it may be wrongly suspected that the diagnosis of CT was made in error. Follow-up of these children has shown a resurgence of IgG levels after the first year (Couvreur 1982).

TRYPANOSOMIASIS

Congenital infection with both forms of African trypanosomiasis (*gambiense* and *rhodesiense*) and with the South American *Trypanosoma cruzi* has been described (Yeager 1983b, Lingam et al 1985). The frequency of congenital infection in endemic areas is not known but the condition is thought to be relatively rare.

Infants congenitally infected with *T. cruzi* may have the typical features of Chagas disease seen in adults, sometimes accompanied by encephalitis associated with hypotonia, poor suck and seizures. A progressive neurodegenerative disorder in a previously normal infant has been described in congenital *T. gambiense* infection (Lingam et al 1985). This child was born in the UK which illustrates the need for diagnostic vigilance in infants with progressive neurological disorders born to mothers who have lived in endemic zones.

Diagnosis is confirmed by isolation of the parasite from the infant's blood although serological tests are also available. The effectiveness of treatment (with suramin and melarsoprol for African trypanosomiasis, nisurtimox for Chagas disease) is unknown; a parasitological 'cure' may be achieved with little effect on clinical outcome.

REFERENCES

Adler S P, Chandrika T, Lawrence L, Baggett J 1983 Cytomegalovirus infections in neonates acquired by blood transfusions. Pediatric Infectious Disease 2: 114–118

Ahlfors K, Ivarsson S, Johnsson T, Svanberg L 1979 A prospective study on congenital and acquired cytomegalovirus infections in infants. Scandinavian Journal of Infectious Diseases 11: 177–178

Ahlfors K, Harris S, Ivarsson S, Svanberg L 1981 Secondary maternal cytomegalovirus infection causing symptomatic congenital infection. New England Journal of Medicine 305: 284

Arvin A M, Yeager A S, Bruhn F W, Grossman M 1982 Neonatal herpes simplex infection in the absence of mucocutaneous lesions. Journal of Pediatrics 100: 715–721

Balfour A H, Harford J P 1985 Detection of specific IgM antibodies to *Toxoplasma gondii* with a commercially available enzyme immunoassay kit system. Journal of Clinical Pathology 38: 679–689

Ballard R A, Drew W L, Hutnagle K 1979 Cytomegalovirus infection in preterm infants. American Journal of Diseases of Children 133: 482–485

Barnes P M, Wheldon D B, Eggerding C, Marshall W C, Leonard J V 1982 Hyperammonaemia and disseminated herpes simplex infection in the neonatal period. Lancet i: 1362–1363

Bates T 1955 Polio in pregnancy, the fetus and the newborn. American Journal of Diseases of Children 90: 189–195

Begg N T, Roebuck M O, Chamberlain R N 1987 Paralytic poliomyelitis in England and Wales 1970–84. Epidemiology & Infection. 99: 97–106

Bell E J, Riding M H, Grist N R 1986 Paralytic poliomyelitis: a forgotten diagnosis? British Medical Journal 293: 193–194

Belman A L, Ultmann M H, Horoupian D et al 1985 Neurological complications in infants and children with acquired immune deficiency syndrome. Annals of Neurology 18(5): 560–566

Bergeisen G H, Bauman R J, Gilmore R L 1986 Neonatal paralytic poliomyelitis. Archives of Neurology 43: 192–194

Bond P R, Caul E O, Usher J, Cohen B J, Clewley J P, Field A M 1986 Intrauterine infection with human parvovirus. Lancet i: 448–449

Bradford Hill A, Doll R, Galloway T M, Hughes J P 1958 Virus diseases in pregnancy and congenital defects. British Journal of Preventive and Social Medicine 12: 1–7

Bray P F, Bale J F, Anderson R E 1981 Progressive neurological disease with cytomegalovirus infection. Annals of Neurology 9: 449–502

Brazin S A, Simkowich J W, Johnson T 1979 Herpes zoster during pregnancy. Obstetrics and Gynecology 513: 175–181

Brunell P A 1967 Varicella zoster infections in pregnancy. Journal of the American Medical Association 199: 315–317

Burton A E, Robinson E T, Harper W F 1984 Fetal damage after accidental polio vaccination of an immune mother. Journal of the Royal College of General Practitioners 34: 390–393

Carne C A, Adler M W 1986 Neurological manifestations of human immunodeficiency virus infection. British Medical Journal 293: 462–463

Carne C A, Smith A, Elkington S G et al 1985 Acute encephalopathy coincident with seroconversion for anti-HTLV-III. Lancet ii: 1206–1208

CDC (Centers for Disease Control) 1985 Education and foster care of children infected with human T-Lymphotropic virus type III/ Lymphadenopathy-associated virus. Morbidity & Mortality Weekly Report 34(34): 517–521

CDC 1986 Rubella and congenital rubella syndrome — United States 1984–1985. Morbidity & Mortality Weekly Report 35: 129–135

CDC 1986 Immunization of children infected with human T-lymphotropic virus type III/lymphadenopathy-associated virus. Morbidity & Mortality Weekly Report 35(38): 1–3

CDC 1987 Acquired immunodeficiency Syndrome (AIDS). Weekly Surveillance Report, United States Aids Program, Jan 12

Chamberlain R N, Christie P N, Holt K S 1983 A study of school children who had identified virus infections of the central nervous system during infancy. Child Care, Health and Development 9: 29–47

Cherry J D 1983 Enteroviruses. In: Remington J S, Klein J (eds) Infectious diseases of the fetus and newborn infant. W B Saunders, Philadelphia, pp 290–335

Chess S 1971 Autism in children with congenital rubella. Journal of Autism and Childhood Schizophrenia 1: 33–47

Chiodo F, Ricchi E, Costigliola P 1986 Vertical transmission of HTLV-III. Lancet i: 739

Chonmaitree T, Menegus M A, Schervish-Swierkosz E M, Schwalenstocker B A 1981 Enterovirus 71 infection: report of an outbreak with two cases of paralysis and a review of the literature. Pediatrics 67(4): 489–492

Committee on Fetus and Newborn 1980 Perinatal herpes simplex virus infection. Pediatrics 66: 147–148

Conboy T, Pass R, Stagno S, Britt W 1986 Intellectual development in school-aged children with asymptomatic congenital cytomegalovirus infection. Pediatrics 77: 801–806

Corey L, Spear P G 1986 Infections with herpes simplex viruses. New England Journal of Medicine 314: 749–757

Couvreur J 1982 Congenital toxoplasmosis: the diagnosis (Colloque international sur l'immunologie dans la toxoplasmose). Lyon Medical, Fondation Marcel Merieux (Suppl Nov 15) 248: 125–132

Dahle A J, McCollister F P, Stagno S, Reynolds D W, Koffman H E 1979 Progressive hearing impairment in children with congenital cytomegalovirus infection. Journal of Speech and Hearing Disorders 44: 220–229

Daffos F et al 1984 Prenatal diagnosis of congenital rubella. Lancet ii: 1–3

Davis G L 1981 In vitro models of viral-induced congenital deafness. American Journal of Otolaryngology 3: 156–160

Desmond M M, Wilson G S, Melrick J J et al 1967 Congenital rubella encephalitis. Journal of Pediatrics 71: 311–331

Desmonts G 1982 Acquired toxoplasmosis in pregnant women: evaluation of the frequency of transmission of toxoplasma and of congenital toxoplasmosis (Colloque international sur l'immunologie dans la toxoplasmose. Lyon Medical, Foundation Marcel Merieux (Suppl Nov 15) 248: 115–124

Desmonts G, Yehudith N, Remington J S 1981 Immunoglobulin M-immunosorbent agglutination assay for diagnosis of infectious diseases: diagnosis of acute congenital and acquired toxoplasma infections. Journal of Clinical Microbiology 14(5): 486–491

Desmonts G, Daffos F, Forestier F, Capella-Pavlovsky M, Thulliez P, Chartier M 1985 Prenatal diagnosis of congenital toxoplasmosis. Lancet i: 500–504

DHSS (Department of Health and Social Security) 1970 Circular 9/70

DHSS 1986 Children at school and problems related to AIDS. HMSO, London

Di Maria H, Courpotin C, Rouzioux C, Cohen D, Rio D, Boussin F 1986 Transplacental transmission of human immunodeficiency virus. Lancet ii: 215–216

Dinwiddie et al 1987 Personal communication

Dudgeon J A 1976 Congenital rubella. Journal of Pediatrics 87: 1078–1086

Dudgeon J A 1976 Congenital rubella. British Medical Bulletin 32: 77–83

Dunkle L M, Schmidt R R, O'Connor D M 1979 Neonatal herpes simplex infection possibly acquired via maternal breast milk. Pediatrics 63: 250–251

Dworsky M, Whitley R, Alford C 1980 Herpes zoster in early infancy. American Journal of Diseases of Children 134: 618–619

Eichenwald H 1960 A study of congenital toxoplasmosis. In: Siim J C (ed) Human toxoplasmosis. Munskgaard, Copenhagen, pp 41–49

Enders G 1985 Varicella zoster virus infection in pregnancy. Progress in Medical Virology 29:166–196

Epstein L G, Leroy R, Sharer L R et al 1986 Neurological manifestations of human immunodeficiency virus infection. Pediatrics 78: 678–687

Farmer K, MacArthur B A, Clay M M 1975 A follow-up study of 15 cases of neonatal meningoencephalitis due to Coxsackie virus B5. Journal of Pediatrics 87(4): 568–571

Feldman H A 1982 Epidemiology of toxoplasma infections. Epidemiologic Reviews 4: 204–213

Fleck D G 1969 Toxoplasmosis. Public Health 83:131–135

Florman A L, Gershon A A, Blackett P R, Nahmias A J 1973 Intrauterine infection with herpes simplex virus: resultant congenital malformations. Journal of the American Medical Association 225: 129–132

Francis D P, Herrmann K L, MacMahon J H, Cahavigny K H, Saunderlin M S 1975 Nosocomial and maternally acquired herpes virus hominis infections. American Journal of Diseases of Children 129: 889–893

Garcia A G P 1963 Fetal infection in chickenpox and alastrim, with histopathologic study of the placenta. Pediatrics 32: 895–901

Gershon A A 1975 Varicella in mother and infant: problems old and new. In: Krugman S, Gershon A A (eds) Infections of the fetus and the newborn infant. AR Liss, New York pp 79–95

Grilner L, Forsgren M, Barr B, Böttiger M, Danielsson L, De Verdier C 1983 Outcome of rubella during pregnancy with special reference to the 17th–24th weeks of gestation. Scandinavian Journal of Infectious Diseases 15: 321–325

Habibi P, Morgan G, Strobel S et al 1986 Clinical features of AIDS in children. Archives of Disease in Childhood 61: 627 (Abstract)

Haentjens M, Sacre L, Demeuter F 1986 Congenital toxoplasmosis after maternal infection before or slightly after conception. Acta Paediatrica Scandinavica 75: 343–345

Hall S M 1983 Congenital toxoplasmosis in England, Wales and Northern Ireland: some epidemiological problems. British Medical Journal 287: 453–455

Hall S M 1986 Toxoplasmosis. British Journal of Small Animal Practice 27: 705–717

Hammerberg O, Watts J, Chernesky M, Luchsinger I, Rawls W 1983 An outbreak of herpes simplex type 1 in an intensive care nursery. Pediatric Infectious Disease 290–294

Hanshaw J B 1983 Cytomegalovirus. In: Remington J S, Klein J (eds) Infectious diseases of the fetus and newborn infant. W B Saunders, Philadelphia, pp 104–142

Hanshaw J B, Dudgeon J A, Marshall W C 1985 Congenital cytomegalovirus. In: Viral diseases of the fetus and newborn. W B Saunders, W A, pp 92–131

Hanshaw J B, Dudgeon J A 1978 Congenital cytomegalovirus. In: Major problems in clinical paediatrics. 17: 97–152

Hanshaw J, Scheiner A, Moxley A, Gaev L, Avel V, Scheiner B 1976 School failure and deafness after 'silent' congenital cytomegalovirus infection. New England Journal of Medicine 295: 468–470

Hatherley L I, Hayes K, Hennessy E M, Jack I 1980a Herpesvirus in an obstetric hospital. I. Herpetic eruptions. Medical Journal of Australia ii: 205–208

Hatherley L I, Hayes K, Jack I 1980b Herpesvirus in an obstetric hospital. II. Asymptomatic virus excretion in staff members. Medical Journal of Australia ii: 273–275

Hayes K, Danks D M, Gila S H, Jack I 1972 Cytomegalovirus in human milk. New England Journal of Medicine 287: 177–178

Haywood A M 1986 Patterns of persistent viral infections. New England Journal of Medicine 315(15): 939–948

Henderson J B, Beattie C P, Hale E G, Wright T 1984 The evaluation of new services: possibilities for prevention of congenital toxoplasmosis. International Journal of Epidemiology 13: 65–72

Hogan M J, Kimura S J, Lewis A, Zweigart P A 1957 Early and delayed ocular manifestations of congenital toxoplasmosis. Transactions of the American Ophthalmology Society 55: 275–296

Hutchinson W M, Dunachie J F, Siim J C, Work K 1969 Life cycle of *Toxoplasma gondii*. British Medical Journal 4: 806

John T J 1984 Immune response of neonates to oral poliomyelitis vaccine. British Medical Journal 289: 881

John T J 1985 Polio vaccination of the newborn. Indian Journal of Pediatrics 52: 385–391

Johnson R T 1968 Hydrocephalus following viral infection: the pathology of aqueductal stenosis developing after experimental mumps virus infection. Journal of Neuropathology and Experimental Neurology 27: 591–606

Johnson R T 1975 Progressive rubella encephalitis. New England Journal of Medicine 292: 1023–1024

Jones P, Watson J G 1986 AIDS. In: Meadow R (ed) Recent advances in paediatrics. Churchill Livingstone, Edinburgh, pp 1–21

Jovaisas E, Koch M A, Schafer A, Stauber M, Lowenthal D 1985 LAV/HTLV-III in 20-week fetus. Lancet ii: 1129

Kilbrick S 1980 What to do with mother, newborn and nursery personnel. Journal of the American Medical Association 243: 157–160

Kinney J S, McCray E, Kaplan J E 1986 Risk factors associated with echovirus II infection in a hospital nursery. Paediatric Infectious Disease 5(2):192–197

Kleinman M B, Schreiner R L, Eitzen H, Lemons J A, Jansen R D 1982 Oral herpesvirus infection in nursery personnel: infection control policy. Pediatrics 70: 609–612

Knott P D, Welply G A C 1984 Serologically proved intrauterine infection with parvovirus. British Medical Journal 289: 1660

Komorous J M, Wheeler C E, Briggamann R A 1977 Intrauterine herpes simplex infections. Archives of Dermatology 113: 918–922

Komrower G M, Williams B L, Stones P B 1955 Lymphocytic choriomeningitis in the newborn. Lancet i: 697–698

Koppe J G, Loewer-Sieger D H, De Roever-Bonnet H 1986 Results of 20-year follow-up of congenital toxoplasmosis. Lancet i: 254–255

Kumar M L. Nankervis G A, Jacobs I B et al 1984 Congenital and postnatally acquired cytomegalovirus infection: long-term follow up. Journal of Pediatrics 104: 674–679

Laforet E G, Lynch C L 1947 Multiple congenital defects following maternal varicella: report of a case. New England Journal of Medicine 236: 534–537

Lancet (Editorial) Herpes simplex — changing patterns. Lancet ii: 1025–1026

Lapointe N, Michaud, J, Pekovic D, Chausseau J P, Dupuy J M 1985 Transplacental transmission of HTLV-III virus. New England Journal of Medicine 312: 1325–1326

Leland D, French M L V, Kleiman M B, Schriener L 1983 The use of TORCH titers. Pediatrics 72: 41–43

Lepow L 1978 Enteroviral meningitis: a reappraisal. Pediatrics 62: 267–269

Lifson A R, Rogers M F 1986 Vertical transmission of human immunodeficiency virus. Lancet ii: 337 (letter)

Light I J 1979 Postnatal acquisition of herpes simplex virus by the newborn infant: a review of the literature. Pediatrics 63: 480–482

Lingam S, Marshall W C, Wilson J, Gould J M, Reinhardt M C, Evans D A 1985 Congenital trypanosomiasis in a child born in London. Developmental Medicine and Child Neurology 27: 664–674

Linneman C C, Buchman T G, Light I J, Ballard J L 1978 Transmission of herpes simplex virus type I in a nursery for the newborn: identification of viral isolates by DNA 'fingerprinting'. Lancet i: 964–966

McCabe R E, Remington J S 1983 The diagnosis and treatment of toxoplasmosis. European Journal of Clinical Microbiology 1983: 95–104

McCracken G H, Shinefield M R, Cobb K, Raunsen A R, Dische M R, Eichenwald M F 1969 Congenital cytomegalic inclusion disease: a longitudinal study of 20 patients. American Journal of Diseases of Children 117: 522–539

MacDonald H, Tobin J O 1978 Congenital cytomegalovirus infection: a collaborative study on epidemiological, clinical and laboratory findings. Developmental Medicine and Child Neurology 20: 471–482

Mann J M, Francis H, Davachi F, Quinn T C 1986a Risk factors for human immunodeficiency virus seropositivity among children 1–24 months old in Kinshasa, Zaire. Lancet ii: 654–657

Mann J M, Francis H, Davochi F et al 1986b Human immunodeficiency virus seroprevalance in pediatric patients 2 to 14 yrs of age at Mama Yemo hospital, Kinshasa, Zaire. Pediatrics 78(4): 673–677

Manson M M, Logan W P O, Loy R M 1960 Rubella and other virus infections in pregnancy. Reports on Public Health and Medical Subjects, No. 101. London, HMSO

Marion R W, Wiznia A A, Hutcheon R G, Rubinstein A 1986 Human T-cell lymphotropic virus type III (HTLV-III) embryopathy. American Journal of Diseases of Children 140: 638–640

Marshall W C 1973 The clinical impact of intrauterine rubella. In: Intrauterine infections. Ciba Foundation, 10 (new series). Associated Scientific Publishers (Elsevier Excerpta Medica, North Holland), Amsterdam, pp 3–22

Martin J A M, Moore W J 1979 Childhood deafness in the European Community. Medicine EUR 6413. Commission of the European Communities, Luxembourg

Meyers J D 1974 Congenital varicella in term infants: risk reconsidered. Journal of Infectious Diseases 129: 215–217

Miller E, Craddock-Watson J E, Pollock T M 1982 Consequences of confirmed maternal rubella at successive stages of pregnancy. Lancet 2: 781–784

Miller E, Hopkinson W M, Cradock-Watson J E, Ridehalgh M K S 1986 Use of anti-varicella zoster immunoglobulin for the prevention of chickenpox in neonates and pregnant women. Public Health Laboratory Service, CDR 86–14

Myers E N, Stool S 1968 Cytomegalic inclusion disease of the inner ear. Laryngoscope 78: 1904–1915

Nagington J, Walker J, Candy G et al 1983 Use of normal immunoglobulin in an Ecovirus 11 outbreak in a special care baby unit. Lancet ii: 443–446

Nahmias A J, Alford C A, Korones S B 1970 Infections of the newborn with herpes virus hominis. Advances in Pediatrics 17: 185–226

Nahmias A J, Josey W E, Naib Z M, Freeman M 1971 Perinatal risk associated with maternal genital herpes simplex virus infection. American Journal of Obstetrics and Gynecology 110: 825–828

Nahmias A J, Keyserling H H, Kerick G 1983 Herpes simplex. In: Remington J S, Klein J O (eds) Infectious diseases of the fetus and newborn infant. W B Saunders, Philadelphia pp 156–190

Nakao T 1970 Prognosis of aseptic meningitis. Developmental Medicine and Child Neurology 12: 680

Naot Y, Desmonts G, Remington J S 1981 IgM enzyme-linked immunosorbent assay test for the diagnosis of congenital toxoplasma infection. Journal of Pediatrics 98: 32–36

Parks W P, Scott G B 1985 Pediatric AIDS: a disease spectrum causally associated with HTLV-III infection. Cancer Research 45: 4659–4661

Parvey L S, Ch'ien L 1980 Neonatal herpes simplex virus infection introduced by fetal monitor scalp electrodes. Pediatrics 65: 1150–1153

Pass R F, Stagno S, Myers G J, Alford C A 1980 Outcome of symptomatic congenital cytomegalovirus infection: results of long-term longitudinal follow-up. Pediatrics 66: 758–762

Pearl K, Preece P, Ades A, Peckham C 1986 Neurodevelopmental assessment after congenital cytomegalovirus infection. Archives of Disease in Childhood 61: 323–326

Peckham C S 1972 A clinical and laboratory study of children exposed in utero to maternal rubella. Archives of Disease in Childhood 47: 571–577

Peckham C 1986 Hearing impairment in childhood. British Medical Bulletin 42(2): 145–149

Peckham C S, Martin J A M, Marshall W C, Dudgeon J A 1979 Congenital rubella deafness: a preventable disease. Lancet i: 258–261

Peckham C, Coleman J C, Hurley R, Chin K S, Henderson K 1983 Cytomegalovirus infection in pregnancy: preliminary finding from a prospective study. Lancet i: 1352–1356

Peckham C S, Johnson C, Ades A, Pearl K, Chin K S 1987 The early acquisition of cytomegalovirus infection. Archives of Diseases in Childhood 62:780–785

Pettersen E J 1984 Transmission of toxoplasmosis via milk from lactating mice. Acta Pathologica Microbiologica Immunologica Scandinavica B 92: 175–176

PHLS (Public Health Laboratory Service) Report 1985 Neonatal meningitis: a review of routine national data 1975–83. British Medical Journal 290: 778–779

PHLS Report 1986 Sexually transmitted disease surveillance in Britain — 1984. British Medical Journal 293: 942–943

PHLS Report 1987 Report from the PHLS Communicable Disease Surveillance Centre. British Medical Journal 294: 361–362

Preece P, Pearl K, Peckham C 1984 Congenital cytomegalovirus. Archives of Disease in Childhood 59: 1120–1126

Probert C G, Sullender W M, Yasukawa L L, Au D S, Yeager A S, Arvin A M 1987 Low risk of herpes simplex virus infections in neonates exposed to the virus at the time of vaginal delivery to mothers with recurrent genital herpes simplex virus infections. New England Journal of Medicine 316: 240–244

Reimen H P O, Meyer M E, Theis J H, Kelso G, Behymer D E 1975 Toxoplasmosis in an infant fed unpasteurised goat milk. Journal of Pediatrics 87: 576–577

Remington J S, Desmonts G 1983 Toxoplasmosis. In: Remington J S, Klein J (eds) Infectious diseases of the fetus and newborn infant, W B Saunders, Philadelphia, pp 144–264

Reynolds D W, Stagno S, Stubbs K G 1974 Inapparent congenital cytomegalovirus infection with elevated cord IgM levels. New England Journal of Medicine 290: 291–296

Reynolds D W, Stagno S, Mosty T S 1980 Maternal cytomegalovirus excretion and perinatal infection. New England Journal of Medicine 302: 1073–1076

Robertson J R, Bucknall A B V, Welsby P D et al 1986 Epidemic of AIDS-related virus (HTLV III/LAV) infection among intra-venous drug abusers. British Medical Journal 292: 527–529

Rogers M F 1985 AIDS in children: a review of the clinical, epidemiologic and public health aspects. Pediatric Infectious Disease 4(3): 230–236

Rubinstein A 1986 Schooling for children with acquired immune deficiency syndrome. Journal of Pediatrics 109(2): 242–244

Rubinstein A, Sicklick M, Gupta A 1983 Acquired immunodeficiency with reversed T4/T8 ratio in infants born to promiscuous and drug-addicted mothers. Journal of the American Medical Association 249: 2350–2356

Ruoss C F, Bourne G L 1972 Toxoplasmosis in pregnancy. Journal of Obstetrics and Gynaecology of the British Commonwealth 79: 1115–1118

Rutter D, Griffiths P, Trompeter R 1985 Cytomegalic inclusion disease after recurrent maternal infection. Lancet ii: 1182

Saigal S, Lunyk O, Larke R P B, Chernesky M A 1982 The outcome in children with congenital cytomegalovirus infection. American Journal of Diseases of Children 136: 896–905

Sathy N, Nair P M, Phillip E, John J 1984 Neonatal poliomyelitis. Indian Journal of Pediatrics 51: 413–414

Saxon S A, Knight W, Reynolds D W, Stagno S, Alford C A 1973 Intellectual deficits in children born with subclinical congenital toxoplasmosis: a preliminary report. Journal of Pediatrics 82: 792–797

Schreiner R L, Kleiman M B, Gresham E L 1979 Maternal oral herpes: isolation policy. Pediatrics 63: 247–249

Sehgal H, Oberoi M 1977 A clinical study of severe form of acute poliomyelitis in children. Indian Journal of Pediatrics 14: 47–52

Seigel M 1973 Congenital malformations following chickenpox, measles, mumps and hepatitis. Journal of the American Medical Association 226: 1521–1524

Sells C J, Carpenter R L, Ray C G 1975 Sequelae of central nervous system enterovirus infection. New England Journal of Medicine 293: 1–4

Sever J, White L R 1968 Intrauterine viral infections. Annual Review of Medicine 19: 471–486

Sheinbergas M M 1976 Hydrocephalus due to prenatal infection with lymphocytic choriomeningitis virus. Infection 4: 185–191

Sheinbergas M M, Kilchauskiene V V, Tulevichiene J P 1984 Prenatal lymphocytic choriomeningitis (LCM): three new cases. Infection 12: 65–66

Singer D B, Rudolph A J, Rosenberg H S, Rawls W F, Bonwik M 1967 Pathology of the congenital rubella syndrome. Journal of Pediatrics 71: 665–675

Smadel J E, Wall M J 1942 Lymphocytic choriomeningitis in the Syrian hamster. Journal of Experimental Medicine 75: 581–591

Smithells R W, Sheppard S, Holzel H, Dickson R 1985 National Congenital Rubella Surveillance Programme. British Medical Journal 291: 40–41

South M A, Tompkins W A F, Morris C R, Rawls W E 1969 Congenital malformations of the central nervous system associated with genital type (type 2) herpes virus. Journal of Pediatrics 75: 13–18

Spector S A, Straube R C 1983 Protean manifestations of perinatal enterovirus infections. Western Journal of Medicine 138(6): 847–851

Sprecher S, Soumerknoff G, Puissant F, Degueldre M 1986 Vertical transmission of HIV in 15 week fetus. Lancet ii: 288–289

Stagno S, Reynolds D W, Amos C S 1977 Auditory and visual defects resulting from symptomatic and subclinical cytomegalovirus and toxoplasma infection. Pediatrics 59: 669–678

Stagno S, Reynolds D W, Pass R F, Alford C A 1980 Breast milk and the risk of cytomegalovirus infection. New England Journal of Medicine 302: 1073–1076

Stagno S, Brasfield D M, Brown M B 1981 Infant pneumonitis associated with cytomegalovirus, chlamydia, pneumocystis and ureaplasma — a prospective study. Pediatrics 68: 322–329

Stagno S, Pass R, Dworsky M 1982 Congenital cytomegalovirus infection: the relative importance of primary and recurrent maternal infection. New England Journal of Medicine 306: 945–949

Stagno S, Pass R F, Dworsky M E, Alford C A 1983 Congenital and perinatal cytomegalovirus infections. Seminars in Perinatology 7: 31–42

Stagno S, Whitley R J 1985 Herpes virus infections in pregnancy. I. Cytomegalovirus and Epstein–Barr virus infections. New England Journal of Medicine 313: 1270–1274

Sullivan-Bolyai J, Hull H F, Wilson C, Corey L 1983 Neonatal herpes simplex virus infection in King County, Washington: increasing incidence and epidemiologic correlates. Journal of the American Medical Association 250: 3059–3062

Sumaya C V, Corman L I 1982 Enteroviral meningitis in early infancy: significance in community outbreaks. Pediatric Infectious Disease 3: 151–154

Thirty L, Spencer-Goldberger S, Jonckheer T 1985 Isolation of AIDS virus from cell-free breast milk of three healthy virus carriers. Lancet ii: 891–892

Townsend J J, Baringer J R, Wolinsky J S 1975 Progressive rubella parenchalitis: late onset after congenital rubella. New England Journal of Medicine 292: 990–993

Ultmann M H, Belman A L, Ruff H A et al 1985 Developmental abnormalities in infants and children with acquired immune deficiency syndrome (AIDS) AIDS-related complex. Developmental Medicine and Child Neurology 27: 563–571

Visintine A, Nahmias A, Whitley R, Alford C 1981 The natural history and epidemiology of neonatal herpes simplex virus infection. In: Nahmias A J, Dowdle W R, Schlnazi R E (eds) The human herpes virus. Elsevier, New York pp 599–600

Vogt M W, Witt D J, Craven D E 1986 Isolation of HTLV-III/LAV from cervical secretions of women at risk for AIDS. Lancet i: 525–527

Weil M L, Habashi H H, Cromer N E, Oshero L S, Lennette E H, Carnay L 1975 Chronic progressive parencephalitis due to rubella virus simulating sclerosing pan encephalitis. New England Journal of Medicine 292: 994–998

Weller T H 1983 Varicella and herpes zoster. New England Journal of Medicine 309: 1362–1368

Weller T H, Hanshaw J B 1964 Virologic and clinical observations on cytomegalic inclusion disease. New England Journal of Medicine 266: 1233–1244

Whitley R J, Nahmias A J, Soong S J, Galasso G G, Fleming C L, Alford C A 1980 Vidarabin therapy of neonatal herpes simplex virus infection. Pediatrics 66: 495–501

Whitley R J, Nahmias A J, Visintine A M, Fleming C L, Alford C A 1980 The natural history of herpes simplex virus infection of mother and newborn. Pediatrics 66: 489–494

Wilfert C M, Thompson R J J, Sunder T R, O'Quinn A, Zeller J, Blacharsh J 1981 Longitudinal assessment of children with enteroviral meningitis during the first three months of life. Pediatrics 67: 811–815

Wilfert C M, Lehrman S N, Katz S L 1983 Enteroviruses and meningitis. Pediatric Infectious Disease 2: 333–341

Williams K A B, Scott J M, MacFarlane D E, Williamson J M W, Elias- Jones T F, Williams H 1981 Congenital toxoplasmosis: a prospective survey in the West of Scotland. Journal of Infection 3: 219–229

Williamson W D, Desmond M M, LaFevers N, Taber L H, Catlin F I, Weaver T G 1982 Symptomatic congenital cytomegalovirus: disorders of language learning and hearing. American Journal of Diseases of Children 136: 902–905

Wilson C B, Remington J S, Stagno S, Reynolds D W 1980a Development of adverse sequelae in children born with subclinical congenital toxoplasma infection. Pediatrics 66: 767–776

Wilson C B, Desmonts G, Couvreur J, Remington J S 1980 Lymphocyte transformation in the diagnosis of congenital toxoplasma infection. New England Journal of Medicine 302: 785–788

Wofsy C B, Cohen J B, Hauer L B et al Isolation of Aids-associated retrovirus from genital secretions of women with antibodies to the virus. Lancet i: 527–529

Wyatt H V 1979 Poliomyelitis in the fetus and the newborn. Clinical Pediatrics 18: 33–38

Yamauchi T, Wilson C, St Geme J W 1974 Transmission of live attenuated mumps virus to human placenta. New England Journal of Medicine 290: 710–712

Yeager A S, Arvin A M, Urbani L J, Kemp J A 1980 Relationship of antibody to outcome in neonatal herpes simplex virus infections. Journal of Infection and Immunity 29: 532–538

Yeager A S, Grumet F C, Hafleigh E B, Arvin A M, Bradley J S 1981 Prevention of transfusion-acquired cytomegalovirus infection in newborn infants. Journal of Pediatrics 98: 281–287

Yeager A S 1983a Viruses uncommonly associated with infection of the fetus and newborn infant. In: Remington J S, Klein J (eds) Infectious diseases of the fetus and newborn infant. W B Saunders, Philadelphia, pp 544–554

Yeager A S 1983b Protozoan and helminth infections. In: Remington J S, Klein J (eds) Infectious diseases of the fetus and newborn infant. W B Saunders, Philadelphia, pp 555–569

Young N A, Gershon A A 1983 Chickenpox, measles and mumps. In: Remington J S, Klein J O (eds) Infectious diseases of the fetus and newborn. W B Saunders, Philadelphia pp 375–427

Ziegler J B, Cooper D A, Johnson R O, Gold J 1985 Postnatal transmission of AIDS-associated retrovirus from mother to infant. Lancet i: 896-899

37. Bacterial and fungal infections

Dr Pamela A. Davies

The damage bacteria can inflict on a host is determined by their numbers and individual characteristics, and by the defence the host is able to muster. When that host is a fetus or newborn infant certain factors unique to this period of life have to be considered. The very gradual maturation of fetal and neonatal defence mechanisms is one; the stage of organ differentiation or growth reached at the time the infection occurs is another, and a third is the state of maternal immune competence.

During pregnancy, infection involving the fetal central nervous system should theoretically have the greatest impact when the infection occurs early, and the conceptus is retained and eventually liveborn. The spectrum of possible end results though ranges (as with other infecting but non-bacterial organisms) through abortion, antenatal fetal death, intrapartum stillbirth, pre-term birth, or neonatal death. Surviving children may or may not have abnormality as a result of the infection. When both parents are healthy in the widest sense, the risk to the developing fetus is negligible. Given these circumstances, and a well-grown infant born normally at full-term, the risk of postnatal infection should be minimal. It is when these favourable conditions are not met that there is potential vulnerability; this chapter considers the possible consequences.

HOST DEFENCE

Comparisons made between the newborn infant and adult where host defence is concerned inevitably lead to the former being dubbed immunocompromised. But this is not strictly true because throughout a normal pregnancy defence mechanisms are maturing so that the emerging baby is able to cope with what should be the first challenge by bacteria, those normally colonizing the birth canal. Fallopian tubes and uterine cavity are sterile, ensuring a safe passage for the fertilized ovum to the endometrium. Later, inside the sac formed by fusion of the amnion and chorion, with the covering decidua capsularis, the developing fetus is surrounded by sterile amniotic fluid which has anti-infective properties. The fetus is further protected by the placenta, which as well as acting as a physical barrier (Fox 1981) has a large mononuclear phagocyte population in the chorionic villi (Wood 1980) and may possess other defence mechanisms.

The essentials of the humoral immune response so important for bacterial infection are derived from the B-cell system and consist of the synthesis and release of antibodies which enhance phagocytosis. Immunoglobulin synthesis of IgM and IgG begins at the end of the third month of gestation and of IgA at about 30 weeks (Gitlin & Biasucci 1969). Levels of IgM and IgA at birth will normally be very low. Only maternal IgG, because of its lower molecular weight, is actively transferred across the placenta. This transfer is quite rapid from about 16 weeks of gestation and at full-term IgG levels in the cord blood are the same as or higher than those of the mother (Kohler & Farr 1966). Synthesis of the humoral mediator complement begins a little before that of IgM but complement levels in cord blood are only half those of the adult (Miller 1978).

The fetus has few circulating white blood cells until the third trimester. Direct vision fetoscopy has recently allowed sampling of fetal blood in 99 cases between 15 and 21 weeks of gestation. The total white blood cell count rose over those 6 weeks from a mean of 1.6 to 2.7 × 10^9/l; and mean counts of neutrophils rose from 113 to 192 × 10^6/l (Millar et al 1985). These very low figures are in agreement with the findings some 20 years earlier following hysterotomy, counts increasing steadily over a gestational age range from 8 to 27 weeks (Thomas & Yoffey 1962, Playfair et al 1963). On the other hand, following abortion, values were roughly four times higher and the cells were predominantly immature forms (Playfair et al 1963). It is not clear from this paper what precise steps were taken to rule out an infective cause for the abortions but whatever the stimulus it appears that the fetus is able to raise its white blood cell count in midtrimester. Experimental work with newborn animals, which seems likely to have relevance for the human baby, suggests that the neutrophil storage pool is rapidly exhausted and that further production of granulocytes from stem cells cannot take place when needed (Christensen et al 1980). The ability of polymorphonuclear leukocytes to reach the site of infection in the human baby after birth — their chemotactic ability — is diminished compared with the adult. In vitro phagocytosis is usually considered normal in the presence of normal concentrations of plasma or serum (Miller & Stiehm 1983).

The cell-mediated immune response derived from the T-cell system is of greater importance for non-bacterial organisms such as intracellularly replicating viruses, fungi and protozoa. However, there are a few intracellularly replicating bacteria: *Listeria monocytogenes*, *Mycobacterium tuberculosis* and *Brucella* sp. In fetal life suppressor rather than helper T-lymphocyte activity is dominant due to maturational differences (Lawton 1984), so the cell-mediated immune response is limited to some extent. Impaired intra-uterine growth too has an adverse effect on cell-mediated immunity (Ferguson et al 1974, Chandra & Matsumura 1979) which may persist for a long period after birth (Ferguson 1978).

The blood cerebrospinal fluid (CSF) barrier is different during fetal and early neonatal life, allowing plasma proteins which may be present in CSF to reach the brain cells. Thus any molecule of sufficiently low weight to cross the placenta may theoretically gain access to the developing brain (see review by Adinolfi 1985). Maturation of the blood–CSF–brain barrier seems to occur quickly after the first 2 or 3 months of postnatal life (Statz & Felgenhauer 1983). It is not yet known whether CSF macrophages function in the same way as or differently from peritoneal and alveolar macrophages, or whether their function can be stimulated artificially. Durack & Perfect (1985) have developed an animal model to study these and related questions of central nervous system defence mechanisms.

Evidence that a good intake of milk from the breast in the first days of life protects against neonatal meningitis is suggestive rather than proved (Winberg & Wessner 1971); but there is ample support for the anti-infective properties of human milk in less-developed areas of the world (Jelliffe & Jelliffe 1978)

Subtle changes in the maternal immune state during pregnancy allow the fetal allograft to survive but there is little evidence of an increased incidence of infections during pregnancy, though recurrences (whether reinfection, relapse, recrudescence or reactivation) may occur (Brabin 1985). Anti-infective properties of amniotic fluid are diminished in poorly nourished African women (Appelbaum et al 1977, Tafari et al 1977). Maternal immune factors have been best studied with regard to the group B streptococcus, the type III variety of which (see 'The infecting organism' p. 430) is most commonly responsible for neonatal group B streptococcal meningitis. Baker & Kasper (1976) showed that infants developing such invasive infections were born to mothers who had low concentrations of antibody to the native type III capsular polysaccharide. Such antibodies are usually of the IgG$_2$ subclass, and any selective maternal deficiency of this nature would thus be reflected in cord blood. Serum antibodies to the K1 antigen of *Escherichia coli* are low in the general population, predominantly of the IgM type (Schiffer et al 1976) and would not cross the placenta. Lastly, the factors governing the numbers and nature of the vaginal bacterial flora are only partly understood (Cohen et al 1984).

EPIDEMIOLOGY AND PATHOGENESIS OF CENTRAL NERVOUS SYSTEM INFECTIONS

Prenatal infection

There are two main routes by which bacterial infection reaches the fetus — transplacentally, via the blood stream, or ascending via the cervix and amniotic sac. Theoretically, it could also reach the fetus from the peritoneal cavity via the Fallopian tubes, or by direct spread from an infected uterine wall. The developing brain is more likely to be primarily involved in transplacental bloodstream infection. However, while the lungs and gastrointestinal tract bear the brunt of ascending infections as the fetus inspires and swallows amniotic fluid, secondary bacteraemia may occur with later central nervous system involvement. It is often assumed that most prenatal infection is blood-borne, while intrapartum infection is nearly always the consequence of ascending infection. Pathologists have acknowledged that it may be difficult to distinguish between the two histologically; ascending infection leads to chorioamnionitis and villous placentitis, while in transplacental infection, involvement of the amniotic sac occurs secondarily (Benirschke & Driscoll 1967, Morison 1970) Reliable estimates of the relative frequency of these two main possibilities are not available but there is much circumstantial evidence to suggest the ascending route is the more important.

When maternal bacteraemia occurs the bacteria will enter the vessels of the placental villi from the uterine arteries and finally (if they survive phagocytosis) may reach the fetal bloodstream via the subamniotic blood vessels of the chorion. That the placenta may occasionally show extensive infection, as with *M. tuberculosis*, when the fetus is uninfected, has been seen as proof of its efficacy as a physical barrier against blood-borne infection. Fox (1981) has warned that this concept may be false. He states that the placenta is actually a preferential site for the localization of invading organisms in animal infections and that in certain experimental infections the organisms may only be able to grow and flourish in placental tissue, and would not survive to establish infection in the non-pregnant state.

Ascending infection leading to chorioamnionitis (in which there is infiltration of amnion and chorion with neutrophil polymorphonuclear leukocytes) is of necessity a histological diagnosis. In the large majority of mothers it causes no symptoms. Unless it is diagnosed fortuitously by amniocentesis it is only evident after delivery and then only if the placenta and membranes are examined microscopically. It occurs in about 11% of all births (Benirschke & Driscoll 1967) but is far more common in pregnancies ending at low gestations (Driscoll 1979, Russell 1979). Although recent surveys of the epidemiological associations of histologically proven chorioamnionitis are not available, there is suggestive evidence from perinatal mortality and other studies that maternal socio-economic disadvantage and pre-term birth are the most important (Naeye & Blanc 1970, Naeye & Peters 1978, 1980).

Intrapartum and postnatal infection

It is sometimes difficult to separate intrapartum central nervous system infection and all studies considering epidemiology and pathogenesis refer to meningitis only — from similar infections acquired after birth. While intrapartum acquired infections have their onset within the first 48 hours of life or at least in the first week, some cases of meningitis occur several weeks after birth due to organisms which are most likely to have been acquired in the birth canal or from the maternal perineum rather than from the environment. This cannot always be proved, however, and maternal hand transmission is always a possibility. In general the associations of the two do not differ greatly and, with the exception of neonatal tetanus and infant botulism considered separately below, are again pre-term birth (less than 37 weeks of gestation) and low birth-weight (less than 2.5 kg). Premature rupture of membranes, intrapartum maternal infection and birth asphyxia are also cited as epidemiological associations of neonatal bacterial meningitis (Klein & Marcy 1983), though care has to be taken to consider birth-weight as an independent variable in assessing their significance; and birth-weight specific analyses have not been made.

Males predominate particularly in meningitis caused by Gram-negative organisms (Washburn et al 1965). Further studies of relative vulnerability of the sexes may need to be made on geographically defined populations within low-birth-weight specific groups where numbers of male to female livebirths differ to be certain to what extent intrapartum and environmentally acquired infections differ in this respect. In the Netherlands a recent study gave the male to female ratio as 1.33:1 for 'neonatal meningitis' which would include both forms (Mulder & Zanen 1984a).

Postnatal central nervous system infections are sometimes acquired in the course of nursery outbreaks, a single infecting source such as a contaminated piece of equipment or medication, or a human carrier being eventually found (Cabrera & Davis 1961, Rance et al 1962, Williams et al 1984). The complex nature of present-day neonatal intensive care increases the possibilities for nosocomial infections of this sort. Recent community outbreaks of listerial infection involving the pregnant woman, fetus or newborn infant have

been traced to consumption of raw vegetables contaminated by silage (Schlech et al 1983), infected pasteurized milk (Fleming et al 1985) and infected cheese (Morbidity and Mortality Weekly Report 1984).

It must be assumed that bacteria causing meningitis or any other CNS infection are derived from those attached to and colonizing mucosal surfaces elsewhere in the body. Considering the wide range of bacteria involved in neonatal meningitis (see later), the most important attachment/colonizing sites are likely to be the nasopharynx and gastrointestinal tract. Animal models may offer some insight into the subsequent sequence of events, although as always extrapolation has to be made with care. *Escherichia coli* meningitis has been studied in the suckling rat and the guinea pig pup (Moxon et al 1977, Glode et al 1977, Sinai et al 1980). The development of meningitis in both models was determined by the magnitude of the bacteraemia; bacteraemia was present for several hours in isolation before meningitis developed. Infant rats have also been used to study *Haemophilus influenzae* meningitis. The organisms penetrated nasopharyngeal subepithelial tissues quickly after intranasal inoculation. Direct invasion of submucosal blood vessels rather than initial clearance by lymphatics with secondary blood vessel entry seemed to occur. Bacteria in the blood were thought to be the offspring of very few survivors. Again the magnitude and duration of the bacteraemia (more than 1000 organisms/ml for more than 6 hours) were essential for the consistent progression to meningitis (Moxon et al 1985).

In the human baby, neonatal meningitis has been reported as occurring in up to a third of bacteraemic infants, being significantly more likely when more than 1000 colony forming units/ml were recovered from the bloodstream (Dietzman et al 1974); two-thirds of infants with meningitis have had proven bacteraemia (Klein & Marcy 1983). Volpe (1981) reviewed evidence to suggest that the blood-borne bacteria localize first in the choroid plexus, a glycogen-rich site in the early days of life, which favours their growth. From there he believes that they enter the ventricular system, circulating with the normal CSF flow to the subarachnoid space. Thus ventriculitis is a very common feature of meningitis. Occasionally bacteria may have a more direct route to the central nervous system, such as in leaking myelomeningocele or congenital dermal sinus (Morison considered the latter a very rare possibility). Morison (1970) has also recorded a few scalp infections which extended through the skull and spread along thrombosed bridging veins. Similar mechanisms have been involved with infected cephalhaematoma and osteomyelitis of the skull. Facial cellulitis (either buccal or orbital) though more common after the neonatal period has also been associated with bacteraemia and meningitis (Baker & Bausher 1986).

Direct extension of infection to the meninges from an infected middle ear or mastoid bone has often been inferred in the pathogenesis of meningitis in older children (Ziai & Haggerty 1958). However, careful histopathological examination of the temporal bones in 16 cases of meningitis aged between 2 and 13 months (mean 6 months) showed no evidence of spread from the tympanomastoid compartment to the intracranial cavity (Eavey et al 1985) but rather the inner ear infection appeared to result from retrograde bacterial invasion from the meninges. There is no clear indication of how often otitis media is present in association with neonatal meningitis and the middle ear is not always examined routinely in neonatal autopsies. Support for the secondary nature of the labyrinthitis is forthcoming from two experimental animal models (Moxon et al 1974, Wiedermann et al 1986).

THE INFECTING ORGANISMS

(See also later for infected CSF shunts.) The infecting organisms differ to some extent before and during birth according to the route of infection — blood-borne or ascending. Pregnant women often have other small children to care for and may be liable to their infections, which are predominantly respiratory or gastrointestinal. Sustained bacteraemia during such infections must, however be extremely rare. Traditionally the organisms classified as bacteria which have been regarded as likely to reach the fetus via the bloodstream are *Treponema pallidum*, *L. monocytogenes* and *M. tuberculosis*. All may reach the developing fetal brain and cause disease there but theoretically any acute systemic bacterial disease leading to bacteraemia may be responsible. Probably far more important numerically are those bacteria gaining ascending access to the amniotic sac, those which colonize the maternal cervix, vagina, the perineum and the rectum. The flora of the lower genital tract in unselected pregnant women includes lactobacilli, corynebacteria and *Staphylococcus epidermidis;* faecal streptococci of groups C, D, E and G may also be found (Hurley et al 1974), and betahaemolytic streptococci of group B are present in 25% or more depending on the population of women studied (Easmon et al 1985), as are yeasts (Cassie & Stevenson 1973). The genital mycoplasmas *Mycoplasma hominis* and *Ureaplasma urealyticum* are present in the genital tract of over half of sexually experienced adults (Taylor-Robinson & McCormack 1980). *E. coli* may be recovered from a few women (Hurley et al 1974) and anaerobes such as *Bacteroides* sp., *Propionibacterium acnes, Peptococcus* and *Peptostreptococcus,* and *Clostridium* sp., have been isolated from cervical cultures immediately after delivery (Brook et al 1979). Some maternally transmitted bacteria and fungi responsible for fetal central nervous system infection are shown in Table 37.1.

A wide variety of organisms have been responsible for neonatal meningitis (acquired intrapartum or after birth) and are shown in Table 37.2. The two most commonly appearing in statutory notifications and voluntary laboratory reports to the Communicable Disease Surveillance Centre (see Fig. 37.1) are *E. coli* and group B streptococcus; *L. monocytogenes* comes a low third (PHLS 1985). However, selective reporting of certain infecting organisms may be a possibility and truly accurate national figures are not yet available. National but similarly acknowledged underreported data from the United States give group B streptococcus as the single most common infecting agent, followed by Gram-negative enteric organisms, *L. monocytogenes*, *H. influenzae*, *Streptococcus pneumoniae* and *Neisseria meningitidis* in that order (Schlech et al 1985). Various geographical differences may exist. While group B streptoccus was only recognized as a cause of bacteraemia and meningitis in Göttingen, Federal Republic of Germany from 1975 onwards (Speer et al 1985), it is still 'conspicuously absent' from Benin, Nigeria where *E. coli* and *Staphylococcus aureus* predominate (Longe et al 1984). *E. coli* was the most common causative organism in Riyadh, Saudi Arabia (Babiker & Taha 1984). A preponderence of *Salmonella* sp. infections were reported from Ibadan, Nigeria some years earlier by Barclay (1971), and these were conspicuous in South America in the United States Neonatal Meningitis Cooperative Study Group trials (McCracken & Mize 1976, McCracken et al 1980, McCracken et al 1984).

E. coli strains causing neonatal meningitis carry the K1 capsular antigen in about three-quarters of the cases; this antigen is similar immunochemically to the capsular polysaccharide of *N. meningitidis* (Schiffer et al 1976). The Netherlands study reported that 88% of the strains causing meningitis in 132 infants carried the K1 antigen and that most of these (80%) belonged to serogroups 07, 018 and 083, or were auto-agglutinable (Mulder et al 1984). Gross et al (1983) tested 131 *E. coli* strains isolated from CSF, of which at least 69 were from newborn infants, to 13 antimicrobial drugs; 41% were resistant to one or more drugs and 34% to three or more. Among the drugs to which resistance was found most often were ampicillin, streptomycin and the sulphonamides.

Group B streptococcal meningitis is caused predominantly by type III strains, whether it occurs early or late. Baker & Edwards (1983) have pointed out that this predilection

Table 37.1 Some maternally transmitted bacteria and fungi responsible for fetal central nervous system infection

Infecting organisms	Selected references
Campylobacter sp.	Eden 1966
Candida albicans	Levin et al 1978
Cryptococcus neoformans	Heath 1950
Haemophilus influenzae	Berczy et al 1973
Listeria monocytogenes	Vawter 1981
Mycobacterium tuberculosis	Huber 1983
Mycoplasma hominis	Christensen et al 1982
Staphylococcus aureus	Crosby et al 1951
Torulopsis glabrata	Quirke et al 1980
Treponema pallidum	Oppenheimer & Dahms 1981

Table 37.2 Some bacteria responsible for meningitis in the first weeks of life

Infecting organisms	Selected references
Gram-positive	
Aerococcus viridans	Nathavitharana et al 1983
Bacillus cereus	Turnbull et al 1977
Listeria monocytogenes	Guin et al 1965, Visintine et al 1977
Mycobacterium tuberculosis	Huber 1983
Staphylococcus aureus	Ziai & Haggerty 1958
Staphylococcus epidermidis	Odio et al 1984
Streptococci	
Group A	Nelson et al 1976
Group B	Baker & Edwards 1983
Group C	Stewardson-Krieger & Gotoff 1977
Group D (enterococcal)	McCracken & Shinefield 1966
Group D (non-enterococcal)	Fikar & Levy 1979
Untypable	Rudensky et al 1978
viridans streptococci	Goldfarb et al 1984
S. mitis	Hellwege et al 1984
S. pneumoniae	McDonald 1972, Tempest 1974, Rhodes et al 1975, Weizer & Heldenberg 1985
Gram-negative	
Acinetobacter sp.*	Yogev 1979, Morgan & Hart 1982, Berkowitz 1982
Aerobacter aerogenes	Berman & Banker 1966, Cussen & Ryan 1967
Aeromonas hydrophila	Unreported case known to author
Alcaligenes faecalis	Bischoff et al 1948
Bacteroides fragilis	Cooke 1975, Dysart et al 1976, Berman et al 1978, Law & Marks 1980
Brucella melitensis	Maschio & Ventura 1967
Campylobacter sp.	Thomas et al 1980, Goossens et al 1986
Citrobacter sp.	Gross et al 1973, Rose 1979, Williams et al 1984
Edwardsiella tarda	Okubadejo & Alausa 1968
Escherichia coli	Headings & Overall 1977, Mulder et al 1984
Flavobacterium meningosepticum	King 1959, Cabrera & Davies 1961, Sugathadasa & Arseculeratne 1963, Maderazo et al 1974
Haemophilus influenzae	Mathies et al 1965
Haemophilus parainfluenzae	Gullekson & Dumoff 1966
Klebsiella pneumoniae	Hill et al 1974
Mycoplasma hominis	Wealthall 1975, Gewitz et al 1979, Siber et al 1977, Hjelm et al 1980, Waites et al 1988
Neisseria gonorrhoeae	Bradford & Kelley 1933, Holmes 1983
Neisseria meningitidis	Stiehm & Damrosch 1966
Pasteurella multocida	Bates et al 1965, Recipe & Neter 1975, Frutos et al 1978, Clapp et al 1986
Plesiomonas shigelloides†	Appelbaum et al 1978, Pahak et al 1983
Proteus mirabilis	Cussen & Ryan 1967, Levy & Ingall 1967
Pseudomonas aeruginosa	Kraus & Hunter 1941, Ziai & Haggerty 1958
Pseudomonas cepacia	Darby 1976
Salmonella sp.	Barclay 1971, Burton et al 1977, Adler & Markowitz 1983, Low et al 1984
Serratia marcescens	Anagnostakis et al 1981
Shigella sp.	Whitfield & Humphries 1967
Ureaplasma urealyticum	Garland & Murton 1987, Waites et al 1988
Vibrio cholerae	Rubin et al 1981

*Included previously *Herellea vaginicola* and *Mima polymorpha*
†Also known as *Aeronomas shigelloides*

of type III strains appears to be restricted to the young infant, since type II strains may predominate in the adult. The reasons for this are not clear, since asymptomatic colonization at all ages, including the neonatal period, is equally distributed between types I (Ia, Ib, Ic),* II and III (Baker & Edwards 1983). Serotype IVb of *L. monocytogenes* has been reported as causing a majority of cases of later onset

meningitis due to that organism (Albritton et al 1976). Both adult and neonatal listerial meningitis was reported more frequently in late summer and early autumn in England and Wales (PHLS 1985); no such seasonal trend was noted in the United States study (Schlech et al 1985). Neonatal bacteraemia due to *H. influenzae* infection has increased in the last decade. Non-typable strains (biotype 4) which are not beta-lactamase producing appear to have an affinity for the maternal genital tract and have been responsible for most cases of early-onset bacteraemia due to this organism.

*Suggested new nomenclature Ia, Ib, Ia (Ia/c) (Henrichsen 1985).

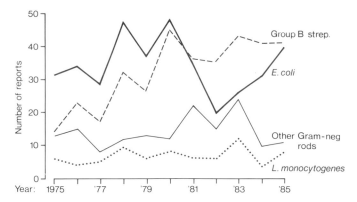

Fig. 37.1 Neonatal meningitis, England and Wales 1975–85. (The numbers are those provided by statutory notification and by voluntary laboratory reports to the Communicable Disease Surveillance Centre; they are acknowledged to be selected and incomplete, and cannot be related to a denominator (courtesy of PHLS 1985).

Neonatal meningitis associated with such bacteraemia, however, occurs less commonly than with group B streptococcal bacteraemia and is more often due to type b strains than to the non-typable variety (Wallace et al 1983). An infant with beta-lactamase positive *H. influenzae* type b meningitis and beta-lactamase negative *H. influenzae* bacteraemia (unfortunately not typed), both concurrent with herpes encephalitis has been reported (Peltola et al 1986). There has also been simultaneous recovery from the CSF of two different strains of *H. influenzae* type b (Stewardson-Krieger & Naidu 1981) and two different strains of *E. coli* (Goldenberg & Neter 1977), as well as a number of case reports dealing with mixed bacterial or bacterial and fungal meningitis (Klein & Marcy 1983, Davies & Gothefors 1984).

PREVALENCE

The extent to which prenatal bacterial infection involves the central nervous system is unknown. This is in sharp contrast to certain viral infections, such as congenital rubella, for which reasonably accurate figures are available. There are probably two main reasons for this. The first and most important must be that the number of different bacteria theoretically capable of causing fetal infection in the first and second trimesters of pregnancy is legion and the application of specific diagnostic tests poses very great problems. The second is that all too often bacterial infection is not considered as a possibility by obstetricians and pathologists in antepartum fetal death or by paediatricians in cases of central nervous system abnormality present at birth, or becoming evident in the months or years after it. The one specific infection for which figures are available is congenital syphilis. Now only 40 or so cases under 2 years of age are recognized annually in the United Kingdom, though this may be an underdiagnosis.

The only reasonably reliable figures for bacterial central nervous system infection presenting in the neonatal period available for a geographically defined population refer to neonatal meningitis. Because of the incomplete system of reporting these also are likely to be an underestimate. Goldacre (1976) in a 5-year review (1969–73) of bacterial meningitis found the prevalence in the first 4 weeks of life in the North West Thames region of London (about 4 million inhabitants) to be 0.26/1000 livebirths when 'congenital or traumatic neuroanatomical lesions' were excluded. The infection was more common in the first week and in the first month of life than in any subsequent week or month. More recently Mulder & Zanen (1984a) gave a minimum prevalence figure of 0.23/1000 livebirths over a later 6-year period (1976–82) for the Netherlands. The figure varied between 0.23 and 0.28 from 1978 onwards, when the figures were considered 'more representative'. These two studies of defined populations may be compared with the United States Collaborative Perinatal Project of several years earlier (1959—66) which involved 12 urban hospitals in different regions and over 53 000 pregnancies. Neonatal meningitis then occurred at a rate of 0.46/1000 livebirths. The figure was 0.37/1000 for infants weighing more than 2.5 kg at birth but 1.36 for those below this weight (Overall 1970).

SPECTRUM OF EFFECTS

Intra-uterine infection

During the period of organ formation there are only two options for recognition of disease as Potter & Craig (1976) have pointed out — congenital malformations or death. That bacteria can gain access to fetal tissue in the first trimester is not in doubt, since Harter & Benirschke (1976) have demonstrated spirochaetes at 9 and 10 weeks of gestation in the offspring of untreated syphilitic women undergoing therapeutic abortion. Inflammatory tissue reaction, however, was absent since the fetus cannot mount any sort of immune response at such an early stage. There seems no reason why other bacteria (particularly those of relatively low virulence such as the genital mycoplasmas) should not similarly gain access, cause anomalous development of the brain, but allow the pregnancy to continue. There is, however, no proof.

Chorioamnionitis has been recognized in up to two-thirds or more of midtrimester abortions (Driscoll 1979, Russell 1979). A mother who developed purulent bronchitis at 18 weeks of gestation aborted some 4 weeks later. Non-capsulated *H. influenzae* were recovered from the fetal brain (Berczy et al 1973) and one can only guess the end result had the pregnancy been retained. Dungal (1961) reported suggestive but unproven confirmation of a specific infection causing central nervous system abnormality. The mother delivered three infants, who successively died between 10 and 18 months of age. All were retarded and thought to have congenital brain malformation. Because of this history, it was arranged that her fourth pregnancy be terminated and a non-viable fetus was delivered by caesarean section. *L. monocytogenes* was cultured from the fluid in the amniotic sac. In a subsequent fifth pregnancy she was treated with oxytetracycline from the third month and later delivered her first healthy normal child. Mental retardation in children has been associated with significantly higher antilisteria titres among those in whom the cause of the retardation was uncertain than among those in whom it was known (Lang 1955). Prenatal meningitis has been reported in a female infant who was found to have hydrocephalus in utero, probably developing between the sixth and seventh months of gestation. Shortly after birth the CSF had a high protein content but no white cells. Subsequently the meninges were explored and homogeneous yellow inflammatory tissue was found from which *S. aureus* was grown in pure culture (Crosby et al 1951).

Morison (1970) has suggested that in prenatal life the pathology of lesions produced depends more on the anatomy of the affected tissue than on the nature of the infecting organism. Blood supply at different stages of gestation must also be important. Prenatal toxoplasmosis for example has been shown to cause hydranencephaly (Altshuler 1973), in which large fluid-filled cavities occupy the position of the absent or nearly absent cerebral hemispheres (Morison 1970). The destroyed regions arc those supplied by the carotid arteries which are entirely responsible for blood reaching the brain in the early embryo; the cerebellum, brainstem and other arcas of brain supplied by the vertebral arteries which develop at a later stage, remain intact (Pape & Wigglesworth 1979). It is conceivable that bacterial infection, gradually overcome as defence mechanisms develop, could leave similar destruction in its wake, but again there is no proof. Many of the bacteria recorded earlier as colonizing the birth canal are of low virulence, and perhaps they should be viewed with greater suspicion. Wigglesworth (1984) has pointed out that it can be virtually impossible to determine whether partly calcified necrotic cerebral lesions seen at autopsy in the neonatal period could be due to a previous intra-uterine infection or to an episode of severe cerebral hypoxia. If severe systemic bacterial disease in pregnancy was accompanied by toxaemia, acidosis and shock, as is known to occur in certain parts of the world with maternal cholera (Hirschhorn et al 1969), such lesions could occur in fetal brain following ischaemia even though the fetus was not directly infected.

The pathology of recognized specific infections has been described in recent reviews. Central nervous system lesions of congenital syphilis usually take second place to those of other organs such as the lung, liver and skeleton. However, Oppenheimer & Dahms (1981) report that at autopsy when carefully sought 'focal mononuclear infiltrates may be found in the pia-arachnoid, in subependymal foci and especially in perivascular locations'. They also point out that dense,

granulomatous inflammatory lesions may be present at the base of the brain, in the choroid plexus, or in the medulla and cord. In survivors these are likely to give rise to the symptoms of congenital neurosyphilis well beyond the first few months of life. The eyes may show a non-specific uveitis or a focal or diffuse mononuclear cell infiltrate of the choroid. In cases of prenatal listeriosis coming to postmorten examination Vawter (1981) has said that purulent meningitis did not occur but that major insults of the central nervous system (subarachnoid haemorrhage, intraventricular haemorrhage, cerebral petechiae and periventricular leukomalacia or massive cerebral necrosis) may all be found in the absence of local listerial inflammation. When, very rarely, tuberculous infection occurs in utero the meninges are invariably involved according to Huber (1983).

Other possible subtle effects, from bacterial toxins rather than bacteria themselves are suggested by experimental animal work. Thus, in endotoxin-treated female rabbits, when trypan blue was used as a marker, the placento–fetal 'barrier' allowed dye to reach various fetal organs, particularly the brain and choroid (McKell et al 1960). Prolonged exposure of the newborn kitten to endotoxin has caused a leukoencephalopathy characterized by astrogliosis which could not be explained by cerebral hypoperfusion (Gilles et al 1976). In the human fetus exposure to bacterial antigen in bacteriuric mothers is believed to be responsible for the fact that, shortly after birth, the infants' lymphocytes, grown in cell culture, show induction of mitosis to *E. coli* antigen. The lymphocytes of control infants born to non-bacteriuric mothers do not behave thus until several weeks from birth have elapsed and they have been exposed to antigen in the course of normal colonization (Brody & Oski 1967, Wallach et al 1969). It has been presumed that the bacteriuric mothers' infants can only have met the infecting organisms before birth if they entered the maternal circulation and reached the intervillous space. Another explanation though is that they reached the amniotic fluid despite intact membranes from a heavily colonized perineum.

There may be two other indirect effects of pregnancy bacterial infections on the fetal central nervous system, possibly to some extent related. Placental villitis of unknown aetiology may be found in 8% of consecutive singleton placentae in pregnancies of over 20 weeks of gestation (Russell 1980); a genuine relationship seems to have been established between such villitis and intra-uterine growth retardation (Knox & Fox 1984, Althabe & Labarrere 1985). Experimental work in the mouse led Coid et al (1978) to suggest that villitis might be caused by transient *E. coli* bacteraemia in women with asymptomatic pregnancy bacteriuria. The brain of the growth-retarded fetus is smaller than normal, though the reduction in size is less than that of other organs (Gruenwald 1974). Follow-up surveys have documented the poorer performance of such children, though environmental causes may be as important as the growth retardation (Neligan et al 1976). It seems likely, but again is quite unproven, that some of the bacteria colonizing the birth canal could be responsible for this villitis. Any such documentation of cause and effect will have to await more sophisticated diagnostic measures than have been used hitherto.

The second indirect effect is intraventricular haemorrhage. Fedrick & Butler (1970) compared 146 neonatal deaths with intraventricular haemorrhage with a control population of 16 994 births. One of the most important factors in the aetiology of the lesions, aside from pre-term birth and growth retardation, was maternal infection before or during delivery.

INTRAPARTUM AND POSTNATAL INFECTION

Neonatal meningitis is the most frequently occurring of central nervous system infections to be diagnosed after birth. Its low prevalence, its epidemiological associations, pathogenesis and causative organisms have been referred to above.

Clinical presentation

Early: those infants with overwhelming intrapartum infection, often due to group B streptococcus, who present with signs within a few hours of birth do so primarily with signs of respiratory distress, often indistinguishable from hyaline membrane disease. Apnoeic episodes and shock may supervene early and despite adequate antimicrobial therapy and supportive measures, death may occur within 24–48 hours of birth. Rather less than one-third of those with intrapartum bacteraemia due to the group B streptococcus develop meningitis (Klein & Marcy 1983) and diagnosis during life rests solely on examination of the CSF.

Later: although the strict definition of the neonatal period is less than 28 days of life, many of the very immature infants now surviving to develop meningitis later may do so after the neonatal period but well before their expected date of delivery. The paucity of signs pointing to the central nervous system in the early days of the illness is doubtless one of the reasons for the continuing high mortality and high morbidity among survivors. Klein & Marcy (1983) analysed the presenting signs from 255 cases of neonatal meningitis studied in six centres in North America and Australia. A raised body temperature (seen in 61%) was the most commonly recorded sign and in descending order of frequency the others were lethargy (50%), anorexia or vomiting (49%), respiratory distress (47%), convulsions (40%), irritability (32%), jaundice, and bulging or full fontanelle (both 28%), diarrhoea (17%), neck stiffness (15%), and apnoea (7%). While some of these 255 cases will have included early-onset meningitis, the non-specific nature of many of these signs,

and the large number of other illnesses presenting similarly which have to be differentiated, will be obvious.

Diagnosis

This rests finally on the isolation of the infecting organism in culture from the CSF. Demonstration of an organism's specific characteristics in CSF may be helpful in confirming the diagnosis. Detection of antigen by counterimmuno-electrophoresis or latex agglutination, antibody by enzyme-linked immunosorbent assay or monoclonal antibody, endotoxin by limulus lysate, or metabolites such as volatile fatty acids by gas–liquid chromatography may be used by laboratories for more rapid information pending the results of culture if the nature of the organism is not obvious on traditional Gram stain (Davies & Gothefors 1984, Philip 1985). However, these tests are by no means routinely available in all hospitals, or throughout the 24-hour period, and tests for antigen or antibody are less helpful when there is no clue to the nature of the infecting organism, and the range of possibilities is so wide. Conventional tests interpreted by a skilled microbiologist from the outset are likely to remain most important in diagnosis. Difficulties with the Gram stain have caused *L. monocytogenes* to appear Gram-negative on occasions, and it has been mistaken most often for *H. influenzae;* coccoid forms are occasionally dismissed as contaminating corynebacteria, or on occasion diagnosed as pneumococci (Seeliger & Finger 1983). The resemblance of *Acinetobacter* to *N. meningitidis* on stain has also been reported (Berkowitz 1982). If the Gram stain is negative, the acridine orange stain may identify the presence of bacteria, particularly if they are within phagocytes, since they stain bright orange (Kleiman et al 1984).

Collection of CSF using a non-styletted needle should be avoided, since a false-positive Gram stain has resulted from skin bacteria carried into the fluid. Also epidermoid spinal cord tumour after lumbar puncture is a theoretical if not an actual possibility following this practice (Halcrow et al 1985). The lumbar CSF pressure should be measured whenever possible, for it can be taken as a measure of intracranial pressure (see p. 377). The collection of CSF, however quickly and swiftly accomplished, will always disturb a small infant. The decision that lumbar puncture is necessary should never be taken lightly. On the other hand early diagnosis of meningitis is essential if morbidity is to be lessened. The ranges of CSF white cell counts, protein and glucose values in the neonatal period vary in the first weeks and with gestational age. Protein values in pre-term infants may be 1 g/l or more in the first weeks of life and over 0.4 g/l but usually under 1 g/l in full-term babies. In 117 sick infants without meningitis, Sarff et al (1976) found the mean CSF white cell count to be 8.4 cells/mm^3 (range 0–32), of which approximately 60% were polymorphonuclear leukocytes. The average CSF protein concentration was 1.15 g/l (range 0.65–1.5) in pre-term and 0.9 g/l (range 0.2–1.7) in full-term babies; CSF/blood glucose ratios were 0.74 and 0.81 respectively. When these results were compared with those from 119 infants with meningitis (only one of whom had a completely normal CSF initially) considerable overlap was evident.

Contamination with red blood cells, which not infrequently occurs in the neonatal period, gives rise to difficulties in diagnosis because the ratio of white blood cells to red blood cells differs from that in peripheral blood and fewer than expected white cells for the number of red cells are found (Osborne & Pizer 1981, Rubenstein & Yogev 1985). Contamination with less than 1.0×10^9 red cells/l did not result in an altered CSF white cell count (Osborne & Pizer 1981). If, however, blood-staining of the CSF is associated with intracranial haemorrhage rather than local trauma due to the tap, there may be a true pleocytosis, raised protein and low CSF glucose value, all secondary to the haemorrhage itself (Volpe 1981). The low CSF glucose value may persist for many weeks, presumably due to some impairment of glucose transport mechanisms. Delays in laboratory examination of CSF have been shown to give a falsely low neutrophil count; this may decrease to 68% ($\pm 10\%$ SEM) and to 50% ($\pm 12\%$) of initial values at one and two hours after collection respectively (Steele et al 1986).

The usefulness of other CSF constituents, such as lactate, lactoferrin, alpha-1-antitrypsin and IgG, in the diagnosis of bacterial meningitis has been studied at other ages but less thoroughly in the neonatal period. On balance it seems unlikely that they will add greatly to accurate diagnosis. Determination of serum C-reactive protein which can be done rapidly by turbidimetry or nephelometry giving an exact quantitative measurement may help to distinguish between bacterial and viral meningitis. In a few older children with epiglottitis and/or bacteraemia, the serum C-reactive protein was positive (well above 20 mg/l) within 12 hours of the onset of symptoms and before positive blood cultures were available (Peltola & Holmberg 1983). Its measurement in the CSF is unreliable (Gray et al 1986, Gutteberg et al 1986).

Treatment

The two most important aspects of treatment are the prompt sterilization of the CSF with antimicrobial drugs and supportive measures aimed at preserving the integrity of the cerebral circulation. Enhancement of the immune response by the addition of intravenous immunoglobulins or granulocyte transfusions is theoretically attractive but much further work needs to be done before either measure has an accepted place.

Meningitis due to Gram-positive organisms. Infection with the group B streptococcus is at present most common; listerial infection is next in frequency, with a range of other organisms seen very occasionally (see Table 37.2).

Table 37.3 Suggested dosage of antibacterial drugs in the neonatal period

Drug	Single dose intravenous (preferred) or intramuscular
Amikacin	7.5 mg/kg
Ampicillin	50 mg/kg
Benzyl penicillin	50 000 IU/kg
Cefotaxime	50 mg/kg
Ceftriaxone	50 mg/kg
Chloramphenicol	12.5–25 mg/kg (smaller dose for pre-term infants)
Gentamicin	2.5 mg/kg
Latamoxef (moxalactam)	50 mg/kg
Vancomycin	15 mg/kg

Frequency of administration:

For term infants (37 weeks of gestation or more). Give above doses every 12 hours in the first 48 hours of life, every 8 hours between 3 days and 2 weeks, and every 6 hours if over 2 weeks. Note: Amikacin, chloramphenicol and gentamicin should not be given more than every 8 hours at any age.
For preterm infants (less than 37 weeks of gestation). This must vary with maturity. Infants of less than 32 weeks of gestation may only need above dose every 18 hours, or occasionally only once daily in the first few days. Most pre-term infants over 32 weeks of gestation can cope with the above dosage every 12 hours in the first week of life, every 8 hours between 1 and 4 weeks, and every 6 hours after that age (amikacin, chloramphenicol and gentamicin excepted, as above).

Rifampicin — there is limited information about dosages in the neonatal period and the drug is usually given orally. A single dose of 10 mg/kg 12 hourly has been used. A tested intravenous preparation may be available in the future.

Benzyl penicillin is the drug of choice for streptococcal pneumococcal and meningococcal meningitis (see Table 37.3 for dosage). McCracken (1985) has reviewed in-vitro and experimental evidence suggesting synergism with drug combinations and advocates a penicillin and an aminoglycoside for initial therapy of Group B Streptococcal meningitis until the CSF is sterile, when benzyl penicillin alone can be continued. If penicillin-tolerant organisms are suspected (these are likely when the ratio of minimal bactericidal concentration to minimal inhibitory concentration is greater than 32) the drug combination should be continued to avoid relapse or recurrence (Siegel et al 1981).

Tolerance of or relative resistance to ampicillin has also been reported for *L. monocytogenes*, and similar in-vitro synergy has been demonstrated for ampicillin with added aminoglycoside. An ampicillin–gentamicin combination would now be the initial treatment of choice, at least until CSF sterilization is certain, when ampicillin alone can be continued (McCracken 1985). Infections with beta-lactamase positive strains of *S. aureus*, *S. epidermidis* or other coagulase-negative staphylococci might best be treated with a cephalosporin such as cefotaxime or ceftriaxone, whose CSF penetration is much superior to that of the isoxazolyl penicillins. Vancomycin and rifampicin must be reserved for strains of these two organisms which are multiply resistant and for some similar strains of enterococci and JK coryneforms, other Gram-positive organisms which are occasionally found colonizing ventriculo-peritoneal shunts for hydrocephalus. The duration of treatment must depend on the clinical response but a minimum of two weeks after sterilization of the CSF has been recommended (McCracken & Nelson 1983). This may be some days before the white cell count, glucose and protein levels have returned to normal; provided the infant is afebrile, gaining weight and showing no new abnormal neurological findings, and has a normal serum C-reactive protein concentration (Peltola et al 1984), not too much concern should be given to continuing pleocytosis.

Meningitis due to Gram-negative organisms, or unknown. Perusal of the literature describing treatment of Gram-negative bacillary neonatal meningitis reveals little unanimity. This is not surprising since the largest neonatal centres see relatively few cases annually and an individual physician may treat an even smaller number. Large series, in which one drug or drug combination has been used to treat one infecting organism are not available; there are many possible such organisms (see Table 37.2) and new drugs are introduced into clinical practice frequently. Thus reliance has rightly come to be placed on co-operative trials involving many centres. However, different standards of care between them and differing time periods between onset of the disease and actual diagnosis and then start of effective treatment pose important variables which cannot be controlled.

The United States Neonatal Meningitis Cooperative Study Group has reported three such trials, all randomized and controlled, comparing treatments for Gram-negative bacillary meningitis. (Despite the Group's title, infants over one month of age were studied and the number of newborn infants included lessened serially.) The first involved 18 centres in North and South America and 117 infants under 2 years old, of whom 98 were under 30 days old (McCracken & Mize 1976). Systemic ampicillin and gentamicin continued for 2 weeks after sterilization of the CSF, or for a minimum of 3 weeks, whichever was longer, plus once daily lumbar intrathecal gentamicin for a minimum of 3 days or until cultures were sterile was not superior to systemic ampicillin and gentamacin alone. The second trial involved 16 United States and South American centres, 71 infants under 1 year of whom 55 were less than 30 days old (McCracken et al 1980). Of the 71 infants, 52 had ventriculitis and these were randomized to two groups, one group receiving intraventricular gentamicin for a minimum of 3 days with systemic ampicillin and gentamacin, the other the systemic drugs only. The study was stopped early because of a significantly higher mortality rate in the intraventricularly treated group. The third trial included 63 infants from 22 centres in the United States, South America and Europe under 1 year of age (48 less than 30 days) who were either treated with systemic ampicillin and moxalactam (latamoxef) — the ampicillin being stopped when the pathogen was positively identified — or with ampicillin and amikacin (McCracken et al 1984). There was no significant difference in mortality between the two treatments (23% vs 15%), despite moxalactam's superior penetration of and bactericidal activity in the CSF. The time taken to sterilize the CSF after starting treatment was 3 days

in both groups. The CSF in meningitis due to Gram-positive organisms on the other hand is usually sterile within 12–24 hours of beginning treatment (McCracken 1972) and this may be the main factor associated with its usually lower mortality rate.

Some have considered chloramphenicol the single drug of choice for neonatal meningitis, at least until the cephalosporins are better evaluated (Mulhall et al 1983). A variety of factors however do not recommend it, at least on theoretical grounds: the ability of babies both to hydrolyse chloramphenicol succinate and to excrete unhydrolysed inactive succinate by the kidneys is very variable, making dosage difficult to judge; the drug is bacteristatic rather than bactericidal for Gram-negative organisms; resistance to it has occurred in the course of treatment; and there is a narrow safety margin (as with the aminoglycosides) between effective and toxic dosage in very ill babies. There is suggestive evidence of antagonism between chloramphenicol and aminoglycosides (Sanderson 1978). At present ampicillin and aminoglycoside (gentamicin or amikacin) have to remain the best tried combination for neonatal bacterial meningitis due to unknown organisms or to gram-negative enteric bacilli; they can be continued for a full three weeks, or for two weeks after the CSF is sterile, whichever is longer. It is likely that when comparative trials are completed ampicillin combined with ceftriaxone (Congeni 1984, Hoogkamp-Korstanje 1985), or cefotaxime (Borderon et al 1985, Hoogkamp-Korstanje 1985, Naqvi Maxwell & Dunkle 1985) or ceftazidime (Blumer et al 1985) may prove as suitable as an alternative. This would obviate the need to monitor serum and CSF concentrations when the potentially toxic aminoglycosides are used.

The apparent harmfulness of intraventricular therapy shown by the second United States Cooperative trial was unexpected. Others had reported favourable results with its use (Lorber 1974, Yeung 1976, Lee et al 1977, Eeckels et al 1980). It is possible that if hydrocephalus is present, as in some cases of meningomyelocele the only way to achieve the concentrations necessary for effective treatment of ventriculitis will be to instill the drug intraventricularly (Stark 1968, Lorber et al 1970, Wright et al 1981). There is evidence though of neurotoxicity following intraventricular therapy with aminoglycoside in the experimental animal (Hodges et al 1981). In addition, porencephalic cysts may occur in the needle track if the drug is instilled by direct puncture (Lorber & Emery 1964, Salmon 1967), and this route should be avoided whenever possible.

Supportive treatment

Other medication. If fits accompany meningitis prompt treatment with a loading dose of phenobarbitone (15–20 mg/kg) intravenously or intramuscularly could be given, followed by a maintenance dose. Non-enzyme inducing drugs should be substituted in the rare event of coincident chloramphenicol therapy. The even more rapid initial action of diazepam (0.1 mg/kg intravenously, repeated if necessary) is preferred by some but hypotension may occur. McCracken (1984) has reviewed older studies in infants and children with regard to steroid treatment for inflammation and oedema of the brain (see also later) and has concluded that it did not significantly improve results. Steroids have been found to be inferior to mannitol in reducing increased intracranial pressure in severe birth asphyxia (Levene & Evans 1985).

Maintenance of cerebral perfusion pressure. Brain oedema may develop in central nervous system infections and such increased intracranial pressure can impair cerebral blood flow, in turn dependent on cerebral perfusion pressure (see p. 378).

Few patients with neonatal meningitis have been treated aggressively for intracranial hypertension and treatment was by no means uniformly successful in maintaining cerebral perfusion pressure; all infants or children in whom it fell to 30 mmHg or below died (Goitein & Tamir 1983, Goitein et al 1983). To what extent such efforts can prevent this fall and so reduce the considerable later morbidity in infants surviving bacterial meningitis is at present unclear. Nevertheless, commonsense dictates that much more attention has to be paid to this aspect of treatment than in the past if sequelae in survivors are to be reduced.

Pathology and complications

Morison (1970) points out that in those few cases where infection extends from a localized skull lesion the infection is unlikely to be confined by the dura mater (as it might be at older ages); instead it involves the pia-arachnoid early. The subarachnoid space may be relatively larger in infancy and considerable amounts of pus can be present there at autopsy if the course has been prolonged and the infecting organism of relatively low virulence. When the exudate is haemorrhagic there is usually localized venous thrombosis but fibrous tissue proliferation, as following subarachnoid haemorrhage is not excessive. Both Morison (1970) and Berman & Banker (1966), the latter reviewing 25 cases of their own, commented that the evolution of meningitis was not essentially different from that in later life.

In the second and third week of illness, however, when plasma cells and lymphocytes would be prominent in the meningeal reaction at other ages, they were sparse. Ventriculitis, blockage of foramina and aqueduct with resulting hydrocephalus, encephalopathy and cerebral infarction were all present. Intense vasculitis leading to haemorrhagic cerebral necrosis has been seen with infection caused by *Proteus* sp. and *Serratia marcescens* (Cussen & Ryan 1967, Shortland-Webb 1968). Morison emphasizes the difficulty of distinguishing whether degenerative changes in the deeper layers of the cortex are due to the meningitis, or to accompanying hypoxia and ischaemia.

Subdural collections of fluid in bacterial meningitis may range from xanthochromic with few white blood cells to grossly purulent and have a higher protein and glucose content than CSF. Although explanations have been put forward for their formation (Rabe 1967), their precise aetiology remains uncertain. None was found by Berman & Banker (1966) in their series of neonatal meningitis collected between 1958 and 1965. Computed tomography, which will detect collections of 30 ml or more, identified their presence in 7% of newborn babies, who were part of a series of older infants and children recorded between 1969 and 1984 (Syrogiannopoulos et al 1986). The peak age for their occurrence was 5 months and the fluid collections were found more frequently with *H. influenzae*, *S. pneumoniae* and *E. coli* infections than with those caused by all other organisms. They have also occurred in the course of group B streptococcal meningitis of both early and later onset (Baker & Edwards 1983). The diagnosis should be suspected if irritability, focal neurological signs, a tense fontanelle and increasing head circumference occur in the course of meningitis. Treatment by aspiration, sometimes repeated, will normally suffice, in addition to the antimicrobial therapy already being given for the underlying infection. Transillumination of the head may be useful, unless the fluid is grossly purulent, or real-time ultrasound, in following resolution.

Other complications recorded, in addition to puncture porencephaly mentioned above, are brain herniation through the anterior fontanelle (Gibson et al 1975), and spinal cord damage (Tal et al 1980). The latter took the form of extensive softening and haemorrhage involving the lower thoracic and lumbo–sacral spinal cord. The nerve cells were necrotic but recognizable. This report also mentioned quadriplegia, sensory loss and lack of sphincter control considered due to similar pathology in two surviving 3-year-olds. Hyponatraemia associated with the syndrome of inappropriate antidiuretic hormone secretion has also been described as occurring in the course of neonatal meningitis (Reynolds et al 1972) but its frequency is uncertain. The safest and most effective treatment is fluid restriction. Brain abscess is considered separately below.

Prognosis

Mortality. Twenty-seven studies of neonatal meningitis recorded in the world literature between 1952 and 1973 were reviewed by Lorber (1974, and personal communication 1983); he found that 470 of 762 (61%) babies 'treated by modern methods in different parts of the world at leading institutions' died. In the defined population of the North West Thames region of London, the case fatality rate for babies under 4 weeks of age born between 1969 and 1973 was 43% (Goldacre 1977). Mortality rates in the three United States Neonatal Meningitis Cooperative Study Group trials involving the years 1971–75, 1976–79, and 1980–82 were 40% (aged 30 days and less), 29% (aged 1 year or less) and 19% (aged less than 1 year) respectively (McCracken & Mize 1976, McCracken et al 1980, McCracken et al 1984). Infants with neural tube defects were not included in any of the studies mentioned so far. A case fatality rate of 27% was recorded for neonatal meningitis throughout the Netherlands between 1976 and 1982 (Mulder & Zanen 1984a); and 24% of the infants less than 28 days old and 11% aged 28 days to 1 year died following proven meningitis in a co-operative study (April 1978–October 1980) from 12 English hospitals (Mulhall et al 1983, De Louvois 1987). Thus insofar as these very differing populations can be compared, an increase in survival has occurred since Lorber's review.

Low birth-weight not surprisingly worsens prognosis; the United States Collaborative Perinatal Project (1959–66) reported that infants weighing less than 2.5 kg at birth were nearly twice as likely to die as those above this weight (Overall 1970). The Netherlands population study showed no significant difference in mortality between meningitis caused by *E. coli* (132 cases) and that caused by group B streptococcus (68 cases); it was 26% and 25% respectively. There was also no difference in mortality rate between early and late onset group B streptococcal meningitis (Mulder et al 1984, Mulder & Zanen 1984b). Factors associated with a good prognosis for survival in neonatal meningitis are a birth-weight above 2.5 kg, age at the time of diagnosis greater than one day, a white blood cell count above 2.0 $\times$ $10^9/l$ and a normal platelet count in the peripheral blood (Eeckels et al 1980). When fat-laden macrophages constituted more than 40% of the white cells in the CSF, the prognosis for mortality was very poor; their appearance in the fluid suggested rising CSF pressure, areas of brain damage, or the development of ventriculitis (Chester et al 1971).

Morbidity. 'A large proportion' of the survivors reviewed by Lorber (1974) had serious physical or intellectual deficits. No long-term detailed follow-up studies involving geographically defined populations are available. Several studies since Lorber's review have reported on infants from individual neonatal units (Fitzhardinge et al 1974, Heckmatt 1976, Haslam et al 1977, Lee et al 1977, Eeckels et al 1980, Edwards et al 1985, Chin & Fitzhardinge 1985, Wald et al 1986). Meningitis was confined to the neonatal period in all but three studies in which the children were aged up to three or six months (Eeckels et al 1980, Edwards et al 1985, Wald et al 1986). Half the reports dealt with infections caused by Gram-negative organisms but group B streptococcal infections only were the subject of four surveys (Haslam et al 1977, Edwards et al 1985, Chin & Fitzhardinge 1985, Wald et al 1986), and one of these included only infants ill in the first week of life (Chin & Fitzhardinge 1985). The length of follow-up and the criteria for judging infants 'normal' were very variable. A total of 189 survivors were examined from an original 308 infants with meningitis. There was a variable loss to follow-up. Approximately one-third were disabled, some very severely. The sequelae reported include mental retardation (from slight to profound), cerebral palsy, hydrocephalus, blindness, deafness and epilepsy. Apparently normal survivors of meningitis occurring in childhood but after the neonatal period have been shown to function significantly less well at school age on a battery of tests when compared with matched controls from the same class (Sell et al 1972) but two of the reports of children surviving group B streptococcal meningitis (Haslam et al 1977, Wald et al 1986) did not find deficiencies in intelligence or academic achievement when comparison was made with sibling controls in the few who had reached school age. Central nervous system infection was found to be a limiting factor in the intelligence of children with myelomeningocele. McLone et al (1982) compared mean intelligence quotients in three groups of 167 such children: those without infection and without hydrocephalus, those shunted for hydrocephalus but without infection, and those shunted who had ventriculitis. The mean intelligence quotient scores were 102, 95 and 72 respectively. Eeckels et al (1980) found that in children under 3 months of age with meningitis, significant risk factors for later disability were metabolic acidosis, onset of treatment over 24 hours after onset of symptoms, age less than 30 days, CSF protein above 3.0 g/l and glucose below 1.7 mmol/l.

Brain abscess

Computed tomography and ultrasonography have undoubtedly contributed to the more frequent recognition and earlier diagnosis of cerebral abscess in the neonatal period and weeks beyond. In the past the condition was recognized rarely, diagnosis was made late and most infants died. The lesions could attain a large size and tended to be poorly encapsulated. The few survivors were often profoundly disabled (Farley 1949, Johnson et al 1953, Butler et al 1957). Prevalence rates for defined populations are not available but it is possible that it is becoming more common, perhaps largely because of a new group of particularly vulnerable infants now surviving, those of extremely low gestations and birth-weights. In a hospital-based population in Texas this appeared to be so at other ages (Samson & Clark 1973) and may reflect the increasing practice of salvage treatments for formerly lethal conditions.

Brain abscess either occurs in the course of meningitis (see earlier for pathogenesis) or following cerebral ischaemia, hypoxia, germinal matrix haemorrhage–intraventricular haemorrhage, bacteraemia and sepsis elsewhere in the body such as adjacent skull bones (Butler et al 1957) or more remotely; the bacteria presumably settle in infarcted or otherwise damaged areas of brain tissue. A congenital cribriform plate defect has been implicated in one infant (Fyfe et al 1983). Cyanotic congenital heart disease rarely seems to have been involved in pathogenesis in infants under 2 years of age (Tingelstad et al 1974).

In the years before computed tomography and ultrasonography, diagnosis was usually made when hydrocephalus became clinically apparent with a full fontanelle and separated skull sutures. Hoffman et al (1970) considered that when the white cell count was raised in peripheral blood in this situation, even though fever was absent, the diagnosis should be strongly suspected. One child who had apparently always been well, presented with a right-sided weakness. Cerebral abscess occurring in the course of meningitis does not necessarily cause any change in state (Spirer et al 1982). The delineation of lesions radiographically in the past was often determined by the injection of thorotrast, with plain skull films, following aspiration of pus after clinical diagnosis. This has been superseded by computed tomography scanning (see Fig. 8.19, p. 133) which, with contrast enhancement and cuts through the entire brain, should not miss multiple lesions, including those in the vertex of the cerebral hemispheres (Fischer et al 1981). Cerebral ultrasonography though less reliable avoids irradiation and can be used serially during the course of meningitis to detect accompanying lesions (as well as developing hydrocephalus).

The most common infecting organisms are Gram-negative and include E. coli, Proteus sp. and Citrobacter sp. However Gram-positive organisms may also be involved and S. aureus, Mycoplasma hominis (Fischer et al 1981) and group B streptococci (Baker & Edwards 1983) have been implicated. In a review of the literature published in 1980, Curless found that in 12 of 16 cases, Citrobacter sp. were causative. These organisms on the other hand were responsible for only 4% of the cases of meningitis in the first of the United States Neonatal Meningitis Cooperative Study trials (McCracken & Mize 1976).

Treatment has traditionally consisted of the appropriate antimicrobial therapy (see earlier), aspiration, often repeated, with final excision. This is discussed in detail in Chapter 47, p. 596). It is possible that earlier detection with the newer diagnostic techniques and prompt effective antimicrobial therapy will allow the lesions to resolve without these more heroic measures (Spirer et al 1982). Prognosis will depend as always in the neonatal period on birth-weight, gestation, speed of diagnosis and prompt effective treatment. When the diagnosis is made late in small and immature infants, disability is predictable.

Infected CSF shunts

Luthardt (1970) reviewed work published between 1959 and 1967 by many authors. Shunt infections occurred in 13.5% of 1540 cases. Bacterial invasion from skin organisms introduced at surgery may account for the majority. Nicholas et al (1970), analysing a small personal series, felt that shunts inserted in infants with myelomeningocele were

no more liable to become infected than those performed for a different aetiology. The infecting organisms are most often coagulase-negative staphylococci. Those strains frequently colonizing shunts have been shown to produce a mucoid slime (Bayston & Penny 1972). The organisms seem able to multiply, possibly using components of the catheter for nutrition, since surface erosion occurs; the slime enhances their adherence to inner and outer surfaces of the catheter and makes them resistant to treatment (Peters et al 1982). *Candida albicans*, enterococci, coryneforms and propionibacteria colonize a small proportion, while *S. aureus* and Gram-negative bacilli are seen rarely and more often cause shunt wound infections, ventriculitis and bacteraemia than internal colonization of the valve or tubing. The propensity for *C. albicans* to form fungal balls frequently leads to blockage (Bayston 1985).

Diagnosis can be difficult if obstruction is not obvious as coagulase-negative staphylococcal infections may be low grade. Continuing serological surveillance (Bayston 1985) or serial C- reactive protein determinations may be helpful. Prompt diagnosis is important for infected ventriculo–peritoneal shunts may lead to frequent operations for shunt infection, while nephropathy and renal failure can result from infected ventriculo–atrial shunts. Review of the recent literature (Bayston 1985) suggests that shunt removal is nearly always essential for effective treatment, though earlier some reported success for prolonged antimicrobial therapy alone in a small number of cases (McLaurin & Dodson 1971). Treatment of any resulting ventriculitis and peritonitis is important before the shunt is put back and external ventricular drainage will be necessary in the intervening period. Antimicrobial therapy likely to be most effective for shunt infections has been referred to elsewhere (see meningitis earlier, and fungal infections later).

Endophthalmitis and panophthalmitis

These potentially very crippling infections have been reported in the course of other infections such as meningitis (Weintraub & Otto 1972, Greene et al 1979, Berger 1981), enteritis (Corman et al 1979), untreated gonococcal ophthalmia (Holmes 1983), or bacteraemia (Burns & Rhodes 1961). Conjunctival scarring caused by tightly fitting face-masks or eye-pads in place during phototherapy has also progressed to endophthalmitis (Cole et al 1980). The infecting organisms recorded in addition to *Neisseria gonorrhoeae* were *Streptococcus pneumoniae* and group B streptococcus (meningitis), *Salmonella enteritidis* (enteritis), and *Pseudomonas aeruginosa* (bacteraemia and conjunctival scarring). Those surviving in these reported cases all had visual impairment or blindness in the affected eye with one exception. This infant with early group B streptococcal meningitis had apparently normal vision at 8 months although a scar was present at the corneoscleral limbus, the site of previous aspiration of vitreous fluid, following which methicillin and dexamethasone had been injected (Berger 1981). Specialist ophthalmic advice should be sought immediately the diagnosis is suspected. Antimicrobial drugs do not always achieve therapeutic concentrations in aqueous and vitreous humour and surgical measures with local instillation may be necessary.

Epidural abscess

This very rarely encountered infection has been recorded in four infants, three of whom survived (Miller & Hesch 1962, Aicardi & Lepintre 1967, Palmer & Kelly 1972, Bergman et al 1983). The infecting organism was *S. aureus* in all cases. In two of the survivors the initial presenting signs in the second and third weeks of life included fever, irritability and crying on handling, and reduced leg movements with depressed knee jerks but exaggerated ankle jerks. Lumbar puncture revealed CSF with a protein content of 24 g/l in one baby; but in the alert second baby only a few drops of thick pus were obtained (Aicardi & Lepintre 1967, Palmer & Kelly 1972). Bilateral decompression laminectomies were performed after myelograms had localized the lesions and abnormal signs disappeared postoperatively. However, kyphosis following this procedure at a very young age is likely. Bergman et al (1983) who reported an infant developing epidural abscess following repeated lumbar punctures during the course of meningitis, successfully treated him without operation. The fourth infant (Miller & Hesch 1962) who presented at 5 weeks of age was recorded as having apparent paralysis of the left arm since birth. At autopsy the abscess was found to extend from C4 to T2. When the diagnosis is suspected, very careful lumbar puncture is recommended. The needle's stylette is removed frequently for inspection while the needle is still in the epidural space and removed altogether if pus is found, to prevent infection of the subarachnoid space.

NEONATAL TETANUS

Tetanus is caused by the potent neurotoxin of *Clostridium tetani*. This anaerobic spore-bearing bacillus is widespread in soil but contamination is highest in warm fertile regions which have large human and animal populations who may carry the organism in their faeces. The effects of toxin on the central rather than the peripheral nervous system are now considered responsible for the clinical features (Adams et al 1969). Although neonatal tetanus is a preventable disease, it has been estimated (collection of accurate figures is impossible) that a million babies die from it annually in certain impoverished areas of the world. Adams et al (1969) cite evidence that a preponderance of males is affected in some areas, though the suggestion that illness and death of the less-esteemed female babies go unrecorded in these societies is always a possibility.

A low oxygen tension is necessary to allow the clostridial spores to germinate, multiply and produce neurotoxin, which is why healthy tissues are not vulnerable; the necrotic umbilical wound, however, provides favourable conditions and this route of entry is considered responsible for nearly all neonatal cases. In some endemic areas the cord may be tied with the contaminated string-like roots of plants (Woodruff et al 1984); in others, soil, ash or dung have been applied to the cut cord (Adams et al 1969). Signs of the disease usually appear towards the end of the first week of life. The shorter the incubation period, the more severe they will be. Constant crying, unusual irritability, and poor feeding may be the initial ones. Fever, trismus, and stiffness sometimes progressing to opisthotonus follow, and finally the tell-tale recurring spasms with flexed extremities and fist clenching may be provoked by the slightest touch or vibration (Marshall 1968, Volpe 1981).

A variably high mortality is reported from many of those areas of the world where neonatal tetanus still occurs. Pulmonary complications (haemorrhage, aspiration pneumonia and bronchopneumonia involving the right upper lobe particularly) and dehydration were the most important causes of death in a series of Iranian infants, 60% of whom survived, reported by Salimpour (1977). In the past, survival has been equated with devoted and skilled nursing and varying schemes of sedation. Cleansing of the wound as at other ages, with removal of necrotic tissue is advised. It is not clear if neutralization of any unfixed toxin with tetanus immunoglobulin has any role. The ability to provide both mechanical ventilation and nutritional support will now reduce mortality to 10% (Smythe et al 1974, Adams et al 1979) but in those areas of the world where tetanus occurs most frequently such treatment is rarely available.

Hygienic care of the umbilical wound at birth will prevent neonatal tetanus. While this is usually available in hospitals and nursing homes in the countries where the disease still occurs on a large scale, many deliveries take place in the home or elsewhere. Woodruff et al (1984), reviewing the situation in the Southern Sudan, felt that prevention could be most effectively achieved there 'by issuing to all midwives and women a simple kit containing a sterile blade, a sterile ligature, two or three sterile adhesive dressings for the stump, and two or three sterile swabs'. They foresaw that publicity about their value, their free availability at health centres, hospitals and dispensaries in much the same way as achieved by UNICEF with packets of rehydration salts for diarrhoea would achieve an enormous saving of lives. It has been shown too that two doses of alum-precipitated tetanus toxoid, given either during pregnancy or up to 4 years previously, will give good protection against neonatal tetanus. Booster immunization at 5-year intervals during the reproductive years may be necessary (Lancet 1983). A surviving affected child needs to be immunized against tetanus in the usual way later because immunity does not follow the neonatal illness (Adams et al 1979).

Long-term disability following neonatal tetanus has been assessed by Teknetzi et al (1983) in 38 survivors examined between 5 and 12 years of age. Four had significant neurological or behavioural abnormality which was presumed to be due to hypoxia during the neonatal illness. The remaining 34 appeared normal.

INFANT BOTULISM

Botulism is the serious illness resulting from the action of a bacterial neurotoxin which blocks acetylcholine release at the neuromuscular junction causing profound muscle weakness. In adults this often-lethal condition has most usually resulted from eating improperly preserved food containing a preformed toxin, of which *Clostridium botulinum* elaborates seven (A–G). This organism's spores are widespread in soil and farm-produce throughout the world. Very occasionally the disease is caused when toxin forms in damaged tissues of a contaminated wound.

The condition was recognized for the first time in young infants in 1976 in the United States (Pickett et al 1976, Midura & Arnon 1976). Unlike the adult cases, toxin (type A or B) formed in vivo, as ingested spores of *C. botulinum* germinated, and the organisms multiplied in the gastrointestinal tract. Honey has been implicated as a source of spores for a small proportion of the infants (Arnon et al 1981). However, it now appears that other clostridial species may also produce botulinal neurotoxin in vivo and infant botulism cases due to type E toxin produced by *C. butyricum* (Aureli et al 1986) and to type F toxin produced by *C. barati* have been described (Hall et al 1985). The newborn infant's gut is colonized with a wide variety of clostridial species other than *C. botulinum* in the weeks after birth (Davies & Gothefors 1984); their numbers, however, are much lower in the breast-fed infant compared with the artificially fed (Olsen 1949). It seems likely that there will be further clarification of the extent to which clostridial species produce neurotoxin in the next decade, particularly now that a few adults have been recognized as having the 'infant' type of botulism (Arnon 1986).

Arnon et al (1981) reviewed the age distribution of all 181 hospitalized cases of infant botulism recognized in the United States between 1976 and 1980. Nearly all were under 6 months of age, with a peak at 2 months; under 5% of the total were recognized in the neonatal period. The infants have usually been previously healthy and the illness has presented with poor feeding, difficulty in swallowing, pooling of oral secretions, a weak cry, and constipation, in addition to generalized hypotonia, diminished or absent tendon reflexes, together with cranial nerve palsies causing squint, ptosis, and facial weakness. The two most dangerous facets of the illness are paralysis of the respiratory muscles; and aspiration of food or secretions. The condition has been recognized as causing sudden infant death syndrome and possibly 5% of such cases are in reality infant botulism, at least in the United States (Arnon et al 1981). It seems likely that the condition may have a wide spectrum, since some healthy infant carriers of *C. botulinum* and its toxin have been identified, as well as some with very mild hypotonia. Breast-feeding seems to protect infants from the more fulminating forms of paralysis.

Diagnosis must rest on the demonstration of botulinal toxin in faeces because in the infant variety it has not commonly been recovered from serum (Arnon 1986). Electromyography and other electrodiagnostic tests will help to make a presumptive diagnosis (Pickett et al 1976, Polin & Brown 1979, Volpe 1981). Treatment consists of respiratory support and if this is available complete recovery should be the rule. Mechanical ventilation has not, however, always been necessary.

FUNGAL INFECTIONS

Reports of fungal infections of the brain in the peri- and neonatal periods are very few compared with those of bacterial infections. They consist often of individual case histories and mostly record infection with *C. albicans*. The few infections acquired during prenatal life, assumed to be of the ascending variety always, are much more likely to involve the lungs and skin than the brain. In recent years the retention of an intra-uterine contraceptive device or a cervical cerclage suture have been recognized as risk factors (Whyte et al 1982).

Levin et al (1978) report the case of a second twin, whose amniotic sac had ruptured 9 days before delivery. The baby was born by the breech and was stillborn, like the first twin. Dense, white striated areas were found along the walls of the lateral ventricles at autopsy. Histological examination revealed spores and hyphae consistent with *Candida* and *C. albicans* was isolated from the maternal vagina. The lungs were apparently uninvolved and the first twin, whose amniotic sac was intact until delivery, was uninfected. A suggestive but unproven case of fetal infection was reported by Burry (1957). An infant weighing 3.4 kg who was slow to breathe and cry at birth required tube feeding because of poor sucking. On the fifth day of life unusual separation of the skull sutures suggested hydrocephalus. After some improvement towards the end of the second week the baby's condition deteriorated and he died eventually at 37 days. Gross hydrocephalus involving the lateral and third ventricles was evident. Sections of exudate at the base of the brain showed marked meningeal thickening with pial adhesions. Irregular masses of partly calcified necrotic material were present and hyphae and fungal spores were found beneath a layer of glial scarring; there was some lymphocyte infiltration around the fungal masses. Cultures had not been made before brain fixation but the presence of septate pseudomycelia and small spores was thought to suggest *C. albicans*. The author felt that the histological appearances and the well-established scarring and calcification suggested an inflammatory process longer than the 5 weeks of postnatal life.

A case of congenital infection due to *Torulopsis glabrata* was reported by Quirke et al (1980). The infant weighed 0.52 kg at approximately 23 weeks of gestation and died one hour after birth. Culture of the CSF (and blood) gave a pure growth of the organism. The leptomeninges were described as congested but otherwise unremarkable and no mention was made of brain histology. Yeast cells were present in the lungs. *Cryptococcus neoformans* infections acquired in the uterus have been reviewed by Miller (1983). A few cases are reported, all with the brain along with other organs showing the encapsulated yeast-like organisms. Hydrocephalus was present in one infant, with numerous granulomata containing calcium scattered over the brain surface. Heath (1950) has described an infant dying at 27 days of age who had a diffuse necrotizing choroidoretinitis and extensive separation of the retina. *Cryptococcus neoformans* was demonstrated in retina and brain.

Postnatally acquired *C. albicans* meningitis is seen either as part of a disseminated candidiasis or secondary to infected ventriculo–atrial or ventriculo–peritoneal shunts. In both cases the infants may be very immature and of low birth-weight; their postnatal course complicated and antimicrobial therapy and indwelling tubes a feature of their care. The case report by Chesney et al (1978) of candidal meningitis in a 1.1 kg pre-term infant who required mechanical ventilation for respiratory distress syndrome, had congestive heart failure associated with a patent ductus arteriosus, was given antibiotics, and required total parenteral nutrition for 20 days because abdominal distension was present, is typical of the complicated course many small babies endure. The authors review 16 other cases from the literature, many with similar histories. Of 17 cases, 5 died. Half of the survivors had hydrocephalus and just over half were retarded. Attention is drawn to the fact that the diagnosis was made late. Culture results were delayed or equivocal because of slow growth of the organism; occasionally it was dismissed as a contaminant. In older and immunocompromised patients, buffy coat smears of blood drawn through central venous catheters has proved to be a rapid method of diagnosis (Ascuitto et al 1985). Only 10 of Chesney and colleagues' 17 cases had positive lumbar CSF cultures; in 3 of those with negative cultures, however, ventricular fluid proved positive. Fungal endophthalmitis may accompany disseminated candidiasis and can be recognized when a vitreous haze with fluffy white lesions are seen on ophthalmoscopy. In one such case the endophthalmitis progressed to bilateral corneal perforations (Michelson et al 1975).

Cerebrospinal fluid shunts colonized by *C. albicans* are often blocked by a fungal mass. A case of cephalosporium meningitis in a full-term infant has been described (Papadatos et al 1969).

Candida brain abscesses, usually multiple and miliary, occasionally larger, unrecognized during life and diagnosed only at postmortem examination, have also been recorded. Haruda et al (1980) describe two cases and presented details of six other in a review of the literature. In contrast with the meningitis cases, only three of the eight infants weighed less than 2.5 kg at birth. Several had had gastrointestinal surgery, with frequent courses of antimicrobial therapy. Central nervous system signs were not a prominent feature. Only one of six blood cultures grew *C. albicans* and CSF cultures when done were all negative, although four of the babies had clinical or laboratory evidence of superficial monilial infection. Two lived for more than 3 months but in others the course was often dramatically short. None was hydrocephalic. After death, multiple small granulomata containing hyphae and yeasts were found in the brain and other organs. In one, a lesion in the left pole of the cerebellum was easily visible to the naked eye. Some well-encapsulated granulomatous abscess cavities contained giant cells, yeast spores and pseudomycelial forms characteristic of *Candida* sp.

Aspergillosis has been reported very rarely indeed (Zimmerman 1955, Akkoyunlu & Yucel 1957, Luke et al 1963, Rhine et al 1986). In three babies the diagnosis was made at necropsy and the brain lesions were part of a disseminated aspergillosis. In one infant who was ill at birth and who received antimicrobial drugs and corticosteroids, *Aspergillus sydowi* was recovered from one of many small brain abscesses after his death at 30 days. A second infant became ill with diarrhoea and respiratory distress at 20 days of age, dying 5 days later. Typical mycelia were found in necrotic areas of the brain. The third infant was born 'minimally hydropic' due to rhesus incompatibility. After a chequered course during which *E. coli* bacteraemia was diagnosed and treated with antimicrobial drugs and corticosteroids, he eventually died at 51 days. Fifteen discrete partially cavitated abscesses were found in both frontal temporal and parietal lobes, measuring between 0.2 and 1.5 cm in diameter (Luke et al 1963). The fourth case, the sole survivor was born at 31 weeks of gestation; her mother had had a Shirodkar suture put in place 4 months previously. The baby's course was complicated, mechanical ventilation being necessary for severe respiratory distress. She was treated with antimicrobial drugs and methylprednisolone. A computed tomography scan at 18 days showed a low-density area in the right frontal region, presumed to be an abscess. By day 25, a repeat scan showed that the lesion occupied one-third of the right parietal and the medial right frontal lobe. Bacterial cultures were all negative. The abscess was aspirated on several occasions from the 26th day and *Aspergillus fumigatus* was grown on two of them. Despite treatment with amphotericin B (and oral flucytosine, later stopped because of the organism's insensitivity), the abscess persisted, and on days 34 and 55 was shown by further scan to involve nearly all the right frontal lobe and some of the left parietal lobe. The left lateral ventricle was dilated. On day 59 the abscess was excised. A shunt became necessary at 8 months. At 2 years this unfortunate child was profoundly developmentally retarded, had fits and a hemiplegia (Rhine et al 1986).

There are few published data about the pharmacokinetics of antifungal drugs in the neonatal period and any recommendations for treatment must be read with this in mind. Amphotericin B and flucytosine, despite their known nephrotoxicity, and hepatotoxity and depressive bone marrow effects respectively, have to remain the drugs of choice for disseminated candidiasis and other fungal infections involving the central nervous system. They are usually prescribed together because of their known in-vitro synergy against *Candida* and in the hope that resistance will be less likely to occur. The imidazole drug, miconazole, cannot be recommended because of its poor penetration into CSF and urine.

Amphotericin B is conventionally given intravenously at a low dose of 0.1–0.25 (mg/kg)/day, and increased gradually to a maximum: of 0.5–1.0 (mg/kg)/day, the smaller doses being for very immature infants. McCracken & Nelson (1983) advise that the dose should be diluted in 5% dextrose and infused over a 4–6 hour period, bottle and tubing being protected from the light by aluminium foil. Flucytosine can be given 6 hourly intravenously, in doses ranging up to 100 (mg/kg)/day. The duration of treatment must always be decided individually, but may be necessary for at least 3–4 weeks. In those cases in which infection is associated with colonized shunts or other indwelling catheters, their removal will be an essential part of successful treatment.

PREVENTION

Prevention of central nervous system infection must always be preferable to treatment, with its all too imperfect results. General principles governing prevention of neonatal bacterial infection have been summarized elsewhere (Davies & Gothefors 1984). Specific attempts are increasingly to the fore, particularly for group B streptococcal infection. Randomized controlled trials in which penicillin has been given to newborn infants within an hour or so of birth have given conflicting results regarding prevention of early-onset infection (Siegel et al 1982, Pyati et al 1983). As infection is often established at the time of birth, attempts to protect the fetus by giving colonized women penicillin in labour are more logical and have been proved effective in selected high-risk pregnancies (Boyer & Gotoff 1986). The logistics of identifying such women in everyday obstetric practice are formidable and this treatment will not prevent later-onset meningitis, the source of much future disability. Increasing attention is therefore being given to the possibility of active immunization of women in their reproductive years with group B streptococcal polysaccharide vaccines (Baker &

Kasper 1985). The use of preparations of immunoglobulin for the infant after birth is another possibility but questions of subclass specificity have to be determined (Givner et al 1987. Similar possibilities for protection against *E. coli* K1 antigen infections are at present less clear.

CONCLUSIONS

Accurate estimates of fetal central nervous system bacterial infections occurring via the transplacental or ascending routes do not exist. Fetal host defences, virtually non-existent in the first trimester, develop only very gradually from the second trimester. Low-grade and undiagnosed infection of the amniotic sac, chorioamnionitis, which must be presumed bacterial in most cases, is present in about 10% of all pregnancies. It is associated with spontaneous abortion or pre-term birth in a much higher proportion. The supposition that ascending bacterial infection could be a cause of brain malformation or later retardation remains untested but as aetiology is unknown in the majority of such cases it must be worthy of serious consideration. Proof will be difficult to establish and will presumably require newer diagnostic techniques.

After birth, those born pre-term, and/or having a complicated neonatal course are most at risk of central nervous system infection. The host defence and environmental factors which allow some women to harbour larger numbers of bacteria in their birth canal are not yet well understood and bacterial meningitis, often maternally transmitted, occurs more commonly in the first week of life than at any other age. No accurate national figures of prevalence in the first 4 weeks of life exist, though one population study provides a minimum figure of 0.26/1000 livebirths. Statutory notifications and the voluntary laboratory reporting system practised in England and Wales, suggest that the group B streptococcus now causes most cases during this period, followed very closely by *Escherichia coli*, with *Listeria monocytogenes* much less common. A very wide variety of other organisms, the majority Gram-negative, comprise the remainder. Although the mortality has fallen as neonatal intensive care is more widely and effectively applied, complications occur in at least a third of survivors. As the number of survivors increases, the number of impaired children, some of them profoundly disabled, will also increase. Much earlier diagnosis, efforts directed at preserving the integrity of the cerebral circulation, and earlier recognition with cerebral ultrasonography, of such complications as brain abscess or developing hydrocephalus, are the factors most likely to improve future results. These will be more important than the advent of new antimicrobial drugs.

The few case histories given show how insidious and ultimately disabling central nervous system infections can be. Prevention must therefore be of prime concern in that period of life encompassing the formation and rapid growth of the brain. Those responsible for newborn nurseries and neonatal intensive care units have to insist on the highest standards of care and vigilance possible if transmission of infection after birth is to be avoided. Future research may increasingly turn to ways of enhancing maternal and hence fetal immunity, as well as the newborn infant's defences against infection.

REFERENCES

Adams E B, Laurence D R, Smith J W G 1969 Tetanus, Blackwell Scientific, Oxford, pp 17–30

Adams J M, Kenny J D, Rudolph A J 1979 Modern management of tetanus neonatorum. Pediatrics 64: 472–477

Adinolfi M 1985 The development of the human blood–CSF–brain barrier. Developmental Medicine and Child Neurology 27: 532–537

Adler S P, Markowitz S M 1983 Failure of moxalactam in the treatment of neonatal sepsis and meningitis from *Salmonella typhimurium*. Journal of Pediatrics 103: 913–916

Aicardi J, Lepintre J 1967 Spinal epidural abscess in 1-month-old child. American Journal of Diseases of Children 114: 665–667

Akkoyunlu A, Yucel F A 1957 Aspergillose broncho-pulmonaire et encéphalo-méningée chez un nouveau-né de 20 jours. Archives Francaises de Pediatrie 14: 615–622

Albritton W L, Wiggins G L, Feeley J C 1976 Neonatal listeriosis: distribution of serotypes in relation to age at onset of disease. Journal of Pediatrics 88: 481–483

Althabe O, Labarrere C 1985 Chronic villitis of unknown aetiology and intrauterine growth-retarded infants of normal and low ponderal index. Placenta 6: 369–373

Altshuler G 1973 Toxoplasmosis as a cause of hydranencephaly. American Journal of Diseases of Children 125: 251–252

Anagnostakis D, Fitsialos J, Koutsia C, Messaritakis J, Matsaniotis N 1981 A nursery outbreak of *Serratia marcescens* infection: evidence of a single source of contamination. American Journal of Diseases of Children 135: 413–414

Appelbaum P C, Holloway Y, Ross S M, Dhupelia L 1977 The effect of amniotic fluid on bacterial growth in three population groups. American Journal of Obstetrics and Gynecology 128: 868–871

Appelbaum P C, Bowen A J, Adhikari M, Robins-Browne R M, Koornhof H J 1978 Neonatal septicemia and meningitis due to *Aeromonas shigelloides*. Journal of Pediatrics 92: 676–677

Arnon S S 1986 Infant botulism: anticipating the second decade. Journal of Infectious Diseases 154: 201–206

Arnon S S, Damus K, Chin J 1981 Infant botulism: epidemiology and relation to sudden infant death syndrome. Epidemiological Reviews 3: 45–66

Ascuitto R J, Gerber M A, Cates K L, Tilton R C 1985 Buffy coat smears of blood drawn through central venous catheters as an aid to rapid diagnosis of systemic fungal infections. Journal of Pediatrics 106: 445–447

Aureli P, Fenicia L, Pasolini B, Gianfranceschi M, McCroskey L M, Hatheway C L 1986 Two cases of type E infant botulism caused by neurotoxigenic *Clostridium butyricum* in Italy. Journal of Infectious Diseases 154: 207–211

Babiker M A, Taha S A 1984 Meningitis in children of Riyadh. Journal of Tropical Medicine and Hygiene 87: 245–248

Baker C J, Edwards M S 1983 Group B streptococcal infections. In: Remington J S, Klein J O (eds) Infectious diseases of the fetus and newborn infant. W B Saunders, Philadelphia, pp 820–881

Baker R C, Bausher J C 1986 Meningitis complicating acute bacteremic facial cellulitis. Pediatric Infectious Disease 5: 421–423

Baker C J, Kasper D L 1976 Correlation of maternal antibody deficiency with susceptibility to neonatal group B streptococcal infection. New England Journal of Medicine 294: 753–756

Baker C J, Kaspar D L 1985 Group B streptococcal vaccines. Reviews of Infectious Diseases 7: 458–467

Barclay N 1971 High frequency of *Salmonella* species as a cause of neonatal meningitis in Ibadan, Nigeria: a review of thirty-eight cases. Acta Paediatrica Scandinavica 60: 540–544

Bates H A, Controni G, Elliott N, Eitzman D V 1965 Septicemia and meningitis in a newborn due to *Pasteurella multocida*. Clinical Pediatrics 4: 668–670

Bayston R 1985 Hydrocephalus shunt infections and their treatment. Journal of Antimicrobial and Chemotherapy 15: 259–261

Bayston R, Penny S R 1972 Excessive production of mucoid substance in *Staphylococcus* S II A: a possible factor in colonisation of Holter shunts. Developmental Medicine and Child Neurology 14 (suppl 27): 25–28

Benirschke K, Driscoll S G 1967 The pathology of the human placenta. Springer-Verlag, Berlin

Berczy J, Fernlund K, Kamme C 1973 *Haemophilus influenzae* in septic abortion. Lancet i: 1197 (letter)

Berger B B 1981 Endophthalmitis complicating group B streptococcal septicemia. American Journal of Ophthalmology 92: 681–684

Bergman I, Wald E R, Meyer J D, Painter M J 1983 Epidural abscess and vertebral osteomyelitis following serial lumbar punctures. Pediatrics 72: 476–480

Berkowitz F E 1982 *Acinetobacter* meningitis — a diagnostic pitfall. A report of 3 cases. South African Medical Journal 61: 448–449

Berman B W, King F H Jr, Rubenstein D S, Long S S 1978 *Bacteroides fragilis* meningitis in a neonate successfully treated with metronidazole. Journal of Pediatrics 93: 793–795

Berman P H, Banker B Q 1966 Neonatal meningitis: a clinical and pathological study of 29 cases. Pediatrics 38: 6–24

Bischoff H W, Recinos A, Anderson W S, Rice E C 1948 *Alkaligenes fecalis* bacteremia and meningitis: report of two cases in newborn infants. Journal of Pediatrics 32: 558–560

Blumer J L, Aronoff S C, Myers C M, O'Brien C A, Klinger J D, Reed M D 1985 Pharmacokinetics and cerebrospinal fluid penetration of ceftazidime in children with meningitis. Developmental Pharmacology and Therapeutics 8: 219–231

Borderon J-C, Despert F, Santini J-J, Laugier J 1985 Traitement des meningites purulentes de l'enfant par cefotaxime. Pediatrie 40: 291–299

Boyer K M, Gotoff S P 1986 Prevention of early-onset neonatal group B streptococcal disease with selective intrapartum chemoprophylaxis. New England Journal of Medicine 314: 1665–1669

Brabin B J 1985 Epidemiology of infection in pregnancy. Reviews of Infectious Diseases 7: 579–603

Bradford W L, Kelley H W 1933 Gonococcic meningitis in a new born infant with review of the literature. American Journal of Diseases of Children 46: 543–549

Brody J I, Oski F 1967 Immunologic memory of the normal and the leukemic lymphocyte. Annals of Internal Medicine 67: 573–578

Brook I, Barrett C T, Brinkman C R III, Martin W J, Finegold S M 1979 Aerobic and anaerobic bacterial flora of the maternal cervix and newborn gastric fluid and conjunctiva: a prospective study. Pediatrics 63: 451–455

Burns R P, Rhodes D H Jr 1961 *Pseudomonas* eye infection as a cause of death in premature infants. Archives of Ophthalmology 65: 517–525

Burry A F 1957 Hydrocephalus after intra-uterine fungal infection. Archives of Disease in Childhood 32: 161–163

Burton B K, Marr T J, Traisman H S, Davis A T 1977 *Salmonella typhi* meningitis in a neonate. American Journal of Diseases of Children 131: 1031

Butler N R, Barrie H, Paine K W E 1957 Cerebral abscess as a complication of neonatal sepsis. Archives of Disease in Childhood 32: 461–465

Cabrera H A, Davis G H 1961 Epidemic meningitis of the newborn caused by *Flavobacteria*. I. Epidemiology and bacteriology. American Journal of Diseases of Children 101: 289–295

Cassie R, Stevenson A 1973 Screening for gonorrhoea, trichomoniasis, moniliasis and syphilis in pregnancy. Journal of Obstetrics and Gynaecology of the British Commonwealth 80: 48–51

Chandra R K, Matsumura T 1979 Ontogenetic development of the immune system and effects of fetal growth retardation. Journal of Perinatal Medicine 7: 279–290

Chesney P J, Justman R A, Bogdanowicz W M 1978 *Candida* meningitis in newborn infants: a review and report of combined amphotericin B–flucytosine therapy. Johns Hopkins Medical Journal 142: 155–160

Chester D C, Emery J L, Penny S R 1971 Fat-laden macrophages in cerebrospinal fluid as an indication of brain damage in children. Journal of Clinical Pathology 24: 753–756

Chin K C, Fitzhardinge P M 1985 Sequelae of early-onset Group B hemolytic streptococcal neonatal meningitis. Journal of Pediatrics 106: 819–822

Christensen K K, Hägerstrand I, Mårdh P-A 1982 Late spontaneous abortion associated with *Mycoplasma hominis:* infection of the fetus. Scandinavian Journal of Infectious Diseases 14: 73–74

Christensen R D, Shigeoka A O, Hill H R, Rothstein G 1980 Circulating and storage neutrophil changes in experimental type II Group B streptococcal sepsis. Pediatric Research 14: 806–808

Clapp D W, Kleiman M B, Reynolds J K, Allen S D 1986 *Pasteurella multocida* meningitis in infancy. An avoidable infection. American Journal of Diseases of Children 140: 444–446

Cohen M S, Black J R, Proctor R A, Sparling P F 1984 Host defences and the vaginal mucosa. A re-evaluation. Scandinavian Journal of Urology and Nephrology (Suppl) 86: 13–22

Coid C R, Sandison H, Slavin G, Altman D G 1978 *Escherichia coli* infection in mice and impaired fetal development. British Journal of Experimental Pathology 59: 292–297

Cole G F, Davies D P, Austin D J 1980 *Pseudomonas* ophthalmia neonatorum: a case of blindness. British Medical Journal 281: 440–441

Congeni B L 1984 Comparison of ceftriaxone and traditional therapy of bacterial meningitis. Antimicrobial Agents and Chemotherapy 25: 40–44

Cooke R W I 1975 *Bacteroides fragilis* septicaemia and meningitis in early infancy. Archives of Disease in Childhood 50: 241–243

Corman L I, Poirier R H, Littlefield C A, Sumaya C V 1979 Endophthalmitis due to *Salmonella enteritidis.* Journal of Pediatrics 95: 1001–1002

Crosby R M N, Mosberg W H Jr, Smith G W 1951 Intrauterine meningitis as a cause of hydrocephalus. Journal of Pediatrics 39: 94–101

Curless R G 1980 Neonatal intracranial abscess: two cases caused by *Citrobacter* and a literature review. Annals of Neurology 8: 269–272

Cussen L J, Ryan G B 1967 Hemorrhagic cerebral necrosis in neonatal infants with enterobacterial meningitis. Journal of Pediatrics 71: 771–776

Darby C P 1976 *Pseudomonas cepacia* meningitis with trimethoprim-sulfamethoxazole. American Journal of Diseases of Children 130: 1365–1366

Davies P A, Gothefors L A 1984 Bacterial infections in the fetus and newborn infant, Vol 26, Major Problems in Clinical Pediatrics. W B Saunders, Philadelphia

De Louvois J 1987 Personal communication

Dietzman D E, Fischer G W, Schoenknecht F D 1974 Neonatal *Escherichia coli* septicemia — bacterial counts in blood. Journal of Pediatrics 85: 128–130

Driscoll S G 1979 Significance of acute chorioamnionitis. Clinical Obstetrics and Gynecology 22: 339–349

Dungal N 1961 Listeriosis in four siblings. Lancet ii: 513–516

Durack D T, Perfect J R 1985 Experimental cryptococcal meningitis: a model for study of defense mechanisms in the central nervous system. In: Sande M A, Smith A L, Root R K (eds) Bacterial meningitis. Churchill Livingstone, Edinburgh, pp 71–82

Dysart N K, Griswold W R, Schanberger J E, Goscienski P J, Chow A W 1976 Meningitis due to *Bacteroides fragilis* in a newborn infant. Journal of Pediatrics 89: 509–510

Easmon C S F, Hastings M J G, Neill J, Bloxham B, Rivers R P A 1985 Is group B streptococcal screening during pregnancy justified? British Journal of Obstetrics and Gynaecology 92: 197–201

Eavey R D, Gao Y-Z, Schuknecht H F, Gonzalez-Pineda M 1985 Otologic features of bacterial meningitis of childhood. Journal of Pediatrics 106: 402–407

Eden A N 1966 Perinatal mortality caused by *Vibrio fetus:* review and analysis. Journal of Pediatrics 68: 297–304

Edwards M S, Rench M A, Haffar A A M, Murphy M A, Desmond M M, Baker C J 1985 Long-term sequelae of Group B streptococcal meningitis in infants. Journal of Pediatrics 106: 717–722

Eeckels R, Corbeel L, de Boeck C et al 1980 Intraventricular and or intralumbar treatment of purulent meningitis in infants. Acta Paediatrica Belgica 33: 243–251

Farley D L B 1949 Cerebral abscess in an infant followed by recovery. Lancet i: 264–266

Fedrick J, Butler N R 1970 Certain causes of neonatal death. II. Intraventricular haemorrhage. Biology of the Neonate 15: 257–290

Ferguson A C 1978 Prolonged impairment of cellular immunity in children with intrauterine growth retardation. Journal of Pediatrics 93: 52–56

Ferguson A C, Lawlor G J Jr, Neumann C G, Oh W, Stiehm E R 1974 Decreased rosett-forming lymphocytes in malnutrition and intrauterine growth retardation. Journal of Pediatrics 85: 717–723

Fikar C R, Levy J 1979 *Streptococcus bovis* meningitis in a neonate. American Journal of Diseases of Children 133: 1149–1150

Fischer E G, McLennan J E, Suzuki Y 1981 Cerebral abscess in children. American Journal of Diseases of Children 135: 746–749

Fitzhardinge P M, Kazemi M, Ramsay M, Stern L 1974 Long-term sequelae of neonatal meningitis. Developmental Medicine and Child Neurology 16: 3–10

Fleming D W, Cocni S L, MacDonald K L et al 1985 Pasteurized milk as a vehicle of infection in an outbreak of listeriosis. New England Journal of Medicine 312: 404–407

Fox H 1981 Placental involvement in maternal systemic infection. Perspectives in Pediatric Pathology 6: 63–81

Frutos A A, Levitsky D, Scott E G, Steele L 1978 A case of septicemia and meningitis in an infant due to *Pasteurella multocida.* Journal of Pediatrics 92: 853

Fyfe D A, Rothner D A, Orlowski J, Cook S A 1983 Recurrent meningitis with brain abscess in infancy. American Journal of Diseases of Children 137: 912–913

Garland S M, Murton L J 1987 Neonatal meningitis caused by *Ureaplasma urealyticum.* Pediatric Infectious Disease Journal 6: 868–870

Gewitz M, Dinwiddie R, Rees L et al 1979 *Mycoplasma hominis:* a cause of neonatal meningitis. Archives of Disease in Childhood 54: 231–233

Gibson N F, Ball M M, Kelsey D S, Morrison L 1975 Anterior fontanelle herniation. Pediatrics 56: 466–469

Gilles F H, Leviton A, Kerr C S 1976 Endotoxin leucoencephalopathy in the telencephalon of the newborn kitten. Journal of The Neurological Sciences 27: 183–191

Gitlin D, Biasucci A 1969 Development of γG, γA, γM, β1C/β1A, C'1 esterase inhibitor, ceruloplasmin, transferin, hemopexin, haptoglobin, fibrinogen, plasminogen, α1-antitrypsin, orosomucoid, β-lipoprotein, α2-macroglobulin, and prealbumin in the human conceptus. Journal of Clinical Investigation 48: 1433–1446

Givner L B, Baker C J, Edwards M S 1987 Type III group B *Streptococcus:* functional interaction with IgG subclass antibodies. Journal of Infectious Diseases 1557: 532–539

Glode M P, Sutton A, Moxon E R, Robbins J B 1977 Pathogenesis of neonatal *Escherichia coli* meningitis: induction of bacteremia and meningitis in infant rats fed *E. coli* K1. Infection and Immunity 16: 75–80

Goitein K J, Tamir I 1983 Cerebral perfusion pressure in central nervous system infections of infancy and childhood. Journal of Pediatrics 103: 40–43

Goitein K J, Amit Y, Mussaffi H 1983 Intracranial pressure in central nervous system infections and cerebral ischaemia of infancy. Archives of Disease in Childhood 58: 184–186

Goldacre M J 1976 Acute bacterial meningitis in childhood: incidence and mortality in a defined population. Lancet i: 28–31

Goldacre M J 1977 Neonatal meningitis. Postgraduate Medical Journal 53: 607–609

Goldenberg R I, Neter E 1977 Meningitis due to two serotypes of *Escherichia coli:* an infant who recovered. American Journal of Diseases of Children 131: 213–214

Goldfarb J, Wormser G P, Glaser J H 1984 Meningitis caused by multiply antibiotic-resistant viridans streptococci. Journal of Pediatrics 105: 891–895

Goossens H, Henocque G, Kremp L et al 1986 Nosocomial outbreak of *Campylobacter jejuni* meningitis in newborn infants. Lancet ii: 146–149

Gray B M, Simmons D R, Mason H, Barnum S, Volanakis J E 1986 Quantitative levels of C-reactive protein in cerebrospinal fluid in patients with bacterial meningitis and other conditions. Journal of Pediatrics 108: 665–670

Greene G R, Carroll W L, Morozumi P A, Ching F C 1979 Endophthalmitis associated with Group-B streptococcal meningitis in an infant. American Journal of Diseases of Children 133: 752–753

Gross R J, Rowe B, Easton J A 1973 Neonatal meningitis caused by *Citrobacter koseri*. Journal of Clinical Pathology 26: 138–139

Gross R J, Ward L R, Threlfall E J, Cheasty T, Rowe B 1983 Drug resistance among *Escherichia coli* strains isolated from cerebrospinal fluid. Journal of Hygiene, Cambridge 90: 195–198

Gruenwald P 1974 Pathology of the deprived fetus and its supply line. In: Elliott K, Knight J (eds) Size at birth. Ciba Foundation Symposium 27 (New Series). Associated Scientific Publishers, Amsterdam, pp 3–19

Guin G H, Gendelman S, Stevens H 1965 Listeriosis of the central nervous system: four affected infants. Clinical Pediatrics 4: 258–263

Gullekson E H, Dumoff M 1966 *Haemophilus parainfluenzae* meningitis in a newborn. Journal of the American Medical Association 198: 1221

Gutteberg T J, Flaegstad T, Jorgensen T 1986 Lactoferrin, C- reactive protein, α-1-antitrypsin and immunoglobulin GA in cerebrospinal fluid in meningitis. Acta Paediatrica Scandinavica 75:569–572

Halcrow S J, Crawford P J, Craft A W 1985 Epidermoid spinal cord tumour after lumbar puncture. Archives of Disease in Childhood 60: 978–979

Hall J D, McCroskey L M, Pincomb B J, Hatheway C L 1985 Isolation of an organism resembling *Clostridium barati* which produces type F botulinal toxin from an infant with botulism. Journal of Clinical Microbiology 21: 654–655

Harter C, Benirschke K 1976 Fetal syphilis in the first trimester American Journal of Obstetrics and Gynecology 124: 705–711

Haruda F, Bergman M A, Headings D 1980 Unrecognised *Candida* brain abscess in infancy: two cases and a review of the literature. Johns Hopkins Medical Journal 147: 182–185

Haslam R H A, Allen J R, Dorsen M M, Kanofsky D L 1977 The sequelae of Group B β-hemolytic streptocccal meningitis in early infancy. American Journal of Diseases of Children 131: 845–849

Headings D L, Overall J C Jr 1977 Outbreak of meningitis in a newborn intensive care unit caused by a single *Escherichia coli* K1 serotype. Journal of Pediatrics 90: 99–102

Heath P 1950 Massive separation of the retina in full-term infants and juveniles. Journal of the American Medical Association 144: 1148–1154

Heckmatt J Z 1976 Coliform meningitis in the newborn. Archives of Disease in Childhood 51: 569–573

Hellwege H H, Ram W, Scherf H, Fock R 1984 Neonatal meningitis caused by *Streptococcus mitis*. Lancet i: 743–744 (letter)

Henrichsen J 1985 Nomenclature of GBS antigens. Antibiotics and Chemotherapy 35: 303–304

Hill H R, Hunt C E, Matsen J M 1974 Nosocomial colonization with *Klebsiella*, type 26, in a neonatal intensive-care unit associated with an outbreak of sepsis, meningitis, and necrotizing enterocolitis. Journal of Pediatrics 85: 415–419

Hirschhorn N, Chowdhury A K M A, Lindenbaum J 1969 Cholera in pregnant women. Lancet i: 1230–1232

Hjelm E, Jonsell G, Linglöf T, Mårdh P-A, Moller B, Sedin G 1980 Meningitis in a newborn infant caused by *Mycoplasma hominis*. Acta Paediatrica Scandinavica 69: 415–418

Hodges G R, Watanabe I, Singer P et al 1981 Central nervous system toxicity of intraventricularly administered gentamicin in adult rabbits. Journal of Infectious Diseases 143: 148–155

Hoffman H J, Hendrick E B, Hiscox J L 1970 Cerebral abscesses in early infancy. Journal of Neurosurgery 33: 172–177

Holmes K K 1983 Gonococcal infections. In: Remington J S, Klein J O (eds) Infectious diseases of the fetus and newborn infant, 2nd ed. W B Saunders, Philadelphia, pp 619–635

Hoogkamp-Korstanje J A A 1985 Activity of cefotaxime and ceftriaxone alone and in combination with penicillin, ampicillin and piperacillin against neonatal meningitis pathogens. Journal of Antimicrobial and Chemotherapy 16: 327–334

Huber G L 1983 Tuberculosis. In: Remington J S, Klein J O (eds) Infectious diseases of the fetus and newborn infant, 2nd ed. W B Saunders, Philadelphia, pp 570–590

Hurley R, Stanley V C, Leask B G S, de Louvois J 1974 Microflora of the vagina during pregnancy. In: Skinner F A, Carr J G (eds) The normal microbial flora of man. Academic Press, London, pp 155–185

Jelliffe D B, Jelliffe E F P 1978 Human milk in the modern world: psychosocial, nutritional, and economic significance. Oxford University Press, Oxford

Johnson G D, Elmore S E Jr, Adams F F Jr 1953 Brain abscess in small infants: report of 3 cases. Journal of the South Carolina Medical Association 49: 281–282

King E O 1959 Studies on a group of previously unclassified bacteria associated with meningitis in infants. American Journal of Clinical Pathology 31: 241–247

Kleiman M B, Reynolds J K, Watts N H, Schreiner R L, Smith J W 1984 Superiority of acridine orange stain versus Gram stain in partially treated bacterial meningitis. Journal of Pediatrics 104: 401–404

Klein J O, Marcy S M 1983 Bacterial sepsis and meningitis. In: Remington J S, Klein J O (eds) Infectious diseases of the fetus and newborn infant, 2nd ed. W B Saunders, Philadelphia, pp 679–735

Knox W F, Fox H 1984 Villitis of unknown aetiology: its incidence and significance in placentae from a British population. Placenta 5: 395–402

Kohler P F, Farr R S 1966 Elevation of cord over maternal IgG immunoglobulin: evidence for an active placental IgG transport. Nature 210: 1070–1071

Kraus E J, Hunter M P 1941 Congenital *Bacillus pyocyaneus* infection. Archives of Pathology 31: 819–824

Lancet 1983 Prevention of neonatal tetanus. Lancet i: 1253–1254

Lang K 1955 Listeria-infektion als mögliche Ursache früh erworbrener Cerebralschäden. Zeitschrift Kinderheilkunde 76: 328–339

Law B J, Marks M I 1980 Excellent outcome of *Bacteroides* meningitis in a newborn treated with metronidazole. Pediatrics 66: 463–465

Lawton A R 1984 Ontogeny of the immune system. In: Ogra P L (ed) Neonatal infections: nutritional and immunologic interactions. Grune & Stratton, Orlando, Florida, pp 3–20

Lee E L, Robinson M J, Thong M L, Puthuchearly S D, Ong T H, Ng K K 1977 Intraventricular chemotherapy in neonatal meningitis. Journal of Pediatrics 91: 991–995

Levene M I, Evans D H 1985 Medical management of raised intracranial pressure after severe birth asphyxia. Archives of Disease in Childhood 60: 12–16

Levin S, Zaidel L, Bernstein D 1978 Intrauterine infection of fetal brain by *Candida*. American Journal of Obstetrics and Gynecology 130: 597–599

Levy H L, Ingall D 1967 Meningitis in neonates due to *Proteus mirabilis*. American Journal of Diseases of Children 114: 320–324

Longe A C, Omene J A, Okolo A A 1984 Neonatal meningitis in Nigerian infants. Acta Paediatrica Scandinavica 73: 447–481

Lorber J 1974 Neonatal bacterial meningitis. Medicine (Medical Education, London) 27: 1579–1582

Lorber J 1983 Personal communication

Lorber J, Emery J L 1964 Intracerebral cysts complicating ventricular needling in hydrocephalic infants: a clinicopathological study. Developmental Medicine and Child Neurology 6: 125–139

Lorber J, Kalhan S C, Mahgrefte B 1970 Treatment of ventriculitis with gentamicin and cloxacillin in infants born with spina bifida. Archives of Disease in Childhood 45: 178–185

Low L C K, Lam B C C, Wong W T, Chan-Lui W Y, Yeung C Y 1984 *Salmonella* meningitis in infancy. Australian Paediatric Journal 20: 225–228

Luke J L, Bolande R P, Gross S 1963 Generalized aspergillosis and *Aspergillus* endocarditis in infancy: report of a case. Pediatrics 31: 115–122

Luthardt T 1970 Bacterial infections in ventriculo–auricular shunt systems. Developmental Medicine and Child Neurology 12 (suppl 22): 105–109

McCracken G H Jr 1972 The rate of bacteriologic response to antimicrobial therapy in neonatal meningitis. American Journal of Diseases of Children 123: 547–553

McCracken G H Jr 1984 Management of bacterial meningitis: current status and future prospects. American Journal of Medicine 76: 215–223

McCracken G H Jr 1985 New developments in the management of neonatal meningitis. In: Sande M A, Smith A L, Root R K (eds) Bacterial meningitis. Churchill Livingstone, Edinburgh, pp 159–166

McCracken G H Jr, Mize S G 1976 A controlled study of intrathecal antibiotic therapy in gram-negative enteric meningitis of infancy: report of the Neonatal Meningitis Cooperative Study Group. Journal of Pediatrics 89: 66–72

McCracken G H Jr, Nelson J D 1983 Antimicrobial therapy for newborns, 2nd ed. Grune & Stratton, New York

McCracken G H Jr, Shinefield H R 1966 Changes in the pattern of neonatal septicemia and meningitis. American Journal of Diseases of Children 112: 33–39

McCracken G H Jr, Mize S G, Threlkeld N 1980 Intraventricular gentamicin therapy in gram-negative bacillary meningitis of infancy: report of the second Neonatal Meningitis Cooperative Study Group. Lancet i: 787–791

McCracken G H Jr, Threlkeld N, Mize S et al 1984 Moxalactam therapy for neonatal meningitis due to gram-negative enteric bacilli: a prospective controlled evaluation. Journal of the American Medical Association 252: 1427–1432

McDonald R 1972 Purulent meningitis in newborn babies: observations and comments based on a series of 82 patients. Clinical Pediatrics 11: 450–454

McKell W M, Helseth H K, Brunson J G 1960 Influence of endotoxin on the placental–fetal barrier. Federation Proceedings 19: 246 (abstract)

McLaurin R L, Dobson D 1971 Infected ventriculo–atrial shunts: some principles of treatment. Developmental Medicine and Child Neurology 13 (suppl 25): 71–76

McLone D G, Czyzewski D, Raimondi A J, Sommers R C 1982 Central nervous system infections as a limiting factor in the intelligence of children with myelomeningocele. Pediatrics 70: 338–342

Maderazo E G, Bassaris H P, Quintiliani R 1974 *Flavobacterium meningosepticum* meningitis in a newborn infant: treatment with intraventricular erythromycin. Journal of Pediatrics 85: 675–676

Marshall F N 1968 Tetanus of the newborn (with special reference to experiences in Haiti, W.I). Advances in Pediatrics 15: 65–110

Maschio C, Ventura T 1967 Granulomatosi Brucellare fetale miliarica con leptomeningite della base dell'encefalo e del midollo spinale. Rivista Anatomia Patologica e di Oncologia 32: 211–230

Mathies A W, Hodgman J, Ivler D 1965 *Haemophilus influenzae* meningitis in a premature infant. Pediatrics 35: 791–792

Michelson P E, Rupp R, Efthimiadis B 1975 Endogenous *Candida* endophthalmitis leading to bilateral corneal perforations. American Journal of Ophthalmology 80: 800–803

Midura T F, Arnon S S 1976 Infant botulism: identification of *Clostridium botulinum* and its toxin in faeces. Lancet ii: 934–936

Millar D S, Davis L R, Rodeck C H, Nicolaides K H, Mibashan R S 1985 Normal blood cell values in the early mid-trimester fetus. Prenatal Diagnosis 5: 367–373

Miller M E 1978 Host defenses in the human neonate. Monographs in Neonatology Grune & Stratton, New York

Miller M E, Stiehm E R 1983 Immunology and resistance to infection. In: Remington J S, Klein J O (eds) Infectious diseases of the fetus and newborn infant. W B Saunders, Philadelphia, pp 27–68

Miller M J 1983 Fungal infections. In: Remington J S, Klein J O (eds) Infectious diseases of the fetus and newborn infant, 2nd ed. W B Saunders, Philadelphia, pp 464–506

Miller W H, Hesch J A 1962 Nontuberculosis spinal epidural abscess: report of a case in a 5-week-old infant. American Journal of Diseases of Children 104:269–275

Morbidity and Mortality Weekly Report 1984 Listeriosis associated with Mexican-style cheese — California 34: 357–359

Morgan M E I, Hart C A 1982 *Acinetobacter* meningitis: acquired infection in a neonatal intensive care unit. Archives of Disease in Childhood 57: 557–559

Morison J E 1970 Foetal and neonatal pathology, 3rd ed. Butterworth, London

Moxon E R, Smith A L, Averill D R, Smith D H 1974 *Haemophilus influenzae* meningitis in infant rates after intranasal inoculation. Journal of Infectious Diseases 129: 154–162

Moxon E R, Glode M P, Sutton A, Robbins J B 1977 The infant rat as a model of bacterial meningitis. Journal of Infectious Diseases 136: 186(S)–190(S)

Moxon E R, Zwahlen A, Rubin L G 1985 Pathogenesis of *Haemophilus influenzae* meningitis: use of a rat model for studying microbial determinants of virulence. In: Sande M A, Smith A L, Root R K

(eds) Bacterial meningitis. Churchill Livingstone, Edinburgh, pp 23–36

Mulder C J J, Zanen H C 1984a A study of 280 cases of neonatal meningitis in The Netherlands. Journal of Infection 9: 177–184

Mulder C J J, Zanen H C 1984b Neonatal Group B streptococcal meningitis. Archives of Disease in Childhood 59: 439–443

Mulder C J J, van Alphen L, Zanen H C 1984 Neonatal meningitis caused by *Escherichia coli* in The Netherlands. Journal of Infectious Diseases 150: 935–940

Mulhall A, de Louvois J, Hurley R 1983 Efficacy of chloramphenicol in the treatment of neonatal and infantile meningitis: a study of 70 cases. Lancet i: 284–287

Naeye R L, Blanc W A 1970 Relation of poverty and race to antenatal infection. New England Journal of Medicine 283: 555–560

Naeye R L, Peters E C 1978 Amniotic fluid infections with intact membranes leading to perinatal death: a prospective study. Pediatrics 61: 171–177

Naeye R L, Peters E C 1980 Causes and consequences of premature rupture of fetal membranes. Lancet i: 192–194

Nathavitharana K A, Arseculeratne S N, Aponso H A, Vijeratnam R, Jayasena L, Navaratnam C 1983 Acute meningitis in early childhood caused by *Aerococcus viridans*. British Medical Journal 286: 1248

Naqvi S H, Maxwell M A, Dunkle L M 1985 Cefotaxime therapy of neonatal gram-negative bacillary meningitis. Pediatric Infectious Disease 4: 499–502

Neligan G A, Kolvin I, Scott D McI, Garside R F 1976 Born too soon or born too small. Clinics in Developmental Medicine, No. 61. Spastics International Medical Publications, London

Nelson J D, Dillon H C Jr, Howard J B 1976 A prolonged nursery epidemic associated with a newly recognised type of Group A streptococcus. Journal of Pediatrics 89: 792–796

Nicholas J L, Kamal I M, Eckstein H B 1970 Immediate shunt replacement in the treatment of bacterial colonisation of Holter valves. Developmental Medicine and Child Neurology 12 (suppl 22): 110–113

Odio C, McCracken G H Jr, Nelson J D 1984 CSF shunt infections in pediatrics. American Journal of Diseases of Children 138: 1103–1108

Okubadejo O A, Alausa K O 1968 Neonatal meningitis caused by *Edwardsiella tarda*. British Medical Journal 3: 357–358

Olsen E 1949 Studies on the intestinal flora of infants. Einar Munksgaard, Copenhagen

Oppenheimer E H, Dahms B B 1981 Congenital syphilis in the fetus and neonate. Perspectives in Pediatric Pathology 6: 115–138

Osborne J P, Pizer B 1981 Effect on the white cell count of contaminating cerebrospinal fluid with blood. Archives of Disease in Childhood 56: 400–401

Overall J C Jr 1970 Neonatal bacterial meningitis: analysis of predisposing factors and outcome compared with matched control subjects. Journal of Pediatrics 76: 499–511

Palmer J J, Kelly W A 1972 Epidural abscess in a 3-week-old infant: case report. Pediatrics 50: 817–820

Papadatos C, Pavlatou M, Alexiou D 1969 Cephalosporium meningitis. Pediatrics 44: 749–751

Pape K E, Wigglesworth J S 1979 Haemorrhage, ischaemia and the perinatal brain. Clinics in Developmental Medicine, Nos 69/70. Spastics International Medical Publications, London

Pathak A, Custer J R, Levy J 1983 Neonatal septicemia and meningitis due to *Plesiomonas shigelloides*. Pediatrics 71: 389–391

Peltola H, Holmberg C 1983 Rapidity of C-reactive protein in detecting potential septicemia. Pediatric Infectious Disease 2: 374–376

Peltola H, Luhtala K, Valmari P 1984 C-reactive protein as a detector of organic complications during recovery from childhood purulent meningitis. Journal of Pediatrics 104: 869–872

Peltola H, Turpeinen M, Koskiniemi M 1986 An infant with simultaneous β-lactamase-positive *Haemophilus influenzae* meningitis and β-lactamase-negative *H. influenzae* septicemia, *Escherichia coli* pyelonephritis, and herpes encephalitis. Acta Paediatrica Scandinavica 75:499–501

Peters G, Locci R, Pulverer G 1982 Adherence and growth of coagulase- negative staphylococci on surfaces of intravenous catheters. Journal of Infectious Diseases 146: 479–482

Philip A G S 1985 Neonatal sepsis and meningitis. G K Hall, Boston

PHLS (Public Health Laboratory Service) Report 1985 Neonatal meningitis: a review of routine national data 1975–83. British Medical Journal 290: 778–779

Pickett J, Berg B, Chaplin E, Brunstetter-Shafer M-A 1976 Syndrome of botulism in infancy: clinical and electrophysiologic study. New England Journal of Medicine 295: 770–772

Playfair J H L, Wolfendale M R, Kay H E M 1963 The leucocytes of peripheral blood in the human foetus. British Journal of Haematology 9: 336–344

Polin R A, Brown L W 1979 Infant botulism. Pediatric Clinics of North America 26: 345–354

Potter E L, Craig J M 1976 Pathology of the fetus and the infant, 3rd ed. Lloyd-Luke (Medical Books), London

Pyati S P, Pildes R S, Jacobs N M et al 1983 Penicillin in infants weighing two kilograms or less with early-onset group B streptococcal disease. New England Journal of Medicine 308: 1383–1389

Quirke P, Hwang W-S, Validen C C 1980 Congenital *Torulopsis glabrata* infection in man. American Journal of Clinical Pathology 73: 137–140

Rabe E F 1967 Subdural effusions in infants. Pediatric Clinics of North America 14: 831–850

Rance C P, Roy T E, Donohue W L, Sepp A, Elder R, Finlayson M 1962 An epidemic of septicemia with meningitis and hemorrhagic encephalitis in premature infants. Journal of Pediatrics 61: 24–32

Repice, J P, Neter E 1975 *Pasteurella multocida* meningitis in an infant with recovery. Journal of Pediatrics 86: 91–93

Reynolds D W, Dweck H S, Cassady G 1972 Inappropriate antidiuretic hormone secretion in a neonate with meningitis. American Journal of Diseases of Children 123: 251–253

Rhine W D, Arvin A M, Stevenson D K 1986 Neonatal aspergillosis: a case report and review of the literature. Clinical Pediatrics 25: 400–403

Rhodes P G, Burry V F, Hall R T, Cox R 1975 Pneumococcal septicemia and meningitis in the neonate. Journal of Pediatrics 86: 593–595

Rose S J 1979 Neonatal meningitis due to *Citrobacter koseri*. Journal of Perinatal Medicine 7: 273–275

Rubenstein J S, Yogev R 1985 What represents pleocytosis in blood-contaminated ('traumatic tap') cerebrospinal fluid in children? Journal of Pediatrics 107: 249–251

Rubin L G, Altman J, Epple L K, Yolken R H 1981 *Vibrio cholerae* meningitis in a neonate. Journal of Pediatrics 98: 940–942

Rudensky B, Finalt M, Isaacson M 1978 Neonatal meningitis and septicemia due to a Lancefield untypable beta hemolytic streptococcus. Journal of Pediatrics 92: 676–677

Russell P 1979 Inflammatory lesions of the human placenta. I. Clinical significance of acute chorioamnionitis. American Journal of Diagnostic Gynecology and Obstetrics 1: 127–137

Russell P 1980 Inflammatory lesions of the human placenta. III. The histopathology of villitis of unknown aetiology. Placenta 1: 227–244

Salimpour R 1977 Cause of death in tetanus neonatorum: study of 233 cases with 54 necropsies. Archives of Disease in Childhood 52: 587–594

Salmon J H 1967 Puncture porencephaly: pathogenesis and prevention. American Journal of Diseases of Children 114: 72–79

Samson D S, Clark K 1973 A current review of brain abscess. American Journal of Medicine 54: 201–210

Sanderson P J 1978 Gentamicin and chloramphenicol in neonatal meningitis. Lancet ii: 210 (letter)

Sarff L D, Platt L H, McCracken G H Jr 1976 Cerebrospinal fluid evaluation in neonates: comparison of high-risk infants with and without meningitis. Journal of Pediatrics 88: 473–477

Schiffer M S, Oliveira E, Glode M P, McCracken G H Jr, Sarff L M, Robbins J B 1976 Relation between invasiveness and the K1 capsular polysaccharide of *Escherichia coli*. Pediatric Research 10: 82–87

Schlech W F III, Lavigne P M, Bortolussi R A et al 1983 Epidemic listerosis — evidence for transmission by food. New England Journal of Medicine 308: 203–206

Schlech W F III, Ward J I, Band J D, Hightower A, Fraser D W, Broome C V 1985 Bacterial meningitis in the United States, 1978 through 1981. The National Bacterial Meningitis Surveillance Study. Journal of the American Medical Association 253: 1749–1754

Seeliger H P R, Finger H 1983 Listeriosis. In: Remington J S, Klein J O (eds) Infectious diseases of the fetus and newborn infant, 2nd ed. W B Saunders, Philadelphia, pp 264–289

Sell S H W, Webb W W, Pate J E, Doyne E O 1972 Psychological

sequelae to bacterial meningitis: two controlled studies. Pediatrics 49: 212–217

Shortland-Webb W R 1968 *Proteus* and coliform meningoencephalitis in neonates. Journal of Clinical Pathology 21: 422–431

Siber G R, Alpert S, Smith A L, Juey-Shien L L, McCormack W M 1977 Neonatal central nervous system infection due to *Mycoplasma hominis*. Journal of Pediatrics 90: 625–627

Siegel J D, Shannon K M, de Passe B M 1981 Recurrent infection associated with penicillin-tolerant Group B streptococci: a report of two cases. Journal of Pediatrics 99: 920–924

Siegel J D, McCracken G H Jr, Threlkeld N, DePasse B M, Rosenfield C R 1982 Single-dose penicillin prophylaxis of neonatal group-B streptococcal disease. Conclusion of a 41 month controlled trial. Lancet i: 1426–1430

Sinai R E, Marks M I, Powell K R, Pai C H 1980 Model of neonatal meningitis caused by *Escherichia coli* K1 in guinea pigs. Journal of Infectious Diseases 141: 193–197

Smythe P M, Bowie M D, Voss T J V 1974 Treatment of tetanus neonatorum with muscle relaxants and intermittent positive-pressure ventilation. British Medical Journal i: 223–226

Speer C P, Hauptmann D, Stubbe P, Gahr M 1985 Neonatal septicemia and meningitis in Göttingen, West Germany. Pediatric Infectious Disease 4: 36–41

Spirer Z, Jurgenson U, Lazewnick R, Reider-Grossvasser I 1982 Complete recovery from an apparent brain abscess treated without neurosurgery: the importance of early CT scanning. Clinical Pediatrics 21: 106–109

Stark G 1968 Treatment of ventriculitis in hydrocephalic infants: intrathecal and intraventricular use of the new penicillins. Developmental Medicine and Child Neurology 12 (suppl 15): 36–44

Statz A, Felgenhauer K 1983 Development of the blood–CSF barrier. Developmental Medicine and Child Neurology 25: 152–161

Steele R W, Marmer D J, O'Brien M D, Tyson S T, Steele C R 1986 Leukocyte survival in cerebrospinal fluid. Journal of Clinical Microbiology 23: 965–966

Stewardson-Krieger P, Gotoff S P 1977 Neonatal meningitis due to Group C beta hemolytic streptococcus. Journal of Pediatrics 90: 103–104

Stewardson-Krieger P, Naidu S 1981 Simultaneous recovery of β-lactamase negative and β-lactamase positive *Haemophilus influenzae* type b from cerebrospinal fluid of a neonate. Pediatrics 68: 253–254

Stiehm E R, Damrosch D S 1966 Neonatal meningococcal meningitis: report of a case acquired in the nursery. Journal of Pediatrics 68: 654–656

Sugathadasa A A, Arseculeratne S N 1963 Neonatal meningitis caused by new serotype of *Flavobacterium meningosepticum*. British Medical Journal i: 37–38

Syrogiannopoulos G A, Nelson J D, McCracken G H Jr 1986 Subdural collections of fluid in acute bacterial meningitis: a review of 136 cases. Pediatric Infectious Disease 5: 343–352

Syrogiannopoulos G A, Olsen K D, Reisch J S, McCracken G H Jr 1987 Dexamethasone in the treatment of experimental *Haemophilus influenzae* type b meningitis. Journal of Infectious Diseases 155: 213–219

Tafari N, Ross S M, Naeye R L, Galask R P, Zaar B 1977 Failure of bacterial growth inhibition by amniotic fluid. American Journal of Obstetrics and Gynecology 128: 187–189

Tal Y, Crichton J U, Dunn H G, Dolman C L 1980 Spinal cord damage: a rare complication of purulent meningitis. Acta Paediatrica Scandinavica 69: 471–474

Taylor-Robinson D, McCormack W M 1980 The genital mycoplasmas. New England Journal of Medicine 302: 1003–1010, 1063–1067

Teknetzi P, Manios S, Katsouyanopoulos V 1983 Neonatal tetanus: long- term residual handicaps. Archives of Disease in Childhood 58: 68–69

Tempest B 1974 Pneumococcal meningitis in mother and neonate. Pediatrics 53: 759–760

Thomas D B, Yoffey J M 1962 Human foetal haemopoiesis. I. The cellular composition of foetal blood. British Journal of Haematology 8: 290–295

Thomas K, Chan K N, Ribeiro C D 1980 *Campylobacter jejuni/coli* meningitis in a neonate. British Medical Journal i: 1301–1302

Tingelstad J B, Young H F, David R B 1974 Brain abscess in an infant with cyanotic congenital heart disease. Pediatrics 54: 113–115

Turnbull P C B, French T A, Dowsett E G 1977 Severe systemic and pyogenic infections with *Bacillus cereus*. British Medical Journal i: 1628–1629

Vawter G F 1981 Perinatal listeriosis. Perspectives in Pediatric Pathology 6: 153–166

Visintine A M, Oleske J M, Nahmias A J 1977 *Listeria monocytogenes* infection in infants and children. American Journal of Diseases of Children 131: 393–397

Volpe J J 1981 Neurology of the Newborn, vol 22. Major Problems in Clinical Pediatrics. W B Saunders, Philadelphia

Waites K B, Rudd P T, Crouse D T et al 1988 Chronic *Ureaplasma urealyticum* and *Mycoplasma hominis* infections of central nervous system in preterm infants. Lancet i: 17–21

Wald E R, Bergman I, Taylor H G, Chiponis D, Porter C, Kubek K 1986 Long-term outcome of Group B streptococcal meningitis. Pediatrics 77: 217–221

Wallace R J Jr, Baker C J, Quinones F J, Hollis D G, Weaver R E, Wiss K 1983 Nontypable *Haemophilus influenzae* (biotype 4) as a neonatal, maternal, and genital pathogen. Reviews of Infectious Diseases 5: 123–136

Wallach E E, Brody J I, Oski F A 1969 Fetal immunization as a consequence of bacilluria during pregnancy. Obstetrics and Gynecology 33: 100–105

Washburn T C, Medearis D N Jr, Childs B 1965 Sex differences in susceptibility to infections. Pediatrics 35: 57–64

Wealthall S R 1975 *Mycoplasma* meningitis in infants with spina bifida. Developmental Medicine and Child Neurology 17(suppl 35): 117–122

Weintraub M I, Otto R N 1972 Pneumococcal meningitis and endophthalmitis in a newborn. Journal of the American Medical Association 219: 1763–1764 (letter)

Weizer S, Heldenberg D 1985 Neonatal sepsis, meningitis and lobar pneumonia due to *Streptococcus pneumoniae*. Harefuah 108: 347–348

Whitfield C, Humphries J M 1967 Meningitis and septicemia due to *Shigellae* in a newborn unit. Journal of Pediatrics 70: 805–806

Whyte R K, Hussain Z, deSa D 1982 Antenatal infections with *Candida* species. Archives of Disease in Childhood 57: 528–535

Wiedermann B L, Hawkins E P, Johnson G S, Lamberth L B, Mason E O, Kaplan S L 1986 Pathogenesis of labyrinthitis associated with *Haemophilus influenzae* type b meningitis in infant rats. Journal of Infectious Diseases 153: 27–32

Wigglesworth J S 1984 Perinatal pathology, Vol 15. Major Problems in Pathology. W B Saunders, Philadelphia

Williams W W, Mariano J, Spurrier M et al 1984 Nosocomial meningitis due to *Citrobacter diversus* in neonates: new aspects of the epidemiology. Journal of Infectious Diseases 150: 229–235

Winberg J, Wessner G 1971 Does breast milk protect against septicaemia in the newborn? Lancet i: 1091–1094

Wood G W 1980 Mononuclear phagocytes in the human placenta. Placenta 1: 113–123

Woodruff A W, Grant J, El Bashir E A, Baya E I, Yugusuk A Z, El Suni A 1984 Neonatal tetanus: mode of infection, prevalence, and prevention in Southern Sudan. Lancet i: 378–379

Wright P F, Kaiser A B, Bowman C M, McKee K T Jr, Trujillo H, McGee Z A 1981 The pharmacokinetics and efficacy of an aminoglycoside administered into the cerebral ventricles in neonates: implications for further evaluation of this route of therapy in meningitis. Journal of Infectious Diseases 143: 141–147

Yeung C Y 1976 Intrathecal antibiotic therapy for neonatal meningitis. Archives of Disease in Childhood 51: 686–690

Yogev R 1979 Ventriculitis from *Acinetobacter calcoaceticus* variant *anitratus*. Journal of Neurology, Neurosurgery and Psychiatry 42: 475–477

Ziai M, Haggerty R J 1958 Neonatal meningitis. New England Journal of Medicine 259: 314–320

Zimmerman L E 1955 Fatal fungus infections complicating other diseases. American Journal of Clinical Pathology 25: 46–65

Metabolic disorders

Biochemical defects causing significant cerebral dysfunction are individually rare conditions but together form a group of great importance to those caring for the fetus and newborn. Great advances have been made in the biochemistry of these disorders which allows assay of the appropriate enzyme from tissue or serum in many of these conditions. Prenatal diagnosis is feasible and accurate in a significant number. In some cases of neonatal disease, early dietary management will alter the course of the illness and allow normal growth and development. The following three chapters review the methods of prenatal diagnosis and the diagnosis and biochemistry (where known) of many of the metabolic disorders presenting in the early months of life. In a book of this size it is impossible to review every condition of this type reported in the literature but Tables 39.2 and 40.1 summarize the relevant features of all the major recognized defects and an approach to diagnosis is discussed in some detail.

38. Prenatal diagnosis of inborn errors

Prof D. M. Danks and Dr J. E. Wraith

Skills in prenatal diagnosis have advanced rapidly since amniocentesis for determination of the fetal karyotype was introduced into general obstetrical practice in the early 1970s (Harrison et al 1984, Milunsky 1986). Changes in ultrasound scanning have been the more spectacular during this period so that it has taken over most of the roles once anticipated for fetoscopy. Micro-analytical procedures for enzyme assay have contributed to progress and the influence of DNA techniques is just now being felt. Skills with a variety of fetal manipulations under ultrasound control are now quite remarkable, with acceptably low complication rates.

A wide range of congenital malformations and genetic diseases can now be diagnosed prenatally. A number of structural defects of the nervous system can be recognized directly by ultrasound scanning and some syndromes which includes brain defects can be diagnosed because of associated physical defects which are detectable on ultrasound. These approaches have been discussed in Section 2. Neural tube defects constitute the most important group of structural nervous system disorders that are diagnosable prenatally and are reviewed in Section 7.

Three important approaches to prenatal diagnosis remain to be discussed. Fetal cells can be obtained by amniocentesis at 16 weeks or by chorion villus sampling at 10 weeks of gestation. The karyotype of these cells can be examined to diagnose any disease caused by visible chromosome imbalance. A wide range of inborn errors of metabolism which affect the brain can be diagnosed by measuring the relevant enzymes in these cells. DNA extracted from these cells can be used to diagnose a number of genetic disorders. A few other genetic disorders are best diagnosed by studies on fetal blood cells or blood plasma which can be obtained by sampling under vision through a fetoscope or by percutaneous fetal venepuncture under ultrasound control.

TECHNIQUES USED TO OBTAIN FETAL SAMPLES

Amniocentesis

Extensive experience has been gained with amniocentesis over the last 15 years and most aspects of the technique are now standardized (Wald 1984). Amniocentesis is performed with local anaesthetic by suprapubic needle puncture under ultrasound control at 16 weeks of gestation. Experienced operators will obtain a satisfactory sample (20 ml with no blood staining) on first puncture in over 95% of cases and at a second puncture in over 99% of cases. Cultivation of fetal amniotic cells will be successful in over 99% of samples and all of these will yield a satisfactory karyotype or be suitable for enzyme assays. The average time in culture to achieve the required number of cells is 2 weeks and almost all samples should yield results in 4 weeks. The frequency of miscarriage induced by the procedure is 0.5 to 1%. All of these figures apply to services in which operators perform at least 100 procedures per annum, have good ultrasound equipment and skills and work in well-organized collaboration with the laboratory handling the sample.

Chorion villus sampling

Experience with chorion villus sampling (CVS) has mounted rapidly over the last 3 years. This procedure is performed at 10 weeks of gestation and involves insertion of a malleable cannula, visible on ultrasound scanning (several different forms are in use), through the cervix advancing its tip to impinge upon the chorion frondosum under ultrasound control and aspirating a portion of this tissue. Immediately the sample is aspirated it must be examined under a dissecting microscope to separate fetal chorionic villi from maternal tissue. An alternative technique of transabdominal needle puncture under ultrasound control has gained popularity recently. It can also be used later in pregnancy.

The statistics about the performance of chorion villus sampling are not as extensive as those for amniocentesis (Simoni et al 1986, Brambati et al 1985). It appears that an experienced operator can expect to obtain a satisfactory sample on first aspiration in about 95% of attempts, and within three attempts in 99% of cases.

Technical success is certainly better than 95% at all stages of the process. Frequency of miscarriage due to the procedure appears to be somewhere between 1 and 3%, against a background of approximately 2% occurrence of spontaneous miscarriage in fetuses known to be alive with a beating heart at 10 weeks of gestation. (This background figure is much lower than had been expected but the experience of the last 5 years has made it clear that most pregnancies which abort in the first trimester are already visibly non-viable on an ultrasound scan performed at 10 weeks.)

Fetal blood sampling and tissue biopsy

Fetoscopy has been used at 18 weeks of gestation to obtain fetal blood. This is a more protracted and complex procedure than those mentioned thus far. Success rate is better than 98% in the hands of a very few extremely experienced operators around the world, who have also achieved miscarriage rates as low as 3 to 5% (Wald 1984). For most other operators the success rate is somewhat lower and the risk somewhat higher.

Fetal blood sampling is now more often achieved by direct needle puncture of a ductus venosus under ultrasound control, a procedure which appears to have a risk of the order of 2% in experienced hands.

Fetal liver biopsy has been performed using a fetoscope and more recently by direct needle puncture. The number of tests performed is too small to discuss success rates or risks.

LABORATORY ANALYSES APPLIED TO FETAL SAMPLES

Chromosome analysis can diagnose all diseases of the fetus caused by chromosome imbalance (Hamerton & Ferguson-Smith 1984). Good-quality banded karyotypes satisfactory for discerning even partial trisomies or monosomies, or translocations, can be obtained from amniotic cells or from CVS. The process is labour intensive but very reliable. The practical problems revolve around the financial resources available for performing these tests and the various methods available for selecting pregnant women at higher than average risk for having a child with a chromosome abnormality.

A large number of enzymes involved in different inborn errors of metabolism can be assayed in amniotic cells or chorion villus sampling (see Ch. 39). The practical limitation is the expression of the gene concerned in the type of cell which is available. Most of the enzymes which break down amino acids or organic acids and most lysosomal enzymes are expressed in these cells and the corresponding diseases can be diagnosed prenatally by enzyme assays. A number of tissue-specific enzymes like phenylalanine hydroxylase, urea cycle enzymes and the brain-specific enzymes cannot be identified by this method.

With amniocentesis, cells must be cultivated until a sufficient number are available to perform the particular assay. Fortunately, many assays have been refined to be applicable to relatively small numbers of cells but the delay in achieving a result can add up to 4 or 5 weeks from obtaining the sample.

Many enzymes can be assayed in uncultured tissue from chorion villus sampling or in cells cultivated from these samples as with amniotic cells or skin fibroblasts. There is also a problem of maternal contamination of the chorion villus sample, especially when assaying an uncultured sample.

Analyses of metabolites in the amniotic fluid itself have proved valuable for some inborn errors of metabolism in which the enzyme assay is particularly difficult (Naylor et al 1980). Precise measurement by isotope dilution techniques using mass spectrometry have been employed to diagnose methylmalonic acidaemia, propionic acidaemia and several other inborn errors of metabolism.

A number of genetic diseases can be diagnosed by testing fetal blood. The laboratory procedures are the same as would be applied to diagnose conditions on blood samples obtained postnatally, except that they have to be miniaturized to cope with the very small volume available — generally 100 µl. Globin-chain synthesis rates can be measured to diagnose thalassaemia and electrophoresis of haemoglobin allows diagnosis of sickle cell and other haemoglobin mutations. Factor VIII or Factor IX can be measured to diagnose haemophilia A or B. Lymphocytes can be stimulated to divide in order to give a rapid method of karyotyping. Lymphocyte function studies can also be performed to diagnose certain immune deficits. It seemed logical to expect that measurement of plasma CPK levels might diagnose Duchenne muscular dystrophy but this has not proved reliable.

Enzyme assays or other tests performed on liver biopsies or skin biopsies are just like those performed on the same tissues obtained postnatally.

The newcomer to the range of techniques for prenatal diagnosis is analysis of DNA. DNA techniques can be used for direct diagnosis of the mutation in a few conditions. Indirect methods using linkage to restriction fragment length polymorphisms (RFLP) have a wider application.

Unfortunately, most mutations comprise single base substitutions in the DNA of the gene concerned. These are very difficult to detect by existing techniques. Some single base substitutions happen to alter a sequence which is recognized by one of the restriction enzymes, producing an additional restriction enzyme cleavage site or abolishing a normally existing cleavage site. Unfortunately this is true for only a small proportion of mutations. Most single base substitutions can be identified only by cloning the mutant gene and sequencing the entire gene. This is a major task and cannot be undertaken on each patient, especially since many different single base substitutions are found among the mutations causing each genetic disease. If a particular single base substitution is very frequent (as is the case in haemoglobin S or in the PiZZ form of alpha-1-antitrypsin deficiency) then a synthetic oligonucleotide can be used to recognize the base substitution in fetal cells. There is a great need for a rapid and simple method of pinpointing the single base substitutions causing genetic diseases.

Some background explanation is needed to introduce the RFLP linkage approach to prenatal diagnosis (Francomano & Kazazian 1986). Restriction endonucleases cut DNA wherever a particular sequence of nucleotide bases occurs. Hundreds of these enzymes have been extracted from different species of bacteria. If one particular enzyme is used, the series of fragments of DNA obtained from each human being will be almost constant. However, the pattern is not absolutely constant because individuals differ slightly in their DNA base sequence, especially in the non-coding regions of DNA, and some of these differences alter enzyme cleavage sites. If enough enzymes are used, a large number of such harmless polymorphic regions of DNA can be identified in normal people. Indeed, an intensive search will nearly always reveal some polymorphic regions around any cloned gene. Figure 38.1 shows the gene which codes for clotting factor IX with its eight coding regions (exons) (a–h) and marks the region recognized by a probe which identifies a 1.8 kb fragment on some X-chromosomes and a 1.3 kb fragment on other X-chromosomes. These are called restriction fragment length polymorphisms (RFLP) because the lengths of the pieces cleaved by enzymes differ. If an individual, heterozygous for a mutant gene, can be shown to have two different forms of a polymorphic region adjacent to that gene, then the two chromosomes of that heterozygote are immediately distinguishable. Two of the results shown in Figure 38.2 come from females heterozygous for this RFLP. Family studies can show which form of the variable region is on the same chromosome as the mutant gene and which accompanies the normal gene (Figs 38.2 and 38.3). The passage of the normal or mutant gene into the offspring can be traced quite reliably by tracing the passage of the adjacent polymorphic region. The risk of error in this process is extremely low when the polymorphic region is within the cloned DNA fragment and right beside the functional gene. This would be true if this RFLP were being used to test for haemophilia B in a family. This probe is also

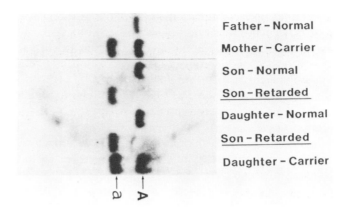

Fig. 38.2 RFLPs from a family with fragile-X mental retardation. In this family the defective gene is associated with 'a'. Mother is a heterozygote for this RFLP.

useful in some families with fragile-X mental retardation (Fig. 38.3). Errors occur when crossing over between the chromosomes happens to occur between the gene of interest and the polymorphic region. Such errors are very rare when this gene probe is used in the diagnosis of factor IX deficiency (haemophilia B).

The same approach can be used starting with a large number of fragments of DNA of unknown function from a particular chromosome and looking for linkage of these fragments to the inheritance of a genetic disease (e.g. fragile-X mental retardation, Duchenne muscular dystrophy). Linkages defined in this way can be used in the same way as the linkages just discussed but carry a higher error rate because the distance between the recognizable segment of DNA and the gene causing the disease is relatively large and poorly measured. The family illustrated in Figure 38.3 was actually tested because of fragile-X mental retardation.

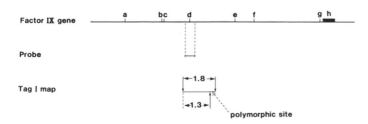

Fig. 38.1 Factor IX gene and gene probe. This probe recognises a 1.8 kb segment on some X-chromosomes and a 1.3 kb segment on other X-chromosomes.

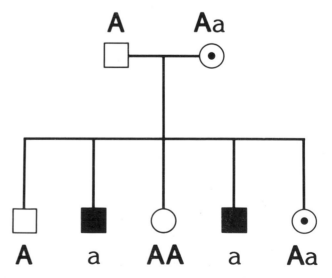

Fig. 38.3 Pedigree of family illustrated in Figure 38.2 with RFLPs showing two affected males and a carrier daughter.

In this family no recombination occurred but recombination has been seen in other families and other probes are now more useful in this condition. Recombination frequencies of 5, 10 or 15% are frequent in this situation and these become the error rates in the diagnostic test.

These DNA tests can be applied to chorion villus samples (CVS) or cultured amniotic cells but CVS is the preferred tissue.

Diseases of neurological interest which can be approached by the latter of these two DNA linkage methods include Duchenne muscular dystrophy, the fragile-X form of mental retardation, myotonic dystrophy and Huntington's disease.

SELECTION OF COUPLES FOR PRENATAL DIAGNOSIS

In inherited conditions due to defects in single genes the couples are selected because of their own previous record of producing children with a particular disease or because of the family history (e.g. in X-linked recessive conditions). Most couples undergoing prenatal diagnosis because of inherited disorders are facing a 1 in 2 or a 1 in 4 risk. In some X-linked conditions women who cannot be clearly defined as carriers or non-carriers may still choose to use a diagnostic test. The linkage type of DNA test cannot be applied in this circumstance but direct tests for the biochemical defect can be applied.

Chromosome translocation carriers are recognized in a similar fashion following investigation of relatives of a trisomic child shown to carry a translocation.

Older women with a moderately increased risk of a chromosomal abnormality because of their age comprise the largest group using prenatal diagnosis. It is difficult to know what age should be chosen as the minimum for testing. Policies vary from country to country according to community attitudes and financial resources. Most countries choose either 37 or 35 years as the cut-off. The prime objective is recognition of Down's syndrome but other autosomal trisomies are also age-dependent and are recognized at increased frequency. The magnitude of risk of producing a liveborn Down's syndrome child was determined quite well by a number of studies performed before the advent of amniocentesis.

These statistics can never be improved because we are no longer seeing the true frequency of Down's syndrome at birth. Over the last 15 years figures describing the frequency of trisomy and other chromosomal abnormalities at 16 weeks of gestation have been accumulated. In due course we will have another batch of figures describing these frequencies at 10 weeks of gestation. The figures at 16 weeks are approximately double the old figures for the frequency at birth. The difference represents trisomic pregnancies which terminate spontaneously between 16 weeks and full-term. An even greater disparity can be expected once the figures

at 10 weeks start to amass. We need to keep clearly in mind that the objective of these procedures is to avoid the birth of children handicapped by these conditions and that these are the figures which should determine our policies.

The availability of RFLP linkage methods of diagnosing diseases like myotonic dystrophy and Huntington's disease before symptoms develop is posing some difficult issues which are being overemphasized at present. When no tests were available it was very easy for the children of a 50-year-old man with Huntington's disease to wish that they could be tested to determine whether or not they had inherited the gene. Now that such testing is becoming possible it is becoming clear that most of these people really meant that they would like to be tested to prove that they do not have the gene. Some baulk at the idea of testing when they realize that they cannot achieve this reassurance without running the risk of learning that they will develop the disease in the future. Careful discussion and counselling can generally help the consultant to decide what to do. The issue is a little more complicated when a parent is shown to carry the gene and then wishes a young child to be tested. One can argue that foreknowledge of the child's genetic status can allow the parent to rear the child with a positive and healthy attitude to the possession of the gene. However, this knowledge may warp the rearing of the child.

CONDITIONS OF SPECIAL NEUROLOGICAL INTEREST

Down's syndrome

Down's syndrome is the most common and best understood of the chromosomal abnormalities. Affected individuals have an additional chromosome 21, giving a total of 47 instead of the normal 46 chromosomes, the error arising because of non-disjunction during meiosis.

In approximately 1–2% of cases, however, the extra chromosome material is not present as a separate chromosome but is due to a translocation of the long arm of chromosome 21 (21q) to another acrocentric chromosome. One of the parents may be a balanced carrier of the translocation and chromosome 14 is most commonly involved in the translocation process. Occasionally a homologous 21q/21q translocation occurs and all liveborn offspring of carriers of this translocation have Down's syndrome. (The monosomy 21 conceptions which also occur die in early development.)

The risk of having an infant with Down's syndrome increases with increasing maternal age — from less than 1 in 1000 at 20 years to 1 in 35 at age 45. Most communities offer prenatal testing by karyotyping on amniotic cells or chorion villus samples but it is difficult to decide the optimum age of introducing the tests. The majority of countries choose either 35 or 37 years as the cut-off point.

Fragile-X

Most of the excess of retarded males over retarded females in the community is due to X-linked genes and it has been estimated that these genes account for about one-fifth of all non-specific retardation in males. A common form of X-linked retardation has been shown to be associated with the cytogenetic finding of a fragile site (seen in culture as a constriction), on the long arm of the X-chromosome (Xq 27–28).

Affected males are retarded, have macro-orchidism, large ears and a prominent chin. About one-third of carrier females have a history of learning difficulties and some are moderately or severely retarded.

Recent work has shown that we still have a lot to learn about the fragile-X syndrome. Not all cells in affected males exhibit the fragile site (usually 30–40%). About 20% of males with the fragile site are not retarded and many obligate female carriers do not show the fragile site at all or show it in only occasional cells. Prenatal diagnosis has been achieved on both amniocytes and fetal blood, the latter proving to be more successful due to the difficulty in demonstrating the fragile site in amniocytes.

Experience with chorion villus sampling is very limited. Linkage analysis using a variety of probes, including that for factor IX gene, has been attempted. Unfortunately this area of the X-chromosome is a recombination 'hot spot' with more recombinants occurring than expected for the length of chromosome involved, thus reducing the diagnostic effectiveness of the probes used.

How should we counsel fragile-X females? If the mother is an obligatory carrier and demonstrates the fragile site her counselling is that of uncomplicated X-linked inheritance — 50% of her sons will be affected and 50% of her daughters will be carriers. We can offer prenatal diagnosis with about 90% confidence using chromosome studies and/or linkage. It is difficult, however, to counsel her mentally normal brothers and sisters — both could still carry the gene but not exhibit the fragile site. A more sensitive indicator of the presence of the gene associated with the fragile-X syndrome is needed before we are in a position to confidently advise these people.

Of all genetic diseases this is currently the one most needing the full skills of an expert clinical geneticist for counselling.

Duchenne muscular dystrophy

Duchenne muscular dystrophy (DMD) is the most frequent of all known fatal X-linked diseases, affecting about 1 in 4000 male livebirths. One-third of all cases arise as new spontaneous mutations.

Affected boys present usually with a progressive gait abnormality or delayed motor milestones with an associated pseudohypertrophy of some muscle groups due to infiltration with fibrous tissue and fat. A significant number will have mild to moderate mental retardation, most will be wheelchair-bound by age 12 and death occurs, usually in adolescence, due to respiratory failure or infection. Girls who carry the affected gene are usually symptomless but may have elevation of the muscle enzyme, creatine kinase (CK). Until recently, carrier identification had been limited to pedigree analysis and serum CK measurement. The selective termination of male fetuses was the only prenatal test which could be offered to carrier females.

A major breakthrough in the prenatal diagnosis of DMD was assignment of the gene to the short arm of the X-chromosome (Xp21). This followed cytogenetic analysis of a number of rare girls with DMD. Some affected females were found to have translocations involving various autosomes but always the same region of the X-chromosome. In other cases, DMD plus other X-linked diseases were found in boys with visible deletions of the X-chromosome — all involving Xp21. Identification of the 'target area' on the X-chromosome was followed by the more detailed mapping of that particular area of the X-chromosome using a number of probes and RFLPs. Initially these probes were too far away to be of general use (>15 centimorgans) as errors due to recombination greatly diminished diagnostic value.

Further research led to isolation of the DMD gene and identification of its product, dystrophin (Koenig et al 1987). The gene is huge and deletions are found in over 50% of cases, making prenatal diagnosis relatively simple (Forrest et al 1987). Errors due to crossing-over within the gene are still a problem in the remaining families. Whilst this exciting and important discovery will soon produce tests of benefit to a large number of families with the DMD gene it is important to remember that one-third of cases are new mutations and thus the disease will continue to affect a significant number of male children.

Myotonic dystrophy

Myotonic dystrophy, inherited as an autosomal dominant, is the most common of the adult-onset muscular dystrophies (see also Ch. 44). The prevalence approaches that for Duchenne muscular dystrophy and all races appear equally affected. A characteristic feature of this disorder is a long insidious course, the disorder being present for many years before diagnosis is established. In contrast to this presentation is a severe neonatal form of myotonic dystrophy, often with a very bad prognosis, affecting some infants of myotonic mothers.

As the disease is an autosomal dominant there is a 1 in 2 risk for the offspring of the patient being affected. As the disorder is so variable in both the age of onset and severity of muscle symptoms it is difficult to counsel apparently healthy children or siblings of an affected patient. The most useful investigations are electromyography and slit lamp examination for lens opacities. A negative test, however, does not exclude the diagnosis in childhood or early adult life although with increasing age a negative test assumes greater significance. Virtually all persons with the gene show abnormalities in these tests by their 50s.

Linkage studies are useful in only a small number of families. Myotonic dystrophy was in fact the first serious autosomal disorder for which linkage was established — to the genes controlling Lutheran blood group antigens and to secretion of ABH blood group substances secretor status. This has been followed by the production of a number of probes which map closer to the actual gene, C3 (7 cM), apolipoprotein CII gene (4 cM) and D1957 (very close), making recombination events less common but, as with all linkage tests, not all families will be informative.

REFERENCES

Brambati B, Simoni G, Fabro S (eds) 1985 Chorionic villus sampling: fetal diagnosis of genetic diseases in the first trimester. Marcel Dekker, New York

Forrest S M, Smith T J, Cross G S et al 1987 Effective strategy for prenatal prediction of Duchenne and Becker muscular dystrophy. Lancet ii: 1294–1296

Francomano C A, Kazazian H H 1986 DNA analysis in genetic disorders. Annual Review of Medicine 37: 377–395

Hamerton J L, Ferguson-Smith M A (eds) 1984 Collaborate studies in prenatal diagnosis of chromosome aberrations. Prenatal Diagnosis 4 (Special Issue): 1–162

Harrison M R, Golbus M S, Filly R A 1984 The unborn patient: prenatal diagnosis and treatment. Grune & Stratton, Orlando

Koenig M, Hoffman E P, Bertelson C J et al 1987 Complete cloning of the Duchenne muscular dystrophy (DMD) CDNA and preliminary genomic organization of the DMD gene in normal and affected individuals. Cell 50: 509–517

Milunsky A (ed) 1986 Genetic Disorders and the Fetus: diagnosis, prevention and treatment, 2nd edn. Plenum Press, New York

Naylor G, Sweetman L, Nyhan W L et al 1980 Isotope dilution analysis of methylcitric acid in amniotic fluid for the prenatal diagnosis of propionic and methylmalonic acidemia. Clinica Chimica Acta 107: 175–183

Simoni G, Gimelli G, Guoco C et al 1986 First trimester fetal karyotyping: one thousand diagnoses. Human Genetics 72: 203–209

Wald N J (ed) 1984 Antenatal and neonatal screening. Oxford University Press, Oxford

39. Inborn errors — diagnosis and management

Prof D. M. Danks, Dr J. E. Wraith and Dr G. K. Brown

Although individually rare, the inborn errors of metabolism as a group constitute a significant problem in neonatal clinical practice. This has increased in recent years with the biochemical definition of a number of new conditions, the effective treatment of some diseases and the development of prenatal diagnosis. In this chapter we focus on those disorders in which neurological abnormalities are prominent. Unless specific references are cited, the reader can obtain further information from Stanbury et al (1983).

Before discussing specific disorders, a few general points about diagnosis and management need to be made. Individual inborn errors of metabolism are rare and experience is important if diagnosis and treatment are to proceed rapidly. Expert labortory services are essential but require interpretation by skilled clinical specialists. Consequently, prompt clinical consultation is important and will generally lead to transfer to a specialized hospital unit. Initial screening tests must be readily available in each region. Clinicians must be encouraged to use screening tests freely and laboratories must be reconciled to a low frequency of abnormal results. More specialized tests are needed in only a small number of supraregional or national reference laboratories.

Throughout this chapter we express a philosophy of very aggressive treatment. Some clinicians feel concerned about this approach and occasionally we are accused of taking the risk of keeping alive a grossly brain-damaged infant. In our experience this is not a problem. After a short period of very energetic treatment one can generally judge the prognosis quite accurately. If the prospect of return to normal cerebral function is poor, one can refrain from employing extraordinary measures in the next acute episode of deterioration. The episodic nature of most inborn errors ensures that treatment can be reassessed at frequent intervals. There is some risk of producing survivors with minor degrees of brain damage but this is true in all acute neonatal illnesses and in all inborn errors that can affect the brain.

PRESENTATION OF INBORN ERRORS OF METABOLISM

Babies with inborn errors of metabolism come to notice in several ways:

Acute, severe illness in the newborn period

The greater part of this chapter concentrates on those inborn errors that present with life-threatening illness in the early neonatal period. A number of clues can be obtained from a careful history, examination and simple bedside tests.

Subacute presentation

A number of infants, especially those with lysosomal storage disease present outside the newborn period. In these infants, visceromegaly and skeletal dysplasia are often associated features. Whilst a life-threatening presentation is rare there is considerable overlap between the two groups and a number of conditions placed in the subacute group can have dramatic neonatal presentation, e.g. hydrops fetalis in the lysosomal storage disorders (Gillan et al 1984) and profound hypotonia in the cerebro–hepato–renal syndrome (Kelley 1983).

Table 39.1 lists those disorders that tend to present in a subacute manner and some of these conditions are discussed in Chapter 40. Intra-uterine protection is not a feature of most of these conditions and in the storage disorders the storage product accumulates throughout gestation. The time of onset of clinical features and their rate of progression vary between and within the conditions.

Dysmorphic features or multiple congenital anomalies

A number of recently described conditions, such as glutaric aciduria type II and 3-hydroxyisobutyryl CoA deacylase deficiency present with multiple congenital abnormality.

Table 39.1 Disorders with subacute presentation in the newborn period

Disorder	Symptoms	Biochemical findings	Enzyme assay	Prenatal diagnosis
Glycogen storage disease type II (Pompe's disease)	Hypotonia, cardiac failure	No consistent abnormality	Fibroblasts, muscle, lymphocytes	Enzyme
Wolman's disease	FTT, developmental delay	↓ Acid lipase	Leukocytes	Adrenal calcification, other variants, enzyme
Hereditary orotic aciduria	FTT, developmental delay, stabismus	↑ Urine orotic acid, ↓ orotidylate-5-decarboxylase, ↓ orotate phosphoribysyl transferase	Erythrocytes	Megaloblastosis
Adenosine deaminase deficiency	Severe combined immune deficiency, motor and mental retardation	↓ Adenosine deaminase	Erythrocytes	Lymphopenia, ↓ gammaglobulin, X-linked, enzyme
3-Methyl glutaconic aciduria	Hypotonia, abnormal movements, mental retardation	Methylglutaconic acid, methylglutaric acid, 3-OH-isovaleric acid	–	–
Fumaric acidaemia	FTT, developmental delay, cerebral atrophy	↑ Fumaric acid ↓ Fumarase	Fibroblasts	Enzyme (Zinn et al 1986)
N-acetyl aspartic aciduria	Severe mental retardation, cerebral atrophy	↑ *N*-Acetylaspartic acid in urine	–	– (Kvittingen et al 1986)
Gangliosidoses	See Chap. 40			
Other lipid disorders	See Chap. 40			
Glycosominoglycan metabolism	See Chap. 40			
Mucolipidoses	See Chap. 40			
Glycoproteinoses	See Chap. 40			
Peroxisomal disorders	See Chap. 40			
Disorders of purines and pyrimidines	See Chap. 40			

FTT = Failure to thrive.

This raises an important principle — that all infants with multiple malformations should be tested by 'metabolic screening'.

In glutaric aciduria type II, the defects include 'Potter type' facies, abnormal kidneys, genitalia and abdominal wall. In addition there is a rapidly lethal illness characterized by severe hypoglycaemia which does not respond to any treatment. The defect is in electron transport flavoprotein or its dehydrogenase, important steps in the electron transport chain (Goodman & Frerman 1984). Affected individuals have the 'sweaty feet' odour of isovaleric acidaemia.

Some of the peroxisomal disorders, e.g. the rhizomelic form of chondrodysplasia punctata, may also present with congenital anomalies.

The one infant described with 3-hydroxyisobutyryl CoA deacylase deficiency had skeletal, cardiac and brain malformations (Brown et al 1982). Disturbed mitochondrial function may interfere with embryogenesis.

Mass screening of the newborn population

In addition to the more dramatic presentations noted above, a large number of infants with inborn errors will be detected in newborn screening programmes. The only inborn error of metabolism that has achieved universal acceptance for mass screening is phenylketonuria. The characteristics of phenylketonuria make it ideal for screening. Treatment is relatively easy and inexpensive. It is relatively frequent (1 in 10 000). Detection and treatment within the first 3–4 weeks of life gives a very good outcome, quite different from the outcome after symptomatic diagnosis. Similar arguments justify screening for hypothyroidism but it is not an inborn error of metabolism.

Mass screening has been suggested for a number of other inborn errors of metabolism but none of these has achieved universal acceptance.

Screening for galactosaemia is carried out by a number of communities. It is much less common than phenylketonuria (1 in 60 000) and a number of babies will have developed acute neonatal illness before the screening test result is back from the laboratory. It is uncertain whether the eventual outcome of babies diagnosed before symptoms develop is any better than that of babies diagnosed quickly, after the onset of symptoms. The same criticisms apply to maple syrup urine disease but are increased by the even lower frequency (1 in 250 000) and the outcome which can be poor even with optimal treatment.

Screening for tyrosinaemia is justified in a small number of communities that have a high incidence of the disorder (e.g. Quebec and Scandinavia) but not elsewhere.

More recently it has been suggested that an assay for biotinidase deficiency should be included on the newborn screen (Heara et al 1986). Whilst the test itself appears satisfactory, the condition is rare and the clinical spectrum not yet fully defined.

Inborn error anticipated because of previous history

Some parents, who have had previously affected infants, find prenatal diagnosis and termination of pregnancy unacceptable. In this situation it is important to plan treatment before birth. In some vitamin-responsive disorders it is possible to treat the fetus before birth by giving large doses of the relevant vitamin to the mother (e.g. in vitamin B12-responsive methylmalonic acidaemia).

In other situations a couple may have lost a previous baby in circumstances suggestive of an inborn error but with no firm diagnosis established. Then, we would arrange transfer of the newborn to the metabolic unit 6–12 hours after delivery. This period allows for some bonding to occur between mother and baby, knowing that most inborn errors do not produce symptoms for 24–48 hours. On arrival the baby is investigated and maintained on a low-protein intake until the results are known. If investigations are negative a normal diet is started and the tests are repeated 48 hours later. This approach allows biochemical diagnosis before symptoms are apparent (Danks 1974).

CLUES TO THE DIAGNOSIS OF SEVERE NEONATAL ILLNESS

The essential points to be noted in the history of any child presenting with an unusual illness in the newborn period are as follows:

1. Is there a history of previous stillbirths or neonatal deaths?
2. Is there a history of parental consanguinity?
3. Was there a period of normality after birth?
4. Has there been a change of feed since birth?
5. Is there any evidence of infection?
6. Has the baby been subject to a fast or surgical procedure?
7. Did the baby improve when feeds were discontinued?
8. Was there a relapse on restarting milk feeds?

With one or two important exceptions (e.g. ornithine carbamyl transferase (OCT) deficiency), inheritance is autosomal recessive. A family history of neonatal death or of parental consanguinity is an important clue. In OCT deficiency there may be a history of male deaths on the maternal side of the family.

Most affected infants are delivered at, or near, full-term in good condition with a normal birth-weight and remain well in the early days of life. Intra-uterine protection from the effects of inherited metabolic disease is due to a number of factors. The fetus is in an anabolic state and this minimizes flux through amino acid degradative pathways and the urea cycle. The placenta effectively haemodialyses the fetus removing toxic metabolites and the fetus is not yet in contact with substances in the diet toxic to infants with a

mutant genotype. There are some important exceptions to the general rule of intra-uterine protection. In non-ketotic hyperglycinaemia and pyridoxine-dependent convulsions, features appear before, at, or soon after birth. The disturbance of neurotransmitter production in these disorders is not greatly influenced by placental function.

Intense catabolism during the first few days of life, together with the initiation of protein-containing feeds, unmasks the metabolic lesion. A change in feeding may be an important precipitating event, e.g. a change from breast-feeding to a higher protein-containing formula or a change from a lactose- to a sucrose-based milk. Detailed information regarding all feeds given since birth is essential — a single bottle of fructose-containing milk can precipitate acute symptoms in hereditary fructose intolerance.

In those infants who escape severe disease in the newborn period, catabolic stress such as infection, surgery or prolonged fasting can precipitate symptoms at some later time. If the infant improves when protein is removed from the diet, only to relapse when milk feeds are recommenced, a metabolic disorder should be suspected.

CLINICAL FEATURES OF SEVERE NEONATAL ILLNESS

Those disorders which present as an acute illness in the newborn period are listed in Table 39.2 together with their main clinical and biochemical findings.

The neonate with a metabolic disorder presents with very non-specific features mimicking a host of more common neonatal problems such as sepsis, cardiorespiratory disease, necrotizing enterocolitis and intracerebral haemorrhage. The correct interpretation of the clinical signs depends upon a high index of suspicion of a metabolic disease in the mind of the clinician managing the child.

INVESTIGATION OF THE SEVERELY ILL NEONATE

Metabolic investigations should proceed urgently, in parallel with other tests for infections and other common neonatal illnesses in very sick infants.

Generally, there is no clue to a specific inborn error and a full 'metabolic screen' should be performed urgently. Occasionally one can get a great deal of help from the history and examination. A male infant, normal at birth, who becomes progressively comatose from day 3 onwards and who comes from a family in which male infants have died early should have an urgent blood ammonia and urinary orotic acid estimation performed. The diagnosis is most likely to be OCT deficiency. In rare cases, a striking odour, may allow one to suspect maple syrup urine disease

Table 39.2 Disorders that may present as a severe illness in the newborn period

Inborn error of metabolism	Symptoms	Biochemical findings	Enzyme assay (tissue)	Comments (prenatal diagnosis)
Urea cycle defects and hyperammonaemia	All have vomiting, drowsiness, coma, hypotonia, convulsions	All have ↑ NH_3		Treatment: Low-protein diet; sodium benzoate, arginine supplement‡
1. *N*-acetyl glutamate deficiency	All have had early acute onset	↑ Transaminases, non-specific amino aciduria, normal orotic acid	Liver	Potential treatment with carbamyl glutamate (–)
2. Carbamyl phosphate synthetase deficiency	All have had early acute onset	As 1	Liver	Death in newborn period (O)
3. Ornithine carbamoyl transferase deficiency	Early acute onset in most males; subacute onset in some females and exceptional males	As 1. *but* ↑ orotic acid	Liver, intestinal mucosa	Treatable(2) as ‡., X-linked. Few males survive (D,O)
4. Citrullinaemia	Early and late onset	↑ Citrulline and orotic acid. Normal argininosuccinic acid	Fibroblasts	Treatable(2) as ‡. (E)
5. Argininosuccinic acidaemia	Early and late onset	↑ Argininosuccinic acid and orotic acid	Fibroblasts, erythrocytes	Treatable(2) as ‡.(E). Trichorrexis nodosa
6. Arginase deficiency	Later onset with retardation, spastic diplegia, liver disease	↑ Arginine	Leucocytes, erythrocytes	Treatable(2), by low-protein diet, sodium benzoate (E)
7. Transient neonatal ↑ NH_3	Early acute onset in premature infants	↑ NH_3 only	–	Treatable(1) as ‡.
8. Hyperlysinaemia/ ammonaemia	Vomiting, seizures, coma, spasticity	Intermittent ↑ NH_3 ↑ lysine	–	Treatable(2) as ‡. (–)
9. Hyperornithinaemia/ homocitrulline/ ammonaemia	Subacute, after protein load	Intermittent ↑ NH_3, ↑ ornithine, ↑ homocitrulline	–	Treatable(2) by low protein diet (–)
10. Lysinuric protein intolerance	As 9.	↓ tubular reabsorption of basic amino acids	–	Treatable(2) by low protein diet (–)
Amino acid and organic acid metabolism				
11. Maple syrup urine disease	Vomiting, convulsions, apnoea, spasticity, coma	A. ↑ Leucine, isoleucine, valine and corresponding α-ketoacids	Leucocytes	Odour, treatable(2) (E)
12. Hypervalinaemia	Vomiting, hypotonia, hyperactivity	A. ↑ Valine	Leucocytes	Treatable(2) (E)
13. Hyperleucineaemia	Seizures, mental retardation	A. ↑ Leucine, isoleucine	Leucocytes	Treatable(2) (E)
14. 3-Hydroxyisobutryl CoA-deacylase deficiency	Multiple malformations	↑ Methacrylyl-cysteine and -cysteamine.	Fibroblasts	No treatment (E)
15. β-Alaninaemia	Lethargy, hypotonia, seizures	↑ β-Alanine, ↑ GABA	–	No treatment (E)
16. Non-ketotic hyperglycinaemia	Lethargy, hypotonia, seizures, severe retardation	↑ Glycine	Liver	Mild cases treated with strychnine. CSF glycine important in diagnosis (O)
17. Isovaleric acidaemia	Lethargy, vomiting, tremor, seizures, apnoea, coma	A. ↑ Isovaleric acid	Fibroblasts	Odour = sweaty feet, neutropenia, treatable 2 (E,O)
18. Hawkinsinuria	Failure to thrive in baby on artificial formula	A. ↑ *p*-Hydroxyphenyl-pyruvic, -lactic, -acetic acids, ↑ Hawkinsin	–	Treatable(1), self-limited illness (–) (Wilcken et al 1981).
19. Tyrosinaemia type I	Failure to thrive, hepatic failure	↑ Tyrosine, ↑ methionine, ↑ succinyl acetone	Fumaryl-acetoacetase	Treatable(2) (O)
20. Propionic acidaemia	As 17.	A. Ketosis, ↑ glycine ↑ propionic acid	Fibroblasts	Neutropenia, thrombycytopenia, treatable(2) (E,O)
21. Multiple carboxylase deficiency	Vomiting, irritability (later deafness, optic atrophy)	A. ↑ β-Methylcrotonyl glycine, ↑ tiglyl glycine, ↑ 3-OH-isovaleric acid	Fibroblasts	Alopecia, skin rash, treatable(1) (E)
22. 3-Methylcrotonyl-glycinuria	Hypotonia, arreflexia	A. ↑ Methylcrotonyl glycine	Fibroblasts	Odour 'Tom Cats' urine. Potentially treatable(2) (E)
23. Methylmalonic acidaemia	As 20.	A. ↑ Glycine, ↑ methylmalonic acid	Fibroblasts	As 20. (E,O)
24. Methylmalonic acidaemia with homocystinuria	Feeding difficulties, seizures	↑ Methylmalonic acid, homocystinuria	Fibroblasts	Megaloblastosis, treatable(2) (O)
25. Glutaric aciduria type I	Hypotonia, abnormal movements, oculogyric crises (generally later infancy)	↑ Glutaric acid	Fibroblasts, leucocytes	No treatment (E)
26. Glutaric aciduria type II	Seizures, hypotonia, coma, hypoglycaemia	A. ↑ Lactate, ↑ 3-OH-butyric, ↑ suberic, adipic, butyric, ↑ isovaleric, 2-PH-glutaric acids	Fibroblasts	Odour = sweaty feet. No treatment. Rapidly lethal in most cases (E)

Table 39.2   Continued

Inborn error of metabolism	Symptoms	Biochemical findings	Enzyme assay (tissue)	Comments (prenatal diagnosis)
27. Ethylmalonic/adipic aciduria	As 26. but milder	A. ↑ Ethylmalonic, ↑ adipic acids	Fibroblasts	May be milder variant of 26. (E)
28. 3-OH-3-methylglutaric	Coma, hypoglycaemia, (generally later onset)	↑ 3-OH-3-Methylglutaric acids	Fibroblasts	Recurrent 'Reyes' syndrome, treatable(1) (E)
29. D-Glyceric aciduria	Hypotonia, seizures, abnormal movements	A. ↑ Glycine, ↑ D-glyceric acid	Fibroblasts, leucocytes	(–)
30. Dicarboxylic aciduria (fatty acyl CoA dehydrogenase deficiency)	Mental retardation, fasting hypoglycaemia	↑ Adipic, ↑ suberic acids	Fibroblasts	Recurrent 'Reyes' syndrome. syndrome, treatable(1) (E)
31. Pyroglutamic aciduria	Mental retardation, failure to thrive	A ↑ Pyroglutamic acid	Fibroblasts, leucocytes	Haemolytic anaemia, no effective treatment (E)
32. 3-Ketothiolase deficiency	Vomiting, lethargy, coma, seizures	↑ Glycine, ↑ NH₃, ↑ 2-methylacetic, ↑ 2-methyl 3-OH-butyric acid	Fibroblasts	Neutropenia, thrombycytopenia, no treatment (E)
33. 2-Hydroxybutyric aciduria	'Cyclic vomiting' (later onset)	↑ 2-Aminobutyric acid	–	Neonatal form not yet described (–)

Carbohydrate metablism

34. Galactosaemia	Vomiting, jaundice, cataracts, hepatic failure, seizures, mental retardation, sepsis common	↑ Bilirubin, ↑ transaminases, ↑ galactose-1-phosphate, renal tubular defects	Erythrocytes	Many variants, treatable(2) (E)
35. Hereditary fructose intolerance	Lethargy, sweating, vomiting, seizures, liver failure	A. ↑ Transaminases, renal tubular defects	Liver	Treatable(1), after exposure to to fructose as 37. (O)
36. Fructose 1-6-diphosphate deficiency	Irritability, hypotonia, coma, apnoea, seizures	A. ↑ Transaminases, ↑ lactate, ↓ glucose	Liver	Treatable(1) (O)
37. Glycogen storage disease, types Ia and b	Irritability, hypotonia, seizures	A. ↑ Lactate, ↑ uric acid, ↑ lipids, ↓ glucose	Liver	Neutropenia, thrombocytopenia, treatable(1) (O)
38. Phosphoenolpyruvate carboxykinase deficiency	Vomiting, drowsiness, hypotonia, hepatomegaly	A. ↑ Lactate, ↓ glucose	Liver	Treatable(2) (–)
39. Pyruvate carboxylase deficiency	As 38	A. ↑ Lactate, ↑ alanine, ↑ NH₃ ↓ glucose	Fibroblasts	Some treatable(2) (thiamine) (E)
40. Pyruvate dehydrogenase deficiency	As 38, 39	As 38, 39	Fibroblasts	Various enzyme defects – some treatable(2) (E)
41. Primary lactic acidosis	As 38, 39, 40	As 38, 39, 40	No enzyme defect demonstrated	Difficult to distinguish from secondary lactic acidosis (–)

Miscellaneous

42. Pyridoxine-dependent seizures	Intractable seizures	–	–	Onset in utero, treatable(1) (–)
43. Sulphite oxidase deficiency	Poor feeding, opistotonus, spasticity, abnormal movements, nystagmus, lens dislocation	↑ Sulphite ↑ S-sulphocysteine, ↑ taurine	Fibroblasts	No treatment (E)
44. Molybdenum cofactor deficiency	As 43. plus renal calculi	As 43. plus ↑ xanthine	Liver, intestinal mucosa	No treatment (E)
45. Transcobalamin II deficiency	Poor feeding, irritability, lethargy, failure to thrive, glossitis, mouth ulcers	Normal B₁₂, ↓ transcobalamin II, ↑ methylmalonic acid	Plasma	Megaloblastosis, treatable(1) (–) (Hakami et al 1971).

Treatable(1) = outcome generally good after early treatment.
Treatable(2) = outcome variable even after early treatment, or uncertain because to few reports.
Prenatal diagnosis: (–) = not available/applicable; (D) = DNA; (E) = enzyme; (O) = other.
Biochemical findings: A = acidosis present.

or isovaleric acidaemia. A skin rash may suggest biotinidase or multiple carboxylase deficiency.

Although techniques vary, most laboratories will require a sample of blood (1–2 ml) and of urine (5–10 ml) to perform a 'metabolic screen'. It is a good principle to collect all urine passed by the infant, record the time collected and then freeze the sample for future analysis. The laboratory tests include urine 'spot' tests, for glucose, other reducing substances, ketones and examination of the urine amino acid and organic acid patterns. In our laboratory high-voltage electrophoresis is used for amino acid analysis, staining first with ninhydrin and then counter-staining with iodoplatinate for sulphur-containing compounds. The origin is then further counter-stained with fast blue B as a screening test for methylmalonic acid. If an abnormal pattern is found, the amino acids in both urine and plasma are determined quantitatively. Gas–liquid chromatography is used for organic acids, with confirmation of abnormal peaks by mass spectrometry. Plasma ammonia is measured and a portion of urine is kept for orotic acid estimation if the plasma ammonia is found to be high.

Infants with lactic acidosis present a difficult problem. It is very difficult to distinguish a primary lactic acidosis due to an inborn error of metabolism from a secondary elevation of lactate due to sepsis, cardiac disease, hypoxia or convulsions. It is necessary to treat the possible underlying causes aggressively whilst trying to separate the two groups. Plasma lactate and pyruvate are extremely sensitive to the method of collection. Venous obstruction by crying, tourniquet or breath-holding can raise levels 2–3 fold. We have generally found that urinary lactate is a very satisfactory way of measuring lactate and monitoring treatment in most cases but have encountered exceptions. In those infants with a secondary lactic acidosis urinary lactate should fall as the child's condition improves with treatment of the underlying disorder. Often, however, the child dies before a clear distinction is made. Then one has to rely on formal assay of the enzymes known to cause lactic acidosis when deficient — an unsatisfactory process because some of the enzymes responsible have not yet been identified.

In many cases the investigations mentioned will provide a definite diagnosis or a suspicion of a particular inborn error and appropriate therapy can begin. Further definition of the condition requires specific enzyme assays, studies of in-vitro cofactor responsiveness and the property of the defective enzyme. These are most often undertaken on cultured skin fibroblasts. In particular circumstances it is useful to repeat the investigations on cerebrospinal fluid (CSF). This is particularly true in non-ketotic hyperglycinaemia which may be associated with minimal or no abnormality of glycine in plasma but with marked elevation in CSF. In addition to this condition we have seen a number of abnormal amino acid patterns in the CSF of children with obscure neurological disease, the findings in the CSF serving as a clue to further studies. Measurement of CSF lactate and pyruvate has assisted us in defining primary lactic acidoses and in recognizing some cases with profound brain involvement but minimal systemic lactate accumulation.

MANAGEMENT

Management whilst awaiting results

General

The severity of symptoms dictates the aggressiveness of management. In infants who have very mild symptoms it is appropriate to discontinue milk feeds once the specimens necessary for the screen have been collected. As it is easy to induce intestinal sugar intolerance in young babies it is prudent to feed 5% dextrose rather than 10% at this stage. In more severe illness, intravenous fluids will be necessary

and 10% dextrose is used except when a primary lactic acidosis is suspected (these conditions may be aggravated by a high-carbohydrate load). Electrolytes and other additives are determined by biochemical results. In those children deteriorating rapidly, aggressive therapy is justified even before a definitive diagnosis has been made. It is of paramount importance to correct acidosis promptly and adequately. In some conditions, e.g. organic acid disorders, this may require very large doses of sodium bicarbonate. Hypernatraemia is a common complication and may necessitate peritoneal dialysis. Attention must be paid to tissue perfusion and oxygenation. Most affected infants will require ventilatory and often inotropic support. Electrolyte balance, calcium and glucose homeostasis must be checked frequently and alterations made as appropriate.

In the acute phase nutrition is confined to dextrose. Most inborn errors are aggravated by catabolism and when acidosis has been corrected, enough glucose should be given to promote anabolism. This usually requires 20% dextrose infused via a central line. Small doses of insulin (0.1 U/kg, 4–6 hourly) may help to initiate anabolism as may the use of lipid solutions which provide a valuable source of calories. The latter is likely to be effective only after an initial improvement has been achieved by the other measures and care needs to be taken, as some conditions are exacerbated by a high-fat diet. Once anabolism is achieved, often marked by a general improvement, increased glucose tolerance and diuresis, protein should be introduced to the diet. We start with 0.5 g/kg for 24 hours and increase daily, by 0.25 to 0.5 mg/kg, if tolerated, to 1.5 g/kg. This, plus 120 calories/kg is sufficient to maintain anabolism; in fact many infants will grow satisfactorily on 1.2 g protein/kg plus appropriate calories. By this stage the infant is usually able to tolerate intragastric feeds but, if not, a parenteral regime can be used.

Removal of toxic metabolites

Peritoneal dialysis or exchange transfusion are essential in the acute management of infants who do not improve rapidly with conservative therapy. This includes those infants who develop hypernatraemia due to excessive bicarbonate requirements. Our policy is to introduce dialysis early as success is unlikely if used as a 'last-ditch' procedure on a moribund infant. Exchange transfusion may be more effective in infants with a bleeding disorder or hepatic failure. In infants with severe hyperammonaemia or a primary organic acid disorder dialysis is likely to be needed for at least 7 days. To minimize the risk of peritoneal infection we prefer the catheter to be inserted surgically via a long subcutaneous tunnel and to use only closed dialysis circuits. Ventilatory support becomes essential when peritoneal dialysis is started, if it has not been initiated for other reasons. We aim to keep dialysis going until anabolism is established and the infant is tolerating nasogastric feeds.

The megavitamin cocktail

Vitamins in pharmacological doses are given to all very sick infants whilst awaiting results. Several inborn errors are known to have vitamin-responsive forms, e.g. vitamin B12 in methylmalonic acidaemia, biotin in multiple carboxylase deficiency and thiamine in maple syrup urine disease. In infants in whom no diagnosis has been established it is reasonable to try a full cocktail in high dosage (Table 39.3). When a diagnosis of an inborn error known to have a vitamin-responsive form is made, that vitamin should be given in a dose about 100 times the daily requirement.

Specific management after diagnosis

For the majority of disorders, treatment is non-specific and relies upon protein restriction. In some, however, more specific regimes are available and this is illustrated in the section on the urea cycle disorders.

In all forms of lactic acidosis muscle paralysis plays a specific role in reducing lactate production. Dietary treatment is difficult as some forms, (e.g. patients with pyruvate dehydrogenase deficiency) are made worse by a low-protein, high-carbohydrate diet whilst others with defects in gluconeogenesis, respond favourably to this regime. Other infants have shown a partial response to a ketogenic diet and dichloracetate.

Management when no diagnosis

If no diagnosis is established it is still worth attempting non-specific therapies such as peritoneal dialysis, protein restriction and the megavitamin cocktail. A number of infants will recover and have no residual disease, a situation analogous to transient hyperammonaemia in pre-term infants.

When no diagnosis is established and death appears inevitable

It is very important to obtain as much information about the child as possible. Autopsy examination is essential. This should be performed soon after death to allow biochemical studies to be carried out on non-autolysed tissues (Perry 1981). The need for autopsy should be discussed with the parents before death and permission obtained at this time; most couples find it easier to discuss this matter before death than after death. A skin fibroblast culture should be established. Tissues obtained after death should be prepared for electron microscopy and portions of liver, kidney, skeletal muscle, cardiac muscle and brain should be frozen quickly and stored at $-70°C$. At the same time a careful examination is made for structural abnormalities of the brain and heart as well as appropriate bacterial and viral cultures.

When the results of the autopsy investigations are known it is important to see the parents and explain the illness and investigation results. If no diagnosis has been established even after autopsy and the infant's illness was suggestive of an inborn error of metabolism, subsequent pregnancies and children should be monitored carefully.

Long-term management

This can involve a specific therapy such as a diet low in branched-chain amino acids in maple syrup urine disease or a non-specific low-protein diet in infants with vitamin-unresponsive forms of the organic acid disorders. In the latter situation the crucial factor is whether or not the child is able to grow within the confines of protein tolerance. A number of infants are in a precarious situation, tolerating just enough protein to allow growth, but the latitude is so slight that any trivial intercurrent infection can produce acute metabolic imbalance. Good judgement is critical in treating these babies. A slightly excessive protein intake may cause a metabolic imbalance which arrests growth. Then, a reduction in protein intake may restore growth. At other times excessive protein restriction may stop growth, with consequent metabolic instability.

To test tolerance it is important to increase protein intake slowly in an inpatient under close biochemical control. After discharge the child should be readmitted during the first two or three episodes of intercurrent illness. This allows one to assess the usefulness of simple therapies, such as diluting feeds and supplementing with oral carbohydrates during mild exacerbations. Severe decompensation needs to be treated as aggressively as the presenting episode. Both parents and doctors gain experience of the child's response to catabolism and are thus able to judge when hospitalization is necessary in future episodes.

Other manoeuvres which help in difficult cases are supplementation with alanine, an important energy resource (Kelts et al 1985), and added carnitine to compensate for the loss in the urine of conjugates, like propionylcarnitine in (for instance) propionic acidaemia (Engel & Rebouche 1984).

Table 39.3 Megavitamin cocktail

Ingredient	mg/day
Vitamin B12	1.0
Biotin	100
Thiamine	50
Riboflavin	50
Nicotinamide	600
Pyridoxine	100
Pantothenic acid	50
Ascorbic acid	3000

A number of the disorders are now considered in a little more detail.

Phenylketonuria

There are a number of conditions associated with an elevation of plasma phenylalanine and all are detected by the newborn screening programme. Of practical importance are 'classical' phenylketonuria due to phenylalanine hydroxylase deficiency and those cases caused by deficiency of the tetrahydrobiopterin cofactor due to defects in synthesis or recycling. One can no longer assume that a positive result on screening indicates phenylalanine hydroxylase deficiency and that one need only decide whether the deficiency is sufficiently severe to require dietary treatment (classical PKU) or not (hyperphenylalaninaemia, HPA). This is further complicated by the fact that infants with cofactor defects may have only marginally elevated phenylalanine levels, which would not warrant dietary treatment in phenylalanine hydroxylase deficiency. In the cofactor-deficient cases, dietary treatment has to be supplemented with neurotransmitter precursors, 5-hydroxytryptophan and L-dopa. It is therefore important to distinguish cofactor defects as quickly as possible. Our policy is to give a tetrahydrobiopterin load intravenously (7.5 mg/kg) as well as examining the urinary pterin excretion of all infants who have a persistently positive screening test.

Also of relevance to this chapter is the syndrome of mental retardation, microcephaly, cardiac defects and poor growth observed in infants born to phenylketonuric mothers (Lenke & Levy 1980). In families with a number of abnormal children it is essential to check the mother for metabolic disease as part of the investigations.

Urea cycle defects

The urea cycle defects (Table 39.2, 1–6), illustrate one or two points that require expansion. OCT deficiency is one of the few conditions presenting as an acute illness in the newborn period that is inherited in an X-linked manner. In affected families there is often a history of early male deaths on the maternal side. Female heterozygotes have a variable degree of illness. Many develop an aversion to protein-rich foods and some develop serious episodes of hyperammonaemia which may cause brain damage or even death (Batshaw et al 1986, Rowe et al 1986). The remainder of the urea cycle defects show autosomal recessive inheritance and occur as severe forms, lethal in the newborn period, or as less severe forms presenting later (as with OCT deficiency).

The clinical features are principally due to the neurotoxicity of ammonia. To lower ammonia levels quickly, peritoneal dialysis or exchange transfusion can be aided by utilizing alternative pathways of waste nitrogen excretion (Batshaw et al 1981). The compounds sodium benzoate and phenylacetic acid are used and amino acid nitrogen is excreted as hippuric acid and phenylacetylglutamine respectively. Use in chronic treatment has made management easier. A low-protein diet is still required and an essential amino acid mixture may be useful in children with a urea cycle defect. Arginine supplementation is necessary because it becomes an essential amino acid in these patients (Brusilow 1984) and arginine deficiency may be responsible for some symptoms. OCT is required for intestinal absorption of arginine, therefore citrulline is used instead of arginine in OCT deficiency.

Prognosis for mental development in severe cases is good only when treatment is started before symptoms develop but the new methods of controlling hyperammonaemia have certainly improved the prognosis.

Transient hyperammonaemia in the newborn period is worthy of mention. The biochemical basis of the disorder is unknown. It is more common in premature infants and is important to recognize because aggressive treatment has led to a normal recovery in infants whose presenting blood ammonia levels have been greater than 1000 μmol/l. Subsequently affected infants tolerate a normal diet, illustrating the transient nature of some metabolic disorders.

Maple syrup urine disease

A deficiency of the branched-chain 2-ketoacid dehydrogenase complex results in an elevation of the branched-chain amino acids, leucine, isoleucine and valine. The urine has the characteristic smell of maple syrup and in the affected infant symptoms are usually present by the end of the first week of life. The infant fails to thrive, vomits and develops convulsions and rigidity. Untreated, stupor, progressive lethargy and coma result, with death the usual outcome. Survivors exhibit severe brain dysfunction with dystonic posturing and profound retardation. A number of variants occur, including intermittent and mild thiamine-responsive forms.

Dietary treatment is difficult as one has to adjust the level of three amino acids in a co-ordinated manner. Over-treatment results in catabolism leading to further instability.

The prognosis in maple syrup urine disease diagnosed after the first week of life is disappointing. Even with early diagnosis and treatment the clinical course is one of frequent readmission to hospital over the early years of life for restabilization but very good results have been achieved in some patients.

Non-ketotic hyperglycinaemia

Glycine encephalopathy or non-ketotic hyperglycinaemia is one of the few disorders in which intra-uterine protection does not occur. Hypotonia and lethargy are present from birth and some mothers have reported decreased fetal movements, suggesting an intrauterine onset. Myoclonic seizures may be prominent with hiccups, opistotonic posturing and progressive deterioration to death. The elevation of glycine is more marked in CSF than in blood, reflecting a primary disturbance of neuronal glycine metabolism. There is no associated increase in urinary organic acids distinguishing the condition from the various ketotic hyperglycinaemias.

As symptoms appear to be due to exaggeration of the inhibitory neuromodulatory role of glycine, treatments which merely modify plasma glycine have little effect on the disease, Strychnine, a specific inhibitor of glycine at synaptic level, has been used with some success in mild cases. Affected individuals tolerate large doses of strychnine without side-effects, adding further support to the proposed pathogenesis.

The biochemical defect involves the glycine cleavage system, responsible for the breakdown of glycine to ammonia, carbon dioxide and formyltetrahydrofolate (Hayasaka et al 1983). In the severe neonatal form of the disease it is debatable whether or not treatment has any effect on outcome and death usually results in the early months of life.

Organic acidaemias

A number of disorders are characterized by impaired catabolism of low-molecular-weight organic acids. These conditions present with a pattern of biochemical abnormality that includes acidosis, hyperglycinaemia and hypoglycaemia. In addition to severe acidosis, clinical features include, vomiting, lethargy and convulsions, leading to apnoea and coma.

Two of the more frequent conditions showing hyperglycinaemia were lumped together as ketotic hyperglycinaemia before the enzyme defects were identified. There is often an associated hyperammonaemia. The underlying biochemical defects are now well understood:

Methylmalonic acidaemia can be subdivided into a number of different categories. This depends on whether the defect is in the methylmalonyl CoA mutase enzyme or in one of the steps in the formation of its cofactor, adenosylcobalamin. If the defect is in the early steps of cobalamin cofactor synthesis there is associated homocystinuria and megaloblastic anaemia. Responsiveness of the defect to vitamin B12 needs to be assessed as treatment is very effective in those with vitamin-responsive forms of the disease and prognosis is excellent, if the injections of vitamin B12 (1000 µg/day) are maintained. In unresponsive forms treatment relies on protein restriction. Frequent exacerbations are common during the early years of life. As with all organic acid disorders mild variants occur and presentation can be at any age.

Propionic acidaemia shares many features with methylmalonic acidaemia. Hyperammonaemia, hypoglycaemia and hyperglycinaemia are more prominent. A number of patients are neutropenic and thrombocytopenic due to a toxic bone-marrow suppression. Propionyl CoA carboxylase activity can be assayed in cultured skin fibroblasts and is deficient in affected infants. Treatment with a low-protein diet is only moderately successful. Children with organic acid defects are often very anorexic and feed poorly. A number will require gavage feeds for long periods.

There are many other organic acidaemias and their features are listed in Table 39.3.

Galactosaemia

The clinical features of 'classical' galactosaemia are due to a deficiency of the enzyme galactose-1-phosphate uridyl transferase. An identical clinical picture can be produced by a generalized deficiency of uridine diphosphate galactose-4-epimerase. (Deficiency of this enzyme in red cells only is harmless.)

Affected infants fail to thrive, vomit and develop progressive liver disease during the first weeks of life. Neurological symptoms are common and a significant number develop *E. coli* sepsis. Cataracts often appear during the first week of life but may be present at birth. Hepatomegaly is usual and renal tubular damage leads to a gross generalized amino aciduria and acidosis.

Long-term treatment with a milk-free diet quickly leads to a reversal of all the clinical signs. Intellectual outcome is usually in the borderline to mildly retarded range, even in those diagnosed and treated early. This may reflect prenatal brain damage. Ovarian failure is frequent in female patients and is thought to be due to a toxic intra-uterine effect of galactose or one of its metabolites.

Pyridoxine-dependent seizures

Pydridoxine-dependent seizures are usually present in the first 24 hours of life. Typically, they are generalized and intractable to normal anticonvulsants. Onset in utero has been reported. However, pyridoxine-dependent seizures may start some days after birth and may fluctuate in severity and/or respond temporarily to standard anticonvulsants (Bankier et al 1983). Exclusion of this diagnosis is necessary in all infants with seizures. This requires administration of 100 mg of pyridoxine by intravenous injection with careful clinical observation or EEG control. Severe drowsiness and depression may follow cessation of the convulsions in patients who truly have the condition. (See also p. 500.)

Lactic acidosis

The neonate with lactic acidosis presents a difficult set of problems. It is very hard to separate, either clinically or biochemically, those infants who have a primary metabolic disorder from those in whom the lactate accumulation is secondary to other events. The majority of cases of primary lactic acidosis remain unexplained in enzymic terms (Robinson et al 1980) and primary lactic acidosis may cause vasoconstriction, arterial thromboses or convulsions, which can lead to a secondary rise in lactate levels.

Other infants may show profound neurological abnormality with evidence of gross brain destruction with only mild degrees of systemic acidosis (Robinson & Sherwood 1984). This emphasizes the importance of measuring CSF levels in infants with possible lactic acidosis.

Some infants will improve on the low-protein, high-carbohydrate regime recommended for most acute inborn errors but others are made much worse by this therapy. This is important to remember in the blind therapy of an undiagnosed inborn error. The infants who improve may have a defect in the gluconeogenic pathway, e.g. fructose-1,6- diphosphatase deficiency. Infants with pyruvate dehydrogenase deficiency deteriorate rapidly with high-carbohydrate feeding. A partial response may also be obtained with a high-fat diet, thiamine or dichloro-acetate.

REFERENCES

Aula P, Autio S, Raivio K O et al 1979 'Salla Disease' a new lysosomal storage disorder. Archives of Neurology 36: 88–94

Bankier A, Turner M, Hopkins I J 1983 Pyridoxine dependent seizures — a wider clinical spectrum. Archives of Disease in Childhood 58: 415–418

Batshaw M L, Thomas G H, Brusilow S W 1981 New approaches to the diagnosis and treatment of inborn errors of urea synthesis. Pediatrics 68: 290–297

Batshaw M L, Msall M, Beaudet A L, Trojak J 1986 Risk of serious illness in heterozygotes for ornithine transcarbamylase deficiency. Journal of Pediatrics 108: 236–241

Brown G K, Hunt S M, Scholem R et al 1982 β-hydroxy isobutyryl coenzyme deacylase deficiency: a defect in valine metabolism associated with physical malformations. Pediatrics 70: 532–538

Brusilow S W 1984 Arginine, an indispensible amino acid for patients with inborn errors of urea synthesis. Journal of Clinical Investigation 74: 2144–2148

Danks D M 1974 Management of newborn babies in whom serious metabolic illness is anticipated. Archives of Disease in Childhood 49: 576–578

Engel A G, Rebouche C J 1984 Carnitine metabolism and inborn errors. Journal of Inherited Metabolic Disease 7 (supp 1): 38–43

Gillan J E, Lowden J A, Gaskin K, Cutz E 1984 Congenital ascites as a presenting sign of lysosomal storage disease. Journal of Pediatrics 104: 225–231

Goodman S I, Frerman F E 1984 Glutaric acidaemia type II (multiple acyl-CoA dehydrogenation deficiency). Journal of Inherited Metabolic Disease 7 (supp 1): 33–37

Hakami N, Neiman P E, Canellos G P, Lazerson J 1971 Neonatal megaloblastic anemia due to inherited transcobalamin II deficiency in two siblings. New England Journal of Medicine 285: 1163–1170

Hayasaka K, Tada K, Kikuchi G, Winter S, Nyhan W L 1983 Nonketotic hyperglycinemia: two patients with primary defects of P-protein and T-protein, respectively, in the glycine cleavage system. Pediatric Research 17: 967–969

Heara G S, Wolf B, Jefferson L G et al 1986 Neonatal screening for biotinidase deficiency: results of a 1-year pilot study. Journal of Pediatrics 108: 40–46

Kelley R I 1983 Review: the cerebro–hepato–renal syndrome of Zellweger, morphologic and metabolic aspects. American Journal of Medical Genetics 16: 503–517

Kelts D G, Ney D, Bay C, Saudubray J-M, Nyhan W 1985 Studies on requirements for aminoacids in infants with disorders of amino acid metabolism. I. Effect of alanine. Pediatric Research 19: 86–91

Kvittingen E A, Guldal G, Borsting S, Skalpe I O, Stokke O, Jellum E 1986 N-Acetylaspartic aciduria in a child with a progressive cerebral atrophy. Clinica Chimica Acta 158: 217–227

Lenke R R, Levy H L 1980 Maternal phenylketonuria and hyperphenylalaninemia: an international survey of the outcome of untreated and treated pregnancies. New England Journal of Medicine 303(21): 1202–1208

Lowden J A, O'Brien J S 1979 Sialidosis: a review of human neuraminidase deficiency. American Journal of Human Genetics 31: 1–18

Perry T L 1981 Autopsy investigation of disorders of amino acid metabolism. In: Barson A J (ed) Laboratory investigation of fetal disease. John Wright, Bristol, pp 429–451

Robinson B H, Sherwood W G 1984 Lactic acidaemia. Journal of Inherited Metabolic Disease 7 (suppl 1): 69–73

Robinson B H, Taylor J, Sherwood W G 1980 The genetic heterogeneity of lactic acidosis: occurrence of recognizable inborn errors of metabolism in a pediatric population with lactic acidosis. Pediatric Research 14: 956–962

Rowe P C, Newman S L, Brusilow S W 1986 Natural history of symptomatic partial ornithine transcarbamylase deficiency. New England Journal of Medicine 314: 541–547

Schutgens R B H, Heymans H S A, Wanders R J A, Bosch H V D, Tager J M 1986 Peroxisomal disorders: a newly recognised group of genetic diseases. European Journal of Pediatrics 144: 430–440

Stanbury J B, Wyngaarden J B, Frederickson D S, Goldstein J L, Brown M S 1983 The metabolic basis of inherited disease, 5th edn. McGraw-Hill, New York

Stevenson R E, Lubinsky M, Taylor H A, Wenger D A, Schroer R J, Olmstead P M 1983 Sialic acid storage disease with sialuria: clinical and biochemical features in the severe infantile type. Pediatrics 72: 441–449

Wilcken B, Hammond J W, Howard N, Bohane T, Hocart C, Halpern B 1981 Hawkinsinuria: a dominantly inherited defect of tyrosine metabolism with severe effects in infancy. New England Journal of Medicine 305: 865–869

Zinn A B, Kerr D S, Hoppel C L 1986 Fumarase deficiency: a new cause of mitochondrial encephalomyopathy. New England Journal of Medicine 315(8): 469–475

40. Degenerative disorders of the infant central nervous system

Dr S. H. Green

There are hundreds of different degenerative diseases affecting the central nervous system (CNS) (Stanbury et al 1983, McKusick 1983), however only a limited number of these are likely to present in early infancy.

The diseases described in this chapter are those where the main presenting features are likely to come well within the first year of life (Adams & Lyons 1982, Brett 1983). These conditions are listed in Table 40.1. The amino acidurias and organic acidurias have already been discussed in Chapter 39.

It is always difficult to date the onset of degenerative disease but those diseases where the presentation is essentially in the second or third year of life where there may have been some early symptoms towards the end of the first year are excluded.

The problem confronting the paediatrician when faced with an infant with an acute or subacute neurological presentation is to 'think' that it might be a neurometabolic disease. The acute presentation, possibly triggered by an infection, may be mistaken for a viral or toxic encephalopathy, especially if partial or temporary recovery takes place e.g. Leigh's encephalopathy. A history of intermittent episodes of coma, ataxia or seizures may be a clue to this condition or an organic acidaemia.

SYMPTOMS

The normal clues to the history of degenerative disease include a period of normality followed by slowing down of progress, plateauing and the regression of skills, and these may be very difficult to detect in early life. Firstly the degeneration may start before there is any certainty about a period of normality; secondly there may be confusion about the early history, especially if this is compounded by perinatal problems; and thirdly mental degeneration, a feature of some of the grey matter degenerations, may not be so obvious in the first year of life, except to an astute observer. Occasionally degeneration may be noted after immunization and wrongly attributed to it.

Visual deficit may not be obvious for quite a few months in the absence of abnormal eye movements. Deafness likewise may not be diagnosed until later in the first year. The pace of development is such that it may mask the degenerative process for a while.

Sometimes a particular pattern gives a clue, e.g. the presence of squint, head retraction and swallowing problems — Gaucher's disease. In other cases a known associated finding, e.g. herniae in the mucopolysaccharidoses, may suggest the diagnosis presymptomatically.

Broadly speaking the amino acid disorders and organic acid disorders present acutely, often in the newborn period. The lysosomal storage diseases tend to manifest themselves a little later with subacute or chronic symptoms but there is an overlap. The recently described peroxisomal disorders (Moser & Goldfischer 1985) may present in the newborn period with symptoms, e.g. hypotonia, which are not all rapidly progressive and previously might have been misdiagnosed as non-neurometabolic stationary encephalopathies.

A history therefore of slow development without specific signs, intermittent episodes of hypotonia, coma and ataxia, failure to achieve expected milestones, unexplained visual problems, co-ordination difficulties, and seizures should alert one to the possibility of a neurometabolic disease in infancy.

There are some major clinical features which of themselves should alert one to the possibility of degenerative CNS disease in the absence of any other obvious cause and these are shown in Table 40.2. Acute (intermittent) coma, collapse, hypotonia, and respiratory problems are much more likely to be due to organic acidurias, amino acidurias or urea cycle disorders than lysosomal disorders.

EXAMINATION AND INVESTIGATION

A full general, neurological and developmental examination is necessary. Individual features do not necessarily give an answer (at an early stage they may be non-specific, at a later stage they may be too diffuse) but a constellation may

Table 40.1 Degenerative disorders of the CNS with onset in the first few months of life

Disorder	Symptoms	Biochemical defect	Enzyme assay	Prenatal diagnosis
Sphingolipidoses				
GM1 generalized gangliosidosis (pseudo-Hurler)	Hypotonia, poor sucking, developmental delay, hepatosplenomegaly, coarse features, CRS	↓ β-Galactosidase	Leucocytes, fibroblasts	Cultured amniotic fluid cells
GM2 gangliosidosis Tay–Sach's disease	Irritability, hypotonia, hyperacusis, regression, CRS, seizures, blindness, spasticity	↓ Hexosaminidase A	Leucocytes, fibroblasts	Cultured amniotic fluid cells
Sandoff's disease	As Tay–Sach's	↓ Hexosaminidase A and B	Leucocytes, fibroblasts	Cultured amniotic fluid cells
Niemann–Pick	Hypotonia, developmental delay, FTT, squint, CRS, hepatomegaly	↓ Sphingomyelinase	Leucocytes, fibroblasts	Cultured amniotic fluid cells
Gaucher's disease type II	Developmental delay and regression, squint, neck retraction, swallowing difficulties, splenomegaly, CRS	↓ Glucocerebrosidase	Leucocytes, fibroblasts	Cultured amniotic fluid cells
Farber's disease	Developmental regression, puffy hands and feet, generalized arthropathy, subcutaneous nodules	↓ Acid ceramidase	Leucocytes, fibroblasts	Cultured amniotic fluid cells
Leukodystrophies				
Metachromatic leukodystrophy	Progressive retardation, spasticity or hypotonia	↓ Arylsulphatase A	Leucocytes, fibroblasts	Cultured amniotic fluid cells
Krabbe's leukodystrophy	Irritability, stiffness, opisthotonus, regression ± seizures, later hypotonia	↓ Galactocerebrosidase	Leucocytes, fibroblasts	Cultured amniotic fluid cells
Pelizaeus–Merzbacher disease (Type I)	X-linked, nystagmus, hypotonia, titubation, ataxia of upper limbs, developmental delay	Unknown	–	None (fetal sexing)
Seitelberger variety (Type II)	More severe and presents in neonatal period	Unknown	–	None (fetal sexing)
Multiple sulphatase deficiency (mucosulphatidosis)	Developmental delay, spasticity with depressed reflexes ± seizures, coarse features, hepatomegaly	↓ Arylsulphatase A, B and C	Leucocytes, fibroblasts	Cultured amniotic fluid cells
Mucopolysaccharidoses				
MPS I (Hurler's disease)	Developmental delay, herniae, corneal clouding	↓ α-Iduronidase, ↑ urinary dermatan and heparan sulphate	Fibroblasts, leucocytes	Glycosaminoglycans in amniotic fluid, cultured amniotic fluid cells
Glycoproteinoses				
Mucolipidosis II (I cell disease)	Coarse features, cloudy cornea, gingival hyperplasia, restricted joint movements	↑ Plasma iduronidase, ↑ plasma glucuronidase, ↑ plasma galactosidase,	Plasma, fibroblasts	Cultured amniotic fluid cells
α-Mannosidosis	As Mucopolysaccharidoses	↓ α-Mannosidase	Leucocytes, fibroblasts	Cultured amniotic fluid cells
α-Fucosidosis	Coarse features, developmental delay, spasticity	↓ α-Fucosidase	Leucocytes, fibroblasts	Cultured amniotic fluid cells
Sialidosis (mucolipidosis I)	Coarse features, CRS, hepatosplenomegaly, developmental delay	Abnormal oligosaccharides, ↓ α-neuraminidase	Fibroblasts (increased fibroblast sialic acid levels)	Cultured amniotic fluid cells
Sialic acid storage disease	Slowly progressive, developmental delay	↑ Sialic acid in blood and urine	–	–
Purine and pyramide metabolic defects				
Lesch–Nyhan disease	X-linked, developmental delay, hypotonia, athetosis	↓ Hypoxanthine guanine phosphoribosyl transferase, ↑ uric acid in blood	Fibroblasts	Cultured amniotic fluid cells
Menkes' disease	X-linked, hypotonia, myoclonic seizures, kinky hair (later),	↓ Serum copper and caeruloplasmin levels	Fibroblasts (copper uptake studies)	Cultured amniotic fluid cells

Table 40.1 Continued

Disorder	Symptoms	Biochemical defect	Enzyme assay	Prenatal diagnosis
Sulphite oxidase deficiency	FTT, hypothermia Seizures, muscular spasms, opisthotonus	↑ Sulphite and thiosulphate in urine	Fibroblasts	Cultured amniotic fluid cells
Peroxisomal disorders	Facial features, hypotonia, seizures, FTT, hepatomegaly	↑ Urinary pipecolic acid, ↓ dihydroxyacetone phosphate acyltransferase, ↓ plasmalogens in erythrocytes, ↑ plasma very long-chain fatty acids, absent peroxisomes	Leucocytes, platelets, fibroblasts, red cells	Cultured amniotic fluid cells
Zellweger's disease	As above	As above	Leucocytes, fibroblasts	Cultured amniotic fluid cells
Infantile Refsum's disease	As above	As above	Leucocytes, fibroblasts	Cultured amniotic fluid cells
Neonatal adrenoleukodystrophy	As above	As above	Leucocytes, fibroblasts	Cultured amniotic fluid cells
Hyperpipecolic acidaemia	See Zellweger's disease	Very high pipecolic acid in urine	Leucocytes, fibroblasts	Cultured amniotic fluid cells
Others				
Leigh's encephalopathy	Variable, hypotonia, abnormal movements, sighing, irregular respirations, dysphagia, FTT, cranial nerve palsies, abnormal ocular movements	Defects in pyruvate metabolism in some infants, ↑ lactate and pyruvate in blood and CSF	–	–
Alper's disease	Seizures, developmental delay or regression, epilepsia partialis continuans, liver failure	–	–	–
Infantile neuraxonal dystrophy	Developmental delay or regression, hypotonia, muscle wasting, cranial nerve palsies	Diagnosed by conjunctival biopsy	–	–
Batten's disease (Early infantile form, Hagberg–Santavuori form)	Developmental regression, blindness ± myoclonic jerks	Diagnosed on rectal biopsy or skin biopsy	–	–
Spongy degeneration Canavan's disease	Developmental delay, hypotonia, optic atrophy, seizures, macrocephaly, excessive crying	Diagnosed by brain biopsy	–	–
Alexander's disease	Developmental delay, macrocephaly, seizures	Diagnosed by brain biopsy	–	–

CRS = cherry-red spot; FTT = failure to thrive.

(vide supra) do so. Particular attention should be paid to the following possible clinical features:

The acuteness of the condition
Extra CNS signs, e.g. herniae, dermatological lesions,
Hepatosplenomegaly
General developmental level
Head size
Visual attention, oculomotor function, ophthalmoscopy
Hair abnormalities
Hypotonia, spasticity, dystonia
Auditory responses, especially to startle
Myoclonus
Abnormal movements, tremor, ataxia, choreoathetosis
Deep tendon reflexes

The following range of tests may be useful and will be referred to in more detail:

Biochemical — acid–base, lactate, pyruvate, urate, oxalate, reducing substances, ammonia, oligosaccharides, glyco-saminoglycans, white cell enzymes, sulphite in urine for sulphite oxidase deficiency.
Biopsies — skin and rectal (for Batten's), skin and muscle for mitochondrial cytopathy, conjunctival biopsy for neuraxonal dystrophy, liver (peroxisomopathy).
Radiology — Skull X-ray, skeletal survey, CAT scan (a

Table 40.2 Guidelines for the identification of CNS degenerative disorders presenting in the first 6 months of life (excluding amino acidurias and organic acidurias). Some features, e.g mental retardation, hypotonia, spasticity and seizures, are not very specific and must be considered with other features. For diagnostic tests see text.

Specific symptoms/signs	Diseases
Acousticomotor response (exaggerated startle)	Tay–Sachs' Sandhoff's Niemann–Pick
Swallowing problems	Gaucher's Multiple sulphatase deficiency Leigh's
Respiratory irregularities	Multiple sulphatase deficiency Leigh's
Oculomotor problems	Leigh's Niemann–Pick Gaucher's Pelizaeus–Merzbacher
Cherry-red spot	Tay–Sachs'

few metabolic diseases may have specific findings e.g. Leigh's, Adrenoleukodystrophy).
Electrophysiological — electro-encephalogram (EEG), electromyogram (EMG), nerve conduction velocity (NCV), electroretinogram (ERG), visual evoked response (VER).

There is no perfectly satisfactory classification for the neurometabolic diseases. As far as possible it is best to classify according to biochemical grouping but some diseases are still poorly understood biochemically and there is not always a 1:1 correspondence between a particular biochemical defect and a symptom complex.

The classification proposed is shown in Table 40.1. No absolutely agreed classification is possible at this stage because the origin of a number of diseases is uncertain: some presenting similarly may have different enzyme defects, and some with apparently identical enzyme defects may have different manifestations.

There are a number of diseases which may have their onset in the later part of the first year with mild signs of development retardation but do not show any characteristic features until the second year of life or later (e.g. late infantile Batten's disease); these diseases are not discussed in any detail.

It is always possible to make a clinical diagnosis very much earlier than usual if the disease is suspected from a family history. In these diseases it is often the mother who makes this observation.

The classical distinction clinically between grey matter diseases presenting with mental degeneration and seizures and white matter disease presenting with spasticity, ataxia and optic atrophy is not easily made in early infancy.

LYSOSOMAL DISEASES

Lysosomes (Stanbury et al 1983, Watts & Gibbs 1986) are one of a number of subcellular organelles (others

are mitochondria and peroxisomes). They degrade certain endogenous and exogenous products of cellular metabolism mainly by hydrolysis of certain carbohydrates, lipids, proteins and lipoproteins. If an enzyme is defective in function the cell becomes stuffed with the substrate of action of the enzyme. This substance accumulates and enlarges, damaging and destroying the cell. In the group of disorders under discussion the central nervous system is involved either on its own or with other organ systems, depending on the distribution in the body of the non-degradable substrate.

Gangliosidoses

The gangliosidoses are a group of neurodegenerative disorders of grey matter in which gangliosides accumulate. These substances consist of sphingosine, hexose, hexosamine and neuraminic acid.

GM2 gangliosidosis, Tay–Sachs' disease

Deficiency of hexosaminidase allows an excess accumulation of ganglioside to be stored in the CNS and elsewhere. A number of diseases are described in which subunits of hexosaminidase activity are deficient (A or B) (Johnson 1983).

Hexosaminidase A deficiency results in classical Tay–Sachs' disease and hexosaminidase A and B deficiency results in Sandhoff disease; both may present early in infancy with a similar clinical picture.

Tay–Sachs' disease occurs relatively more frequently in Ashkenazi Jews but overall in the UK any infant with the disorder is much more likely to be non-Jewish because of the relatively small percentage (1%) of Ashkenazi Jews in the UK.

Presentation often occurs before 6 months but not usually in the immediate neonatal period. Irritability, hyperacusis, a slowing down of acquired skills and hypotonia are the early signs. A cherry-red spot in the fundus is to be expected but is not pathognomonic as it occurs in other conditions. There is no visceromegaly. Further deterioration is accompanied by frequent seizures and spasticity. Blindness supervenes (the ERG is retained and the VER becomes abnormal). The head becomes large and death usually occurs before the age of 3 years. Confirmation of the diagnosis is by demonstrating the absence of hexosaminidase A activity in the leukocytes or fibroblasts. There is no specific therapy.

Sandhoff disease, which is due to a deficiency in hexosaminidase A and B subunit activity, has a similar clinical picture but may have a slight visceromegaly. Many late-onset variants occur (Adams & Green 1986).

Generalized gangliosidosis (GM1)

This disease is due to beta-galactosidase defiency (O'Brien et al 1965) and occurs in three forms, only one of which is likely to be present in the first 6 months of life. In GM1 type 1 (pseudo-Hurler) there may be hypotonia and poor sucking early in infancy. Development is slow with the appearance of hepatosplenomegaly. Coarsening of facial features resembles that in Hurler's disease (hence the name). There is skeletal dysplasia and occasionally a cherry-red spot. Other variants occasionally occur, e.g. with dystonia, but these do not usually present so early. Urinary oligosaccharide thin-layer chromatography is often useful in detecting this disorder. Diagnosis is confirmed by demonstrating the absence of beta-galactosidase activity in leukocytes. As with Tay–Sachs' disease, prenatal diagnosis is possible by analysis of cultured cells from amniotic fluid (Lowden et al 1973).

Niemann–Pick disease

In this condition there is deficiency of sphingomyelinase with accumulation of sphingomyelin in the CNS and elsewhere. There are a number of subtypes with varying clinical pictures, some non-neurological, occurring at different ages (Crocker & Farber 1958). The infantile type is one of the most commonly encountered forms. There may be very slow development from birth with hepatomegaly and failure to thrive. Occasionally there is jaundice (rare in other diseases in this group). Squints are common and the retinae may show a cherry-red spot in 25% of cases. Corneal and lens opacities occur. Hypotonia becomes apparent, progressing to spasticity and accompanied by myoclonic seizures. Death may occur within the first year. On average these children survive until about 2 years of age.

There is a generalized distribution of lipid-laden foam cells throughout the CNS and reticulo–endothelial system. Bone-marrow aspirate may show such lipid-laden cells which stain specifically and may help to confirm the diagnosis (Adams & Lyon 1982) but a normal aspirate does not exclude the diagnosis. Final confirmation in subtypes A and B is by enzyme assay in leukocytes or fibroblasts (Beaudet & Manschrek 1982) showing a sphingomyelinase deficiency. Prenatal diagnosis is possible as with the gangliosidoses.

Gaucher's disease

There are several forms presenting at different ages. They all have a defect in glucocerebrosidase. The so-called Type II is the one which may occur in infancy (Verity & Montasir 1977). Delayed development from the start or psychomotor retardation after a few months may be apparent. The spleen is more enlarged than the liver. Squints, swallowing problems and head retraction occur (Fig. 40.1). Fits occur but not as a major feature. Again, as with Niemann–Pick disease, a cherry-red spot may be seen. Anaemia and thrombocytopenia occur. Gaucher cells may be found in the bone-marrow and can be easily distinguished from Niemann–Pick cells. There is a strongly positive acid phosphatase reaction within the cells and acid phosphatase is elevated in blood. The definitive diagnosis is by demonstrating gluococerebrosidase deficiency in leukocytes

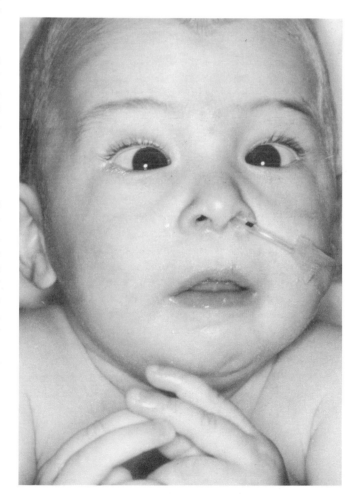

Fig. 40.1 Gaucher's disease.

or fibroblasts. Prenatal diagnosis is possible (Schneider et al 1972). Apart from correcting anaemia and control of fits there is no specific treatment and death occurs early. Splenectomy is not of any proven value.

Farber's disease

This rare metabolic disease is an inborn error of ceramide metabolism (Pavone et al 1980). Onset is in the first few weeks of life. There is swelling of the hands and feet, a hoarse cry, a generalized arthropathy and subcutaneous nodules over bony parts. Mental and motor deterioration occur. Pyramidal signs may come later. Diagnosis is suggested by the clinical picture and confirmed biopsy of the nodules which show granulomas with PAS-positive material. A deficiency of acid ceramidase has been found and prenatal diagnosis is available (Stanbury et al 1983). Death occurs in early infancy.

LEUKODYSTROPHIES

Metachromatic leukodystrophy

Although in some ways the archetypal leukodystrophy, and one of the most common of the lysosomal disorders, metachromatic leukodystrophy (MLD) presents very rarely in early infancy (McFaul et al 1982). It is mentioned because it is one of the common disorders in this group. The disease is well known to be due to a deficiency of arylsulphatase A which allows the accumulation of sulphatide. The pathological picture is one of diffuse demyelination with metachromatic staining. The classical presentation with hypertonia progressing to hypotonia with depressed reflexes is not usually seen in infancy. However, it is worth considering the diagnosis in any infant with progressive retardation, and spasticity or hypotonia, without any other explanation.

Prenatal diagnosis is available for this condition. Recently some success has been reported with marrow transplantation as a therapeutic measure but the results are too early to assess definitely (Bayever et al 1985).

All cases in which MLD is suspected at an early age should have urinary glycosaminoglycans measured because of the possibility of multiple sulphatase deficiency.

Krabbe's disease

The leukodystrophies classically present with more long tract involvement and less in the way of psychomotor retardation than does the grey matter degeneration. In the first year of life this distinction is not so clear cut. Nevertheless the presentation of Krabbe's is different from that of the other neurovisceral storage diseases. The enzyme deficiency is known to be in galactocerebrosidase.

The most typical picture in infancy is of an irritable child who cries excessively. The child is stiff and this progresses to episodes of opisthotonos. Regression becomes more obvious towards 6 months with head retraction, stiffness and occasionally exaggerated startle to noise. Later in the first year hypotonia with depressed reflexes may supervene and be associated with a gross demyelinating peripheral neuropathy. Seizures are not common.

Pathologically there is widespread demyelination of the CNS and peripheral nerve system with globoid cells occurring in pericapillary areas.

Diagnostic suspicion is raised in an infant with progressive CNS degeneration, depressed reflexes and slow nerve conductions and a raised CSF protein. The definitive test is demonstration of lack of galactocerebrosidase in fibroblasts or leukocytes (Martin et al 1981). Death occurs in the infantile type. Prenatal diagnosis is available.

Pelizaeus–Merzbacher

This is a leukodystrophy where the underlying enzymatic defect is unknown. The clinical picture of the classical Type I is essentially of a male infant (the disease is considered to be X-linked recessive) who presents in infancy with abnormally jerky eye movements. Horizontal nystagmus and tracking difficulties are seen (and should be distinguished from the wandering eye movements of the blind and the more bizzare movements of Leigh's encephalopathy). These are accompanied or followed by hypotonia, titubation and ataxic movements of the arms. Sitting may be delayed or never achieved. Degeneration is slow and although visual failure, spasticity and mental deterioration occur these are not usually noted in infancy. Children may survive with this condition for many years and progressive degeneration is slow.

There exists a more severe variety (Type II Seitelberger) (Ulrich & Herschkowitz 1977) where presentation is in the neonatal period. Nystagmus, gross involuntary movement and spasticity of the lower limbs are the main features. There is little developmental progress. This type may be X-linked recessive. Sporadic transitional types may occur.

Pathologically there is atrophy of the cerebellum and cortex with accumulation of sudanophilic lipid. CT scanning may help by confirming atrophy but the diagnosis is essentially clinical after the exclusion of other known diseases. There is no diagnostic test and therefore no prenatal test as yet available.

Multiple sulphatase deficiency (mucosulphatidosis)

This condition can be regarded as a variant of metachromatic leukodystrophy in which more than one specific sulphatase is deficient. This gives rise to an accumulation of sulphatide, acid mucopolysaccharides and cholesterol sulphate in the brain, liver and kidney. The presenting features occur much earlier than in MLD and have clinical features more akin to the mucopolysaccharidoses.

The condition is rare, development may be normal for the first year or may be very slow from the start. A neonatal case has been described (Vamos et al 1981). As in other leukodystrophies there may be a combination of spasticity with depressed reflexes (and slowed nerve conduction). Seizures are not a particular feature. Early coarsening of the facial features may be noted, hands may be stubby with short fingers, and there is hepatomegaly. X-ray of the thoraco–lumbar spine shows mild changes of dyostosis. There is from early on a fine icthyosis.

There is slow progression with bulbar paresis, spasticity, deafness and optic atrophy. The patient may survive in this state for a number of years.

Diagnostic tests include elevated CSF protein, increased levels of mucopolysaccharides (heparan and dermatan sulphate) in urine, and metachromatic staining in nerve biopsy of Schwann cells. Confirmation is by demonstrating deficiency of arylsulphatases A, B and C. As with known enzyme deficiencies which are autosomal recessive, prenatal diagnosis is available in specialized centres.

OTHER STORAGE DISEASES

The mucopolysaccharidoses, the glycoproteinoses and the sialic acid storage diseases show some features in common.

These are all storage diseases, mostly autosomal recessive with a relatively slow evolution of psychomotor retardation, coarsening of the features and hepatomegaly. Seizures are not a major feature of the majority although there are exceptions. The early signs are often more subtle than some of the diseases so far discussed and often the time of onset is only realized to be relatively early in infancy retrospectively.

MUCOPOLYSACCHARIDOSES

There are seven different subtypes within this well-known clinical group according to McKusick's classification (McKusick 1983). Few of these are recognized in early infancy but the following may present as early as 6 months.

Hurler's disease (MPS I)

This autosomal recessive condition is due to a deficiency of alpha-iduronidase (Bach et al 1972) and has been estimated to have an incidence of 1 in 100 000 (Lowry & Renwick 1971). Dermatan and heparan sulphate accumulate in the CNS and elsewhere and gangliosides accumulate in neurones. The early signs may be snorting breathing, snoring,

inguinal and umbilical herniae, a barrel-shaped chest and psychomotor slowing. The classical gargoyle like features are not usually present before one year of age. Hepatomegaly may or may not be present early. Clouding of the corneas may be apparent on slit lamp examination.

There may be early radiological changes, a J-shaped sella, rounded dorso–lumbar vertebral bodies, broad ribs and wide shafts of long bones but these signs may be subtle in infancy.

Confirmation of the diagnosis is by determining the pattern of urinary excretion of mucopolysaccharides (dermatan and heparan sulphate in Hurler's disease) or by the demonstration of the absence of alpha-iduronidase in fibroblasts or leucocytes. It is in this group of diseases that enzyme replacement therapy has been tried (marrow transplant) with, it is claimed, limited success (Lancet 1986).

The other mucopolysaccharides II–VII very rarely present in early infancy with neurological signs (although occasionally Sly's Type II disease may present in early infancy with severe retardation and hydrops fetalis, Beaudet et al 1975).

Identification of glycosaminoglycans in amniotic fluid can be as accurate as specific enzyme analysis for prenatal diagnosis (Mossman & Patrick 1982).

GLYCOPROTEINOSES

These disorders combine certain features of the gangliosidoses and the mucopolysaccharidoses and resemble clinically the latter. They are inherited as autosomal recessive but the main one that merits consideration in infancy is mucolipidosis Type II or I Cell Disease (Milla 1978).

Mucolipidosis II

This condition is clinically similar to Hurler's disease but often evident from birth. The coarse features are evident early in life with gingival hyperplasia, congenital dislocation of the hips, restricted joint movements and thickened skin. Nasal discharge is common, corneas are cloudy, kyphosis and hepatomegaly may appear later. Retardation is less easy to detect in the first year of life although this becomes evident later on.

A number of different lysosomal hydrolases are deficient in fibroblasts, whilst these enzymes are grossly elevated in plasma (alpha-iduronidase, beta-glucuronidase, beta-galactosidase; Leroy et al 1972). There is slow progression of the disease with death in early childhood. As with other diseases in this group, prenatal dignosis is available.

Alpha-mannosidosis

This is another disorder of glycoprotein degradation due to the absence of alpha-mannosidase. The clinical picture is very like that of the mucopolysaccharidoses with coarse features, deafness, hepatomegaly and skeletal dysplasia. It should be considered in the differential diagnosis of Hurler-like conditions in the first 6 months of life. It is a rare condition. Vacuolated lymphocytes may be seen; urinary oligosaccharide thin-layer chromatography is often useful in detecting this disease but the definitive diagnosis is by assay of mannosidase in cultured leukocytes or fibroblasts (Taylor et al 1975).

Alpha-fucosidosis

This disease due to the absence of alpha-fucosidase may present in the first year of life with retardation, coarse features and spasticity. As with cystic fibrosis there is a marked increase in the chloride of the sweat and the child may 'taste' salty. There is rapid progression to death over the next few years. Urinary oligosaccharide thin-layer chromatography may be useful in detecting this disorder and the enzyme deficiency may be detected in cultured fibroblasts or leukocytes. Again this is a rare condition.

Sialidosis (Mucolipidosis I)

Another disorder of glycoprotein degradation is sialidosis. This disease, relatively recently delineated (Lowden & O'Brien 1979), exists in two forms Type II (mucolipidosis Type I) being an infantile form. The basic deficiency is of the enzyme alpha-neuraminidase.

Clinical presentation may be at birth with visceromegaly and coarse features, or rarely in the first year of life, with mental retardation, myoclonus, ataxia, a cherry-red spot and dyostosis multiplex. The features of neuraminidase deficiency are variable and a number of different symptoms have been described. Urinary oligosaccharide thin-layer chromatography is often useful in detecting this disease. In some patients there is a co-existing deficiency of galactosidase (which may present like GM1) or N-acetylgalactosamine-6-sulphatase, and in the latter case the children present with a Morquio-like condition (Glossl et al 1984).

SIALIC ACID STORAGE DISEASE

This is an unusual type of disease in that it may only be slowly progressive. Sialic acid is excreted in the urine and is found to be elevated in the blood and fibroblasts. No specific enzyme deficiency has been identified. In one variety (Salla disease) (Aula et al 1979), more common in Finland, the features are coarse facies, developmental delay, ataxia and spasticity. The exact classification of this group remains in doubt.

DISORDERS OF PURINE AND PYRIMIDINE METABOLISM

Lesch–Nyhan syndrome

This well-known disorder of purine metabolism is due to deficiency of hypoxanthine–guanine phosphoribosyl-transferase (HGPRT), leading to hyperuricaemia (Lesch & Nyhan 1964). A number of genetic varieties are now known (Wilson et al 1983). It is an X-linked recessive condition and the classical feature in the older child is that of self-destructive biting. However, the condition may present early with signs that are more subtle. Motor and mental retardation, hypotonia and athetosis may manifest as early as 6–9 months. It is the presence of early athetosis of unexplained origin that should be the clue to investigation. Orange-stained nappies due to the crystals of urate formation should also arouse suspicion.

Uric acid screening should be routine for all males with developmental delay, especially with abnormal movement. Confirmation of the diagnosis is by finding hyperuricaemia and the specific deficiency HGPRT in fibroblasts. The mechanism whereby the condition causes symptoms is unknown. Allopurinol does not affect the neurological progress but may relieve hyperuricaemia. The disease slowly progresses with severe athetosis and self-destructive behaviour which causes great problems in management later on. Death usually occurs towards the end of the first or the beginning of the second decade. Prenatal diagnosis has been available for some time.

MENKES' DISEASE

This is a degenerative disease of grey matter due to a defect in copper metabolism (Danks et al 1972). Copper levels are low in the liver and brain but raised in other tissues. The exact defect is unknown but copper becomes unavailable for the synthesis of caeruloplasmin and other enzymes. This sex-linked condition has an incidence of between 1 in 50 000 and 1 in 100 000 and may present very early in infancy. Hypotonia in the newborn period followed soon by refractory myoclonic like seizures should arouse suspicion. These children feed poorly and hypothermia may be a problem, so they fail to thrive. The typical facial appearance is not always obvious for a few months, and the steely or kinky hair is not usually noted to be abnormal for a few weeks (Fig. 40.2). It is the stubbliness and roughness of the hair which should arouse suspicion. The abnormalities monilethrix, pili torti and trichorrhexis nodosa are very characteristic, although not specifically pathognomonic. They are best demonstrated by scanning electron microscopy (Taylor & Green 1981). Radiographs show metaphyseal spurring of the long bones.

The evolution of the condition is that of profound retardation of development, hypotonia, further refractory

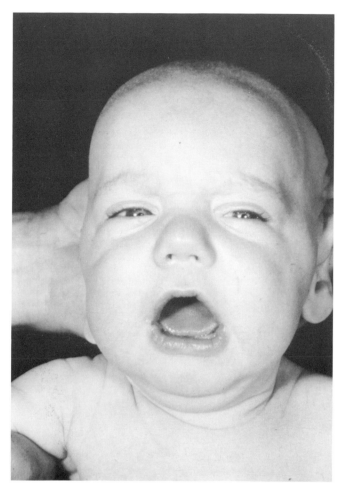

Fig. 40.2 Menkes' disease

seizures. These children may fail to thrive and often succumb in the first year of life, although some survive longer. Diagnosis is by the clinical history, confirmation of low copper and caeroloplasmin levels, and the typical scanning EM of hair.

No specific enzyme defect is known but copper uptake studies may be useful in prenatal diagnosis and carrier-state detection (Horn et al 1978). It may also be possible to detect carriers by examining the hair of the affected child's mother by electron microscopy (Collie et al 1978, Taylor & Green 1981).

Therapy of the condition by copper infusion has been tried without clinical success (Grover & Scrutton 1975, Garnica 1984). Death usually occurs in late infancy but occasionally cases have been reported with relatively prolonged survival.

SULPHITE OXIDASE DEFICIENCY

This is a very rare metabolic disease. Only a few cases have been reported but the condition may present in the neonatal period with seizures, muscular spasms and opisthotonos.

Sulphite and thiosulphate are markedly increased in the urine. Amino acid screening shows *S*-sulphocystine in the urine but this is not primarily an amino acid disorder. Sulphite oxidase is dependent on molybdenum as a cofactor and this could be a theoretical approach to treatment (Shih et al 1977).

This disease should be considered in the early onset of seizures with reduced responses where other routine screening is negative.

PEROXISOMAL DISORDERS

Although not all truly degenerative, these disorders give rise to a group of symptoms very similar to those discussed above. They are a group of conditions that have been described relatively recently (Moser & Goldfischer 1985) in which there is a defect in the functioning of the subcellular organelles — peroxisomes (Schutgens et al 1986). These structures were first reported in 1969 (DeDuve 1969) and their relationship to a variety of human diseases is at the moment of writing being unfolded. Some of these diseases give rise to progressive CNS degeneration in infancy, hence it is important to recognize the symptom complexes that may lead to their diagnosis.

Although the purpose of this chapter is not basically biochemical, as peroxisomal disorders are so new their functions will be briefly listed. They include:

Breakdown of very long-chain fatty acids
Biosynthesis of ether phospholipids important for plasmalogen function
Biosynthesis of bile acids
Catabolism of pipecolic acid
Catabolism of dicarboxylic acids
Catabolism of phytanic acid
Oxidation of polyamines
Breakdown of long/medium-chain fatty acids
Hydrogen peroxide degradation

A number of different disorders affecting the central nervous system, not previously thought to be connected, have been shown to be due to peroxisomal disorders. Some of these are due to impairment of a single peroxisomal function and others are due to multiple defects. Those due to a single impairment include X-linked adrenoleukodystrophy, adult Refsum's disease, acatalasaemia and chondrodysplasia punctata (Rhizomelic form). Only the last of these presents in infancy.

Those peroxisomal disorders which have multiple defects include Zellweger's syndrome, pseudo-Zellweger's syndrome, infantile Refsum's disease, neonatal adrenoleukodystrophy and hyperpipecolic acidaemia. At present it is not exactly clear whether the last three are absolutely distinct genetic entities.

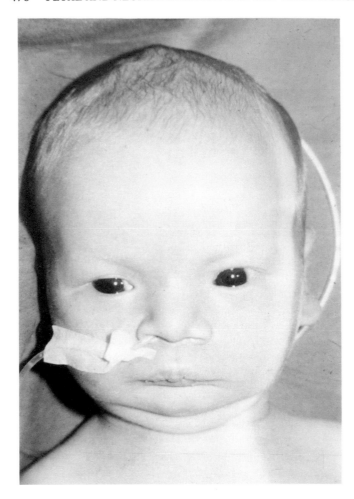
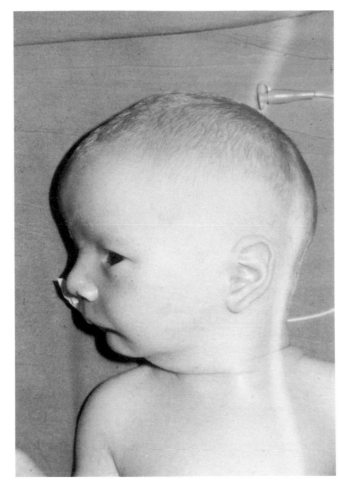

Fig. 40.3 Zellweger's syndrome

For the clinician the main features which should draw the attention to this group of conditions are:

Neonatal hypotonia
Seizures
Psychomotor retardation
Dysmorphic features
Hepatic enlargement
Failure to thrive
Retinal dysfunction — suspected because of blindness

Zellweger's syndrome

Zellweger's syndrome is the archetype of this group of disorders and was known for some considerable time before it was realized that it was a peroxisomal disorder (Bowen et al 1964).

The main features are hypotonia present from birth, seizures which may be early in onset and refractory, failure to thrive and variable hepatomegaly. The dysmorphic features are subtle but, as in many syndromes, after seeing a case they become easier to recognize. They include a high-domed forehead, external ear abnormalities, large fontanelle, flat occiput, micrognathia, shallow supra-orbital ridges, epicanthic folds, low broad nasal root, and peri-orbital oedema with redundant neck folds (Fig. 40.3). These children usually die in early infancy. The brain at postmortem shows an abnormal convolutional pattern with microgyria, heterotopic cortex, ectopic neurones and olivary dysplasia.

Investigations at a ward-level which are helpful include X-rays of the knees which show patella calcification, liver function tests which may be abnormal, serum iron which is occasionally elevated, and pipecolic acid excreted in the urine.

More specific laboratory tests (done only in specialized units) include the estimation of dihydroxyacetone phosphate acyltransferase (DHAPAT) in leucocytes, plasmalogens in erythrocytes and DHAPAT and the catalase latency test in fibroblasts. Tests of plasmalogen synthesis, raised levels of plasma long-chain fatty acids, estimation of bile acid metabolites, and (in survivors of greater than 6 months) phytanic acid can also be done. None of these tests is specific as a number of different enzymes are thought to be defective.

In pseudo-Zellweger's disease (Goldfischer et al 1986) (an extremely rare condition) the clinical picture is similar but the liver is not enlarged and there is no patella calcification. Peroxisomal function appears to be normal but the peroxisomes themselves may be of abnormal size. The underlying defect is unknown.

In infantile Refsum's disease (Schutgens et al 1986) the clinical picture is similar but in addition there is a definite retinopathy which may manifest itself as visual dysfunction. (A depressed electroretinogram would be a confirmatory finding.) There is usually hepatic fibrosis.

In neonatal adrenoleukodystrophy (Schutgens et al 1986) the disease is truly progressive. The symptoms again are very similar to those in Zellweger's disease and different from the later problems in X-linked adrenoleukodystrophy. This disease is autosomal recessive.

It is not absolutely certain if hyperpipecolic acidaemia is a separate entity. Again the symptoms are similar to the above with, as the name suggests, high levels of pipecolic acid being excreted.

All of the above diseases are fatal within the first few years of life. There is no specific therapy as yet. Prenatal diagnosis is available for Zellweger's syndrome and X-linked adrenoleukodystrophy and may be available for other disorders in this group in the near future.

OTHER DISEASE OF UNCERTAIN ORIGIN

Leigh's disease

Although Leigh's disease probably represents a number of different genetic entities, at the moment it serves the purpose of describing a clinical picture which although variable is important to recognize, not least because of possible therapeutic intervention. The pathology of this condition is that of symmetrical vascular lesions throughout the brainstem, basal ganglia and thalamus (Dayan et al 1970); the origin of this is unknown. Some infants with Leigh's have been found to have defects in the metabolism of pyruvate. Pyruvate carboxylase (Hommes et al 1968) and pyruvate dehydrogenase (Robinson & Sherwood 1975) have been shown in individual cases to be deficient and cases have been shown to be associated with a mitochondrial cytopathy (Crosby & Chou 1974).

Of the degenerative diseases seen in the first year of life, Leigh's disease is one of the most common, although experience varies from country to country. The onset is nearly always in the first year, often by 4 months of age and may even present in the neonatal period. There is a wide variety of presenting symptoms and the initial features may be acute, apparently triggered by non-specific infection. The condition may be self-limiting or may be followed by deterioration which may be chronic or stepwise downhill with varying plateaus. In the absence of known amino acidurias and organic acidurias this is a relatively unusual pattern and should make one suspect Leigh's.

The typical features include hypotonia, abnormal movements (later becoming athetoid), sighing or irregular respirations with periods of hyperventilation and apnoea, swallowing difficulties which may contribute to failure to thrive, and other cranial nerve palsies. Abnormal eye movements occur. These are not simply the wandering nystagmoid eye movements of the blind but include complex nystagmoid movements which may be horizontal, rotary or vertical, ocular flutter, gaze palsies and oculomotor paresis. Seizures are not a common feature in infancy, optic atrophy may develop later and there may be evidence of a peripheral neuropathy (depressed reflexes and delayed nerve conduction studies). CT scan may show hypodense symmetrical lesions in the region of the basal ganglia.

Lactate and pyruvate are sometimes elevated in the blood and CSF. A number of specific tests have been suggested in the past but none have proved very useful. Final confirmation is only by the typical postmortem findings.

Most cases of the disease are likely to be autosomal recessive and as yet there is no prenatal test. The course of the disease may be very prolonged with periods of stabilization.

Various cofactors, lipoic acid, vitamin B6, thiamine have been tried without any proof of success. The natural history of the disease makes assessment of therapy difficult.

It is likely we are dealing here with a syndrome complex with more than one cause. The literature is confused because of different definitions of the syndrome, some pathological and some clinical and in only a few have specific enzyme defects been determined.

Alpers' disease

Like Leigh's disease (see earlier) Alpers' disease (progressive degeneration of cerebral grey matter, Alpers 1960) probably represents more than one neurological disorder. The literature on Alper's disease is sometimes confusing and conflicting but in general the presentation is in infancy with seizures and an intermittent downhill course and there is diffuse non-specific destruction of cortical neurones. However, there has been described recently a condition known as 'progressive neuronal degeneration with hepatic failure' (Harding et al 1986) which seems to be a specific entity within the Alpers' spectrum. This condition presents with seizures which start suddenly and may have a myoclonic or generalized pattern. These seizures progress over months and are often refractory to therapy. Epilepsia partialis continuans may appear (this sign is otherwise very unusual in neurometabolic disease), there is progressive psychomotor retardation and in the preterminal phase hepatic involvement becomes apparent. The liver may be noticeably enlarged and jaundice supervenes. Liver failure may be a terminal event. Serum enzymes indicative of liver damage (alanine transaminase and aspartate transaminase) become raised.

It has been suggested that liver involvement may be the result of anti-epileptic drugs (Green 1984) but there is no evidence that drugs are responsible for the whole disease. The pathology of the liver shows a microvesicular steatosis and in the brain there is widespread proliferation and loss of neurones particularly affecting the visual cortex.

There are no specific biochemical tests yet available and the genetics of the condition are as yet unknown, although it is likely to be autosomal recessive.

Infantile neuraxonal dystrophy

The disease is as yet of unknown origin, although it is probably due to a defective enzyme. Both the central neuraxis and the peripheral nerves are involved. The latter may be shown on biopsy to have specific swellings (spheroid bodies) along the length of the axons. Three different clinical pictures emerge, only one of which (Seitelberger's disease, Seitelberger 1971) presents in infancy.

The clinical picture is that of CNS degeneration with mental retardation and long tract signs accompanied by hypotonia and peripheral wasting. Facial nerve paresis, oculomotor paresis and optic atrophy may occur. Deterioration with dementia follows.

Nerve conduction studies and EMG show denervation but relatively normal speeds of conduction and the CSF protein is raised. One convenient method of diagnosis is by conjunctival biopsy which may demonstrate the spheroid bodies in nerve endings (Arsenio-Nunes & Goutières 1978). The disease is slowly progressive with death in early childhood. No prenatal diagnosis is yet available.

Batten's disease

There is some variation in terminology in this group of central nervous system degenerative diseases. The term Batten's is best used for the whole group — alternatively known as neuronal ceroid lipofuscinosis because of the storage material found in the central nervous system and elsewhere. An enzyme deficiency has not been identified but it is thought that some defect of cellular oxidation causes accumulation of what is essentially a degradation product or 'wear and tear pigment' (there is an unconfirmed suggestion that dolichol metabolism may be disturbed). There is an early infantile, a late infantile and a juvenile form.

Early infantile Batten's disease (Hagberg–Santuavuori)

This variety of Batten's disease (neuronal ceroid lipofuscinosis) is the rarest of the three variants in the UK, although relatively more common in Finland (Haltia et al 1973). It may present in the second half of the first year of life with progressive psychomotor retardation without any obvious features. Blindness may slowly supervene (the ERG is extinguished and the VER diminished). The head stops growing and myoclonic jerks appear although sometimes these do not present until the second year of life.

It is a relatively rare disease in this country and as the signs early on are not very specific it is easily missed. The EEG is abnormal before seizures appear — it is chaotic and irregular and gradually becomes lower in amplitude as the disease progresses.

Diagnosis is confirmed by biopsy of rectum or skin and the demonstration under electron microscopy of electron-dense bodies described as 'Finnish Snowballs'. The disease is relentlessly progressive after the first year and unfortunately no specific therapy is available; nor is prenatal diagnosis yet a practical possibility.

Spongy degenerations

Both Canavan's disease and Alexander's disease are examples of spongiform leukodystrophies which may present early in infancy. Canavan's is autosomal recessive, while the genetic origin of Alexander's disease is unclear.

Canavan's disease

There is early onset of developmental delay with hypotonia, visual failure due to optic atrophy and seizures in this disease. Symptoms may start in the first few months and macrocephaly is a striking feature. The delay, visual problems and large head often make the clinician suspect hydrocephalus. Nystagmus may be a clue to optic atrophy. Excessive, apparently unprovoked, crying may be a striking feature. Hypotonia and listlessness give way to spasticity and relentless progress to a decorticate state. These children regress with gross deterioration, blindness and spasticity. It is said to be most common in Ashkenazi Jews but non-Jewish children may be affected (Hogan & Richardson 1965).

The diagnosis is essentially clinical but may be confirmed by brain biopsy (Boltshauser & Wilson 1976). CSF protein may be raised and the EEG non-specifically abnormal. The most characteristic finding is the CT scan picture which shows widespread attenuation of subcortical white matter, external and internal capsules and thalami. There is no specific test and therefore no prenatal diagnosis.

Alexander's disease

This disease is probably rarer than Canavan's disease. There are few symptoms other than psychomotor retardation amounting to an arrest of development; seizures and spasticity may supervene. An enlarging head is a constant sign. CT scan shows low attenuation of white matter, particularly in the frontal areas, and ventricular dilatation.

There is no specific marker that can be identified in life. Seizures become more prominent later on and death occurs early in childhood. This condition is one of the few where it may be justified to do a brain biopsy. The typical findings include the so-called 'Rosenthal' fibres (Boltshauser & Wilson 1976).

SPECIFIC THERAPIES

There are very few specific therapies available in this group discussed. Copper therapy has been tried in Menkes' disease without success (Grover & Scrutton 1975, Garnica 1984). The possibility of the use of molybdenum in sulphite oxidase deficiency exists (Shih et al 1977).

Marrow transplantation has been performed in a few centres in different countries (Lancet 1986). Claims have been made for limited success with MLD (Bayever et al 1985). The most experience, however, is with the mucopolysaccharides in the UK. Not all the data of analysis are yet available and the results are not yet clear. Although successes have been claimed with Hurler's disease (Hobbs et al 1981) it is my impression from the literature and from colleagues that there is no hard and fast evidence that the transferred enzyme gets into the CNS and persists. Physical reduction of liver size and clearing of corneal clouding has been shown (Hobbs et al 1981). It is much more difficult to evaluate the improvement of intellectual status over a short period. Moreover, the procedure is available in only a few specialized centres, requires a compatible donor, is expensive, and has a very high morbidity and mortality. At the moment it must be considered experimental therapy.

DISCUSSION

Even though there is as yet no evidence of any specific therapy in the CNS degenerative diseases discussed, it is very important to try and make a diagnosis, and to do this accurately, efficiently and as early as possible. Diagnosis is important for management, prognosis and counselling and is essential for prenatal diagnosis with a particular family. It may later on serve as a starting point for therapy should that become available.

The management of the progressive diseases is fraught with difficulty for the clinician. Firstly the time from symptoms to diagnosis may be prolonged, causing anxiety in the family. This may occur because of the confusing clinical picture that presents and the rarity of individual diseases which have to be thought about before they can be diagnosed. Sometimes the symptoms are wrongly ascribed to perinatal encephalopathies or the consequence of infantile spasms. Some diseases in this group are only slowly progressive without gross symptomatology and development masks psychomotor retardation. An acute deterioration may be, for example in Leigh's disease, wrongly attributed to a virus encephalopathy.

The very act of diagnosis sometimes gives relief to some parents (at least to those who have been aware that there is something wrong). Supportive therapy must include management of seizures, often very difficult, reduction of spasticity and sometimes sedation. Most important is an excellent standard of nursing care both in hospital and at home. Facilities for shared care and respite care should be provided. The management problems of the dying child with all the social, emotional and nursing implications have been a concern of those working in the field over the last few years. This has led to number of approaches based on support groups, specialized home nursing, and hospices for children.

The diagnosis of this group of conditions should always be confirmed pathologically or biochemically. As these tests are not available in non-specialized laboratories the diagnosis should be confirmed by a specialist laboratory and that the same laboratory should be involved in the prenatal diagnosis of any further pregnancies. This will to some extent avoid difficulties caused by variations in enzyme assays between laboratories.

Other non-metabolic causes of CNS degeneration must be considered in the differential diagnosis of the metabolic diseases. Progressive epilepsy, particularly myoclonic, may be due to a number of different epileptic encephalopathies (Aicardi 1986). Progressive psychomotor retardation with hypotonia or spasticity may occasionally be due to diffuse tumours of the CNS. Post-infective (viral) encephalopathies may occasionally be progressive, e.g. progressive polio encephalitis.

Rett's syndrome, probably a relatively common condition in girls causing developmental regression, loss of communication skills, ataxia and abnormal hand movements, may just be recognized at 6–9 months, although classically it presents in the second year of life. The cause is unknown (Kerr & Stephenson 1985).

The newly described group of diseases due to mitochondrial disorders (mitochondrial cytopathies) usually present with some form of progressive neuromuscular syndrome in early childhood, associated with retinitis pigmentosa, ataxia and mental retardation. Occasionally the presentation may be in the first year of life with acute neurological symptoms. Some cases of Leigh's syndrome may be examples of mitochondrial cytopathy. The presence of a high resting lactate in the serum would be suggestive. Diagnosis is by muscle biopsy and the use of special staining and biochemical techniques. The diagnosis is confirmed by the finding of abnormal mitochondria on electron microscopy and specialized analysis of the specific enzyme defect in the respiratory chain of mitochondria (Clark et al 1984).

For a detailed review of prenatal diagnosis see Golbus 1982.

ACKNOWLEDGEMENTS

Grateful thanks are expressed to Dr George Gray (Senior Biochemist), Miss Mary-Anne Edwards (Senior Biochemist) and Mrs Anne Green (Top Grade Biochemist), Department of Clinical Chemistry, Children's Hospital, Birmingham for their helpful comments in the preparation of this chapter.

REFERENCES

Adams C, Green S 1986 Late-onset hexosaminidase A and hexosaminidase A and B deficiency: family study and review. Developmental Medicine and Child Neurology 28: 236–243

Adams R D, Lyon G R 1982 Neurology of hereditary metabolic disease of children. Hemisphere Publishing, Washington

Aicardi J 1986 Epilepsy in children (International Review of Child Neurology Series). Raven Press, New York

Alpers B J 1960 Progressive cerebral degeneration of infancy. Journal of Mental and Nervous Diseases 130: 442–448

Arsenio-Nunes M L, Goutières F 1978 Diagnosis of infantile neuraxonal dystrophy by conjunctival biopsy. Journal of Neurology, Neurosurgery and Psychiatry 41: 511–515

Aula P, Autio S, Raivio K O et al 1979 'Salla disease': a new lysosomal storage disease. Archives of Neurology 36: 88–94

Bach G, Friedman R, Weissman B, Neufeld E 1972 The defect in the Hurler and Scheie Syndromes: deficiency of alpha-L-iduronidase. Proceedings of the National Academy of Sciences USA 69: 2048–2051

Bayever E, Ladisch S, Philippart M et al 1985 Bone-marrow transplantation for metachromatic leucodystrophy. Lancet ii: 471–473

Beaudet A L, Manschrek A A 1982 Metabolism of sphingomyelin by intact cultured fibroblasts: differentiation of Niemann–Pick disease types A and B. Biochemical and Biophysical Research Communications 105: 14–19

Beaudet A L, DiFerrante N M, Ferry G D, Nichols B L, Mullins C E 1975 Variation in the phenotype expression of beta-glucuronidase deficiency. Journal of Pediatrics 86: 338–394

Boltshauser E, Wilson J 1976 Value of brain biopsy in neurodegenerative disease in childhood. Archives of Disease in Childhood 51: 264–268

Bowen P, Lee C S N, Zellweger H, Lindenberg R 1964 A familial syndrome of multiple congenital defects. Bulletin of the Johns Hopkins Hospital 114: 402–414

Brett E M (ed) 1983 Paediatric neurology. Churchill Livingstone, Edinburgh

Clark J B, Hayes D J, Morgan-Hughes J A, Byrne E 1984 Mitochondrial myopathies: disorders of the respiratory chain and oxidative phosphorylation. Journal of Inherited Metabolic Diseases 7 (suppl 1): 62–68

Collie W R, Moore C M, Goka T J, Howell R R 1978 Pili torti as marker for carriers of Menkes' disease. Lancet i: 607–608

Crocker A C, Farber S 1958 Niemann–Pick disease: a review of 18 patients. Medicine (Baltimore) 37: 1–95

Crosby T W and Chou S M 1974 'Ragged-Red' fibres in Leigh's disease. Neurology 24: 49–54

Danks D M, Campbell P E, Stevens B J, Mayne V, Cartwright E 1972 Menkes' kinky hair syndrome: an inherited defect in copper absorption with widespread effects. Pediatrics 50: 188–201

Dayan A D, Ockenden B G, Crome L 1970 Necrotising encephalomyelopathy of Leigh: neuropathological findings in 8 cases. Archives of Disease in Childhood 45: 39–48

DeDuve C 1969 The peroxisome: a new cytoplasmic organelle. Proceedings of the Royal Society of London (B) 173: 71–83

Garnica A D 1984 The failure of parenteral copper therapy in Menkes' kinky hair syndrome. European Journal of Pediatrics 142: 98–102

Glossl J, Kresse H, Mendla K, Cantz M, Rosenkranz W 1984 Partial deficiency of glycoprotein neuraminidase in some patients with Morquio disease Type A. Pediatric Research 18: 302–305

Golbus M S 1982 The current scope of antenatal diagnosis. Hospital Practice 17: 179–186

Goldfischer S, Collins J, Rapin I et al 1986 Pseudo–Zellweger syndrome: deficiencies in several peroxisomal oxidative activities. Journal of Pediatrics 108: 25–32

Green S H 1984 Sodium valproate and routine liver function tests. Archives of Disease in Childhood 59: 813–814

Grover W D, Scrutton M C 1975 Copper infusion therapy in trichopoliostrophy. Journal of Pediatrics 86: 216–220

Haltia M, Rapola J, Santavuori P 1973 Infantile type of so-called neuronal ceroid lipofuscinosis. Acta Neuropathologica 26: 157–170

Harding B N, Egger J, Portman B, Erdohazi M 1986 Progressive neuronal degeneration of childhood with liver disease. Brain 109: 181–206

Hobbs J R, Hugh-Jones K, Barrett A J et al 1981 Reversal of clinical features of Hurler's disease and biochemical improvement after treatment by bone-marrow transplantation. Lancet ii: 709–712

Hogan G R, Richardson E P 1965 Spongy degeneration of the nervous system (Canavan's disease): report of a case in an Irish–American family. Pediatrics 35: 284–294

Hommes F A, Polman H A, Reerink J D 1968 Leigh's encephalo-myelopathy: an inborn error of gluconeogenesis. Archives of Disease in Childhood 43: 423–426

Horn N, Heydorn K, Damsgaard E, Tygstrup I, Vestermark S (1978) Is Menkes' syndrome a copper storage disorder? Clinical Genetics 14: 186–187

Johnson W G 1983 Genetic heterogeneity of the hexosaminidase deficiency diseases. Research Publications Association for Research in Nervous and Mental Disease 60: 215–237

Kerr A M, Stephenson J B P 1985 Rett's syndrome in the West of Scotland. British Medical Journal 291: 579–582

Lancet (Leading article) 1986 Bone marrow transplantation of neurovisceral storage disorders. Lancet ii: 788–789

Leroy J G, Ho H W, MacBrinn M C, Zielka K, Jacob J, O'Brien J S 1972 I-cell: biochemical studies. Pediatric Research 6: 752–757

Lesch M, Nyhan W L 1964 A familial disorder of uric acid metabolism and central nervous system function. American Journal of Medicine 36: 561–570

Lowden J A, O'Brien J S 1979 Sialidosis: a review of human neuraminidase deficiency. American Journal of Human Genetics 31: 1–18

Lowden J A, Cutz E, Conen P E, Rudd N, Doron T 1973 Prenatal diagnosis of GMI gangliosidosis. New England Journal of Medicine 288: 225–228

Lowry R B, Renwick H G 1971 Relative frequency of the Hurler and Hunter syndromes. New England Journal of Medicine 284: 221–222

McFaul R, Cavanagh N, Lake B D, Stephens R, Whitfield A E 1982 Metachromatic leucodystrophy: review of 38 cases. Archives of Disease in Childhood 57: 168–175

McKusick V 1983 Metabolic basis of inherited diseases. Johns Hopkins University Press, Baltimore

Martin J J, Leroy J G, Centerick C, Libert J, Dodinval P, Martin L 1981 Fetal Krabbe leukodystrophy: a morphological study of two cases. Acta Neuropathologica 53: 87–91

Milla P J 1978 I-cell disease. Archives of Disease in Childhood 53: 513–515

Moser H W, Goldfischer S L 1985 The peroxisomal disorders. Hospital Practice (Office Edition) 20: 61–70

Mossman J, Patrick A D 1982 Prenatal diagnosis of mucopolysaccharidoses by two-dimensional electrophoresis of amniotic fluid glycosaminoglycans. Prenatal Diagnosis 2: 169-176

O'Brien J S, Stern M B, Landing B H, O'Brien J K, Donnell G N 1965 Generalised gangliosidosis: another inborn error of ganglioside metabolism? American Journal of Diseases of Children 109: 338–346

Pavone L, Moser H W, Mollica F, Reitno C, Durand P 1980 Farber's lipogranulomatosis: ceramide deficiency and prolonged survival in three relatives. Johns Hopkins Medical Journal 147: 193–196

Robinson B H, Sherwood W G 1975 Pyruvate dehydrogenase phosphatase deficiency: a cause of congenital chronic lactic acidosis in infancy. Pediatric Research 9: 935–939

Schneider E L, Ellis W G, Brady R O, McCulloch J R, Epstein C J 1972 Infantile (type II) Gaucher's disease: in utero diagnosis and foetal pathology. Journal of Pediatrics 81: 1134–1139

Schutgens R B H, Heymans H S A, Wanders R J A, Bosch H, Tager J M 1986 Peroxisomal disorders: a newly recognised group of genetic diseases. European Journal of Pediatrics 144: 430–440

Seitelberger F 1971 Neuropathological conditions related to neuraxonal dystrophy. Acta Neuropathologica (Suppl) 5: 17–19

Shih V E, Abrams I F, Johnson J L, Mudd S H 1977 Sulphite oxidase deficiency. New England Journal of Medicine 297: 1022–1028

Stanbury J B, Wyngaarden J B, Frederickson J B, Goldstein J L, Brown M S 1983 Metabolic basis of inherited disease, 5th edn. MacGraw-Hill, New York

Taylor C J, Green S H 1981 Menkes' Syndrome (trichopoliodystrophy): use of scanning electron-microscope in diagnosis and carrier identification. Journal of Developmental Medicine and Child Neurology 23: 361–368

Taylor H A, Thomas G H, Aylsworth A et al 1975 Mannosidosis: deficiency of a specific alpha-mannosidase component in cultured fibroblasts. Clinica Chimica Acta 59: 93–99

Ulrich J, Herschkowitz N 1977 Seitelberger's connatal form of Pelizaeus–Merzbacher disease: case report; clinical, pathological and biochemical findings. Acta Neuropathologica 40: 129–136

Vamos E, Liebaers I, Bousard N, Libert J, Perlmutter N 1981 Multiple Sulphatase deficiency with early onset. Journal of Inherited Metabolic Diseases 4: 103–104

Verity M A, Montasir M 1977 Infantile Gaucher's disease: neuropathology, acid hydrolase activities and negative staining observations. Neuropaediatrie 8: 89–100

Watts R W E, Gibbs D A 1986 Lysosomal storage diseases: biochemical and clinical aspects. Taylor & Francis, London

Wilson J M, Young A B, Kelley W N 1983 Hypoxanthine–guanine phosphoribosyltransferase deficiency: the molecular basis of the clinical syndromes. New England Journal of Medicine 309: 900–910

Seizure disorders

41. Seizure disorders

Dr J. K. Brown and Dr R. A. Minns

The newborn infant has a limited repertoire of signs and symptoms with which he can respond to dysfunction of his central nervous system. A fit is one of the most common presentations of disease involving the central nervous system of the newborn and is much more specific than other symptoms and signs such as apnoeic attacks or feeding difficulty which may have their origin in diseases of other organs than the brain.

The brain is in a stage of rapid maturation around the time of birth and so not only do normal neurological findings change rapidly but the manner in which a particular pathology manifests may also change. Static pathology may result in a dynamic clinical picture which may give the appearance of a progressive disorder, the change being due to progressive brain maturation rather than progress in the pathology. The type of seizure may also vary with the age of the child and is not specific to the pathology, this has given rise to the idea of epileptic syndromes such as West's syndrome, Lennox–Gastaut or Ohtahara syndrome, all of which arise, for example from a cortical dysplasia, i.e. a static pathology (Brown & Livingston 1985). In the newborn most fits are symptomatic of some underlying pathology but one cannot assume because a fit is focal in nature that it represents focal pathology — it can be due to a generalized biochemical disturbance.

The importance of seizures in the newborn is not only that they indicate an acute disturbance in the brain at that particular time but failure to control the seizure may result in an increase in brain damage so that an antenatal event such as hypoxia-ischaemia from a placenta or cord problem is compounded by postnatal consumptive asphyxia from uncontrolled seizures. There has been a tendency to become obsessed with the long-term sequelae of a neonatal seizure and although prognostic of a statistically significant risk in terms of future mental handicap and cerebral palsy the importance of a seizure lies in its indication that there is something immediately wrong with the brain which requires investigation and treatment (Brown & Minns 1980).

INCIDENCE OF SEIZURES

One cannot give a useful or meaningful figure for the incidence of seizures because of changing patterns of disease and the non-comparability of different neonatal populations. In the past an incidence as high as 16/1000 deliveries was recorded in the Simpson Maternity Pavilion in Edinburgh but 55% of these infants were having convulsions due to simple neonatal tetany or hypocalcaemia. With the lowering of the phosphate content of feeds this group dramatically diminished. If this metabolic group is excluded, one had an incidence of 8/1000 due to the other multitude of causes which will be discussed later. Intrapartum asphyxia in the full-term infant was responsible for 3/1000 livebirths (Brown 1973). This figure of 8/1000 has now halved within the same population with the total incidence of all fits around 3–4/1000 livebirths. Burke (1954) reported an incidence of 5.3/1000 and Craig (1960) an incidence of 8/1000 livebirths. Keen & Lee (1973) found 112 infants with fits over a 39-month period with an incidence of 12.2/1000 but this was at a time when, like Edinburgh, hypocalcaemia was playing a significant role. Dennis (1978) from Oxford suggested a low rate of 4.2/1000 could be achieved whilst the remarkably low figure of 1.6/1000 was reported recently from Dublin (Derham et al 1985). These figures, however, cannot be compared from unit to unit as some neonatal units take only tertiary referrals from a very wide area. Some only take the small pre-term infant requiring ventilation, and others take all infants from a given population, and so the populations from which the studies are taken are not comparable.

The number of infants with a fit due to perinatal asphyxia has fallen with the use of fetal monitoring. The number of infants with meningitis will vary according to the group of mothers who carry group B streptococcus or the use of parenteral nutrition or broad-spectrum antibiotic policies predisposing to *Klebsiella* meningitis. 'Fifth day' fits appear to be common in Australia and yet other units do not appear to see them (Goldberg 1983). In addition to these factors there are difficulties in defining a seizure, in that some units would label every infant with tonic decerebration as suffering from a fit and others would include all the excitable behaviour patterns that one sees in recovery from asphyxia, as subtle seizures. With this variation in population and the definition of what constitutes a fit, straight comparison of one unit with another becomes a meaningless exercise. Follow-up of infants with seizures is, however, vital as this is a very important means of quality control for the individual intensive care unit to show that morbidity is decreasing with improvements in treatment. The importance of this was seen in a recent 10-year review from Melbourne where the overall incidence of neonatal convulsions was found to have risen from 2/1000 to 8.6/1000 and this has pointed the direction for further investigation and research.

DEFINITIONS

The terms convulsion, fit and seizure, tend to be used loosely. Seizure should be used as a generic term for any paroxysmal event which may or may not be a fit. A convulsion in the older child usually signifies a tonic–clonic attack. One does not see the typical grand mal tonic–clonic, generalized seizure in the newborn and so the term convulsion tends to be used synonymously with either a tonic or a generalized clonic fit. We reserve the term 'fit' or ictus for the clinical manifestation of a cerebral arrhythmia. We regard the cerebral arrhythmias in a similar way to the cardiac arrhythmias as disorders of the electrical activity within the brain. A fit need not arise in the cerebral cortex, e.g. in spinal epilepsy one may see rhythmic myoclonic jerks arising from an isolated cord segment in children with a type II cord involvement in myelomeningocele. Electrical discharges may arise in the brainstem, basal ganglia or cortex. The electro-encephalogram is theoretically the best method of studying cerebral arrhythmias, in the same way that the electrocardiogram is the best way of studying cardiac arrhythmias. The problem arises in that the electrode placement only allows examination of a very limited part of the neocortex.

One can consider arrhythmias of the central nervous system as acute, recurrent or continuous. Acute arrhythmias arise in association with an acute encephalopathy, such as trauma, asphyxia, encephalitis, meningitis or metabolic upsets and they indicate an acute disease of the nervous system complicated by a disorder or rhythm. This does not mean that there is going to be a continuing recurrent problem of seizures unless ongoing brain damage results. Recurrent arrhythmias are what we conventionally regard as the epilepsies. Most fits in the newborn period are acute arrhythmias and disappear within a week or so of birth only to return if there is a chronic brain damage syndrome. Abnormalities in the structure of the cerebral cortex (i.e. the cortical dysplasias) may have resulted in fits in utero as well as after birth (i.e. a recurrent arrhythmia) and they can be regarded, therefore, as true neonatal epilepsy.

Continuous arrhythmia is synonymous with status epilepticus. This may be convulsive or non-convulsive or may constitute electrical status without clinical status. We are beginning to appreciate that non-convulsive status epilepticus is not all that uncommon in these small infants and many infants with infantile spasms are in essence in non-convulsive status, the infantile spasms merely being a different sort of seizure which draws attention to the condition.

TYPES OF SEIZURE

The international classification of epilepsy is not helpful in the description of seizure types in the newborn period. Fits occurring in utero pose a particular problem although they may be visualized by antenatal ultrasound. Often the diagnosis is retrospective and when the mother sees the movements that the infant is making postnatally she associates these with fetal movements she felt before birth. Intra-uterine fits are particularly likely to occur with vitamin B6-dependency and the cortical dysplasias.

Types of seizure, such as the absence seizure, psychomotor, akinetic, and tonic–clonic, do not occur or are very difficult to recognize in the newborn infant. Most fits in the newborn period are recognized because of motor phenomena and can be accommodated into one of four main categories (Brown & Minns 1980):

1. Tonic
2. Clonic
   a. Focal
   b. Multifocal
   c. Generalized (bilateral)
3. Fragmentary seizures
   a. Motor
   b. Ophthalmic
   c. Loss of awareness
   d. Apnoea/cyanosis
4. Myoclonic

Tonic seizures

These are in essence a functional electrical decerebration, the infant usually assuming the decerebrate posture with the neck retracted and arms and legs extended. Occasionally one does see the decorticate posture but this is less common as the infant's central nervous system does not possess the maturation of basal ganglia necessarily to sustain the common type of decorticate posturing. Respiration usually ceases in an attack and the episode may be heightened by inspiration. Most episodes last less than one minute. The EEG in true tonic seizures is abnormal, since we regard this as functionally electrical decerebration and the abnormality may consist of runs of spikes which may be asymmetrical, or show runs of slow waves. Occasionally a tonic seizure may be accompanied by focal spikes confined to one hemisphere on the EEG.

Difficulty in diagnosis arises as an identical decerebrate posture may arise from release of the reticulospinal pathways with true decerebrate rigidity (in reality decerebrate spasticity). This is usually due to midbrain compression from raised intracranial pressure. This is seen at its maximum in the infant with untreated hydrocephalus who develops sunsetting, central neurogenic hyperventilation, and repeated episodes of tonic decerebrate extension due to fluctuations in intracranial pressure. One should not regard these tonic decerebrate attacks as being fits but difficulty will continue until monitoring of intracranial pressure and blood flow in the small premature infant becomes more routine. The absence of EEG abnormalities (although conventional montages may not detect seizure activity in the orbital or temporal lobe without nasopharyngeal leads) together with the poor response to anticonvulsants in many of these infants suggests that they are being wrongly classified as fits. The difficulty is compounded by the fact that rising intracranial pressure will also increase the possibility of having seizures from a pre-existing cortical abnormality.

True tonic seizures are seen most commonly in the first 24 hours in infants who have sustained intrapartum hypoxic–ischaemic brain damage.

Clonic seizures

A clonic seizure consists of a rhythmic jerking of one part of the body which is commonly at a frequency of one or three cycles per second. This is a cortical seizure and is less common before 36 weeks of gestation. In our experience a true clonic seizure is always accompanied by a spike discharge in the corresponding hemisphere with the electrical discharge being at the same speed as the clinical ictus. There often appears to be quite a delay between the spike and the clinical jerk. Placement of the electrodes is important and will be discussed later; one may appear to have a normal EEG in the presence of a clonic fit if vertex electrodes are not used as a routine.

Focal clonic seizures are seen in infants with birth injury and asphyxia as well as those with metabolic disease such as hypocalcaemia and hypoglycaemia. The clonic fit does not follow a tonic phase and two clonic fits may occur together at different rates, starting and stopping at different times due to independent foci in different parts of the brain. A focal clonic seizure may also be followed by a Todd's (localized) paresis lasting for several hours when there is diminished movement of the affected side, i.e. the normal doggy paddling and cycling movements are reduced, or there is loss of the normal neonatal flexor tone on that side. Baby

movements which may appear random can be classified into identifiable groups (Weggeman et al 1987). Focal infarcts, contusions, hamartomas, arteriovenous malformations and focal intracerebral bleeding can result in focal seizures in the newborn. They are diagnosed more frequently since the advent of new imaging techniques; an ultrasound scan should be performed on all infants with a focal seizure (Levene & Trounce 1986).

Focal clonic seizures

These are rhythmic jerkings of the arm, leg or face on one side of the body. The fit remains localized to that particular part of the body and if there are several seizures they always occur in the same area. The frequency of the jerking may vary between individual fits or may suddenly change during the course of a single seizure. Partial status epilepticus may occur and is characteristically thought to point to focal localization in the brain. Bilard et al 1982 have reported focal status, e.g. from localized brain lesions such as infarcts, haematomas, occasionally bacterial meningitis, and arteriovenous malformations such as Sturge–Weber and incontinentia pigmenti.

Multifocal clonic seizures

This is the name given to a group of seizures which affect different parts of the body at different times, i.e. the right arm may be predominantly involved in one seizure and the left leg in a subsequent seizure. This type of seizure indicates diffuse hyperexcitability of the cortex and is the type that is seen in metabolic disease such as hypocalcaemia and hypomagnesaemia or diffuse cortical abnormalities such as the cortical dysplasias. They are occasionally seen also in the recovery phase of asphyxia.

Generalized clonic seizures

Most seizures reported by nursing staff are generalized but in a study of over 50 infants in whom the seizure occurred whilst under EEG monitoring it was found that over 95% commenced with a focal origin and then spread to become bilateral. Primary generalized seizures for all practical purposes do not occur in the neonate. Spread tends to occur from vertex to vertex and once the jerking becomes bilateral and rhythmic then consciousness is lost and there may be interruption of respiratory rhythm with cyanosis. The number of generalized seizures reported in any series will, therefore, depend upon the accuracy of the observation, whether EEG monitoring was available and whether the start of the fit was witnessed. Spread of the seizure to become generalized requires a degree of CNS maturation and so this is characteristically a type of fit seen in the full-term infant.

Fragmentary seizures (subtle seizures)

We have already discussed the importance of defining what is meant by a fit, so that every paroxysmal behaviour disturbance in the newborn is not labelled as a seizure. This is discussed more fully in the section on the differential diagnosis of a fit. If the nervous system of the infant is in a high state of arousal, e.g. in the hyperexcitable recovery phase after a period of intrapartum asphyxia or if the mother has been taking CNS depressant drugs, such as barbiturates, benzodiazepines or heroin, or alternatively, if the baby is in a high state of arousal from hunger drive, as for example in intra-uterine malnutrition, there is an increase in the amount of motor activity. The infant can show tremor, clonus, startles, stretches, cycling movements and grimacing. The postasphyxial infant also shows athetoid movements, adder tonguing, tonic mouth opening or abnormal eye movements. Some authorities argue that all these movements should be regarded as a form of subtle seizures. Most so-called brainstem (fragmentary) fits are due to release phenomena secondary to epileptic activity arising in the cortex rather than necessarily indicating epileptic discharges within the pons or medulla (see p. 495). Arguments that the EEG may be normal or show minimal activity because the epilepsy is arising in the brainstem cannot be discounted, but the onus of proof must rest upon finding evidence of such discharge, if we are to treat the infant with large doses of anticonvulsant drugs to which this type of seizure does not necessarily respond.

Subtle motor seizures

We do not deny that brainstem release phenomena such as adopting an asymmetrical tonic neck reflex position (adversive attack) repeated startles (infantile spasms), or sudden episodes of doggy paddling, cycling, mouthing, tongue rolling, cannot occur as seizures. One can see these ictal behaviours occurring in the presence of well-established cortical epileptic spikes. Equally episodes of apnoea or cyanosis may represent the only manifestation of a seizure but if this is not accompanied by evidence of epileptic activity on the electro-encephalogram one must be very wary of missing other potentially more easily treatable causes. The most difficult clinical situation is the diagnosis of subtle seizures in the very small pre-term infant.

Loss of awareness seizures

Loss of awareness without any motor manifestations is well-recognized as the absence of seizure in the older child. We do not usually see classical absences in the first year of life but that is not to say that loss of awareness may not be the only manifestation of a seizure. In the infant suffering from the infantile spasm syndrome, loss of awareness with development of autistic features is often the first complaint by the mother and may precede the actual development of the spasms which eventually persuades the doctor that the child has a seizure disorder. In the normal types of tonic or clonic seizure, loss of awareness occurs when the fit becomes generalized. However, occasionally it becomes apparent to nursing staff or skilled EEG technicians that the infant appears glazed ('not with it') and there is increasing concern that it may be showing so-called non-convulsive status with loss of awareness and marked epilepsy on the EEG. This is easily missed if EEG monitoring is not performed over a prolonged period using, for example, a 24-hour tape-monitor or continuous oscilloscope montage of the EEG.

Ophthalmic fits

The eyes may show sudden tonic deviation with nystagmoid movements in association with a fixed asymmetrical tonic neck posture in adversive seizures. Deviation of the head and eyes is not uncommon with other types of fit. One may occasionally see fluttering of the eyelids with horizontal deviation of the eyes and a jerking form of subtle seizures as well as in the recovery phase of asphyxia. It is sometimes difficult to be sure if sudden onset of abnormal eye movements indicates a seizure; for example, the sudden hippus with alternating dilatation and constriction of the pupil and tonic downward movement of the eyes which occurs in raised intracranial pressure before the development of true sunsetting and a subsequent third-nerve palsy. Metabolic disease such as Leigh's encephalopathy can be associated with severe eye movement abnormalities and the so-called dancing-eyes syndrome may be the herald of a latent neuroblastoma. Hyperventilation with bizzare eye movements are seen clasically in Joubert's syndrome (p. 241).

Myoclonic fits

Myoclonus is conventionally divided into axial myoclonus and limb myoclonus. In a clonic seizure the jerking is rhythmic, repeated and often lateralized. In limb myoclonus, both arms or both legs jerk together, timing of the movement often appearing random rather than the regular rhythm at 1 or 3 c/s seen in the clonic seizure. Occasionally one sees so-called metronomic myoclonus when a jerk may occur every 10 seconds. Axial myoclonus indicates that the axial musculature is involved and this produces either flexion of the trunk or head-nodding episodes. Myoclonus usually indicates diffuse cerebral disease and occurs only in the terminal phase of very severe asphyxia, diffuse cortical dysplasia, degenerative disease or often later merges into the intractable epileptic syndromes of Otahara, West or Lennox–Gastaut.

DIFFERENTIAL DIAGNOSIS OF A FIT

We have already mentioned several release phenomena which can occur in pathological states such as tonic extension with decerebrate posturing, uninhibited primitive reflexes, e.g. an obligatory asymmetrical tonic neck reflex, adder tonguing, mouthing and doggy paddling, and the difficulty in deciding whether these behaviours constitute a fit. To complicate matters further the normal infant may show other paroxysmal changes in behaviour which may also cause confusion.

Startles

An infant may show sudden startles with flexion of the arms and legs. Startles are particularly likely in premature babies and any newborn may have sleep startles during non-eye movement (REM) sleep. Since the EEG during non-eye movement (REM) sleep shows the classical tracé alternans or burst suppression picture. During the bursts there may be very sharp elements looking like spikes or spike and waves. It may be very difficult to be sure whether sudden myoclonic movements are epileptic or not.

Moro reflex

This consists of four components in the fully mature infant — abduction and extension of the arms followed by adduction and flexion. This is usually a phasic response with rapid abduction and extension but a tonic component sustaining the arms in rigid extension for several seconds is occasionally seen in the neurologically abnormal infant — resembling a tonic fit. Peiper (1963) pointed out that the startle reflex is a flexor reflex and the Moro reflex an extensor one and the two are not synonymous.

Stretches

The normally flexed lower limbs may suddenly extend in rigid extension with dorsiflexion of the big toes and fanning of the toes, i.e. a spontaneous Babinski response. These stretches are normal in the immature infant and may also be seen in the very hungry small-for-gestational-age infant or in hypocalcaemia.

Dystonic episodes

The premature baby as he approaches full-term may show an abnormal pattern of extensor tone rather than the development of the flexed adducted posture of the normal full-term infant. Handling of the infant, suspension in space or contact with an extensor surface, can result in the infant arching and appearing to become opisthotonic. These extensor spasms may be an initial manifestation of a dystonic cerebral palsy or simply the so-called transient dystonia of prematurity.

Congenital athetosis

Infants whose mothers have been taking phenothiazine drugs, some perfectly normal infants, and infants after mild asphyxia may show a pattern of so-called congenital athetosis. In this the nares dilate and constrict, the tongue shows adder or protrusion and withdrawal movements, fingers are hyperextended individually and flexed as if the infant was piano playing, pronation on supination movements may be made, and the big toes are widely abducted and adducted with spontaneous Babinski movements.

The hyperalert infant

The infant who is very hungry, particularly that with intra-uterine malnutrition and starvation, or the infant with mild hypoglycaemia may show a very high level of arousal and jitteriness. The feeding reflexes are very marked so that the infant roots on stimulus, even over the vertex of the skull. He shows side to side movements of the mouth with constant rooting. The mouth opens with any contact from the cardinal points reflex. There is continuing cycling, doggy paddling, crawling and in the prone position the infant may appear to crawl round his incubator, excoriating his knees. The doggy paddling and cycling movements are part of intra-uterine swimming movements, used in hatching behaviour to enable the infant to swim into the vertex position. They are recognized in normal pregnancies as movements against the abdominal wall at one per second, which 'medical' mothers can mistakenly diagnose as fits in their own fetus.

The jittery baby

The pyramidal tract in the full-term infant is not myelinated and one major function of the pyramidal tract is inhibition of spinal reflexes. These are relatively uninhibited with alpha–gamma imbalance and so the peripheral monosynaptic spinal reflexes tend to respond in a mass way to the level of central arousal. Arousing factors such as thirst (including hyponatraemia) and hunger (including hypoglycaemia) may result in an infant who not only shows an increase in the level of basic muscle tone and increase in progression movements as above but in addition will show an increase in peripheral neuromuscular hyperexcitability. The tendon reflexes are brisk with marked crossed adductor response (Fig. 41.1). There is jaw clonus, ankle clonus and hamstring clonus. Spontaneous movements of the infant can set off spontaneous clonus at 6–10 c/s (Fig. 41.2) so that a Moro reflex for example may initiate marked finger and jaw tremor and this is accompanied by brisk finger jerks. Crying may initiate jaw clonus and the hyperventilation

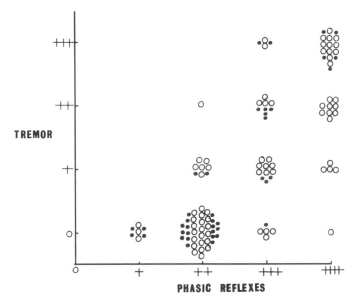

Fig. 41.1 The relationship between tremor and phasic reflexes. Note that tremor is much more common when peripheral reflexes are exaggerated. Hypocalcaemic infants (circle), normal control infants (filled circle).

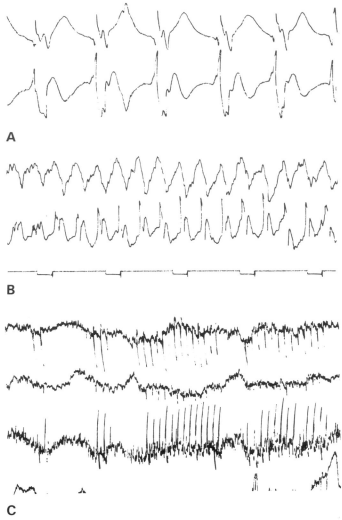

Fig. 41.2 The electrical frequencies of seizures and tremors. (**a**) seizure discharge at 1 cycle/s; (**b**) seizure discharge at 3 cycles/s; and (**c**) tremor at 10 cycles/s. Note the time-scale below trace (**b**).

and mild alkalosis that is associated with prolonged crying may make the jitteriness worse. The spontaneous tremor or clonus always results from sudden stretching of the muscle and it can be abolished by simply flexing or relieving tension on the affected muscle.

The movement that causes particular confusion between clonus and a fit is hamstring clonus. If one flexes the hip so that the thigh is on the abdomen and then suddenly extends the leg at the knee, the hamstrings can be set into an oscillating circuit which is much slower than ankle clonus, finger tremor or jaw clonus and appears to be a rhythmic 3 c/s fit. If one simply flexes the leg this stops and sudden extension will start it again.

Apart from arousing factors in a hyperalert infant anything else which increases neuromuscular excitation will increase the jitteriness, e.g. recovery from asphyxia, hypocalcaemia or hypomagnesaemia (see Table 41.1). If the infant has been depressed by maternal drugs, such as phenobarbitone or heroin, then withdrawal of these results in an overswing with temporary neurotransmitter imbalance and again this can result in a very jittery baby. Tremor of the limbs not associated with peripheral neuromuscular excitability, i.e. with brisk reflexes and clonus, is of much more sinister import and so-called central tremor may represent either a true seizure or is seen in very severe hypoxic–ischaemic brain damage often as a terminal event.

In summary, a jittery baby is usually seen in association with a hyperalert state (normal) but jitteriness with a hypoalert state should always be considered abnormal and central jitteriness without peripheral hyperexcitability (i.e. without brisk jerks) only occurs in extremis.

Apnoeic attacks

Apnoea may occur with generalization of a focal seizure, i.e. when it becomes bilateral. It is common with tonic seizures. Certain subtle seizures may be associated with apnoea or sudden rapid breathing as the only manifestation

Table 41.1 Causes of the jittery baby

Hunger and intra-uterine starvation
Mild hypoglycaemia
Thirst
Hypernatraemia
Water intoxication
Rebound from asphyxia
Hypocalcaemia/hypomagnesaemia
Blood in CSF
Thyrotoxic mother
Mother on narcotics or phenobarbitone
Alcohol withdrawal

of the seizure. The causes of apnoea or apnoeic attacks may include abnormalities of many systems such as primary lung disease, cardiac failure, septicaemia, hypoglycaemia, respiratory depressant drugs and aspiration syndromes, as well as primary CNS disease. Apnoea may result from raised intracranial pressure due to cerebral oedema, hydrocephalus or from intracerebral haemorrhage. Of infants with intrapartum hypoxia, 60% will have apnoeic or cyanotic attacks. These need not represent a seizure but are due to the structural damage and selective vulnerability of the brainstem. Detailed polygraphic and physiological monitoring are necessary before one can be sure of the primary aetiology of an apnoeic attack.

Neonatal hyperkineseis

In the acute stage of asphyxia the infant is apathetic, hypotonic with bulbar paresis, diminished movement and abnormal sleep state and shows generalized CNS depression. After 12–24 hours in the average case, this depression is replaced by a phase of hyperexcitability when the infant may show signs of becoming jittery with ankle, jaw and hand clonus. There is a gradual increase in muscle tone, so that the infant shows marked extensor hypertonus or decerebrate posturing (postasphyxial rigidity); mouthing, adder tonguing, eye rolling, athetoid hand movements, hyperventilation and clonic seizures may all occur.

Extensor spasms

We have already discussed the differentiation of tonic seizures from release of decerebrate rigidity with those due to loss of inhibition from electrical paralysis. Extensor spasms due to cerebral oedema occurring in asphyxia, metabolic disease such as galactosaemia, maple syrup urine disease, water intoxication, proprionic acidaemia, or raised pressure from an intracerebral bleed or hydrocephalus should not be regarded as the same mechanisms as true tonic fits. Extensor hypertonus and extensor spasms have already been mentioned in the dystonic premature infant — those with postasphyxial rigidity, severe hypocalcaemia, neonatal tetanus and parenchymatous brain damage as well as from

meningoencephalitis or kernicterus (Table 41.2). It may not always be easy in the individual case to be sure which is the predominant mechanism, e.g. the infant who has been asphyxiated may show true tonic fits or decerebration from cerebral oedema (either vasogenic oedema due to the loss of autoregulation or osmotic oedema from inappropriate ADH secretion). He may also have heightened extensor tone (postasphyxial rigidity) and have associated secondary hypocalcaemia with tetanic extension or even primary midbrain damage. The clinical assessment must remain to some extent guesswork unless continuous EEG monitoring, intracranial pressure monitoring and sequential blood-flow studies are available.

PATHOPHYSIOLOGY OF NEONATAL FITS

Before we outline the causes of fits in the newborn it is necessary to consider the mechanisms whereby a neurone can be made to fire in order to act as a focus and so initiate a seizure, and also to consider factors which may influence spread of the seizure discharge.

Origin of the epileptic spike focus

Neurones can be considered to fall into two distinct groups. Firstly, those that show a tonic discharge and under normal circumstances will fire continuously. These neurones are needed for the continuous oscillating circuits involved in control of respiration, vasomotor tone, EEG rhythms, arousal, etc. The second type of neurone only fires when stimulated. This brings us to two basic concepts within neurophysiology — inhibition and excitation. Those neurones with a tendency to fire spontaneously would normally be controlled by inhibitory circuits to regulate the rate of firing and to switch them on or off. Failure of this inhibition would result in continuous spontaneous firing. The second type of neurone would normally fire when excited. A further complication is added by virtue of the fact that the neurones which only fire when excited, e.g. the Purkinje cells of the cerebellum, may themselves be inhibitory neurones, so that excitation of a Purkinje cell

Table 41.2   Causes of extensor hypertonus in the neonate

Postasphyxial rigidity
Dystonia of prematurity
Hypocalcaemia, alkalosis, tetany
Kernicterus
Encephalitis, e.g echovirus 11
Cerebral oedema
    Toxic, e.g propionic acidaemia, maple syrup urine disease, galactosaemia, ? hexochlorophane.
    Water intoxication, e.g hypo-osmolar intravenous fluids, inappropriae ADH secretion,
        postasphyxial, septicaemia, meningitis, trauma
        Vasogenic
Raised intracranial pressure, e.g hydrocephalus, intraventricular haemorrhage, subdural
    haematoma, cerebral abscess, tumour

results in inhibition of the cerebral cortex. A neurone may fire, therefore, due to a defect in inhibition or facilitation.

Figure 41.3 represents a neurone. This will fire through the axon (a) when its cell body is stimulated. Changes in sodium (e.g. hyponatraemia) or in potassium (e.g. hyperkalaemia), a decrease in ionized calcium or a decrease in magnesium, or alternatively a change in pH (e.g. alkalosis) may all result in spontaneous depolarization and firing of the neurone without cell body stimulation. This may occur at all levels of the central nervous system causing tetany, release of primitive reflexes, extensor hypertonus or convulsions.

The excitability of the neurone is also controlled by the cartridge (c) which spirals around the apical dendrite. The reticular formation can act through this cartridge, switching on or off the neurone's response to stimulation of its other dendrites or the surface of the cell body. The reticular arousal system increases sensitivity of the neurone so that other stimuli may more easily trigger off discharge along the axon. The reticular inhibitory system will tend to damp down or switch off the response. The balance between arousal or inhibition can, therefore, vary the response of the cell to a given stimulus.

When there has been chronic damping of the reticular formation, e.g. due to endorphin receptor block by the chronic use of opiates or effect of barbiturate therapy, then sudden withdrawal of these will leave an imbalance with relative arousal and excitation. Sleep deprivation also accounts for similar changes in convulsive threshold.

Stimulation of inhibitory synapses on the surface of the cell, e.g. those utilizing gamma-aminobutyric acid (GABA) as their neurotransmitter, will also lessen the ease of depolarization of the cell. Factors which decrease GABA production such as vitamin B6 deficiency, may cause fits. Alternatively use of benzodiazepine drugs, GABA transaminase inhibitors, or gabinergic drugs mimicking the effects of stimulation of the GABA pathways will all increase the inhibition of the cell and decrease the likelihood of seizures and so are used as anticonvulsants.

Excitatory synapses from excitatory neurones, utilize glutamate or acetylcholine as their neurotransmitter. The metabolic pathways which remove endogenous ammonia do so by converting glutamate to glutamine. Owing to the metabolic relationship of glutamate (an excitator) to gamma-aminobutyric acid (an inhibitor) there exists a metabolic circuit controlling the balance of excitation of inhibition (Fig. 41.4). Excess of glutamine or ammonia tends to increase excitation of the cell. Ammonia may be raised in the premature infant with a high protein intake or associated with liver dysfunction after asphyxia as well as the genetic hyperammonaemias. A supply of energy for the cell derives from glucose and utilizes the formation of

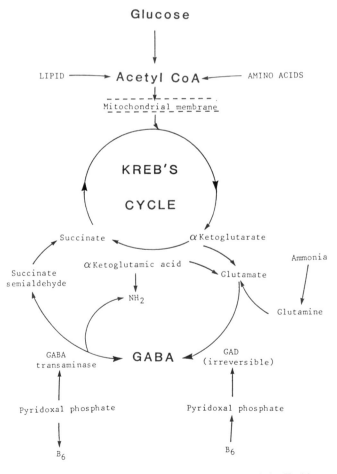

Fig. 41.4 The relationship between the GABA shunt and the Kreb's cycle. There is a close metabolic relationship between glutamate (an excitatory neurotransmitter) and GABA (an inhibitory neurotransmitter). GAD = glutamic acid dehydrogenase.

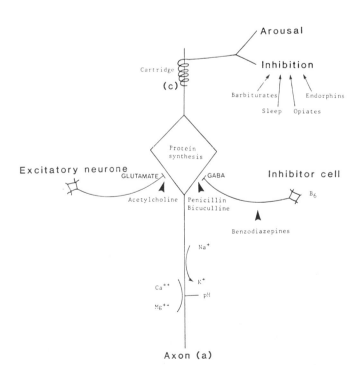

Fig. 41.3 Representation of a neurone showing the various ways that the cell may be excited to cause an electrical discharge (depalorization).

ATP. It is necessary to maintain depolarization of the cellular membranes and so keep the ionic pumps in working order. Failure to the system from hypoglycaemia or mild asphyxia may again lead to spontaneous depolarization of the cell and may cause fits.

From this brief description it can be seen that a vast number of conditions, e.g. sleep deprivation, barbiturate withdrawal, opiate withdrawal, hypoglycaemia, hypoxaemia, hypocalcaemia, hypomagnesaemia, hyponatraemia alkalosis, all result in seizures (Table 41.3). Isolation of a neurone from its neighbours (e.g. in an area of brain damage) can result in it firing in a tonic manner due to removal of inhibition or isolation of excitatory neurones.

Recruitment (the epileptic spike)

When a single neurone discharges, this is the equivalent of fibrillation potential in elecromyography and is not likely to cause any problems. A group of neurones must be recruited and fire together synchronously to produce an action potential which is a compound of a group of neurones firing together, i.e. the epileptic spike. If excitation is increased or there is loss of inhibition in a group of adjacent neurones within the same module in the cerebral cortex, they would tend to synchronize so that if one fires the whole unit may fire together, i.e. a sort of epileptic neuronal unit. Certain parts of the brain (e.g. the hippocampus) are more easily excited than others and certain parts of the cerebral cortex (e.g. the frontal lobes) are more likely to become epileptic than the parietal lobes.

Table 41.3 Possible mechanisms for epileptic discharges

Depolarization of the cell membrane
    Hypocalcaemia
    Hypomagnesaemia
    Hyponatraemia
    Alkalosis
    Hyperkalaemia

Reticular system
    Sleep deprivation
    Barbiturate withdrawal
    Heroin withdrawal
    Analeptics (nikethemide, xanthines)
    Postasphyxial hyperexcitable states

Neurotransmitter effects
    Inhibitory
        Vitamin B6 deficiency
        Vitamin B6 dependency
        Phenothiazine poisoning
    Excitatory
        Glutamate
        Acetylcholine
        Hyperammonaemia
        Experimental bicuculline
        Overdose of intrathecal penicillin

Energy supply
    Hypoxia
    Hypoglycaemia

Spread of the spike focus to cause a fit

A fit is the clinical manifestation of an electrical cerebral arrhythmia and may arise in two basic ways. First, local electrical excitation of part of the brain may result in symptoms as if that part of the brain were being stimulated. This is easy to appreciate in the focal clonic seizure affecting either face, arm or leg, when one sees on the EEG a rhythmically discharging spike focus at an identical frequency in the corresponding part of the brain to the clinical fit. In the older child this may result in disorders of speech, hallucinations, abnormal behaviour, or sensations. In the neonate, diagnosis is usually restricted to motor phenomena.

Should the focal epileptic discharge spread within the cerebral cortex (rather than local excitation of part of the brain) it may result in more extensive electrical paralysis. If the part of the brain so paralysed normally kept some lower centre inhibited, the loss of inhibition may result in release phenomena, e.g. release of primitive reflexes, abnormal muscle tone and behaviours. A tonic seizure can be regarded as release of midbrain decerebrate rigidity due to electrical paralysis of the cortical pathways, normally keeping it under control. The release of obligatory asymmetrical tonic neck reflexes, doggy paddling, cycling, mouthing, sucking, grimacing, adder tonguing, nystagmus, startle reflexes or Moro reflexes can be regarded in a similar way. These are due to release from inhibition and not due to stimulation of a part of the brain, so the origin of the ictal behaviour may be organized at a distance from the actual epileptic process, i.e. one may see brainstem phenomena as a result of cortical seizures, due to release of the brainstem from normal cortical control rather than epilepsy arising primarily in the stem itself.

This leads us to further considerations of how the electrical discharge spreads within the brain and why and how it stops. Spread within the cerebral cortex (i.e. the neocortex) is slow even in the mature infant and not more than 4 mm/s, so that there is a very slow Jacksonian march. Each module of the cerebreal cortex is connected with a mirror module on the opposite side via the corpus callosum. In the neonate, myelination has occurred initially in the leg area and, therefore, spread is easy from one vertex area to the other through the myelinated pathways via the corpus callosum. This is well demonstrated on the EEG when one may see a spike spreading from the vertex area of one side to the other. There is a very slow subsequent spread down to the hand and mouth area so that one may clinically see a visible time lag.

There are two other methods of spread, firstly, the cerebral cortex (neocortex) but not the temporal lobe (archicortex) is connected in a specific manner to the various thalamic nuclei. It is thought that the genetic tendency to spread and synchronize at 3 c/s involves these thalamic circuits. It does not appear that this genetic predisposition applies in the newborn period, although it certainly plays a major role by the end of the first year in the genesis of febrile convulsions.

The other method of spread is from the archicortex, i.e. the temporal lobe through the limbic system and then via connections to the reticular formation, so that any discharge would tend to occur into the limbic or reticular formation producing loss of consciousness or awareness and cognitive change; generalization would then occur to the neocortex via the reticular formation.

The only supportive information about spread within the cortex in the newborn period is that it does appear to occur and is slow. It is also apparent that genetic factors important in later epilepsy are not important in the newborn, apart from spread of seizure discharge. Myelination of the white matter occurs to a particular part of the brain and corpus callosum, e.g. infants with the Aicardi syndrome may have fits or hypsarrhythmia occurring independently within the two hemispheres.

The concept of 'kindling' also deserves mention. That is to say that if a part of the cerebral cortex receives a constant bombardment of electrical activity from discharging neurones on the opposite side; this may eventually result in a new independent focus being kindled. It would appear, therefore, that if an area of cortex is constantly activated by a discharge from neurones elsewhere within the brain this results in a lowered threshold, i.e. an increased excitation of what was otherwise a normal part of the brain. This is the rationale for the prophylactic use of anticonvulsants; if one seizure has occurred then the brain is more susceptible to a seizure, whilst if seizure activity can be controlled then the threshold rises so that hopefully seizures are less likely to arise spontaneously. We do not know why a fit once started does not continue indefinitely. There appears to be a system within the brain whereby it can 'shut down' to stop all excess electrical activity and this can be seen on PET scans as a spreading wave of inhibition. Failure of this mechanism would result in status epilepticus.

ANATOMICAL BRAIN DEVELOPMENT

The difference in the external appearance of the brain between the premature and the newborn infant is a gross demonstration of the rate of anatomical brain maturation. The brain at birth in the full-term neonate weighs around 340 g and at 4 years, 1340 g, showing that there is continued rapid growth in the postnatal period. Birth being a variable event between 26 and 43 weeks of gestation, means that the stage of brain maturation at birth can be very different and this accounts for differences in the clinical type of seizure, the EEG changes associated with a seizure and the convulsive threshold, i.e. the ease with which a given aetiology produces a fit. The neurological examination also

varies, so that one cannot talk in terms of the typical 'neurological examination of the newborn' (see Ch. 3).

The spread of the epileptic discharge within the brain also depends upon the stage of anatomical maturation and this is discussed in detail in Part 1 of this book. In summary, by the end of the first trimester the cerebral cortex is very thin and consists of a layer of undifferentiated neuroblasts which have migrated from deeper structures. In the second trimester the cortex expands and the gyral pattern of the brain becomes more apparent instead of the smooth outer surface of the premature baby. Neurones and glia are now differentiated, the cortex assumes its six layers and long pathways are developed. By full-term some myelination beings in the leg area and the occipital cortex. This functional and anatomical development permits extension of the epileptic discharge and an example of this is the vertex spread with progressive myelination.

If development is arrested at the stage of cell division or migration then the cerebral cortex may have an abnormal architecture and groups of cells that have not completed their migration may be found in the future white matter i.e. heterotopia. If the cells differentiate and become electrically active but are not connected to the normal excitatory and inhibitory pathways, then they may act as a source of epileptic activity. The cells in heterotopic positions may also take on neoplastic change. This is seen particularly in tuberosclerosis, Von Recklinghausen's disease, fetal alcohol syndrome and Zellweger's syndrome.

THE EFFECTS OF NEONATAL SEIZURES

The effect of a seizure can be considered under three main headings — the effect on the cell, the effect on the organ and the effect on the organism.

Effects at the cell level

Discharging neurones require energy to sustain the discharge which depends in the first instance upon the cell's energy supply from the production of ATP. One would, therefore, postulate an increase in glucose consumption, oxygen consumption and lactic acid production, together with a rise in intracellular sodium and an increase in extracellular potassium. Local ammonia concentration rises and ammonia concentration can be regarded as a good indicator of the adequacy of mitochondrial function. Plum's group has confirmed these postulates and found that brain oxidative metabolism increased by some 300–400% and that lactate rose within brain cells during experimentally induced seizures (Beresford et al 1969). There is a decrease in the concentration of ATP and high-energy phosphate (i.e. of phosphocreatinine) together with a corresponding increase in the amount of ADP. The increase in ADP results in stimulation of glycolysis at the phosphofructokinase step that is converting glucose to pyruvate and it also acts on NAD to form NADH. These metabolic changes can be studied using PET scanning or magnetic resonance spectroscopy (see Section 5) which allows us to look at glucose and oxygen consumption as well as intracellular compounds such as ADP, ATP, phosphoethanolamine and phosphocreatine in the intact human infant brain.

Apart from the effect of a fit on energy metabolism of the cell, it has been increasingly recognized that there is also a profound effect upon protein metabolism. Dwyer et al 1986 have found that both generalized and focal seizures dissociate brain polyribosomes and severely inhibit brain protein synthesis in experimental animals. Nissl is reduced after a period of epileptic discharge of a neurone. Cyclic AMP rises and may in turn interfere with protein synthesis so that RNA is significantly reduced, there is ribosome breakdown and protein synthesis stops. DNA synthesis is also inhibited and it is felt that this may have an effect upon brain development in the rapidly growing brain when active mitosis and protein synthesis is so important (Wasterlain 1978). Cyclic guanine monophosphate is also increased in the brain during seizures, as is cyclic AMP. Cyclic GMP encourages maintenance of a fit.

Immature rats receiving supramaximal electrical seizures can be shown to have a significant reduction in brain weight and cell numbers. Animals who convulse between the 9th and 18th day of life undergo a reduction in birth weight, brain protein and brain RNA content without a fall in the brain DNA. The largely non-miotic brain of older animals shows no such changes in brain weight as a result of induced fits. This has led to the concept that the immature brain may be more vulnerable to damage from severe seizures than the non-growing brain of the older animals.

Damage to neurones can theoretically occur in several ways.

1. If a cell continues to be excited (e.g. from glutamate) this results in an increase in energy demands. If this cannot be met then permanent cell damage may occur (excitotoxicity).
2. Owing to consumptive asphyxia when the oxygen supply to the cell fails to meet demand there is marked intracellular acidosis and rupture of lysosomes, causing autodigestion.
3. There may be production of free radicals (e.g. epoxides) which cause cell damage.
4. Blockage of protein synthesis occurs and, therefore, of production of essential enzymes within the cell.
5. Membrane leak of extracellular calcium into the cell may disrupt metabolism.

Effects at organ level

The increased production of lactate and CO_2 results in a local increase in blood flow and regional cerebral vasodilatation. This enables an increased supply of blood containing oxygen, glucose and nutrients to reach the metabolically hyperactive part of the epileptic brain. Maintenance of circulation is essential to remove lactate and prevent very severe acidosis as well as providing nutrients to sustain the energy demand. The cells must also be able to get rid of metabolic water produced from glycolysis, otherwise cellular oedema results. Local damage to the vascular endothelium from anoxia and ischaemia encourages the development of vasogenic oedema. If brain swelling as a result of this oedema continues, it will cause a rise in intracranial pressure which can in turn diminish cerebral blood flow and so establish a vicious circle, producing progressive anoxic–ischaemic brain damage (Minns & Brown 1978).

Effects at organismal level

A fit is usually accompanied by a massive sympathetic discharge ('sympathetic storm') which stimulates glycogenolysis and, therefore, the maintenance of blood sugar by the breakdown of liver glycogen. Cardiac output is increased, blood pressure is increased (Lou & Friis-Hansen 1979) and this, along with the local metabolic effects of the seizure within the brain, allows the massive increase in cerebral perfusion which is necessary to compensate for seizure activity. If there is ongoing muscle activity due to muscle contraction (either from tonic or clonic seizures) then competition for oxygen and blood flow occurs between brain and muscle. The muscle also produces large quantities of lactic acid. If the seizure continues unabated, eventually, the oxygen demands of brain and muscle, together with increasing acidosis, result in decompensation. In the compensated phase, the cerebral metabolic rate for oxygen and glucose is increased 2–3 fold (Meldrum 1978) and the cerebro–arterio–venous difference for oxygen is maintained; if decompensation occurs this difference increases. With the development of cerebral oedema together with the effects of hypoxia and hyperkalaemia on the myocardium, causing a fall in blood pressure together with the low P_{a,O_2}, metabolic acidosis and eventually depletion of liver glycogen with hypoglycaemia, severe brain and other tissue damage results. This may be measured as a rise in creatinine phosphokinase from muscle, a rise in transaminase enzymes from liver and increasing lactate and hypoxanthine in the CSF.

It will be apparent that seizure activity may, therefore, result in damage to focal areas of neurones due to the effects on protein metabolism and energy supply, to selective areas of brain from consumptive asphyxia or the development of cerebral oedema, and to the whole brain when the infant reaches the stage of decompensation. In the child, towards the end of the first year of life, it would appear that, seizures lasting more than 20 minutes are associated with signs of decompensation. In the neonate the physiological mechanisms to withstand asphyxia are better-developed having been prepared for the physiological asphyxia which occurs during normal delivery. The brain is able to utilize ketone bodies and also has a better supply of intracellular glycogen than in the older child. However, we have no reason to believe that the newborn is better able to withstand status epilepticus without damage than the older infant.

AETIOLOGY OF NEONATAL FITS

Fits in the newborn are for all practical purposes always symptomatic of some underlying disease rather than due to a genetic predisposition of a low convulsive threshold. (Hopkins 1972, Brown 1973, Dennis 1978, Levene & Trounce 1986). Often several factors interact, e.g. a disease state, genetic predisposition, the stage of maturation of the brain and biological rhythms; these will all determine if and when a fit occurs. The number of possible causes embraces the whole of neonatal medicine. The more common conditions are listed in Table 41.4, and their frequency shown in Table 41.5.

Genetic factors

The dominantly inherited tendency to synchronize and generalize at 3 c/s is important in febrile convulsions, petit mal and some of the idiopathic epilepsies but does not appear to operate in the newborn period. There is a relatively rare genetic syndrome of dominantly inherited benign familial neonatal fits in which parents and grandparents will usually give a history of fits confined to the neonatal period occurring mostly on the 2nd and 3rd day of life. There may be one, two or scores of fits lasting for the first few weeks of life which subsequently frequently disappear with normal psychomotor development. In approximately 14% of cases epilepsy develops later either in infancy, childhood or adulthood (Plovin 1985). In these infants all biochemical tests and imaging are normal.

A family history of neonatal seizures may be due to transmission of an autosomal recessive metabolic disease such galactosaemia, maple syrup urine disease or one of

Table 41.4 The major cause of convulsions in the first month of life

Asphyxia

Metabolic
  Alkalosis
  Hypocalcaemia
  Hypomagnesaemia
  Hypoglycaemia
  Hyponatraemia
  Water intoxication
  Neurodegenerative conditions (see Ch. 40)
  Hypernatraemia
  Hyperbilirubinaemia
  Pyridoxine dependency
  Galactosaemia
  Amino acidurias (Ch. 39)
  Organic acidurias (Ch. 39)

Intracranial haemorrhage (see Section 8)

Infections
  Bacterial and fungal (see Ch. 37)
  Viral and protozoal (see Ch. 36)

Genetic
  Familial neonatal convulsions
  Neurodermatoses (neurofibromatosis, incontinentia pigmentii, tuberose sclerosis)
  Chromosomal abnormalities
  Congenital cerebral malformations and dysplasias (see Ch. 19)
  Alper's cortical degeneration of infancy
  Neurodegenerative disorders (see Ch. 40)

Miscellaneous
  'Fifth day fits'
  Compression head injury without haemorrhage
  Fetal alcohol syndrome
  Ectodermal dysplasia with hyperpyrexia
  Drugs, (opiates, nikethamide, xanthines, cycloserine, phenothiazines, lignocaine)
  Narcotic withdrawal
  Neoplasms and cysts

the organic acidurias, such as proprionic acidurias. Structural defects may be transmitted by autosomal dominant inheritance, e.g. tuberosclerosis or Von Recklinghausen's disease. A disorder which occurs in several members of a family is not necessarily genetic, i.e. familial incidence may be due to an abnormal intra-uterine environment. This is seen in fetal alcohol syndrome and the infants of mothers who are narcotic addicts or who themselves suffer from

Table 41.5 Causes of fits in the neonatal period (%)

Cause	Brown 1973 ($n = 65$)	Brown 1980 ($n = 61$)	Painter 1981 ($n = 77$)	Ment 1982 ($n = 116$)	Dennis 1978 ($n = 56$)
Asphyxia	35	40	56	32	} 46
Intracranial haemorrhage	32	31	23	33	
Infection	17	10	3	11	10
Metabolic	10[a]	5[b]	0	6	40[c]
Malformation	6	5	0	5	16
Idiopathic	0	6.5	16.5	3	10
Other	0	0.5	1.5	10	0

[a]Excluding 75 cases of hypocalcaemia; [b]excluding 38 cases of hypocalcaemia; [c]including 14 cases of hypocalcaemia, i.e. neonatal tetany. Secondary metabolic disturbances classed according to primary cause.

phenylketonuria (Zelson et al 1971, Desmond et al 1972). Some genetic disorders which causes brain damage have an intermediary mechanism and are, therefore, potentially amenable to therapy. In this group one must include not only galactosaemia, maple syrup urine disease and phenylketonuria but also rhesus immunization with the risk of hyperbilirubinaemia and kernicterus.

Hypoxic–ischaemic encephalopathy

The problems of perinatal asphyxia are considered in detail in Chapter 9. Because of the difficulty in defining asphyxia in simple terms relating to obstetrics, biochemistry or neonatal behaviour we have found the concept of symptomatic neonatal asphyxia useful in clinical practice. One should not use an Apgar score alone as an indication of asphyxia. It does not correlate with oxygen saturation in the blood and it may be influenced by maternal factors (e.g. drugs or acidosis). The fetus has a 'built-in' physiological compensatory mechanism to allow it to withstand the 'normal' degree of hypoxia at birth, so that placental insufficiency, cord prolapse or fetal distress need not necessarily result in any significant damage to the baby. We have already stressed that the infant has a limited repertoire of signs and symptoms with which he can manifest CNS disease and so one cannot take any type of abnormal behaviour in the newborn period as being specific for asphyxia. Conditions such as the infant of the mother with dystrophia myotonica or the Prader Willi syndrome may not show normal intra-uterine movements and are therefore more likely to be delivered by breech. There may then be problems at birth; the baby can be flat at birth and is neurologically abnormal but the difficulties all relate to his prenatal disease.

For these reasons we accept a diagnosis of 'symptomatic neonatal asphyxia' depending on three parameters.

1. A condition in the mother, or complications of pregnancy, likely to cause asphyxia in the fetus.
2. A measured parameter to show that asphyxia is present.
3. Abnormal behaviour or result of investigations in the newborn period to show that cerebral asphyxia was present.

If one defines asphyxia purely by means of an Apgar score or the need for resuscitation by endotracheal intubation and artificial ventilation, then up to 50/1000 would be regarded as asphyxiated, only 10% of infants defined in these terms will subsequently have any symptoms to suggest that they have suffered from any significant 'cerebral asphyxia'. About 3 infants out of every 1000 deliveries will have a fit attributable to asphyxia, i.e. about 50% of infants with symptomatic neonatal asphyxia will have a fit (Brown 1976), compared with only 6% if one defines asphyxia on the basis of Apgar score or intubation alone.

The fits may be of any type — tonic, clonic, or myoclonic. Tonic fits are particularly common in the first 24 hours when the infant has decreased conscious level and is hypotonic, with bulbar palsy and varying degrees of ophthalmoplegia. As extensor hypertonus begins to appear with hyperventilation and jitteriness, the clonic type of seizure becomes more common.

Complications of asphyxia, such as hypocalcaemia, hyponatraemia and hypoglycaemia, may also trigger fits. Tonic fits appearing in the first 24 hours of life have prognostic significance at the $P<0.01$ level in relation to long-term handicap, whilst clonic fits in the second 24 hours do not have prognostic significance. Of seizures associated with perinatal asphyxia, 90% occur in the first 72 hours.

Intracranial haemorrhage

Bleeding into the perinatal brain is a common event and the various types of intracranial haemorrhage are discussed in Section 8. Seizures may occur as a result of any type of bleed. Tonic seizures associated with intraventricular haemorrhage may be due to a true fit or may be due to fluctuating intracranial pressure changes with a structural decerebration. Recent studies of infants with fits have shown that primary intracerebral haemorrhage is not as rare as was previously diagnosed when relying on postmortem studies. In some cases these may be due to microvascular malformations but in other cases represent haemorrhage into an infarct possibly secondary to a placental embolus (perinatal stroke p. 334). A fit may be the sole presentation in the neonate of an intracerebral bleed.

Infection

Infection as a cause of a fit can be due to infection in utero or postnatal infection. Meningitis due to E. coli (Berman & Banker 1966), group B streptococci (Barton et al 1973) or listeria monocytogenes may be present at birth or some time during the neonatal period. Infants with bacterial septicaemia may develop a cortical thrombophlebitis which again may present with fits. Virus infections in utero, e.g. with rubella (Peckham 1972), cytomegalovirus (Hanshaw 1971), herpes simplex and HIV infection, may cause an illness presenting with fits in the neonatal period. Alternatively, virus infection acquired at the end of pregnancy as occurs with echovirus 11 may also result in an acute viral encephalitis. Transplacentally acquired toxoplasmosis may also present as neonatal fits.

Gastroenteritis in the neonatal period can be associated with fits due to a wide variety of different mechanisms, e.g. Salmonella infection may be associated with a neonatal Salmonella meningitis, which can be particularly intractable and associated with hydrocephalus. Certain organisms such as Campylobacter and Shigella produce neurotoxins which themselves may cause a toxic encephalopathy. Dehydration may cause hyperviscosity syndromes with venous thrombosis. Secondary metabolic disturbances may show as hyponatraemia, hypernatraemia, hypomagnesaemia, hypokalaemia and hypocalcaemia. This emphasizes how one must be aware of different mechanisms whereby a fit can occur in association with an infection.

Metabolic disease

Hyponatraemia due to water intoxication from inappropriate secretion of antidiuretic hormone is seen in any stressed infant but particularly those suffering from asphyxia, meningitis or septicaemia. True salt depletion causing hyponatraemia is seen in the various sorts of congenital adrenal hyperplasia. Hypernatraemia is most likely to occur due to injudicious use of sodium bicarbonate, confusion of salt and sugar, high sodium milks or hypernatraemic dehydration from gastroenteritis. Hypoglycaemia has many primary causes (disorders of glycogen metabolism, other inborn errors of metabolism, light for dates infants, infants of diabetic mothers etc.) but may also occur secondary to existing brain damage (complicating asphyxia, kernicterus, meningitis). Certain congenital malformations eg. septo-optic dysplasia or other causes of congenital hypopituitarism may also present with hypoglycaemia. Thus hypoglycaemia may cause brain damage or brain damage may cause hypoglycaemia. Disturbances of calcium metabolism were very common in the past, when up to half of all fits in the neonatal period were due to neonatal tetany. The modification of cows' milk formula to reduce the phosphate content has caused a dramatic reduction in primary hypocalcaemic fits. Calcium metabolism in the newborn has been extensively reviewed by Forfar (1976) and David & Annast (1974).

Hypocalcaemia

Hypocalcaemia will complicate any stressful condition such as severe asphyxia, respiratory distress syndrome, intra-uterine growth retardation, the infant of the diabetic mother, severe infection, artificial ventilation, or neonatal surgery (Robertson & Smith 1975). This type of hypocalcaemia is often referred to as early hypocalcaemia. It occurs in the first 24 hours of life and is associated with a normal or low phosphate concentration.

Hypoglycaemia may also result from certain diseases of calcium metabolism in the *mother* such as hypoparathyroidism, hyperparathyroidism, steatorrhoea, Phenytoin ingestion or Vitamin D deficiency, (Friis and Sardemann 1977) or diseases in the *infant*, such as the Di George syndrome, specific magnesium malabsorption syndrome (Skyberg ct al 1968), citrate-binding from exchange transfusion, or true hypoparathyroidism in the infant (Friedman & Hatcher 1967, Paunier et al 1965, Radde et al 1972). In these cases the hypocalcaemia is more prolonged and is

resistent to treatment. In all cases of neonatal hypocalcaemia maternal calcium and phosphorus concentrations should be measured.

The third type of hypocalcaemia consists of classical neonatal tetany. In a typical case, a normal, fully grown, mature infant, born at full-term, after an uneventful pregnancy and delivery shows an uneventful postnatal course until the fifth to seventh day of life. Then, and often during a feed, the mother notices a rhythmic, clonic movement of the face, arm and leg on one side. This may happen once or several hundred times. The infant is usually not distressed, unconscious or cyanosed as long as the fits remain unilateral. The infant is always on an artificial feed, and most frequently born in the spring months. Examination of the blood biochemistry confirms hypocalcaemia, hyperphosphataemia and hypomagnesaemia. CSF concentrations of calcium and magnesium are also significantly reduced. The infant is often stiff, extended and jittery but with a normal alert conscious state.

Various inborn errors of metabolism may present in the newborn period as fits, e.g. galactosaemia, certain organic acidurias (such as proprionic acidaemia, Vigevano et al 1982), disorders of amino acid metabolism (such as maple syrup urine disease) and D-glyceric acidaemia (Brandt et al 1974); certain types of glycogen storage disease may present in the newborn period with hypoglycaemia. (Grandgeorge et al 1980). Hyperammonaemia can also be incriminated in seizures and again this may result from several different disease processes, such as the inborn errors of metabolism (e.g. ornithine transcarbamalase deficiency (OTC) associated with parenteral nutrition), or be due to high-protein feeding in the presence of liver damage (e.g. in the small, pre-term infant or following severe asphyxia).

Pyridoxine deficiency (see also p. 467)

A rare cause of seizures, and one which deserves mention because it illustrates a basic disorder in brain metabolism, is the seizure disorder resulting from abnormalities in metabolism of pyridoxine, i.e. vitamin B6 (Minns 1986). Pyridoxine (or pyridoxol) specifically refers to 3-hydroxy-4, 5-bis(hydroxymethyl)-2-methylpyridine. Dietary vitamin B6 is largely metabolized to pyridoxol and the main urinary metabolite is 4-pyridoxic acid. Pyridoxine is involved in a vast number of enzyme reactions acting as co-enzyme. These include transaminations, decarboxylations, deaminations and other reactions involving brain amino acids, as well as being involved in lipid nucleic acid and glycogen metabolism. Pyridoxine may be deficient in the diet and one well-known infant feed was manufactured with insufficient pyridoxine content with resultant convulsions in the infants fed on the formula.

Excessive pyridoxine intake, e.g. if used to prevent vomiting, may then result in a relative deficiency in the infant with pyridoxine withdrawal. Certain drugs, such as isoniazid may interfere with the metabolism of pyridoxine. In the neonate pyridoxine deficiency is most likely to occur in infants fed on the formula containing insufficient pyridoxine. Normally there is six times the content of pyridoxine in cows milk that there is in breast milk. The placenta concentrates pyridoxine in the fetus compared with maternal blood concentrations. Vitamin B6 present in milk is, however, a heat-labile compound and can be depleted during the manufacturing process. Pyridoxal phosphate is required by the enzyme glutamic acid decarboxylase in the synthesis of gamma-aminobutyric acid (GABA). Deficiency of pyridoxine would, therefore, result in absence of the co-enzyme required for the synthesis of GABA and the subsequent depletion of GABA (which is the major inhibitory neurotransmitter), resulting in convulsions. In deficiency-states these convulsions will respond to physiological doses of pyridoxine.

There appears to be an inborn error of metabolism in which a much higher concentration of co-enzyme is required for the normal functioning of glutamic acid decarboxylase. This is a familial disorder in which fits may commence in utero and following delivery the infant is irritable with an intractable seizure disorder and abnormal EEG. Intravenous administration of pharmacological doses of vitamin B6 (e.g. 100 mg) results in rapid cessation of the seizures and restoration of the EEG to normality. The actual pool of pyridoxine in the body is normal in pyridoxine dependency and the only way to prove the diagnosis is by the therapeutic response to pharmacological doses of pyridoxine. Care must be taken, however, that resuscitation facilities are to hand as large doses of intravenous pyridoxine are not without hazard and occasionally profound hypotonia and weakness of respiratory muscles may result. It is believed that in pyridoxine deficiency there is a genetic defect with the binding of pyridoxine to its apoenzyme, glutamate decarboxylase. Bankier et al (1983) stress that many of these infants may appear to have been asphyxiated at birth and if one is not alert to the situation it is easy to regard the fits as due to intractable epilepsy secondary to intrapartum asphyxial brain damage. They recommend that a neonate with intractable seizures, even if there is well-documented birth asphyxia, should be given 100 mg of intravenous pyridoxine and be observed for 30 minutes. They accept that a response may take up to an hour but then seizures will disappear sometimes for several weeks before recurring.

Toxic causes

The classical toxic encephalopathy seen in the newborn period is that of bilirubin encephalopathy resulting in kernicterus (see p. 547). Endogenous toxins from liver failure, renal failure or inborn errors of metabolism may also cause fits as already described. Toxins may be produced in the gut, as for example in the case of *Shigella* and possibly *Campylobacter* infection. Exogenously administered toxins usually consist of the use of drugs, so that fits may occur in infants as a result of heroin addiction in the mother (Herzlinger et al 1977). Barbiturate withdrawal seizures may also occur if the mother has been taking barbiturates before delivery. The fetal alcohol syndrome (alcohol embryopathy) results in intra-uterine and postnatal growth retardation, microcephaly, craniofacial dysmorphism with other internal and external malformations and anomalies of genitalia. At least one-quarter will have abnormal EEGs and fits with hyperexcitability (Majewski 1985). Fits may also result from the use of lignocaine, as in paracervical block (O'Meara & Brazie 1968); the administration of analeptics, such as nikethamide; the use of morphine; overdosage with aminophylline used to prevent apnoeic attacks; and the use of certain drugs to terminate cardiac arrhythmias. Penicillin, if given in an overdose intrathecally, will cause severe intractable seizures, and occasionally cloxacillin necessary to treat ventriculitis in children with hydrocephalus may result in fits at the necessary therapeutic dosage.

Congenital malformations of the brain

Malformations of the central nervous system may consist of gross defects in organization such as holoprosencephaly, or the absence of parts of the brain such as cerebellar agenesis or agenesis of the corpus callosum. Agenesis of the corpus callosum may be associated with an intractable seizure disorder in the Aicardi syndrome. Suspicion of this is enhanced by the finding of colobomata of the retina and the diagnosis is less likely to be missed if cerebral ultrasound examination is made of all infants with convulsions. Destructive lesions such as porencephaly are associated with fits because of the mechanism of production, e.g. coalescence of cystic periventricular leukomalacia, extension of the subependymal bleed or liquefaction of an infarct from a perinatal stroke. Hydrocephalus is accompanied by seizures surprisingly infrequently if intracranial pressure is properly monitored and treated so that tonic decerebrate attacks are not confused with fits.

The most common cause of intractable seizures in the newborn period is that associated with cortical dysplasia. This may occur as part of a more generalized malformation such as holoprosencephaly or in association with occipital encephaloceles. Dysplasia of the cerebral cortex is also seen in fetal alcohol syndrome, Zellweger's syndrome, tuberose sclerosis, Von Recklinghausen's disease and chromosome disorder (e.g. 13 trisomy, 8 trisomy) but fits are uncommon in infants with Down's syndrome.

The fits associated with cortical dysplasia may occur in utero. They are often the most intractable of all the neonatal seizure disorders, becoming obvious within 24–48 hours of birth. They are associated with severe anticonvulsant resistance and often eventually merge into one of the other epileptic syndromes of the young infant and child, i.e. early or neonatal myoclonic encephalopathy, Otahara syndrome, West's syndrome and eventually the Lennox–Gastaut syndrome. The presence of cortical dysplasia may be suspected by an abnormality of the eye, since the retina is derived from the optic vesicle and outgrowth of the primitive brain. Eye abnormalities may range from coloboma, or phakomata to anophthalmia as seen for example in the Aicardi syndrome, tuberose sclerosis and neurofibromatosis.

Early myoclonic encephalopathy has its onset in the neonatal period and consists of fragmentary or massive myoclonus, partial motor seizures or infantile spasms. The EEG shows a prehypsarrhythmic pattern evolving to atypical hypsarrhythmia later. All these infants are neurologically abnormal and up to 50% die in infancy (Aicardi 1985). This condition should be seen as a syndrome due to pathological malformation within the CNS, as shown by abnormal neuronal migration, heterotopia, megalencephaly, etc. Differential diagnosis of a primary disorder of development of the cerebral cortex from a degenerative disorder (polio dystrophy) of early onset (acute infantile form) can be difficult. Seizures which may present in the newborn period can be due to infantile Gaucher's disease, Krabbe's leukodystrophy, Niemann–Pick disease and type 1 glycogenosis (see Ch. 40). Certain diseases such as incontinentia pigmenti may present as a transient vesicular rash in one infant or severe intractable fits with microcephaly and severe mental retardation at the other extreme. We do not know if this is a genetic disease with sex-linked dominant inheritance or due to intra-uterine infection. Another of the neurodermatoses, the Sturge–Weber syndrome, also falls into this group. Apart from the cortical dysplasia, there may be a progressive degeneration in the cerebral cortex with calcification. Much of the apparent progressive nature of the condition, in particular the onset of hemiplegia, is related to poorly controlled fits.

Miscellaneous

There is a group of disorders, some of which have a known aetiology others of which remain idiopathic, which may result in seizures of the newborn period. Ectodermal dysplasia can be associated with fits and with hyperpyrexia. Congenital neoplasms such as hamartomas, teratomas or congenital lipomas may be the source of intractable seizures. An entity which seems to be increasingly documented is that of so-called 'idiopathic fifth day fits' (benign ideopathic neonatal convulsions). These were first described from Australia, on moving to a new maternity hospital. Although abnormalities of zinc metabolism have been postulated no actual aetiology has been convincingly demonstrated in these infants; the circumstances suggested an environmental factor and the outcome is favourable.

INVESTIGATION OF THE INFANT WITH FITS

All infants who have fits in the newborn period should have certain investigations performed as a routine. Plasma glucose, calcium and magnesium should be measured, together with sodium, potassium and acid–base status. An ultrasound examination should nowadays be mandatory in all infants for evidence of infarction, intracranial haemorrhage, or malformation. If positive it may be used to be followed by CT or MRI scan. The question of lumbar puncture is more difficult, as certainly all infants who have an onset of seizures beyond 48 hours of life should have examination of the cerebrospinal fluid performed to exclude infection. Lumbar puncture will aid diagnosis of subarachnoid haemorrhage and assessment of the degree of asphyxia (by measuring lactate and hypoxanthine). In infants, the unfused sutures and readily expandable skull mean that there is not the same hazard from the lumbar puncture as in the older child.

In infants with unexplained seizures, a much wider list of investigations including estimation of plasma amino acids, examination of the urine for an organic aciduria and detailed investigation for intra-uterine infection with toxoplasma, rubella, cytomegalovirus, HIV and herpes simplex may be necessary. Recently Wyatt et al (1986) have used near-infrared spectrophotometry (NIR) for detecting abnormal responses in cerebral oxygenation and haemodynamics in sick newborns, especially with birth asphyxia.

Electro-encephalography in the newborn

The EEG can be recorded from scalp electrodes and displayed in real-time by the usual technique of 8- or 16-channel pen write-out. The size of the infants head means that 8 channels are usually sufficient in the neonatal period. The usual length of record in the older child is 20–30 minutes but all neonates should be recorded through at least one phase of sleep, i.e. 60 minutes. Alternatively, the EEG trace may be stored on tape over a prolonged period (24 hours or several hours) to include several periods of sleep. The EEG can be exhibited on a cathode ray oscilloscope as a continuous rhythm strip (Eyre 1983) in infants suspected of having status epilepticus, non-convulsive status, or used to monitor the effects of drugs. This can be combined with a continuous Fourier or Berg analysis of the waveform which is then written as an analysis of the waves from the right and left sides of the brain. More recently computerized colour scans of the EEG activity can be produced (brain mapping). The use of CFM (cerebral function monitor) may be particularly useful in prolonged monitoring of 'silent seizures' (Hellstrom-Westas et al 1985). The electro-encephalogram is useful in localizing the origin of seizures and in proving that odd behaviours are of ictal origin. EEG techniques, particularly continuous monitoring, are discussed in detail in Chapter 13.

Interpretation of EEG

The record is scanned overall for an assessment of the background activity in relation to maturity of the infant as discussed in Chapter 13. Any asymmetry of background must be gross, as mild asymmetries are common. Episodic sleep activity may not be synchronous and is often asymmetrical. Short runs of asymmetrical theta or delta rhythms which would be significant in the older child do not have the same significance. Sleep spindles are not well developed but quasi-spindling may be misinterpreted as epileptic. Persistent flattening in an area of dead brain, as for example following infarction or in the presence of brain abcess, does show in the neonatal period. Persisting slow wave foci also occur over areas of infarction.

The full-term infant is less difficult to interpret than the pre-term infant in that by full-term the brain can produce well-differentiated spikes or spike and wave activity. The spikes may consist of a single spike and wave or be polyphasic and may show PLEDS (paroxysmal lateralizing epileptic discharges) or classical phase reversal. Spikes may be single or rhythmic at 1 or 3 c/s and can certainly change from one frequency to another during a seizure. Spikes last less than 60 microseconds and reach an amplitude of 300 volts. If the discharge spreads, it does so within the same hemisphere and then from one vertex to the opposite vertex (Fig. 41.5). Mirror spread from temporal lobe to temporal lobe is not seen. Spikes may arise at random from all parts of the hemisphere and from both hemispheres (Fig. 41.6) and a picture of hypsarrhythmia can be seen even with relatively benign conditions such as severe hypocalcaemia. The discharge is often extremely 'pulsed' and is synchronous in all leads. When a convulsion is focal, the spike focus is always over the corresponding area of brain and at the

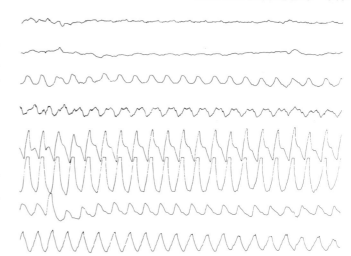

Fig. 41.6 Generalized spike and wave epileptic discharge with random spikes.

same frequency. If the electrodes are placed slightly distant to the focus it appears more blunted and M-shaped.

Epileptic foci appear to arise more commonly in the right hemisphere (76%) than the left hemisphere (24%). Although a fit can be accompanied by runs of slow waves (Fig. 41.7), single spike asymmetry, or immaturity of the EEG, these form a less secure basis for the diagnosis that the episodes are epileptic than the classical spike. In a group of infants with hypocalcaemia recorded some years ago, we studied 53 infants who had fits during EEG monitoring and no single infant had a clonic seizure without this being accompanied by a cortical spike.

In infants with fits due to asphyxia or birth injury, 54 recordings done as soon as possible after the indexed seizure, showed that 40% had an epileptic record of spikes.

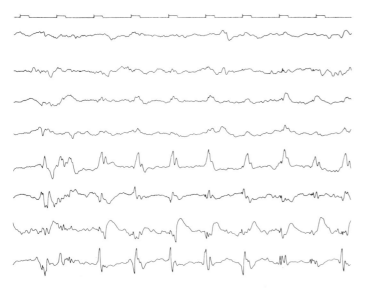

Fig. 41.5 A focal epileptic discharge of 1 c/s arising in the left hemisphere and spreading from left to right vertex with a slow wave component but little other spread within the right hemisphere.

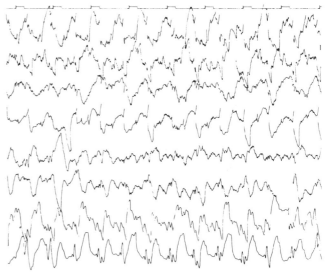

Fig. 41.7 A regular pulsed epileptic discharge of slow waves rather than spikes.

The resting record is more often abnormal in the asphyxiated infant and may be abnormally flat or show asymmetries and paroxysmal theta rhythms. Tonic fits may occur with a spike discharge, a flat EEG or large-amplitude slow waves. Sudden paroxysmal behaviour changes such as cylcing, or sucking are more often accompanied by slow waves than spikes. Sudden cessation of respiration can be accompanied by focal cortical discharge, slow waves or spikes and we have also seen sudden paroxysms of deep hyperventilation accompanied by focal spikes and generalized slow waves. Records have confirmed that lip smacking, sucking, opening and closing one eye, rapid respiration, cessation of respiration, hyperventilation, tongue protrusion, cycling and an assumption of the tonic neck pattern may all occur as ictal episodes in a brain-damaged baby with corresponding paroxysmal changes in the EEG. Multifocal asynchronous spikes have also been seen accompanying a central type of 'jitter'. Runs of faster (alpha fits) are also seen when there is a rhythmic run at 6–10 hertz.

The EEG on the first day of life in the full-term infant is a useful indicator of early cerebral injury (Pezzani et al 1986). However, the EEG is not recommended as a good prognostic tool as it may show gross abnormalities in relatively benign biochemical disorders and appear unremarkable in the presence of severe asphyxia. If one takes infants with asphyxia and then uses the EEG to help prognosis this is slightly better than taking a number of random EEGs and trying to prognosticate from blind analysis of the record. If the interictal EEG shows a very flat record or persisting burst suppression or multifocal seizure discharge of more than 10 seconds with abnormal background activity (Amiel-Tison & Ellison 1986, Holmes et al 1982) this has a bad prognosis; it may merge into the Otahara syndrome.

MANAGEMENT OF THE INFANT WITH FITS

General management

The infant will in many cases be seriously ill from the condition of which the fits are a symptom (e.g. birth trauma, asphyxia, septicaemia, meningitis or certain metabolic diseases) and many are immature of very-low-birth-weight. It is more convenient to nurse all infants with fits in an incubator, without clothes, so that fits are easily witnessed and the number and type recorded. An apnoea mattress is desirable as apnoea may occur in many of the conditions which give rise to fits, as well as being the clinical presentation of a fit. Blood gas and acid–base state should be monitored in all ill infants or if the fits are accompanied by apnoea or cyanosis. Hypoxaemia can occur in many acute neurological diseases without frank respiratory failure (i.e. normal P_{a,CO_2}).

The brain requires more energy to sustain a fit. Failure to supply adequate oxygen can result in a consumptive asphyxia. An increased FiO_2 is required in any prolonged fit. Blood glucose should be monitored 4 hourly (by dextrostix) in all seizures since hypoglycaemia not only causes fits but recurrent seizures may cause hyper- or hypoglycaemia. Experimental evidence from newborn animals has shown that glucose given before seizures reduces the chance of brain damage (Wasterlain & Duffy 1975). The importance of monitoring serum calcium and magnesium in all neonatal fits has already been indicated.

Cerebral oedema can complicate birth trauma, asphyxia, infections and some inborn errors of metabolism and these cases may need treatment by fluid restriction, mannitol or dexamethasone. The neonate with a severe brain insult is incapable of excreting a water load due to either inappropriate ADH secretion or simple water intoxication from excess intravenous fluids, and dilution hyponatraemia may occur. Fluids should be restricted to 60% of maintenance requirements in the acute stage of convulsive illness in the absence of dehydration. Body temperature may vary in both directions, hypothermia is seen in many of the diseases which cause fits, recurrent fits may swing this in the opposite direction causing hyperthermia and the asphyxiated infant can be poikilothermic. A thermocouple feedback to the incubator is necessary.

Treatment of fits can be considered as specific when there is a single therapeutic agent which is used to reverse a specific metabolic deficiency, i.e. glucose, calcium, magnesium, pyridoxine; or non-specific when anticonvulsants such as phenobarbitone, phenytoin or benzodiazepines, are indicated.

Specific treatment of fits

Glucose

Hypoglycaemia should be anticipated in 'at risk' groups of infants such as pre-term and small-for-dates infants, infants of diabetic mothers, and those with severe rhesus disease or symptomatic asphyxia. Routine blood glucose estimations should be commenced at birth and repeated every 4 hours using the dextrostix method on blood obtained by heel prick (Chantler et al 1967). Every infant with a fit should have a check dextrostix at the time of the fit and a fasting blood glucose performed later if it is not satisfactory so as not to miss cases of reactive hypoglycaemia. If hypoglycaemia is present it should be terminated by an intravenous bolus of glucose 20% (0.5–1.0 g/kg body weight i.e. 2–4 ml/kg 20%, or 1–2 ml 50%) followed by glucose–electrolyte solution to prevent recurrence. If the blood glucose concentration is raised above the renal tubular capacity to excrete it, an osmotic diuresis can cause serious dehydration in small infants.

If hypoglycaemia persists, detailed investigation of insulin concentration, lactate, alanine and urine for ketone bodies is needed. Hypoglycaemia in an infant of a diabetic mother may have a poor prognosis unless diagnosed and treated promptly (Holden & Freeman 1975).

Calcium

Prevention is the ideal by ensuring that mothers get an adequate supply of vitamin D during pregnancy (at least 800 units per day) and that the infants do not have their parathyroid function stressed by having to try and cope with a high phosphate load from an unmodified milk. In the case of simple uncomplicated neonatal tetany, the infant should first of all be placed on a modified milk if not already taking one. Oral calcium is difficult to administer since susbtances such as calcium chloride with readily available ionic calcium can cause severe bowel upset with blood in the stool. This could lead to a misdiagnosis of necrotizing enterocolitis. It is usual to use the less-irritant but less-effective calcium gluconate (5–10 ml before each feed).

The use of intravenous injections of calcium gluconate are usually ineffective, short-lived, and not without danger. Intravenous calcium should only be given when fits are severe, recurrent and associated with chronic hypocalcaemia. If indicated it should be given under ECG control as bradycardia, P-wave inversion or very erratic sinus activity may occur. The serum calcium is rarely significantly elevated 30 minutes after a single intravenous injection.

In the case of early hypocalcaemia (usually with a normal or low phosphate), associated with asphyxia, small-for-dates infants or mechanical ventilation, electrolyte fluid balance and correction of hypocalcaemia is usually sufficient; oral calcium supplements are occasionally necessary.

Magnesium

The difficulties encountered with calcium administration mean that the more general acceptance of the use of magnesium has greatly helped the therapeutic problem (Cockburn et al 1973). Two injections of 50% magnesium sulphate are given by intramuscular injection in a dose of 0.2 mg/kg. This dose should not be repeated until the calcium and magnesium concentrations have been remeasured, as hypermagnesaemia has a curare-like effect and produces a floppy infant (reversed by giving calcium). In most cases two doses of intramuscular magnesium are all that is required, especially as cases now tend to be milder since most infants are fed on modified milks. Magnesium has been shown to be more effective than oral calcium or phenobarbitone in neonatal tetanic convulsions (Turner 1974). Magnesium is necessary for calcium absorption and the serum calcium rises as a result of the magnesium therapy (Cockburn et al 1973).

Pyridoxine

In pyridoxine-dependency there is no immediate test which is of help, such as plasma pyridoxal phosphate, tryptophan loading tests. In practice it is therefore more usual to try a therapeutic trial of the vitamin. This needs to be done under continuous EEG monitoring. The dosage should be large — at least 50–100 mg given intravenously or intramuscularly. The response is usually dramatic and resuscitation facilities must be at hand in case of the rare side-effect of severe hypotonia and respiratory embarrassment.

Pyridoxine-deficiency is very rare in the neonatal period when smaller physiological doses of pyridoxine such as 5.0 mg are used. It is thought that the normal full-term infant requires about 0.2 mg pyridoxine per day and with an intake below 0.1 mg fits may occur. Breast milk is not rich in pyridoxine but contains well above the minimum in a normal 24-hour feed volume. Cows milk is relatively rich with more than twice the amount found in breast milk. Pyridoxine can, however, be destroyed in certain heat processes used in making milk for artificial feeding. In these cases pyridoxal phosphate concentrations in the plasma are low and tryptophan load tests are abnormal.

Pyridoxine is also used therapeutically in certain inborn errors of metabolism such as homocystinuria and cystathioninuria. Pyridoxine needs to be continued indefinitely in infants with pyridoxine-dependency and the inborn errors.

ANTICONVULSANT TREATMENT OF NON-SPECIFIC FITS

Before considering the individual anticonvulsant drugs used in the neonatal period it is necessary to consider some of the pharmacological and pharmacokinetic principles which distinguish the neonate from the older child. For any drug we need to consider several variables: pharmaceutical preparation, mode of administration, dose, absorption, protein binding, distribution, tissue penetration, metabolism and excretion.

Pharmaceutical preparation

Oral preparations must of necessity be in liquid form and this may pose problems; for example, phenobarbitone and benzodiazepines may not be stable in solution. Phenobarbitone is available in the commercial form as phenobarbitone elixir BP, which has an alcohol base sufficiently concentrated to render the preparation inflammable. Parenteral preparations such as phenytoin are very irritant and alkaline and, if they extravasate into the tissues when given intravenously, may cause wide tissue necrosis. If given into umbilical vessels there is a danger of provoking arterial spasm. Benzodiazepines show a great affinity for plastic given in intravenous infusion; most of the drug may adhere to the plastic in the drip set.

Mode of administration

Intramuscular injection in the infant is not reliable.

In many cases the thickness of subcutaneous fat means that intramuscular injections are given subcutaneously. Absorption is correspondingly poorer and there is a risk of localized tissue necrosis with ulceration, as with the use of paraldehyde and phenytoin. The upper quadrant of the buttock is not safe in the neonate, as the sciatic nerve may show a variable course and injections (particularly of paraldehyde) may result in sciatic nerve palsy. The intravenous route is the most commonly used route for initiating therapy in order to administer loading doses, followed by oral maintenance therapy.

Dosage

After a decision has been made to commence treatment with an anticonvulsant drug and the most appropriate drug has been chosen, one has to decide how much, how often and for how long. Dosages in the neonatal period are rarely arrived at in a scientific way, by in-depth study of the pharmacology and pharmacokinetics of the drug. There is a tendency either to scale down the adult dose and change it into a mg/kg equivalent, or to wait until the first paper is published and the drug firm then adopts the recommended dosage. The result has been that, with many substances used in the neonatal period, dosages have varied by as much as 100% between the initial use of the drug and it becoming established in clinical practice. Because of the widely varying pharmacokinetics between different newborn infants, the only certain way of assessing dosage of a drug is to monitor the blood level. Any drug that is potentially toxic, such as the aminoglycoside antibiotics, aminophylline, digoxin or anticonvulsant drugs, should be monitored by regular assay of plasma concentration.

The rate of metabolism of drugs varies, so that one may need to give benzodiazepine drugs very regularly throughout the 24 hours, whilst phenobarbitone may be given (when in a steady state) once per day. It is more usual to divide the dose of most anticonvulsant drugs to at least twice daily, as the peak levels from acute absorption may present with toxic effects in the neonate, e.g. a large dose of barbiturate may depress respiration or prevent the infant from breast feeding.

The duration of therapy depends upon the condition being treated. For example, an infant who has had fits due to perinatal asphyxia rarely has seizures after the fifth day of life. This is because the infant has in effect an acute arrhythmia, rather than a chronic epilepsy. It is usual therefore to tail off the anticonvulsants after 3 weeks of treatment. Infants with fits due to cortical dysplasia may require continued therapy from the neonatal period throughout the whole of childhood as they have in effect an intractable neonatal epilepsy.

Absorption

Gastric-emptying time and intestinal transit times vary between different infants and may depend in part upon the type of feed. The infant who has been parenterally fed may for a period have a temporary steatorrhoea. Gastric-emptying times may be prolonged without any pathological pylorospasm.

Protein binding

The plasma albumen concentration is not constant and depends upon the maturity of the infant and whether there has been intra-uterine malnutrition. It also tends to drop over the first 2 weeks after birth and then gradually rises again. The amount of protein available for binding is therefore variable compared with that in the older child or adult. The degree of protein-binding varies between different drugs. Phenobarbitone is normally 30–45% protein-bound. Bilirubin also competes for binding sites on the albumen so that in the presence of jaundice 70% of the phenobarbitone may be unbound.

Distribution

The distribution of the drug depends upon its protein binding, ionization, penetration into the extracellular fluid and then penetration into tissue (including brain, liver, kidney, muscle and particularly subcutaneous fat). The amount of fat in the neonate, although it appears podgy, is small compared with other ages and may be very small in infants with intra-uterine malnutrition.

The premature infant consists of about 48% extracellular water, the full-term infant about 45%, the infant at 1 year 25%, and by 14 years 17%. This difference in the amount of extracellular fluid and in the amount of fat means that the volumes of distribution for drugs are different from those in the older child. Certain anticonvulsants, such as phenytoin, penetrate fat very readily and a large amount of the dose can easily be taken up by the fat from the bloodstream.

Tissue penetration

For anticonvulsants tissue penetration is synonymous with penetration into the brain. The more lipid-soluble a drug the more easily it penetrates into the brain. This also depends upon its degree of ionization. Brain to plasma ratios rise with gestational age; the more protein binding (i.e. the higher the plasma proteins), the lower the brain to plasma ratio. There is no accumulation of drugs, particularly of phenobarbitone, in the brain with chronicity of therapy (Table 41.6). Distribution between grey and white matter

Table 41.6   Brain penetration of anticonvulsants (from Painter et al 1981)

Phenobarbitone	0.5–0.91	0.71 +/− 0.21 (Grey = White)
Phenytoin	0.75–1.5	1.28 +/− 0.32 (White > Grey)

is thought to be the same, although the brainstem may show higher concentrations than the cortex. Acidosis causing a lowering of pH affecting the ionization of the drug, together with gestational age and protein binding, are the three factors that are likely to influence the amount of the drug, even if correctly administered, which can penetrate into the brain (Ramsay et al 1979).

Metabolism

The drug may be excreted by the kidney without any metabolism, or it may undergo metabolic change in the liver and then be excreted directly through the kidney or after recirculation through the entero–hepatic circulation. Since there is renal immaturity and the kidney may also be affected by the same disease which is causing the fits, especially in cases of hypoxic–ischaemic encephalopathy, renal excretion of the drug is unpredictable.

Equally unpredictable is detoxification in the liver, especially if this requires glucuronidation (Table 41.7). It is well known that glucronyltransferase is immature but when it does switch on there may be competition by bilirubin or oestriol from the mother for the metabolic pathway. The transporting proteins, i.e. the ligands, may show low concentration. Hydroxylation mechanisms required (for example for phenytoin) may be equally immature. Although these enzyme systems switch on after birth the metabolism of a drug will depend, therefore, upon its penetration into the hepatocyte, its transport within the hepatocyte, whether the enzyme is switched on, whether there is competitive inhibition and whether there has been enzyme induction before birth. For example, this would happen if the mother had been given phenobarbitone before the infant was born. For this reason drugs may have a very prolonged half-life in the first week of life and the same dose may be extremely rapidly metabolized in the second week of life.

Excretion

We have already mentioned the difficulties in excreting drugs via the kidney. Drugs (such as paraldehyde) which are excreted via the lungs may be impeded in the presence of respiratory distress syndrome. Drugs excreted in the bile and reabsorbed via the entero–hepatic circulation will vary in excretion — dependent again upon intestinal transit time, type of feed, use of parenteral nutrition, or the presence of infection.

It will be apparent that since we are not always sure of the correct dose of drug, we cannot be sure of its absorption: it may be more or less protein-bound, depending upon the presence of jaundice and concentration of albumen. Metabolism of a drug depends upon the maturity of liver enzymes; its penetration into brain depends upon maturity and pH and excretion depends upon maturation of kidney and entero–hepatic circulation. One cannot guess or measure each of these variables in any given infant and so one should not be utilizing anticonvulsant therapy in the neonatal period without adequate facilities for regular monitoring of plasma concentrations (Table 41.8).

ANTICONVULSANT TREATMENT OF NEONATAL FITS

Drugs used in older children (such as carbamazepine and sodium valproate) are not used routinely in the newborn period. Their effects, however, may be seen in the newborn of mothers taking carbamazepine and valproate during pregnancy. These babies are born with significantly smaller head circumferences than the normal population. Carbamazepine appears to be the safest anticonvulsant taken in pregnancy from a point of view of teratogenic effects. The main standby of therapy is still phenobarbitone, with phenytoin as back-up therapy, and benzodiazepine drugs as the other group most commonly used for long-term therapy.

Phenobarbitone

Indications

Phenobarbitone is still the most commonly prescribed drug for infants with fits not due to a specific metabolic abnormality, requiring glucose, calcium, pyridoxine, etc. It is a drug of first choice in infants whose fits are thought to be due to asphyxia, birth trauma, infection, congenital malformation, intracranial haemorrhage, or metabolic disturbances without specific replacement therapy, e.g. kernicterus. It is also used for 'cerebral protection' in hypoxic–ischaemic encephalopathy and in the treatment of jaundice. It has been used in the past as a method of trying to prevent intraventricular haemorrhage (p. 320).

Table 41.7 Processes in the metabolism of drugs in the liver

Phase 1	Hydroxylation
	Deamination
	Dehalogenation
	Dealkylation
	Hydrolysis (e.g. of esters)
Phase 2	Conjugation — Glucuronide
	— Sulphate
	— Methylation
	— Acetylation

Table 41.8 Some reasons for the unpredictable serum levels of drugs used in the neonatal period

Esterase rise over the first year of life
Conjugation is not functional
Cytochrome P-450 is 50% of adult values
Ligandin is 20% of adult values

Passive maternal transfer

Phenobarbitone was the most common drug taken by epileptic mothers and studies have shown that it crosses the placenta rapidly, achieving equilibrium between the maternal and fetal blood (Ploman & Persson 1957). Chronic administration can result in enzyme induction in the fetus and withdrawl symptoms may occur, the infant becoming very jittery and irritable when it is stopped. In 100 epileptic mothers (Table 41.9) studies in the Simpson Memorial Maternity Pavilion, 10 infants only were irritable and jittery and 6 showed the typical withdrawal syndrome; this compared to 3 out of 97 control infants who were irritable and jittery and none who had symptoms of withdrawal.

Pharmaceutical preparations

Phenobarbitone is available as an oral elixir which has an alcohol base, although some hospitals make their own aqueous suspension which is less stable. The usual concentration is 15 mg phenobarbitone to 5 ml elixir. There is a parenteral preparation of phenobarbitone which is available in three sizes of 15, 30 and 60 mg in 1 ml of solution which can be used undiluted for intramuscular injection but is diluted for intravenous use.

Metabolism

Phenobarbitone is hydroxylated by the microsomal fraction in the liver and then excreted as a conjugate but 25% can be excreted unchanged in the urine (Figs 41.8 and 41.9). The effect of phenobarbitone in causing enzyme induction has led to its use in trying to mature microsomal glucuronyltransferase and to its administration to mothers before birth as well as the infant after birth, to try and reduce the incidence of jaundice in the newborn (Maisels) 1972). Whilst well-established in the older child, there is no convincing evidence that it enhances degradation of other drugs in the newborn, e.g. phenytoin (Rane et al 1973).

The rate of elimination of phenobarbitone in the neonate appears to be related to the duration of exposure (Melchior et al 1967). Phenobarbitone given to the mother, although causing enzyme induction in the fetus, nevertheless may take several weeks after birth before all its metabolites are excreted (Hill et al 1977, Draffan et al 1976). Metabolism in the first week of life is half the rate of the adult but this is followed by an overswing so that by the end of the next week it is twice as rapid as the adult with the half-life in the region of 47 hours; i.e. the half-life may be 100 hours in the first week and 50 hours in the second week but this hides the fact that at the extreme, the half-life of phenobarbitone in the first week can be as long as 400 hours (Heinze & Kampffmeyer 1971; Table 41.10). It is dangerous, therefore, to place an infant on a set dose of, for example, 8 mg/kg or 15 mg/bd as was sometimes indiscriminately suggested in the past. This results in only a very slow build-up to anticonvulsant levels to stop the fits but may also be followed by dangerous accumulation. The dosages used in the neonate would be considered enormous in the

Table 41.9 Symptoms compatible with drug withdrawal in infants of drug-treated mothers compared with control mothers

	Number of infants	Feeding problems, vomiting, weight loss	Jitteriness, tremor, excessive crying	Full withdrawal symptomatology
Epileptic mothers	100	19	10	6
Control mothers	97	4	3	0

Table 41.10 Half-life and degree of protein-binding of phenobarbitone at different ages

	Protein binding (%)	Half-life (h)
Newborn	28–43	45–500
After first week		30–100
Infant/toddler	46–48	20–133
Adult	36–38	60–180

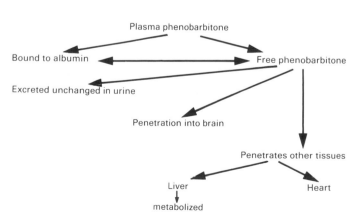

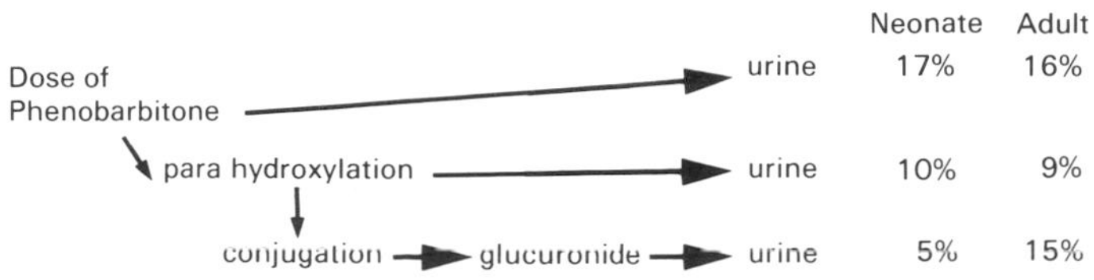

Fig. 41.8 Metabolism of phenobarbitone in the newborn infant.

Fig. 41.9 Metabolic fate of urinary excreted phenobarbitone. Over an 8-day period 32% of the phenobarbitone is excreted in the urine of a neonate compared with 39% in an adult. Note that poor conjugation is not the rate-limiting step. (From Boreus et al 1978.)

adult if administered on the same mg/kg basis (Sevensmark & Buchtal 1964).

Dosage

In infants given oral phenobarbitone after birth for the treatment of hyperbilirubinaemia, a steady-state as far as plasma concentration is concerned is not reached in the first week of life (Wallin et al 1974). Using intramuscular therapy in a dose of 6 mg/kg/day, the plasma concentration only reaches therapeutic (anticonvulsant) levels after the first week of administration. If the dose is increased by 10 mg/kg, therapeutic levels are not achieved until after 24 hours and sometimes 72 hours. Intravenous administration of 10 mg/kg is well tolerated and quickly achieves levels in the low therapeutic range (Ouvrier & Goldsmith 1978).

Failure of phenobarbitone to control fits in the first 24 hours is therefore more likely to be due to failure to achieve adequate blood levels. Oral and intramuscular therapy cannot be relied upon to give adequate plasma concentration rapidly, so that intravenous therapy is necessary. On the other hand, resultant drowsiness, hypotonia, lack of movement and feeding difficulty may be misdiagnosed as due to brain damage from perinatal asphyxia when they are due to accumulation of barbiturate. It is usual practice now to give a loading dose of 15–20 mg/kg which gives a good high initial level, followed over the next 24 hours by maintenance therapy of 6–8 mg/kg/day until the monitored blood concentrations are available. After the initial 24 hour loading, it is often only necessary to administer 1–2 mg/kg/day for the next 5 days, as the decay of the blood concentration may be very slow due to slow metabolism and excretion (Table 41.11). The dosage is likely subsequently to need increasing in the second week of life.

Therapeutic range

Difficulties are compounded by the fact that we are not sure that the therapeutic ranges established for older children apply in the newborn period. The usual range that one tries to achieve is in the region of 15–30 mg/ml (65–120 μmol/l) but higher concentrations may be required in severe convulsions or for cerebral protection (Pippinger & Rosen 1975, Buchtal & Lennox-Buchtal 1972).

Table 41.11 Summary of phenobarbitone penetration into the brain

Brain/plasma ratio rises with gestational age
The higher the plasma proteins, the lower the brain/plasma ratio
There is no accumulation of drug with chronicity of therapy
Penetration is influenced by degree of acidosis
Equal concentration in both grey and white matter
Possibly better penetration into the brainstem than cortex

Phenytoin

Indications

Phenytoin is used as a back-up or second-line drug to phenobarbitone in the newborn period, most often in infants with intractable fits or status epilepticus secondary to hypoxic–ischaemic encephalopathy or cortical dysplasia. It is a highly effective anticonvulsant when used in the correct dosage.

Pharmaceutical preparations

Phenytoin is available as an oral suspension of 30 mg in 5 ml which can be further diluted with syrup, and as a parenteral preparation of 250 mg in 5 ml.

Administration

It is usual to commence with intravenous therapy and this should be given very slowly under ECG control due to the effect of phenytoin as a myocardial depressant. Care should be taken with the injection, as already outlined, because of the irritant nature of the solvent and the risk of tissue necrosis if extravasation occurs. For the same reason it must never be used intramuscularly, as it crystallizes out in the muscle and is not absorbed (Willensky & Lowden 1973). Oral administration after initial intravenous loading is to be preferred in infants who are able to absorb normally from the gut.

Dosage

An initial intravenous loading dose of 15 mg/kg is commonly used. This can be given as an initial dose of 10 mg/kg followed by a further dose of 5 mg/kg, one hour later. This prevents very high initial levels with possible myocardial toxicity but maintains the blood level at the time when it would begin to fall due to absorption into body fat. The half-life is again so variable that no fixed maintenance dosage regime is possible without monitoring plasma concentrations. An initial maintenance routine of 8 mg/kg in the first 24 hours will usually need to be modified once plasma concentration is available, as the maintenance therapy can then vary from as little as 3 mg/kg/24 hours to as much as 25 mg/kg. The drug needs to be given in divided doses throughout the 24 hours or wide swings in plasma concentrations may occur. The once-daily dose regime of the adult is not applicable in the newborn.

Metabolism

Laughnan et al (1977) studied the metabolism of phenytoin in the newborn and found the plasma half-life of diphenyl-hydantoin in the full-term infant to be prolonged and variable — 20.7 ± 11.6 hours in the first week of life and 7.6 ± 3.5 hours after the first week. In the small premature infant, the half-life is even longer at 75.4 ± 64.5 hours. The premature infant is therefore especially likely to accumulate the drug and develop acute toxicity.

The usual process of metabolism of 50–70% of administered phenytoin is by a cytochrome P-450 dependent hydroxylation (Rane et al 1973, Neims et al 1976) and this step can occur in many tissues, not being confined to liver. Phenytoin is hydroxylated but is also excreted in part as a glucuronide (Rane et al 1973), a process which does occur in the liver and is well known to be immature in the small infant (Neims et al 1976).

The infant does have a higher free phenytoin of 10.6% ± 1.4 compared to the adult 7.4% ± 0.7 (Rane et al 1973). In premature infants the brain concentration is not as high as one might expect, considering the very high blood levels, but in the presence of inflammation the concentration can be very high. CSF concentration may to some extent reflect concentrations in cerebral tissues but blood/CSF ratios are probably not the same as blood/brain due to the changing blood and CSF protein. However, CSF studies in 26 patients (Schulte 1977) with raised plasma concentrations showed significantly higher CSF levels ($P<0.005$) than when plasma concentration was normal. Much more work is needed on the toxic effect of high plasma concentrations alone and the factors that influence actual brain concentration of drugs. The pharmacokinetics of phenytoin are as follows:

Loading dose of 15 mg/kg intravenously
May need further booster to achieve control of fits
Oral dosage of 12 mg/kg did not achieve therapeutic blood levels
Volume distribution not related to gestational age so the same dose given independent of maturity
Metabolism changes in the second week of life or with infection
Dose to maintain blood level varies from 3 to 24 mg/kg/day.

Blood levels

While we have to assume that the 'normal' plasma phenytoin range in the infant is the same (40–80 μmol/l) as in the older child, as established by Buchtal et al (1960), we do not know if this is the case. It has been suggested that with the lower plasma albumen concentration, a range of 24–56 μmol/l may be more appropriate. A concentration of at least 20 μmol/l is necessary for anticonvulsant effect in the full-term newborn infant.

Toxicity

Toxicity may not be obvious and the first sign may be an increase in the number of fits or a cardiac arrhythmia.

The infant only occasionally shows nystagmus and cannot show ataxia or gum hypertrophy. That overdose of anticonvulsants can cause fits should always be borne in mind. A further matter of concern is that an unstable intermediary compound may be formed which is difficult to detect, i.e. an epoxide. These epoxides may bind to cellular DNA and interfere with the read-out of the base sequence.

This could be important in the aetiology of congenital malformations but also since the brain grows by 1000 g in the first 4 years of life we must be aware constantly of the effect of all chronically administered drugs on brain growth as well as their potential teratogenicity and carcinogenicity.

Interference with folate metabolism can also theoretically jeopardize normal brain growth and in older children it has been shown to cause a type of degenerative brain disease (Vallarta et al 1974).

Phenytoin crosses the placenta and concentrations in umbilical artery and vein approach those found in maternal serum (Baughman & Randinitis 1970, Rane et al 1973). It has been incriminated as a possible cause of congenital malformations, especially cleft palate (Monson et al 1973).

The infant may therefore receive phenytoin transplacentally before he is born (Baughman & Randinitis 1970), therapeutically after birth, or in breast milk in a mother taking the drug (Rasmussen 1973). The amount in breast milk is about 40% of the maternal plasma concentration (Mirkin 1971, Rane et al 1973) and this would give the average infant a dose of 2 to 4 mg a day. If the infant is not itself taking the drug, present knowledge suggests that it will not cause harm. However, caution dictates that until the effect of the drug on brain growth is actually known, its administration for 6 months during the time of maximum brain growth, a time when other metabolic upsets such as hypothyroidism and phenylketonuria have a permanent and irreversible effect, may be unwise. Chronic phenytoin ingestion could theoretically damage the development of Purkinje cells, in view of the drug's high affinity for them.

Occasionally cases of a permanent cerebellar ataxia due to drug toxicity are seen in the older child (Valsamis & Mancall 1973). However, if this was a major hazard one might have expected a high incidence of ataxia to have been reported in infants of epileptic mothers taking phenytoin during the whole of pregnancy and then breast feeding. It is further suggested that phenytoin taken by mothers during pregnancy could damage the optic nerves of the developing fetus (Hoyte & Billson 1978).

Studies on the teratogenic effects of the drug have shown that the incidence of cleft palate is 10/1000 in mothers taking anticonvulsant drugs as compared to 1.5/1000 in the general population. Epileptic mothers not taking anticonvulsant drugs do not have a higher incidence of congenital malformation than the general population. It is thought that phenytoin and phenobarbitone together are additive in their risk (Monson et al 1973, Fedrick 1973).

Mountain (1970) has suggested that phenytoin can

cause a bleeding diathesis due to deficiency of the vitamin K-dependent factors II, VII, IX and X in the neonate. Rickets due to interference with vitamin D metabolism by phenytoin is well recognized in older age groups. Two infants with fits in the newborn period due to refractory hypocalcaemia have been described and the hypocalcaemia was ascribed to maternal phenytoin, causing a relative lack of vitamin D in the mother (Friis & Sardemann 1977). There is not enough evidence at present on the risks of anticonvulsants to warrant changing the medication in an anticonvulsant-dependent mother.

Benzodiazepines

Indications

Diazepam may be used for the rapid termination of status epilepticus or frequent recurrent seizures in the newborn and is effective. It is not commonly used for long-term medication. Nitrazepam is also in relatively common use in the newborn period for the intractable neonatal epilepsies, e.g. associated with cortical dysplasia. Benzodiazepine drugs work by enhancing the synaptic sensitivity to endogenous GABA. Clonazepam (0.25 mg loading dose in full-term infants and 0.1 mg daily) has been used in the newborn to treat severe fits with some success (Levene 1987).

Pharmaceutical preparations

The most common preparation of diazepam used is the 10 mg ampoule which is available in two forms: one as a clear solution using propylene glycol as solvent and the other as soya bean oil emulsion which is less irritant and thus causes less discomfort on injection. A rectal preparation is available as 'stesolid' in a 5 mg plastic dispenser. The manufacturer claims that the plastic is treated so as not to absorb the drug. Diazepam used intramuscularly is too slow and erratic in absorption to recommend its use in seizure control.

Nitrazepam is now commercially available as an oral suspension containing 2.5 mg in 5 ml. It is tolerated well by infants, who seem to like the taste. A syringe is needed to measure the dose and the mixture needs to be well shaken to ensure uniformity of dose

Metabolism

Benzodiazepines have a high protein-binding capacity, over 95% being protein-bound. The relatively higher values for volume of distribution of these drugs suggest that relatively higher concentrations exist in tissues, than in plasma, compared with other anticonvulsants. This may account for the rapid fall in blood level after a single intravenous bolus injection, which explains the short duration of its anticonvulsant action.

Although benzodiazepines penetrate brain very rapidly, showing a clinical effect in seconds, penetration into CSF is poor (about 2%; Kangas et al 1974).

The rapid penetration into tissues such as the brain is due to the very high lipid solubility, especially of diazepam. If displaced from plasma protein-binding sites, as may happen due to displacement by bilirubin, the free benzodiazepine is quickly taken up by the tissues. Release from tissues and subsequent metabolism may be very slow and persist for 10 days. Metabolism is by the liver and involves glucuronidation. Some benzodiazepines require prior hydroxylation, which may lead to slow metabolism. This does not apply to nitrazepam which undergoes nitroreduction before glucuronidation.

Blood levels

There is no good relation between blood level and clinical effect and the estimation of benzodiazepine concentrations is not available in most routine laboratories so blood level is not used as a guide to dosage.

Dosage and use

The usual dose in status epilepticus is 1.0 mg given intravenously (0.3 mg/kg) and this can be repeated if seizures return (McMorris & McWilliams 1969, Smith & Mosotti 1971). Continuous infusion of diazepam is not usually practicable as the dilution required means a large volume of fluid needs to be administered and the drug tends to adhere to plastic in the giving set making dosage regulation unpredictable.

Benzodiazepine sensitivity can be tested by injecting diazepam during EEG monitoring, provided that the EEG shows a marked dysrrhythmia. This may cause return of the EEG to normal but, rarely, has the opposite effect and makes the epileptic activity worse. Fast beta activity appears in the EEG of older infants but in the full-term neonate diazepam may produce runs of sleep spindle-like activity. Rectal diazepam can be used in a dose of 0.5 mg/kg and is effective in about 3 minutes.

Nitrazepam is used in a dose starting with 0.5 mg bd and can be increased usually to 1.0 mg bd but it is well tolerated and is better given as multiple small doses than infrequent large ones.

Toxicity

Diazepam may cause dangerous respiratory depression if combined with a barbiturate. It is short-lived, dosage is difficult to assess, and the solvent vehicle may compete for bilirubin-binding sites and increase the risk of kernicterus (Volpe 1977). Most of these disadvantages apply at any age in childhood and not just to the newborn. Rectal diazepam can cause respiratory depression and marked hypotonia. Any respiratory depression is easily diagnosed in the newborn and we have not found this to be a real problem in practice. Sedation occurs during the first few days of treatment with nitrazepam.

Diazepam is believed to cross the placenta and reach equilibrium between maternal and fetal blood (Scanlon 1974). Diazepam is very frequently given to the mother during labour and appreciable amounts may therefore reach the infant who may be drowsy, hypotonic and hypothermic. He only slowly metabolizes it and diazepam or its metabolite desmethyldiazepam may be still detected 10 days after a single dose given to the mother (Morselli et al 1973, Eliot et al 1974). Diazepam is also excreted in breast milk and can cause drowsiness in the baby but the ratio in maternal blood to milk is only 10 to 1 (Erkkola & Kanto 1972); this is probably because the drug is highly protein-bound.

Thus many infants may receive diazepam in other ways than its use in status epilepticus without any obvious side effects. The risk of the solvent competing for bilirubin binding sites and precipitating kernicterus should be borne in mind when treating fits in a jaundiced infant but this has not proved in practice to be a major obstacle to therapy.

Paraldehyde

Paraldehyde is a much maligned, extremely useful and very effective anticonvulsant which has the added advantage of being one of the few drugs which are rapidly absorbed on intramuscular injection. In recurrent bouts of seizures it can be given by repeated intramuscular injection and the modern plastipak-type syringes do not dissolve. Ampoules do not deteriorate like the older multidose vials but should be fresh and not exposed to sunlight. When given intramuscularly paraldehyde is remarkably free of pharmacological side effects. It should never be given intravenously in the neonatal period, as it may cause pneumonitis and hepatic necrosis. It should also be avoided in severe respiratory distress syndrome as it is excreted via the lungs. It does not cause respiratory depression and its use is not prejudiced by previous phenobarbitone administration. The only risk in its use is the irritant effect and possible sterile abscess formation. It should never be given into the buttock in the neonate, as the sciatic nerve is not constant in position, but should be given deeply into the lateral side of the thigh, usually in a dose of 0.5 ml in the first instance (0.2 ml/kg).

Lignocaine

The most important maxim in the treatment of intractable or recurrent seizures is that the physician should use as few drugs as possible and only those with which he is familiar. Lignocaine is popular in Scandinavia and, in the hands of certain physicians, it appears effective. In the wrong dose it is a myocardial depressant and can result in an increased number of seizures. The dose recommended is 1.0 mg/kg and this should be administered under ECG control.

Chlormethiozole

This is not a drug in routine use in the newborn but recent reports suggest that it may have a limited place for neonatal status epilepticus which is resistant to conventional treatments. It has been used for this purpose as a chlormethiozole infusion (Miller & Kovar 1983).

PROGNOSIS

There are many reports on the long-term effects of neonatal seizures (Burke 1954, Craig 1960, Keith 1964, Tibbles & Pritchard 1965, Schulte 1966, McInery & Schubert 1969, Rose & Lombroso 1970, Brown et al 1972, Dennis 1978). Most authors have found an overall poor prognosis of about 50% (48–70%) dying or having significant persisting neurological or intellectual handicap. If we exclude fits secondary to neonatal tetany, mortality in 123 cases in the Simpson Maternity Pavilion was 17%; this gives an overall mortality rate of 1/1000 births.

The incidence of neonatal seizures in the past was as high as 12/1000 liveborn infants and approximately 1.5/1000 infants went on to long-term epilepsy (Forfar et al 1972). Follow-up statistics for infants with neonatal seizures who develop long-term sequelae of epilepsy, cerebral palsy or mental handicap do, of course, depend upon the cause of the seizures (Knauss & Marshall 1977). Late hypocalcaemia or simple neonatal tetany has an excellent prognosis with no mortality and no long-term sequelae in virtually 100% of cases, apart from enamel hypoplasia of the teeth. In hypocalcaemia, secondary to intrapartum asphyxia, the prognosis is poor. As many as 50% may have sequelae. With better neonatal care there is no doubt that in perinatal asphyxia, for example, only 12% of infants with fits now, have long-term sequelae compared with 46% 10 years ago, and the total number of infants presenting with fits has reduced. It is difficult to know how much this reflects the improvements in neonatology with earlier diagnosis and more aggressive treatment or whether it reflects better obstetrics with a shorter period of asphyxia in utero.

The worst prognosis is in infants known to be brain damaged with fits associated with a cortical dysplasia or when brain damage is proved by imaging techniques, for example, demonstrating periventricular leukomalacia. There is no evidence that brief seizures themselves leave any lasting damage as seen in infants with hypocalcaemia or benign dominantly inherited neonatal seizures. This is not to say that prolonged or recurrent seizures do not significantly increase the risk of long-term brain damage, especially in the infant with an already compromised brain from asphyxia, raised intracranial pressure or decreased cerebral blood flow. Seizures remain one of the most treatable aspects of neonatal neurology for improving quality of survival.

REFERENCES

Aicardi J 1985 Early myoclonic encephalopathy in epileptic syndromes in infancy, childhood, and adolescence. In: Roger J, Dravet C, Bureau M, Dreifuss J E, Wolf P (ed) Benign neonatal convulsions (familial and non-familial). John Libbey Eurotext

Albani M, Schulte F J 1977 Phenytoin concentration in cerebrospinal fluid and brain tissue. Neuropadiatre (Suppl) 8: 488 (abstract)

Amiel-Tison C, Ellison P 1986 Birth asphyxia in the full-term newborn: early assessment and outcome. Developmental Medicine and Child Neurology 28: 671–682

Bankier A, Turner M, Hopkins I J 1983 Pyridoxine dependent seizures: a wider clinical spectrum. Archives of Disease in Childhood 58: 415–418

Barton L L, Feigin R D, Lins R 1973 Group B beta hemolytic streptococcal meningitis in infants. Journal of Pediatrics 82(4): 719–723

Baughman F A Jr, Randinitis E J 1970 Passage of diphenylhydantoin across the placenta. Journal of the American Medical Association 213: 466

Beresford H R, Posner J B, Plum F 1969 Changes in brain lactate during induced cerebral seizures. Archives of Neurology 20: 243–248

Berman P H, Banker B Q 1966 Neonatal meningitis. Pediatrics 28: 6–24

Billard C, Dulac O, Diebler C 1982 Ramollissement cérébral ischémique du nouveau-né: une étiologie possible des états de mal convulsifs néonatals. Archives Francaises de Pediatrie 39: 677–683

Boréus L O, Jalling B, Kallberg N 1975 Clinical pharmacology of phenobarbital in the neonatal period. In: Morselli P L, Garattini S, Serieni F (eds) Basic and therapeutic aspects of perinatal pharmacology. Raven Press, New York, p 331

Brandt N V, Rassmussen K, Brandt S, Schonheyder F 1974 D-Glyceric acidemia with hyperglycinemia: a new inborn error of metabolism. British Medical Journal 4: 334

Brown J K 1973 Convulsions in the newborn period. Developmental Medicine and Child Neurology 15(6): 823–846

Brown J K 1976 Infants damaged during birth. In: Hull D (ed) Recent advances in paediatrics. Churchill Livingston, Edinburgh, pp 36–88

Brown J K, Livingston S 1985 The malignant epilepsies of childhood: West's syndrome and Lennox–Gastaut syndrome. In: Ross E, Reynolds E (eds) Paediatric perspectives in epilepsy. John Wiley & Sons, pp 29–39

Brown J K, Minns R A 1980 Epilepsy in neonates. In: Tyrer J H (ed) The treatment of epilepsy, current status of modern therapy, Vol. 5. MTP Press, England, pp 161–202

Brown J K, Cockburn F, Forfar J O 1972 Clinical and chemical correlates in convulsions of the newborn. Lancet: 135–139

Buchtal F, Lennox-Buchtal M A 1972 Phenobarbital: relation of serum concentration to control of seizures. In: Woodburn D M, Penry J K, Schmidt R P (eds) Anti-epileptic drugs. Raven Press, New York, pp 335–344

Buchtal F, Svensmark O, Schiller P J 1960 Clinical and electro-encephalographic correlation with serum levels of diphenylhydantoin. Archives of Neurology 2: 624–630

Burke J B 1954 The prognostic significance of neonatal convulsions. Archives of Disease in Childhood 29: 342–345

Chantler C, Baum J D, Normal D A 1967 Dextrostix in the diagnosis of neonatal hypoglycaemia. Lancet i: 1395–1396

Cockburn F, Brown J K, Belton N R et al 1973 Neonatal convulsions associated with primary disturbance of calcium, phosphorus, and magnesium metabolism. Archives of Disease in Childhood 48: 99

Craig W S 1960 Convulsive movements occurring in the first ten days of life. Archives of Disease in Childhood 35: 336–343

David L, Anast S 1974 Calcium metabolism in newborn infants: the interrelationship of parathyroid function and calcium, magnesium, and phosphorus metabolism in normal, 'sick' and hypocalcemic newborns. Journal of Clinical Investigation 54(2): 287–296

Della Bernadina B, Akardi J, Goutieres F, Plovin P 1979 Glycine encephalopathy. Neuropadiatric 10: 209–225

Dennis J 1978 Neonatal convulsions: aetiology, late neonatal status and long-term outcome. Developmental Medicine and Child Neurology 20(2): 143–158

Derham R J, Matthews T G, Clarke T A 1985 Early seizures indicate quality and perinatal care. Archives of Disease in Childhood 60: 809–813

Desmond M M, Schwanecke R P, Wilson G S, Yatsunaga S, Burgdorff I 1972 Maternal barbituarate utilization and neonatal withdrawal symptomatology. Journal of Pediatrics 80: 190

Draffan G H, Dollery C T, Davies D S et al 1976 Maternal and neonatal elimination of amylobarbital after treatment of the mother with barbiturates during late pregnancy. Clinical Pharmacology and Therapeutics 19: 271–275

Dwyer B E, Wasterlain C G, Fujikawa D G, Yamada L 1986 Brain protein metabolism in epilepsy. Advances in Neurology 44: 903–918

Eliot B W, Hill J G, Cole A P, Hailey D M 1974 Continuous pethidine/diazepam infusion during labour and its effects on the newborn. British Journal of Obstetrics and Gynaecology 82: 126

Erkkola R, Kanto J 1972 Diazepam and breast-feeding. Lancet i: 1235

Eyre J A, Oozeer R C, Wilkinson A R 1983 Diagnosis of neonatal seizure by continuous recording and rapid analysis of the electro-encephalogram. Archives of Disease in Childhood 58: 785–790

Forfar J O 1976 Normal and abnormal calcium phosphorus and magnesium metabolism in the perinatal period. Clinics in Endocrinology and Metabolism 5(1): 123–148

Forfar J O, Brown J K, Cockburn F 1972 Early infantile convulsions and later epilepsy. In: Parsonage M J (ed) Prevention of epilepsy and its consequences. International Bureau for Epilepsy, London

Fredrick J 1973 Epilepsy and pregnancy: a report from the Oxford Record Linkage Study. British Medical Journal 2: 442–448

Friedman M, Hatcher G 1967 Primary hypomagnesemia with secondary hypocalcaemia in an infant. Lancet i: 703

Friis B, Sardemann H 1977 Neonatal hypocalcaemia after intrauterine exposure to anticonvulsant drugs (Short reports). Archives of Disease in Childhood 52: 239–247

Goldberg H J 1983 Neonatal convulsions — a 10-year review. Archives of Disease in Childhood 58: 976–978

Grandgeorge D, Favier A, Bost M et al 1980 L'acidémie D-glycérique a propos d'une nouvelle observation anatomo-clinique. Archives Francaises de Pediatrie 37: 577–584

Hamilton P A, Cady E B, Wyatt J S, Hope P L, Delpy P T, Reynolds E O R 1986 Impaired energy metabolism in brains of newborn infants with increased cerebral echodensities. Lancet i: 1242–1246

Hanshaw J B Congenital cytomegalovirus infection: a 15-year perspective. Journal of Infectious Diseases 123: 555–561

Heinze E, Kampffmeyer H G 1971 Biological half-life of phenobarbital in human babies. Klinische Wochenschrift 49: 1146–1147

Hellstrom-Westas L, Rosen I, Svenningsen N M 1985 Silent seizures in sick infants in early life: diagnosis by continuous cerebral function monitoring. Acta Paediatrica Scandinavia 74: 741–748

Herzlinger R A, Kandall S R, Vaughan H G 1977 Neonatal seizures associated with narcotic withdrawal. Journal of Pediatrics 91: 638

Hill R M, Verniaud, W M, Morgan N F, Nowlin J, Glazener L J, Horning M G 1977 Urinary excretion of phenobarbital in a neonate having withdrawal symptoms. American Journal of Diseases of Children 131: 546

Holden K R, Freeman J M 1975 Neonatal seizures and their treatment (Symposium on drug therapy in the neonate). Clinics in Perinatology 2: 3–13

Holmes G, Rowe J, Hafford J, Schmidt R, Testa M, Zimmerman A 1982 Prognostic value of the electroencephalogram in neonatal asphyxia. Electroencephalographgy and Clinical Neurophysiology 53: 60–72

Hopkins I J 1972 Seizures in the first week of life: a study of aetiological factors. Medical Journal of Australia 2: 647–651

Hoyte C S, Billson F A 1978 Maternal anticonvulsants and optic nerve hypoplasia. British Journal of Ophthalmology 62: 3–6

Kangas L, Kanto J, Surtola T 1974 CSF concentration and serum protein binding of diazepam and N. De Methyl Diazepam. Acta Pharmacologica et Toxicologica 35 (suppl 1)

Keen J H, Lee D 1973 Sequelae of neonatal convulsions: a study in 112 infants. Archives of Disease in Childhood 48: 542

Keith H M 1964 Convulsions in children undr 3 years of age: a study of prognosis. Mayo Clinic Proceedings 39: 895–907

Knauss T A, Marshall R E 1977 Seizures in a neonatal intensive care unit. Developmental Medicine and Child Neurology 19: 719–728

Levene M I 1987 Neonatal neurology. Current Reviews in Paediatrics, No. 3. Churchill Livingstone, Edinburgh

Levene M I, Trounce J Q 1986 Cause of neonatal convulsions: towards more precise diagnosis. Archives of Disease in Childhood 61: 78–87

Lou H C, Friis-Hansen B 1979 Arterial blood pressure elevations during motor activity and epileptic seizures in the newborn. Acta Paediatrica Scandinavia 68: 803

Loughlan P M, Greenwald A, Purton W W, Arandra J V, Watters G, Neims A H 1977 Pharmacokinetic observations of phenytoin disposition in the newborn and young infant. Archives of Disease in Childhood 52: 302–309

McInery T K, Schubert W K 1969 Prognosis of neonatal seizures. American Journal of Diseases of Children 117: 261

McMorris S, McWilliams P K A 1969 Status epilepticus in infants and young children treated with parenteral diazepam. Archives of Disease in Childhood 44: 604

Maisels M J 1972 Bilirubin: on understanding and influencing its metabolism in the newborn infant. Pediatric Clinics of North America 19(2): 447–502

Majewski F 1985 Two teratogens of major importance: alcohol and anticonvulsants. In: Arune M, Suzuki Y, Yabwucki H (eds) The developing brain and its disorders. Karger

Melchior J C, Svensmark O, Trolle D 1967 Placental transfer of phenobarbitone in epileptic women, and elimination in newborns. Lancet ii: 860–861

Meldrum B 1978 Physiological changes during prolonged seizures and epileptic brain damage. Neuropediatrie 9(3): 203–212

Miller P, Kovar I 1983 Chlormethiazole in the treatment of neonatal status epilepticus. Postgraduate Medical Journal 59(698): 801–802

Minns R A 1980 Vitamin B6 deficiency and dependency. Developmental Medicine and Child Neurology 22: 795–798

Minns R A, Brown J K 1978 Intracranial pressure changes associated with childhood seizures. Developmental Medicine and Child Neurology 20: 561–569

Mirkin B L 1971 Diphenylhydantoin: placental transport, fetal localization, neonatal metabolism and possible tetratogenic effects. Journal of Pediatrics 78: 329–337

Monselli P L, Principi N, Tognoni G et al 1973 Diazepam elimination in premature and full-term infants and children. Journal of Perinatal Medicine 1: 133–141

Monson R R, Rosenberg L, Hartz S C, Shapiro S, Heinonen O P, Slone D 1973 Diphenylhydantoin and selected congenital malformations. New England Journal of Medicine 289: 1049–1052

Mountain K R, Hirsch J, Gallus A S 1970 Neonatal coagulation defect due to anticonvulsant drug treatment in pregnancy. Lancet i: 265–268

Neims A H, Warner M, Loughnan P M, Aranda J V 1976 Developmental aspects of the hepatic cytochrome P450 monooxygenase system. Annual Review of Pharmacology and Toxicology 16: 427–446

O'Meara O P, Brazie J V 1968 Neonatal intoxication after paracervical block. New England Journal of Medicine 278: 1127

Ouvrier R A, Goldsmith R 1978 Phenobarbitone dosage in the neonate. Brain and Development 3: 194–202

Paunier L, Radde I C, Kooh S W, Fraser D 1965 Primary hypomagnesemia with secondary hypocalcaemia. Journal of Pediatrics 67: 945

Peckham C S 1972 Clinical and laboratory study of children exposed in utero to maternal rubella. Archives of Disease in Childhood 47: 571–577

Peiper A 1963 Cerebral function in infancy and childhood. (Trans. 3rd rev. German edn by B. Nagler and H. Nagler.) Pitman Medical, London

Pezzani C, Radvanyi-Bouvet M F, Relier J P, Monod N 1986 Neonatal electroencephalography during the first 24 hours of life in full-term newborn infants. Neuropediatrics 17: 11–18

Pippenger C E, Rosen T S 1975 Phenobarbital plasma levels in neonates (Symposium on drug therapy in the neonate). Clinics in Perinatology 2(1): 111–115

Ploman L, Persson B H 1957 On the transfer of barbiturates to the human foetus and their accumulation in some of the vital organs. Journal of Obstetrics and Gynaecology of the British Commonwealth 64: 706–711

Plovin P 1985 Epileptic syndromes in infants, childhood and adolescence. In: Roget J, Dravet C, Bureau M, Dreifus F E, Wolf P (eds) Benign neonatal convulsions (familial and non-familial). John Libbey Emotext

Purpura D P 1974 Dendritic spine 'dysgenesis' and mental retardation. Science 186: 1126

Purpura D P, Shofer R J, Hougepian E M et al 1964 Comparative ontogenesis of structure–function relations in cerebral and cerebellar cortex. Progress in Brain Research 4: 187

Radde I C, Parkinson D K, Höffken B, Appiah K E, Hanley W B 1972 Calcium ion activity in the sick neonate: effect of bicarbonate administration and exchange transfusion. Pediatric Research 6: 43–49

Ramsay R E, Hammond E J, Perchalski R J, Wilder J 1979 Brain uptake of phenytoin, phenobarbital and diazepam. Archives of Neurology 36: 535

Rane A, Lunde P K M, Jalling B, Yaffe S T, Sjöqvist F 1971 Plasma protein binding of DPH in normal and hyperbilirubinaemic infants. Journal of Pediatrics 78: 877–882

Rane A, Garle M, Borga O, Sjöqvist F 1973 Plasma disappearance of transplacentally transferred diphenythydantoin in the newborn studied by mass fragmentography. Clinical and Pharmacology and Therapeutics 15: 39–45

Rasmussen F 1973 The mechanism of drug secretion into milk. In: Dietary lipids and post-natal development. Raven Press, New York

Robertson N R C, Smith M A 1975 Early neonatal hypocalcaemia. Archives of Disease in Childhood 50: 604

Rose A L, Lombroso C T Neonatal seizure states: a study of clinical, pathological and electroencephalographic features in 137 full-term babies with a long-term follow-up. Pediatrics 45: 404–425

Scanlon J W 1974 Obstetric anaesthesia as a neonatal risk factor in normal labor and delivery. Clinics in Perinatology 1: 465–482

Schulte F J 1966 Neonatal convulsions and their relation to epilepsy in early childhood. Developmental Medicine and Child Neurology 8: 381–392

Sevensmark O, Buchtal F 1964 Diphenylhydantoin and phenobarbital serum levels in children. American Journal of Diseases of Children 108: 82–87

Skyberg D, Stromme J H, Besbakken R, Harnaes K 1968 Neonatal hypomagnesemia with selective malabsorption of magnesium — a clinical entity. Scandinavian Journal of Clinical and Laboratory Investigation 21: 355–363

Smith B T, Masotti R E 1971 Intravenous diazepam in the treatment of prolonged seizure activity in neonates and infants. Developmental Medicine and Child Neurology 13: 630

Tibbles J A R, Prichard J S 1965 The prognostic value of the electroencephalogram in neonatal convulsions. Pediatrics 35: 778–786

Turner T 1974 Comparison of phenobarbitone magnesium sulphate and calcium gluconate in treatment of neonatal hypocalcaemia convulsions. Archives of Disease in Childhood 49: 244

Vallarta J M, Bell D B, Reichert A 1974 Progressive encephalopathy due to chronic hydantoin intoxication. American Journal of Diseases of Children 128: 27–34

Valmis M P, Mancall E M 1973 Toxic cerebellar degeneration. Human Pathology 4: 513–520

Vigevano F, Maccagnani F, Bertini E et al 1982 Encefalopatia mioclonia precoce associata ad alti livelli di acido propionico nel siero. Boll. Lega. It. Epil. 39: 181–182

Volpe J J 1977 Neonatal seizures (Symposium on neonatal neurology). Clinics in Perinatology, March. W B Saunders

Wallin A, Jalling B, Boreus L O 1974 Plasma concentrations of phenobarbital in the newborn during prophylaxis for neonatal hyperbilirubinaemia. Journal of Pediatrics 85: 392–397

Wasterlain C G 1978 Neonatal seizures and brain growth. Neuropediatrie 9(3): 213–228

Wasterlain C G, Duffy T E 1975 Neonatal status epilepticus: decrease in brain glucose without decrease in blood glucose. Neurology 25: 365

Weggemann T, Brown J K, Fulford G E, Minns R A 1987 A study of normal baby movements. Child Care, Health and Development 13: 41–58

Wilensky A J, Lowden J A 1973 Inadequate serum levels after intravenous administration of diphenylhydantoin. Neurology 23: 318–324

Wyatt J S, Delpy P T, Cope M, Wray S, Reynolds E O R 1986 Quantification of cerebral oxygenation and haemodynamics in sick newborn infants by near infrared spectrophotometry. Lancet ii: 1063–1065

Zelson C, Rubio E, Wasserman E 1971 Neonatal narcotic addiction. Pediatrics 48: 178

The special senses

42. Disorders of vision

Prof A. R. Fielder

This chapter is concerned with disorders affecting the eye, vision, and abnormalities of eye movement. Other ocular disorders such as congenital cataract and buphthalmos are not considered. In view of the rapid development taking place during infancy various aspects of normal development are reviewed. For many clinicians certain aspects may be considered irrelevant but they are included as detailed comments on eye movements and visual development are relevant to clinical practice and it is hoped that the limited information contained herein and the references quoted will provide a basis for further study. Necessarily the consideration of individual conditions is brief and the references selective, not exhaustive. The chapter is divided into two main sections: eye movements — normal and abnormal; and vision — normal and abnormal.

EYE MOVEMENTS

NORMAL EYE MOVEMENTS

This is a field most clinicians find complex and intimidating, a feeling heightened by our lack of knowledge both of the normal development of eye movements and the natural history of many common disorders of ocular motility such as congenital nystagmus and congenital convergent strabismus.

Eye movement patterns must be studied carefully: failure of one eye to abduct may be due to a sixth nerve palsy, whereas failure of both eyes to look to one side could signify either a gaze or saccadic palsy. These three possibilities have different important implications.

In this section a brief description of the various types of eye movements is given. For more detailed accounts there are several recent reviews (Hoyt et al 1982, Leigh & Zee 1983, Boothe et al 1985, Fielder 1985).

Embryology of the extra-ocular muscles

The extra-ocular muscles are formed as condensations of mesoderm which begin to differentiate at 6 weeks of gestation and are fully formed by 12 weeks. By this time the ocular motor nerves have reached their destination. In contrast, the supranuclear eye movement system responsible for feeding information to the brainstem ocular motor nuclei is not fully developed until after full-term.

Fetal eye movements

Eye movements can be detected, using ultrasonography, from 16 weeks of gestation (Birnholz 1981, Prechtl & Nijhuis 1983, Inoue et al 1986). Initially these are simply slow changes of eye position but later they become faster. Rapid eye movements are seen between 30 and 33 weeks and are organized into periods of activity, which after 36 weeks are related to fetal behavioural state (see also Chapter 6).

TYPES OF EYE MOVEMENT

Conjugate eye movement are movements of both eyes in the same direction and are also called versions. In disjugate movements both eyes move in opposite directions and these are called vergence movements. Conjugate movements include pursuit, saccadic, optokinetic and vestibulo–ocular eye movements. Pursuit movements enable the eyes to follow a relatively slow-moving target and as the image is maintained on the fovea of the retina the target is seen clearly. If the object moves too fast for the pursuit system a catch-up saccade is required to refixate the image back onto the fovea. Saccades are fast movements which allow us to change our direction of visual interest and direct the object of interest on to the fovea. Both optokinetic and vestibulo–ocular movements co-ordinate head and eye movements during body movements. Each type of eye movement is subserved by a separate supranuclear system but all share a final common infranuclear pathway from the ocular motor nuclei to the eye muscles.

Eye movements in infancy

The distinction between normal and abnormal eye movements in the neonatal period is not easy to make and is also considered in the section dealing with abnormal movements.

Ocular alignment and excursion

The eyes of neonates are commonly divergent (Fig. 42.1) particularly if they are born prematurely (Rethy 1969). Recently Nixon et al (1985) examined 1219 alert neonates for strabismus and found no deviation in 593 but 398 (32.7%) were divergent and 40 (3.2%) convergent. Comparing pre-term with full-term neonates they found a higher incidence of constant divergence in the former suggesting that in the normal course of development eyes are initially divergent but this diminishes over the ensuing few weeks. Surprisingly there is almost no information regarding the extent of the neonatal ocular excursion but horizontal gaze probably develops before vertical (Jones, quoted by McGinnis 1930).

Pursuit movements

The pursuit system enables the eyes to follow a moving target accurately and smoothly. Until recently it was thought that the neonate was incapable of such movements. It has now been shown that smooth eye and head movements can be performed but only if the target is slow-moving (Kremenitzer et al 1979, Roucoux et al 1983). If the velocity of the target is increased, jerky (saccadic) tracking supervenes.

Tests of pursuit involve following a slow-moving target, or the slow phase of optokinetic nystagmus (see later).

Saccadic movements

The saccadic system allows us to change our direction of visual interest and place the new object of regard on to the

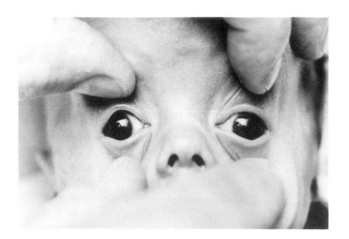

Fig. 42.1 The divergent eyes of a pre-term infant.

fovea. An everyday example is the shifting of gaze from the end of one line to the beginning of the next whilst reading. Saccades are rapid movements and the example given is a voluntary movement but saccades also include reflex changes of fixation and the fast phases of all forms of nystagmus (vestibular and optokinetic nystagmus).

Adults can change fixation from looking straight ahead to a target in the periphery of the visual field by one saccade (a slight approximation). The infant achieves this by means of multiple hypometric saccades, taking longer both to start the movement and reach the target (Regal et al 1983, Roucoux et al 1983). Infants also rely more on co-ordinated head and eye movements than do adults when shifting gaze. By the age of one year the saccadic system has developed, enabling a change of fixation on to an eccentric target to be achieved by using a single saccade. Clinically these changes are easily observed: for example, it takes much longer to attract the visual interest of a neonate to a novel stimulus in the periphery of the visual field compared with a 9-month-old infant. The fast phases of the various types of nystagmus are considered later.

Tests of saccadic function involve inducing refixation eye movements. The fast phase of nystagmus as in optokinetic nystagmus and on rotation.

Optokinetic nystagmus (OKN)

This response is elicited by moving a striped tape or drum across the field of vision. It is characterized by a slow following phase in the direction of the moving stripe followed by a fast corrective phase in the opposite direction, returning the eye to its original position. Functionally OKN is linked to the vestibulo-ocular reflex (VOR) and co-ordinates head and eye movements, ensuring clear vision during body movements such as running or walking up stairs. With both eyes open, both slow and fast phases of OKN can be elicited from the first day of life in the full-term infant (McGinnis 1930, Gorman et al 1957). However, whether the slow phase at this age is a true smooth pursuit movement (as it is in the adult) or merely the slow component of the OKN response (these two may not necessarily be the same) is unknown.

So far we have considered the OKN response obtained binocularly. Before the age of 3 months an OKN response can be obtained when the tape is moved in a temporal to nasal direction but not in a nasal to temporal direction when each eye is tested separately. After 3 months this OKN asymmetry disappears due to the establishment of binocular vision (Braddick & Atkinson 1983). For the pre-term infant the transition from asymmetrical to symmetrical OKN occurs later postnatally, corresponding to about 3 months corrected age (Van Hof-Van Duin & Mohn 1984a). Persistence of monocular OKN asymmetry beyond this age may be associated with strabismus.

The pathways involved in the OKN response are poorly

understood (Braddick & Atkinson 1983, Van Hof-Van Duin and Mohn 1983). The temporal-to-nasal response is probably mediated to a large extent subcortically, whereas the nasal-to-temporal response requires a functioning cortex.

Despite the many seemingly intimidating complexities surrounding the neuro-anatomy and functions of this response, OKN is of considerable value in routine clinical practice.

Tests of OKN. I prefer a tape (white tapes 1.5 m long, with either red squares 5×5 cm or cartoon pictures of similar size) to a drum, as it occupies more of the baby's visual environment than the standard drum and is more portable. The tape should be moved slowly in both horizontal and vertical directions, the responses being recorded separately as 0 to ++++. The clinical uses of OKN include:

1. Vision assessment. A valuable but crude indication that vision is present. However, this is a test of visibility, not resolution (see later). It is also important to be aware of the extremely rare possibility of a positive response in cortical blindness (Van Hof-Van Duin & Mohn 1983).
2. Eye movements. OKN is a test of both pursuit and saccadic systems, and of binocular eye movements. This is a simple means of detecting subtle slowness of the adducting eye in internuclear ophthalmoplegia.
3. Nystagmus. In congenital nystagmus the OKN responses horizontally are characteristically inverted (see later) but normal vertically. This is useful diagnostically and distinct from the variable nystagmoid movements associated with reduced vision in which no OKN response can be elicited in any direction.

Vestibulo–ocular reflexes (VOR)

The VOR ensure that the visual image remains stationary on the retina during head and body movements. Acceleration induces a movement of endolymph in the semicircular canals from which impulses are conveyed by the vestibular nerve to the brainstem and via the medial longitudinal fasciculus to the ocular motor nuclei. Thus a head movement induces an ocular movement, a response which is often modified by vision.

Tests of the VOR. Clinically these are done in three ways: doll's head manoeuvre and rotational and caloric testing.

1. Doll's head manoeuvre. Eye movements are observed whilst passively turning the infant's head. In infancy, before vision has developed sufficiently to suppress this response, or in the comatose patient, head rotation induces a conjugate ocular deviation towards the opposite side: head to the left, eyes to the right (Fig. 42.2). A normal response indicates an intact vestibular apparatus and ocular motor system including the nuclei and peripheral nerves. The doll's head manoeuvre can therefore be used to detect limitation of ocular movements due to a gaze or cranial nerve palsy. This

test does not give any information about the pursuit or saccadic systems.

2. Rotational tests. These fall into two groups which induce different responses:
a. Barany chair rotation. In this laboratory technique the infant is rotated about his own vertical axis and this induces an ocular deviation in the direction opposite to the direction of rotation, as in the doll's head manoeuvre (Eviatar et al 1974). In the premature infant only a slow tonic deviation is induced but with increasing gestational age a recovery fast phase develops (producing nystagmus).
b. Rotation at arm's length. For this method of rotation the infant is held upright at arm's length with the head inclined slightly forward. This procedure, commonly used in clinical practice, induces a tonic ocular deviation in the direction of the movement (as if the infant is looking ahead): rotation to the right, eyes deviate to the right (Fig. 42.3); in the older infant nystagmus occurs. This response using a different axis of rotation induces a movement in the opposite direction to that seen using the Barany method.

Whichever method is used, rotation of the premature infant induces a tonic deviation alone and the fast phase (nystagmus) does not develop until about 45 weeks of postmenstrual age (Mitchell & Cambon 1969, Eviatar et al 1979, Ornitz et al 1979, Rossi et al 1979, Donat et al 1980, Cordero et al 1983). An exception to these findings has been reported by Pendleton & Paine (1961) who demonstrated a fast phase in pre-term infants as early as 33 weeks of postmenstrual age. Behavioural state can influence this test; a fast phase elicited when the infant is awake may not be present when drowsy.

Once the age at which nystagmus occurs has been reached, postrotatory nystagmus, in the opposite direction to that occurring during rotation, is seen. Its duration depends upon gestational age, behavioural state, whether

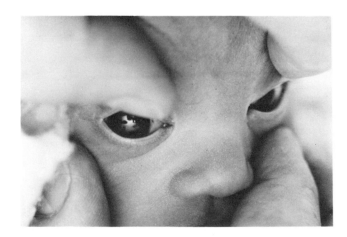

Fig. 42.2 Doll's head manoeuvre: head turn to the left induces a deviation of the eyes to the right.

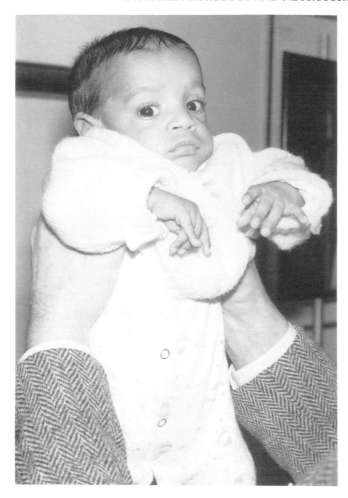

Fig. 42.3 Rotation at arm's length. This baby is being rotated to his right, his eyes deviate to the right — the opposite direction to that seen in the doll's head manoeuvre.

the test is performed in the dark, and the stage of visual development (Mitchell & Cambon 1969, Ornitz et al 1979, Cordero et al 1983) but in the alert sighted infant it should cease within 5 seconds.

Rotation at arm's length is simple to perform and provides a great deal of clinically useful information on: vision, the saccadic system, the vestibular system, and ocular motor nuclei and infranuclear pathways.

Thus, rotation of the premature infant induces a full ocular deviation because at this age vision is not sufficiently developed to modify the VOR. With increasing age and visual development, vision dampens the VOR and hence the rotational excursion decreases. In clinical terms severely reduced vision can be suspected if rotation after 3 months of age induce an inordinately large rotational excursion and postrotatory nystagmus persisting for more than 5 seconds. This test is also a simple method of evaluating the range of eye movements in infancy and distinguishing a sixth nerve palsy from concomitant convergent squint.

3. Caloric tests. Donat et al (1980) confirmed the observation that the pre-term infant cannot generate the fast phase of nystagmus. They observed, on caloric testing, an internuclear ophthalmoplegia in some normal premature infants indicating immaturity of the medial longitudinal fasciculus, i.e. the brainstem communication between the vestibular apparatus and the ocular motor nuclei. As the doll's head manoeuvre always induced complete excursion they considered caloric testing to be a sensitive test of brainstem interconnections.

Vergence movements

The eye movements considered so far have all been conjugate. Convergence to near targets is clearly dysjugate and cannot be consistently demonstrated until 2 months of age (Ling 1942, Aslin 1977). Fusion, the response to a base-out prism is not established until 6 months (Aslin 1977). Pre-term infants probably show a delay in the development of fusion commensurate with gestational age (Coakes et al 1979).

Tests of vergence involve observing convergence and divergence when an object is brought nearer or taken further away.

ABNORMAL EYE MOVEMENTS

Some of the disorders mentioned here persist throughout life but the emphasis will be directed towards those aspects relating particularly to the neonatal period and early infancy; details of examination are adequately covered in other texts. Eye movement disorders can be divided into three groups; nuclear and infranuclear disorders, supranuclear disorders, nystagmus and related oscillations. Many of these conditions have important neurological or ophthalmological associations which are not always immediately obvious.

Nuclear and infranuclear disorders

These disorders limit the movement of one eye, whereas supranuclear abnormalities affect the movement of both eyes. Conditions involving the peripheral nerves, in the cavernous sinus, orbit, and the extra-ocular muscles, as in myasthenia are all included in this category. This chapter concentrates entirely on strabismus.

Strabismus

It has already been noted that about 33% of neonates are divergent (Fig. 42.1) (Rethy 1969, Nixon et al 1985) and 3% are convergent. These deviations tend to be relatively small and the eyes of both groups tend to become normally aligned over the next few weeks.

The so-called congenital esotropia (convergent strabismus) is rarely, if ever, present at birth (Nixon et al 1985) but develops within the first 6 months of life and is therefore more appropriately called infantile esotropia. Abduction is often initially considered to be limited but by rotating the infant at arm's length or performing the doll's head manoeuvre full excursions can be elicited differentiating infantile esotropia from a true sixth nerve palsy.

Paralytic squints, either congenital or acquired, are not common in early infancy. Congenital palsies may be due to maldevelopment of the cranial nerve nuclei or nerves, or prenatal infection, although in most the aetiology is unknown. The role of birth trauma has probably been overemphasized. A true sixth nerve palsy as an isolated anomaly can very rarely be present at birth as a very large angle esotropia and this characteristically resolves spontaneously over a few weeks. An acquired cranial nerve palsy usually denotes a significant neurological disorder such as hydrocephalus, intracranial inflammation, tumour, neurodegenerative disorder and trauma (Harcourt 1983) and clearly may develop at any age. Although the signs of a third or sixth nerve palsy are relatively obvious, a congenital fourth nerve palsy can easily be missed in early infancy, and indeed may not be detected for several years until a compensatory head tilt is noted.

Squint may be the presenting feature of an infant with severe ophthalmic pathology. A blind eye may diverge or less commonly converge (Fig. 42.4), although this usually becomes apparent later in childhood. The paediatrician should also be wary of the divergent squint persistent after the neonatal period as it may be the first sign of a severe bilateral visual deficit.

The prevalence of concomitant squint in the general population is about 2–3% but occurs more commonly in children who have suffered brain damage (Von Noorden 1985), or are experiencing developmental problems (Bankes 1974). Pre-term birth is also associated with an increased incidence of squint from 11 to 19% (Kitchen et al 1980, Kushner 1982, Keith & Kitchen 1983).

In most instances squint has no significant associations, however, the possibility of co-existent or causative neurological or ophthalmological pathology must always be borne in mind and every infant should have a detailed ophthalmic assessment and neurological work-up if indicated.

Supranuclear disorders

In contrast to the infranuclear pathways which mediate the movements of one eye, the supranuclear centres and pathways govern the movements of both eyes in unison: pursuit, saccadic, vestibulo–ocular, OKN and vergence movements. According to the site of the lesion the various types of movement are affected differentially but in all the

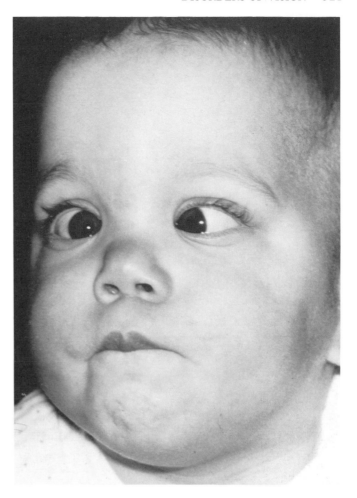

Fig. 42.4 Left convergent squint due to ocular pathology. Cicatricial retinopathy of prematurity has severely affected the vision of the left eye.

retention of some infranuclear movement and its bilaterality distinguishes supranuclear from infranuclear disorders.

Saccadic palsy

This is not uncommon in infancy and is usually the result of an intracranial haemorrhage in the neonatal period affecting either the frontal cortex or the fronto–mesencephalic pathway as this descends to the brainstem (Trounce et al 1985). In saccadic palsy the eyes deviate to the side of the lesion (Fig. 42.5); thus ipsilateral but not contralateral saccades can be elicited. Pursuit and the slow phase of the VOR are both unaffected if the lesion is above the brainstem.

Pursuit disorders

Isolated abnormalities of pursuit but not saccades are rare.

Disorders of optokinetic nystagmus

As stated earlier, OKN can be affected by disorders of pursuit, saccades, brainstem connections (internuclear

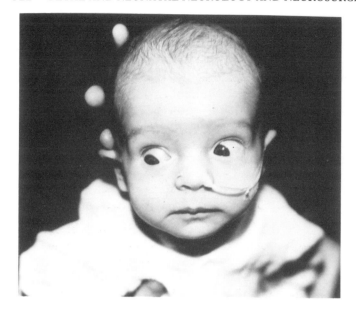

Fig. 42.5 Neonatal thalamic haemorrhage. Ocular signs include 'sunsetting', skew deviation (left eye is higher than the right) and a tonic deviation of the eyes to the right (saccadic paresis).

ophthalmoplegia) and muscle pareses. This test can be particularly helpful in distinguishing a hemianopia resulting from a lesion of the occipital and parietal lobes. In the former the OKN response is intact, whereas in the latter the slow phase of the OKN response is present but there is no fast phase when the tape is moved to the side of the lesion, i.e. from the hemianopic to the normal field.

Gaze palsy

In gaze paresis both saccadic and pursuit function are affected, and depending on the site also the vestibulo–ocular reflex. Most gaze palsies are caused by brainstem pathology where the various supranuclear eye movement pathways are close together. Horizontal gaze palsy may be congenital, as an isolated anomaly (Hoyt et al 1977) or in association with other abnormalities, e.g. in the Klippel–Feil or Mobius syndromes. Brainstem glioma may produce an acquired palsy. In neonates, vertical gaze palsies are more common than horizontal. Up- gaze is usually affected more than down-gaze and the eyes may deviate down — 'sunsetting' sign (Fig. 42.5). Eyelid retraction is common, although occasionally ptosis is present. Transient downward deviation of the eyes can occur in healthy neonates (Hoyt et al 1980) but an up-gaze gaze abnormality is usually indicative of a midbrain lesion, e.g. tumour, neurodegenerative disorder, encephalitis or hydrocephalus. This last is the most common cause of an up-gaze paresis in early infancy and the signs, according to Swash (1976), are due to hydrocephalic distortion of the posterior commissure. Recently, up- gaze palsy has been reported in pre-term infants who sustained intraventricular haemorrhages (Tamura & Hoyt 1987).

These infants showed tonic downwards ocular deviations and convergent squints due to haemorrhage in thalamic and mesencephalic structures.

Congenital ocular motor apraxia (COMA)

In COMA, horizontal saccades to command are defective. Consequently the affected child cannot shift gaze to either side voluntarily, and in order to look from one object to another has to insert a jerky head thrust characteristic of COMA (Cogan 1952, 1966). The head thrust, which is in the direction of the target, uses the VOR to drive the eyes to the opposite side of the orbit. The head movement carries on past the target dragging the eyes with it until they are aligned on the target; the head then moves slowly back as the eyes remain fixated. Although primarily a defect of saccades, slow pursuit is also affected especially in early infancy. These abnormalities are entirely confined to horizontal movements; all types of vertical movement are normal.

This fairly uncommon condition is mentioned here because of its mode of presentation in infancy, the frequency of neurodevelopmental problems and structural CNS malformations. The head thrust does not develop until about 6 months of age. Before this the infant may be suspected to be blind as he will not show any visual interest in objects placed to one side and no horizontal following movements can be demonstrated. At this early age the diagnosis can be suspected if the OKN response is absent horizontally but normal vertically. Also, rotation induces nystagmus if performed in the vertical but not in the horizontal meridian. After the head thrust has developed the diagnosis is obvious, although over the years signs subside considerably.

Motor delay is probably universal in infancy and lessens but does not necessarily completely resolve with time. Conceptual delay, particularly with speech, is common in these children (Fielder et al 1986b).

Structural CNS abnormalities are common, particularly agenesis of the corpus callosum and cerebellum. However, in view of the occurrence of these anomalies without COMA, it is possible that COMA forms part of a spectrum of neurological malformation which may at times involve the corpus callosum and/or the cerebellum. But these may simply be markers indicative of early CNS maldevelopment and not an integral part of the mechanism of COMA.

Neonatal eye movements

As already mentioned, eye movements, which would be considered abnormal and even warrant urgent neuro–ophthalmic investigation in the older child, are quite common in the neonate, particularly if pre-term. Bursts of eye movements may be seen through closed eyelids but are most commonly seen when the infant is turned or disturbed.

Tonic downwards deviation, up- or down-beat nystagmus and nystagmus in other directions are commonly observed. Ocular flutter, opsoclonus (bursts of saccades) and skew deviations are less commonly seen. There is essentially no information on the prevalence and possible significance of these neonatal eye movements, or indeed whether they should even be considered abnormal. Dubowitz et al (1981) reported a strong correlation between intraventricular haemorrhage and roving eye movements. Hoyt et al (1980) examined 242 full-term neonates, without neurological abnormalities, and observed downward deviations (5 infants), opsoclonus (9) and skew deviation (22). Five of those with a skew deviation later developed a squint.

Nystagmus

The rhythmic oscillation of the eyes — nystagmus — has always baffled clinicians, mainly because there is no clinically ideal classification. The jargon currently used to describe this movement also contributes to this confusion. The pathophysiology of nystagmus is beyond the scope of this book, instead a few aspects of clinical relevance are mentioned. For detailed accounts the reader is referred to existing excellent texts (Glaser 1978, Leigh & Zee 1983). Our understanding of nystagmus in early infancy is not helped by a serious lack of information about the natural history of several common conditions, such as congenital nystagmus, and our relative ignorance about the underlying mechanisms of certain neonatal eye movement patterns. In this section only those nystagmus types relevant to the first 6 months of life are considered.

Physiological nystagmus

The various nystagmus types, including rotational, caloric and optokinetic have already been discussed. Remember the normal development of the response being tested before considering the abnormal.

Central nervous system conditions

Not surprisingly nystagmus can occur in many CNS conditions. These include cerebellar, brainstem and vestibular lesions. In the adult these often produce predictable specific types of nystagmus which point to a particular anatomical location, whereas in the infant features tend to be more variable, less predictable, and consequently have less diagnostic value (Daroff et al 1978). Clearly nystagmus due to a CNS cause may be apparent at any age; thus nystagmus observed within the first week or so of life is more likely to have a CNS basis, although occasionally congenital nystagmus can be present at this time. Dubowitz et al (1981) observed roving eye movements some time after the development of germinal matrix haemorrhage – intraventricular haemorrhage in pre-term infants.

Sensory deprivation nystagmus

Bilaterally reduced vision in infancy and early childhood leads to nystagmus only if the lesion involves the anterior visual pathway. Consequently, nystagmus is not a feature of cortical blindness (Whiting et al 1985). Any condition of the anterior visual pathway sufficient to preclude normal visual development will cause sensory deprivation nystagmus. These conditions include: corneal scarring, albinism, achromatopsia, aniridia, congenital cataracts, and optic nerve pathology including atrophy and hypoplasia.

Nystagmus due to a visual deficit does not develop until about 3 months of age and presents clinically in two forms:

1. Wandering eye movements associated with blindness.
2. Nystagmus which is clinically indistinguishable from or very similar to congenital nystagmus.

Blindness. As mentioned, severe visual deprivation before the age of 2 years, and sometimes later, results in nystagmus. In this case the eye movements are slow, large in amplitude and variable in direction.

Nystagmus indistinguishable from congenital nystagmus. Conditions such as albinism, achromatopsia and aniridia cause a visual defect, but not blindness, and result in nystagmus which is either similar or identical to that seen in congenital nystagmus. As mentioned, the oscillation usually starts at about 3 months. Occasionally the movement may be vertical on presentation (Hoyt & Gelbart 1984) but this subsequently becomes horizontally directed, as is the rule in congenital nystagmus. As the ocular findings in many of these conditions are subtle and easily missed, it is essential that congenital nystagmus is a diagnosis of exclusion, made only after all other possibilities have been eliminated (see later). The clinical severity of certain conditions may vary between patients: thus, Leber's amaurosis or optic nerve hypoplasia may both cause either blindness and nystagmus of the blind or, if less severe, reduced vision and a congenital nystagmus picture. Two conditions deserve special mention: albinism and achromatopsia.

Albinism. This is straightforward to diagnose in most instances but can be difficult early on, especially in the infant from a blond family or the X-linked ocular form. As will be discussed later, albinos may present in early infancy with reduced vision which subsequently improves (delayed visual maturation), sometimes even before the nystagmus has commenced. Slit-lamp examination is essential and the finding of the typical carrier retinal picture in the mother or sister of a suspected ocular albino is diagnostic.

Achromatopsia. Achromatopsia is a congenital absence of retinal cones and is inherited as an autosomal recessive trait but rarely correctly diagnosed in the first year of life. Retinal cones function optimally in bright light and subserve fine discrimination (acuity) and colour vision. The infant with achromatopsia (complete colour blindness) presents with photosensitivity and poor vision, particularly under conditions of bright illumination. Visual function improves when the illumination is reduced. Visual acuity is reduced (about 6/60 in the older child) and colour vision is severely affected. Crudely, achromatopsia may be considered the opposite of rod disorders such as retinitis pigmentosa in which night vision and the peripheral visual field are affected before visual acuity. However, this analogy should not be pursued further as achromatopsia is not progressive, unlike many rod disorders. Nystagmus in achromatopsia closely resembles congenital nystagmus but the amplitude tends to be less (Yee et al 1981). Ocular examination is essentially negative in infancy; colour vision testing is impossible at this age and the diagnosis can only be established by electroretinography (ERG) at 30 Hz (Figs 42.6 and 42.7).

Congenital nystagmus

This term should be reserved for nystagmus presenting in infancy which is not associated with any other ocular abnormality (Daroff et al 1978). The term motor nystagmus is sometimes used to avoid confusion with nystagmus due to a sensory defect. The condition may be inherited as a dominant, recessive or X-linked disorder. Despite its name the onset is usually at about 6 weeks or age but occasionally is observed immediately after birth. Sometimes, if associated with delayed visual maturation (see later), it does not develop for a few months, until the vision improves.

In congenital nystagmus the oscillation is binocular, symmetrical and beats horizontally in all positions of gaze, except for the rare vertical variant. The movement is dampened by convergence and often increases on lateral gaze. Vertical OKN is normal but horizontal OKN is commonly, though not invariably, inverted (a fast phase in the direction of the tape, effectively reducing the response). Head nodding is present in some patients but this probably develops later on in childhood. Other aspects such as the null position will not be covered here. Making a diagnosis can be difficult, particularly as during early infancy congenital nystagmus may be variable and the characteristics just mentioned not apparent. Furthermore, as many other forms of nystagmus with ocular or neurological associations mimic this condition, the diagnosis of congenital nystagmus must be one of exclusion.

Spasmus nutans

This syndrome consists of nystagmus, head nodding and torticollis, and commences between 4 and 18 months of age. Not all features are present at one time; thus the head nod may be present before the nystagmus and vice versa. Although the nystagmus is usually bilateral, it can be grossly asymmetrical and may be either horizontal or vertical. Like congenital nystagmus, spasmus nutans is a diagnosis of exclusion. As occasionally patients with these signs harbour intracranial tumours (Antony et al 1980), full assessment is

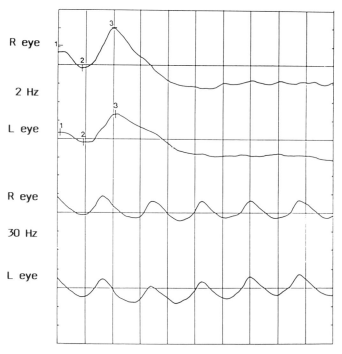

Fig. 42.6 ERG traces at 2 Hz (rod and cone response) and 30 Hz (cone response alone). These are normal responses obtained from a 2-year-old child without sedation using skin electrodes.

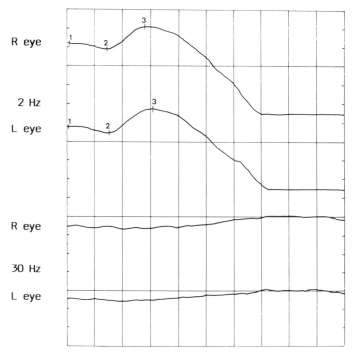

Fig. 42.7 ERG traces from a child with achromatopsia. A response is obtained at 2 Hz indicating the presence of rod photoreceptors but not at 30 Hz due to an absence of retinal cones.

mandatory. Spasmus nutans resolves spontaneously usually within 1–2 years but can sometimes take longer.

Asymmetric nystagmus

Nystagmus which is either totally monocular or grossly asymmetric between the two eyes may be seen in infancy; both can occur in spasmus nutans. Recently Farmer & Hoyt (1984) emphasized the frequency of mononuclear nystagmus in infants with chiasmal tumours. Vision was commonly but not invariably reduced in one eye. However, they did not consider that the visual deficit per se accounted for the nystagmus as visual loss does not commonly lead to monocular nystagmus in early childhood. Monocular blindness can cause monocular nystagmus but the latter usually develops later in life. Unfortunately, as there are no clinical features which distinguish absolutely infants with spasmus nutans from those with chiasmal tumours, full neurological and neuroradiological investigations are necessary.

Special nystagmus types

There are many other types of nystagmus which cannot be considered here but may have important neurological implications, such as downbeat, upbeat, see-saw, dissociated (e.g. in internuclear ophthalmoplegia), ocular bobbing, and retraction nystagmus.

The investigation of nystagmus

As nystagmus may signify a serious neurological or ocular disorder it must always be taken seriously. The age at onset can be a useful diagnostic clue. The pattern of eye movement must be carefully evaluated by recording the direction (convention dictates this to be in the direction of the fast phase), amplitude and frequency of the nystagmus in the nine positions of gaze. This ensures that the clinician has studied the eye movement pattern carefully. The distinction between pendular and jerk nystagmus is not diagnostically helpful as both may exist in the same patient, in different positions of gaze. Accurate diagnosis is rarely possible from the observation of the pattern of nystagmus alone. It is essential, therefore, that every infant with nystagmus has a detailed, but appropriate, paediatric and ophthalmological examination. Neuroradiological investigation is often necessary. As has been mentioned, in certain ocular conditions the eye examination may be normal or near-normal, in which case a diagnosis can only be established by an ERG. This may be performed simply without sedation (Fielder 1979) in most infants and the stimulus frequencies should be 2 Hz (which elicits a combined rod and cone response) and 30 Hz (cone response alone) (Figs 42.6 and 42.7).

VISION

NORMAL DEVELOPMENT

The rapid development of vision in the first few months of life is one of the most rewarding features of infancy, although its quantitative assessment has always been a considerable challenge to clinicians. In this section only brief mention is made of the qualitative assessment of visual function, emphasis being on the quantitative measurement of visual acuity, particularly the recently developed adaptation of the preferential looking technique — the acuity card procedure.

Qualitative aspects of visual development

Many infant's responses have a visual basis and consequently provide a useful, qualitative indication of visual development. This topic has been reviewed recently (Van Hof-Van Duin & Mohn 1984a).

Blink reflex

The blink reflex to a bright light is said to be present from 28 weeks of postmenstrual age (PMA) (Robinson 1966) and in almost all full-term and pre-term babies at 40 weeks of PMA (Kurtzberg et al 1979). A response does not invariably indicate the presence of vision, as a blink reflex has been observed in hydranencephaly with absence of the visual cortex (Aylward et al 1978).

Awareness and fixation

From 30 weeks of PMA there are periods of awareness during which visual fixation occurs and these periods naturally increase with increasing age (Hack et al 1981).

Orientation

Head turning to a diffuse light can be demonstrated from about 32 weeks of PMA (Robinson 1966) and is elicited in most by full-term (Goldie & Hopkins 1964). After 36 weeks of PMA there is no significant difference between pre-term and full-term infants (Robinson 1966), although Ferrari et al (1983) have reported that pre-term infants examined around 40 weeks of PMA are significantly poorer in orientation.

Following

Using a red ball, Brazelton et al (1966) detected following in 57% of normal infants at full-term. Dubowitz et al (1980) found a red woollen ball to be a better stimulus and were able to elicit following from 31 weeks of PMA (see Ch. 3). Vehrs & Baum (1970) in testing pre-term and full-term neonates around full-term considered a flashing light to be a more effective stimulus than either a red ball or diffuse light. Kurtzberg et al (1979) found reduced following in pre-term infants at 40 weeks of PMA compared to full-term neonates but this was not confirmed by Ruff et al (1982) who could not detect differences between these two groups at 44 and 48 weeks of PMA, except in neurologically abnormal pre-term infants who performed less well. As mentioned in the section on eye movements, following movements can only be elicited to a slowly moving target.

Optokinetic nystagmus

A binocular response to an OKN stimulus can be elicited at full-term (Kremenitzer et al 1979) and in over half of pre-term infants (Kiff & Lepard 1966), although in this study the degree of prematurity was not stated. This topic has been discussed elsewhere in this chapter.

Visual threat response

Eyelid closure to an approaching threatening object does not develop until about 16 weeks of corrected age for full-term and pre-term infants. When performing this test it is important to avoid tactile stimulation, e.g. a rush of air (Van Hof-Van Duin & Mohn 1984a).

Reaching

Visually directed reaching with one hand is first seen from about 2½ months (White et al 1964).

Smiling

Obviously, as vision can be an important component of this response, failure to smile by 6 weeks of age may signify a serious visual defect.

Other visual functions

Pupil reactions

Although present from 31 weeks of gestation (Robinson 1966) the pupillary reactions are clinically difficult to assess in neonates and infants and care must be taken to ensure that light and near reactions are not also active.

Colour vision

At 2 months of age infants are probably tritanopic, i.e. lacking the blue mechanism, but by 3 months colour vision is similar to that in adults (Boothe et al 1985).

Visual field

At birth the visual field is approximately 30 degrees on either side of the horizontal and this reaches adult proportions by about one year of age (Mohn et al 1986).

DEVELOPMENT OF VISUAL ACUITY — METHODS OF MEASUREMENT

Resolution and visibility

An appreciation of the distinction between resolution and visibility is an essential prerequisite to the evaluation of the visual aspects of a patient's history of tests of visual function. Resolution is the ability to distinguish two points or lines, (e.g. black and white stripes) or the details of a Snellen letter (strictly speaking the Snellen test is a measure of recognition, i.e. resolution and the ability to recognize the shape of a letter), whereas visibility is the ability to see a single object such as a white Stycar ball on a black background. These functions are quite different and must not be equated. Tests of vision which employ visibility tend to seriously overestimate vision when compared with resolution acuities. Thus a parent's observation that a child can see a very small sweet is merely a comment on visibility and does not preclude a serious defect of resolution. Tests of visibility include Stycar balls, Catford drum, identification of sweets etc.; whereas Snellen and related acuity tests, grating acuities, such as preferential looking, and the acuity card procedure, test resolution.

BEHAVIOURAL METHODS — PREFERENTIAL LOOKING

The preferential looking (PL) technique of measuring visual acuity in infants arose from the observation by Fantz some 30 years ago that patterned objects are visually interesting to infants. In PL the infant is usually presented simultaneously with two stimuli: one containing black and white stripes (gratings) whilst the other is homogeneous grey and matched for brightness with the grating so that, if blurred sufficiently to make the stripes indistinguishable, both stimuli appear to be equally grey and bright. These are then encased by a grey screen to minimize patient distraction. The observer situated behind the screen, looks at the infant through a peep-hole midway between the patterned and homogeneous stimuli. Based on the infant's looking behaviour following stimulus presentation, the observer is forced to decide which side contains the grating (the observer is ignorant of the pattern location). During the test the spatial frequency of the grating is increased (stripes become finer) in steps and the side of pattern presentation varied. The finest grating to induce a consistent looking response is considered to represent the infant's visual acuity. There are a number of procedural modifications of this technique (e.g. operant preferential looking and the diagnostic grating procedure). Unfortunately these are all tedious and time-consuming to perform and consequently have not been incorporated into routine clinical use. These disadvantages should not, however, disguise the fact that laboratory PL-based studies have added greatly to our knowledge of normal visual development and vision in many pathological conditions.

Fortunately this situation has changed with the latest PL modification — the acuity card procedure (ACP) (McDonald et al 1985) and a similar test employed by Dubowitz and co-workers (Dubowitz et al 1980, Morante et al 1982). In standard PL the stimuli are usually presented on TV screens but in the ACP are mounted, in pairs, on a series of cards. These are presented through a large aperture in a grey cardboard screen (Fig. 42.8). The whole apparatus, often made of card, is easily portable. This procedure has several advantages over standard PL techniques: it is rapid to perform (2 to 6 minutes for binocular testing) and fixation can be confirmed by a small sideways movement of the card. The large aperture in the screen keeps the tester and infant in close proximity (sitting on a parent's lap 36 cm from the stimulus) between presentations, and enables interest and attention to be maintained by toys. The older child may prefer to point at the grating and the correct identification of horizontally and vertically orientated stripes can be used to prevent guessing and ensure that the grafting has been correctly identified. It is advisable, in most instances, to use the surrounding screen to minimize distraction. However, under certain circumstances this can be discarded, for example when the patient is lying in bed, in the neonatal intensive care unit, or when testing the mentally retarded child (Fig. 42.9). The test is applicable to all ages from the

pre-term infant onwards. The success rate from six studies was reviewed recently by Teller et al (1986) and varied according to age: 80% in neonates, 100% from 12 weeks to 12 months and after 30 months, and down to 75% between 18 and 24 months.

Inevitably the ACP has certain disadvantages: as the tester often knows the location of the grating (but this need not be so) the test is more subjective than formal PL, although published results of ACP and PL correlate well (Teller et al 1986). Matching the luminance of the two stimuli is critical to ensure that the patient is not simply responding to brightness rather than resolving the grating. Judging looking patterns in the presence of nystagmus is not easy. Field defects may 'interfere' with testing if the stimulus is inadvertently presented into the defective field. The infant with the rare condition, congenital ocular motor apraxia, being unable to execute horizontal refixation movements, cannot perform ACP unless the cards are presented vertically. More important problems are encountered when measuring monocular acuities and in older children controversy exists over the accuracy of gratings in general compared with Snellen acuities in amblyopia (Mayer et al 1984, Moseley et al 1988).

Despite these problems the introduction of the ACP is an exciting and important development for the clinician; for the first time there is a reliable test of visual acuity (i.e. resolution, not visibility) which can be used quickly and easily in the clinical situation, even in neonates (Dobson et

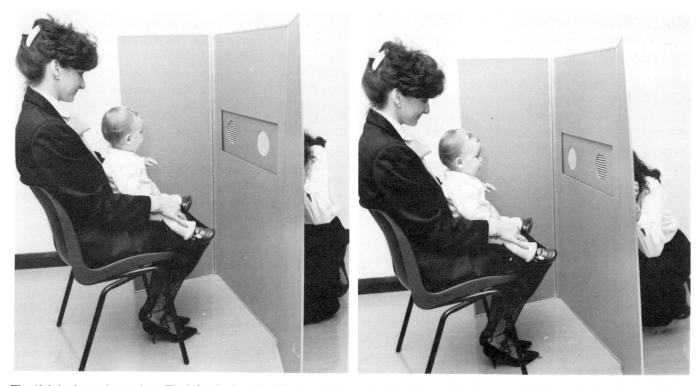

Fig. 42.8 Acuity card procedure. The infant is clearly looking towards the grating (the side panel has been turned sideways for the photograph.)

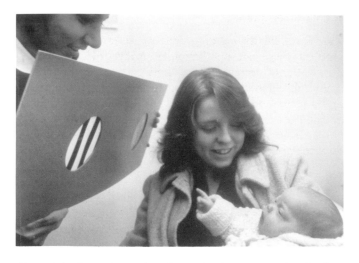

Fig. 42.9 Acuity card procedure. In certain circumstances the stimulus cards may be used without the surrounding apparatus.

al 1987). Furthermore the success rate is high and enables the detailed and repeated evaluation of a large population for whom no other test is applicable.

According to PL-based studies, including the ACP, vision improves at a rate of one cycle per degree per month and does not reach adult levels of 30 cycles until 3–5 years of age (Atkinson & Braddick 1983, Dobson 1983, Boothe et al 1985, Teller et al 1986). Grating acuities are measured in cycles per degree, i.e. the number of pairs of black and white stripes per degree of visual angle. Thus the infant whose vision is developing normally sees 3 cycles/degree (6/60) at 3 months, 6 cycles/degree (6/30) at 6 months and 12 cycles/degree (6/18) at one year of age.

Optokinetic nystagmus

This response has been used to measure visual acuity (Gorman et al 1957, Kiff & Lepard 1966) although recently this technique has attracted relatively little interest. It is noteworthy that the Catford drum, because it elicits a to-and-fro smooth pursuit movement, does not, as is usually quoted, employ OKN. Hoyt (1986a) has recently outlined the limitations of OKN as a clinically viable test.

Visual evoked potentials

This subject has already been dealt with in Chapter 16 but a few aspects need to be mentioned. Both the flash (Fielder et al 1983) and pattern VEP (Moskowitz & Sokol 1983) reflect visual pathway maturation. However, only the latter, as it contains an edge, can be used to measure acuity. Pattern reversal VEP estimates of infant visual acuity indicate that adult levels are reached by about 6 months (Marg et al 1976, Sokol 1978). However, in a study by De Vreis-Khoe & Spekreijse (1982), using a pattern-onset stimulus, this level was not achieved until about 4 years of age.

The VEP : PL discrepancy

The foregoing sections have shown that adult acuity levels are reached by about 6 months using most VEP studies but not until 3–5 years using PL. The basis of this discrepancy has not been fully resolved but it is interesting to note that foveal development takes much longer than originally thought, maturity not being reached until between 15 and 45 months after birth (Hendrickson & Yuodelis 1984) corresponding closer to PL than VEP results. One exception is the VEP study of De Vreis-Khoe & Spekreijse (1982) which correlates with both anatomical and PL data.

The PL : Snellen acuity discrepancy

The clinician, already confused by the discrepancy between behavioural and evoked potential acuity estimates, is now confronted with another discrepancy: PL grating acuities may be significantly better than Snellen acuities in certain clinical conditions, particularly amblyopia (Mayer et al 1984). This difference, which also is not fully understood but may be due partly to methodological differences in measuring PL and Snellen acuities (Moseley et al 1988), does not negate the value of either test but does indicate the need for further research. In any case, Snellen acuity is not relevant for the age group under consideration in this book but the issue remains: does PL overestimate acuity in certain ocular conditions, and if so by how much? Despite these problems it should not be forgotten that the ACP is the only quantitative test of vision which can be used simply and rapidly in the clinical situation and gives far more information than existing qualitative tests. Its value in recording visual development and assessing the infant who appears not to see well is not in question.

Visual development of pre-term infants

At full-term, the vision of the pre-term infant is lower than that of a full-term counterpart (Morante et al 1982). It remains so until about 30 weeks (Van Hof-Van Duin et al 1983, Van Hof-Van Duin & Mohn 1984a) if postnatal age is used as the parameter. However, when corrected for the degree of prematurity, pre-term and full-term infants behave similarly (Dobson et al 1980, Van Hof-Van Duin et al 1983, Van Hof-Van Duin & Mohn 1984a, Brown & Yamamoto 1986). These results show that, very broadly speaking, premature birth neither hastens nor retards visual development in infancy. However, Sebris et al (1984) reported that although many 3–4-year-old pre-term children had visual acuities within the normal range, on average, their acuities were lower than those born at full-term. This finding has also been reported in the older expremature child (Fledelius 1981). Neurologically abnormal pre-term infants may show a delay in visual acuity maturation (Placzek et al 1985).

ABNORMALITIES OF VISION

Except for the relatively uncommon instance of the obviously blind infant, one of the most difficult clinical problems is the identification of the child harbouring a visual deficit. Measuring visual acuity is obviously ideal but not always possible, qualitative tests are often quite inadequate and as yet preferential looking tests, such as the acuity card procedure (ACP), are not universally available. Under these circumstances and in the absence of a reliable objective measure, a carefully taken history is often more informative than the subsequent clinical examination. Concern voluntarily expressed by a parent must always be taken seriously as this is rarely unfounded and usually more reliable than most qualitative tests of vision. Seeming lack of concern must, however, be treated with caution as it does not necessarily indicate that all is well. This attitude can be adopted for a number of reasons. First, a low expectancy is generally held for vision in very early infancy. Second, anxiety may be hidden until the mother's fear that her baby has defective vision is either allayed or confirmed by medical staff, following which she may pour out a detailed account accurately describing reduced vision dating back to very early infancy. Third, information may be witheld for fear of biasing the professional towards an unfavourable verdict.

The visual pathway abnormalities to be considered in this section are divided into those affecting the anterior (eye to optic chiasm) and posterior (optic tracts to visual cortex) portions. Only neuro-ophthalmic conditions are considered and problems such as cataract and retinopathy of prematurity are omitted. The conditions listed are representative and not exhaustive and individual topics will necessarily be dealt with only briefly.

Disorders of the anterior visual pathway

Characteristically, lesions of the anterior visual pathway (i.e. as far back as the optic chiasm) sufficient to reduce vision bilaterally in early life lead to nystagmus and afferent pupillary defects. The latter can be difficult to test clinically in infants and children.

Electroretinography in infancy

In several conditions, in the absence of ophthalmoscopic signs, an electroretinogram (ERG) is essential to distinguish retinal pathology from that elsewhere in the visual pathway. As mentioned earlier, this can be performed without sedation, using lid or conjunctival gold-foil electrodes, at stimulus rates of 2 Hz (producing rod and cone responses) and 30 Hz (producing only a cone response (Fig. 42.6)). Performed this way it is probably advisable to consider the ERG obtained as qualitative rather than quantitative but in most clinical instances this is adequate.

Retinal disorders

Several retinal disorders produce a severe visual defect. Some of these are ophthalmoscopically obvious such as retinopathy of prematurity or chorioretinal scarring. Other conditions such as achromatopsia (see p. 523) and the tapeto–retinal degenerations (including Leber's amaurosis) are not associated with ophthalmoscopically visible signs, at least in early infancy. In these conditions a precise diagnosis can only be established by an ERG.

The cherry-red spot

This classic but rarely seen sign results from storage of abnormal substances in the retinal ganglion cells. As these cells are abundant around the macula but are absent from the very centre the fovea is red and its surround white. This subtle sign, which fades with time, is seen in a number of conditions including: Tay Sach's, Sandhoff's, Niemann-Pick and Farber's diseases, metachromatic leukodystrophy and the mucolipidoses. These are discussed in detail in Chapter 40.

Optic nerve disorders

Optic atrophy

This ophthalmoscopic sign can be difficult to make if mild and it is important to recall that the optic disc appearance alone does not indicate the amount of visual function. Optic atrophy (particularly if associated with retinal arteriolar attenuation) may be the only visible sign of serious retinal disease, for instance in Leber's amaurosis or the Laurence–Moon–Biedl syndrome. Only by an ERG can retinal involvement be diagnosed or eliminated.

Optic nerve damage secondary to retinal disease is referred to as consecutive or ascending atrophy. Damage to the optic radiation and visual cortex can cause trans-synaptic degeneration and a descending type of optic atrophy but this response is confined to visual pathway insults before and during early infancy.

Hereditary optic atrophy. Behr's optic atrophy is an autosomal recessive condition in which optic atrophy is associated with mild mental retardation, hypertonia and ataxia. Onset may be within the first year of life. Whether isolated recessive optic atrophy is a true entity is uncertain.

Other hereditary optic atrophies such as Leber's optic neuropathy, dominant optic atrophy and the DIDMOAD syndrome all present after the first year of life and are not considered here.

Retinal disease. Tapeto–retinal degenerations such as Leber's amaurosis, Laurence-Moon-Biedl and Zellweger's syndromes may all cause optic atrophy.

Intra-uterine disease. Optic atrophy may occur following intra-uterine infections, asphyxia and cerebral malformations.

Perinatal damage. It is well established that optic atrophy can result from neonatal events. Birth trauma very rarely leads to unilateral nerve damage. Birth asphyxia is sometimes associated with optic atrophy which may be trans-synaptic, resulting from damage to the postgeniculate pathway. This is a feature of the immature visual system alone and may result from perinatal brain asphyxia or malformation, e.g. holoprosencephaly, porencephaly and hydranencephaly.

Inflammatory. Severe meningoencephalitis in infancy may cause optic atrophy.

Compression. Hydrocephalus, by stretching or compression, can lead to optic atrophy. Tumours may compress the chiasm or nerve (e.g. craniopharyngioma) or involve the anterior visual pathway (glioma).

Metabolic. This includes the lipid storage diseases (e.g. Tay Sach's disease), Leigh's subacute necrotizing encephalopathy and osteopetrosis.

Optic nerve hypoplasia

This is a relatively common congenital anomaly of the optic nerve. Typically, the optic disc is small, surrounded by a peripapillary pigmented ring (Fig. 42.10), the retinal vessels are slightly tortuous and the nerve fibre layer is thinned (Frisen & Holmegaard 1978, Skarf & Hoyt 1984). As none of these signs is pathognomonic, mild optic nerve hypoplasia (ONH) may be difficult to diagnose — the disc may be of normal size and examination of the nerve fibre layer is not feasible in infancy. To add to this difficulty the double-ring sign is quite common in the 'normal' premature infant.

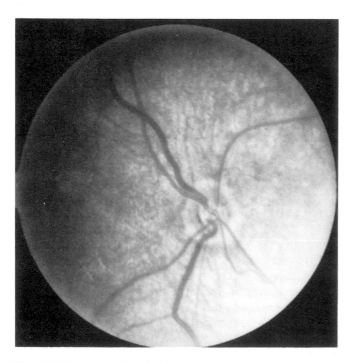

Fig. 42.10 Optic nerve hypoplasia.

The pathogenesis of ONH is not known but may represent a non-specific manifestation of damage to the developing visual system (Frisen & Holmegaard 1978). Not surprisingly, therefore, a degree of optic atrophy often co-exists. Thus ONH may be associated, particularly if bilateral, with a large variety of ocular or systemic abnormalities (Margalith et al 1984, Skarf & Hoyt 1984). Structural CNS abnormalities associated with ONH include absence of the septum pellucidum, hydranencephaly, porencephaly, holoprosencephaly, cerebral atrophy and cystic subcortical leukomalacia, and may therefore be occasionally detected on routine examination of neurologically abnormal neonates (Fielder et al 1986b).

Neuro-endocrine dysfunction occurs in 20 to 30% cases of ONH, with or without a structural neurological anomaly. As this does not become apparent until about 2–5 years of age, continued surveillance is necessary. Growth, thyroid and gonadotrophin hormones may all be affected, and diabetes insipidus has been reported (Margalith et al 1984, 1985, Skarf & Hoyt 1984, Costin & Murphree 1985). Transient neonatal cholestatic jaundice and hypoglycaemia are reported associations (Stanhope et al 1984) but it is not known whether these are the patients liable to develop other neuro-endocrine problems later.

Whilst CT scanning may not be necessary in the older patient (Skarf & Hoyt 1984), for the infant it is important to determine the extent of neurological involvement in order to anticipate possible future developmental problems. At this early age the identification of structural CNS abnormalities can be simply performed by cranial ultrasound (Fielder et al 1986a).

Other congenital abnormalities of the optic disc

Abnormalities such as colobomas, the morning glory syndrome and pits are well covered by ophthalmic texts (e.g. Brown & Tasman 1983) and are not considered here.

Posterior visual pathway disorders

In contrast to anterior visual pathway conditions, which are characteristically associated with nystagmus and afferent pupillary defects, disorders of the posterior visual pathway do not affect the pupil responses and nystagmus is not a feature. As a proviso to the last comment, many posterior visual pathway disorders are the consequence of widespread neurological damage. Under these circumstances nystagmus may be present but is not due to the visual deficit per se, exhibits a different pattern, and is usually poorly sustained.

Delayed visual maturation

Clinicians have known for years that the sight of a blind infant may later improve. First described by Beauvieux in 1926, the term delayed visual maturation (DVM) was introduced by Illingworth in 1961. This is probably the most common cause of a severe bilateral visual defect in early infancy and at its simplest, DVM is an isolated defect with subsequent complete and permanent visual improvement. Unfortunately as Beauvieux recognized (1947) not all infants with DVM do so well. Although a degree of visual improvement by definition occurs in all, some with associated ocular and/or neurological problems behave differently clinically (Fielder et al 1985b — Figure 42.11) and suffer a permanent visual defect dependent upon the underlying pathology.

Uemera et al (1981) expanded upon Beauvieux's observations and divided DVM into three categories:

1. DVM as an isolated anomaly
2. DVM associated with mental retardation
3. DVM associated with ocular abnormalities.

DVM as an isolated anomaly. In this type of DVM the infant presents with severely reduced or absent vision. There are no abnormal signs on examination, other than those attributable to the visual defect (e.g. ocular divergence). Nystagmus is not present. The ERG is always normal, and the flash VEP may range from absent to normal. The time of visual improvement ranges from about 10 to 20 weeks and is rarely later. Characteristically this change is rapid, often occuring over only a few days

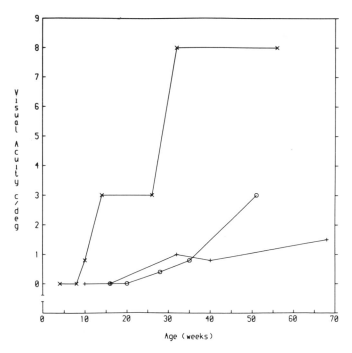

Fig. 42.11 Delayed visual maturation. The top trace (×–×) is an example of type 1, in which DVM is the sole abnormality. Visual recovery is rapid and complete. Type 2 (O–O) is a mentally retarded infant whose vision gradually but only incompletely improved. Type 3 (+–+) is an infant with Leber's amaurosis who was initially completely blind. Subsequently his vision improved to a level which permits navigation. Note that all these results were obtained under the age of 1¼ years, at a time when no other test is possible.

or a week or so, and the subsequent visual acuity development is normal. Although DVM is considered the sole abnormality in this group, a significant number are either born prematurely or suffer perinatal problems, on occasion resulting in permanent, usually mild, neurological sequelae including squint.

DVM associated with mental retardation. That blind, mentally retarded infants may later improve visually is well known. However, in contrast to the first type of DVM the improvement is often slow, occurring over weeks and months rather than days. The eventual level of vision achieved is obviously governed by the amount of visual pathway damage. Nystagmus, consequent upon associated neurological damage may be present in this group. Again the ERG is always normal and the VEP variably affected.

DVM associated with ocular disease. This is the least understood type of DVM. Ophthalmologists have known for years the dangers of giving too gloomy a prognosis on the infant with a severe, permanent ocular abnormality (e.g. optic nerve hypoplasia or even Leber's amaurosis). Unfortunately, in the absence of a suitable vision test and until the advent of the acuity card procedure, this improvement could not be quantified and recorded.

This third type of DVM is observed in two forms. In the first there is an identified and severe ocular defect such as optic nerve hypoplasia. The hallmark of the second form is the finding of a visual deficit far greater than can be accounted for by the presence of the ocular abnormality alone. Examples of the second group include congenital nystagmus and albinism. The albino infant may be initially blind and the onset of nystagmus coincides with the visual improvement. The infant with congenital nystagmus may present similarly although during the period of blindness chaotic eye movements may be seen, only settling to the characteristic congenital nystagmus pattern when the visual improvement has occurred.

The natural history of this type of DVM is not well understood but appears to exhibit more variability than when DVM is the sole abnormality. Of course, the degree of visual improvement is governed by the underlying ocular abnormality. It is imperative that the clinician does not anticipate improvement, for not all children with ocular abnormalities show improvement. The effect of false optimism on the parents is far more damaging than the joy of unexpected improvement, even if limited.

Nystagmus may be a feature of the last two types of DVM but not the first. Not surprisingly, depending on the nature of the ocular problem, the ERG may be reduced in some patients with the ocular form of DVM.

The pathogenesis of DVM. This is unknown (Fielder et al 1985b) and is not discussed in detail here. As the ERG is normal a defect in the retina is most improbable and a defect in myelination is unlikely to be the whole story. The evidence at present points either to a cortical or subcortical defect. In connection with the latter it is interesting to note the suggestion that the VEP in early infancy may have a subcortical origin (Dubowitz et al 1986, see also Ch. 3). As a number of these infants have experienced problems in the neonatal period there is a possibility that a subtle neurological insult may be a factor in some cases of DVM and it is pertinent to recall the observation that neurologically abnormal pre-term infants may show delayed acuity maturation (Placzek et al 1985). It is not known whether the spectrum of DVM ranging from DVM as an isolated anomaly, to associated involvement with other ocular and neurological conditions, can be accounted for by a single pathogenesis or whether each type of DVM is a distinct entity.

Cortical blindness

Many clinicians use the term cortical blindness to describe a patient totally and permanently blind but with a normal ocular examination including preservation of the pupillary responses. Fortunately for the child this is far from true, as a degree of visual recovery is the rule. Unfortunately for the clinician attempting to make a diagnosis, however, the cortically blind child has often suffered widespread brain damage and may exhibit many diverse CNS and ocular signs (Whiting et al 1985).

The causes of cortical blindness include:

Prenatal: malformations, intra-uterine infection and toxaemia.
Perinatal: hypoxic–ischaemic episodes as in neonatal asphyxia and intracerebral haemorrhage, hypoglycaemia, meningitis and encephalitis.
Acquired: meningitis, encephalitis, cardiac arrest, neuro-degenerative disorders, trauma, cortical vein thrombosis and shunt failure.

Clinical assessment of these patients is often difficult and as many have suffered diffuse brain damage, co-existent ophthalmic and neurological signs are common (Whiting

et al 1985). The absence of nystagmus is an important clue to cortical involvement with the qualification already made that poorly sustained CNS nystagmus may be present. Vision assessment is usually possible during infancy but infrequently after this age (Van Hof-Van Duin & Mohn 1984b).

The VEP to a flash stimulus is not always abnormal in cortical blindness, and was so in less than half of the patients reported by Whiting et al (1985). Frank & Torres (1979) were unable to detect a significant difference between the VEPs of normal and cortically blind children. These findings have reduced the value of this test as a means of investigation in cortical visual problems.

The clinical course of cortical blindness is extremely variable and is determined to a certain extent by its aetiology. Hoyt (1986b) was unable to establish any correlation between the duration of the blindness and the extent of the visual recovery. However, total recovery within a few hours has been observed in children who suffered 'trivial' head trauma (Griffith & Dodge 1968). Visual improvement is not anticipated in patients with neurodegenerative disorders and the prognosis following bacterial meningitis is worse than for other causes (Ackroyd 1984). Thus, complete recovery has been reported following head injury (Griffith & Dodge 1968) and cardiac arrest (Weinberger et al 1962) but in only 50% of patients with bacterial meningitis (Ackroyd 1984).

Cortical blindness is rarely permanent although it should be emphasized that the degree of improvement is often incomplete (Hoyt 1986b); for this reason the designation cortical visual impairment is more appropriate (Whiting et al 1985). Visual improvement may take from a few hours to more than two years and begins first with light perception and then the ability to follow objects. Eye-to-eye contact is often lacking and visual function may vary from hour to hour. Most children achieve at least navigational vision although severe visual-perceptual difficulties sometimes persist.

REFERENCES

Ackroyd R S 1984 Cortical blindness following bacterial meningitis: a case report with reassessment of prognosis and aetiology. Developmental Medicine and Child Neurology 26: 227–230
Antony J H, Ouvrier R A, Wise G 1980 Spasmus nutans: a mistaken identity. Archives of Neurology 37: 373–375
Aslin R N 1977 Development of binocular fixation in human infants. Journal of Experimental Psychology 23: 133–150
Atkinson J, Braddick O 1983 Assessment of visual acuity in infancy and early childhood. Acta Ophthalmologica (Copenhagen) (Suppl) 157: 18–26
Aylward G P, Lazzara A, Meyer J 1978 Behavioural characteristics of a hydranencephalic infant. Developmental Medicine and Child Neurology 20: 211–217
Bankes J L K 1974 Eye defects of mentally handicapped children. British Medical Journal 2: 533–535
Beauvieux J 1926 La pseudo-atrophie optique des nouveaux-nes (dysgenesie myelinique des voies optiques). Annales d'Oculistique 163: 881–921

Beauvieux M 1947 La cecite apparente chez le nouveau-ne la pseudo-atrophie grise du nerf optique. Archives Ophtalmologie (Paris) 7: 241–249
Birnholz J C 1981 The development of human fetal eye movement patterns. Science 213: 679–681
Boothe R G, Dobson V, Teller D Y 1985 Postnatal development of vision in human and nonhuman primates. Annual Review of Neurosciences 8: 495–545
Braddick O, Atkinson J 1983 Some recent findings on the development of human binocularity: a review. Behavioural Brain Research 10: 141–150
Brazelton T B, Scholl M L, Robey J S 1966 Visual responses in the newborn. Pediatrics 37: 284–290
Brown A M, Yamamoto M 1986 Visual acuity in newborn and preterm infants measured with grating acuity cards. American Journal of Ophthalmology 102: 245–253
Brown G, Tasman W 1983 Congenital anomalies of the optic disc. Grune & Stratton, New York.
Coakes R L, Clothier C, Wilson A 1979 Binocular reflexes in the first 6

months of life: preliminary results of a study of normal infants. Child Care, Health and Development 5: 405–408

Cogan D G 1952 A type of congenital ocular motor apraxia presenting jerky head movements. Transactions of the American Academy of Ophthalmology and Otolaryngology 56: 853–862

Cogan D G 1966 Congenital ocular motor apraxia. Canadian Journal of Ophthalmology 1: 253–260

Cordero L, Clark D L, Urrutia J G 1983 Postrotatory nystagmus in the full-term and premature infant. International Journal of Pediatric Otorhinolaryngology 5: 47–57

Costin G, Murphree A L 1985 Hypothalamic–pituitary function in children with optic nerve hypoplasia. American Journal of Diseases of Children 139: 249–254

Daroff R B, Todd Troost B, Dell'Osso L F 1978 In: Glaser J S (ed) Neuro-ophthalmology. Harper & Row, Hagerstown, pp 201–244

De Vries-Khoe L H, Spekreijse H 1982 Maturation of luminance and pattern EPs in man. In: Niemeyer G (ed) Documenta Ophthalmologica Proceedings Series, Vol. 31. Techniques in Clinical Electrophysiology. Huber, The Hague, pp 461–475

Dobson V 1983 Clinical applications of preferential looking measures of visual acuity. Behavioural Brain Research 10: 25–38

Dobson V, Mayer D L, Lee C P 1980 Visual acuity screening of preterm infants. Investigative Ophthalmology and Visual Science 19: 1498–1504

Dobson V, Schwartz T L, Sandstrom D J, Michel L 1987 Binocular visual acuity of neonates: the acuity card procedure. Developmental Medicine and Child Neurology 29: 199–206

Donat J F G, Donat J R, Lay K S 1980 Changing response to caloric stimulation with gestational age in infants. Neurology 30: 776–778

Dubowitz L M S, Dubowitz V, Morante A, Verghote M 1980 Visual function in the preterm and fullterm newborn infant. Developmental Medicine and Child Neurology 22: 465–475

Dubowitz L M S, Levene M I, Morante A, Palmer P, Dubowitz V 1981 Neurologic signs in neonatal intraventricular hemorrhage: a correlation with real-time ultrasound. Journal of Pediatrics 99: 127–133

Dubowitz L M S, Mushin J, De Vries L, Arden G B 1986 Visual function in the newborn infant: is it cortically mediated? Lancet i: 1139–1141

Eviatar L, Eviatar A, Naray I 1974 Maturation of neurovestibular responses in infants. Developmental Medicine and Child Neurology 16: 435–446

Eviatar L, Miranda S, Eviatar A, Freeman K, Borkowski M 1979 Development of nystagmus in response to vestibular stimulation in infants. Annals of Neurology 5: 508–514

Farmer J, Hoyt C S 1984 Monocular nystagmus in infancy and early childhood. American Journal of Ophthalmology 98: 504–509

Ferrari F, Grosoli M V, Fontana G, Cavazzuti G B 1983 Neurobehavioural comparison of low-risk preterm and fullterm infants at term conceptual age. Developmental Medicine and Child Neurology 25: 450–458

Fielder A R 1979 Simple pediatric ocular electrodiagnosis. In: Smith J L (ed) Neuro-ophthalmology (Focus 1980). Masson, New York, pp 217–227

Fielder A R 1985 Neonatal eye movements: normal and abnormal. British Orthoptic Journal 42: 10–15

Fielder A R, Harper M W, Higgins J E, Clarke C M, Corrigan D 1983 The reliability of the VEP in infancy. Ophthalmic Paediatrics and Genetics 3: 73–82

Fielder A R, Levene M I, Trounce J Q, Tanner M S 1986a Optic nerve hypoplasia in infancy. Journal of the Royal Society of Medicine 79: 25–29

Fielder A R, Russell-Eggitt I R, Dodd K L, Mellor D H 1985b Delayed visual maturation. Transactions of the Ophthalmological Societies of the United Kingdom 104: 653–661

Fielder A R, Gresty M A, Dodd K L, Mellor D H, Levene M I 1986b Congenital ocular motor apraxia. Transactions of the Ophthalmological Societies of the United Kingdom 105: 589–598

Fledelius H C 1981 Ophthalmic changes from 10 to 18 years. A longitudinal study of sequels to low birth weight. II. Visual acuity. Acta Ophthalmologica 59: 64–70

Frank Y, Torres F 1979 Visual evoked potentials in the evaluation of 'cortical blindness' in children. Annals of Neurology 6: 126–129

Frisen L, Holmegaard L 1978 Spectrum of optic nerve hypoplasia. British Journal of Ophthalmology 62: 7–15

Glaser J S, 1978 Neuro-ophthalmology. Harper & Row, Hagerstown

Goldie L, Hopkins I J 1964 Head turning towards diffuse light in the neurological examination of newborn infants. Brain 87: 665–672

Gorman J J, Cogan D G, Gellis S S 1957 An apparatus for grading the visual acuity of infants on the basis of opticokinetic nystagmus. Pediatrics 19: 1088–1092

Griffith J G, Dodge P R 1968 Transient blindness following head injury in children. New England Journal of Medicine 278: 648–651

Hack M, Muszynski S Y, Miranda S B 1981 State of awakeness during visual fixation in preterm infants. Pediatrics 68: 87–92

Harcourt B 1983 Guidelines in the management of incomitant strabismus in children. In: Wybar K, Taylor D (eds) Pediatric ophthalmology: current aspects. Marcel Dekker, New York, pp 341–355

Hendrickson A E, Youdelis C 1984 The morphological development of the human fovea. Ophthalmology 91: 603–612

Hoyt C S 1986a Objective techniques of visual acuity assessment in infancy. Pediatric Ophthalmology and Strabismus: Transactions of the New Orleans Academy of Ophthalmology. Raven Press, New York, pp 7–13

Hoyt C S 1986b Cortical blindness in infancy. Pediatric Ophthalmology and Strabismus: Transactions of the New Orleans Academy of Ophthalmology. Raven Press, New York, pp 235–243

Hoyt C S, Billson F A, Taylor H 1977 Isolated unilateral gaze palsy. Journal of Pediatric Ophthalmology 14: 343–345

Hoyt C S, Mousel D K, Weber A A 1980 Transient supranuclear disturbances of gaze in healthy neonates. American Journal of Ophthalmology 89: 708–713

Hoyt C S, Nickel B L, Billson F A 1982 Ophthalmological examination of the infant: developmental aspects. Survey of Ophthalmology 26: 177–189

Hoyt C S, Gelbart S S 1984 Vertical nystagmus in infants with congenital ocular abnormalities. Ophthalmic Paediatrics and Genetics 4: 155–162

Illingworth R S 1961 Delayed visual maturation. Archives of Disease in Childhood 36: 407–409

Inoue M, Koyanagi T, Nakahara H, Hara K, Hori E, Nakano H 1986 Functional development of human eye movement in utero assessed quantitatively with real-time ultrasound. American Journal of Obstetrics and Gynecology 155: 170–174

Keith C G, Kitchen W H 1983 Ocular morbidity in infants of very low birth weight. British Journal of Ophthalmology 67: 302–305

Kiff R D, Lepard C 1966 Visual response of premature infants. Archives of Ophthalmology 75: 631–633

Kitchen W H, Ryan M M, Rickards A, McDougall A B, Billson F A, Keir E H, Naylor F D 1980 A longitudinal study of very-low-birthweight infants. IV. An overview of performance at eight years of age. Developmental Medicine and Child Neurology 22: 172–188

Kremenitzer J P, Vaughan H G, Kurtzberg D, Dowling K 1979 Smooth-pursuit eye movements in the newborn infant. Child Development 50: 442–448

Kurtzberg D, Vaughan H G, Daum C, Grellong B A, Albin S, Rotkin L 1979 Neurobehavioural performance of low-birthweight infants at 40 weeks conceptual age: comparison with normal fullterm infants. Developmental Medicine and Child Neurology 21: 590–607

Kushner B J 1982 Strabismus and amblyopia associated with regressed retinopathy of prematurity. Archives of Ophthalmology 100: 256–261

Leigh J R, Zee D S 1983 The neurology of eye movements. F A Davis, Philadelphia

Ling B-C 1942 A genetic study of sustained visual fixation and associated behaviour in the human infant from birth to six months. Journal of Genetic Psychology 61: 227–277

McDonald M A, Dobson V, Sebris S L, Baitch L, Varner D, Teller D Y 1985 The acuity card procedure: a rapid test of infant acuity. Investigative Ophthalmology and Visual Science 26: 1158–1162

McGinnis J M 1930 Eye-movements and optic nystagmus in early infancy. Genetic Psychology Monographs 8: 321–427

Marg E, Freeman D N, Peltzman P, Goldstein P J 1976 Visual acuity development in human infants: evoked potential measurements. Investigative Ophthalmology 15: 150–153

Margalith D, Jan J E, McCormick A Q, Tze W J, Laponte J 1984 Clinical spectrum of congenital optic nerve hypoplasia: a review of 51 patients. Developmental Medicine and Child Neurology 26: 311–322

Margalith D, Tze W J, Jan J E 1985 Congenital optic nerve hypoplasia with hypothalamic–pituitary dysplasia. American Journal of Diseases of Children 139: 361–366

Mayer D L, Fulton A B, Rodier D 1984 Grating and recognition acuities of pediatric patients. Ophthalmology 91: 947–953

Mitchell T, Cambon K 1969 Vestibular response in the neonate and infant. Archives of Otolaryngology 90: 40–41

Mohn G, Dobson V, Schwartz T, Van Hof-Van Duin J 1986 The visual field of human infants: kinetic perimetry. Behavioural Brain Research 20: 122

Morante A, Dubowitz L M S, Levene M I, Dubowitz V 1982 The development of visual function in normal and neurologically abnormal preterm and fullterm infants. Developmental Medicine and Child Neurology 24: 771–784

Moseley M J, Fielder A R, Thompson J R, Minshull C, Price D 1988 Grating and recognition acuities of young amblyopes. British Journal of Ophthalmology 72: 50–54

Moskowitz A, Sokol S 1983 Developmental changes in the human visual system as reflected by the latency of the pattern reversal VEP. Electroencephalography and Clinical Neurophysiology 56: 1–15

Nixon R B, Helveston E M, Miller K, Archer S M, Ellis F D 1985 Incidence of strabismus in neonates. American Journal of Ophthalmology 100: 798–801

Ornitz E M, Atwell C W, Walter D O, Hartmann E E, Kaplan A R 1979 The maturation of vestibular nystagmus in infancy and childhood. Acta Otolaryngology 88: 244–256

Pendleton M E, Paine R S 1961 Vestibular nystagmus in newborn infants. Neurology 11: 450–458

Placzek M, Mushin J, Dubowitz L M S 1985 Maturation of the visual evoked response and its correlation with visual acuity in preterm infants. Developmental Medicine and Child Neurology 27: 448–454

Prechtl H F R, Nijhuis J G 1983 Eye movements in the human fetus and newborn. Behavioural Brain Research 10: 119–124

Regal D M, Ashmead D H, Salapatek P 1983 The coordination of eye and head movements during early infancy: a selective review. Behavioural Brain Research 10: 125–132

Rethy I 1969 Development of the simultaneous fixation from the divergent anatomic eye-position of the neonate. Journal of Pediatric Ophthalmology 6: 92–96

Robinson R J 1966 Assessment of gestational age by neurological examination. Archives of Disease in Childhood 41: 437–447

Rossi L N, Pignataro O, Nino L M, Gaini R, Sambataro G, Oldini C 1979 Maturation of vestibular responses: preliminary report. Developmental Medicine and Child Neurology 21: 217–224

Roucoux A, Culee C, Roucoux M 1983 Development of fixation and pursuit eye movements in human infants. Behavioural Brain Research 10: 133–140

Ruff H A, Lawson K R, Kurtzberg D, McCarton-Daum C, Vaughan H G 1982 Visual following of moving objects by full-term and preterm infants. Journal of Pediatric Psychology 7: 375–386

Sebris S L, Dobson V, Hartmann E E 1984 Assessment and prediction of visual acuity in 3-to 4-year-old children born prior to term. Human Neurobiology 3: 87–92

Skarf B, Hoyt C S 1984 Optic nerve hypoplasia in children. Archives of Ophthalmology 102: 62–67

Sokol S 1978 Measurement of infant visual acuity from pattern reversal evoked potentials. Vision Research 18: 33–39

Stanhope R, Preece M A, Brooke C G D 1984 Hypoplastic optic nerves and pituitary dysfunction. Archives of Disease in Childhood 59: 111–114

Swash M 1976 Disorders of ocular movement in hydrocephalus. Proceedings of the Royal Society of Medicine 69: 480–483

Tamura E E, Hoyt C S 1987 Oculomotor consequences of intraventricular hemorrhages in premature infants. Archives of Ophthalmology 105: 533–535

Teller D Y, McDonald M A, Preston K, Sebris S L, Dobson V 1986 Assessment of visual acuity in infants and children: the acuity card procedure. Developmental Medicine and Child Neurology 28: 779–789

Trounce J Q, Dodd K L, Fawer C-L, Fielder A R, Punt J, Levene M I 1985 Primary thalamic haemorrhage in the newborn: a new clinical entity. Lancet i: 190–192

Uemera Y, Oguchi Y, Katsumi O 1981 Visual developmental delay. Ophthalmic Paediatrics and Genetics 1: 49–58

Van Hof-Van Duin J, Mohn G 1983 Optokinetic and spontaneous nystagmus in children with neurological disorders. Behavioural Brain Research 10: 163–176

Van Hof-Van Duin J, Mohn G 1984a Vision in the preterm infant. In: Continuity of neural functions from prenatal to postnatal life. Clinics in Developmental Medicine, No 94. Spastics International Medical Oxford, pp 93–114

Van Hof-Van Duin J, Mohn G 1984b Visual defects in children after cerebral hypoxia. Behavioural Brain Research 14: 147–155

Van Hof-Van Duin J, Mohn G, Petter W P F, Mettau J W, Baerts W 1983 Preferential looking in preterm infants. Behavioural Brain Research 10: 47–50

Vehrs S, Baum D 1970 A test of visual responses in the newborn. Developmental Medicine and Child Neurology 12: 772–774

Von Noorden G K 1985 In: Burian-Von Noorden's Binocular vision and ocular motility: theory and management of strabismus. C V Mosby, St Louis

Weinberger H A, Van der Woude R, Maier H C 1962 Prognosis of cortical blindness following cardiac arrest in children. Journal of the American Medical Association 179: 126–129

White B L, Castle P, Held R 1964 Observations on the development of visually-directed reaching. Child Development 35: 349–364

Whiting S, Jan J E, Wong F K H, Flodmark O, Farrell K, McCormick A Q 1985 Permanent cortical visual impairment in children. Developmental Medicine and Child Neurology 27: 730–739

Yee R D, Baloh R W, Honrubia V 1981 Eye movement abnormalities in rod monochromacy. Ophthalmology 88: 1010–1018

43. Disorders of hearing

Dr K. Thiringer

Hearing is essential for the acquisition of speech, the most important means of human communication. The normal child is born to a sound-rich world conveying both verbal and non-verbal information, leading to balanced development both emotionally and intellectually. In contrast to this, the hearing impaired/deaf child enters a world of silence or an environment with limited 'sound experience', which restricts both communication and development.

Early diagnosis and management of hearing impairment is therefore essential if subsequent speech is to be as normal as possible. Equally important are efforts directed to further understanding the causes and research into the prevention of deafness. The prevention of hearing impairment caused by rhesus immunization (Queenan 1986) and immunization to prevent rubella embryopathy illustrate the triumph of preventive medicine within the field. Hearing impairment caused by these two factors is expected to diminish further in the future. For those already damaged, early diagnosis and fitting of hearing aids with appropriate auditory training is essential. This will hopefully prevent the delayed speech development, behavioural disturbances and poor educational performance, which often occur in children with impaired hearing.

DEVELOPMENT OF HEARING

The auricle, auditory canal and middle ear are derived from the two first branchial arches during the embryonic period, while the inner ear is derived from the hindbrain. At 11 weeks from conception the cochlea has reached its adult form of two-and-one-half turns and at 16 weeks it has reached its adult size. The hair cells and organ of Corti differentiate from the base of the cochlear duct towards the apex 11 weeks postconception and the inner ear structures are fully developed by 25 weeks. The primitive origins of the eighth cranial nerve are present from the fourth week, and after 12 weeks the nerve has differentiated into acoustic and vestibular parts. By 26 weeks the ossicles of the middle ear are fully ossified. The last structure to be fully developed is the cartilaginous part of the outer ear, and the mastoid air spaces are not complete until well after birth.

The fetus lives in a sound-rich environment. The maternal heart, uterine and placental blood vessels and bowel sounds provide a low-frequency symphony of around 85 dB (Walker et al 1971). The attenuation of external sound has been measured to 16–35 dB in the fetal sheep (Armitage et al 1980), which means that sound of above 65 dB often penetrates the uterus. Fetal hearing has been ascertained by ultrasound registration of fetal movement, changes in breathing and heart rate pattern, in response to sound stimuli from 22 weeks (Leader et al 1982). Birnholz & Benacerraf (1983) registered blink-startle responses from 24 weeks sporadically and from 28 weeks consistently. Auditory evoked responses have been recorded from the fetal brain during labour (Scibetta et al 1971). Accordingly the fetus can both listen and handle auditory information in an intelligent way (Drife 1985). Several investigators (DeCasper & Fifer 1980, Kolata 1984, Querleu et al 1984) have found that the fetus is able to differentiate certain sounds, prefers his mother's voice to others and listens more readily to a text previously presented to him. Another indication of the intact fetal nervous system function is habituation of response to vibrotactile stimuli found in the majority of normal fetuses (Leader et al 1982). In this study female fetuses responded 2 weeks earlier than males.

These findings provide evidence for the integrity of the fetal ear well before birth as well as the functioning of the central auditory pathways. Alerting to a bell was registered as change in heart and respiratory rate only or with facial and body movements by Allen & Capute (1986) in extremely premature infants from 25 weeks of gestational age. The majority of the infants appeared to habituate to the bell during their first examination at one week of age. The fetal sound response has also been used experimentally as a test of fetal well-being (Grimwade et al 1971, Serafini et al 1984), although the difference in the response due to different sleep–wake states may make the interpretation of the results difficult (Schmidt et al 1985).

Aeration of the middle ear, which takes place within

some hours from birth, does not seem to be needed for sound perception in the fetus. Measurements of middle ear compliance in newborns aged from 2 to 10 hours have shown relative mobility of these structures (Keith 1975). Eustachian tube function was also found to be intact. The presence of some residual unresolved mesenchymal tissue in the middle ear may explain why occasionally some children do not respond to sound in the first few weeks of life.

CLASSIFICATION OF HEARING IMPAIRMENT

Hearing impairment (HI) can be broadly classified as conductive, sensorineural and mixed (Fig. 43.1). Atresia of the external auditory meatus and/or abnormalities of the auditory canal and middle ear structures result in conductive deafness, which is usually quite severe but does not alter sound quality and is often possible to treat by surgery or hearing aids. Conductive HI usually affects all frequencies equally, while sensorineural HI generally more often affects high-frequency sounds. This is why moderate sensorineural HI may be more handicapping than severe conductive loss. Consonants are of higher frequency and lower intensity than vowels (see Fig. 43.2), which makes them harder to appreciate in children with impaired hearing.

If the damage to the ear is multifocal there will be a combination of conductive and sensorineural HI, which is called a 'mixed' loss. Mixed HI is often a sequel of chronic otitis media.

Sensorineural HI (SNHI) can be further divided into cochlear, retrocochlear and central damage. The cochlear damage may be localized to the lymphatic spaces, the organ of Corti and the dendrites and cell body of neurones in the cochlear nuclei. However, differentiation of damage within the first neurone is not in practice possible, and all eighth nerve cell damage is regarded as retrocochlear. Injuries above the level of the cochlear nuclei lead to a clinically different type of HI and are referred to as central HI. The central auditory pathways are shown in Fig. 15.2, p. 198.

HI can be present at birth (congenital) or be of delayed onset and may be progressive. The human ear can hear frequencies between 20 and 20 000 Hz, but frequencies between 300 and 3000 lie in the most crucial range for acquisition of normal speech. The severity of HI is defined according to international agreement as the mean decibel (dB) hearing loss at frequencies 0.5, 1.0 and 2.0 kHz in the better ear. Figure 43.2 shows the auditory threshold and the loudness level of some sounds often experienced. For simplicity, hearing losses up to 30 dB may be regarded as slight, up to 60 dB as moderate and above 60 dB as severe. Hearing aids are usually required for more than 30–40 dB hearing loss. In practice losses above 60 dB represent significant deafness. If no sound can be detected with the highest amplification, then the person is considered to be totally deaf.

INCIDENCE OF HEARING IMPAIRMENT

In Europe 0.7 to 1.5/1000 8-year-old children born in 1969 had HI above 40 dB (Commission of European Communities 1979). In Sweden 4.2/1000 6-year-olds, born in 1970–74 in Gothenburg were found to have some form of HI (Table 43.1). When monaural loss (1.2/1000) and HI below 40 dB (1.6/1000) were subtracted, the prevalence of severe HI was found to be 1.4/1000. This is close to the 1/1000 incidence reported from Manchester in 4-year-olds (Newton 1985). The 1971 National Census of the Deaf Population of the United States reported the prevalence of 'inability to hear or understand speech' as

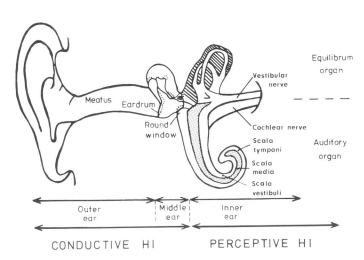

Fig. 43.1 Classification of hearing impairment according to site of lesion.

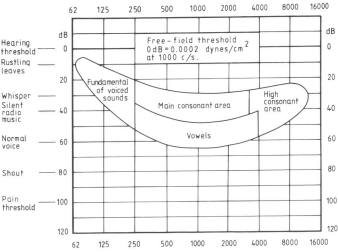

Fig. 43.2 The average speech spectrum within an audiogram in terms of main formant areas (male voices at 1 m distance from lips). Ordinate corresponds to hearing loss or sensation level in dB relative to the standardized free-field threshold. (Modified from Fant 1959.)

Table 43.1 Prevalence of hearing impairment among preschool children in Gothenburg born in 1970–74 (study period 1970–January 1981)

	Total livebirths 1970–74 (*n* = 30 559)	Child population 0–5 years, 1 Jan. 1975 (*n* = 27 425
All hearing impairment	3.8	4.2
Conductive loss	0.5	0.6
Monaural loss/deafness	1.0	1.2
Degree of impairment (dB)		
<40	1.4	1.6
41–60	0.6	0.6
61–100	0.5	0.6
>100	0.3	0.3

All frequencies given in cases/1000.
(Reproduced with permission from Thiringer et al 1984.)

1/1000 in children below the age of 3 and this figure rose to 2.03/1000 in young people below the age of 19 (Riko et al 1985). Feinmesser et al (1982) found the incidence of HI in Israeli children over 5 years to be 1.7/1000.

The ratio of conductive to sensorineural deafness was found to be 1:7 in the Gothenburg study (Thiringer et al 1984) and the male to female ratio was 1.7:1. The Manchester study, which only considered bilateral SNHI, also found a slight preponderance for males (54%), which was statistically more frequent if the aetiology of the HI was perinatal, while females were more frequently present in the group where the HI was associated with chromosomal abnormality (Newton 1985).

METHODS OF NEWBORN AND INFANT HEARING ASSESSMENT

There is a variety of different methods for auditory screening as well as ascertaining the degree of the HI.

Newborn auditory screening

The question of newborn auditory screening is controversial. For many years it was thought that, because the babbling of the HI child is very similar to that of the hearing child, the first 6 months of life was not critical for language acquisition. New research has shown that the human species even at the fetal stage can differentiate between different voices. The babbling of the HI child decreases in its range of vocalizations at a very early age and then arrests so that it does not acquire the sophisticated aspects of sound production such as intonational contour (Menyuk 1977). According to recent evidence severely-to-profoundly deaf infants do not proceed from 'marginal babble' (Oller 1980) to 'canonical babble', which is regarded as a crucial step in the emergence of a capacity for speech. Deaf infants also produce a larger proportion of glottal sequences in their babble compared with hearing infants (Oller 1984). These

findings indicate that auditory feedback may be crucially important for later language development and emphasize the need for remedial procedures as early as possible.

On the other hand, the frequency of HI above 40 d HL (hearing level) is rare at about 1/1000 (Downs & Hemenway 1969, Simmons 1980) in apparently normal newborns and the methods of newborn screening are laborious and often require skilled personnel and expensive instrumentation. According to this, the Joint Committee on Newborn Hearing Screening of the USA (1974) did not recommend routine newborn hearing screening but stated that infants at risk should be identified by means of history and physical examination.

Nevertheless, there are some reports of successful screening in newborns. Downs & Hemenway (1969) screened 17 000 newborns using a warble 3000 Hz tone at 90 dB SPL (sound pressure level) and recorded blink, face and/or body movements. Of the 500 suspect cases, 15 turned out to have HI, which shows a specificity of less than 3%.

Crib-o-gram

In 1974 Simmons & Russ described the Crib-o-gram — a completely automated multichannel method, which records a baby's heart rate, respiration, and other movements or cessation of movements in response to a 93 dB narrow-band noise sound. The test is positive if the infant responds within 2–5 seconds after the test sound. By 1978 they had tested 10 891 newborns: of 986 infants who failed the initial test, 27 were found eventually to have HI. This gives a 4.2% specificity for the test, however, some infants were lost or were not yet retested (Simmons 1978). Screening of graduates from a neonatal intensive care unit gave a 7.4% specificity and the frequency of HI found was 1:52 (Simmons 1980).

Auditory response cradle

The Linco–Bennett auditory response cradle (ARC) is a microprocessor controlled device for neonatal auditory screening developed in England. It records the baby's movements and respiration when sounds are presented and also during 'blank' trials. The microprocessor evaluates the response and passes or fails the infant. The stimulus is a 2600 Hz high pass noise of 85 dB SPL. Bhattacharya et al (1984) used the cradle to screen 5553 selected at-risk newborns, of which 88 failed a first and second test. Of those 88 infants, 15 were subsequently diagnosed as having HI, and one infant with HI passed the test. McCormick et al (1984) tested 396 special care unit babies and of 79 who failed, 6 were diagnosed as deaf. Again, one infant with severe bilateral HI passed the test. They have subsequently modified the computer algorithm and conclude that the test is too labour intensive and unrealistic for mass screening purposes but has considerable potential as an objective method for newborn auditory screening of high-risk groups.

Brainstem evoked responses (BSER)

These responses are recorded by scalp electrodes following sound stimuli, and will be discussed more as a method for auditory testing. The origin and characteristics of the response is described in Chapter 15. The computer-averaged signal has been extensively studied during the last years and normal amplitudes and latencies of the different wave components as well as normal hearing thresholds have been defined for normal neonates at different gestational ages (Despland & Galambos 1980, Lary et al 1985). Finitzo-Hieber (1981) found the latency of wave V (originating from the inferior colliculus, Fig. 15.2) to be the most useful measure of hearing function.

Screening risk populations, like those from neonatal intensive care units with BSER has been suggested by the American Academy of Pediatrics, Joint Committee on Infant Hearing 1982, either by observation of behaviour or recording electrophysiological response to sound. Schulman-Galambos & Galambos (1979) tested with brainstem evoked response audiometry (BERA) 50 graduates from an intensive care unit and found a 2% incidence of HI. They concluded that BSER is an objective and reliable method, which unquestionably meets the criteria for newborn hearing screening. However, the complexity and cost of the test makes it unsuitable for use in normal newborns. By 1984 Galambos et al had tested 1613 high-risk infants with BERA and of 16% not passing the test, 54% were retested. Permanent HI could be identified in 8–10% of the original total, with approximately 4% having bilateral severe HI and requiring hearing aids. At present in the USA, a voluntary organization performs BERA on all graduates from neonatal intensive care with a machine called Synap and some help from trained experts interpreting the registrations.

Sanders et al (1985) summarized the results of five BERA screening programmes in high-risk infants in Canada. Depending on the failure criteria used (between 25 dB and 40 dB and normal wave morphology), 10–30% of these infants failed the test initially and 10% went on showing some abnormalities of hearing on follow-up tests at 2–5 months of age. Between 2 and 4% had moderate to profound HI. In two of these studies, neonatal screening tests with behavioural methods, Crib-o-gram and BERA were compared for sensitivity and specificity. False-positive tests were frequent with behavioural screening (50.5 and 86.1% in 'at risk' and neonatal intensive care infants, respectively, compared with 23 and 8.2% for BERA). The Crib-o-gram detected HI in 100% if the BERA pass level was set to 50 dB HL (hearing level), and 59.1% if the pass level was 30 dB HL. The specificity of the Crib-o-gram was found to be 71% (Durieux-Smith & Jacobson 1985).

In addition to diagnosing HI, auditory evoked responses may provide information about brainstem abnormalities in the newborn, as typical BSER configurations may be associated with specific neurological problems (Kileny & Robertson 1985).

Infant auditory screening

For a more general assessment of the infant's hearing response (or in the newborn response) the acoustic blink reflex (ABR) the 'wake-test' may be used. Wedenberg (1956) has standardized the test and found that a 105–115 dB sound pressure level (SPL) is necessary to elicit the ABR over the frequency range of 0.5 to 4 kHz during the first 10 days of life in the normal infant. To wake the infant he found that 70–75 dB SPL was necessary in the 0.5 to 3 kHz range. If the infant blinks or awakes, a profound HI can be excluded, but a negative response does not always mean HI. Infants who are crying, laughing or sleeping deeply and those with facial nerve paresis will not respond.

In Sweden, an auditory response assessment (the BOEL-test) has been used for screening infants of 8 months ± 14 days of age (Stensland-Junker 1972). This is a simple form of a distraction test, modified to suit screening purposes, and tests the infant's capacity for visual and auditory attention together with its communicative ability.

Methods for hearing assessment

The most frequently used methods for hearing assessment are summarized according to age in months at which we regard them as suitable (or possible) to use, in Table 43.2.

Electrophysiological methods

Auditory evoked responses are described in Chapter 15. They are of three general types: early latency (within 10 ms following the stimulus), middle latency (10–50 ms after the stimulus) and late latency. Electrocochleography (ECoG) and auditory brainstem response (ABR) are early latency types. ECoG requires sedation of the infant and is mainly used in special centres for research purposes. ABR is a very useful complement to other tests of HI, especially in the newborn and mentally retarded child when psycho-acoustical tests are not possible. In children below 6 months of age, ABR is easy to perform during sleep and provides information not only about auditory thresholds but also about the functional state of the brainstem auditory neurones. The damage can be localized as cochlear or retrocochlear. However, there are some limitations and technical errors. High stimulus repetition rate may depress the infant ABR; infants with severe neonatal asphyxia may have poor response because of brainstem depression other than auditory; and when clicks are used as stimulus, the

Table 43.2 Methods for hearing assessment of children

Hearing test	Age (months)														
	1	2	3	4	5	6	7	8	9	10	11	12	24	36	48
Psycho-acoustical tests															
Respiration audiometry															
Behaviour-observation audiometry															
Visual reinforcement audiometry															
Play audiometry															
Electrophysiological audiometry															
Electrocochleography															
Auditory brainstem response															
40 Hz middle latency response															
Cortical response audiometry															
Acoustic impedance															
Tympanometry															
Acoustic reflex															
Spoken voice test															
Test for reaction level															
Picture identification															
Word repetition															

test does not detect low-frequency HI. Riko et al (1985) have, therefore, used bandstop masked tonepip ABR at 40 dB HL (hearing level) or less at 0.5 kHz and think that this place-specific, low-frequency ABR audiometry is more sufficient than click testing.

A special type of middle latency response, the 40 Hz middle latency response (Galambos et al 1981) for hearing threshold assessments was used by Kankkunen & Rosenhall (1985). It is easy to perform on newborns and threshold measurements cover the frequency range from 0.25 to 8.0 kHz. The sensitivity of middle latency response audiometry for detecting a hearing loss was 100% and the specificity for recognizing normal hearing was 91%. There was a good concordance with thresholds obtained by psycho-acoustical tests. The disadvantages of the method were that the thresholds in sleeping children were elevated by about 40 dB and the test took one hour, if all frequencies were tested. Cortical response audiometry (CRA) is a test of late latency response audiometry. It is used for diagnosis of psychogenic HI and is less suitable for testing children than other evoked response audiometry methods.

Psycho-acoustical methods

Respiration audiometry. This test is one of many using the registration of changes in resting state of the infant to auditory stimuli. Earlier described by Rousey (1964) and Bradford (1975), it has been used in a modified form, by recording changes in breathing impedance by electrodes attached to the chest (Fig. 43.3). Hearing threshold for frequencies from 0.5 to 4.0 kHz are tested in infants from 0 to 4 months of age. In infants below 6 months the test gave

excellent recordings in 53%, good in 38% and usable in 9%. The test performer must be skilled in audiometry and with children. The room has to be silent and the child comfortable. Tone level is increased gradually until response (usually diminished respiration) is noted. The operator then quickly changes to the next frequency, as speed is essential in the performance of the test, which can be completed in 15–30 minutes. If the test is prolonged, the child loses interest and will not respond.

Behaviour-observation audiometry This method applies the same principles as respiration audiometry but the responses (respiratory, movement or sound) are observed and noted. This test also requires skilled personnel and quiet surroundings.

Visual reinforcement audiometry (Lidén & Kankkunen 1969), play audiometry (Barr 1955), picture identification and word repetition are methods for testing the hearing of older infants (Table 43.2).

Methods for testing middle ear function

Middle ear function is tested by measuring its acoustic impedance. Two of the methods, namely tympanometry and acoustic reflex threshold (ART) measurements require no co-operation and can be carried out in the newborn period. Tympanometry gives reliable information about pressure in the middle ear, and thereby about middle ear disease. It should always be performed before testing ART. The threshold SPL (sound pressure level) for eliciting ART is about 85 dB at 0.5– 4.0 kHz. The 95% variation limit for one-year-olds was measured as 70–99 dB HL at 1.0 kHz (Kankkunen & Lidén 1984). The method should not be used alone for identifying HI, as it only detects 60% of

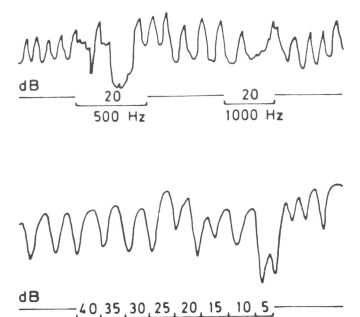

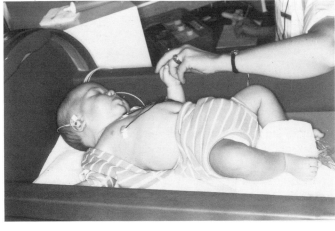

Fig. 43.3 Respiration audiometry in a 3-month-old infant. The breathing pattern changes clearly upon stimulation with faint tones (**a**). Stimulation with tones of decreasing intensity causes wider fluctuations (**b**). The changes in the breathing are clearest at low intensity levels. (Reproduced with permission from Kankkunen & Liden 1977.)

children with HI. The specificity of the method is, however, about 90%. The reflex should, accordingly, be used with great caution for the prediction of hearing level in the young paediatric population (Kankkunen & Lidén 1984).

AETIOLOGIES OF HEARING IMPAIRMENT

It is important to discover the cause of hearing impairment (HI) in order to indicate prognosis and risk of recurrence in subsequent children. It may also be possible to direct research into prevention. Unfortunately, in a number of cases, recognition of a precise cause of the HI is not possible. This emphasizes the need for assessment of the deaf child on a multidisciplinary basis leading to a holistic view of the problems. Besides assessment by the audiologist and otolaryngologist, the HI child should be evaluated by a paediatrician (preferably with special training in neuropaediatrics) and an ophthalmologist. Titres for virological diagnosis, ECG and urine sample for haematuria and proteinuria are routine examinations in the child with HI. Thyroid function tests, skull X-ray and chromosome analysis should be performed in special cases, as well as psychological assessment, when associated mental retardation is suspected.

Factors recognized to cause HI may be divided into those operating prenatally, perinatally and postnatally (Table 43.3). The Gothenburg study of 146 children with HI born between 1970 and 1979 (Thiringer et al 1984) revealed a prenatal cause in 61%, perinatal in 9% and postnatal in 18%, while 12% were of unknown origin. Similar results

were obtained from Manchester (Newton 1985), concerning 111 children with SNHI born 1977–80 (Table 43.3).

Genetic hearing loss

Genetic aetiology for HI has been noted by several authors as the single most important cause of HI (Königsmark & Gorlin 1976, Fraser 1976, Feinmesser et al 1978, Thiringer et al 1984), being present in 30–55% of cases. The frequency of hereditary deafness has been estimated as 1–3 in 6000 infants. A positive family history for HI seems also to play a role as a predisposing factor when other damaging influences (infection, noise, jaundice, asphyxia, ototoxic drugs) operate (Anderson et al 1970). Positive family history for HI (defined as HI of unknown origin before the age of 50 in the parents, siblings or cousins, or in the parents' and grandparents' siblings or first cousins) occurred in 17% of a normal hearing population of 14-year-olds in Sweden (Klockhoff & Lyttkens 1982). Amongst a newborn population with anterior ear tags, 29% had close relatives with HI (Kankkunen & Thiringer 1986) and among children with anterior ear tags and HI, 78% had a positive family history of deafness.

Single gene defects are responsible for most familial deafness, through the exact number of genes causing deafness is not known. About 60% of these genes show autosomal recessive inheritance, 25% autosomal dominant inheritance and 1–2% X-linked recessive inheritance. McKusick (1976) has listed over 100 clearly defined syndromes conveyed by Mendelian inheritance. The HI may be conductive or sensorineural, congenital or of delayed onset, and may affect preferentially the high-, low- or mid-frequency areas. About 50% of hereditary deafness occurs without any associated anomalies. However, many types of hereditary hearing loss can be associated with anomalies of the external ear, integumentary system (skin, hair, nails, teeth) and visual, nervous, skeletal, urinary and endocrine systems. The different syndromes are listed in extensive reviews by Königsmark (1969a,b,c), Jaffe & Königsmark (1977) and Caldarelli (1977). Some of them are present from birth and will be briefly described.

All anomalies associated with the ear (malformed pinna, pre-auricular pits, atresia of the external meatus) should alert the neonatologist to the possibility of HI. One example of anomaly, which is usually considered innocent, is pre-auricular ear tag. Yet, in a study of 180 newborns we found an increased rate of mild to moderate sensorineural HI associated with this condition (Kankkunen & Thiringer 1986).

Conductive HI is a part of various craniofacial and cervical syndromes, such as the Treacher–Collin's syndrome (Fig. 43.4; mandibulo–facial dysostosis with characteristic anomalies of the face and outer ears — documented autosomal heredity in 50% of the cases), hemifacial microsomia (Fig. 43.5); usually unilateral mandibular and maxillary hypoplasia, macrostomia, microtia and various external ear malformations including meatal atresia — most cases are sporadic but some show autosomal dominant or recessive inheritance, Crouzon's disease (Fig. 43.6; cranio–facial dysostosis with bilateral exophtalmos, divergent strabismus, hypertelorism, maxillary hypoplasia and relative prognathism, parrot-beak nose, high arched or cleft palate and increased intracranial pressure, — autosomal dominant inheritance) and Klippel–Feil's syndrome (Fig. 43.7; short neck, various external ear anomalies, causing all types of HI — type I autosomal dominant, type II autosomal recessive and type III sporadic).

Other inherited conditions associated with HI are listed in Table 43.4.

Multifactorial inheritance is attributed to the combination of polygenic inheritance and environmental factors and is a major factor in the aetiology of many common single malformations, like cleft lip and palate (Smith & Aase 1970). This type of inheritance is responsible for most

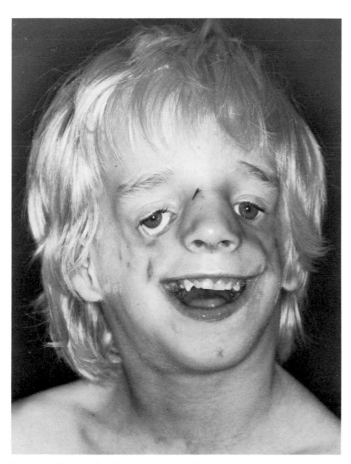

Fig. 43.4 Treacher–Collin's syndrome. Bilateral incipient facial clefts, aplasia of corpus zygomaticus, incipient coloboma of eyelids and poorly developed mandible. (Provided by Dr Lauritzen, Dept Plastic Surgery, Gothenburg and reproduced by kind permission of the patient.)

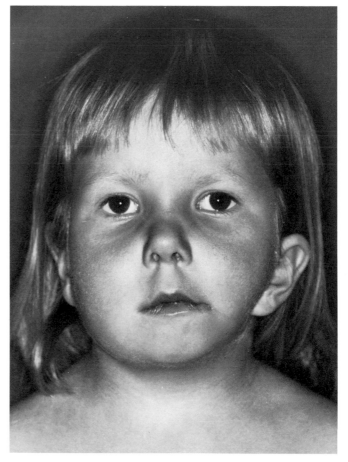

Fig. 43.5 Hemifacial microsomia — underdeveloped left lower face. (Provided by Dr Lauritzen, Dept Plastic Surgery, Gothenburg and reproduced by kind permission of the patient.)

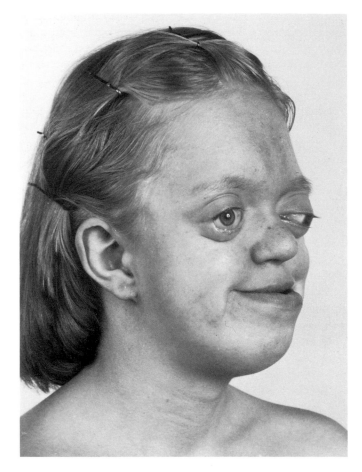

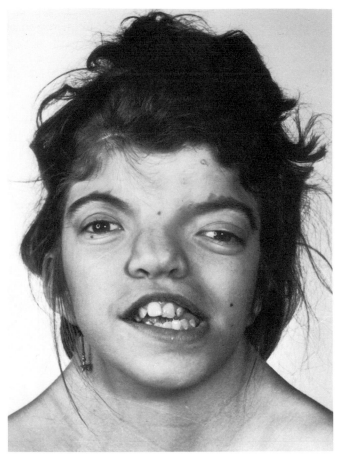

Fig. 43.6 Crouzon's disease in a 13-year-old girl. Middle part of face poorly developed. Flat orbitae and turricephaly. (Provided by Dr Lauritzen, Dept Plastic Surgery, Gothenburg and reproduced by kind permission of the patient.)

Fig. 43.7 Klippel–Feil's syndrome. Bilateral webbed neck. (Provided by Dr Lauritzen, Dept Plastic Surgery, Gothenburg and reproduced by kind permission of the patient.)

genetic diseases. While all types of disease have been found as a result of multifactorial inheritance, none has been described for HI. It has, however, been found that a family predisposition for HI is an important factor for HI caused by infections (Anderson et al 1970) and noise (Klockhoff & Lyttkens 1982) and is most probably a factor involved in the causation of perinatal HI by ototoxic drugs, hyperbilirubinaemia and so on.

Chromosomal defects, including Turner's (45, X0), Klinefelter's (47, XXY), Edward's (47, XX or XY+18) and Pataús syndrome (47, XX or XY + 13), may have HI as part of the disease. Children with Down's syndrome (47, XX or XY+21) are at risk for both sensorineural and conductive HI as they often suffer from recurrent otitis media. Balkany et al (1979) found SNHI in 10–35% of children and young adults with Down's syndrome and conductive HI in up to 83% of such children.

Prenatal acquired disorders

The main factors operating during the fetal period are infections, drugs and alcohol. Generally, the earlier in preg-

nancy the noxious agent occurs to the mother/fetus, the more pronounced the damage with more severe and multiple abnormalities, but some toxic factors like drugs and alcohol may exert their influence throughout pregnancy.

Congenital infections

Rubella and cytomegalovirus (CMV) are the best-known and most common infective causes of congenital HI. In rare instances syphilis, toxoplasmosis, Epstein–Barr virus, varicella and herpes virus have been reported as teratogenic to the ear. Viruses may also damage the inner ear postnatally, the most common being the unilateral deafness caused by mumps. The histological appearance may be similar in the pre- and postnatally damaged cochlea with viral invasion either by the haematogenous or cerebrospinal route, leading to the Mondini or Scheibe type of defect. In the former the intrascalar septi and the osseous spiral laminae are destroyed with resulting damage to the hair cells. In the latter there is extensive neuronal destruction with degeneration and sometimes ossification of the cochlea (Linthicum 1978).

Rubella (See p. 408). The notorious damage to the

Table 43.3 Aetiology of hearing impairment (HI): distribution of cases by probable aetiologies in two cohorts (Thiringer et al 1984, Newton 1985)

Prenatal aetiologies	(Thiringer)	(Newton)
Hereditary HI	77 (53%)	28 (25%)
Autosomal dominant		
Autosomal recessive		
X-linked		
Chromosomal		5 (4.5%)
Rubella	8 (5.5%)	12 (11%)
Cytomegalovirus	1 (0.7%)	3 (3%)
Other viral infections of pregnancy		
Ototoxic drugs, alcohol fetopathy	3 (2%)	
	89 (61%)	48 (43.5%)
Perinatal aetiologies	13 (9%)	15 (13.5%)
Postnatal aetiologies	26 (18%)	5 (4.5%)
Unknown aetiology	18 (12%)	43 (38.5%)
Total	146	111

fetus which follows first trimester maternal rubella was first recognized in Australia by Gregg (1941) and Swan et al (1943). The classic triad of malformations affecting the heart, eye and ear was described. Until recently rubella has been the most important viral cause of HI. In some years rubella has been found to cause up to 50% of all congenital HI in Stockholm (Fig. 43.8). Following the isolation of the virus in 1962 and the production of an effective vaccine, world-wide vaccination programmes began in the 1970s. In Sweden, general vaccination of schoolgirls and susceptible newly delivered women was instituted in 1974 and from 1981 infants at 18 months receive a combined mumps–measles–rubella immunization, which was repeated at 13 years of age. As a consequence, no HI due to rubella has been reported since 1981 at the Karolinska Hospital (Barr personal communication 1986). Similar policies for vaccination are in use in the USA, UK and Australia. The Swedish experience with immunization is encouraging, no side-effects of any magnitude or fetal infection have been reported and the immunity seems to be of long duration (Barr 1982).

Hearing loss can result from fetal infection as late as the 25th week but is much more common when infection occurs during the first trimester. The incidence of HI has been reported to be 10–50% if rubella occurs early in pregnancy. Frequently HI is the only manifestation of the disease. The HI caused by rubella is usually moderately severe to profound, uni- or bilateral and often affects the higher frequencies only. It is often congenital but may progress

Table 43.4 Inherited conditions in which congenital or early onset of deafness is a prominent feature

Condition	Features	Inheritance
Achondroplasia	Short-limbed dwarfism. Conductive or mixed hearing impairment due to middle ear ossicle deformities	Dominant Sporadic cases mutational
Alport's syndrome	Progressive nephritis, proteinuria, haematuria, sensorineural hearing impairment	Dominant, males more severely affected
Apert's syndrome (acrocephalosyndactyly)	Cranial synostosis, syndactyly of hand and feet, face malformations	Dominant and sporadic cases
Goldenhar's syndrome (oculo–auriculo–vertebral dysplasia)	A variant of hemifacial microsomia, facial malformation and eye finding: epibulbar dermoids, coloboma, cataracts, spinal defects	Variable
Jervell and Lange-Nielsen's syndrome	Prolonged QT interval with risk of asystole and sudden death	Recessive (heterozygotes diagnosed by the ECG abnormality)
Leopard syndrome	Multiple lentigines, cardiac abnormalities, facial features	Dominant
Lewis' syndrome	Congenital pulmonary stenosis	
Madelung's deformity	Malformation of radius, ulna and carpal bones	Dominant
Marshall's syndrome	Congenital myopia, cataract, saddle nose, progressive congenital hearing impairment	Dominant
Mucopolysaccharidoses (Hunter and Hurler)	Characteristic facies, corneal, cardiac and multiple musculo-skeletal anomalies	Autosomal or X-linked recessive
Osteogenesis imperfecta	Large skull, multiple fractures of the long bones, blue sclerae	Dominant
Osteopetrosis (Albers–Schönberg)	Skeletal anomalies of the skull with secondary effects due to nerve compression	Variable
Pendred's syndrome	Congenital deafness, pubertal goiter	Recessive
Usher's syndrome	Retinitis pigmentosa, congenital hearing impairment	Recessive
Wardenburg syndrome	White forelock of hair, heterochromia iridis	Dominant

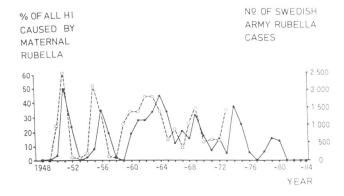

Fig. 43.8 Percentage of congenital rubella deafness in children registered at Karolinska Hospital, Stockholm ------ and number of rubella cases reported among Swedish army personnel ———. (Reproduced with permission of Prof. Barr.)

(Kankkunen 1982), especially if there is a familial risk for HI (Anderson et al 1970). Central auditory imperception (Ames et al 1970) and severe behavioural disturbances may further complicate the situation and make the rubella-damaged HI child dependent on multidisciplinary therapy of the highest calibre. The eye lesion is classically a retinopathy showing the typical 'salt and pepper' appearance but this does not significantly impair the child's vision. Infantile autism has also been reported to follow congenital rubella infection. The diagnosis of the cause of HI in congenital rubella is sometimes difficult because subclincial rubella without rash may result in isolated HI without other anomalies. The diagnosis by serology and virus isolation is discussed in Chapter 36.

Cytomegalovirus (See p. 409). CMV is a ubiquitous infectious agent, causing problems mainly in immunosuppressed individuals and in the fetus. The rate of maternal immunity varies between 25 and 100% (data from 1978 for Manchester and the Ivory Coast respectively) depending on geographical location and socio-economic status. Around 1% of pregnant women seroconvert during pregnancy as a sign of primary infection (Ahlfors et al 1982, Griffiths & Baboonian 1984). Approximately 12.5% of the mothers excrete virus from the cervix in the third trimester (Stagno et al 1975), in contrast to 1.6% during the first trimester, which indicates a reactivation of this infection during the later part of pregnancy and a suppression in the first. Fetal infection (diagnosed as CMV isolated from urine during the first 3 weeks of life) occurs in about 1% of neonates. Of the fetal infections, 24 to 60% occur after secondary or reactivated maternal CMV infection (Ahlfors et al 1982, Preece et al 1984) and infants with symptomatic congenital CMV infection leading to neurological sequelae have been reported after recurrent maternal CMV infection (Ahlfors et al 1981, Peckham et al 1983, Preece et al 1984). Only 10–20% of the infected infants show symptoms and these may be severe, with microcephaly, intracranial periventricular calcification, rash, hepatosplenomegaly, jaundice, chorioretinitis,

sensorineural HI and mental retardation. The hearing defect is usually bilateral, moderate to profound and may progress (Stagno et al 1977, Dahle et al 1979, Williamson et al 1982). HI is diagnosed in about 15% of asymptomatic infants and in approximately 30% of symptomatic infants. Hanshow (1982) reviewed the results of three North American studies (Reynolds et al 1974, Hanshow et al 1976, Saigal et al 1982) reporting on 32 956 infants and found the incidence of HI due to congenital CMV to be 0.6/1000 births. CMV now appears to be the major cause of non-hereditary congenital HI in the developed world. Immunization against CMV is, however, a controversial issue, since a large proportion of the infected babies are born to immune mothers. Treatment with antiviral medication is currently not available and as reinfection may cause congenital abnormalities its value is disputed.

Drugs

The incidence of bilateral meatal atresia among children examined at the Karolinksa Hospital in Stockholm increased from 1.4% to 9.5% during the years of thalidomide availability (1959–62) (Barr 1982). Other drugs reported to damage hearing are streptomycin and aminoglycosides, especially when given in combination with diuretics or ethacrynic acid. Cases with deafness or malformations of the hearing organ have been reported occasionally after excessive intake of the antimalarial drugs quinine and cloroquine.

Intra-uterine growth retardation

As intra-uterine growth retardation is not a disease but a symptom of many different conditions affecting the fetus, its connections with HI is related to the aetiology of the growth retardation. Generally, small-for-gestational-age (SGA) babies have elevated risks for neurological sequelae (Fitzhardinge & Steven 1972, Sabel et al 1972, Butler 1974, Hagberg et al 1976). In the Gothenburg study (Thiringer et al 1984) infants who were SGA were at increased risk for HI (Table 43.5). Sensorineural HI (SNHI) was present in 1 of 170 SGA infants. However, of the 6 SGA infants with HI, 3 had rubella, 1 mumps and 3 a positive family history with similar HI in close relatives. Fitzhardinge & Steven (1972) found one child with HI among 87 full-term SGA children tested and Drillien (1972) reported a single child with HI out of 27 SGA infants with birth-weight <2000 g.

Perinatal causes of hearing impairment

HI thought to have originated from the perinatal period was reported in 13.5 and 9% of 111 and 146 children with HI in Manchester and Gothenburg respectively (Newton 1985, Thiringer et al 1984). Males were most frequently affected (80–90%). HI of perinatal origin is often associated with other neurological handicaps, which was the case in 50 and

30% in the above-mentioned studies respectively. The type of HI is often recorded as high-frequency loss, though a 'flat' type of hearing loss has also been observed.

Various potentially damaging factors in the perinatal period are listed in Table 43.5 together with the incidence of SNHI found in children with the risk factors born between 1970 and 1979 in Gothenburg. Children treated in the neonatal intensive care unit are clearly at risk, as they usually have a combination of several risk factors. When studying ABR abnormalities in very-low-birth-weight (VLBW) infants nursed in intensive care units, 18% were abnormal before discharge; the proportion decreasing to 8% at 4 months (Cox et al 1984). Of 12 risk factors no single one, with the exception perhaps of intracranial haemorrhage, was predictive of ABR abnormality. Combined risk factors were, on the other hand, highly predictive (Schulte & Stennert 1978, Cox et al 1984). In clinical studies of survivors of neonatal intensive care, significant predictors of HI were hypoxia caused by apnoeic spells, IRDS or perinatal asphyxia (Simmons 1980, Hope et al 1981, Anagnostakis et al 1982, Thiringer et al 1984, Bergman et al 1985), intracranial haemorrhage (Marshall et al 1980, Cox et al 1984), high bilirubin level (Bergman et al 1985, Clarke et al 1986), time in incubator (Clarke et al 1986), hyponatraemia (Bergman et al 1985) and prolonged perfusion of the cochlea with blood low in pH (Galambos & Despland 1980).

Some of these risk factors are now discussed in detail.

Birth trauma

Neither vacuum extraction nor breech delivery was associated with increased rate of SNHI in the Gothenburg study (Table 43.5). High frequency of traumatic haemorrhage into the inner ear was found by Buch (1966) in combination with difficult delivery, especially in the pre-term infant. Intracranial haemorrhage may extend into the inner ear (Spector et al 1978) and it has found to be a risk factor for HI by several investigators (Cox et al 1984, Marshall et al 1980).

Asphyxia

Compared with adults, thalamic and brainstem nuclei in the newborn infant are more frequently damaged by anoxic–ischaemic encephalopathy (Myers 1975, Leech & Alvord 1977, Pape & Wigglesworth 1979). Hall (1964) found, in a careful study of infants who died of neonatal asphyxia, no damage to the cochlea or the organ of Corti but an extensive (20–60%) loss of neurones in the cochlear nuclei, the extent correlating with the duration of asphyxia. The cell loss was most pronounced in the dorsal nucleus, corresponding to high-frequency hearing loss. Hypoxia occurs mainly in two situations: in severe birth asphyxia, usually preceded by fetal distress, and in the pre-term baby with apnoea and/or Idiopathic Respiratory Distress Syndrome, usually requiring mechanical ventilation. Studies from the UK and USA of very severely asphyxiated newborns, defined as 10 minutes to spontaneous respiration or Apgar <4 at 5 and 10 minutes respectively (D'Souza et al 1981, Thomson et al 1977, Nelson & Ellenberg 1981) show the frequency of HI to be 3.5–4%. Asphyxia of milder degree, defined as Apgar <7 at 1 or 5 minutes did not seem to increase the rate of HI in our study (Table 43.5). Neonatal intensive care, on the other hand, especially when the infant was mechanically ventilated, was the most important perinatal risk factor, giving HI in 1 of 41 and 1 of 27 infants respectively. The prevalence of HI among graduates from neonatal intensive care reported from various neonatal centres varied between 1 in 52 and 1 in 11 (Abramovich et al 1979, Simmons 1980, Thompson & Folsom 1981, Anagnostakis et al 1982). Sell et al (1985) found 8 children with SNHI among 40 infants who had persistent fetal circulation (PFC), a condition in which chronic hypoxia is frequent.

Table 43.5 Incidence rates of sensorineural hearing impairment (SNHI) in children with perinatal risk-factors born in Gothenburg in 1970–79

Group	No. in group	No. with SNHI	Incidence of SNHI (%)	P
All newborn infants	56 334	124	2.2	
Caesarean section	4 466	9	2.0	
Vacuum extraction	3 279	11	3.4	
Breech delivery	2 190	5	2.3	
Low birth-weight	2 333	10	4.3 (1:233)	0.04
Very low birth-weight	227	3	13.2 (1:75)	0.014
Asphyxia				
Apgar score <7 at 1 min	3 192	5	1.9	
Apgar score <7 at 5 min	1 011	2	2.0	
Small for dates	1 008	6	5.9 (1:170)	0.025
Hyperbilirubinaemia >250 μM	5 752	13	2.3	
Exchange transfusion	100	1	10.0	
Neonatal intensive care	124	3	24.0 (1:41)	0.003

Numbers for low birth-weight, very low birth-weight and intensive-care infants refer to surviving cases.
P-values for Fisher's exact test stand for comparison with incidence of SNHI in the total newborn population.
(Reproduced with permission from Thiringer et al 1984.)

Prematurity

The incidence of SNHI is reported to be 1 in 233 for infants of birth-weight <2500 g and 1 in 75 for infants of birth-weight <1500 g born in Gothenburg in 1970–79 (Table 43.5). Bjerre (1975) found HI in 1 in 68 low-birth-weight (LBW) infants born in Malmö in 1966. The Vancouver study (1958–65) included infants with birth-weight mainly below 2000 g and HI above 40 dB occurred in 1 in 17 infants (Clarke et al 1986). Respiratory problems were encountered in all 8 children with bilateral HI.

Generally, the more premature the baby and the more severely ill, the greater the risk of HI. A total of 3.6% of infants born in Melbourne (1966–70) with birth-weights mainly between 1000 and 1500 g were subsequently found to have HI (Kitchen et al 1980). In London, 9% of VLBW children born in 1966–72 and who received intensive care had HI (Abramovich et al 1979). The same incidence (9%) was reported from Athens in children <1800 g born in 1971–73 (Anagnostakis et al 1982). In Pittsburgh, 9.7% of VLBW infants born in 1976–80 had HI (Bergman et al 1985), and of those with neonatal seizures 16.7% were subsequently found to have HI. Infants surviving both VLBW and seizures were at greatest risk (28.6%). Generally, comparisons between different units are difficult to make because of different definitions of the population investigated as well as what is considered to be significant HI.

The HI of the premature infant who received intensive care is often of the high-frequency type but 'flat' curves are also frequently found (Bergman et al 1985). They are considered to be present from birth but in two of three ventilatory-treated babies in our study the HI was of delayed onset.

Ototoxic drugs

Aminoglycosides are potentially nephro- and ototoxic. The use of streptomycin in tuberculosis treatment has been abandoned because of its toxicity to the eighth cranial nerve. In neonatal medicine the switch to kanamycin was due to the emergence of streptomycin-resistant enterobacteria by the end of the 1950s. Kanamycin is now replaced by the new aminoglycosides gentamicin, tobramycin, netilmicin and amikacin, which are used in different countries depending on local tradition and availability.

Tyberghein (1962) looked at guinea pig cochlear microphonics and found neomycin to be extremely toxic, streptomycin and kanamycin sulphate moderately toxic, and kanamycin monopantothenate non-toxic. In adults the average frequency of cochlear toxicity was 13.9% for amikacin, 8.3% for gentamicin, 6.1% for tobramycin and 2.4% for netilmicin, as reported in 63 clinical trials (Kahlmeter & Dahlager 1984). However, in two large, prospective, controlled studies in the neonate, Eichenwald (1966) and Finitzo-Hieber et al (1985) did not find any ototoxic effects of streptomycin, kanamycin, netilmicin and amikacin if given in therapeutic doses. There was a high incidence of transitory auditory abnormalities as measured by the ABR, which was also reported by Bernard (1981) in the form of delayed maturation of wave V latency (see Ch. 15).

Antibiotic treatment did not predict HI in the Vancouver study (Clarke et al 1986), nor could we find a single case of HI attributable to aminoglycoside treatment in Gothenburg (Thiringer et al 1984). The conclusion must be that current practices with frequent measurements of serum concentrations of the potentially ototoxic antibiotics seem to be safe.

Transient deafness has been reported after treatment with frusemide (furosemide) (Mudge 1980) and it may potentiate the ototoxic effect of the aminoglycosides.

Incubator noise

HI can be the result of both acute and chronic noise exposure as both the intensity and duration of noise has to be considered when discussing the effect. Noise-induced HI is mostly pronounced around 3.0 to 6.0 kHz. Histopathology shows breakage of the tectorial membrane and endolymph-induced damage to hair cells. In chronic noise exposure constriction of the vessels of the cochlea has been observed.

Incubator noise is 58 to 80 dB with the frequency distribution mainly below 0.5 kHz (Falk & Farmer 1973, Blennow et al 1974). Slamming incubator doors may produce 90 to 100 dB. Young animals have been found to be more susceptible to noise (Douek et al 1976) and in animal studies Dayal et al (1971) and Jauhiainen et al (1972) found a combined ototoxic effect of aminoglycosides and noise. Winkel et al (1978), however, could not confirm this in LBW infants nursed in incubators and receiving kanamycin. Although 80 dB has never been shown to cause HI in adults, they found small 'noise dips' at 4.0 kHz in 52% of babies nursed in incubators, but this was not considered significant for normal hearing. They support the recommendation of the American Academy of Pediatrics (Committee on Environmental Hazards 1974) to develop quieter incubators and to advise the physician to limit the use of ototoxic drugs.

Infection

Serious neonatal infection (sepsis/meningitis) occurs in 1/1000 newborns and much more frequently in pre-terms. Histopathologically, the infection can cause inflammation of the auditory nerve, cochlear damage and/or suppurative labyrinthitis. The reported incidence of postmeningitic HI varies between 5 and 40% (Lancet 1986). Postnatal HI due to meningitis is responsible for 5 to 10% of all childhood HI (Thiringer et al 1984, Newton 1985, Lancet 1986). The causal organisms most commonly associated with HI are group-B streptococci and *E. coli* in the neonatal period and *Haemophilus influenzae*, *Neisseria meningitides* and pneumococci in older infants. Viral meningitis has also rarely been found to cause HI. We have seen HI after neonatal Coxsackie B virus infection but the virus best-known to cause HI is mumps. Hearing impairment following mumps is caused by direct viral infection of the inner ear and is not a complication of mumps meningitis. The deafness is most commonly unilateral. In Sweden and the USA this virus is included in the vaccination programme of 18-month-olds but is not routinely undertaken in the UK.

Postmeningitic HI is often severe, of mixed frequencies, commonly bilateral and often results in total deafness. All children with meningitis should be assessed by an audiologist some months after the infection. The HI can show improvement within the first 6 months and children should be retested. The addition of other handicaps after meningitis, such as blindness, motor disability and impairment of the vestibulary organ may require special assessment and specially skilled testers.

Hyperbilirubinaemia

About 110 years ago Orth first described the yellow staining of parts of the brains of children dying from neonatal jaundice and in 1903 Schmorl coined the term 'kernicterus' to describe the phenomenom. The Rh-factor was discovered in 1940 by Landsteiner and Weiner and about the same time (1941) Phelps observed the association of choreoathetosis and HI when studying cerebral palsy. He also recognized that HI mainly affected the higher frequencies. In 1944 Coquet described deafness as a sequel to neonatal jaundice and in 1950 Goodhill noted the clinical association of moderate bilateral perceptive deafness, athetoid CP and a history of erythroblastosis. Also in 1950, Allen et al demonstrated the benefit of exchange transfusion and in 1954 they showed the value of pre-term delivery for decreasing mortality and morbidity. Methods of diagnosis and prevention were further developed by Liley (1961, 1963), who advocated intra-uterine transfusions to treat severe forms of the condition. The use of Rh immunoglobu-lin has further reduced the problem but has not entirely eradicated it. Today, a few cases of Rh-immunization still occur and hyperbilirubinaemia, especially in the pre-term baby, remains a major concern.

Bilirubin encephalopathy. The term bilirubin encephalo-pathy (BE) is presently more commonly used for the condition formerly called 'kernicterus'. It is now rare in full-term babies and in the pre-term infant it is not seen in its typical form. The markedly jaundiced infant becomes lethargic, hypotonic, feeds poorly and subsequent-ly develops hypertonia progressing to opisthotonus, fever, high-pitched cry and convulsions. If the infant survives after a seemingly normal period, the typical sequelae of choreoathetosis, paralysis of upward gaze, high-frequency HI, swallowing difficulties, grimacing and dysarthria occur. Usually there is little or no mental retardation.

Bilirubin toxicity. Unconjugated bilirubin has been shown to be toxic to a number of cell functions in vitro, namely cellular respiration, protein synthesis and enzyme activity (Zetterström & Ernster 1956, Schutta & Johnson 1971, Thaler 1971, Rasmussen & Wennberg 1972, Greenfield & Majumdar 1974). The common damaging mechanism may be lipid peroxidation of mitochondrial and cellular membranes (Jew & Williams 1977, Hackney 1980) in view of the great affinity of bilirubin for sphingomyelin (Nagaoka & Cowger 1978) and gangliosides (Weil & Menkes 1975). Differences in adult and infant grey matter gangliosides may explain the marked cytotoxicity of bilirubin in the newborn.

Bilirubin entry into the brain. It has been difficult to produce kernicterus in newborn animal models by infusing bilirubin. Monkeys had to be asphyxiated before bilirubin infusion to cause kernicterus (Lucey et al 1964) or the blood–brain barrier had to be opened by the injection of hypertonic solution into the internal carotid artery of the young adult rat (Levine et al 1982). However, Diamond & Schmid (1966) produced severe neurological damage leading to coma by infusing unbound bilirubin to the level of 100 μmol/l into newborn guinea pigs.

Thus, until recently, it has been thought that only the unbound fraction of bilirubin would pass to the brain. Because of the variation in the level of that fraction at the same total-bilirubin level, the prediction of neurological damage has been difficult. Cashore & Oh (1982) found no differences in any clinical parameters or bilirubin and albu-min concentrations between kernicteric and non- kernicteric pre-term infants coming to postmortem, apart from their level of unbound bilirubin and bilirubin binding capacity and affinity.

The difficulties in measuring unconjugated bilirubin and the absence of cranial ultrasound measurements, as well as the great variation in bilirubin measurements from different laboratories, make many studies of little value. Albumin–bilirubin binding in sera from sick, small, premature infants was found to be profoundly depressed for prolonged periods, lasting at least one month (Ritter & Kenny 1986). Considering this, it is conceivable that kernicterus can be present at low bilirubin concentrations in these babies (Gartner et al 1970). Additional damage can result from the flow of albumin-bound bilirubin into the brain in the presence of an open blood–brain barrier. This is more likely to occur in combination with acidosis, asphyxia, or other insults like haemorrhage and the injection of hypertonic solutions.

Site of brain damage. Even if the full-blown clinical picture of kernicterus is not seen in our wards, we still see at autopsy the yellow staining of the brain, mainly in pre-term infants. The prevalence of kernicterus in at-risk neonates varied between 25 and 7% at gestational ages of 21–24 and 33–40 weeks (Ahdab-Barmada 1984). The gross yellow staining and the microscopic pattern of bilirubin encephalopathy cannot always be found in the same patient but there may be (microscopically) a spongy appearance, which may reflect underlying diffuse damage to the brain from a variety of insults (Turkel 1983). Other investigators (Ahdab-Barmada & Moosy 1984), however, still see the characteristic microscopic damage of BE to neurones in susceptible grey nuclei; the localization being somewhat different to that of the sites of the anoxic–ischaemic encephalopathy, as damage is not seen in the cerebral cortex or periventricular white matter. Instead, the globus pallidus, subthalamic nucleus, the H2–3 sector of the hippocampus, several nuclei of the midbrain (inferior colliculus, interstitial nucleus of Cajal, third nerve nuclei) and pons (locus ceruleus, sixth and seventh nerve nuclei), the vestibular and cochlear nuclei of the medulla and the cerebellum are involved (Ahdab-Barmada 1983, Sarnat 1984).

The areas involved relating to the auditory system are the medial geniculate body, inferior colliculus and the cochlear nuclei. The distribution of the damage to the dorsal cochlear nuclei would correspond to the high-frequency HI (Fenwick 1974). Also, the ventral cochlear nuclei were found to show histological neuronal disease (Ahdab-Barmada & Moosey 1984) which would explain the flat HI found in some pre-term infants.

Sequelae of hyperbilirubinaemia. Athetosis as a sequel to kernicterus has not been registered in Gothenburg since 1954 and in the western Swedish region since 1962 (Hagberg et al 1975). We are now dealing with the more subtle diagnosis of developmental outcome after neonatal hyperbilirubinaemia. Maisels (1983) reviewed 63 clinical studies of human infants over the previous 30 years and came to the following conclusions. For pre-term infants with serum bilirubin in the region 300–340 μmol/l (18–20 mg/dl) there is an increased risk of kernicterus but perhaps not adverse development. In the presence of additional damaging mechanisms this might not apply but lower levels of bilirubin may cause kernicterus. The results of large follow-up studies of full-term infants with hyperbilirubinaemia (Scheidt et al 1977, bilirubin >170 μmol/l; Rubin et al 1979, bilirubin >270 μmol/l) are contradictory. Impaired development or motor performance has been present at one assessment but disappears at a later age. The study methods may cause problems in comparing results, sample sizes may be too small and other confounding variables may be present. Only one study was designed as a randomized, controlled trial (Wishingrad et al 1965).

HI following hyperbilirubinaemia. The association of hyperbilirubinaemia and HI after the introduction of exchange transfusion and other methods of preventing jaundice in the newborn is also a controversial area. Keaster et al (1969) reported a 4.2% incidence of HI in 405 patients with haemolytic disease of the newborn, 351 of them with exchange transfusion. The exchange transfusion level was 340 μmol/l (20 mg/dl). Athetosis appeared in

infants with bilirubin levels >510 μmol/l (30 mg/dl). Though the association of HI and hyperbilirubinaemia was strong, all but one infant also received streptomycin as part of the exchange transfusion. Valaes et al (1980) in a case-control study of 233 jaundiced infants found no differences in neurological assessment but an increase of SNHI in those with bilirubin >200 μmol/l (12 mg/dl). In the Gothenburg study (Thiringer et al 1984) the incidence of SNHI among children with bilirubin >250 μmol/l (15 mg/dl) was not different from the overall incidence of SNHI (2.2/1000). The only infant receiving an exchange transfusion among 146 children with HI was a 1150 g, 26 week baby, whose brother and both grandfathers had HI. In Norway, Nilsen et al (1984) studied a cohort of 55 18-year-olds, who had neonatal jaundice with bilirubin >255 μmol/l and did not find any differences compared to the total population of Norwegian conscripts regarding physical or mental health, vision, hearing and general intelligence. Only 7 with positive Coombs' test and hyperbilirubinaemia more than 5 days had a lower mean intelligence.

Bradford et al (1985) followed 117 infants at <33 weeks of gestation and found 9 with SNHI at one year of age. The mean total plasma bilirubin concentration of the infants with birth-weight between 940 and 1735 g was 228 μmol/l (range 180–348 μmol/l). Of the 9 infants, 6 had germinal matrix haemorrhage–intraventricular haemorrhage (GMH–IVH) and one had generalized cerebral atrophy. The infant with the normal scan had Down's syndrome. All infants were mechanically ventilated.

The study of De Vries et al (1985) classified 99 infants at <34 weeks of gestation and with bilirubin level >240 μmol/l (>14 mg/dl) into high- and low-risk according to the presence of birth asphyxia, mechanical ventilation, pneumothorax, infection, persistent fetal circulation and/or PDA requiring treatment, infection hypoglycaemia and GMH–IVH. Only in infants with birth-weights less than 1500 g did the risk factors result in significantly higher numbers of SNHI, while in infants with birth-weights greater than 1500 g the combination of hyperbilirubinaemia of this grade and other risk factors seemed to carry little risk. The 12 deaf infants had a significantly longer period of hyperbilirubinaemia and a greater number of acidotic episodes.

Guidelines for treatment. Full-term babies in Sweden are treated with phototherapy at a total serum bilirubin level of 350 μmol/l (20 mg/dl), if no risk factors are present. Exchange transfusion is performed at 425 μmol/l (25 mg/dl). Rh or ABO-immunized babies are treated prophylactically with phototherapy and exchange transfusion is performed at 170 μmol/l before the age of 12 hours, at 240 μmol/l at 24 hours and 340 μmol/l at 36 hours.

LBW infants receive phototherapy at 250 μmol/l at birth-weight 2000–2500 g, 200 μmol/l at 1500–2000 g and 150 μmol/l at 1000–1500 g. Limits are lowered by

50 μmol/l for each weight group when further risk factors are present in addition to hyperbilirubinaemia. Infants below 1000 g are prophylactically treated with phototherapy for the first 3 days of life.

The biliburin levels for exchange transfusion are different in the UK and USA. In the UK, a level equivalent to 10 times the gestational age in weeks is sometimes taken (28 weeks = 280 μmol/l) (De Vries et al 1985). The American Academy of Pediatrics (1977) recommends a much lower level: 1% of the birth-weight in grams in mg/dl (1000 g = 10 mg/dl = 170 μmol/l). The latter regimen has been used in Sweden with some modifications. Serum bilirubin in LBW infants is never allowed to increase above 350 μmol/l.

In view of the difficulties in predicting bilirubin toxicity, especially in the high-risk pre-term neonate, the above guidelines are at most useful approximations for treatment levels. Therapy (phototherapy and exchange transfusion) must be decided individually for infants, taking all risk factors into consideration.

PERINATAL RISK CRITERIA FOR HEARING ASSESSMENT

Newborn hearing screening and testing is either laborious and requires extensive equipment (ECoG, ARC, Crib-o-gram) or gives a high false-positive rate (psycho-acoustical tests). The selection of high-risk groups for screening or testing has resulted in early detection of HI, if the criteria for inclusion are adequate.

For babies born in Gothenburg during the 1970s we have used a liberal perinatal high-risk list, as seen in Table 43.6. According to the list 6.3% (3530 infants) of the newborn population were tested; 41 (1.2%) of the referred infants were subsequently diagnosed as having HI. After an analysis of the cause–effect relationship of the listed potentially damaging factors (Thiringer et al 1984) the perinatal risk criteria were revised to include the following groups:

1. positive family history of HI
2. rubella or other viral infections during the first half of pregnancy
3. malformations of the ear, face, syndrome-like appearance, chromosomal defects and fetal alcohol syndrome
4. asphyxia requiring >10 minutes of resuscitation
5. all intensive care-treated neonates
6. VLBW infants
7. culture-positive neonatal sepsis/meningitis.

After revision of the risk criteria, the neonatal referrals decreased from 6.3 to 1.5% of the newborns and the proportion of infants having HI increased from 1.2 to 9% of the referrals. The incidence of HI >40 dB HL was virtually the same in the two populations (1.4 and 1.1/1000) but the age at which detection was complete was 5 years in

children born in 1970–79 as opposed to one year in children born in 1982–84 (Table 43.7). This is to be compared to the mean age of identification of the HI in the Manchester study, which was 23.3 months (Bellman 1986) or hearing impairment incidence of 1/1000, averaging 25 db HL or more, for children born in 1977, and diagnosed by 5 years of age (Newton 1985). In Gothenburg, the initiator of the test was the neonatologist in 32% of the diagnosed cases. At the same time, new guidelines were introduced at the well-baby clinics with more intense information to parents and four questionnaires, of which one at 8 months of age is administered to every family and the three others at 2 to 10 weeks, 3 to 6 months and 18 months of age available if there is any doubt about the child's hearing. A screening test with tone-generator or BOEL (see Methods) was carried out at 8–9 months of age. The practice of this programme (Kankkunen 1986) resulted in the detection of HI increasing from 15 to 44%. In the remaining 24% of cases the HI was suspected by the general practitioner or the parent in equal numbers (Table 43.8).

The tests used for the detection of the HI were respiration and observation audiometry at 3–8 months

Table 43.6 High-risk criteria for referral from maternity hospitals in Gothenburg for hearing assessment during 1970–81. (For revised criteria see text)

1. Family history of hearing loss
2. Rubella or other viral disease during first half of pregnancy
3. Malformation of face and ears
4. Low birth-weight
5. Serum bilirubin >340 μM (20 mg/dl) in infants >2500 g and >250 μM (15 mg/dl) in low birth-weight infants
6. Birth asphyxia (Apgar <7 at 1 min or later)
7. Neurological symptoms of cerebral origin lasting >24 h
8. Infants of diabetic mothers
9. Hypoglycaemia
10. Treatment with ototoxic drugs
11. Neonatal infection

(Reproduced with permission from Thiringer et al 1984.)

Table 43.7 The level of hearing loss in one-year-old children born in 1982–83, as diagnosed 1982–84 (livebiths 9952)

Hearing loss	n
<25 dB HL	13
25–40 dB HL	13
41–60 dB HL	5
61–100 dB HL	1
>100 dB HL	2
Deaf	3
Unilateral HL	4
Total	41
HL/1000	4.1
HL >40 dB HL/1000	1.1

HL = hearing level
(Modified from Kankkunen 1986.)

Table 43.8 Initiator in detection of hearing loss in children born in 1970–81 and 1982–83

Referral from:	Children born 1970–81 (n = 141) %	Children born 1982–83 (n = 41) %
Postnatal/neonatal units	35	32
Well-baby clinics	15	44
Paediatric clinics	15	12
Otolaryngologist	3	–
Parents	32	12

(Modified from Kankkunen 1986.)

of age, tympanometry and 40 Hz MLR audiometry (see Methods) when needed. Some children will also be tested subsequently with visual reinforcement audiometry and play-audiometry if there is any doubt about the grade of the HI or if there is a suspicion of progression.

The programme used by us is very similar to that described by Feinmesser et al (1982) in Israel. The perinatal risk criteria there also include apnoea and cyanosis, Apgar score 1–4 (time not given), hyperbilirubinaemia above 340 μmol/l and exchange transfusion. These criteria apply to 7% of the neonates. According to the Position Statement of the American Academy of Pediatrics (1982) screening, optimally by 3 months of age but not later than 6 months of age, should be carried out in at-risk infants. Their list of risk items also includes seven damaging factors, differing from those suggested by us in only one item — they list hyperbilirubinaemia at levels exceeding indications for exchange transfusion, while the Gothenburg list proposes that all intensive care babies be tested.

The suggestion of screening neonatal risk populations, like those who have been in intensive care units, with ABR (Schulman-Galambos & Galambos 1979, Bradford 1985) or the auditory response cradle (McCormick et al 1984) or all newborns with the Crib-o-gram is sensible if the facilities and skilled personnel are available. However, retesting between 1 and 2 years of age may be indicated in certain groups of high-risk infants. Recently, high-risk infants requiring prolonged ventilatory treatment resulting in chronic lung disease have been found to have significant hearing loss despite normal ABR at the time of discharge from the neonatal intensive care unit (Nield et al 1986).

In summary, it seems that heredity is an important factor in the causation of HI in childhood, followed by postnatal causes, mainly of infectious origin. The good news is that some of the former perinatal risk factors, like rubella and hyperbilirubinaemia caused by Rh-immunization may not be with us for many more years. Perinatal risk factors of unknown origin (malformations and syndromes) may be clarified by more intense research as well as factors known but not yet fully preventable, like those which operate in VLBW infants.

ACKNOWLEDGEMENTS

The part on methods of hearing assessment was written after discussions with and help from Aira Kankkunen, Audiologist, to whom the author wants to express her sincere thanks for pleasant collaboration. The part on genetic hearing loss was written with valuable help from Dr Jan Wahlström, Head of the Genetic Laboratory at the Eastern Hospital. My sincere thanks to Dr Malcolm Levene for revising the English, to Margareta Rydén for typing the tables and to Kajsa Gullman for drawing the figures. Above all thanks to my family who took care of themselves and me.

REFERENCES

Abramovich S J, Gregory S, Slemick M, Stewart A 1979 Hearing loss in very low birthweight infants treated with neonatal intensive care. Archives of Disease in Childhood 54: 421–426

Ahdab-Barmada M 1983 Neonatal kernicterus: neuropathologic diagnosis. In: Hyperbilirubinemia in the newborn (Report of the Eighty-Fifth Ross Conference on Pediatric Research). Ross Laboratories, Ohio, pp 2–8

Ahdab-Barmada M, Moosey J 1984 The neuropathology of kernicterus in the premature neonate: diagnostic problems. Journal of Neuropathology and Neurology 43: 45–56

Ahlfors K, Harris S, Ivarsson S-A, Svanberg L 1981 Secondary maternal cytomegalovirus infection causing symptomatic congenital infection. New England Journal of Medicine 305: 284

Ahlfors K, Ivarsson S-A, Johnsson T, Svanberg L 1982 Primary and secondary maternal cytomegalovirus infections and their relation to congenital infection. Acta Paediatrica Scandinavica 71: 109–113

American Academy of Pediatrics, Committee on Environmental Hazards 1974 Noise pollution: neonatal aspects. Pediatrics 54: 476–479

American Academy of Pediatrics 1977 Standards and Recommendations for Hospital Care of Newborn Infants, 6th edn. American Academy of Pediatrics, Evanston, p 95

American Academy of Pediatrics, Joint Committee on Infant Hearing 1982 Position statement. Pediatrics 70: 496–497

Allen F H Jr, Diamond L K, Vaughan V C 1950 Erythroblastosis fetalis. VI. Prevention of kernicterus. American Journal of Diseases of Children 80: 779–791

Allen F H Jr, Diamond L K, Jones A R 1954 Erythroblastosis fetalis. IX. The problems of stillbirth. New England Journal of Medicine 251: 453–459

Allen M C, Capute A J 1986 Assessment of early auditory and visual abilities of extremely premature infants. Developmental Medicine and Child Neurology 28: 458–466

Ames M D, Plotkin S A, Winchester R A, Atkins T E 1970 Central auditory imperception — a significant factor in congenital rubella deafness. Journal of the American Medical Association 213: 419–421

Anagnostakis D, Petmezakis J, Papazissis G, Messaritakis J, Matsaniotis N 1982 Hearing loss in low-birth weight infants. American Journal of Diseases of Children 136: 602–604

Anderson H, Barr B, Wedenberg E 1970 Genetic disposition: a prerequisite for maternal rubella deafness. Archives of Otolaryngology 91: 141–147

Armitage S E, Baldwin B A, Vince M A 1980 The fetal sound environment of sheep. Science 208: 1173–1174

Balkany T J, Downs M P, Jafek B W, Krajicek M J 1979 Hearing in Down's syndrome: a treatable handicap more common than generally recognized. Clinical Pediatrics 18: 116–118

Barr B 1955 Pure tone audiometry for preschool children. Acta Oto-laryngologica (Suppl) 121: 1–84

Barr B 1982 Teratogenic hearing loss. Audiology 21: 111–127

Barr B 1986 Personal communication

Bellman S 1986 Hearing screening in infancy. Archives of Disease in Childhood 61: 637–638

Bergman I, Hirsch R P, Fria T J, Shapiro S M, Holzman I, Painter M J 1985 Cause of hearing loss in the high-risk premature infant. Journal of Pediatrics 106: 95–101

Bernard P A 1981 Freedom from ototoxicity in aminoglycoside treated neonates: a mistaken notion. Laryngoscope XCI (12): 1985–1994

Bhattacharya J, Bennet M J, Tucker S M 1984 Long term follow up of newborns tested with the auditory response cradle. Archives of Disease in Childhood 59: 504–511

Birnholz J C, Benecerraf B R 1983 The development of human fetal hearing. Science 222: 516–518

Bjerre I 1975 Neurological investigation of 5-year-old children with low birth-weight. Acta Paediatrica Scandinavica 64: 859–864

Blennow G, Svenningsen N W, Almquist B 1974 Noise levels in infant incubators: adverse effects? Pediatrics 53: 29–32

Bradford L 1975 Respiration audiometry. In: Bradford L (ed) Physiological measures of the audio-vestibular system. Academic Press, New York

Bradford B C, Baudin J, Conway M J, Hazell J W P, Stewart A L, Reynolds E O R 1985 Identification of sensory neural hearing loss in very preterm infants by brainstem auditory evoked potentials. Archives of Disease in Childhood 60: 105–109

Buch N H 1966 The inner ear of newborn infants: a histopathological study. Journal of Laryngology and Otology 80: 765–777

Butler N R 1974 Risk factors in human intrauterine growth retardation. Ciba Foundation Symposium 27: 379–382

Cashore W J, Oh W 1982 Unbound bilirubin and kernicterus in low-birth- weight infants. Pediatrics 69 (4): 481–485

Caldarelli D D 1977 Congenital middle ear anomalies associated with cranio–facial and skeletal syndromes. In: Jaffe B F (ed) Hearing loss in children. University Park Press, Baltimore, pp 310–340

Clarke B R, Conry R F, Dunn H G 1986 Hearing impairment and associated factors. In: Dunn H G (ed) Sequelae of low birthweight: the Vancouver study. Clinics in Developmental Medicine, No. 95/96. MacKeith Press, London, pp147–167

Commission of the European Communities 1979 Childhood deafness in the European Community. EUR Report 6413. European Commission, Luxembourg

Coquet M 1944 Les séquelles neurologiques tardives de l'ictére nucléaire. Annales de Pediatrie 163: 83–104

Cox L C, Hack M, Metz D A 1984 Auditory brain stem response abnormalities in the very low birthweight infant: incidence and risk factors. Ear and Hearing 5: 47–51

Dahle A J, McCollister F P, Stagno S, Reynolds D W, Hoffman H E 1979 Progressive hearing impairment in children with congenital cytomegalovirus infection. Journal of Speech and Hearing Disorders 44: 220–226

Dayal Vijay S, Kokshanian A, Mitchell D P 1971 Combined effects of noise and kanamycin. Annals of Otology, Rhinology and Laryngology 80: 897–902

De Casper A J, Fifer W P 1980 Of human bonding: newborns prefer their mothers' voices. Science 208: 1174–1176

Despland P A, Galambos R 1980 The auditory brainstem response (ABR) is a useful diagnostic tool in the intensive care nursery. Pediatric Research 14: 154–158

De Vries L S, Lary S, Dubowitz L M S 1985 Relationship of serum bilirubin levels to ototoxicity and deafness in high-risk low-birth-weight infants. Pediatrics 76: 351–354

Diamond I, Schmid R 1966 Experimental bilirubin encephalopathy: the mode of entry of bilirubin ^{14}C into the central nervous system. Journal of Clinical Investigation 45: 678

Douek E, Bannister L H, Dodson H C, Ashcroft P, Humphries K N 1976 Effects of incubator noise on the cochlea of the newborn. Lancet ii: 1110–1113

Downs M J, Hemenway W 1969 Report on the hearing screening of 17 000 neonates. International Audiology 8: 72–76.

Drife J O 1985 Can the fetus listen and learn? British Journal of Obstetrics and Gynaecology 92: 777–779

Drillien C M 1972 Aetiology and outcome in low-birthweight infants. Developmental Medicine and Child Neurology 14: 563–574

D'Souza S W, McCartney E, Nolan M, Taylor I H 1981 Hearing, speech, and language in survivors of severe perinatal asphyxia. Archives of Disease in Childhood 56: 245–252

Durieux-Smith A, Jacobson J T 1985 Comparison of auditory brainstem response and behavioral screening in neonates. Journal of Otolaryngology (Suppl) 15: 47–53

Eichenwald H F 1966 Some observations on dosage and toxicity of kanamycin in premature and full-term infants. Annals of the New York Academy of Sciences 132: 984–991

Falk S A, Farmer J C 1973 Incubator noise and possible deafness. Archives of Otolaryngology 97: 385–387

Fant G 1959 Acoustic analysis and synthesis of speech with application to Swedish. Ericsson Technics No. 1

Feinmesser M, Tell L, Levi H 1978 Deafness in early childhood in Jerusalem. Journal of the Israel Medical Association 95: 192–194

Feinmesser M, Tell L, Levi H 1982 Follow-up of 40 000 infants screened for hearing defect. Audiology 21: 197–203

Fenwick J D 1974 Neonatal jaundice as a cause of deafness. Meeting of the British Society of Audiology, 20th September

Finitzo-Hieber T 1981 Auditory brainstem response in assessment of infants treated with aminoglycoside antibiotics. In: Lerner S A, Matz C J, Hawkins J E (eds) Aminoglycoside ototoxicity. Little Brown, Boston

Finitzo-Hieber T, McCracken G H Jr, Brown K C 1985 Prospective controlled evaluation of auditory function in neonates given netilmicin or amikacin. Journal of Pediatrics 106: 129–136

Fitzhardinge P M, Steven E M 1972 The small-for-date infant. II. Neurological and intellectual sequelae. Pediatrics 50: 50–57

Fraser G R 1976 The causes of profound deafness in childhood. Johns Hopkins University Press, Baltimore

Galambos R, Despland P A 1980 The auditory brainstem response (ABR) evaluates risk factors for hearing loss. Pediatric Research 14: 159–163

Galambos R, Makeig S, Talmachoff P J 1981 A 40-Hz auditory potential recorded from the human scalp. Proceedings of the National Academy of Sciences of the USA 78: 2643–2648

Galambos R, Hicks G E, Wilson M J 1984 The auditory brainstem response reliably predicts hearing loss in graduates of a tertiary intensive care nursery. Ear and Hearing 5: 254–260

Gartner L, Snyder R, Chabon R et al 1970 Kernicterus: high incidence in premature infants with low serum bilirubin concentrations. Pediatrics 54: 906–917

Goodhill V 1950 Nuclear deafness and the nerve deaf child: the importance of the Rh factor. Transactions of the American Academy of Ophthalmology and Otolaryngology 54: 671–687

Greenfield S, Majumdar A P N 1974 Bilirubin encephalopathy: effect on protein synthesis in the brain of the Gunn rat. Journal of the Neurological Sciences 22: 83–89

Gregg N M 1941 Congenital cataract following German measles in the mother. Transactions of the Ophthalmological Society of Australia 3: 34–45

Griffiths P D, Baboonian C 1984 A prospective study of primary cytomegalovirus infection during pregnancy: final report. British Journal of Obstetrics and Gynaecology 91: 307–315

Grimwade J C, Walker D W, Bartlett M, Gordon S, Wood C 1971 Human fetal heart rate change and movement in response to sound and vibration. American Journal of Obstetrics and Gynecology 109: 86–90

Hackney D D 1980 Photodynamic action of bilirubin on the inner mitochondrial membrane. Biochemical and Biophysical Research Communications 94: 875–880

Hagberg B, Hagberg G, Olow I 1975 The changing panorama of cerebral palsy in Sweden 1954–1970. II. Analysis of the various syndromes. Acta Paediatrica Scandinavica 64: 193–200

Hagberg B, Hagberg G, Olow I 1976 The changing panorama of cerebral palsy in Sweden 1954–1970. III. The importance of foetal deprivation of supply. Acta Paediatrica Scandinavica 65: 403–408

Hanshow J B 1982 On deafness, cytomegalovirus and neonatal screening. American Journal Diseases of Children 136: 886–887

Hanshow J B, Scheiner A P, Moxley A et al 1976 CNS effects of 'silent' cytomegalovirus infection. New England Journal of Medicine 296: 468–470

Hall F G 1964 The cochlea and cochlear nuclei in neonatal asphyxia. Acta Oto-laryngologica (Suppl) 194: 1–93

Hope P L, Hazell J W P, Stewart A L 1981 Sensori-neural hearing loss in the very low birthweight survivor. In: Proceedings of the Scientific

Meeting of the British Association of Audiological Physicians and Community Paediatric Group. Department of Audiology, University of Manchester

Jaffe B F, Königsmark B W 1977 Genetic hearing loss. In: Jaffe B F (ed) Hearing loss in children. University Park Press, Baltimore, pp 348–366

Jauhiainen T, Kohonen A, Jauhiainen M 1972 Combined effect of noise and neomycin on the cochlea. Acta Oto-laryngologica 73: 387–390

Jew J, Williams T 1977 Ultrasound aspects of bilirubin encephalopathy in cochlear nuclei of the Gunn rat. Journal of Anatomy 124: 599–614

Kahlmeter G, Dahlager I 1984 Aminoglycoside toxicity — a review of clinical studies published between 1975–1982. Journal of Antimicrobial Chemotherapy 13 (Suppl): A 9–22

Kankkunen A 1982 Pre-school children with impaired hearing in Göteborg 1964–1980. Acta Oto-laryngologica (Suppl) 391: 1–124

Kankkunen A 1986 Effective programme for early diagnosis of hearing impairments in children. Läkartidningen 83: 523–527

Kankkunen A, Lidén G 1977 Respiration audiometry. Scandinavian Audiology 6: 81–86

Kankkunen A, Lidén G 1984 Ipsilateral acoustic reflex thresholds in neonates and in normal-hearing and hearing-impaired pre-school children. Scandinavian Audiology 13: 139–144

Kankkunen A, Rosenhall U 1985 Comparison between thresholds obtained with pure-tone audiometry and the 40-Hz middle latency response. Scandinavian Audiology 14: 99–104

Kankkunen A, Thiringer K 1987 Hearing impairment in connection with pre-auricular tags. Acta Paediatrica Scandinavica 76: 143–146

Keaster J, Hyman C B, Harris I 1969 Hearing problems subsequent to neonatal hemolytic disease or hyperbilirubinemia. American Journal of Diseases of Children 117: 406–410

Keith R W, 1975 Middle ear function in neonates. Archives of Otolaryngology 101: 376–379

Kileny P, Robertson C M T 1985 Neurological aspects of infant hearing assessment. Journal of Otolaryngology (Suppl) 14: 34–39

Kitchen W H, Ryan M M, Rickards A et al 1980 A longitudinal study of very low-birthweight infants. IV. An overview of performance at eight years of age. Developmental Medicine and Child Neurology 22: 172–188

Klockhoff I, Lyttkens L 1982 Hearing defects of noise trauma type with lack of noise exposure. Scandinavian Audiology 11: 257–260

Kolata G 1984 Studying hearing in the womb. Science 225: 302–303

Königsmark B W 1969a Hereditary deafness in man (part 1). New England Journal of Medicine 281: 713–720

Königsmark B W 1969b Hereditary deafness in man (part 2). New England Journal of Medicine 281: 775–778

Königsmark B W 1969c Hereditary deafness in man (part 3). New England Journal of Medicine 281: 827–832

Königsmark B W, Gorlin R J 1976 Genetic and metabolic deafness. Saunders, Philadelphia

Lancet (Editorial) 1986 Deafness after meningitis. Lancet i: 134–135

Lary S, Briassoulis G, de Vries L, Dubowitz L M S, Dubowitz V 1985 Hearing threshold in preterm and term infants by auditory brainstem response. Journal of Pediatrics 4: 593–599

Leader L R, Baillie P, Martin B, Vermeulen E 1982 The assessment and significance of habituation to a repeated stimulus by the human fetus. Early Human Development 7: 211–219

Leech R W, Alvord E C Jr 1977 Anoxic–ischemic encephalopathy in the human neonatal period. Archives of Neurology 34: 109–113

Levine R, Fredericks W, Rapoport S 1982 Entry of bilirubin into the brain due to opening of the blood–brain barrier. Pediatrics 69: 255–259

Lidén G, Kankkunen A 1969 Visual reinforcement audiometry. Acta Oto-laryngologica 67: 281–292

Liley A W 1961 Liquor amnii analysis in management of the pregnancy complicated by the rhesus sensitization. American Journal of Obstetrics and Gynecology 82: 1359–1370

Liley A W 1963 Intrauterine transfusion of fetus in haemolytic disease. British Medical Journal 2: 1107–1109

Linthicum F H 1978 Viral causes of sensorineural hearing loss. Otolaryngologic Clinics of North America 11: 29–34

Lucey J, Hibbard E, Behrman R et al 1964 Kernicterus in asphyxiated newborn rhesus monkeys. Experimental Neurology 9: 43–58

McCormick B, Curnock D A, Spavins F 1984 Auditory screening of special care neonates using the auditory response cradle. Archives of Disease in Childhood 59: 1168–1172

McKusick V A 1976 Mendelian inheritance in man. Johns Hopkins University Press, Baltimore

Maisels M J 1983 Clinical studies of the sequelae of hyperbilirubinemia. (Report of the Eighty-Fifth Ross Conference on Pediatric Research). Ross Laboratories, Ohio, pp 26–38

Marshall R E, Reichert T J, Kerley S M, Davis H 1980 Auditory function in newborn intensive care unit patients revealed by auditory brain-stem potentials. Journal of Pediatrics 96: 731–735

Menyuk P 1977 Effects of hearing loss on language acquisition on the babbling stage. In: Jaffe B F (ed) Hearing loss in children. University Park Press, Baltimore, pp 621–629

Mudge G H 1980 Diuretics and other agents employed in the mobilization of the edema fluid. In: Goodman L S, Gilman A (eds) The pharmacological basis of therapeutics, 6th edn. Macmillan, New York

Myers R E 1975 Fetal asphyxia due to umbilical cord compression: metabolic and brain-pathologic consequences. Biology of the Neonate 26: 21–43

Nagaoka S, Cowger M L 1978 Interaction of bilirubin with lipids studied by fluorescence quenching method. Journal of Biology and Chemistry 253: 2005–2011

Nelson K B, Ellenberg J H 1981 Apgar scores as predictors of chronic neurologic disability. Pediatrics 68: 36–44

Newton V 1985 Aetiology of bilateral sensori-neural hearing loss in young children. Journal of Laryngology and Otology (Suppl) 10: 1–57

Nield T A, Schrier S, Ramos A D, Platzker A C G, Warburton D 1986 Unexpected hearing loss in high-risk infants. Pediatrics 78: 417–422

Nilsen S T, Finne P H, Bergsjö P, Stamnes O 1984 Males with neonatal hyperbilirubinemia examined at 18 years of age. Acta Paediatrica Scandinavica 73: 176–180

Oller D K 1980 The emergence of the sounds of speech in infancy. In: Yeni-Komshian G H, Kawanagh J F, Ferguson C A (eds) Child phonology, Vol I. Academic Press, New York, pp 93–112

Oller D K 1984 Metaphonology and infant vocalizations. In: Lindblom B, Zetterström R (eds) Precursors of early speech (Proceedings of an International Symposium held at the Wenner-Gren Center, Stockholm 1984). Stockton Press, New York, pp 21–63

Pape K E, Wigglesworth J S 1979 Haemorrhage, ischemia and the perinatal brain. Clinics in Developmental Medicine, Nos 69/70. Spastics International Medical/Heinemann Medical, London

Peckham C S, Coleman J C, Hurley R, Shin Chin K, Hendersen K, Preece P M 1983 Cytomegalovirus infection in pregnancy: preliminary findings from a prospective study. Lancet i: 1352–1355

Phelps W M 1941 The management of cerebral palsies. Journal of the American Medical Association 117: 1621–1625

Preece P M, Pearl K N, Peckham C S 1984 Congenital cytomegalovirus infection. Archives of Disease in Childhood 59: 1120–1126

Queenan J T 1986 Erythroblastosis fetalis: closing the circle (Editorial). New England Journal of Medicine 314: 1448–1449

Querleu D, Lefebvre C, Titran M, Renard X, Morillion M, Crepin G 1984 Reactivite du nouveau-ne de moins de deux heures de vie a la voix maternelle. Journal de Gynecologie, Obstetrique et Biologie de la Reproduction 13: 125–134

Rasmussen L F, Wennberg R P 1972 Pharmacologic modification of bilirubin toxicity in tissue culture cells. Research communications of Chemistry, Pathology and Pharmacology 3: 567–578

Reynolds D W, Stagno S, Stubbe K G et al 1974 Congenital cytomegalovirus infection: relation to auditory and mental deficiency. New England Journal of Medicine 290: 291–296

Riko K, Hyde M L, Alberti P W 1985 Hearing loss in early infancy: incidence, detection and assessment. Laryngoscope 95: 137–145

Ritter D A, Kenny J D 1986 Bilirubin binding in premature infants from birth to 3 months. Archives of Disease in Childhood 61: 352–356

Rousey C 1964 Changes in respiration as a function of auditory stimuli. Journal of Auditory Research 4: 107–114

Rubin R A, Balow B, Fisch R O 1979 Neonatal serum bilirubin levels related to cognitive development at ages 4 through 7 years. Journal of Pediatrics 94: 601–603

Sabel K G, Olegård R, Victorin L 1972 Remaining sequelae with modern perinatal care. Pediatrics 57: 652–658

Saigal S, Lunyk O, Bayce Larke R P, Chernesky M A 1982 The outcome in children with congenital cytomegalovirus infection. American Journal of Diseases of Children 135: 895–901

Sanders R, Durieux-Smith A, Hyde M, Jacobson J, Kileny P, Murnane O 1985 Incidence of hearing loss in high risk and intensive care nursery infants. Journal of Otolaryngology (Suppl) 14: 28–33

Sarnat M 1984 Neonatal bilirubin encephalopathy. In: Harvey B, Sarnat M (eds) Topics in neonatal neurology. Grune & Stratton, Orlando, pp 109–136

Scheidt P C, Mellits E D, Hardy J B 1977 Toxicity to bilirubin in neonates: infant development during first year in relation to maximum neonatal serum bilirubin concentration. Journal of Pediatrics 91: 292–297

Schmidt W, Boos R, Auer J G, Schulze S 1985 Fetal behavioural states and controlled sound stimulation. Early Human Development 12: 145–153

Schulman-Galambos C, Galambos R 1979 Brain stem evoked response audiometry in newborn hearing screening. Archives of Otolaryngology 105: 86–90

Schulte F J, Stennert E 1978 Hearing defects in preterm infants. Archives of Disease in Childhood 53: 269–270

Schutta H S, Johnson L 1971 Electron microscopic observations on acute bilirubin encephalopathy in Gunn rats induced by sulfadimethoxine. Laboratory Investigations 24: 82–89

Scibetta J J, Rosen M G, Hochberg C J, Chik L 1971 Human fetal brain response to sound during labor. American Journal of Obstetrics and Gynecology 109: 82–85

Sell E J, Gaines J A, Gluckman G, Williams E 1985 Persistent fetal circulation — Neurodevelopment outcome. American Journal of Diseases in Childhood 139: 25–28

Serafini P, Lindsay M B J, Nagey D A, Pupkin M J, Tseng P, Crenshaw C 1984 Antepartum fetal heart rate response to sound stimulation: acoustic stimulation test. Year Book of Obstetrics and Gynecology 1985, pp 186–187

Simmons F B 1978 Identification of hearing loss in infants and young children. Otolaryngologic Clinics of North America 11: 19–28

Simmons F B, 1980 Patterns of deafness in newborns. Laryngoscope 90: 448–453

Simmons F B, Russ F N 1974 Automated newborn hearing screening, the Crib-o-gram. Archives of Otolaryngology 100: 1–7

Smith D W, Aase J M 1970 Polygenic inheritance of certain common malformations. Journal of Pediatrics 76: 653–659

Spector G, Pettit W, Davis G, Strauss M, Rauchbach E 1978 Fetal respiratory distress causing CNS and inner ear hemorrhage. Laryngoscope 88: 764–768

Stagno S, Reynolds D W, Tsiantos A et al 1975 Cervical cytomegalovirus excretion in pregnant and nonpregnant women: suppression in early gestation. Journal of Infectious Diseases 131: 522–527

Stagno S, Reynolds D W, Amos C et al 1977 Auditory and visual defects resulting from symptomatic and subclinical cytomegaloviral and toxoplasma infections. Pediatrics 59: 669–678

Stensland-Junker K 1972 Selective attention in infants and consecutive communicative behavior. Acta Paediatrica Scandinavica (Suppl) 231: 13–137

Swan C, Tostevin A L, Moore B, Mayo H, Black G H B 1943 Congenital defects in infants following infectious diseases during pregnancy with special reference to the relationship between German measles and cataract, deaf-mutism, heart disease and microcephaly and to the period of pregnancy in which the occurrence of rubella is followed by congenital abnormalities. Medical Journal of Australia 2: 201–210

Thaler M M 1971 Bilirubin toxicity in hepatoma cells. Nature: New Biology 230: 218–219

Thiringer K, Kankkunen A, Liden G, Niklasson A 1984 Perinatal risk factors in the aetiology of hearing loss in preschool children. Developmental Medicine and Child Neurology 26: 799–807

Thompson G, Folsom G 1981 Hearing assessment of at risk infants: current status of audiometry in young infants. Clinical Pediatrics 20: 257–261

Thomson A J, Searle M, Russell G 1977 Quality of survival after severe birth asphyxia. Archives of Disease in Childhood 52: 620–626

Tyberghein J 1962 Influence of some streptomyces antibiotics on the cochlear microphonics in the guinea pig. Acta Oto-laryngologica (Suppl) 171: 1–56

Turkel S B 1983 Clinical and pathologic correlations with kernicterus and pulmonary hyaline membranes: hyperbilirubinemia in the newborn (Report of the Eighty-Fifth Ross Conference on Pediatric Research). Ross Laboratories, Ohio, pp 11–16

Valaes T, Kipouros K, Petmezaki S et al 1980 Effectiveness and safety of prenatal phenobarbital for prevention of neonatal jaundice. Pediatric Research 14: 947–952

Walker D, Grimwade J, Wood C 1971 Intrauterine noise: a component of the fetal environment. American Journal of Obstetrics and Gynecology 109: 91–95

Wedenberg E 1956 Auditory tests on newborn infants. Acta Oto-laryngologica 46: 446–461

Weil M L, Menkes J H 1975 Bilirubin interaction with ganglioside: possible mechanism in kernicterus. Pediatric Research 9: 791–793

Williamson W D, Desmond M M, LaFevers N, Taber L H, Catlin F I, Weaver T G 1982 Symptomatic congenital cytomegalovirus: disorders of language, learning and hearing. American Journal of Diseases of Children 136: 902–905

Winkel S, Bonding P, Kildegård Larsen P, Roosen J 1978 Possible effects of kanamycin and incubation in newborn children with low birth weight. Acta Paediatrica Scandinavica 67: 709–715

Wishingrad L, Cornblath M, Takaluwa T et al 1965 Studies of non-hemolytic hyperbilirubinemia in premature infants. I. Prospective randomized selection for exchange transfusion in premature infants. Pediatrics 36: 162

Zetterström R, Ernster L 1956 Bilirubin, an uncoupler of oxidative phosphorylation in isolated mitochondria. Nature 178: 1335–1337

Neuromuscular disorders

44. Neuromuscular disorders

Dr J. Heckmatt and Prof V. Dubowitz

Although the neuromuscular disorders in infancy and childhood have had extensive coverage in recent publications (Dubowitz 1978, 1980, 1985), this chapter concentrates on those specific to the neonatal period, and provides a problem-orientated approach as well as dealing with each disorder individually.

CLINICAL PROBLEMS

Clinical presentation

Table 44.1 details the main features of the various neuromuscular disorders that present in infancy with hypotonia plus other problems, and contrasts them with the non-neuromuscular disorders that may present in a similar fashion. In the Table, an attempt is made to indicate the relative importance of various signs and laboratory abnormalities.

A neuromuscular disorder should be suspected when the infant has a problem, such as hypotonia, feeding difficulty or persistent ventilatory failure but insufficient central nervous system (CNS) or lung involvement to apparently account for it. Important clues are: (1) delayed quickening and poor fetal movements throughout the pregnancy or normal movements initially but reduction later, (2) polyhydramnios suggesting involvement of the muscles of swallowing, (3) a family history of neonatal death and stillbirth, (4) a history of possible or definite neuromuscular disease in the mother and other members of the family, and (5) thin ribs on the chest X-ray, suggesting poor respiratory muscle movement in utero.

On examination of the baby there may be important associated abnormalities, such as overt facial weakness, ophthalmoplegia, limited limb movement and lack of antigravity power on stimulation of the limbs. These physical signs may be difficult to assess on one single occasion if the baby is severely ill (e.g. on a ventilator) and repeated examination is often useful. It is not always easy to differentiate a CNS from a neuromuscular disorder, especially as the baby may have overt CNS involvement (e.g. seizures, hydrocephalus, intraventricular haemorrhage/periventricular leukomalacia) in association with a neuromuscular disorder, and this may not always relate to severe birth asphyxia. Furthermore, a baby with neuromuscular disease may have reasonable power in the limbs and still have severe respiratory muscle weakness.

The timing of the clinical onset

Some disorders may already have an antenatal onset, others present in the immediate newborn period and others are delayed for hours or days after birth. For example, myotonic dystrophy is associated with an antenatal onset (Table 44.1), while neonatal myasthenia usually presents a few hours after birth and the mitochondrial myopathies present a few days or weeks after birth. Spinal muscular atrophy is also characterized by a period of normality before the onset of weakness. This onset may be gradual or sudden, and in utero or any time after birth.

The family

Most neuromuscular disorders are genetic and establishing a pattern of inheritance is important in the differential diagnosis. There may be subclinical manifestations in dominant and X-linked disorders. For example, myotonic dystrophy is inherited as an autosomal dominant trait. In many cases the mother, who is always affected, and other affected family members may be unaware they have the disease. It is therefore important to inquire about any family history that would indicate myotonic dystrophy, in particular presenile cataract, muscle stiffness, progressive weakness, frontal baldness and early death from cardio–respiratory disease. In addition family members should be examined personally for abnormal physical signs, such as facial weakness (which may consist only of inability to bury the eyelashes), wasting of the facial muscles (especially the temporalis and the sternomastoids), percussion myotonia of the tongue and hands, and relaxation myotonia of the hands.

The other neuromuscular disorder that should be

Table 44.1 Differential diagnosis of neuromuscular disease in the neonatal period presenting as hypotonia and other problems

	Diminished fetal movements	Polyhydramnios	Birth asphyxia	Persistant ventilatory failure	Distribution of respiratory muscle weakness	Facial weakness	Ptosis	Ophthalmoplegia	Proximal muscle paralysis	Fixed bilateral talipes	Arthrogryposis	Feeding difficulties	Tendon jerks	Distended bladder	Seizures	Hepatomegaly	Persistent metabolic acidosis	Hyperammonaemia	Abnormal smell	Genetics
Muscular dystrophy																				
Myotonic	++	++	++	+	G/D	++	++	(+)	+	+	(−)	++	(−)	−	(−)	−	−	−	−	AD(m)
Congenital	+	(+)	(+)	(+)	G/D	+	(+)	−	+	++	++	+	(−)	−	(+)	−	−	−	−	(AR)
Myasthenia gravis																				
Neonatal	−	−	(+)	*	G/D	+	(+)	(+)	+	−	−	+	(−)	−	−	−	−	−	−	−(m)
Congenital	(+)	(−)	−	(*)	(−)	+	+	+	(+)	−	−	(+)	(−)	−	−	−	−	−	−	(AR)
Familial	(+)	(+)	(+)	*	G/D	(+)	(+)	−	+	−	−	+	(−)	−	−	−	−	−	−	(AR)
Congenital myopathy																				
Nemaline	+	+	+	(+)	G/D	+	(+)	(−)	+	(+)	(−)	+	(−)	−	−	−	−	−	−	(AR)
Centronuclear	++	++	++	++	G/D	++	++	+	++	+	(−)	++	(−)	−	(−)	−	−	−	−	(XLR)
Mitochondrial	(−)	−	−	*	G	+	+	(+)	+	−	(+)	+	(+)	−	(+)	+	++	−		AR/XLR
Neurogenic weakness																				
Spinal muscular atrophy	+	(−)	(−)	(−)	I/G	(−)	−	−	++	(−)	−	(+)	−	−	−	−	−	−	−	AR
Spinal cord transection	−	−	++	(+l)	I/G(l)	−	−	−	+(l)	−	−	+	−	++	(−)	−	−	−	−	−
Non-neuromuscular																				
Prader–Willi syndrome	(+)	(+)	−	−	−	(+)	−	−	−	−	−	++	+	−	−	−	−	−	−	−(15)
Organic acidurias	−	−	−	*	(G)	(+)	(+)	−	(+)	−	−	++	(−)	−	+	+	++	+	+	AR
Urea cycle defects	−	−	−	*	(G)	−	−	−	(+)	−	−	+	(−)	−	+	−	(−)	++	−	AR
Peroxisomal disorders	−	−	(−)	(−)	−	−	−	−	(+)	−	−	+	(−)	−	++	(+)	−	−	−	AR
Neonatal sepsis	−	−	(+)	*	−	−	−	−	−	−	−	+	+	−	(+)	(−)	(+)	(+)	−	−
IVH/PVH/PVL	−	−	(+)	*	−	−	−	−	−	−	−	+	+	−	(+)	−	−	−	−	−

KEY:
Ventilatory failure: *=may present with sudden collapse.
Distribution of respiratory muscle weakness: G=global, D=diaphragmatic, I=intercostal.
Genetics: AR=autosomal recessive, XLR=X-linked recessive, AD=autosomal dominant, (15) = deletion or translocation chromosome 15, (m)=mother affected.
Clinical and laboratory features: ++ = frequently present and striking, + = often present, (+) = sometimes present, (−) = usually absent, − = always absent.
IVH=intraventricular haemorrhage, PVH=periventricular haemorrhage, PVL=periventricular leukomalacia (l)=depends on the level of the spinal cord lesion.

excluded in the mother is myasthenia gravis, which may lead to transient neonatal myasthenia due to passive transfer of antibody across the placenta. Severe centronuclear myopathy, which is characterized by a similar clinical presentation to myotonic dystrophy in the newborn, is X-linked recessive and there may be a family history of stillbirth and neonatal death stretching back several generations.

Clinical examination

Overt facial weakness is characteristic of myotonic dystrophy and centronuclear myopathy but also often occurs in other congenital myopathies such as nemaline myopathy and congenital muscular dystrophy. External ophthalmoplegia is a feature of centronuclear myopathy. In the severe type of spinal muscular atrophy, the facies are usually normal and the infant is likely to be quite bright and able to follow with the eyes despite being very weak generally. Tongue fasciculation at rest is a characteristic feature of spinal muscular atrophy. While spinal muscular atrophy is highly likely to be associated with severe paralysis, other neuromuscular disorders such as myotonic dystrophy and congenital muscular dystrophy are more variable.

The distribution of the respiratory muscle weakness is important. It may be diaphragmatic with abdominal paradox in the myasthenias, the dystrophies and the congenital myopathies; while in spinal muscular atrophy the weakness is mainly intercostal, the breathing pattern is abdominal and the rib cage moves paradoxically with the abdomen.

Fixed bilateral talipes is associated with congenital myotonic dystrophy and myotubular myopathy. Arthrogryposis (i.e. contractures of several joints) is associated with congenital dystrophy and certain neurogenic disorders. Fixed joint contractures are not a feature of severe spinal muscular atrophy.

INVESTIGATIONS

The serum creatine kinase (CK) activity is increased in cord blood up to 1000 units as measured by the 'European' recommended method (Moss et al 1981; normal levels for adults <200 ui/l). This increased activity reflects muscle damage during labour and usually comes down in the first 10 days of life. Measurement of serum CK activity is likely to be of most value in preclinical Duchenne's muscular dystrophy, where it will be markedly elevated (several thousand units); in congenital muscular dystrophy the elevation is moderate and variable and only occurs in about half the patients. Motor nerve conduction study will reveal an absent motor action potential in spinal muscular atrophy due to the extensive denervation. If myasthenia gravis is suspected, then repetitive stimulation of the peripheral nerve may show decrement in the motor action potential. Slow nerve conduction velocity may point to a hereditary motor neuropathy which may rarely present in early infancy.

An electromyograph (EMG) can be useful in identifying abnormality in the muscle and distinguishes between myopathic and neurogenic disorders. Fibrillation potentials at rest suggest extensive denervation and may be seen in spinal muscular atrophy. On contraction of the muscle, small polyphasic motor units without obvious 'drop-out' suggests a myopathy while the presence of large units with 'gaps' in between them ('reduced interference pattern') suggests a neuropathy. The EMG is useful in diagnosis and differential diagnosis of neuromuscular disorders in infancy. However, in the neonatal period interpretation can be difficult as the severely weak baby often makes little spontaneous movement. If there is any suggestion that the infant may have myotonic dystrophy, then one should do an EMG on both parents (and particularly the mother) looking for myotonic discharges. The favoured site for this is the first dorsal interosseus muscle of the hand.

Ultrasound imaging of muscle is a new technique we have introduced as a diagnostic screen; it detects diseased muscle on the basis of increased echogenicity. Although it is useful in floppy infants from about the age of 3 months onwards, its application in the newborn period is limited at present by poor resolution. Recently we have demonstrated with ultrasound imaging striking selective involvement within the quadriceps muscle usually with sparing of the rectus femoris and marked involvement of the vasti. This is of considerable practical importance when taking a biopsy. In two infants we have been able to confirm the selective muscle involvement histologically, by performing a concurrent biopsy of affected and unaffected muscle in the thigh with the Bergstrom needle (see later and Heckmatt & Dubowitz 1987).

Muscle biopsy is done using a 4 mm Bergstrom needle. This technique has had a high success rate since 1982 with only one failure in 30 infants when performed in the first 2 months of life. In the case of the one failure, a repeat needle biopsy obtained a good sample. The success rate is as high as in older children, despite the small size of the patient. This is because there has been no chance for muscle atrophy, nor extensive replacement of muscle by fat and connective tissue to occur, and also because the size of the individual muscle fibres is small and only a relatively small sample is needed. Needle muscle biopsy is done under local anaesthetic in the cot or incubator, and the critically sick newborn can readily have the investigation with minimal disturbance. A detailed description of the technique is given in Heckmatt et al (1984).

It is important to be aware of the value and limitations of muscle biopsy in the newborn period. Muscle biopsy will show unequivocal abnormality in the congenital myopathies which have specific structural changes but may appear normal in spinal muscular atrophy (prepathological stage) or show universal atrophy (i.e. very small fibres at about 10 μm) without the characteristic large fibres (Dubowitz 1978). Muscle biopsy is usually normal in infants with myotonic dystrophy but may show identical appearances to centronuclear myopathy (Farkas et al 1974).

Table 44.2 gives a diagnostic breakdown of the muscle biopsies done on babies presenting in the neonatal period in the years 1982 to 1986, in relation to the presenting problems. During the same period, 10 neonates were seen with myotonic dystrophy of whom 5 had prolonged ventilatory failure, but only one had a muscle biopsy because in all of them the diagnosis was made on examination of the mother. Centronuclear myopathy was also associated with ventilatory failure. Three babies presented with prolonged and severe ventilatory failure and had generalized weakness. However, they had a normal muscle biopsy and there was no evidence for myotonic dystrophy in either parent, although this remains a possible diagnosis. All three died and one came to a detailed postmortem. Histochemical examination of other muscles, including those of respiration, and examination of the CNS failed to identify a specific lesion; comprehensive biochemical studies were also normal.

Cranial ultrasound which is a routine procedure in neonatal intensive care units, identifies intracranial abnormalities, such as haemorrhage and ischaemic lesions, and also ventricular dilatation, which is a common associated feature in myotonic dystrophy and centronuclear myopathy.

MANAGEMENT

The major problem of management presented by these disorders is that of ventilatory failure and deciding a

Table 44.2 Muscle biopsies in the first month of life

Diagnosis	No.	Presenting problem
Congenital muscular dystrophy	9	Ventilatory failure (2), arthrogryposis (3), floppy infant (4)
Myotubular myopathy	4	Ventilatory failure (4)
Spinal muscular atrophy	4	Floppy infant (3), ventilatory failure (1)
Mitochondrial myopathy myopathy	1	Progressive weakness and ventilatory failure
Nemaline myopathy	1	Floppy infant
Continuous muscle fibre activity	1	Progressive muscle stiffness and ventilatory impairment
Normal muscle	10	Arthrogryposis (2), ventilatory failure (myotonic dystrophy) (1), Floppy infant — Prader–Willi syndrome (2) and primary CNS problem (2), ventilatory failure (no specific diagnosis made) (3)

prognosis and how long to continue giving ventilatory support. It will be necessary to take into account any CNS complication, such as progressive ventricular dilatation. In myotonic dystrophy, there is a trend for improvement in muscle power and a reasonable chance of the infant becoming independent of the ventilator (see later). If an infant with spinal muscular atrophy is put on a ventilator, it may be extremely difficult to wean him off, but most infants with this disorder have sufficient diaphragm function to cope without ventilatory support. The other disorders are more variable but in myotubular myopathy and congenital muscular dystrophy there is a trend for improvement although it is slow, and a tracheostomy may be necessary for long-term respiratory management.

There now follows a systematic description of the various neuromuscular disorders that affect the neonate.

THE MUSCULAR DYSTROPHIES

Congenital myotonic dystrophy

The first description of congenital myotonic dystrophy was by Vanier (1960) of 6 children between the ages of 9 months and 13 years, all of whom had presented as floppy infants; 4 had had feeding difficulty, and 3 had bilateral talipes. Vanier pointed out the severe facial muscle weakness and wasting (particularly of the sternomastoids leading to a long 'swan-like' neck), nasal speech and mental retardation. The mothers in all the cases were affected but only had minimal signs of the disease. In two families the maternal uncles were severely affected and in one family both the mother and maternal grandmother had presenile cataracts.

Another important early report was that by Dodge et al (1965) of five definite cases. The bilateral facial weakness had led to severe feeding difficulties in infancy and this was accompanied by marked generalized weakness and hypotonia. One girl had an affected 4-year-old brother who had been admitted at the age of 2 months for eventration of the diaphragm associated with partial collapse of the right lung; he had been cyanosed as an infant but had sucked better than his sister and had good limb strength and reflex activity.

Harper (1975a,b) reported an extensive survey of all available cases in Britian. He emphasized the polyhydramnios and reduced fetal movements and suggested a high incidence of missed cases as there was an elevated neonatal mortality (16%) in liveborn siblings. Of the 70 cases in his study, the mean IQ was only 66.1. However, there was no correlation with respiratory problems, suggesting a prenatal cause for the mental deficiency. In all cases the mother was affected, and Harper postulated that an intra-uterine factor must be operating, in addition to the gene that has to be present to have the disease.

Outside the neonatal period, most cases with the congenital type survive but few become independent, Of 46 congenital cases followed-up retrospectively, only 4 had died but of the 42 survivors, only 2 were in normal education, and only one was gainfully employed. Testicular atrophy was evident in all affected males at puberty (O'Brien & Harper 1984).

Table 44.3 summarizes our experience of 10 patients who presented in the neonatal period. In general these were more severely affected than previous reported cases which reflects referral to our neonatal intensive care unit. The extent of the weakness was variable but most had some antigravity power in the limbs. There was no direct relationship with limb power and degree of respiratory muscle involvement and the baby with the best limb power was the longest on the ventilator (112 days) because of elevation of the diaphragm which required plication. The 8 infants who had cranial ultrasound showed ventricular dilatation. In 3 of these this was present on the first day of life without evidence for intraventricular haemorrhage, suggesting an antenatal cause (Regev et al 1987). Three of the infants had gastrointestinal stasis with bile-stained aspirate requiring a period of intravenous feeding (duration 2 to 7 weeks). A typical case is illustrated in Fig. 44.1.

Percussion myotonia of the tongue, facial weakness and myotonic discharge on the EMG were demonstrated in all 10 mothers. Clinical myotonia of the hands was more variable. Three mothers had been previously diagnosed, two on the basis of an affected baby, one born to the same mother and

Table 44.3 Congenital myotonic dystrophy: presenting features

Patient	Gestation (weeks)	Birth weight (kg)	Fetal movements	Hydramnios	Apgar score (1/5/10 mins)	IPPV* (days)	Talipes
D.C.	32	1.8	?	–		–	–
B.P.	34	1.7	reduced	+	4/5	31	+
C.McC.	34	1.8	?	+		16	+
K.E.	34	2.2	?	+	1/5/10	1	+
C.T.	35	1.3	reduced	–	2/4	112	–
S.Bl.	35	2.3	reduced	+	4/5/5	12	–
E.H.	36	1.9	reduced	+	6/7/8	>49	+
S.Bo.	38	2.7	reduced	–	0/3/4	1	–
R.G.	40	2.7	?	–	1/7/5	–	–
J.W-B.	40	4.0	reduced	+	1/7/4	–	+

*IPPV=intermittent positive pressure ventilation.

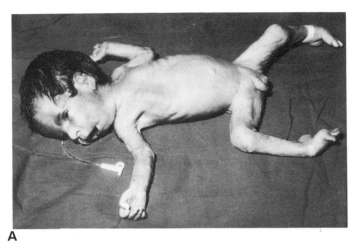

A

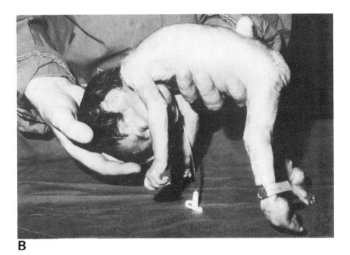

B

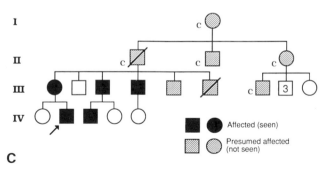

C

Fig. 44.1 (**a** and **b**) Infant with congenital myotonic dystrophy admitted at the age of 20 days, having been ventilator-dependent from birth till 15 days without overt lung problem. He was born at 34 weeks of gestation (birth-weight 1.8 kg), by elective caesarian section for breech presentation. On examination, he was generally hypotonic with fixed bilateral talipes equino-varus. He had a large head with wide open fontanelles and parted sutures and ultrasound scan showed bilateral ventricular dilatation. The mother had definite signs of the disease although she had not been previously diagnosed. (**c**) On investigation of the family, two maternal uncles (III 3 and 4) and one cousin (IV 3) were affected with facial weakness, myotonia and a positive EMG. Two uncles (III 5 and 6) were not available but one was said to have frontal baldness and the other to have some stiffness of the hands. One of these uncles subsequently died following dental anaesthesia, possibly due to undue sensitivity to muscle relaxants and an unsuspecting anaesthetist. There was a history of presenile cataract in several relatives on the maternal grandfather's side of the family.

one to an aunt. In only one case had the mother previously presented with symptoms of myotonia, and this had led to the diagnosis in other members of her family. In all cases there was a strongly suggestive family history, apart from evidence of disease in the mother. In these 10 families, we were personally able to confirm the diagnosis beyond doubt in 7 previously undiagnosed adults, apart from the mothers, and were suspicious about a further 5, either on the basis of presenile cataract (3 cases), or frontal baldness with probable facial muscle wasting (2 cases) but without other physical signs, or abnormality on the EMG.

Congenital muscular dystrophy

This is an important group of neuromuscular disorders characterized by weakness, usually from birth, and a muscle biopsy showing striking pathological changes similar to muscular dystrophy (Vassella et al 1967, Donner et al 1975, Dubowitz 1980). Table 44.2 shows that, in our experience, only myotonic dystrophy was diagnosed more frequently in the newborn period. Facial weakness is frequently present but not as severe or striking as that in congenital myotonic dystrophy. Many will have contractures at birth, sometimes extensive arthrogryposis (see later), and will show a tendency to develop contractures during infancy. It is particularly important to recognize these patients and start a programme of active treatment of the contractures in infancy to try and improve the range of joint mobility. Despite severe change on the muscle biopsy there is rarely progression of the muscle weakness and the child usually shows an improvement with time (see Fig. 44.2).

A few patients have respiratory involvement at birth. A feature of this condition is that the disease process may pick out certain muscles, including those of respiration, leaving others relatively spared (see Fig. 44.3). Other patients may present as a floppy infant. A further group presents later in the first or second years of life with motor delay, having not apparently had any recognized problem in infancy.

Congenital muscular dystrophy may be associated with CNS involvement, in particular mental retardation and seizures, reviewed recently by Echenne et al (1986).

THE CONGENITAL MYOPATHIES

These disorders are associated with a structural abnormality within the muscle fibre. They can all present in the neonatal period as a floppy infant. Only centronuclear and nemaline myopathy are described here, however, because of their propensity to severe respiratory problems.

Congenital centronuclear (myotubular) myopathy

There are three clinical and genetic subtypes: (1) a severe X-linked type, presenting in the neonatal period with birth

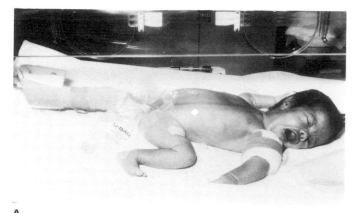

A

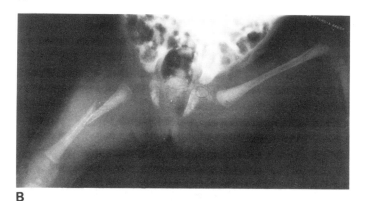

B

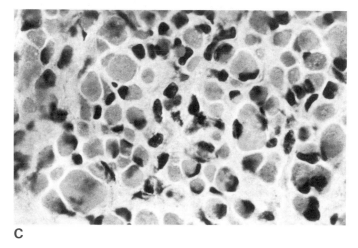

C

Fig. 44.2 (a) A 5-day-old girl with congenital muscular dystrophy. She was born at elective caesarean section at 39 weeks of gestation but sustained a fracture of the femur during delivery (birth-weight 2.3 kg), and subsequently a fracture of the left humerus during normal nursing care. On examination she had probable mild facial weakness and no antigravity power in the limbs. A brother had also been affected, had been born with fractures of all four limbs and had died on the first day of life of intracranial haemorrhage. He had been suspected of having osteogenesis imperfecta. (b) The girl's X-ray shows slender bones but only minimal osteoporosis. Her serum CK was normal (28 iu/l). (c) Needle muscle biopsy at 5 days of age showed unequivocal pathological change with variability in fibre size, proliferation of endomyseum and some cellular infiltration. The poor bone development was presumably secondary to the weak muscles. Following an intensive programme of regular passive stretching of all joints and early mobilization in a standing frame, she was walking independently by the age of 4 years in light-weight knee–ankle–foot orthoses and there were no further fractures.

asphyxia and persistent ventilatory failure and associated skeletal muscle weakness; (2) a less severe infantile type, which is probably autosomal recessive; and (3) a mild juvenile or adult type, which is autosomal dominant in some cases. We have recently reviewed the clinical, pathological and genetic features in 8 unrelated patients with this disorder (Heckmatt et al 1985).

The principle pathological feature (irrespective of the genetics) is the presence of large central nuclei in fibres of both types. Only a proportion of the fibres show the central nuclei in transverse section because they are spaced out along the fibres with gaps in between them. The central area of the fibres is devoid of myofibrils but occupied by mitochondria and glycogen. Histochemical stains show a large proportion of fibres with central aggregation of stain with the NADH-TR and PAS reactions and 'holes' in the centre of the fibres on the ATPase reaction due to the absence of myofibres. These striking histochemical changes are particularly prominent in infants with the X-linked type. There is a pathological variant which has been described under the title 'type 1 fibre hypotrophy with central nuclei' in which the affected fibres are principally type 1 and markedly reduced in size. There does not seem to be any fundamental clinical distinction in this pathological subtype, which has been described in both the severe X-linked type and milder cases.

Severe X-linked type

This was first described by Van Wijngaarden et al (1969) in a large Dutch family and later by Barth et al (1975) in another large Dutch family. In the family described by Van Wijngaarden et al, the index case was a 2-year-old boy who had been cyanosed at birth and had presented as a floppy infant. He was of normal intelligence but was unable to sit or stand and had bilateral ptosis and limitation of vertical eye movements. There were 4 live males in two generations, aged from 18 months to 33 years, all of whom had been severely asphyxiated at birth, and 3 other males all probably affected who had died, 2 in the neonatal period of asphyxia and respiratory complications and one at 5-years-old of pneumonia. In the report by Barth et al, all 13 affected males died shortly after birth and the authors stressed the decreased fetal movements, hydramnios, and birth asphyxia. Other similar X-linked cases have been described (Meyers et al 1974, Askanas et al 1979, Heckmatt et al 1985).

From the point of view of genetic counselling, it is sometimes possible to detect abnormality in the muscle biopsy of some carriers. Two out of 3 obligate carriers investigated by Van Wijngaarden et al, and 4 out of 5 investigated by Barth et al, had 'myotubes' scattered amongst normal muscle fibres.

In our series, there were 2 definite (Fig. 44.4), and 3 probable X-linked recessive cases, all with virtually identical

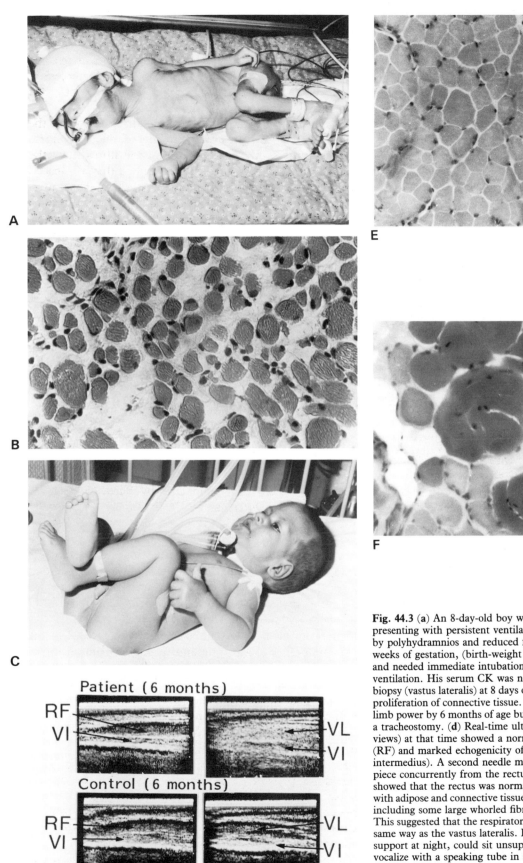

Fig. 44.3 (**a**) An 8-day-old boy with congenital muscular dystrophy presenting with persistent ventilatory failure. Pregnancy was complicated by polyhydramnios and reduced fetal movements. He was born at 34 weeks of gestation, (birth-weight 1.6 kg). He was severely asphyxiated and needed immediate intubation and intermittent positive-pressure ventilation. His serum CK was normal (66 iu/l). (**b**) Needle muscle biopsy (vastus lateralis) at 8 days of age showed variability in fibre size and proliferation of connective tissue. (**c**) There was a marked improvement in limb power by 6 months of age but he still needed ventilation and had had a tracheostomy. (**d**) Real-time ultrasound scans of the thigh (longitudinal views) at that time showed a normal appearance of the rectus femoris (RF) and marked echogenicity of the vastus lateralis (VL) (VI = vastus intermedius). A second needle muscle biopsy was performed, taking a piece concurrently from the rectus femoris and the vastus lateralis. This showed that the rectus was normal (**e**) while the vastus was abnormal (**f**), with adipose and connective tissue proliferation and variability in fibre size, including some large whorled fibres with multiple internal nuclei (H&E). This suggested that the respiratory muscles were selectively affected in the same way as the vastus lateralis. By 13 months he only needed ventilatory support at night, could sit unsupported and stand with support, and vocalize with a speaking tube in situ. At 15 months of age he had a sudden respiratory and cardiac arrest while having tracheostomy care, suffering irreversable brain damage, and died the following day.

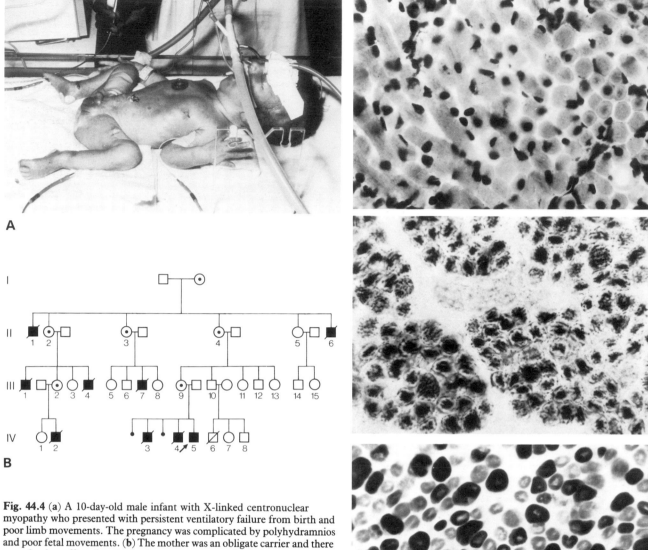

Fig. 44.4 (a) A 10-day-old male infant with X-linked centronuclear myopathy who presented with persistent ventilatory failure from birth and poor limb movements. The pregnancy was complicated by polyhydramnios and poor fetal movements. (b) The mother was an obligate carrier and there were 8 other affected males in three generations, all of whom were either stillborn or had died in the neonatal period. She had mild facial weakness with difficulty burying eyelashes but she had no evidence of myotonia (Heckmatt et al 1985). (c) Needle muscle biopsy (quadriceps) from the patient at 10 days of age showed prominent central nuclei in about 40% of fibres (H&E). (d) The NADH-Tr reaction showed central aggregation of stain in virtually all fibres. (e) The ATPase 9.5 showed a clear zone in the centre of many fibres.

presentation. All 5 had the following features: severe birth asphyxia, swallowing difficulties, ophthalmoplegia and facial diplegia, and 4 had persistent ventilatory failure from the first day of life. Abnormality of muscle morphology at light microscope level was seen in only one of the mothers and consisted of many focal areas with variability in fibre size, internal nuclei and adipose tissue. In this case, the maternal aunt also had variation in fibre size and 24% of nuclei were internal. We presumed on the basis of these biopsies that the inheritance was X-linked recessive and both the mother and the aunt were carriers. In the other cases, muscle biopsy of the mothers showed abnormalities on detailed quantitation similar in type to that found in Duchenne's muscular dystrophy carriers, but there were no striking abnormalities of morphology or central nuclei (see Heckmatt et al 1985).

Intracranial ventricular dilatation was a feature in these infants, as it is in congenital myotonic dystrophy, and in one there was progressive ventricular dilation.

Nemaline myopathy

This congenital myopathy is of variable severity and inheritance and may present in the neonatal period. The rods are easily overlooked on the haematoxylin and eosin section and readily demonstrated with the Gomori trichrome, being a striking red colour in contrast to the blue– green of the muscle fibres. There may be two populations of fibres, one hypertrophic and the other atrophic, and the rods are mainly in the atrophic fibres.

The first severe infantile case was reported by Shafiq et al (1967) in a 15-week-old male infant, who presented with generalized hypotonia and difficulty in feeding. The infant's main problem was the accumulation of secretions, which tended to obstruct and compromise his airway. His face was expressionless but moved symmetrically on crying. He had had multiple episodes of pneumonitis and atelectasis, and at 4 months a feeding gastrostomy was performed. Subsequently his muscle power improved but he died at the age of 10 months from a fulminating pneumonia. Postmortem showed involvement of the tongue, diaphragm and pharynx, in addition to variable involvement of the skeletal muscles.

Kuitunen et al (1972) described two unrelated children who had been weak from birth with sucking difficulty — both improved and had eventually became ambulant. Neustein (1973) reported three affected siblings who had been floppy from birth. The first had died at 3 months of age, the second at 2 days, and the third at 11 months, probably from respiratory causes in each case. All had reduced fetal movements in utero. The third sibling had a detailed autopsy and involvement of skeletal muscle was widespread. In this family the inheritance seemed to be autosomal recessive.

More recently there have been reports of nemaline myopathy presenting as ventilatory failure in the newborn. Norton et al (1983) reported two infants, one a girl born at 35 weeks of gestation who had persistent ventilatory failure with no improvement, and ventilatory support was discontinued after 3 months. Tsujihata et al (1983) reported a female infant, born at 37 weeks of gestation, who was hypotonic from birth, failed to establish effective respiration and required ventilatory support, and subsequently died at the age of 3 months. Autopsy again revealed widespread involvement of skeletal muscles, particularly the diaphragm.

MYASTHENIA GRAVIS

Autoimmune

Neonatal myasthenia gravis is a transient disorder occurring in about 12% of the offspring of myasthenic mothers. Namba et al (1970) did a detailed review of 82 cases from the literature and included two of their own. The infants presented usually within a few hours of birth, or at the very latest the first 72 hours, with feeding difficulty, generalized weakness, poor respiratory effort and inability to handle pharyngeal secretions. At least half had facial weakness characterized by 'mask-like' facies and infrequent

blinking and staring; 15% had ptosis, and 8% decreased ocular movements. Virtually all cases reviewed responded to anticholinesterases. Some of the patients had repetitive stimulation, at 5 to 20 Hz, which showed a decrement in the amplitude of the motor action potential. Nine died, and in six who came to autopsy the cause was respiratory failure, with atelectasis and pneumonia. The mean duration of illness was 18 days, with a maximum of 7 weeks.

Neonatal myasthenia cannot be related to duration or severity of maternal disease, to any alteration in the maternal symptoms during pregnancy, or to thymectomy. It is associated with acetylcholine receptor (AChR) antibody, which is passively transferred across the placenta in both affected and unaffected babies but is more persistent in the serum of affected babies. Exchange transfusion is said to be of no value in the management of the baby (Lefvert & Osterman 1983), which is contrary to what might be expected, considering the undoubted response to plasma exchange in most adults.

An equivocal response to anticholinesterase medication does not exclude the diagnosis, as demonstrated by Rowland (1955) in an otherwise typical case. We have also recently seen a baby with neonatal myasthenia whose response to medication was equivocal (see Fig. 44.5). In this case maternal AChR antibody could not be demonstrated and we suggested that the putative antibody was to diaphragmatic antigen determinants not shared by calf muscle AChR (Heckmatt et al 1987).

Non-autoimmune

There are two clinical types of non-autoimmune myasthenia, so-called 'familial' and 'congenital' (Vincent et al 1981). The classification is confusing as congenital myasthenia is also familial. The familial infantile type is characterized by episodes of severe respiratory and feeding difficulties at birth or during infancy. Extra-ocular movements are normal and patients show a good response to anticholinesterase treatment and a high remission rate. Although the disease occurs frequently in siblings it is not present in the mother and inheritance is probably autosomal recessive. Congenital myasthenia usually develops before the age of 2 years and in many cases symptoms have been present at birth or in utero. Males tend to be affected more than females and affected siblings are frequently encountered, which also suggests autosomal recessive inheritance. Ocular muscles are the most commonly affected but severe weakness of bulbar, trunk and limb muscles can occur. The symptoms tend to be non-progressive and, in contrast to the familial type, anticholinesterase is not always beneficial and remission is unusual. Thymectomy has been performed in a few cases but has been of doubtful benefit. It is occasionally associated with congenital arthrogryposis (Smit & Barth 1980, Teyssier et al 1982).

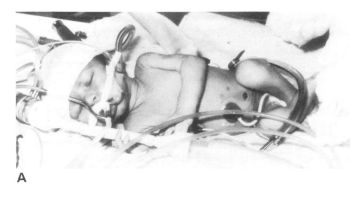

A

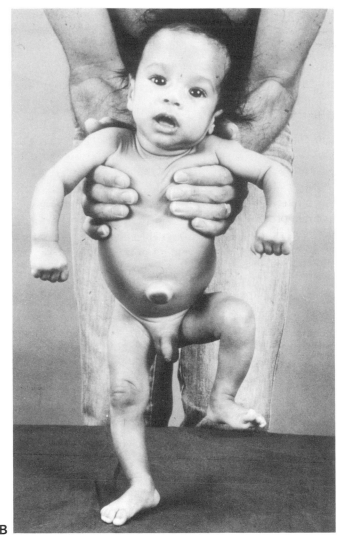

B

Fig. 44.5 (a) A 10-day-old boy with transient neonatal myasthenia. Atypical presentation at birth with diaphragmatic and pharyngeal paralysis in the presence of normal limb and facial movements. The mother had a similar pattern of muscle involvement and developed ventilatory failure postpartum, due to severe diaphragm weakness, responding eventually to plasma exchange and immunosuppressive medication. The baby presented at birth because the mother was not on anticholinesterase medication; this is transferred passively across the placenta and has some transient protective effect. Magnetometry of the rib cage and abdomen, and repetitive stimulation of the peripheral nerve, were both suggestive of muscle fatigue (Heckmatt et al 1987). By 6 weeks of age the baby had made a complete recovery. (b) The infant attempting to stand at the age of 6 months.

Conomy et al (1975) reported an 18-month-old boy with familial infantile myasthenia who had recurrent episodes of choking from the age of 2 weeks, who responded dramatically to edrophonium, and whose sister had had delayed motor milestones and 'bedroom eyes' and had died suddenly during a respiratory infection at the age of 15 months. Robertson et al (1980) reported a 14-year-old boy who had had repeated episodes of severe apnoea from the neonatal period which resolved at around the age of 2 years. Marked fatiguabilty had persisted and there was mild proximal weakness. He had responded to prostigmine which was first tried at the age of 4 years. An older brother had had similar episodes of apnoea which also ceased at the age of 2 years. On repetitive stimulation, there was a marked decrement in the size of the motor action potential in the biceps. Albers et al (1984) reported a clinically atypical infant who had to be ventilated from one week of age and who failed to respond to anticholinesterase but showed a striking decrement in the motor action potential on repetitive stimulation at 2 Hz. The baby died at the age

of 8 months of pneumonia. The authors suggested a failure of resynthesis, mobilization or storage of acetylcholine.

Vincent et al (1981) reported 5 male patients, including 2 brothers, aged 13 to 25 years with congenital myasthenia gravis. Three had an onset at birth with feeding difficulty, ptosis and facial involvement and 2 had an onset before 2 years. Four had oculomotor paralysis but none had major respiratory involvement. The response to anticholinesterases was variable but 3 showed a definite improvement. The authors performed end-plate electrophysiology on intercostal muscle biopsies and found a variety of pre- and postsynaptic defects suggesting that congenital myasthenia is a heterogeneous condition.

Infantile botulism enters into the differential diagnosis of myasthenia, and results from colonization of the infant's bowel with the organism *Clostridium botulinum* and production of toxin. Affected infants are aged from 2 weeks to 6 months, with a median onset at 10 weeks. There is profound weakness of skeletal and bulbar muscles with the danger of respiratory arrest. Ptosis is common; extra-ocular movements are usually normal but the pupils are dilated and respond poorly to light. The majority of reported cases have been from the USA (Lancet 1986).

METABOLIC DISORDERS OF MUSCLE

Mitochondrial myopathies

The mitochondrial myopathies that present in the first few weeks of life can be divided into three clinical and genetic subtypes: a 'benign' type, of unknown genetic aetiology and two progressive, fatal or 'severe' types, one autosomal recessive and one X-linked recessive. In general, presentation is with progressive muscle weakness after a period of apparent normality and these infants may be mistakenly diagnosed as spinal muscular atrophy.

Benign type

This was first described by Jerusalem et al in 1973 who coined the term 'mitochondrial–lipid–glycogen storage' myopathy to describe the appearances of the muscle at biopsy with excess glycogen deposition, striking lipid vacuolation and large abnormal mitochondria with sparse cristae. The patient was a 7-week-old girl with profound weakness, macroglossia and hepatomegaly. There had been no birth asphyxia but during the neonatal period she had had feeding and respiratory difficulty and a weak cry. She subsequently improved and the macroglossia resolved. By 9 months of age she could swallow soft foods and by 20 months she was able to sit independently. A repeat muscle biopsy at 22 months showed striking resolution, with only 4% of the fibres containing vacuolation at light level, and reduction in the numbers of abnormal mitochondria.

Di Mauro et al (1983) subsequently described a second case in a 2-week-old boy with profound generalized weakness, hypotonia, hyporeflexia, macroglossia and severe lactic acidosis, but no hepatomegaly. He was sitting by 13 months and walking independently by 16 months. There was reduced activity of cytochrome c oxidase which was reversed by 36 months of age. Later studies showed that immunologically reactive enzyme protein was present (Zeviani et al 1985).

Fatal type

Autosomal recessive. This is probably the most common type. One of the first reports was by Van Biervliet et al (1977) of a boy admitted at 7 weeks of age with increasing weakness, who was normal at birth although his fetal movements had been diminished. He needed artificial ventilation soon after admission and died at 13 weeks of age. There was a profound lactic acidaemia, and also a DeToni–Fanconi–Debre renal tubular defect (amino aciduria, glycosuria, hyperphosphaturia and polyuria).

Subsequent reports have confirmed the above features. In addition, there is often facial weakness, ptosis, a feeding problem and 'failure to thrive'. Presentation may be any time during the first few weeks of life. Cardiomyopathy is not usually prominent. Muscle biopsy shows vacuolated fibres which contain lipid droplets. The trichrome stain shows either clumps of granular red-staining material dispersed throughout the sarcoplasm of many fibres or 'ragged-red' fibres with striking red-staining and disruption of the fibres. There is often a slight increase in PAS-positive glycogen. Electron microscopy shows giant mitochondria with disordered cristae. In all cases a functional defect of the respiratory chain has been demonstrated in the muscle mitochondria, consistently involving cytochrome c oxidase, and often cytochromes b and aa_3, and in one case immunologically reactive cytochrome c oxidase was shown to be markedly decreased (Zeviani et al 1985). Free and bound carnitine levels in the muscle have been variable.

The inheritance seems to be autosomal recessive, as either sex may be affected and there is often a history of a sibling dying in infancy following a similar clinical course (Di Mauro et al 1980, Heimann-Patterson et al 1982). Most mitochondrial proteins are coded by nuclear DNA but a few are coded by mitochondrial DNA, for example three (I to III) of the seven subunits that go to make up cytochrome c oxidase. Mitochondrial DNA is maternally inherited but to date there has been no evidence for mitochondrial disease affecting the mothers of these infants. Furthermore, in the case described by Minchom et al (1983), the mother had normal muscle cytochrome c oxidase activity. Presumably the defect or defects in these infants involves cytochrome subunits encoded by nuclear DNA. In the case described by Boustany et al (1983), a female second cousin, related through the maternal grandfather, had died at 9 months of age with a mitochondrial hepatopathy.

X-linked recessive. Barth et al (1983) described a large pedigree with an X-linked disease characterized by dilated cardiomyopathy, neutropenia and skeletal myopathy. The propositus was normal at birth but presented on the third day of life with grunting respirations and acidosis. A brother was similarly affected, and neutropenia was documented in his cord blood. A cousin had recurrent skin eruptions and moderate skeletal muscle weakness and seemed to respond to oral carnitine although there was no improvement in the neutropenia. He was alive at 42 months, while all the other affected males had died in infancy or early childhood from cardiorespiratory failure or sepsis. A respiratory chain defect was identified, also involving cytochromes c, b and aa_3. Carriers could not be identified by clinical or laboratory examination, although muscle biopsies were not done.

Pompe's disease (glycogenosis type 2)

This is a fatal autosomal recessive disorder characterized by deficiency of acid alpha-glucosidase and the lysosomal accumulation of glycogen. Presentation is usually between the ages of 3 to 6 months with either cardiorespiratory failure or severe progressive hypotonia but abnormality may extend back to the neonatal period, in particular the cardiomegaly (Burton 1987). There is likely to be skin pallor, hepatomegaly, macroglossia, and possibly some skeletal muscle hypertrophy. The EMG is a useful screening investigation showing pseudomyotonic discharges; peripheral blood leukocytes should show the presence of glycogen granules.

Muscle biopsy shows marked vacuolation of the muscle fibres and increased glycogen but no lipid accumulation. The enzyme can be assayed in skin fibroblasts, amniotic fluid cells, and trophoblasts (Besancon et al 1985). Rapid prenatal diagnosis can also be made by electron microscopy of uncultured amniotic fluid cells (Hug et al 1984). There is also a juvenile or adult form which presents either with skeletal muscle weakness or diaphragmatic paralysis.

Glycogenosis type 3

This disorder presents with hepatomegaly, hypoglycaemia and ketosis. Time of presentation is variable but may be at birth. The defective enzyme is the glycogen debrancher amylo-1,6-glucosidase. There is usually mild hypotonia and muscle biopsy is likely to show some glycogen accumulation. It seems to be unusual for muscle manifestations to be detected before the patient is ambulant (Slonim et al 1984).

Infantile phosphorylase deficiency

Di Mauro & Hartlage (1978) described an infant who had progressive feeding difficulties and respiratory impairment from the age of 4 weeks and died at the age of 13 weeks. Muscle biopsy showed subsarcolemmal vacuoles containing glycogen, and phosphorylase activity could not be detected while activity of the other glycogenolytic enzymes was normal.

OTHER NEUROMUSCULAR DISORDERS

Arthrogryposis

This disorder is defined as congenital non-progressive limitation of movement in two or more joints in different body areas (Hageman & Willemse 1983). It is not a diagnosis as such but a symptom complex and the potential and result of several different types of pathological process. There is general agreement that the final mechanism is immobility in utero. This might be produced by restriction of the fetus, or inability of the fetus to move due to some failure of the motor system.

Hall (1985) states that affected limbs are, on average, 20% shorter than expected for gestational age, while the trunk and head are of normal size, which suggests part of normal limb growth relates to forces engendered by use. Catch-up may occur during vigorous use of limbs and also a return to normal size of lungs, and cranio–facial structures. Hall states that return of range of motion could occur up to one year (in our experience this is a conservative estimate) and relative increases in strength of the muscle for many years.

Prolonged oligohydramnios or a bicornute uterus might be a cause in some cases (Fig. 44.6). It has been generally assumed that very few are due to primary muscle disease. After an extensive review of the literature, Swinyard (1982) estimated that the proportion was only 10– 15%. In a study of the spinal cord of 11 infants with arthrogryposis, Clauren & Hall (1983) found a reduction in the number of alpha motor neurones and an increase in the numbers

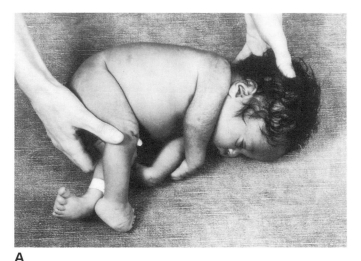

A

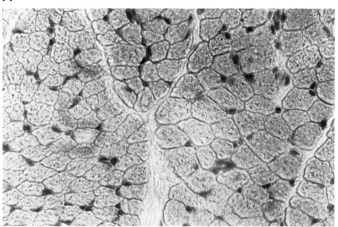

B

Fig. 44.6 (a) A 2-day-old boy, born at full-term with arthrogryposis. Continuous drainage of liquor occurred from the sixth month of pregnancy and fetal movements diminished from that time. He was delivered at full-term. Note the flexion deformities of the fingers and wrists and equinus deformities of the feet but no hip and knee contractures. Shoulder abduction was limited and elbows were held in extension. The muscles of the shoulders were atrophic but there seemed to be reasonable power of the hip and thigh muscles. The trunk seemed normal but there was excessive head lag. The facies was normal. (b) Needle muscle biopsy at 2 days of age (quadriceps) was normal. The arthrogryposis was thought to be due to intra-uterine restriction secondary to the oligohydramnios.

of small neurones in all but one, and CNS involvement in three. These results cannot be applied to all arthrogryposis patients, as those who die may be a selected population. The Pena–Shokeir syndrome of multiple ankyloses, facial abnormalities, pulmonary hypoplasia and cryptorchidism, has been associated with problems in brain formation and loss of anterior horn cells in the spinal cord but a primary muscle disorder could also have the same clinical end result (Moerman et al 1983).

There have been relatively few reports of EMG and muscle studies done systematically in arthrogryposis, particularly with modern histochemical techniques. One such study was by Strehl & Vanasse (1985) in 22 patients and they found 10 with a neurogenic cause (5 spinal origin, 2 cerebral origin and 3 mixed), and 9 myopathic (3 congenital muscular dystrophy, 3 congenital myotonic dystrophy, 1 fibre type disproportion and 2 non-specific myopathy). One had an inherited malformation syndrome and in 2 the cause was unknown. They stated that precise diagnosis would have been impossible without needle muscle biopsy. This is more in accord with our own experience, where the most common associated neuromuscular disorder is congenital muscular dystrophy (see Fig. 44.7).

Spinal muscular atrophy

This important group of disorders can be divided into three clinical subtypes: (1) severe, in which the infant is very weak, never acquires the ability to sit, has severe respiratory muscle weakness and dies usually before the age of one year of an intercurrent respiratory infection; (2) intermediate, in which the infant acquires the ability to sit and usually survives but with complications such as scoliosis; and (3) mild, in which the child is able to walk (for a detailed discussion of the clinical classification see Dubowitz (1978)). In general, those presenting in the neonatal period will have the severe type but the age of onset of symptoms is not an absolute guide to disease severity. The severe type is generally known as Werdnig–Hoffman disease but this term is sometimes applied by clinicians to all grades of severity of disease which is a source of confusion and erroneous prognosis.

Although spinal muscular atrophy is the most common cause of severe paralysis in infancy, because of the preservation of diaphragm function, ventilatory failure in the newborn period is extremely uncommon. The one neonate we have seen with this complication had not been asphyxiated at birth but had been placed on a ventilator at the age of 8 days before transfer to us. In addition to the extensive paralysis of the limbs and distinctive breathing pattern, other useful pointers to the diagnosis are the characteristic 'jug-handle' posturing of the upper limbs with internal rotation of the shoulders and pronation of the forearms, tongue fasciculation and the bright alert facies (Brandt 1950) (Fig. 44.8).

When there is a short history of weakness and the muscle biopsy is normal or shows only universal atrophy, the nerve conduction study is useful because it will show an absent or greatly diminished amplitude of the motor action potential, whereas in the myopathies the motor action potential is usually of reasonable size (>0.5 mV). The EMG may show some fibrillation potentials at rest, and isolated motor units of normal size and configuration on volition, but will not show the classical changes of reinnervation (i.e. large isolated motor units).

Spinal muscular atrophy is autosomal recessive and the severity in affected siblings is usually similar but occasionally there may be marked discordance in severity.

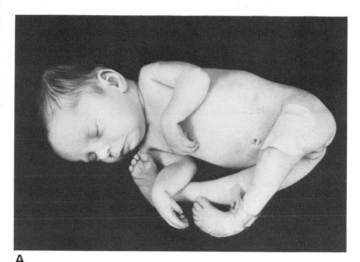

A

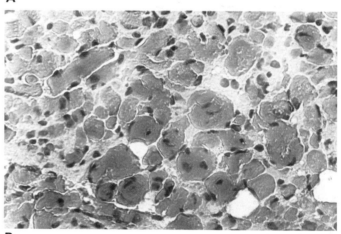

B

Fig. 44.7 A 2-week-old girl with arthrogryposis and generalized hypotonia. Fetal movements were reduced throughout pregnancy and there was oligohydramnios and poor fetal growth. The baby was delivered at full-term (birth-weight 2 kg) and adopted a 'fetal' position with the arms tucked under the chin and the legs flexed at the hips, the left against the chest and the right along the trunk behind the arm. There were no spontaneous movements of the limbs. She sucked well, however, and there were no breathing difficulties. She had fixed flexion contractures of both elbows, 30° flexion contractures of both wrists, dislocated right hip, right genu recurvatum and severe bilateral talipes. Her serum CK was normal (107 iu/l). (**b**) Needle muscle biopsy at 2 weeks of age (quadriceps) showed dystrophic change. She had bilateral talectomy to correct the talipes at the age of 19 months and is now standing regularly in a frame.

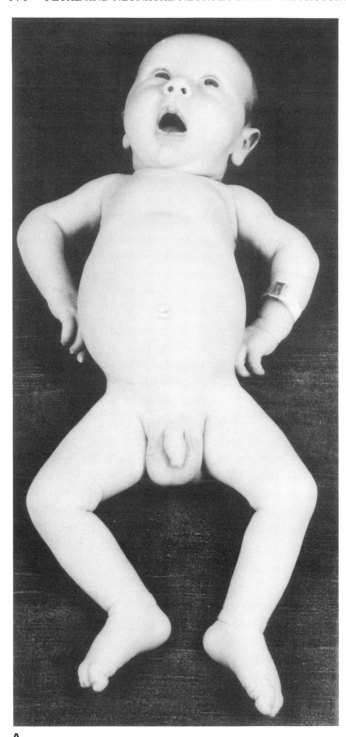

A

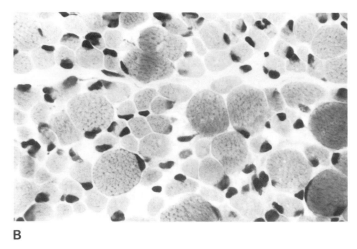

B

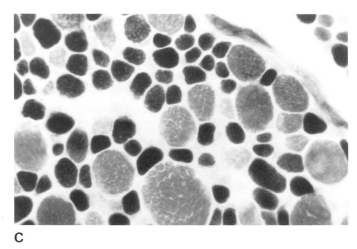

C

Fig. 44.8 (a) A 4-week-old boy with severe spinal muscular atrophy. There was insidious onset of weakness with poor limb movement and internal rotation of the arms. Fetal movements were normal and movements seemed normal at birth. Note the typical frog posture and alert facies. Tongue fasciculation was present. Motor nerve conduction (peroneal nerve) showed a markedly reduced motor action potential at 0.05 mV (normal >0.5 mV). EMG of the quadriceps showed fasciculation potentials at rest but no activity on volition. (b) Needle muscle biopsy (quadriceps) at 4 weeks of age showed variability in fibre size (H&E). (c) The larger fibres were all type 1, suggestive of some reinnervation (ATPase 9.5).

Spinal cord transection

This is now rare but enters into the differential diagnosis of any paralysed baby. The exact signs depend on the level of the lesion, in particular there are various postural abnormalities of the upper limbs including the 'Thorburn posture' characterized by abduction at the shoulders and flexion of the elbows and wrists in association with damage to the lower cervical and upper thoracic cord. A high cervical lesion will lead to ventilatory failure. The injury is usually associated with breech presentation with difficulty delivering the after-coming head and the obstetrician may report a loud 'snap' from within the birth canal. The baby is likely to be shocked at birth and need intubation. On examination, the legs will be flaccid and there will be bladder distention (Byers 1975). (See also Ch. 35.)

Stiff baby syndrome (continuous muscle fibre activity)

Klein et al (1972) described a congenital disorder resembling the 'stiff-man syndrome' in 10 individuals from three generations of one family. The most striking findings occurred in infancy and consisted of extreme rigidity either preventing vaginal delivery or developing a few hours after birth. Although all affected members of the family lost the rigidity during the first 2 years of life and gained good function, they suffered sudden spasms of stiffness when encountering unexpected physical contact, or sudden movement. The EMG performed in 2 of the infants, showed continuous electrical activity, and this abnormal activity was abolished by diazepam, which also seemed to be of some symptomatic benefit. This disorder is probably identical to 'startle disease' or 'hyperekplexia' (Lingam et al 1981).

Black et al (1972) described what seems to be a different syndrome of progressive generalized muscle stiffness in an infant in whom there was no family history. The baby died of pneumonia at 30 days of age. Autopsy revealed reactive astrocytosis in the cerebrum and axonal swelling in the peripheral nerves.

NON-NEUROMUSCULAR DISORDERS

Prader–Willi syndrome

This is a relatively common disorder with an estimated incidence of 1 in 10 000. It occurs in all races. It was originally described by Prader et al (1956) who reported 5 patients with adiposity, short stature, mental subnormality and undescended testes in the males. The presentation is frequently in the neonatal period with extreme hypotonia and lethargy. There is also a marked swallowing defect in the absence of any associated respiratory problems, in contrast to conditions such as myotonic dystrophy or myotubular myopathy which have both. With time the hypotonia resolves and all these children become ambulant. The problems with hyperphagia and obesity usually start after that.

There is a characteristic facies, with a high forehead, narrow bifrontal diameter, upslanting almond-shaped palpebral fissures, and triangular mouth with thin upper lip. Squint is present in approximately two-thirds and there are small hands and feet, which may be more apparent in later childhood. The facies may be more distinctively abnormal when the infant is crying, as these infants tend to screw up the face in a particular way. The striking feature about these infants, in comparison with those with neuromuscular disorders, is that the severity of the hypotonia is disproportionate to the intermittently good antigravity movements, which may be observed.

There is no neuromuscular involvement, the EMG, nerve conduction velocity and muscle biopsy are normal, and diagnosis is primarily clinical. Routine chromosome analysis is usually normal in these patients and Prader–Willi syndrome seems to be a sporadic disorder. A few families may be at high risk, however, because they carry a balanced translocation which may appear as an unbalanced chromosome 15 abnormality in their offspring (Berry et al 1981). Using new high-resolution prometaphase banding techniques, a small deletion on the long arm of chromosome 15 (15q12) has now been reported in about 50% of cases in several studies (Ledbetter et al 1982, Fear et al 1985). The chromosome that has undergone the deletion is thought to be of paternal origin (Butler et al 1983).

Metabolic disorders

Metabolic disorders not primarily involving muscle are the other big group of conditions that present as the floppy infant. It is not possible to give more than a brief outline here, and they are also listed in Table 44.1 (see also Section 11.)

Organic acidurias and urea cycle defects

In the neonatal period, these disorders may present acutely with a weak cry and suck, seizures and diminishing level of consciousness and rapid progression with shallow respirations, cyanosis and hypotonia, sometimes alternating with decerebrate posturing and opisthotonus. There is a symptom-free interval varying from one to several days before presentation and the signs are often precipitated by the onset of protein intake or any condition associated with catabolism such as infection. There will be a metabolic acidosis, usually a ketoacidosis, hypoglycaemia and hyperammonaemia (found particularly in disorders of the urea cycle). Odour of the urine can be diagnostic, e.g. in maple syrup urine disease or isovalericacidaemia. (See also Ch. 39).

Peroxisomopathies

This is a new group of genetic disorders, associated with cranio–facial dysmorphism (often present at birth in Zellweger's syndrome), severe hypotonia, a poor suck, epileptic seizures and hepatomegaly. There is progressive deterioration and if presentation is in early infancy, survival beyond a year is unusual. Diagnosis may require detailed examination of serum bile acids but it is worth estimating white cell dihydroacetonephosphate acetyltransferase activity and performing an X-ray of the knee for calcification as a diagnostic screen (Schutgens et al 1986). (See also p. 478.)

CONCLUSION

This description will hopefully alert the clinician to the wide range of neuromuscular and non-neuromuscular disorders that may present in the neonatal period with hypotonia and other problems. The most important requirement is a good clinical assessment of the baby, the mother and sometimes other family members. This will give guidance as to the appropriate investigations to establish a definitive diagnosis.

ACKNOWLEDGEMENTS

We are grateful to Mrs Karen Davidson for the high quality of the illustrations and to Dr Carlos De Souza for help in drawing up Table 44.1.

REFERENCES

Albers J W, Faulkner J A, Dorovini-Zis K, Barald K F, Must R E, Ball R D 1984 Abnormal neuromuscular transmission in an infantile myasthenic syndrome. Annals of Neurology 16: 28–34

Askanas V, Engel W K, Reddy N B et al 1979 X-linked recessive congenital muscle fibre hypotrophy with central nuclei. Archives of Neurology 36: 604–609

Barth P G, van Wijingaarden G K, Bethlem J 1975 X-linked myotubular myopathy with fatal neonatal asphyxia. Neurology 25: 531–536

Barth P G, Scholte H R, Berden J A et al 1983 X-linked mitochondrial disease affecting cardiac muscle, skeletal muscle and neutrophil leukocytoses. Journal of the Neurological Sciences 62: 327–355

Barry A C, Whittingham A J, Neville B G R 1981 Chromosome 15 in floppy infants. Archives of Disease in Childhood 56: 882–885

Besancon A-M, Castelnau L, Nicolesco H, Dumez Y, Poenaru L 1985 Prenatal diagnosis of glycogenosis type II (Pompe's disease) using chorionic villi biopsy. Clinical Genetics 27: 479–482

Black J T, Garcia-Mullin R, Good E, Brown S 1972 Muscle rigidity in a newborn due to continuous peripheral nerve hyperactivity. Archives of Neurology 27: 413–425

Boustany R N, Aprille J R, Halperin J, Levy H, DeLong G R 1983 Mitochondrial cytochrome deficiency presenting as a myopathy with hypotonia, external ophthalmoplegia, and lactic acidosis in an infant and as fatal hepatopathy in a second cousin. Annals of Neurology 14: 462–470

Brandt S 1950 Course and symptoms of progressive infantile muscular atrophy: a follow-up study of 112 cases in Denmark. Archives of Neurology and Psychiatry 62: 221–228

Burton B K 1987 Inborn errors of metabolism: the clinical diagnosis in early infancy. Pediatrics 79: 359–369

Butler M G, Palmer C G 1983 Parental origin of chromosome 15 deletion in Prader–Willi syndrome. Lancet i: 1285–1286

Byers R K 1975 Spinal-cord injuries during birth. Development Medicine and Child Neurology 17: 103–110

Clauren S K, Hall J G 1983 Neuropathological findings in the spinal cords of 10 infants with arthrogryposis. Journal of the Neurological Sciences 58: 89–102

Conomy J P, Levinsohn M, Fanaroff A 1975 Familial infantile myasthenia gravis: a cause of sudden death in young children. Journal of Pediatrics 87: 428–430

Di Mauro S, Hartlage P L 1978 Fatal infantile form of muscle phosphorylase deficiency. Neurology 28: 1124–1129

Di Mauro S, Mendell J R, Sahenk Z et al 1980 Fatal infantile mitochondrial myopathy and renal dysfunction due to cytochrome-c-oxidase deficiency. Neurology 30: 795–804

Di Mauro S, Nicholson J F, Hays A P et al 1983 Benign infantile mitochondrial myopathy due to reversible cytochrome c oxidase deficiency. Annals of Neurology 14: 226–234

Dodge P R, Gamstorp I, Byers R K, Russell P 1965 Myotonic dystrophy in infancy and childhood. Pediatrics 35: 3–19

Donner M, Rapola J, Somer H 1975 Congenital muscular dystrophy: a clinico–pathological and follow-up study of 15 patients. Neuropediatrie 6: 239–258

Dubowitz V 1978 Muscle disorders in childhood. W B Saunders, London

Dubowitz V 1980 The floppy infant, 2nd ed. Heinemann, London

Dubowitz V 1985 Muscle biopsy, a practical approach. Bailliere Tindall, London

Echenne, Arthurs M, Billard J 1986 Congenital muscular dystrophy and cerebral CT scan anomalies: results of a collaborative study of the Societe de neurologie infantile. Journal of the Neurological Sciences 75: 7–22

Farkas E, Tome F M S, Fardeau M, Arsenio-Nunes M L, Dreyfus P, Diebler M F 1974 Histochemical and ultrastructural study of muscle biopsies in 3 cases of dystrophia myotonica in the newborn child. Journal of the Neurological Sciences 21: 273–288

Fear C N, Mutton D E, Berry A C, Heckmatt J Z, Dubowitz V 1985 Chromosome 15 in Prader–Willi syndrome. Developmental Medicine and Child Neurology 27: 305–311

Hageman G, Willemse J 1983 Arthrogryposis multiplex congenita. Neuropediatrics 14: 6–11

Hall J G 1985 In utero movement and use of limbs are necessary for normal growth: a study of individuals with arthrogryposis. Progress in Clinical and Biological Research 200: 155–162

Harper P S 1975a Congenital myotonic dystrophy in Britain. II. Genetic basis. Archives of Disease in Childhood 50: 514–521

Harper P S 1975b Congenital myotonic dystrophy in Britain. I. Clinical aspects. Archives of Disease in Childhood 50: 505–513

Heckmatt J Z, Dubowitz V 1987 Ultrasound imaging and directed needle biopsy in the diagnosis of selective involvement in neuromuscular disease. Journal of Child Neurology 2: 205–213

Heckmatt J Z, Moosa A, Hutson C, Maunder-Sewry C A, Dubowitz V 1984 Diagnostic needle muscle biopsy, a practical and reliable alternative to open biopsy. Archives of Disease in Childhood 59: 528–532

Heckmatt J Z, Sewry C A, Hodes D, Dubowitz V 1985 Congenital centronuclear (myotubular) myopathy: a clinical and genetic study in eight children. Brain 108: 941–964

Heckmatt J Z, Placzek M, Thompson A H, Dubowitz V, Watson G 1987 An unusual case of neonatal myasthenia, with selective diaphragmatic and pharyngeal involvement, and absent acetylcholine receptor antibodies. Journal of Child Neurology 2: 63–66

Heiman-Patterson T D, Bonilla E, Di Mauro S, Foreman J, Schotland D L 1982 Cytochrome-c-oxidase deficiency in a floppy infant. Neurology 32: 898–900

Hug G, Soukup S, Ryan M, Chuck G 1984 Rapid prenatal diagnosis of glycogen-storage disease type II by electron microscopy of uncultured amniotic-fluid cells. New England Journal of Medicine 310: 1018–1022

Jerusalem F, Angelini C, Engel A G, Groover R V 1973 Mitochondria–lipid–glycogen (MLG) disease of muscle. Archives of Neurology 9: 162–169

Klein R, Haddow J E, DeLuca C 1972 Familial congenital disorder resembling stiff-man syndrome. American Journal of Diseases of Children 124: 730–731

Kuitunen P, Rapola J, Noponen A L, Donner M 1972 Nemaline myopathy. Acta Paediatrica Scandinavica 61: 353–361

Lancet (Editorial) 1986 Infant botulism. Lancet ii: 1256–1257

Ledbetter D H, Mascarello J T, Riccardi V M et al 1982 Chromosome 15 abnormalities and the Prader–Willi syndrome: follow-up report of 40 cases. American Journal of Human Genetics 34: 278–285

Lefvert A K, Osterman P O 1983 Newborn infants to myasthenic mothers: a clinical study and an investigation of acetylcholine receptor antibodies in 17 children. Neurology 33: 133–138

Lingam S, Wilson J, Hart E W 1981 Hereditary stiff baby syndrome. American Journal of Diseases of Children 135: 909–911

Meyers K R, Golomb H M, Hansen J L, McKusick V A 1974 Familial neuromuscular disease with 'myotubes'. Clinical Genetics 5: 327–337

Minchom P E, Dormer R L, Hughes I A et al 1983 Fatal infantile mitochondrial myopathy due to cytochrome c oxidase deficiency. Journal of the Neurological Sciences 60: 453–463

Moerman Ph, Fryns J P, Goddeeris P, Lauweryns J M 1983 Multiple ankyloses, facial anomalies, and pulmonary hypoplasia associated with severe antenatal spinal muscular atrophy. Journal of Pediatrics 103: 238–241

Moss D W, Whitaker K B, Paramar C et al 1981 Activity of creatine kinase in sera from healthy women, carriers of Duchenne muscular dystrophy and cord blood, determined by the 'European' method with NAC-EDTA activation. Clinical Chimica Acta 116: 209–216

Namba T, Brown S B, Grob D 1970 Neonatal myasthenia gravis: report of two cases and review of the literature. Pediatrics 45: 488–504

Neustein H B 1973 Nemaline myopathy, a family study with three autopsied cases. Archives of Pathology 96: 192–195

Norton P, Ellison P, Sulaiman A R, Harb J 1983 Nemaline myopathy in the neonate. Neurology 33: 351–356

O'Brien J A, Harper P S 1984 Course prognosis and complications of childhood onset myotomic dystrophy. Developmental Medicine and Child Neurology 26: 62–67

Prader A, Labhart A, Willi H 1956 Ein syndrom von adipositas, kleinwuchs, kryptorchismus und oligophrenie nach myatonieartigm zustand im neugeborenenalter. Schweizerische Medizinische Wochenschrift 86: 1260–1261

Regev R, de Vries L S, Heckmatt J Z, Dubowitz V 1987 Cerebral ventricular dilation in congenital myotonic dystrophy. Journal of Pediatrics 111: 372–376

Robertson W C, Chun R W M, Kornguth S E 1980 Familial infantile myasthenia. Archives of Neurology 37: 117–119

Rowland I P 1955 Prostigmine responsiveness and the diagnosis of myasthenia gravis. Neurology 5: 612–624

Schutgens R H B, Heymans H S A, Wanders R J A, v.d. Bosch H, Tager J M 1986 Peroxisomal disorders: a newly recognised group of genetic diseases. European Journal of Pediatrics 144: 430–440

Shafiq S A, Dubowitz V, Hart de C Peterson, Milhorat A T 1967 Nemaline myopathy: report of a fatal case, with histochemical and electron microscopic studies. Brain 90: 817–828

Slonim A E, Coleman R A, Moses W S 1984 Myopathy and growth failure in debrancher enzyme deficiency: improvement with high-protein nocturnal enteral therapy. Journal of Pediatrics 105: 906–911

Smit L M E, Barth P G 1980 Arthrogryposis multiplex congenita due to congenital myasthenia. Developmental Medicine and Child Neurology 22: 371–373

Strehl E, Vanasse M 1985 EMG and needle muscle biopsy studies in arthrogryposis multiplex congenita. Neuropediatrics 16: 225–227

Swinyard C A 1982 Concepts of multiple congenital contractures in man and animals. Teratology 25: 247–258

Teyssier G, Damon G, Bertheas M F, Freycon F, Lauras B 1982 Congenital myasthenia and arthrogryposis: apropos of 2 cases manifesting at birth. Pediatrie 37: 295–298

Tsujihata M, Shimomura C, Yoshimura T, Akira S, Teruyuki O, Tsuji Y, Nagataki S, Matsuo T 1983 Fatal neonatal myopathy; a case report. Journal of Neurosurgery and Psychiatry 46: 856–859

Van Biervliet J P G M, Bruinvis L, Fetting D et al 1977 Hereditary mitochondrial myopathy with lactic acidaemia, a DeToni–Fanconi–Debre syndrome, and a defective respiratory chain in voluntary muscles. Pediatric Research 11: 1088–1093

Vanier T M 1960 Dystrophia myotonica in childhood. British Medical Journal ii: 1284–1288

Van Wijngaarden G K, Fleury P, Bethlem J, Hugo Meijer A E F 1969 Familial 'myotubular' myopathy. Neurology 19: 901–908

Vassella F, Mumenthaler M, Rossi E, Moser H, Weissmann U 1967 Dei kongenitale muskel-dystrophie. Deutsche Zeitschrift fur Nervenheikunde 190: 349–374

Vincent A, Cull-Candy S Q, Newsom-Davis J, Trautmann A, Molenaar P C, Polak R L 1981 Congenital myasthenia: end plate acetylcholine receptors and electrophysiology in five cases. Muscle and Nerve 4: 306–318

Zeviani M, Nonaka I, Bonilla E et al 1985 Fatal infantile mitochondrial myopathy and renal dysfunction caused by cytochrome c oxidase deficiency: immunological studies in a new patient. Annals of Neurology 17: 414–417

Neurosurgery

Advances in prenatal and postnatal diagnostic imaging, and in neonatal supportive therapy and anaesthesia provide the paediatric neurosurgeon with increasing opportunities for making operative interventions in younger and smaller babies. It is the purpose of these chapters to describe those conditions which present in the perinatal period and which should be recognized by the obstetrician and neonatal physician and referred for neurosurgical advice on appropriate management. Many of these conditions will require close and continuing collaboration between physician and surgeon because of the immature state of the child, concomitant medical aspects, and the need for careful developmental monitoring. Furthermore, management often involves several specialists and good lines of communication are essential. A combined neurology and neurosurgery clinic dedicated to neonates, as operated by this writer and his co-editor, is the ideal setting for such collaboration. Clearly, once a neural abnormality is discovered in a neonate there is considerable parental anxiety and it is crucial that prompt assessment, accurate diagnosis, concise plan of management, realistic prognosis and sympathetic explanation are forthcoming without unreasonable delay.

As elsewhere in fetal and neonatal medicine there are many points of uncertainty both on medical and ethical grounds which will only be resolved by careful collaborative studies conducted by neonatal physicians and neurosurgeons who must concern themselves with the long-term consequences of their activities.

45. Management of fetal ventriculomegaly

Dr R. J. Hudgins, Dr M. S. B. Edwards
and Dr M. S. Golbus

The prognosis for patients with untreated hydrocephalus is poor. Lawrence & Coats (1962) reviewed 182 unoperated cases of hydrocephalus in patients under the age of 13 who were followed for over 20 years by one surgeon, Wylie McKissock. They found that 46% were alive with hydrocephalus arrested spontaneously, 5% had progressive hydrocephalus, and 49% had died. Of the survivors, 73% had IQs of more than 50. Lawrence and Coates calculated that the acutarial life expectancy of survival into adulthood was 26%.

With the development of successful postnatal shunting systems in the 1950s, the numerous technical improvements in those systems over the last several decades, and the development of high-resolution ultrasonography and computerized tomography (CT) scanning, the mortality and morbidity associated with hydrocephalus have declined considerably. McCullough & Balzer-Martin (1982) followed 37 patients with congenital hydrocephalus shunted after delivery: 86% survived to 16 years of age and approximately two-thirds had normal or near-normal intellectual capacity (median IQ of 96).

The development of high-resolution ultrasonography has allowed accurate evaluation of the prenatal neural axis (see Ch. 7 for review), and has led to the hope that in-utero treatment of fetal ventriculomegaly would improve neurological outcome beyond that possible with postnatal shunting. Numerous publications have described the experience first with serial percutaneous ventricular punctures and then with ventriculo–amniotic (V–A) shunting both in experimental models and in the clinical setting (Birnholtz & Frigoletto 1981, Michejda & Hodgen 1981, Clewell et al 1982, Frigoletto et al 1982, Glick et al 1984, Manning et al 1984, 1986). In this chapter we discuss the pathophysiology, diagnosis, natural history, and treatment of in-utero ventriculomegaly.

PATHOPHYSIOLOGY

Cerebrospinal fluid (CSF) is actively produced by an energy-dependent mechanism, primarily by the choroid plexuses that lie within the ventricular system. A significant but unknown amount is formed by flow across the cerebral capillaries and then by bulk flow through the brain parenchyma into the ventricles. An extraordinary amount of CSF (374–936 ml/day) is produced in the newborn (Vintzileus et al 1983).

CSF flows from the lateral ventricles through the foramena of Monroe into the third ventricle. It then moves through the aqueduct of Sylvius, the narrowest and thus most vulnerable section of the pathway, into the fourth ventricle. From there, CSF passes through the midline foramen of Magendie and the lateral, paired foramena of Luschka to reach the spinal subarachnoid space of the cisterna magna and the basal cisterns, and on over the convexity of the brain. The flow of CSF is generated by venous and/or arterial pulsations of the brain and choroid plexuses.

Absorption of CSF occurs at the arachnoid granulations present along the large dural venous sinuses and at the dorsal root ganglia in the spinal subarachnoid space. These granulations act passively as one-way valves that allow CSF to flow into the venous system when CSF pressure is greater than intravenous pressure. This system is capable of absorbing five times the amount of CSF produced.

Hydrocephalus occurs when CSF flow or absorption is obstructed or impaired. Burton (1979) reviewed 205 consecutive cases of congenital hydrocephalus seen over a 10-year period at the Children's Memorial Hospital in Chicago. She found that hydrocephalus was caused by stenosis at the aqueduct of Sylvius in 43% of patients, by communicating hydrocephalus (with blockage distal to the ventricular system) in 38%, Dandy–Walker syndrome in 13%, and obstruction of flow secondary to other anatomical lesions in 6%. Infants with neural tube defects, intracranial haemorrhage, meningitis, or tumour were excluded from this study. In rare instances, hydrocephalus may be caused by overproduction of CSF secondary to a choroid plexus tumour.

Damage to cerebral tissue occurs most readily when hydrocephalus is acute and severe but chronic hydrocephalus may also cause cerebral injury. The initial damage is confined primarily to the periventricular white matter and consists of flattening and destruction of the ependymal lining; oedema and destruction of nerve fibres are found in subependymal white matter (Weller et al 1978). This destructive process is of special importance in the fetus because primitive cells destined to differentiate into neurones are found in this region and damage to subependymal germ cells in utero may result in subsequent cortical neuronal depletion. As oedema subsides, the ependymal surface is partially reconstituted and gliosis of the subependymal white matter develops.

Progressive hydrocephalus leads to compression and eventually to thinning of neural tissue, occasionally leaving only a thin mantle of residual cortical brain. That brain tissue may reconstitute itself to a significant extent after this marked thinning is a well known but little understood fact. The cranial sutures are open in the fetus and progressive enlargement of the ventricles leads to enlargement of the calvarium. The head may become so large that vaginal delivery is precluded.

It is necessary to differentiate between ventriculomegaly and hydrocephalus. Ventriculomegaly simply means enlargement of the ventricles and may be caused by increased intraventricular pressure secondary to obstruction of CSF flow and absorption, in which case hydrocephalus is the proper term; or it may be the result of passive enlargement caused by atrophy of the parenchyma. A progressive increase in head size suggests that hydrocephalus is causative but hydrocephalus cannot be ruled out if the size of the head is not increasing. This distinction may be difficult to make clinically but is obviously important both for treatment and prognosis.

DIAGNOSIS

The development of grey scale, B-mode, real-time imaging and focused transducers has greatly improved the resolution of obstetric ultrasonography (Wright 1981). This has allowed more precise visualization of anatomical detail, has aided in the diagnosis of pathological conditions such as ventriculomegaly, and has made it possible to obtain sequential images during the development of ventriculomegaly (Fig. 45.1). The appearance of ventriculomegaly can be appreciated only if the normal developmental features of the fetal ventricular system and cranium are understood. This is described in detail in Section 2 and will be only briefly reiterated here.

The fetal skull can be seen on sonograms at about 8 weeks after conception. At that time it consists largely of fluid-filled cerebral vesicles that will become the lateral ventricles; by week 12, they can be seen on sonograms as filling the cranial vault and containing the highly echogenic choroid plexus. The cerebral mantle is thin and is difficult to distinguish because of its low echogenicity.

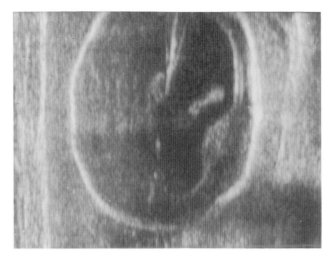

Fig. 45.1 High-resolution ultrasonogram showing marked hydrocephalus. Choroid plexus is seen as an area of high echogenicity in the lateral ventricle.

By 15 weeks the lateral ventricles are easily seen and are filled with echogenic choroid plexus. The occipital horns cannot be seen at this point in development; the anterior horn is the only component of the ventricular system that is not filled with choroid plexus. By 20 weeks of gestation, the size of the lateral ventricles has decreased in relation to the transverse intracranial dimension but remains full of choroid plexus. The temporal horns may be seen and the slit-like third ventricle and the thalamus may be recognized. The aqueduct of Sylvius also may be seen as a bright echo midway between the cerebral peduncles and toward the posterior aspect of the midbrain. The brainstem and basilar cisterns are located by the presence of pulsating vasculature. After 24 weeks, the ventricles progressively become smaller until they are slit-like. A cavum septi pellucidi is often recognized between the anterior portion of the lateral ventricles. The brain undergoes little structural change other than increased cortical convolutions.

The diagnosis of hydrocephalus may be made as early as the twelfth week when the ventricles are normally filled with choroid plexus. Hydrocephalus is detected by a relative shrinkage of the choroid plexus in relation to the ventricle; that is, as the ventricle enlarges it is no longer filled with echogenic choroid plexus. This finding is diagnostic for ventricular enlargement until 20–24 weeks of gestation, at which time the choroid plexus is a less reliable indicator of ventricular enlargement.

Many measurements have been proposed to detect ventricular dilatation. In the most frequently used method, the distance from the lateral wall of the ventricle to the midline is compared with the hemispheric width (LVW/HW ratio). Unfortunately, the large standard deviations associated with this ratio make it insensitive to early ventricular dilatation. It also varies depending on the plane of section in which the sonogram is obtained.

A more sensitive measure of ventricular dilatation described by Fiske et al (1981) is displacement of the medial wall of the lateral ventricle towards the midline. Displacement may be detected at approximately 22 weeks and occurs before the lateral ventricular wall is displaced from the midline, thus changing the LVW/HW ratio. By the third trimester the ventricles should be slit-like and therefore the diagnosis of hydrocephalus becomes less difficult. If hydrocephalus is detected, a thorough ultrasonographic examination should be made for associated abnormalities such as spina bifida, encephaloceles, and abnormal posterior fossa CSF collections (Dandy–Walker malformation or arachnoid cyst). Amniocentesis or fetal blood sampling should be performed to rule out chromosomal abnormalities (unbalanced translocation, trisomy 13, trisomy 18), to determine the sex of the fetus (X-linked aqueductal stenosis), and to determine the amniotic fluid alpha-fetoprotein level, which should be elevated in the presence of open neural tube defects. Finally, maternal serum and amniotic fluid should be tested to rule out congenital infections such as rubella, toxoplasmosis, cytomegalovirus, and syphilis.

NATURAL HISTORY

Until recently, the natural history of fetal ventriculomegaly has been poorly defined and prognosis was determined by extrapolation from data for newborns with hydrocephalus. This method is obviously inaccurate because selection is biased toward infants who survive and may not include those fetuses with severe hydrocephalus and/or other severe systemic disorders. Chervenak et al (1985) published the Yale University experience with 53 cases of autopsy, or ultrasound documented cases of fetal ventriculomegaly. Ultrasound diagnoses were made using standard normograms for the lateral ventricle-to-hemispheric width ratio. Hydrocephalus was isolated in only 17% of cases and associated with other anatomical abnormalities in 83%. Spina bifida was the most commonly associated abnormality ($n = 15$) but abnormalities in the neurological skeletal, respiratory and reproductive systems were also identified. Chromosomal abnormalities were detected in 5 cases. Although diagnostic accuracy improved during the course of the study, in 14 cases (26%) the diagnosis of significant associated abnormalities was not made in the antepartum period.

In the Yale study, management of fetuses depended upon gestational age at the time of diagnosis and the presence or absence of associated abnormalities. Management consisted of termination of pregnancy (26%), cephalocentesis and caesarean section (4%), caesarean section alone (34%), cephalocentesis and vaginal delivery (17%), and vaginal delivery alone (17%). The outcomes were spontaneous abortion (26%), intrapartum death (15%),

postnatal death (30%), and survival (28%). Fetuses died in 10 of 11 instances in which cephalocentesis was performed.

Ventriculo–atrial (V–A) shunting was performed in two fetuses. In the first, a shunt was placed at 27½ weeks of gestation after progressive hydrocephalus had been documented but no other abnormalities had been seen on sonograms. The shunt malfunctioned between 4½ and 6½ weeks after placement and the child was delivered one week later by caesarean section. The infant was found to have hypoplastic digits of both hands and feet. A ventriculo-peritoneal (V–P) shunt was placed on the third day of life; at 10 months of age, the child was reported to have moderate mental and motor delay.

In the second case, a V–A shunt was placed at 29½ weeks gestation in a fetus with hydrocephalus and a large midline intracranial arachnoid cyst. Despite shunting, the size of the head and ventricles continued to increase. The child was delivered by caesarean section at 37 weeks of gestation and the shunt catheter was found to be entirely intracranial. A V–P shunt was placed 3 days after delivery. At 9 months of age, the infant was reported to have severe mental and motor delay.

Chervenak et al (1985) concluded that the accurate antenatal assessment of abnormalities associated with hydrocephalus is essential to determine proper care. They felt that the value of V–A shunting was uncertain and should be limited to cases of isolated hydrocephalus in which progressive ventriculomegaly has been documented and the fetus is too immature to deliver for postpartum shunting. Finally, they concluded that fetuses with isolated hydrocephalus and macrocephaly are best delivered by caesarean section.

Since we published our experience with 24 human fetuses with ventriculomegaly documented by antenatal ultrasonography (Glick et al 1984a), we have evaluated 23 additional cases, and will discuss our experience with 47 fetuses followed over a 5-year period. The diagnosis of ventriculomegaly included not only ventricular measurements but also the size of the choroid plexus relative to the transverse diameter of the ventricular body. All fetuses were followed by serial ultrasound examinations and a careful search was made for associated abnormalities. The diagnosis was often made early in pregnancy, the earliest at 13 weeks. When associated abnormalities were detected, the parents were offered the options of termination of pregnancy or vaginal delivery after cephalocentesis (depending upon gestational age). Because this option was chosen by 19 families, our series does not fully represent the pure natural history of fetal ventriculomegaly but, considering the legal and ethical issues involved, may represent the best available documentation of the natural history of this disease.

Ventriculomegaly was associated with other severe abnormalities in 20 fetuses. In 19 of these cases the family elected for termination of pregnancy. Cephalocentesis was necessary in 4 cases to effect vaginal delivery; none of these fetuses survived. One family did not elect to have termination of pregnancy or cephalocentesis and therefore a caesarean section was necessary at full-term for dystocia of the fetal head. The neonate survived for 30 minutes after delivery and, although the family refused autopsy, the infant was found upon examination immediately after birth to have hydrocephalus, congenital heart disease, oesophageal atresia, and cleft palate.

In 5 other fetuses, ventriculomegaly was detected late in pregnancy. In each case there was an associated abnormality such as myelomeningocele, cranial hydrops, hydronephrosis, encephalocele, and polycystic kidneys. These fetuses were treated with routine obstetric management and none survived.

Of the remaining 22 fetuses, ventriculomegaly was not thought to be associated with any other severe systemic abnormalities. Ventriculomegaly remained stable throughout gestation in 19, progressed in 2, and gradually resolved in one fetus who had mild ventricular enlargement.

Of the 19 children with stable ventriculomegaly, 9 had signs of increased intracranial pressure at birth or within the first 6 months of life and all underwent V–P shunting. With a median follow-up of 3.5 years, 6 of these children are mentally normal, one child with a myelomeningocele who was developing normally at one year of age died of urinary sepsis, 2 have mild developmental delay, and one is severely retarded.

Ten of the 19 children with stable ventriculomegaly in utero did not require placement of a shunt. Five had no signs of increased intracranial pressure at birth; with a median follow-up of 3 years, all have radiographical evidence of stable ventriculomegaly and all are developmentally normal. The remaining 5 children all have underlying cerebral parenchymal abnormalities (septo-optic dysplasia, agenesis of the corpus callosum) or abnormalities that preclude normal development (temporal porencephalic cyst and cardiac abnormalities, chromosomal abnormalities, amniotic band disruption complex). One child with a chromosomal abnormality (47, XX+, isodic, (14)(21)) died at 3 months of age.

The child whose ventriculomegaly resolved in utero is neurologically normal at 3½ years of age and has no evidence of ventriculomegaly on follow-up CT scans. The two infants with progressive in-utero ventriculomegaly were shunted after delivery and both are developmentally normal.

In summary, of 22 fetuses thought to have isolated ventriculomegaly, 14 (64%) are developmentally normal; 9 required a V–P shunt. Two of the shunted fetuses are mildly delayed. Six are severely delayed.

We were unable to identify a group of fetuses who would have benefited from in-utero shunting. Even the two fetuses with progressive ventriculomegaly and no associated abnormalities would not have benefited from in-utero shunting. We agree with Chervenak et al (1985) that even in the hands of an expert ultrasonographer, all associated abnormalities

cannot be identified. In our series, four fetuses with what we believed to be isolated ventriculomegaly had other abnormalities identified after delivery, such as agenesis of the corpus callosum (2), absence of the septum pellucidum, and septo-optic dysplasia.

Serlo et al (1986) reported results of 38 fetuses with hydrocephalus diagnosed over a 5-year period (1978–83). Five were diagnosed before 20 weeks of gestation and all of these pregnancies were terminated. Of the remaining 33 fetuses, 23 were noted to have severe associated abnormalities that were lethal. Of these, 2 died in utero, 12 during vaginal delivery, 5 during the first week of life, and the remaining 4 died by 9 months of age. All were treated 'conservatively', that is, without taking into consideration diagnostic information about the fetus while planning the safest maternal obstetric care.

Ten fetuses had no characteristics that suggested a poor prognosis. Eight were delivered by caesarean section and two were delivered vaginally. Nine required shunt placement after delivery. Six of these children had normal or near-normal development and six were severely retarded. Serlo et al (1986) conclude that fetal hydrocephalus is frequently associated with severe, lethal abnormalities and that termination of pregnancy should be recommended in these cases. They felt that only a minority of fetuses were suitable for antenatal therapy, although none was treated antenatally in their series.

Outcome of fetal ventriculomegaly has been discussed by three other groups. Cochrane et al (1984) reported 41 cases from four Canadian universities. In most instances, the diagnosis was made late in pregnancy, with 32 of 41 cases detected after 30 weeks of gestation. Pregnancy was not terminated in any instance and delivery requiring cephalocentesis was used in only three instances. The prognosis for a normal outcome in this series was poor: 22% of fetuses were stillborn, 30% who were not treated died, 13% died after treatment (V–P shunting), 28% have delayed developmental milestones, and only 7.5% are normal. Other CNS abnormalities were found in 75% of fetuses. In contrast to our experience, Cochrane et al report that most of their cases exhibited progressive ventricular dilatation with macrocephaly.

Pretorius et al (1985) reviewed 40 cases of fetal ventriculomegaly seen at the University of Colorado. Of these, 34 fetuses died: 9 were aborted, 7 were delivered after cephalocentesis and all died, 5 died of infection, 4 had multiple abnormalities that led to death, 3 died in utero, 2 died of respiratory failure, and 4 died of unknown causes. Only 3 of the 6 survivors were neurologically normal.

Williamson et al (1984) reported 30 cases from the University of Iowa Hospitals. There were only 5 survivors: 3 infants with myelomeningocele who were shunted after birth, one infant with communicating hydrocephalus who was shunted after birth and is functionally normal, and one infant with microcephaly and probable congenital rubella syndrome who has considerable neurological and mental impairment. They tabulated an extensive list of abnormalities in non-survivors, including endocardial cushion defects, bilateral renal hypoplasia, transposition of great vessels, pulmonary hypoplasia, and Pierre–Robin anomaly.

The following conclusions can be drawn from this information:

1. fetal ventriculomegaly may be diagnosed early in gestation (13 weeks);
2. in most instances, fetal hydrocephalus is associated with other severe abnormalities;
3. even in the hands of an expert ultrasonographer, some systemic and central nervous system abnormalities associated with ventriculomegaly cannot be detected;
4. despite the results of Cochrane et al (1984), the occurrence of progressive ventriculomegaly in utero is probably unusual (2 of 47 in our series);
5. the prognosis for ventriculomegaly diagnosed in utero is poor;
6. no group of fetuses has been identified in which in-utero V–A shunting would be of clear benefit.

RESEARCH

Possibly because of the technical difficulties inherent in developing and maintaining a fetal animal model of hydrocephalus, there have been few laboratory studies of the efficacy of in-utero shunting (Michejda & Hodgen 1981, Glick et al 1984). Michejda and Hodgen reported the production of fetal hydrocephalus in Rhesus monkeys and the results of treatment by the hydrocephalic antenatal vent for intra-uterine treatment (HAVIT). Hydrocephalus and neural tube defects were induced by the intramuscular injection of triamcinolone acetonide (10 mg/kg) in the gravid Rhesus monkey on days 21, 23, and 25 of pregnancy. Hydrocephalus was confirmed by X-ray, ultrasonography, and fetoscopy

A hysterotomy was performed between gestational days 115 and 125 and intracranial pressure was monitored by insertion of a pressure monitor into the lateral ventricle. In normal control monkey fetuses, intraventricular pressure was in the range of 45–55 mmH$_2$O but was greater than 100 mmH$_2$O in hydrocephalic fetuses.

The HAVIT was developed in an effort to treat increased intracranial pressure in utero. The stainless steel device has a ball-and-spring flow valve that allows drainage of CSF into the amniotic fluid when intracranial pressure exceeds 60 mmH$_2$O. The device is placed at hysterotomy performed in the late second or early third trimester, when the cranial bones in the monkey fetus are sufficiently ossified to allow the device to be anchored firmly by threading it into the skull. Periodic X-rays were obtained to ensure that the HAVIT remained in place; no mention is made of the use of ultrasonography or other methods to assess continuing function of the device. All shunted infant monkeys were delivered by caesarean section.

Unfortunately, results are not tabulated but Michejda & Hodgen (1981) state that control hydrocephalic Rhesus monkeys manifested intra-uterine growth retardation, had confirmed severe hydrocephalus, frequent seizures, progressive motor weakness, and often died within 10–14 days after delivery. In contrast, most (no numbers were given) of the treated monkeys showed progressive physical dexterity, grew at near-normal rates, and did not die. Michejda and Hodgen concluded that fetal hydrocephalus could be diagnosed and treated in utero.

In the other major experimental study of in-utero treatment of hydrocephalus (Nakayama et al 1983, Glick et al 1984b, Edwards 1986), we developed a model in both fetal lambs and Rhesus monkeys. The gravid sheep uterus was surgically exposed, the posterior atlanto–occipital membrane identified by palpation through the thin uterine wall, and 0.5–2.0 cc of 2% kaolin was injected into the cisterna magna of the fetus. At approximately 20 days after kaolin injection, one of three different shunting procedures was performed: ventriculo–amniotic (V–A), ventriculo–right atrial (V–RA), or ventriculo–pleural (V–PL). A standard multiholed ventricular catheter and a distal catheter with a one-way, low-pressure slit valve were used. Delivery was performed at full-term by caesarean section and viability was determined two hours after birth. Animals were sacrificed and their brains were submitted for gross and microscopic pathological examinations.

In unshunted control lambs, intracranial pressure increased linearly ($r = 0.94$) from the time of kaolin injection until full-term. Unshunted lambs had enlarged heads and bulging anterior fontanelles. On gross inspection, it was found that the anatomy of the surface of the cerebral hemispheres was distorted and marked ventriculomegaly was present in all instances. An inflammatory infiltrate caused by the kaolin was found in the leptomeninges around the brainstem and cerebellum, and occasionally extended into the fourth ventricle and aqueduct of Sylvius.

In contrast, most shunted fetal lambs had a more normal head size, overriding sutures, preservation of the anatomy of cerebral hemispheres, and ventricles of normal size. The viability at 2 hours after delivery was significantly greater for shunted (70%) than for unshunted (14%) lambs. Interestingly, an intense inflammatory response was found in the ependymal lining of the lateral ventricle and the ventricular CSF spaces were often obliterated by dense adhesions. This was thought to be caused by reflux of kaolin from the cisterna magna into the lateral and third ventricles in shunted animals. In Rhesus monkeys, shunting did not significantly alter the histopathology, probably because of a high incidence of shunt malfunction. Subdural haematomas and hygromas, shunt infection, and improper shunt tip placement occurred in both groups of animals.

Based on these results, we have concluded that in-utero shunting improved overall survival and reduced gross ventriculomegaly in the animal model but that significant complications were associated with the shunting procedure. The pathophysiology of fetal hydrocephalus and the technique of shunting should be more vigorously explored in animal models before being used to treat human fetuses in utero.

CLINICAL EXPERIENCE

The first experiences with in-utero drainage of CSF in hydrocephalic fetuses were performed to reduce the size of the fetuses' head in order to effect safe vaginal delivery (Larson & Banner 1966) and not for the treatment of ventriculomegaly per se. In 1966, Barke et al reported the first case of fetal ventriculomegaly confirmed by roentgenograms in a full-term fetus with hydrocephalus. Using an 18-gauge spinal needle inserted through the cervix into the ventricle, an air ventriculogram was obtained that confirmed the diagnosis of hydrocephalus. The day after the ventriculogram was obtained, the child was delivered stillborn transvaginally. Several other case reports of fetal ventriculograms were then published. Robertson et al (1969) used nitrous oxide to visualize ventriculomegaly, and Miller et al (1974) reported visualizing ventriculomegaly in a fetus whose ventricle was accidentally punctured and infused with a radio-opaque agent (50% Triognost) during an amniogram.

Kellner et (1980) reported obtaining a transabdominal, ultrasonically guided ventriculogram using air in a 36-week-old fetus. Because amniocentesis had shown an L/S ratio of 1.69, it was decided that delivery should not be attempted, and that if it could be documented that cortical damage was not severe, a valve-regulated V–A shunt would be placed. The ventriculogram showed the absence of cortex in the parietal and occipital regions and therefore it was felt that the fetus was not a good candidate for in-utero shunting. The infant was delivered stillborn at 39 weeks after transvaginal cephalocentesis. Multiple abnormalities were noted at autopsy.

Birnholz & Frigoletto (1981) were the first to report the use of serial percutaneous cephalocentesis to treat in-utero hydrocephalus. The diagnosis of hydrocephalus was made at 24 weeks of gestation in what was considered to be an otherwise normal male fetus. Under continuous ultrasound guidance, serial percutaneous cephalocenteses were performed beginning at 25 weeks and continuing at 1–2 week intervals until the child was delivered by caesarean section at 34 weeks. Five taps were performed. Postnatal ultrasound and cranial CT scans showed asymmetrical hydrocephalus, a posterior midline cyst, and absence of the corpus callosum. A V–P shunt was inserted. The child was subsequently found to have Becker's muscular dystrophy and has remained developmentally retarded and suffers from a seizure disorder.

It seemed that in-utero hydrocephalus might be better treated by continuous rather than intermittent drainage of CSF. The first instances of treating human fetuses by prenatal V–A shunting were reported by Clewell et al (1982) and by Frigoletto et al (1982). Clewell et al reported the insertion of a V–A shunt in a 23-week-old male fetus; there was a family history of X-linked aqueductal stenosis and no other abnormalities could be seen on ultrasonograms. A silastic V–A shunt with a unidirectional, flow-limiting valve was placed transabdominally with ultrasound guidance through the posterior parietal skull and brain into the lateral ventricle. Ultrasonograms obtained after insertion showed decreases in the size of the ventricles, the LVW/HW ratio, and the biparietal diameter. The thickness of the cortical mantle had also increased. The shunt malfunctioned between 32 and 34 weeks of gestation, as indicated by an increase in the size of the ventricles, and the infant was delivered by caesarean section. The shunt was found to be occluded by tissue that had grown into the lumen and valve. A V–P shunt was placed. At the last follow-up (52 weeks of postmenstrual age), the infant had poor head control, contractures of the hands, and did not follow objects, but had developed a social smile.

Frigoletto et al (1982) attempted placement of a V–A shunt in a 23-week-old fetus whose only other known abnormality was a facial cleft. The catheter was inserted through a thin-walled, 13-gauge needle; the valve portion of the catheter jammed in the needle after CSF had been withdrawn. The catheter was lost in the maternal peritoneal cavity when the needle was withdrawn from the fetal ventricle. Subsequently, a second catheter was placed without difficulty. Serial ultrasonograms showed that there was a slight but progressive increase in the size of the ventricles; therefore, a valveless piece of silastic tubing was placed into the ventricle. The result was an evident and progressive decrease in the size of the ventricles.

Because of transcervical leakage of amniotic fluid, the infant was delivered by caesarean section at 28 weeks of gestation. CSF was observed to be dripping freely from the valveless silastic tube but not from the valved catheter. A V–P shunt was inserted at 2 weeks of age. The infant's course was complicated by diabetes insipidus, seizures and possibly sepsis and he died of a cardiac arrest at 5½ weeks of age. Frigoletto et al (1982) speculated that amniotic fluid had refluxed into the ventricular system through the valveless silastic tubing, which might produce aseptic ventriculitis. There was no 'indirect evidence' of this complication and a CSF cell count was not reported nor was an autopsy performed.

During the year in which these reports appeared, the Kroc Foundation sponsored a conference entitled 'Unborn: management of the fetus with a correctable congenital defect', for workers active in the field of fetal treatment. Participants, including ourselves, reviewed the available experimental and clinical research on the treatment of fetuses, one aspect of which was the treatment of fetal hydrocephalus. The experience gained in treating 8 fetuses by in-utero V–A shunting was discussed. A decrease in ventricular size was seen in 7 fetuses and the dislodgement and malfunctioning of shunts required revision in 3 fetuses: 6 survived and had V–P shunts placed after delivery. Efficacy could not be determined without long-term follow-up. A registry of treated cases was established to allow evaluation of the 'benefits and liabilities' of fetal surgery. The participants felt that in-utero shunting should be attempted only if the fetus had progressive ventriculomegaly, was too immature for delivery and placement of a shunt postnatally, had a normal karyotype, and had no other severe abnormalities identified on ultrasonograms.

Even as case reports of V–A shunting continued to be published (Depp et al 1983), many experts called for restraint. Venes (1983) called for a moratorium on in-utero shunting. Among the reasons that led to her opinion were: 1. there was little or no evidence for a correlation between the size of the ventricle and eventual psychomotor development that could justify in-utero shunting; 2. because CSF flow may be necessary for the development of CSF pathways, placement of a shunt in utero too early in gestation could cause reversible hydrocephalus to become irreversible; 3. it was unwise to place shunts in utero when the natural history of fetal hydrocephalus was not well defined. Venes (1983) suggested that intra-uterine shunting in humans be halted until these questions were answered.

These calls for restraint dampened the initial fervour for in-utero shunting. Thus the International Fetal Surgery Registry, which included 29 centres in 7 countries, recorded only 41 attempts at in-utero ventricular decompression between 1982 and 1985 (Manning et al 1986). Of the 41 registered attempts at treatment, which represents the largest compilation of fetuses treated for hydrocephalus, 39 fetuses were treated with V–A shunting and 2 were treated by serial ventricular puncture. A silastic shunt with a one-way valve was used in most instances. The mean gestational age at diagnosis was 25 weeks, and the mean gestational age at treatment was 27 weeks.

Seven of the fetuses died (17%), one before and six after birth. The one stillborn fetus died as the result of needle trauma to the brainstem at the time of V–A shunt placement. Three of the six postpartum deaths were the result of premature labour proved or presumed secondary to chorioamnionitis from shunt placement. Thus, there was a procedure-related mortality of 10%.

The 34 surviving infants were followed for 8.2 ± 5.8 months: 12 infants, all with aqueductal stenosis, were normal (35%); 22 have various degrees of neurological and systemic deficits — 4 are mildly to moderately handicapped (12%) while 18 were classified as having severe deficits and

gross delay in developmental milestones (53%, IQ less than 50). Other significant non-CNS abnormalities were found in 22% of infants. The group of fetuses with aqueductal stenosis appeared to gain the most benefit from in-utero shunting. A comparison of outcome in this group with the natural history of fetal aqueductal stenosis treated after delivery, however, suggests that fetal intervention may improve survival without improving functional outcome.

RECOMMENDED MANAGEMENT

It is clear that the optimum management of fetuses with hydrocephalus remains to be determined. Before improvements can be made in devices for and techniques of V–A shunting, it will be necessary to have a better understanding of the natural history of fetal ventriculomegaly and improve our ability to diagnose in utero other abnormalities associated with ventricular enlargement. Despite these limitations, we have formulated the following approach to treatment that is based on the best information currently available (Fig. 45.2).

After the diagnosis of fetal ventriculomegaly has been made, a high-resolution ultrasonogram screening examination should be performed to identify any associated abnormalities. An amniocentesis should be performed to determine the presence or absence of chromosomal abnormalities, alpha-fetoprotein and acetylcholinesterase levels, and to obtain fluid for analysis for the presence or absence of rubella and cytomegalovirus. If ventriculomegaly is severe, if there are significant associated abnormalities, or if there is evidence of intra-uterine infection, aggressive treatment may not be appropriate. In the absence of these factors, fetuses are followed by weekly sonograms. If the size of the ventricles remains stable, the fetus is followed to full-term. If there is cephalo–pelvic disproportion at full-term, caesarean section is the preferred form of delivery. The neonate is evaluated at birth by ultrasound, CT, or magnetic resonance imaging (MRI) and a decision on treatment is made. If hydrocephalus is not confirmed at the initial evaluation, the infant is followed clinically and by serial ultrasonography for signs of hydrocephalus that may occur many months after delivery. Should hydrocephalus develop, a shunting procedure is performed.

If progressive ventriculomegaly is documented by serial ultrasonography, the choice of treatment depends on gestational age and an assessment of the viability of the fetus. In a fetus older than 32 weeks of gestational age, pre-term caesarean section is performed and a postnatal shunt is placed. For fetuses less than 32 weeks of gestational age, the risk of pulmonary immaturity should be weighed against the potential damage that may be caused by progressive ventriculomegaly. At present, we think that there is no evidence to justify placement of a shunt in utero.

Parents should be informed of the current knowledge

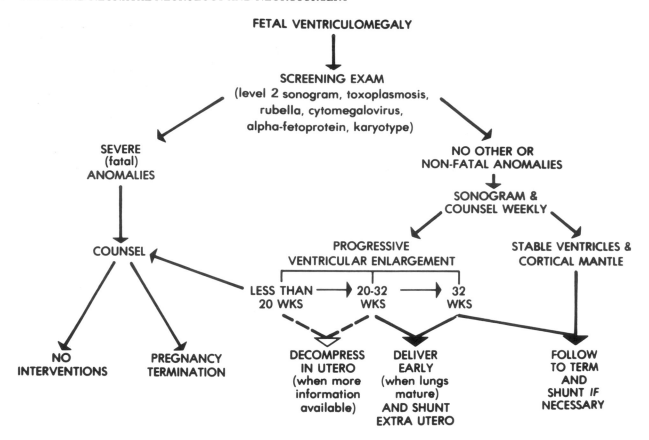

Fig. 45.2 A recommended approach to the management of ventriculomegaly in the fetus. Journal of Pediatrics 105: 97–108

of the natural history of fetal hydrocephalus, the possible aetiology of hydrocephalus in their particular case, the presence or absence of associated abnormalities, and the therapeutic alternatives that include termination of pregnancy for a previable fetus. Emotional support from social workers and/or clergy should be made available to the family. Management should be based on the decision of the parents after consultation with physicians familiar with congenital neurological disorders.

SUMMARY

The aetiology of fetal hydrocephalus is variable and the pathogenesis and natural history are not fully defined. A significant number of fetuses will have severe associated abnormalities that will preclude a functional existence. Ultrasonography is the standard for diagnosis of in-utero hydrocephalus but, even in the best of hands, may not reveal all associated abnormalities. While the results of research in animal models are encouraging, clinical experience with in-utero treatment of hydrocephalus has been disappointing. Difficulties include selection of the appropriate fetus for shunting and the development of reliable shunting systems. Until these problems have been solved, the optimum treatment is delivery of the fetus at a time consistent with available neonatal care, followed by placement of a ventricular shunt in the neonate.

REFERENCES

Barke M W, Scarbough J I, O'Gorman L 1966 Intrauterine ventriculography of the hydrocephalic fetus. Obstetrics and Gynecology 28: 568–570

Birnholz J C, Frigoletto F D 1981 Antenatal treatment of hydrocephalus. New England Journal of Medicine 303: 1021–1023

Burton B K 1979 Recurrence risks for congenital hydrocephalus. Clinical Genetics 16: 47–53

Chervenak F A, Berkowitz R L, Tortura M, Hubbins J C 1985 The management of fetal hydrocephalus. American Journal of Obstetrics and Gynecology 151: 933–942

Clewell W H, Johnson M L, Meier P R et al 1982 A surgical approach to the treatment of fetal hydrocephalus. New England Journal of Medicine 306: 1320–1325

Cochrane D D, Myles S T, Nimrod C, Still D K, Sugarman R G, Wittmann B K 1984 Intrauterine hydrocephalus and ventriculomegaly: associated anomalies and fetal outcome. Canadian Journal of Neurological Sciences 12: 51–59

Depp R, Sabbagha R E, Brown J T, Tamura R K, Reedy N J 1983 Fetal surgery for hydrocephalus: successful in utero ventriculoamniotic shunt for Dandy–Walker syndrome. Obstetrics and Gynecology 61: 710–714

Edwards M S B 1986 An evaluation of the in utero neurosurgical treatment of ventriculomegaly. Clinical Neurosurgery 33: 347–357

Fiske C E, Filly R A, Callen P W 1981 Sonographic measurement of lateral ventricular width in early ventricular dilation. Journal of Clinical Ultrasonography 9: 303–307

Frigoletto F D, Birnholz J C, Greene M F 1982 Antenatal treatment of hydrocephalus by ventriculoamniotic shunting. New England Journal of Medicine 248: 2496–2497

Glick P L, Harrison M R, Nakayama D K et al 1984a Management of ventriculomegaly in the fetus. Journal of Pediatrics 105: 97–108

Glick P L, Harrison M R, Halks-Miller M et al 1984b Correction of congenital hydrocephalus in utero. II. Efficacy of in utero shunting. Journal of Pediatric Surgery 19: 870–881

Kellner K R, Cruz A C, Gelman S R, Vries J K, Spellancy W N 1980 Percutaneous fetal ventriculography. Journal of Reproductive Medicine 24: 225–228

Larson S L, Banner E A 1966 Hydrocephalus: a 30 year survey. Obstetrics and Gynecology 28: 571–577

Lawrence K M, Coates S 1962 The natural history of hydrocephalus. Archives of Disease in Childhood 37: 345–362

McCullogh D C, Balzer-Martin C A 1982 Current prognosis in overt neonatal hydrocephalus. Journal of Neurosurgery 57: 378–383

Manning F A, Lange I R, Morrison I, Harman C 1984 Treatment of the fetus in utero: evolving concepts. Clinics in Obstetrics and Gynaecology 27: 378–390

Manning F A, Harrison M R, Rodeck C 1986 Catheter shunts for fetal hydronephrosis and hydrocephalus. New England Journal of Medicine 315: 336–340

Michejda M, Hodgen G D 1981 In utero diagnosis and treatment of non-human primate fetal skeletal anomalies. I. Hydrocephalus. Journal of the American Medical Association 246: 1093–1109

Miller P, Grünstein S, Gogol G, Simon J 1974 Accidental intrauterine ventriculography during termination of mid trimester pregnancy by boero technique. Neuroradiology 7: 283–285

Nakayama D K, Harrison M R, Berger M S, Chinn D H, Halks-Miller M, Edwards M S 1983 Correction of congenital hydrocephalus in utero. I. The model: intracisternal kaolin produces hydrocephalus in fetal lambs and rhesus monkeys. Journal of Pediatric Surgery 18: 331–338

Pretorius D H, Davis K, Manco-Johnson M L, Manchester D, Meier P R, Clewell W H 1985 Clinical course of hydrocephalus: 40 cases. American Journal of Radiology 144: 827–831

Robertson C H, Lund R R, Soroosh F, Cheatham G R 1969 Percutaneous fetal ventriculography. Obstetrics and Gynecology 34: 841–846

Serlo W, Kirkinen P, Jouppila P, Herva R 1986 Prognostic signs in fetal hydrocephalus. Childs Nervous System 2: 93–97

Venes J L 1983 Management of intrauterine hydrocephalus. Journal of Neurosurgery 58: 793–794 (letter)

Vintzileus A M, Ingardia C J, Nochimson D J 1983 Congenital hydrocephalus: a review and protocol for perinatal management. Obstetrics and Gynecology 62: 539–549

Weller R O, Mitchell J, Griffin R L, Garkner M J 1978 The effects of hydrocephalus upon the developing brain. Journal of the Neurological Sciences 36: 383–402

Williamson R A, Schauberger C W, Varner M W, Aschenbrener C A 1984 Heterogeneity of prenatal onset hydrocephalus: management and counseling implications. American Journal of Medical Genetics 17: 497–508

46. Hydrocephalus

Mr J. Punt

Hydrocephalus is an abnormal accumulation of cerebro-spinal fluid within the cerebral ventricles and cranial subarachnoid space due to an imbalance between production and absorption of cerebrospinal fluid, or to an obstruction to the flow of cerebrospinal fluid. In practice virtually all cases of hydrocephalus seen in humans are due to an obstruc-tive lesion (Russell 1949). The term non-communicating hydrocephalus describes those conditions in which the obstructive lesion is so placed that there is no free communi-cation between the ventricular system and the subarachnoid space. The term communicating hydrocephalus describes those conditions in which the obstructive lesion is outside the brain, thus allowing communication between the cerebral ventricles and at least part of the subarachnoid space. These distinctions are of importance with regard to the differing aetiologies, the radiological appearances and the therapeutic possibilities. Posthaemorrhagic ventricular dilatation, which in some cases progresses to hydrocephalus is discussed separately in Chapter 31.

AETIOLOGY AND PATHOLOGY

The overall incidence of infantile hydrocephalus is given as 3 to 4 per 1000 live births (Milhorat 1978) but this is almost certainly an underestimate. As an isolated congenital disorder the incidence is 0.9 to 1.5 per 1000 births and when associated with myelomeningocele it is 1.3 to 2.9 per 1000 births (Myrianthopoulos & Kurland 1961).

A simple, but practical, classification into those cases due to, or associated with, a cerebral malformation as opposed to those cases due to an acquired lesion is given in Table 46.1. Hydrocephalus has been noted in a large number of syndromes (see p. 251, Ch. 20) but a genetic aetiology for this condition is uncommon. The best-known inherited form of hydrocephalus is the rare X-linked recessive variety (Bickers & Adams 1949, Edwards 1961, Edwards et al 1961) in which a form of aqueduct stenosis described only in males and transmitted by a female carrier occurs. X-linked hydrocephalus accounts for less than 2% of all cases of congenital hydrocephalus. The aetiology of the acquired lesions is usually self-evident.

Aqueduct stenosis

This is by far the most common cause of neonatal hydro-cephalus occurring as a result of cerebral malformation and it accounts for two-thirds of all cases (Milhorat 1972). The apparent pathology in the majority is either stenosis, gliosis or forking of the aqueduct; a simple obstruction is the exception (Russell 1949). There are arguments in favour of at least some cases of aqueduct stenosis being secondary to compression of the midbrain by hydrocephalus which is ini-tially communicating but later produces midbrain distortion (Williams 1973). Aqueduct stenosis is seen in many children with hydrocephalus in association with the dysraphic states, both spinal and cranial (MacFarlane & Maloney 1957). Intraventricular haemorrhage and ventriculitis may lead to aqueductal scarring and closure. The end result is dilatation of the lateral and third ventricles.

Table 46.1 Classification of neonatal hydrocephalus

Malformations
  Aqueduct stenosis
  Dandy–Walker syndrome
  Chiari malformation
  Encephalocele
  Major cerebral malformations (e.g. holoprosencephaly)
  Skull deformities (e.g. craniosynostosis)
Acquired lesions
  Posthaemorrhagic
  Postmeningitic and ventriculitis
  Neoplastic masses
  Non-neoplastic masses

Dandy–Walker syndrome

This condition is also discussed in detail in Chapter 19. It accounts for approximately 13% of cases of neonatal hydrocephalus due to cerebral malformation (Burton 1979). The entire ventricular system is enlarged in association with atresia of the foramina of Luschka and Magendie (Dandy & Blackfan 1914, Dandy 1921, Taggart & Walker 1942). The frequent association of other concomitant cerebral malformations (Hart et al 1972) implies a much more complex pathology than originally envisaged. Congenital absence of the cerebellar vermis and failure of normal regressive processes in the posterior medullary velum leading to cyst formation at the caudal end of the fourth ventricle is now regarded as a more acceptable explanation (Benda 1954). Malformations of the cerebral gyri, agenesis of the corpus callosum and abnormalities of the brainstem are frequently present (Hart et al 1972). Associated extraneuraxial anomalies include heart defects (Huong et al 1975), sclerocornea (March & Chalkley 1974) and renal abnormalities (D'Argostino et al 1963). The Dandy–Walker malformation is recorded in siblings (Nova 1979) and in identical twins (Jenkyn et al 1981).

Hydrocephalus is seen in the majority of children with myelomeningocele and in 60 to 70% of children with occipital encephalocele. Both of these conditions are usually seen in association with the Chiari malformations (p. 271). Hydrocephalus is also observed in many children with major cerebral malformations such as holoprosencephaly (De Myer 1977).

Hydrocephalus of varying degrees and clinical significance is seen in association with some forms of craniosynostosis, usually the cranio–facial dysmorphisms (Fishman et al 1971, Renier et al 1982), platybasia (Sajid & Copple 1968), osteogenesis imperfecta (Frank et al 1982), achondroplasia (Priestley & Lorber 1981) and Hurler's syndrome (Neuhauser et al 1968).

Hydrocephalus may also result from the ependymitis and leptomeningeal scarring that follows intracranial haemorrhage due to parturitional trauma (see Ch. 35) or germinal matrix haemorrhage (see Ch. 28). Intra-uterine infection with toxoplasmosis or cytomegalovirus (Milhorat 1972) or neonatal meningitis (see Ch. 36 and 37) are also potent causes of perinatal hydrocephalus. Other rare causes of hydrocephalus in the fetus and neonate include neoplastic or hamartomatous mass lesions.

CLINICAL FEATURES

The first clinical indication is usually discovery of an abnormally large head circumference at or shortly after birth, or abnormally rapid increases in head growth during the neonatal period either in an otherwise normal baby or in one known to be at risk of developing hydrocephalus. It is important to realize that such a finding merely indicates raised intracranial pressure and does not allow any assumptions to be made about the cause of the raised intracranial pressure, whatever the clinical background. Furthermore, both constitutional macrocephaly and the acceleration in head growth seen in previously malnourished babies who are 'catching up' may be clinically indistinguishable from the macrocephaly of raised intracranial pressure. Megalencephaly, hydranencephaly and certain degenerative disorders, notably Alexander's disease (p. 481), all display macrocephaly.

Later symptoms include bulging of the anterior fontanelle, sutural diastasis, dilatation of scalp veins, irritability, vomiting, sixth nerve palsies, downward deviation of the eyes, bradycardias and bradypnoea. Again these symptoms merely indicate raised intracranial pressure and not the underlying cause.

If the diagnosis is not made in the neonatal period then relative spasticity of the lower limbs or an ataxic gait disturbance may be seen in infancy and childhood. Papilloedema, with or without consecutive optic atrophy, is not a major feature in the neonatal period.

Hydrocephalus in the neonate rarely causes rapidly progressive raised intracranial pressure and the baby with severely advanced intracranial hypertension should be regarded as having a more sinister condition such as chronic subdural effusion, brain abscess or tumour. Epileptic seizures are not a feature of hydrocephalus.

Increasingly, hydrocephalus is discovered by ultrasound scanning in asymptomatic babies in the pre- and postnatal period. Furthermore, ultrasound is used to follow those children at risk of developing progressive ventriculomegaly following germinal matrix or other intracranial haemorrhage, meningitis, or closure of myelomeningocele or encephalocele.

DIAGNOSIS

The great majority of cases can be diagnosed immediately and simply by ultrasound scanning through the anterior fontanelle as described in Chapter 9. Rarely computerized tomography (CT) scanning and magnetic resonance imaging (MRI) will be required to resolve diagnostic difficulties. The very occasional case of hydranencephaly may be resolved only on cerebral angiography. Some cases of hydrocephalus in association with intracranial cysts may require CT ventriculography following shunt insertion. Radio-isotope ventriculography has been described in Chapter 31 as a means of distinguishing between communicating and non-communicating hydrocephalus.

MANAGEMENT

The management of hydrocephalus in the special circumstances of the child still in utero, following germinal matrix haemorrhage and in association with acute pyogenic meningitis and ventriculitis, has been discussed in detail in Chapter 45 and will not be reiterated; neither will the non-surgical management which is reviewed in Chapter 31. This chapter is concerned with the surgical aspects of management.

The objective in the surgical management of infantile hydrocephalus is the symptomatic relief of raised intracranial pressure so as to minimize the risks of neurological handicap, developmental delay and unsightly macrocephaly. Experiments on laboratory animals showing ultrastructural changes in the periventricular tissues notwithstanding (Weller & Wisniewski 1969, Weller et al 1971, Wozniak et al 1975), neuronal destruction is a late consequence of hydrocephalus. The finding of ventriculomegaly by imaging techniques is not therefore in itself an indication for surgical intervention; there needs to be either radiological evidence of progression or clinical evidence of adverse effects attributable to the hydrocephalus. In particular, in the case of premature babies with posthaemorrhagic ventriculomegaly following germinal matrix haemorrhage, it is unproven whether early surgical intervention, based purely on ultrasound appearances, influences the neurological outcome.

As essentially all human hydrocephalus is obstructive in nature, the ideal remedy would be removal of the obstruction; however, with the exception of the very occasional cerebral tumour this is rarely feasible.

Choroid plexectomy

This was first described in 1918 (Dandy 1918) as an open procedure and, more recently, introduced by endoscopic coagulation (Scarff 1979). It usually is a dangerous and unsuccessful procedure.

Third ventriculostomy

This technique, originally devised in 1922 by Dandy, has also again found favour with some (Hoffman et al 1981) in the treatment of aqueductal stenosis but has not gained universal popularity; when successful it carries the great advantage of obviating the need for a ventricular shunt.

Ventricular shunt

The mainstay of modern management of infantile hydrocephalus is the ventricular shunt, introduced in 1951 (Nulsen & Spitz 1961, Pudenz 1980). The decision to insert a shunt should result from a close collaboration between the physician and the surgeon, who should agree that the benefit that may accrue outweighs the risks of complications for any particular child. Similarly the timing of operation is a point of clinical nicety, especially in the premature baby with posthaemorrhagic ventriculomegaly or the child with neonatal meningitis. In both cases temporizing by medical means such as acetazolamide or lumbar puncture taps may be valuable, allowing the general condition of the baby to improve. This may permit the infant to be temporarily discharged from the neonatal intensive care unit with its potentially hazardous bacterial environment and achieve a short period at home with the parents. Prolonged medical treatment rarely avoids a shunt altogether except in babies with posthaemorrhagic ventriculomegaly (see Ch. 31).

In the period immediately before shunting it is crucial that the condition of the child's skin is considered; scalp vein needles must be avoided, especially in the posterior part of the head. Napkin rashes, and in particular any candidal infection, must be eradicated; the skin along the proposed path of the shunt, usually the anterior chest and abdominal wall, must be left entirely free of monitoring electrodes as these damage the epidermis and increase bacterial contamination. Any other focus of infection must be controlled, as all of these factors greatly increase the risk of shunt infection (Renier et al 1984).

The physician, and indeed the inexperienced surgeon, may be justifiably bewildered by the wide variety of shunt devices now available and by lengthy debates on the physical characteristics of their performance (Portnoy 1982). These considerations can be safely ignored; in practice the surgeon should gain familiarity with one, preferably simple, device and stick with it. Of much greater importance is the choice of the route of shunting. Although ventriculo–atrial shunting was the first to be regularly successful, the need for regular revision due to growth of the child and the serious nature of the complications experienced with this route, especially nephritis, systemic sepsis, venous thrombosis, and fatal pulmonary hypertension (Forrest & Cooper 1968, Strenger 1963, Nugent et al 1966), render this route highly undesirable. In essence ventriculo–peritoneal shunts require fewer revisions and the late complications are much less serious. This is the only route that should be employed in children (Keucher & Mealey 1979).

The operative surgery of shunt insertion will not be considered, except to state a personal opinion that shunt surgery, especially in infants, should be carried out by experienced and interested surgeons and operations should be conducted swiftly so as to minimize the risk of colonization of the shunt and to reduce heat loss from the baby. Operations should be performed in a properly equipped operating room rather than a sideroom adjacent to the neonatal intensive care unit and there must be facilities on site for continuing appropriate medical care of the baby, including respiratory support for premature babies. As with all neonatal surgery the highest anaesthetic skills are mandatory.

Lumbo–peritoneal shunting is advocated by some for the treatment of children with communicating hydrocephalus (Hoffman et al 1976). Early complications are relatively few but late complications can be tiresome, including spinal deformity, arachnoiditis and slit ventricles. It is not widely performed in infancy.

Postoperatively the child is handled and fed normally. Some premature babies who have only recently become ventilator-independent may require a few days of assisted ventilation. Routine follow-up scans are not required if the child remains well and without signs of intracranial hypertension. The shunt track is examined daily for the first week; bruising is permissible but any inflammation indicates an acute infection and only immediate shunt removal will prevent potentially damaging ventriculitis. Malnourished premature babies should be provided with protection when lying on the side of the shunt for several weeks and prolonged pressure on the cranial end should be avoided otherwise decubitus ulceration may result with inevitable shunt infection.

Follow-up should occur jointly with the neurosurgeon and the physician, preferably in a combined clinic. The parents should be instructed throughout on the changing symptoms of shunt malfunction, as the child matures. Shunt revision is only undertaken for symptomatic malfunction. Routine digital pumping by parents and attendants is unnecessary and undesirable.

COMPLICATIONS

The catalogue of shunt complications is extensive and well documented (Keucher & Mealey 1979) and includes obstruction, infection, ulceration of the overlying skin, perforation of viscera, disconnection of components, fracture of tubing, subdural effusions, slit ventricles, secondary craniosynostosis, peritoneal cyst formation and many others. Only the most frequently encountered and the most significant will be considered here.

Obstruction

Obstruction of the shunt occurring soon after insertion most frequently results from poor positioning of the ventricular catheter. Early re-opening of the wound (within 10 days of surgery) is deprecated as infection of the shunt will inevitably result: it is preferable to insert a second shunt through fresh incisions. Early obstruction of the peritoneal end may result from extraperitoneal placement of the tubing. Late obstruction of the peritoneal end will occur with growth if only short peritoneal catheters are used: I insert the same total length of peritoneal catheter into all infants

as into older children and have not, as yet, encountered any disadvantages from this practice.

Infection

This is the most serious complication encountered in infancy as, even in the absence of frank ventriculitis, it relates strongly to poor ultimate intellect (McLone et al 1982). Infection rates of up to 20% (Renier et al 1984) are reported and for premature babies I have encountered those who privately acknowledge rates of up to 50% in this group. In the most fortunate hands the incidence has, however, declined and rates of less than 3% are now achieved by specialist paediatric neurosurgeons (O'Brien et al 1979). Identifiable aetiological factors include very young age, poor skin condition, intercurrent sites of infection and technical inexperience on behalf of the surgeon (Renier et al 1984). Acute postoperative infection is heralded by malaise, fever and occasionally seizures and can be confirmed by examination of cerebrospinal fluid aspirated from the shunt reservoir. Chronic colonization most frequently presents as intermittent shunt malfunction, perhaps accompanied by mild fever. Cerebrospinal fluid taken from the shunt may be sterile and the causative organism may only be obtained by culture of the shunt tubing. The finding of a loculus of fluid around the tip of the peritoneal catheter is highly suggestive of colonization, as are frequent unexplained episodes of malfunction. Blood cultures are usually unhelpful in the diagnosis of colonized ventriculo–peritoneal shunts.

Although treatment of shunt infection by intensive intravenous and intrashunt antibiotics without shunt removal has been successful for some surgeons (Wald & McLaurin 1980) most practitioners have found the technique to be associated with an unacceptably high failure rate (Forward et al 1983). The majority of cases are treated by shunt removal, intravenous antibiotics and shunt reinsertion through fresh incisions after an interval. It is important to obtain accurate microbiological diagnosis and to employ high doses of antibiotics likely to penetrate the blood–cerebrospinal fluid barrier (Frane & McLaurin 1982). For the occasional child in whom further shunt surgery would be most undesirable, medical treatment may be attempted. The prerequisites for this form of treatment are that the shunt is functioning, there should be no loose, free-floating items of shunt hardware, accurate microbiological diagnosis and antibiotic sensitivities are available, and high-dose antibiotics (intravenous and intrashunt) are administered until the cerebrospinal fluid becomes bactericidal to the infecting organism at a titre of 1:8 when tested in vitro. At least two antibiotics should be used and treatment continued for three weeks from the time of achieving bactericidal levels in the cerebrospinal fluid. Traditional therapy by removal, interval antibiotics and reinsertion is frequently simpler, quicker and cheaper.

The infecting organism is usually *Staphylococcus epidermidis*, occasionally *Staphylococcus aureus* and less frequently coliforms, *Pseudomonas*, *Klebsiella* or *Candida*. Premature babies on neonatal intensive care units may well harbour multiply resistant organisms.

The slit-ventricle syndrome

This is a late complication of ventricular shunting occurring in approximately 5% of children; it is particularly common in those shunted in very early life and appears to relate to chronic over-drainage of the ventricles with subsequent stiffening of the ventricular walls so that ventriculomegaly does not occur in the face of shunt malfunction. These children typically deteriorate very rapidly if the shunt obstructs. A useful therapeutic manoeuvre is subtemporal decompression which reduces the frequency of obstruction and makes revision of the ventricular catheter easier by permitting slight ventricular dilatation (Epstein et al 1978).

Trapped ventricle

Isolated dilatation of a trapped ventricle may occur in hydrocephalus, resulting from germinal matrix haemorrhage (Eller & Pasternak 1985), from neonatal meningitis (Kalsbeck et al 1980) and in association with myelomeningocele (Scotti et al 1980). Either lateral or fourth ventricles may be affected. The symptoms include recurrence of raised intracranial pressure, accentuation of pre-existing focal neurological signs and the appearance of a brainstem syndrome. The condition emphasizes the importance of full radiological evaluation of children with shunts at times of recurrent or new neurological symptoms.

OUTCOME

Since the introduction of modern shunting devices and with greater understanding of shunt complications and management, 95% of shunted children survive for 10 years and 70% of these have normal intelligence (Milhorat 1972). This report, however, did not include significant numbers of infants shunted for posthaemorrhagic hydrocephalus. Of those who have impaired intellect, neurodevelopmental delay or frank neurological handicap, the deficits relate either to shunt complications, especially infection (McLone et al 1982), or to the process that has produced the hydrocephalus. In this regard neonates who have suffered Grade III or Grade IV intraventricular haemorrhage, or pyogenic meningitis, fare relatively badly (see Ch. 28 and 37). Children with aqueductal stenosis have an excellent prognosis while those with Dandy–Walker syndrome do badly, 70% having a degree of mental handicap with an IQ less than 83 (Sawaya & McLaurin 1981). Although the thickness of the cerebral mantle correlates variably with ultimate intellectual function, it appears that for most children with hydrocephalus uncomplicated by other factors, IQ will be normal if a cerebral mantle of 3 cm or more is achieved by the age of four or five months (Nulsen & Rekate 1982).

It should be fully appreciated that although many of the processes that produce hydrocephalus in the neonatal period carry a significant risk of handicap, the option of not placing a shunt in the face of progressive and symptomatic ventriculomegaly is usually not a realistic one. The neonatal neurosurgeon must accept that shunt placement in such children can be an important palliative measure and should not reject them out of hand because of the likelihood of a less than perfect developmental outcome.

REFERENCES

Benda C E 1954 The Dandy–Walker syndrome or the so-called atresia of the foramen Magendie. Journal of Neuropathology and Experimental Neurology 13: 14–29

Burton B K 1979 Recurrence risks for congenital hydrocephalus. Clinical Genetics 16: 47–53

D'Agostino A N, Kernohan J W, Brown J R 1963 The Dandy–Walker syndrome. Journal of Neuropathology and Experimental Neurology 22: 450–470

Dandy W E 1918 Extirpation of the choroid plexus of the lateral ventricles in communicating hydrocephalus. Annals of Surgery 68: 569–579

Dandy W E 1921 The diagnosis and treatment of hydrocephalus due to occlusions of the foramina of Magendie and Luschka. Surgery, Gynecology and Obstetrics 32: 112–124

Dandy W E 1922 An operative procedure for hydrocephalus. Johns Hopkins Hospital Bulletin 33: 189

Dandy W E, Blackfan K D 1914 Internal hydrocephalus: an experimental clinical and pathological study. American Journal of Diseases of Children 8: 406–482

De Myer W 1977 Holoprosencephaly (cyclopia–arrhinencephaly). In: Vinken P J, Bruyn G W (eds) Congenital malformations of the brain and skull, Part I. Handbook of Clinical Neurology, Vol. 30. Elsevier, Amsterdam, pp 431–478

Edwards J H 1961 The syndrome of sex-linked hydrocephalus. Archives of Disease in Childhood 36: 486–493

Edwards J H, Norman R M, Roberts J M 1961 Sex-linked hydrocephalus: report of a family with 15 affected members. Archives of Disease in Childhood 36: 482–485

Eller T W, Pasternak J F 1985 Isolated ventricles following intraventricular hemorrhage. Journal of Neurosurgery 62: 357–362

Epstein F, Marlin A E, Wald A 1978 Chronic headache in the shunt-dependent adolescent with nearly normal ventricular volume: diagnosis and treatment. Neurosurgery 3: 351–355

Fishman M A, Hogan G R, Dodge P R 1971 The concurrence of hydrocephalus and craniosynostosis. Journal of Neurosurgery 34: 621–629

Forrest D M, Cooper D G N 1968 Complications of ventriculo–atrial shunts: a review of 455 cases. Journal of Neurosurgery 29: 506–512

Forward K R, Fewer D, Stiver H G 1983 Cerebrospinal fluid shunt infections: a review of 35 infections in 32 patients. Journal of Neurosurgery 59: 389–394

Frane P T, McLaurin R L 1982 Antibiotic therapy in central nervous system infections. In: Pediatric neurosurgery: surgery of the developing nervous system. Grune & Stratton, New York, pp 591–599

Frank E, Bersert, Tew J M Jr 1982 Basilar impression and platybasia in osteogenesis imperfecta tarda. Surgical Neurology 17: 116–119

Hart M N, Malumud N, Ellis W G 1972 The Dandy–Walker syndrome: a clinicopathological study based on 28 cases. Neurology 22: 771–780

Hoffman H J, Hendrick E B, Humphreys R P 1976 New lumboperitoneal shunt for communicating hydrocephalus (technical note). Journal of Neurosurgery 44: 258–261

Hoffman H J, Harwood-Nash D, Gilday D L, Crauen M A 1981 Percutaneous third ventriculostomy in the management of non-communicating hydrocephalus. In: Concepts in pediatric neurosurgery, Vol. I (American Society for Pediatric Neurosurgery). Karger, Basel, pp 87–106

Huong T T, Goldblatt E, Simpson D A 1975 Dandy–Walker syndrome associated with congenital heart defects: report of three cases. Developmental Medicine and Child Neurology 17 (suppl 35): 35–41

Jenkyn L R, Roberts D W, Merlis A L, Razycki A A, Nordgren R F L 1981 Dandy–Walker malformation in identical twins. Neurology (New York) 31: 337–341

Kalsbeck J E, DeSouza A L, Kleiman M B, Goodman J M, Franken E A 1980 Compartmentalization of the cerebral ventricles as a sequela of neonatal meningitis. Journal of Neurosurgery 52: 547–552

Keucher T R, Mealey J Jr 1979 Longterm results after ventriculoatrial and ventriculoperitoneal shunting for infantile hydrocephalus. Journal of Neurosurgery 50: 179–186

MacFarlane A, Maloney A F J 1957 The appearance of the aqueduct and its relationship to hydrocephalus in the Arnold–Chiari malformation. Brain 80: 479–491

McLone D, Czyzewski D, Raimondi A J 1982 The effects of complications on intellectual function in 173 children with myelomeningocele. Cited by Reigel D J Spina bifida, in Pediatric neurosurgery: surgery of the developing nervous system. Grune & Stratton, New York, pp 23–47

March W F, Chalkley T H F 1974 Sclerocornea associated with Dandy–Walker cyst. American Journal of Ophthalmology 78: 54–57

Milhorat T H 1972 In: Hydrocephalus and the cerebrospinal fluid. Williams & Wilkins, Baltimore

Milhorat T H 1978 In: Pediatric neurosurgery. Daris, Philadelphia

Myrianthopoulos N C, Kurland L T 1961 Present concepts of the epidemiology and genetics of hydrocephalus. In: Fields W J, Desmond M M (eds) Disorders of the developing nervous system. Charles Thomas, Springfield, Illinois, pp 187–202

Neuhauser E B D, Griscom N T, Gilles N H, Crocker A C 1968 Arachnoid cysts in the Hurler–Hunter syndrome (Kystes arachnoidicus dans le syndrome de Hurler–Hunter). Annals de Radiologie (Paris) II: 453–469

Nova H R 1979 Familial communicating hydrocephalus, posterior cerebellar agenesis, mega cisterna magna, and port wine nevi: report of five members of one family. Journal of Neurosurgery 51: 862–865

Nugent G R, Lucas R, Judy M, Bloor B M, Warden H 1966 Thromboembolic complications of ventriculoatrial shunts: angiographic and pathologic correlation. Journal of Neurosurgery 24: 34–42

Nulsen F E, Rekate H L 1982 Results of treatment for hydrocephalus as a guide to future management. In: Pediatric neurosurgery: surgery of the developing nervous system. Grune & Stratton, New York, pp 229–241

Nulsen F E, Spitz E B 1951 Treatment of hydrocephalus by direct shunt from ventricle to jugular vein. Surgical Forums 2: 399–403

O'Brien M, Parent A, Davis B 1979 Management of ventricular shunt infections. Child's Brain 5: 304–309

Portnoy H D 1982 Hydrodynamics of shunts. In: Choux M (ed) Problems in shunts. Monographs in Neural Sciences, Vol. 8. Karger, Basel, pp 173–183

Priestley B L, Lorber J 1987 Ventricular size and intelligence in achondroplasia. Zeitschrift fur Kinderchirurgie und Grenzgebiete 34: 320–326

Pudenz R H 1980 The surgical treatment of hydrocephalus: an historical view. Surgical Neurology 15: 15–26

Renier D, Sainte-Rose C, Marchac D, Hirsch J F 1982 Intracranial pressure in craniosynostosis. Journal of Neurosurgery 57: 370–377

Renier D, Lacombe J, Pierre-Kahn A, Sainte-Rose C, Hirsch J F 1984 Factors causing shunt infection: computer analysis of 1174 operations. Journal of Neurosurgery 61: 1072–1078

Russell D S 1949 Observations on the pathology of hydrocephalus. Special Reports and Services of the Medical Research Council, No. 265. HMSO, London

Sajid M H, Copple P J 1968 Familial aqueductal stenosis and basilar impression. Neurology (Minneap.) 18: 260–262

Sawaya R, McLaurin R L 1981 Dandy–Walker syndrome: clinical analysis of 23 cases. Journal of Neurosurgery 55: 89–98

Scarff J E 1970 The treatment of non-obstructive (communicating) hydrocephalus by endoscopic cauterization of the choroid plexuses. Journal of Neurosurgery 33: 1–18

Scotti G, Musgrave M A, Fitz C R, Harwood-Nash D C 1980 The isolated fourth ventricle in children: CT and clinical review of 16 cases. American Journal of Radiology 135: 1233–1238

Strenger L 1963 Complications of ventriculovenous shunts. Journal of Neurosurgery 20: 219–224

Taggart J K Jr, Walker A E 1942 Congenital atresia of the foramens of Luschka and Magendie. Archives of Neurology and Psychiatry 48: 583–612

Ward S L, McLaurin R L 1980 Cerebrospinal fluid antibiotic levels during treatment of shunt infections. Journal of Neurosurgery 52: 41–46

Weller R O, Wisniewski H 1969 Histological and ultrastructural changes with experimental hydrocephalus in adult rabbits. Brain 92: 819–828

Weller R O, Wisniewski H, Shulman K, Terry R D 1971 Experimental hydrocephalus in young dogs: histological and ultrastructural study of the brain tissue damage. Journal of Neuropathology and Experimental Neurology 30: 613–627

Williams B 1973 Is aqueduct stenosis a result of hydrocephalus? Brain 96: 399–412

Wozniak M, McLone D G, Raimondi A J 1975 Micro- and macrovascular changes as the direct cause of parenchymal destruction in congenital murine hydrocephalus. Journal of Neurosurgery 43: 535–545

47. Congenital defects, vascular malformations and other lesions

Mr J. Punt

SCALP AND SKULL ABNORMALITIES

Aplasia cutis congenita

This is an unusual condition first described in 1826 (Campbell 1826) in which a variably sized scalp defect is associated with an underlying skull defect in 20% of cases and skin defects on the trunk and limbs in 25% of cases (Vinocur et al 1976). The aetiology is unknown although familial cases, usually autosomal dominant and more rarely recessive, are recorded (McMurray et al 1977). In those with multiple congenital anomalies chromosomal abnormalities may be found, as in trisomy D in which 35% of cases have aplasia cutis. There is a known association with monozygotic fetus papyraceous (Mannino et al 1977). The scalp lesions are usually 1–2 cm in size and situated over the parietal part of the vertex (Fig. 47.1); they may be multiple and very extensive. If the skull is absent the dura is also frequently missing, arachnoid forming the base of the lesion. Associated anomalies may affect many systems including the brain (holoprosencephaly, hydrocephalus), spinal cord (myelomeningocele), skull base (aplastic sphenoid wing), genitourinary system (absent and polycystic kidneys, ambiguous genitalia, double uterus) and limb bones (Cutlip et al 1967).

The principal concerns are the dangers of infection and haemorrhage; the latter may prove fatal if the superior sagittal sinus is involved. Excision and primary repair, using complex full-thickness skin grafts if necessary, have been advised in the past, followed by cranioplasty at a later age to repair the skull defect. These procedures, hampered by the limited availability of donor sites in the neonate, have not infrequently been complicated by meningitis, haemorrhage, occlusion of the superior sagittal sinus, cortical damage and a surgical mortality of up to 30%. Conservative management with dressings kept moist with sterile saline has proved successful even for huge full-thickness lesions, spontaneous healing of skin and skull defects being observed (Muakkassa et al 1982). This approach, fastidiously avoiding desiccation, is I think favourable. Any remaining bone defect can be repaired at the age of 5 years by calvarial grafting.

Congenital skull defects

The most frequently encountered congenital skull defects are parietal foramina which occur less than once in 25 000 live births (Robinson 1962). The cause is unknown. The anomaly consists of symmetrically placed, paired defects 1–2 cm in diameter at the site of emissary veins on either side of the midline in the mid- to posterior parietal region.

Over the first 5 years of life the defects become relatively smaller as the rest of the calvarium grows. They have no

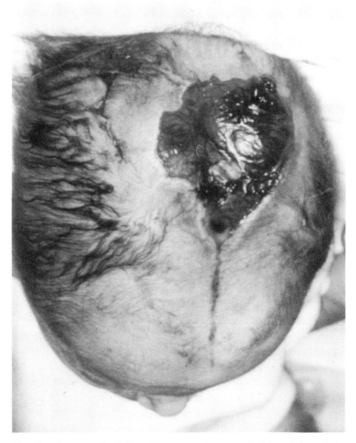

Fig. 47.1 Large scalp defect. There was also an underlying defect of the skull and agenesis of the corpus callosum.

serious significance but reassurance is required, especially if pulsatile venous channels are prominent. If anxiety persists, especially regarding the risk of injury, the defects can be closed at the age of 3–5 years using calvarial grafts.

Agenesis of the sphenoid wing is a rare abnormality producing painless, pulsatile and usually mild and non-progressive proptosis (Dandy 1929, Le Wald 1933). This occurs as mesodermal manifestations of neurofibromatosis in 50% of cases (Matson 1969). The lesion is usually of cosmetic significance only and if desired can be repaired at craniotomy at or after the age of 5 years. Cranioplasty using autogenous ribs or calvarium is performed: it is crucial to plicate the underlying middle fossa dura to avoid erosion of the bone graft.

Dermoid cysts and sinuses

Incomplete separation of the epithelial ectoderm in the fourth week of gestation results in a lesion lined with stratified squamous epithelium and containing hair follicles and sebaceous and sweat glands (Lekias & Stokes 1970).

Continuous production of sebaceous matter and epithelial desquamation produces a slowly expanding lesion with or without an associated discharging skin sinus. When skin sinus is present, superadded infection produces inflammatory changes which significantly reduce the possibilities for total excision and eradication. In those with an intradural component, recurrent episodes of meningitis, septic or chemical, may occur. Dermoids may occupy all or any of the layers of the neuraxis from the skin to the brain and it is this possibility of intracranial extension that occasions concern and demands proper neurosurgical attention. The risk of intracranial extension relates to the site of the lesion, principally those lesions occurring over the occipital bone, at the nasion and along the line of the nose. For lesions in these sites nothing less than full neuroradiological evaluation with CT of the brain and skull base is adequate. Under no circumstances should partial excision of the cutaneous element alone by a general, plastic or ear, nose and throat surgeon be permitted as this regularly precipitates serious intracranial sepsis if an unrecognized intracranial portion is left behind. Excision should be performed by a neurosurgeon fully prepared to pursue the lesion intracranially to its anatomical conclusion. In occipital dermoid sinuses the track always takes a caudal direction and may even traverse the brainstem.

The most common location is over the anterior fontanelle, especially in black children (Wong et al 1986). Happily dermoids at this site never extend intradurally and can be safely excised without any prior special investigation (Pannell et al 1982). Care should be taken, however, to avoid damaging the superior sagittal sinus which lies in the underlying skull defect. Although typically midline, dermoids are also seen over the parietal eminence, at the lateral canthus of the orbit and over the root of the mastoid

process, usually at the site of cranial sutures (Pannell et al 1982). Investigation, where indicated, and elective excision are recommended in the first few months of life. Clinically indistinguishable lesions that I have encountered at the anterior fontanelle include histiocytosis and angiofibroma.

Craniosynostosis

Craniosynostosis describes a very wide range of conditions in which one or more of the cranial sutures becomes functionally obliterated or ossified at a premature stage in the growth of the skull with the result that, during the most rapid period of brain growth in the first 6 months of extra-uterine life, the skull vault expands asymmetrically (Virchow 1851). The resultant deformity is characteristic of the pattern of sutural fusion involved.

In the most complex forms the facial skeleton is also implicated and the more correct term cranio–facial dysmorphism applies. The cause is unknown but primary abnormality of the skull base commencing in utero and producing abnormal tensile forces in the convexity dura has been suggested (Moss 1959). There are at least 17 syndromes of cranio–facial dysmorphism with differing genetic characteristics and a wide range of associated somatic anomalies (Hoffman 1979).

The overall incidence of all forms of craniosynostosis is 1 in 2000 of the population (Andersson 1977). Sagittal synostosis occurs four times as frequently in males as in females; coronal synostosis affects females slightly more often than males. Caucasians considerably outnumber black- and yellow-skinned children.

Isolated sagittal synotosis comprises 60% of all cases; unilateral coronal synostosis 18%; bilateral coronal synostosis 12%; metopic synostosis 4%: involvement of three or more sutures occurs in 18% of cases (Matson 1969). Lambdoid synostosis has only more recently been fully recognized (Hinter et al 1984).

Appropriate management commences with recognition of the condition shortly after birth. This depends essentially upon the clinical acumen of the neonatal physician who must not succumb to the temptation to attribute the deformity to moulding, forceps delivery, cephalhaematoma or prematurity through a misguided desire to reassure the parents that their newborn is normal. Plain skull radiographs, occasionally supplemented by radio-isotope bone imaging with technetium, will demonstrate the synostosed sutures but the most profitable investigation is an informed neurosurgical opinion, which should be obtained early in the neonatal period so that the parents may receive the correct advice and appropriately timed surgical treatment may be planned.

The deformities are characteristic: sagittal synostosis produces a long scaphocephalic head, often narrow posteriorly, with bulging of the frontal bones and a palpable, and often visible, ridge along the line of the sagittal suture (Fig.

47.2a). Unilateral coronal synostosis leads to plagiocephaly with asymmetrical flattening of the forehead, supra-orbital recession and deviation of the nasion; bilateral coronal synostosis results in brachycephaly with an elevated forehead which (Fig. 47.2b), in the cranio–facial dysmorphisms, is associated with ocular hypertelorism, proptosis, midface deformity and frequent concomitant peripheral anomalies (such as polysyndactyly) in up to 60% of cases.

Metopic synostosis causes a keel-shaped forehead deformity called trigonocephaly. Lambdoid synostosis produces flattening of the affected side of the back of the head and when unilateral the compensatory expansion of the ipsilateral frontal bone may be mistaken for a contralateral coronal synostosis; the pinnae are asymmetrical. Cranioscoliosis is a benign but confusing condition (quite different from craniosynostosis) recognized by viewing the child's head from above and appreciating that one half of the cranium, including the maxilla, is further forward than its fellows but the two halves are symmetrical. No treatment is required, or indeed is effective. In the very rare total craniostenosis the head circumference is very small and there may be severe proptosis. A variant of this condition in which all the sutures are closed (except the squamosal suture) produces the bizarre clover-leaf skull deformity in which there is pronounced bulging of the temporal bones.

Further investigation with computerized tomography (CT) scanning of the brain and skull base is only required for those children with bilateral coronal synostosis and cranio–facial dysmorphism. It provides further documentation of the skull base anatomy and any associated hydrocephalus or cerebral malformation.

Advanced computer software packages have been developed to produce three-dimensional bone images which can be used for planning operative strategies in the more complex cases.

It is important to appreciate that only in bilateral coronal synostosis (especially when part of a cranio–facial dysmorphism), or in total craniostenosis and clover-leaf

skull is there a major risk of retardation of brain growth; some cranio–facial syndromes are associated with severe proptosis placing the eyes at risk. Hydrocephalus contributes to raised intracranial pressure in some cranio–facial syndromes. Raised intracranial pressure has been documented in many of these more complex conditions but only rarely in cases of fusion of a single suture (Hirsch et al 1981). The parents of the child with simple sagittal, unilateral coronal or lambdoid synostosis can be reassured that brain growth and intellectual development should be normal.

The principle of treatment is to open the fused suture releasing the restrained portion of the skull, capitalizing on the rapid growth of the brain to remould the head into a normal shape. To this end early surgery brings the best results. For all cases, except the cranio–facial dysmorphic syndromes, surgery is advised as soon as the child has regained birth-weight.

The major prerequisites are therefore: prompt diagnosis and referral in the neonatal period; skilled anaesthesia and diligent postoperative nursing to ensure adequate blood volume replacement; and a good surgical technique to minimize blood loss and operating time.

Sagittal and lambdoid synostosis are treated by excision of the affected suture and wide craniectomy with insertion of silastic sheets over the cut bone edges (Shillito 1973, Muakkassa et al 1984). For lambdoid synostosis some surgeons advocate resection of the lateral end of the petrous bone to unhitch the dura (Rekate 1985) but this is probably unnecessary.

Simple unilateral or bilateral coronal synostosis without hypertelorism or facial deformity responds well to lateral canthal advancement (Hoffman & Mohr 1976) in which excision of the affected coronal suture is combined with a craniectomy into the middle cranial fossa, creation of a free frontal bone flap and mobilization of the supra-orbital margin.

The cranio–facial dysmorphisms are treated by more complex combined techniques as introduced by Tessier (1967) in which multiple osteotomies to correct hypertelorism and the maxillary deformities are combined with forehead advancement. These procedures are the domain of highly specialized cranio–facial teams and are best postponed until infancy or early childhood.

Extensive multiple sutural closure and total craniostenosis are treated by morcellation craniotomy in which extensive free calvarial flaps are mobilized and prevented from refusing by interposition of silastic sheeting.

The cosmetic results of appropriate treatment are now excellent. The recognition of raised intracranial pressure, and the treatment of hydrocephalus in some cases, has led to preservation of intellectual potential. No excuse is made for reiterating the necessity for early diagnosis and neurosurgical referral and if in doubt the neonatal physician should not hesitate to seek an informed and interested opinion.

a   **b**

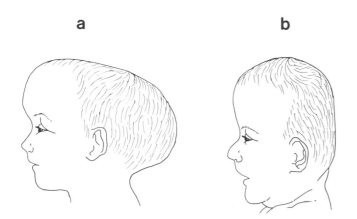

Fig. 47.2 Typical head configuration in craniosynostosis. (**a**) Sagittal craniosynostosis with scaphocephaly. (**b**) Bilateral coronal synostosis showing the characteristic brachycephalic head shape.

INTRACRANIAL INFECTIONS

Consequences of meningitis

The major aspects of neonatal meningitis have been covered in Section 10 and here only those aspects will be considered in which neurosurgical involvement is required. Such consequences are particularly frequent when pyogenic meningitis occurs in the first 2 months of life (Overall 1970) and sequelae are especially severe in the pre-term and low-birth-weight baby (Karan 1986).

Hydrocephalus

This is observed in 30% of cases of neonatal meningitis at some stage of the illness (Karan 1986). It may occur as an early phenomenon when it is usually indicative of either a partially treated infection or an infection with an unusual organism such as listeria, *Salmonella*, active toxoplasmosis or fungi.

Clinical recognition of an unusual degree of tenseness of the fontanelle, abnormally large head circumference or particularly poor neurological state indicates the need for cranial ultrasound examination which reveals the ventriculomegaly. The management consists of establishment of an accurate microbiological diagnosis by examination of lumbar and ventricular CSF and introduction of intravenous antibiotics in high and prolonged dosage. Unless there is frank ventriculitis, as judged by the cell count and glucose level in the ventricular CSF, there is no advantage in giving intraventricular antibiotics to all cases (McCracken & Mize 1976, McCracken 1977). Ventricular shunting is often not required and in any event should be delayed until the child is less acutely ill and preferably until the infection is controlled. If, however, raised intracranial pressure from progressive ventriculomegaly becomes a clinical problem in the acute stage then control by anterior fontanelle punctures or by placement of a ventriculostomy reservoir is preferable to an external ventricular drain with its attendant hazards of further infection with other organisms. When hydrocephalus is recognized early in the illness the child should be monitored by cranial ultrasound every 5–7 days during the acute phase.

Hydrocephalus may also develop after 1–2 weeks of intravenous chemotherapy when it is usually associated with persistent, or intermittent, fever and malaise and it is then almost invariably a manifestation of ventriculitis which, if not promptly recognized and treated appropriately, is a common cause of therapeutic failure (Salmon 1972). Assessment of the ventricular CSF in terms of cell count, glucose level, Gram stain and culture is vital, together with a review of the chemotherapy with an interested and involved microbiologist (see Ch. 37). Microorganisms may continue to multiply in, and be cultured from, the ventricular CSF even when the lumbar CSF is sterile (McCracken 1977, Salmon 1972). Intraventricular antibiotics are given by daily intraventricular instillation either through the anterior fontanelle or through a ventriculostomy reservoir and, if indicated, the intravenous antibiotics are changed or augmented. The ventricular CSF is examined to establish that bactericidal levels of antibiotics to the child's own organism have been achieved. When this is established antibiotics are continued by both intravenous and intraventricular routes for 2 weeks. The daily removal of 10 to 20 ml of CSF usually controls the intracranial pressure: the fontanelle punctures are made on alternate sides on alternate days and it is important to place a suture across the puncture sites to prevent leakage of CSF and secondary infection.

When 2 weeks of therapy is completed and if there has been a satisfactory response in terms of fever resolution, CSF cell count and the general state of the baby, then all chemotherapy is stopped and both lumbar and ventricular CSF re-examined after 48 hours. If ventricular shunting is required to control progressive ventriculomegaly it can be proceeded with at this stage.

Finally, hydrocephalus, manifested by an abnormally rapid rate of head growth and other signs of raised intracranial pressure, may occur over the months following successful antibacterial treatment of pyogenic meningitis as a result of fibrosis of the leptomeninges consequent upon purulent exudate in the basal cisterns in the acute stage (Volpe 1981). Ventricular shunt placement is indicated without delay, beyond confirming the diagnosis by cranial ultrasound examination. During treatment of any neonate with meningitis it is important to avoid the placement of intravenous cannulae into scalp veins, especially over the posterior half of the cranuim, as this will render the scalp in a poor condition for shunt placement should this become necessary.

The prognosis in terms of neurodevelopmental sequelae relates to the extent of cerebral infarction rather than to the occurrence of hydrocephalus (Albanese et al 1981) but overall 65% make a good recovery (McCracken 1972, 1977).

The management of the hydrocephalus may be complicated by the development of compartmentalization of the ventricular system due to ependymitis (Berman & Banker 1966, Kalsbeck et al 1980). This possibility should always be considered when a child returns with recrudescence of raised intracranial pressure following shunt placement and should not be mistaken for shunt malfunction. The need for accurate evaluation by cranial ultrasound, complemented by CT scanning and even CT ventriculography, is emphasized.

Subdural effusions

These are relatively commonly seen on cranial ultrasound examination of neonates in the convalescent phase of pyogenic meningitis, being found in up to 50% of cases. Medically and surgically significant effusions are, however, relatively infrequent and complicate only about 5% of cases (Milhorat 1978). They present with persistent fever, irritability and seizures, or with signs of raised intracranial pressure, or with a combination of these symptoms. Diagnosis by cranial ultrasound may be difficult with machines of less than optimum quality and the interposition of a water-bag to increase the distance between the probe and the fontanelle may be useful. CT scanning with contrast enhancement may be required in equivocal cases. In the first instance treatment is by subdural puncture through the anterior fontanelle.

If, unusually, organisms are seen in the fluid obtained on Gram stain or subsequently cultured, then appropriate intravenous antibiotics are continued for at least a further 3 weeks. The majority of postmeningitic subdural effusions will resolve on a regimen of subdural taps which are performed on alternate sides of the anterior fontanelle on alternate days as, although the effusions are almost always bilateral, there is usually free communication across the midline. An 18 gauge needle is used and the puncture sites closed with sutures on each occasion. Up to 50 ml can usually be drained without disturbing the baby. Those effusions which do not resolve after 2 weeks of daily taps will require insertion of a subdural shunt, as will most effusions of a depth greater than 2 or 3 cm. Subdural shunting, either into the peritoneum or into the pleural cavity, using a simple non-valved tube without a reservoir is highly effective (Till 1968). In very small neonates or premature babies who have suffered pneumothoraces or other pulmonary complications, the peritoneal cavity should be used rather than the pleural cavity as pleural effusions may result. A unilateral shunt usually suffices. The shunt is inserted away from any site that might later be needed for placement of a ventricular shunt should hydrocephalus occur. Outcome relates to the degree of cerebral infarction sustained from the acute meningitis.

Subdural empyema

This is a much less frequent consequence of neonatal meningitis than is subdural effusion. I restrict the use of the term empyema to those cases in which there is frank pus in the subdural space. The condition presents during the course of antibacterial chemotherapy for pyogenic meningitis, or within 2–3 weeks of stopping treatment. The clinical features are raised intracranial pressure, persistent fever and malaise, lethargic behaviour, seizures and hemiparesis. CT scan shows a low-attenuation extracerebral collection with a characteristic enhancing rim over the surface of the brain (Curless 1985). Subdural taps through the anterior fontanelle may produce turbid fluid containing a preponderance of polymorphonuclear leukocytes but often is surprisingly unproductive. Gram stain and culture are usually negative. In most cases the fluid is thin enough to be removed by subdural taps with an 18 gauge needle; repeated taps and appropriate intravenous antibiotics suffice (Curless 1985). Occasionally the pus is too thick to be drained in this way, forming an extensive slough with the consistency of institutional scrambled egg over the cerebral hemispheres. In these cases evacuation at craniotomy is indicated. This is a very major undertaking in a sick baby and demands a combination of swift surgery and skilful anaesthesia.

Following evacuation, appropriate antibiotics in maximum intravenous dosage are continued for 3 weeks, together with anticonvulsants if indicated by continuing seizures, although often the seizures regress following drainage. CT is repeated weekly until the lesions are clearly resolving. Very frequently the initial postoperative CT shows alarming enhancement of the surface of the brain with appearances suggestive of extensive subcortical infarction but this is transient and not necessarily indicative of severe irretrievable neurological damage. A mortality of 50% has been recorded (Farmer & Wise 1973) but more recently the mortality has fallen considerably (Curless 1985). Serious neurological sequelae occur in about 25% of cases and include microcephaly, diplegia and developmental retardation (Jacobson & Farmer 1981, Curless 1985) but for the majority a good recovery is possible. Aggressive surgical intervention is therefore indicated.

Intracerebral abscess (see also Ch. 37, p. 438)

Brain abscesses in neonates are the result of bacteraemia occurring during or shortly after birth. In many cases the source of the infecting organism is never identified, though the predominance of Gram-negative organisms tends to implicate the mother's genital tract and in one-third of cases the same organism can be cultured both from the abscess and from the mother's urine.

The occasional case can be traced to peripheral sepsis in soft tissues or the umbilicus. Spread to the brain is haematogenous. Typically brain abscesses in neonates are large with thin walls and particularly extensive cerebral oedema (Arseni et al 1966). Rupture into the subarachnoid space with resultant meningitis or into the ventricles with pyocephalus may occur (Izquierdo et al 1978). Although infantile brain abscess has been known for a long time (Holt 1898, Farley 1949) the condition was difficult to recognize until the advent of CT (see Fig. 8.19) and ultrasound scanning; previously the diagnosis was usually made by chance in the course of a ventricular puncture. Hopefully the more widespread application of ultrasound scanning will lead to earlier diagnosis.

The clinical features are those of raised intracranial pressure, with or without fever, meningeal irritation or fits. Lumbar puncture is undesirable because of the considerable risk of precipitating brain shifts and deterioration (Garfield 1969) but it will often have been performed to investigate a clinical diagnosis of meningitis. Clearly any neonate in whom there are atypical features of meningitis should undergo ultrasound examination.

The mainstays of treatment are: the establishment of

an accurate microbiological diagnosis from pus obtained from the abscess or, failing that, from cultures of the baby's blood and the mother's genitourinary tract; control of raised intracranial pressure by aspiration of pus from the abscess, either through the fontanelle or through a burr hole; control of sepsis by appropriate antibiotics in high intravenous dosage; and suppression of seizures by phenobarbitone and paraldehyde. If there is a well-formed abscess cavity, repeated daily aspirations should continue until the cavity has collapsed; this can be monitored by ultrasound or CT scans. Intracavitary antibiotics are not needed unless there has been intraventricular rupture. Intravenous antibiotics continue until there is satisfactory reduction in the size of the lesion and never for less than 3 weeks. Because rupture into the ventricular system is quite common, hydrocephalus frequently results (Hoffman et al 1970) and ventriculo–peritoneal shunt placement may be required once the ventricular CSF is clear. The occasional baby in whom there is no well-formed cavity has a septic cerebritis (Enzman et al 1979, 1982) and is best treated with antibiotics alone on a 'best guess' basis without surgical aspiration (Daniels et al 1985); the same applies to those with multiple small abscesses or lesions in inaccessible sites such as the brainstem (Rosenblum et al 1980). Surgical excision is rarely needed.

The outcome has been poor in the past (Munslow et al 1957, Hoffman et al 1970) but hopefully will improve with more prompt recognition through heightened clinical awareness lowering the threshold for application of the modern investigative imaging (Rosenblum et al 1978). The degree of cerebral infarction associated with the abscess and any additional morbidity from shunt-dependent hydrocephalus still make neonatal brain abscess a formidable condition in which good team work between neonatal physician, microbiologist, neurosurgeon and neuroradiologist is central to successful management.

VASCULAR MALFORMATIONS

Intracranial aneurysms

Although often presumed to be congenital in origin, presentation in the neonatal period is exceptional. Interestingly, no incidental aneurysm or arterio–venous malformation was discovered in 10 000 cerebral angiograms performed at the Hospital for Sick Children, Toronto (Harwood-Nash & Fitz 1976) nor in an autopsy study which included 3000 children (Housepian & Pool 1938). Only a handful of cases are reported from the neonatal period (Newcomb & Munns 1949, Jones & Shearburn 1961, Pickering et al 1970, Grode et al 1978, McLellan et al 1986) at ages ranging from a few hours (Newcomb & Munns 1949) to 6 weeks (McLellan et al 1986).

Presentation is usually with a spontaneous intra-cranial haemorrhage precipitating irritability and seizures; a bulging fontanelle, retinal haemorrhages, low haemoglobin and blood-stained CSF obtained at lumbar puncture to exclude meningitis. These features may misleadingly suggest non-accidental injury but the pattern of intracranial haemorrhage on CT scan characterizes the source as spontaneous rather than traumatic (McLellan et al 1986). Cerebral angiography should be performed urgently lest a further haemorrhage leads to neurological deterioration (Storrs et al 1982).

When the child is in a stable state, with any fits controlled, craniotomy is performed and the aneurysm is excluded from the circulation by clipping to forestall further haemorrhage.

The results of aggressive surgical management, including developmental follow-up, have been good in the few cases that have been operated upon (Grode et al 1978, McLellan et al 1986). Aneurysms have been encountered on the middle cerebral artery (Jones & Shearburn 1961, Grode et al 1978, McLellan et al 1986), the posterior cerebral artery (Newcomb & Munns 1949) and the posterior inferior cerebellar artery (Pickering et al 1970).

More frequent use of cranial ultrasound and CT scanning will inevitably reveal similar cases in the future and in this regard the characteristics of intracranial aneurysms discovered later in infancy are noteworthy. They frequently present with seizures, are often located peripherally on the cerebral circulation rather than on the circle of Willis, and size greater than 1 cm is not unusual (Crisostomo et al 1986).

Intracranial arterio–venous malformations

Although arterio–venous malformation is twice as common as aneurysm as a cause of spontaneous intracranial haemorrhage in childhood (Humphreys 1982), only 4% of childhood arterio–venous malformations occur in infancy (Shapiro 1985) and virtually none of these in the neonatal period. Two cases of intraventricular haemorrhage in full-term babies aged 4 days (Schum et al 1979) and 2 weeks (Heafner et al 1985) are on record. In both cases small arterio–venous malformations in the wall of the third ventricle fed by the posterior choroidal artery were demonstrated angiographically. One child underwent excision of the malformation by the transcallosal route with normal neurological and developmental progress at 8 months (Heafner et al 1985).

These lesions must be excessively rare and my practice is to reserve angiography for those babies in whom the site of the haemorrhage or the appearances on a high-definition, contrast-enhanced CT scan after the haematoma has resolved, indicate the possibility of an underlying arterio-venous malformation being disclosed. Certainly this does not seem to be the case with primary thalamic haemorrhage in full-term babies (Trounce et al 1985). A cerebral tumour (p. 597) is a more likely structural cause of spontaneous intracranial haemorrhage in a neonate than is an arterio-venous malformation.

Vein of Galen malformations

These rare congenital vascular anomalies, barely 200 of which have been reported in the literature, result from fistulous connections that develop near the embryonic choroidal plexuses of the 20–40 mm embryo (Padget 1956). The consequent high-flow arterio–venous shunt between branches of the anterior, middle, posterior and superior cerebellar arteries and the vein of Galen leads to progressive aneurysmal dilatation of the vein of Galen whose wall becomes thick and tough. Two distinct types of malformation are recognized: primary, in which large arteries feed directly into the aneurysmal sac; and secondary, in which an arterio–venous malformation in the adjacent cerebral or cerebellar hemispheres, brainstem or tentorium drains via the galenic vein which thus becomes dilated.

The clinical features differ quite characteristically with the age at presentation (Gold et al 1964). Neonates present in the first few hours after birth with severe and progressive high-output congestive cardiac failure (Silverman et al 1959), soon complicated by pulmonary hypertension and myocardial ischaemia (Hoffman et al 1983). Infants present either with abnormal head size, due to hydrocephalus, and are found to have cardiomegaly; or with mild neonatal cardiac failure resolving spontaneously or with treatment, and within the first few months of life progressive abnormal head growth and a cranial bruit are observed. Children aged over 2 years with this condition may be discovered in the course of investigation of macrocephaly. In adolescence or adult life, headaches, subarachnoid haemorrhage or the incidental finding of pathological, ring-shaped, pineal region calcification lead to diagnosis. Contrast ultrasound or CT scans (see Fig. 8.23) will confirm the diagnosis.

In the neonate the prognosis is abysmal, the majority dying of intractable heart failure and the only survivors having severe neurological deficits due to gross ischaemic damage in the surrounding brain (Norman & Beckcr 1974). Having confirmed the diagnosis, often first revealed at the time of cardiac catheter studies, the only appropriate management is an attempt to control the cardiac failure by medical measures in the vain hope that the child will weather the storm into the infant period.

For those presenting in infancy the correct management is an accurate assessment of cardiac function, even if there has been no previous cardiac failure, with a precise estimation of blood volume, followed by insertion of a ventriculo–peritoneal shunt to control hydrocephalus as a prelude to surgical closure of the fistula at craniotomy. The peri-operative haemodynamic management is complicated and has to take into account the risks of precipitating cardiac failure due to the already expanded blood volume, and of myocardial ischaemia which may progress to infarction if

hypotension occurs accidentally or by misguided intent. Postoperatively, seizures and persistent subdural effusions have been the major complications.

For older children and adolescents the only measure that is usually required is ventricular shunt placement to treat hydrocephalus.

Overall the outcome for neonates with this condition remains very poor but for infants there is a distinct possibility of good-quality survival (Amacher & Shillito 1973, Hoffman et al 1982). Interventional radiology to partially close the fistula, as an adjunct to open surgery is a hope for the future but its role is currently ill-defined (Berenstein & Epstein 1982).

TUMOURS OF THE CENTRAL NERVOUS SYSTEM

Neoplasms of any type are very rare in the neonatal period accounting for 6.24 deaths per million live births (Fraumeni & Miller 1969), but CNS tumours must still be remembered in the differential diagnosis of raised intracranial pressure and of paraplegia.

Intracranial tumours

Intracranial tumours present at birth, or producing symptoms in the first few months of life, are correctly regarded as true congenital tumours (Arnstein et al 1951, Solitaire & Krigman 1964) and they account for 0.5 to 1.5% of all childhood brain tumours (Bodian & Lawson 1953, Sato et al 1975, Jooma & Kendall 1982). This scarcity notwithstanding, 200 cases have been available for systematic review (Wakai et al 1984). An incidence of 0.34 per million live births has been estimated (Fraumeni & Miller 1969).

Unlike in older children, 70% of neonatal brain tumours are supratentorial and only 30% infratentorial. The supratentorial tumours are as often hemispheric in location as they are midline and the infratentorial lesions are uniformly related to the fourth ventricle (Jooma et al 1984). Also, 36.5% are teratomas and of the rest 50% are of neuro-epithelial origin of which the most frequent are medulloblastoma (12%), astrocytoma (10%), choroid plexus tumour (8%) and ependymoma (7%).

There is no overall sex predilection but females predominate with medulloblastomas and males with ependymomas (Wakai et al 1984). Of affected babies, 12% have associated congenital anomalies, although there is no particular pattern except for epignathus in about 15% of those with teratomas. Neonatal medulloblastoma has been recorded in siblings of different pregnancies (Belamaric & Chan 1969) and also in identical twins (Grienpentrog & Pauly 1957).

Presentation is with symptoms of raised intracranial pressure which is characteristically more severe and more rapidly progressive than that encountered in non-tumoural hydrocephalus or subdural effusion. Macrocephaly may be of such degree as to cause dystocia in 18% of cases. 15% present with spontaneous intracranial haemorrhage, 18% are stillborn and 14% are premature (Wakai et al 1984).

The diagnosis of brain tumour is suggested by the appearance on ultrasound scanning and is confirmed by CT scanning (see also Fig. 8.17) or magnetic resonance imaging. The occasional non-tumoural congenital malformation may create diagnostic difficulty, especially if associated with hydrocephalus. Typically these neonatal tumours are very large, heterogenous and variably enhancing on CT (Fig. 47.3). Prenatal diagnosis is likely to become more frequent as imaging techniques improve.

In most cases craniotomy is advisable, if only to establish a histological diagnosis. In those children with severely raised intracranial pressure from hydrocephalus, a ventriculo–peritoneal shunt will provide a few days of respite in which to improve the child's nutritional state and thereby minimize complications. Both surgeon and anaesthetist must be fully prepared for major haemorrhage amounting to one or two whole-blood volumes. When the diagnosis is made in utero, delivery by elective caesarean section is probably the safest policy, especially if there is considerable macrocephaly, if only to minimize the risk of intracranial haemorrhage into the tumour.

With the exception of benign astrocytomas of the cerebral hemispheres and choroid plexus tumours, which in skilled hands are amenable to curative excision, the outcome is poor, most babies being dead within a year: the teratomas

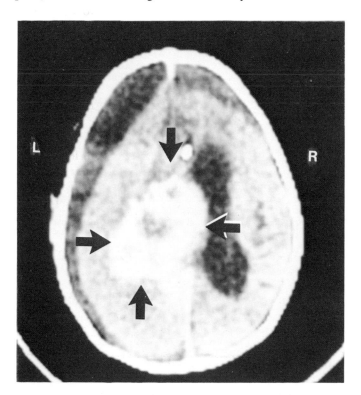

Fig. 47.3 Primitive neuro-epithelial tumour (arrowed) in a young infant. There is subdural effusion on the left side. (Reproduced by courtesy of Dr Rosemary Shannon.)

are almost uniformly highly malignant (Sato et al 1984, Jooma et al 1984, Wakai et al 1984, Ellams et al 1986). The dire neurodevelopmental consequences of irradiation of the immature brain preclude the administration of radiotherapy (Jooma et al 1984). It remains to be seen whether combination chemotherapy as an adjuvant to radical surgical extirpation has anything to offer.

Spinal tumours

Spinal tumours are exceptionally rare in the neonatal period but should still be suspected in any child without features of spinal dysraphism who has congenital paraplegia, or who develops progressive paraparesis or sphincter disturbance. The majority are dumb-bell, or hour-glass, neuroblastomas (Punt et al 1980) but occasional gliomas (Parkinson et al 1954), schwannomas (Elliott 1884) and leukaemic deposits (Mosberg 1951) are encountered. The occasional child with an intramedullary astrocytoma has symptoms originating in infancy but recognition in the neonatal period is exceptional.

Plain spine radiographs may show expansion of the spinal canal and, in the case of neuroblastoma, a paraspinal soft tissue mass, with or without tumour calcification. The definitive diagnosis is made by CT myelography, MRI or ultrasound. Elevated levels of urinary catecholamines indicate neuroblastoma.

Surgical decompression at laminectomy is indicated to forestall further neurological deterioration and to obtain tissue for histological diagnosis. In the case of neuroblastoma, the paraspinal element is treated with appropriate chemotherapy and secondary excision of the residuum.

The outcome is dependent upon the nature of the tumour and the neurological state of presentation, those with congenital paraplegia being left with severe sensorimotor and sphincter deficits that require the same combined services of orthopaedic and urological surgeons as those with spinal dysraphism. For those with neuroblastoma the prospect for survival is excellent as with most children with the disease in the first year of life (Punt et al 1980).

REFERENCES

Albanese V, Tomasello F, Sampaulo S 1981 Multiloculated hydrocephalus in infants. Neurosurgery 8: 641–646

Amacher A L, Shillito J Jr 1973 The syndromes and surgical treatment of aneurysms of the great vein of Galen. Journal of Neurosurgery 39: 88–98

Anderson H 1977 Craniosynostosis. In: Vinken P J, Bruyn G W (eds) Handbook of Clinical Neurology, Vol. 30, Part 1: Congenital malformations of the brain and skull. Elsevier, Amsterdam, pp 219–233

Arnstein L H, Boldrey E, Naffzigger H C 1951 A case report and survey of brain tumours during the neonatal period. Journal of Neurosurgery 8: 315–319

Arseni C, Horvath L, Dumitrescu L 1966 Cerebral abscesses in children. Acta Neurochirurgica (Wien) 14: 197–224

Belarmaric J, Chan S 1969 Medulloblastoma in newborn sisters. Journal of Neurosurgery 30: 76–79

Berenstein A, Epstein F 1982 Vein of Galen malformations: combined neurosurgical and neuroradiologic intervention. In: Pediatric neurosurgery: surgery of the developing nervous system. Grune & Stratton, New York, pp 637–647

Berman P H, Banker B Q 1966 Neonatal meningitis: a clinical and pathological study of 39 cases. Pediatrics 38: 6–24

Elliott G R 1884 Neurofibroma complicating spina bifida. Med Rec NY 25: 194–195

Enzman D R, Britt R H, Yeager A S 1979 Experimental brain abscess evolution: computed tomographic and neuropathologic correlation. Radiology 133: 113–122

Enzman D R, Britt R H, Lyons B, Carroll B, Wilson D A, Buxton J 1982 High resolution ultrasound evaluation of experimental brain abscess evolution: comparison with computed tomography and neuropathology. Radiology 142: 95–102

Farley D L B 1949 Cerebral abscess in an infant followed by recovery. Lancet i: 264–266

Farmer T W, Wise G R 1973 Subdural empyema in infants, children and adults. Neurology (Minneap) 23: 254–261

Fraumeni J F, Miller R W 1969 Cancer deaths in the newborn. American Journal of Diseases of Children 117: 186–189

Garfield J S 1969 Management of supratentorial abscess: a review of 200 cases. British Medical Journal 2: 7–11

Gold A P, Rawsohoff J, Carter S 1964 Vein of Galen malformation. Acta Neurologica Scandinavica (Suppl) 11: 5–31

Grienpentrog F, Pauly H 1957 Intra- und extrakranielle, fruhmanifeste Medulloblastome bei erbgleichen Zwillingen. Zentralblatt fur Neurochirurgie 17: 129–139

Grode M L, Saunders M, Carton C A 1978 Subarachnoid hemorrhage secondary to ruptured aneurysms in infants. Report of two cases. Journal of Neurosurgery 49: 898–902

Harwood-Nash D C, Fitz C R 1976 In: Neuroradiology in infants and children, Vol 3. C V Mosby, St Louis, pp 906–913

Heafner M D, Duncan C C, Kier E L et al 1985 Intraventricular hemorrhage in a term neonate secondary to a third ventricular arteriovenous malformation. Journal of Neurosurgery 63: 640–643

Hinton D R, Becker L E, Muakkassa K F, Hoffman H J 1984 Lambdoid suture: normal development and pathology of 'synostosis'. Journal of Neurosurgery 61: 333–339

Hirsch J, Renier D, Saint-Rose C 1981 Intracranial pressure in craniostenosis. Ninth meeting of the International Society for Pediatric Neurosurgery, Budapest, Hungary, 20–22 July 1981

Hoffman H J, Mohr G 1976 Lateral canthal advancement of the supraorbital margin: a new corrective technique in the treatment of coronal synostosis. Journal of Neurosurgery 45: 376–381

Hoffman H J, Hendrick E B, Hiscox J L 1970 Cerebral abscesses in early infancy. Journal of Neurosurgery 33: 172–177

Hoffman H J, Chuang S, Hendrick E B, Humphreys R P 1982 Aneurysms of the vein of Galen. Journal of Neurosurgery 57: 316–322

Hoffman H J, Chuang S, Hendrick E B 1983 Aneurysms of the vein of Galen. In: Raimondi A J (ed) Concepts in pediatric neurosurgery, No. 3. S Karger, Basel, pp 52–74

Holt L E 1898 A report of 5 cases of abscesses of the brain in infants, together with a summary of 27 collected cases in infants and very young children. Archives of Pediatrics 15: 81

Housepian E M, Pool J L 1958 A systematic analysis of intracranial aneurysms from the autopsy file of the Presbyterian Hospital 1914–1956. Journal of Neuropathology and Experimental Neurology 17: 409–423

Humphreys R P 1982 Arteriovenous malformations of the brain and spinal cord. In: Pediatric neurosurgery: surgery of the developing nervous system. Grune & Stratton, New York, pp 625–635

Izquierdo J M, Sanz F, Coca J M 1978 Pyocephalus of the new-born child. Child's Brain 4: 129–136

Jacobson P L, Farmer T W 1981 Subdural empyema complicating meningitis in infants. Neurology (NY) 31: 190–193

Jones R K, Shearburn E W 1961 Intracranial aneurysms in a four week old infant: diagnosis by angiography and successful operation. Journal of Neurosurgery 18: 122–124

Jooma R, Kendall B E 1982 Intracranial tumours in the first year of life. Neuroradiology 23: 267–274

Jooma R, Kendall B E, Hayward R D 1984 Intracranial tumours in neonates: a report of seventeen cases. Surgical Neurology 21: 165–170

Kalsbeck J E, DeSousa A L, Kleiman M B, Goodman J M, Franken

E A 1980 Compartmentalization of the cerebral ventricles as a sequel of neonatal meningitis. Journal of Neurosurgery 52: 547–552

Karan S 1986 Purulent meningitis in the newborn. Child's Nervous System 2: 26–31

Lekias J, Stokes B 1970 Dermoid lesions of the central nervous system in childhood. Australian and New Zealand Journal of Surgery 39: 335–340

Le Wald L T 1933 Congenital absence of the superior orbital wall associated with pulsatile exophthalmos: report of four cases. American Journal of Roentgenology 30: 756–764

McCracken G H Jr 1977 Intraventricular treatment of neonatal meningitis due to gram-negative bacilli. Journal of Pediatrics 91: 1037–1038

McCracken G H Jr, Mize S G 1976 A controlled study of intrathecal antibiotic therapy in gram negative enteric meningitis of infancy. Journal of Pediatrics 89: 66–72

McLellan N J, Prasad R, Punt J 1986 Spontaneous subhyaloid and retinal haemorrhages in an infant. Archives of Disease in Childhood 61: 1130–1132

McMurray B R, Martin L W, Dignan P S, Fogelson M H 1977 Hereditary aphasia cutis congenita and associated defects: three instances in one family and a survey of reported cases. Clinical Pediatrics 16: 610–614

Mannino F L, Jones K L, Benirschke K 1977 Congenital skin defects and fetus papyraceous. Journal of Pediatrics 91: 559–564

Matson D D 1969 Congenital defects of the scalp and skull. In: Neurosurgery of infancy and childhood, 2nd edn. Charles C Thomas, Springfield, Illinois, pp 168–178

Milhorat T H 1978 In: Pediatric Neurosurgery. Davis, Philadelphia, pp 352–356

Mosberg W H 1951 Spinal tumours diagnosed during the first year of life: with report of a case. Journal of Neurosurgery 8: 220–224

Moss M L 1959 The pathogenesis of premature cranial synostosis in man. Acta Anatomica (Basel) 37: 351

Muakkassa K F, King R B, Stark D B 1982 Nonsurgical approach to congenital scalp and skull defects. Journal of Neurosurgery 56: 711–715

Muakkassa K F, Hoffman H J, Hinton D R, Hendrick E B, Humphreys R P, Ash J 1984 Lambdoid synostosis. 2. Review of cases managed at The Hospital for Sick Children 1972–1982. Journal of Neurosurgery 61: 340–347

Munslow R A, Stovall V S, Price R D, Kohler C M 1957 Brain abscess in infants. Journal of Pediatrics 51: 74–79

Newcomb A L, Munns G F 1949 Rupture of aneurysm of the circle of Willis in the newborn. Pediatrics 3: 769–772

Norman M G, Becker L E 1974 Cerebral damage in neonates resulting from arteriovenous malformation of vein of Galen. Journal of Neurology, Neurosurgery and Psychiatry 37: 252–258

Overall J C Jr 1970 Neonatal bacterial meningitis: analysis of predisposing factors and outcome compared with matched control subjects. Journal of Pediatrics 76: 499–511

Padget D H 1956 The cranial venous system in man with reference to development, adult configuration, and relation to the arteries. American Journal of Anatomy 98: 307–355

Pannell B W, Hendrick E B, Hoffman H J, Humphreys R P 1982 Dermoid cysts of the anterior fontanelle. Neurosurgery 10: 317–323

Parkinson D, Medovy H, Mitchell J R 1954 Spinal cord tumour in a newborn. Journal of Neurosurgery 11: 629–632

Pickering K, Hogan G R, Gilbert E F 1970 Aneurysm of the posterior inferior cerebellar artery: rupture in a newborn. American Journal of Diseases of Children 119: 155–158

Punt J, Pritchard J, Pincott J, Till K 1980 Neuroblastoma: a review of 21 cases presenting with spinal cord compression. Cancer 45: 3095–3101

Rekate H L 1985 Lambdoid suture synostosis. Journal of Neurosurgery 62: 185 (letter)

Robinson R G 1962 Congenital perforations of the skull in relation to the parietal bone. Journal of Neurosurgery 19: 153–158

Rosenblum M L, Hoff J T, Norman D, Weinstein P R, Pitts L 1978 Decreased mortality from brain abscesses since advent of computerised tomography. Journal of Neurosurgery 49: 658–668

Rosenblum M L, Hoff J T, Norman D, Edwards M S, Berg B O 1980 Nonoperative treatment of brain abscesses in selected high risk patients. Journal of Neurosurgery 52: 217–225

Salmon J H 1972 Ventriculitis complicating meningitis. American Journal of Diseases of Children 124: 35–38

Sato O, Tamura A, Sano K 1964 Brain tumours of early infants. Child's Brain 1: 121–125

Sato T, Shimodaa, Takahashi T et al 1984 Congenital anaplastic ependymoma: a case report of familial glioma. Child's Brain 11: 342–348

Schum T R, Meyer G A, Grausz J P, Glaspey J C 1979 Neonatal intraventricular hemorrhage due to an intracranial arteriovenous malformation: a case report. Pediatrics 64: 242–244

Shapiro K 1985 Subarachnoid hemorrhages in children. In: Fein J M, Flamm E S (eds) Cerebrovascular surgery, Vol. 3. Springer-Verlag, New York, pp 941–965

Shillito J 1973 A new cranial suture appearing in the site of craniectomy for synostosis. Radiology 107: 83–88

Silverman B K, Brekzt T, Craig J, Nadas A S 1959 Congestive failure in the newborn caused by cerebral arteriovenous fistula. American Journal of Diseases of Children 89: 539–543

Solitaire G B, Krigman M R 1964 Congenital intracranial neoplasm. Journal of Neuropathology and Experimental Neurology 2: 280–292

Storrs B B, Humphreys R P, Hendrick E B, Hoffman H J 1982 Intracranial aneurysms in the pediatric age group. Child's Brain 9: 358–361

Tessier P 1967 Osteotomies totales de la face, syndrome de Crouzon, syndrome d'Apert, oxycephalies, scaphocephalies, turricephalies. Annales de Chirurgie Plastique 12: 273–286

Till K 1968 Subdural haematoma and effusion in infancy. British Medical Journal 2: 400–402

Trounce J Q, Fawer C-L, Punt J, Dodd K L, Fielder A R, Levene M I 1985 Primary thalamic haemorrhage in the newborn: a new clinical entity. Lancet i: 190–192

Vinocur C D, Weintraub W H, Wilensky R T, Coran A G, Dingman R O 1976 Surgical management of aplasia cutis congenita. Archives of Surgery 111: 1160–1164

Virchow R 1851 Uber den Cretisimus, Namentlich in Franken und uber pathologische Schadel formen. Verh Phys-Med Ges Wurzburg 2: 230

Volpe J J 1981 Neurology of newborn. Saunders, Philadelphia, pp 747–802

Wakai S, Arai T, Nagai M 1984 Congenital brain tumours. Surgical Neurology 21: 597–609

Wong T, Wann S, Lee L 1986 Congenital dermoid cysts of the anterior fontanelle in Chinese children. Child's Nervous System 2: 175–178

Ethical dilemmas of diagnosis and intervention

48. Ethical dilemmas of diagnosis and intervention

Dr P. Barbor

Ethics may be defined as the Science of Morals; morals are concerned with the right or wrong conduct or duty to one's neighbour which must be confirmed or justified by conscience if not by law. The words are often used synonymously and this has a rational basis as the Greek word *ethos* and the Latin word *mores*, both mean habits or customs (*Encyclopaedia Britannica*).

This chapter is concerned with the ethical dilemmas that confront all those who care for families during and immediately after pregnancy. The dilemmas have become more acute because of the massive advances in intra-uterine diagnosis and neonatal care that have been made possible by modern medical technology. All concerned take pride in these advances but there is a darker side to the story. For some babies, months of intensive care end in failure with all the social, emotional and financial stress on the family that this must entail; for others successful intensive care heralds a lifetime of severe impairment. Recently both the lay public (Rachels 1975, Stinson & Stinson 1981) and professional persons (Duff & Campbell 1976, Kennedy 1981, Campbell 1982, Bissenden 1986) have expressed concern at the apparently indiscriminate use of modern technology without a more sophisticated Code of Law and Ethics governing its use. The inevitable sequel to such concern is to suggest that a Code of Law and Ethics would define which infants would be selected not to receive the full panoply of modern medicine but would be allowed to die. For a variety of reasons it is extremely unlikely that such a Code will appear. Code or no Code, obstetricians, paediatricians, neurosurgeons and all who care for the fetus and newborn have to evolve a modus vivendi, a way of coping with the ethical dilemmas that surround the use of modern technology.

It could be suggested that there are three moral philosophical points to be taken into consideration. These are fully discussed in *Causing death and saving lives* (Glover 1977), *Doctors talking* (Autton 1985) and *Should the baby live?* (Kuhse & Singer 1985).

The principle of the sanctity of life

'Most of us think it is wrong to kill people. Some think it is wrong in all circumstances, while others think that in special circumstances (say, in a just war or in self defence) some killing may be justified. But even those who do not think killing is always wrong normally think that a special justification is needed. The assumption is that killing can at best only be justified to avoid a greater evil . . . ' (Glover 1977).

There are doctors and nurses as well as some highly articulate pressure groups who feel that not only is it wrong in all circumstances to take life but it is equally wrong to withhold maximal treatment for any child. Doctors practising what can be called 'conviction medicine' may hold views that cannot be altered by information concerning the prognosis as to the quality of life or by parental wishes. Doctors practising 'consensus medicine' may feel that their actions are influenced by parental wishes and prognosis, and that withdrawing maximal treatment can be seen as 'justified in order to avoid a greater evil', the greater evil being an unacceptable quality of life.

Quality of life

A clear assessment of the acceptability or otherwise of a quality of life is probably impossible (Glover 1977) and yet an assessment is being made many times every year in antenatal clinics and in neonatal units. Pregnancies are terminated because of certain medical conditions and the law permits this, presumably on the grounds that the quality of life that the fetus would enjoy is unacceptable (Crawford 1983) (see Abortion Act quoted under Antenatal diagnosis).

Duff & Campbell (1973) have articulated what most of the medical profession have long understood and accepted: 'in our view the most important medical criterion is the degree of abnormality, disease or damage to the central nervous system, especially the brain. If there is little or no prospect of brain function sufficient to allow a personal life of meaning and quality or no potential for development in harmony with Fletchers' indicators of humanhood, non-treatment seems the prudent course of action'. On the whole this is consistent with the views held by most people with whom the author has discussed the problem.

Having said that, it is well known to all who work in neonatal or obstetric units that every child and its family are different. Two babies with apparently similar medical conditions may have different decisions made about them. Because of other factors related to parental wishes and beliefs, we would suggest that this is not immoral as is suggested by Sherlock (1979) but shows a sensitivity to all factors surrounding the baby's future. Fletchers' 'tentative profile of man' suggests that positive criteria for humanhood would include minimal intelligence, self awareness, self control, a sense of time, a sense of futurity and a sense of the past, the capability to relate to others, concern for others, communication, control of existence, and curiosity (Fletcher 1972). This may be too philosophical to be of great value when decisions are being made at the bedside but perhaps it incorporates much of what we are thinking in assessing the quality of life.

When such decisions come to be taken this is done only after much discussion with the family and with all the health professionals involved. The decisions are tragic and difficult and rely very much upon mutual trust and respect between all concerned.

Acts of commission and omission

Terminating a pregnancy according to the strict criteria laid down by the Abortion Act of 1967 is condoned by law. An act of commission is performed bringing about the death of a fetus that otherwise might have lived. Switching off a ventilator when a baby has very severe brain damage may bring about the death of the baby. Although the means of keeping the baby alive a little longer are available, the baby's death is hastened as a result of an act of omission (Autton 1985).

In the case of severely handicapped infants it could be argued that there is no significant moral difference between acts of commission and omission. This is lucidly argued by Jonathan Glover 'In many instances it is not absolutely clear what the boundary between killing and simply withholding treatment is . . . . The central point is that in assessing the morality of two things people do or fail to do there are two plausible candidates which make a moral difference. One is a difference in consequences, the other possible candidate is a difference in a person's intention. Now in many of the cases where there are two possible strategies for bringing about death there is the same consequence and the same intention in each case . . . . I find it extraordinarily hard to see why, in a case where the intention and consequences are equivalent, we should attach any moral significance to

what particular course of activity or non-activity happened to be adopted . . . . That is not to say of course there is never any place for the distinction between killing and failing to save life' (Glover 1977).

When Norman Autton discussed the same issue with Professor Ian Kennedy, two points were made that will be familiar to all who care for the very sick: 'But what people would argue, who are engaged in terminal care is that they do not withhold treatment, they change treatment. They change it from a treatment for the living, to a treatment for the dying. Secondly, is it really necessary to hasten death, so that in effect you really have to kill the patient? I would have thought the answer is very rarely. After all the doctor already has the moral tool of the double effect theory, that is to say that although his primary intention is to relieve suffering, it may also be the case that death is also intended, in that it will predictably follow from the course of treatment adopted. But if it is intended as a secondary effect, this may be morally justified' (Autton 1985).

This is of course the way medicine is practised in the terminally sick. The aims of treatment are changed from cure to care. Care involves controlling pain. Morphia controls pain but may also expedite death.

In summary, all who care for newborn babies have the greatest respect for life and spend much of their time trying to save lives. However, most feel that there are occasions when a baby has a right to die, that it is right to allow a baby to die and in some cases to hasten death in order to avoid a greater evil, this being an unacceptable quality of life. All would agree that it is impossible to define an acceptable quality of life; many doctors would accept the criteria given by Campbell (1982) and Duff (1976) in reply to Sherlock (1979).

Although our views, which are similar to those of many other doctors, are stated simply here, this does not imply that the dilemmas we all face are other than horrendous and tragic.

There are three occasions when abnormalities of the central nervous system may be diagnosed and decisions about a child's future may be made: antenatally; at and immediately after delivery; and after prolonged intensive care.

ANTENATAL DIAGNOSIS

The purpose of diagnosing an abnormality of the central nervous system as early as possible in pregnancy is to recognize an abnormality of sufficient severity to warrant termination of the pregnancy.

Section 1(i)(b) of the 1967 UK Abortion Act describes one of the grounds for termination as ' . . . a substantial risk that if the child were born it would suffer from such physical or mental abnormalities as to be seriously handicapped'. The judgement as to what is a 'substantial risk' and what is 'seriously handicapped' is left to the doctor and patient.

Before proceeding with antenatal diagnosis, informed consent is required. Counselling of parents at this stage will help them to make decisions. Relatively few obstetricians will undertake antenatal diagnosis to prepare a woman for the birth of a handicapped child. The purpose of antenatal diagnosis can be explained and the prognosis of the lesions likely to be found discussed in some detail, as well as the hazard of the investigations.

The principal methods of antenatal diagnosis are as follows:

Screening of maternal blood for alpha-fetoprotein (AFP)

This is usually done between 16 and 20 weeks. The gestational age is confirmed by ultrasound, as the AFP levels are dependent upon an accurate assessment of this (see Ch. 24).

Ultrasound

This is usually carried out at 16 weeks. There are no known hazards attached to its use. It is particularly effective in diagnosing structural abnormalities but this requires a higher level of skill than the routine obstetric ultrasound examination. It is possible to detect some central nervous system defects, e.g. anencephaly, encephalocele, spina bifida cystica, severe hydrocephaly, microcephaly and ventriculomegaly (see Ch. 25).

When a serious abnormality is diagnosed, the decision to terminate is likely to be made on the basis of the prognosis. If a child is shown to be anencephalic or severely hydrocephalic, death is likely to occur soon after birth. Spina bifida is discussed in detail in Section 7 but on the whole it is common for parents to request termination if spina bifida is diagnosed in utero. Ventriculomegaly, however, is more difficult. If at the time the ultrasound is done it is already extreme, or is associated with other severe malformations or there is evidence of intra-uterine toxoplasmosis, cytomegalovirus or herpes simplex infection, termination is usually offered. But if it is not extreme and the fetus is otherwise normal, i.e. normal karyotype, AFP and viral cultures, the fetus is serially assessed with ultrasound. Most cases do not progress. If they do and 32 weeks of gestation is reached, labour is induced and an early shunt operation is performed.

Because ultrasound is apparently free from hazard and is fairly routine it may be that counselling of parents takes place after the ultrasound has been done. In the case of the lesions described above it would be usual for the obstetrician to offer termination.

Amniocentesis

As a rule amniocentesis is used when there is an indication for doing so, rather than routinely. In a neurological context it is used when the maternal alpha-fetoprotein is raised and to look for chromosomal abnormalities, such as Down's syndrome or trisomy 13 or 18. There are hazards attached to amniocentesis. The MRC multicentre study (1978) found an increase in fetal loss of 1.0–1.5% and a further increase of 1.0–1.5% risk of postural deformities such as talipes, congenital dislocation of the hip, respiratory difficulties and antepartum haemorrhage — all probably due to amniotic fluid leakage. This is thought to be an overestimate now, and most units report a figure of no higher than 1%.

The purpose of amniocentesis is to look for specific abnormalities in the fetus in order to terminate the pregnancy if the abnormality is found. Counselling of parents always precedes such an invasive investigation as amniocentesis — the hazards of the investigation are discussed and also the action to be taken when the findings are known. Most obstetricians feel that it would not be justified to carry out amniocentesis unless termination was planned if the findings were sufficiently abnormal. Parents have to give informed consent and have the right to decide not to have a termination.

Chorionic villus sampling

This can be carried out between the 9th and 11th week of gestation. Its safety and reliability are still being assessed but for many diseases it promises great hope for the future. Although it is useful for chromosomal abnormalities (e.g. trisomies 21, 13 and 18) and for biochemical abnormalities, it is not as helpful in structural neurological abnormalities as ultrasound. It carries a risk of abortion of about 4%.

Fetoscopy

This is a highly specialized procedure and rarely performed today. It is possible to examine the face and limbs and to take fetal blood but it is seldom, if ever, used in neurological disorders.

In summary, it is possible to diagnose antenatally most of the severe neurological disorders which would cause the child, if born, to be seriously handicapped. In some, such as anencephaly and hydrocephaly, the baby usually dies soon after birth; in others it is suggested that the child would be severely handicapped within the meaning of the British Act. As antenatal diagnosis becomes more sophisticated and more parents take advantage of this and agree to the termination of pregnancy, fewer and fewer babies are being born with these severe abnormalities.

DIAGNOSIS AT AND IMMEDIATELY AFTER DELIVERY

Despite the availability of antenatal diagnosis many children with spina bifida are born in the UK each year. Before the

1950s it seems likely that most died from infection. During the 1960s a policy of operating on all children with spina bifida, by covering the spinal defect soon after birth, was adopted by the Sheffield team of Lorber, Zachary and Sharrard. World-wide this policy had a profound effect but was not adopted by all centres. It provided important information on the future of babies operated on soon after birth (Lorber 1972).

Over 12 years, 848 children were operated on. Exactly half of them died, 75% of these within the first year. Of the 424 survivors, 6 had no handicap and 73 a moderate degree of handicap; 345 (80%) had severe handicaps and one-third of them were retarded, many severely.

On the basis of these results Dr Lorber altered his policy and the majority of centres in the UK and Australia now follow his recommendations on selective treatment. Using these criteria (see below) Lorber demonstrated that in the group that was studied not a single moderately handicapped child or one with no handicap would have been lost. One great difficulty is that the physical handicaps do not assist in predicting the IQ. Some babies with the severest physical handicaps had normal IQs.

Adopting a policy of treating selected children according to the criteria will mean that about 75% of children with spina bifida will not receive treatment. This means no surgery, no antibiotics, nursing care, feeding on demand and analgesics. Although this may sound clinically tidy, as a policy it causes ethical dilemmas of frightening proportions concerning the sanctity of life, the quality of life and acts of omission and commission as discussed briefly earlier. These dilemmas are discussed in detail in *Should the baby live?* by Helga Kuhse and Peter Singer (1985).

When a child with spina bifida is born, a full assessment is carried out either by a paediatrician or by paediatrician and neurosurgeon separately. The formal criteria put forward by Lorber are: severe paraplegia, gross enlargement of the head, kyphosis, and associated gross congenital anomalies or major birth injuries. If one or more of these adverse criteria are present the position is discussed in detail with both parents together. After providing information on the child's likely future and on the possible courses of action and the result of these, many doctors like to leave parents on their own so that they can find out clearly what each is thinking. They then return after a few minutes to reach a decision with the parents. It has been suggested (Duff & Campbell 1973) that at this stage parents may be so overwrought that they cannot be expected to make a rational decision. It is not our experience that this is so (Duff & Campbell 1973, Lorber 1972). Once the decision is made, whether it is to treat or to allow to die, much support will be needed both in the hospital and on returning home. This support may be provided by the general practitioner and practice nurse or by an experienced hospital social worker and paediatric liaison sister in the home and by the paediatrician in the hospital.

DIAGNOSIS AFTER PROLONGED INTENSIVE CARE

The heart-rending account given by Roger and Peggy Stinson (1982) should be obligatory reading for all who care for the very premature and low-birth-weight babies. After six months of intensive care Andrew Stinson died. At the time of his death he suffered from bronchopulmonary dysplasia, retinopathy of prematurity, numerous infections, septicaemias and pneumonias, numerous fractured bones from nutritional rickets, an iatrogenic cleft palate, pulmonary hypertension, gangrene of muscle in the right leg, enlarged ventricles, microcephaly and severe developmental delay. This catalogue of largely iatrogenic disasters is of course only one side of the story. The other side demonstrates outstanding success in saving many very small babies for whom survival only a few years ago was unthinkable.

The high-technology medicine that is practised in neonatal units with great success runs the risk of becoming 'disease orientated'. Each problem as it arises is attacked with all the skill and technology that is available. In this way advances in the use of medical technology are brought about, but at a price, for the fear is that this approach dehumanized patients (Duff & Campbell 1976). A 'person orientated' approach accepts that there is a quality of life that is worse than death. This approach protects the patient and the family from cruel and painful treatment but it may run the risk of being illegal. Doctors are concerned primarily with caring for their patients and their families, not with the law. The pleas made by the Stinsons was that the Code of Law and Ethics governing the use of modern medical technology should become more sophisticated. It is not the wish of any doctor to violate the law in these circumstances but there is a feeling that the law is lagging behind the very difficult situations that are arising (British Medical Journal 1986).

The main complaint that the Stinsons made was not that their child was allowed to die, rather the reverse in fact, but that they were apparently excluded from most of the decisions made. The usual sequence of events in a neonatal unit is that medical information is given to parents, often daily, parental wishes and views are sought and then a medical decision is made which will usually coincide with parental wishes. On occasions they do not and then doctors or social service departments have had recourse to the courts. At the moment the courts have usually found in favour of prolonging life irrespective of its quality. Campbell's main comment on the Stinson case (Stinson 1981) was the apparent lack of clear leadership. Neonatal intensive care is so complex that it demands team work of the highest order. The views of all concerned, the family, junior doctors and nurses of all levels are sought. Clear leadership with discussion throughout to ensure that the skills, knowledge and technology are applied with sensitivity towards the family and the child, would seem to be an integral part of good neonatal care. This is particularly relevant when caring for a baby at the very limits of viability.

It has been suggested that in as many as one-fifth of all deaths that occur in a neonatal unit a conscious decision has been taken to allow the child to die rather than to continue treatment in the way described by the Stinsons. As a rule it is possible to investigate a neonate and to demonstrate that the lungs will not function adequately without ventilation, or that the brain has been so damaged that a worthwhile life cannot be anticipated. The advances made in the diagnostic value of ultrasound examination on the neonatal brain have been of great significance in making these decisions.

As a result of the investigations and the assessment of the child and the family and after hearing the views of the staff, who have been caring for the child and will be caring for the child and family afterwards, a decision will be made by the consultant. With good communications throughout, parents have usually come to expect and even want a decision to be made; sometimes this decision will be to allow the child to die.

Ideally what now happens is that all the machinery, the ventilator, the monitoring devices and the intravenous lines are removed and the child is placed in the mother's arms with the father and if appropriate brothers and sisters, all together in a quiet room or secluded area in the unit. Duff & Campbell (1976) quote a father as saying that the scene of mother and dying child was one of sublime beauty despite its occurrence in the midst of tragedy. It is very much our experience that when a child is allowed to die in this way the word beautiful is often used to describe the event although it might seem anything but beautiful to others.

Our views are not new. We believe that in providing the best medical care for a family there occasionally comes a time when the quality of life to be expected is worse than death, that a child has earned a right to die (British Medical Journal 1981). We also believe that when this tragic decision is reached that there is no morally significant difference between allowing a child to die and helping the child to die peacefully.

We also believe strongly that decisions of this sort demand medical leadership of a high order. The decision will be based on medical information but will be heavily influenced by the views of parents and staff. It is not an ideal solution and there probably is no ideal solution, but we hope it might be seen as the most sensitive in a tragic situation. Our views coincide closely with those propounded during the last 10 years by Duff & Campbell (1976), Campbell (1982), Lorber (1972) and Kuhse & Singer (1985) and are accepted by many of our colleagues.

REFERENCES

Autton N 1985 Doctors talking. A R Mowbray, Oxford
Bissenden J G 1986 Ethical aspects of neonatal care. Archives of Disease in Childhood 61: 639–641
British Medical Journal (Leading Article) 1981 The right to live and the right to die. British Medical Journal 283: 569–570
British Medical Journal (Leading Article) 1986 In the rear and limping a little: ethics and law in medicine. British Medical Journal 292: 1028
Campbell A G M 1982 Which infants should not receive intensive care? Archives of Disease in Childhood 57: 569–571
Crawford M d'A 1983 Ethical and legal aspects of antenatal diagnosis. British Medical Bulletin 39: 310–315
Duff R S, Campbell A G M 1973 Moral and ethical dilemmas in the special care nursery. New England Journal of Medicine 289: 890–894
Duff R S, Campbell A G M 1976 On deciding the care of severely handicapped or dying persons; with particular reference to infants. Paediatrics 57: 487–493

Fletcher J 1972 Indicators of humanhood: a tentative profile of man. Hastings Centre Report 2: 1–4
Glover J 1977 Causing death and saving lives. Penguin, London
Kennedy I 1981 Unmasking medicine. George Allen & Unwin, London (Reith Lectures)
Kuhse H, Singer P 1985 Should the baby live? Oxford University Press, Oxford
Lorber J 1972 Spina bifida cystica. Archives of Disease in Childhood 47: 854
MRC Working Party on Amniocentesis 1978 British Journal of Obstetrics and Gynaecology 85 (suppl 2): 1–41
Rachels J 1975 Active and passive euthanasia. New England Journal of Medicine 292: 78–80
Sherlock R 1979 Selective non-treatment of newborns. Journal of Medical Ethics 5: 139–142
Stinson R & Stinson P 1981 On the death of a baby. Journal of Medical Ethics 7: 5–18

Index